Advanced Point-of-Care Ultrasound

Michael Gottlieb • Nova Panebianco
Editors

Advanced Point-of-Care Ultrasound

A Comprehensive Review

Springer

Editors
Michael Gottlieb
Department of Emergency Medicine
Rush University Medical Center
Chicago, IL, USA

Nova Panebianco
Department of Emergency Medicine
University of Pennsylvania
Philadelphia, PA, USA

ISBN 978-3-031-85307-4 ISBN 978-3-031-85308-1 (eBook)
https://doi.org/10.1007/978-3-031-85308-1

This Springer imprint is published by the registered company Springer Nature Switzerland AG
The registered company address is: Gewerbestrasse 11, 6330 Cham, Switzerland

I would like to dedicate this book to my wife Vicki and daughters Chloe and Emily, without whose love and support this would not have been possible.
—MG
Seeing with sound is a passion that wouldn't have been possible without the teachers that invested in my education, or the enduring love and support from my husband Jeffery, and daughters Soleil, Selene, and Celeste.
—NP

Preface

Point-of-care ultrasound (POCUS) has transformed the practice of medicine, evolving from a supplementary diagnostic tool to an integral part of patient care. Over the past several decades, the field of POCUS has rapidly advanced, pushing the boundaries of how and where ultrasound can be used. Once confined to radiology suites, POCUS is now utilized at the bedside across a growing number of medical specialties and settings. From the emergency department to the operating room, from outpatient clinics to rural and global health environments, POCUS has become a critical skill for physicians seeking to make real-time clinical decisions.

This book, *Advanced Point-of-Care Ultrasound: A Comprehensive Review*, was conceived with these developments in mind. While a wealth of resources exists for beginners, few texts address the needs of advanced users. This book fills that gap, balancing core foundational knowledge with advanced techniques, applications, and innovations. It is designed for experienced practitioners who are already proficient in POCUS basics but are eager to deepen their fund of knowledge of advanced applications.

A unique aspect of this book is its specialty-agnostic approach. Recognizing that POCUS has become a multidisciplinary tool, we aim to provide value to a diverse range of practitioners, including anesthesiology, critical care, emergency medicine, family practice, internal medicine, and surgeons, among others. In doing so, we have also hand-selected leading experts across a wide range of specialties to serve as authors and section editors. Whether you are interested in trauma, critical care resuscitation, musculoskeletal injuries, procedural guidance, or the wealth of other POCUS applications, this book offers insights and techniques to enhance your practice.

The chapters are designed to be both practical and detailed, with topics spanning from essential physics principles to advanced applications like transesophageal echocardiography (TEE), nerve blocks, and integrated resuscitation protocols. Specialty-specific areas, such as obstetric and gynecologic ultrasound, are included alongside emerging topics like global health applications, artificial intelligence, and ultrasound-guided procedural innovations. By blending established practices with cutting-edge developments, this book ensures readers are equipped to stay at the forefront of POCUS practice.

In addition to its clinical focus, this text explores nonclinical but equally critical dimensions of POCUS, particularly for POCUS educators and leaders. Chapters on education, research, diversity, equity, and inclusion (DEI), as well as system management and information technology, address the broader ecosystem required to optimize ultrasound's impact. These areas are often overlooked in traditional texts, yet they are vital for fostering sustainable growth, equitable access, and continuous innovation in the field.

Whether you are performing an advanced cardiac assessment, supervising a trainee through a nerve block, or implementing ultrasound protocols in a global health setting, this textbook can be a one-stop resource. We hope this book will serve as a trusted tool as you continue to elevate your own POCUS practice and of those around you.

Chicago, IL, USA — Michael Gottlieb

Philadelphia, PA, USA — Nova Panebianco

Contents

Editors, Section Editors and Contributors

Editors

Michael Gottlieb Department of Emergency Medicine, Rush University Medical Center, Chicago, IL, USA

Nova Panebianco Department of Emergency Medicine, University of Pennsylvania, Philadelphia, PA, USA

Section Editors

Stephen Alerhand Department of Emergency Medicine, Rutgers New Jersey Medical School, Newark, NJ, USA

Cameron Baston Department of Medicine, University of Pennsylvania, Philadelphia, PA, USA

Sara Damewood Department of Emergency Medicine, University of Wisconsin, Madison, WI, USA

Meghan Herbst Department of Emergency Medicine, University of Connecticut School of Medicine, Farmington, CT, USA

Jeff Kramer Department of Emergency Medicine, University of Pennsylvania, Philadelphia, PA, USA

Irene Ma Division of General Internal Medicine, Department of Medicine, University of Calgary, Calgary, AB, Canada

Kevin Piro Division of Hospital Medicine, Division of General Internal Medicine, Department of Medicine, Oregon Health & Science University, Portland, OR, USA

Lynn Roppolo Department of Emergency Medicine, John Peter Smith Hospital, Fort Worth, TX, USA

Contributors

Josie Acuña Department of Emergency Medicine, University of Arizona, Tucson, AZ, USA

Srikar Adhikari Department of Emergency Medicine, University of Arizona, Tucson, AZ, USA

Robert James Adrian Department of Emergency Medicine, Christchurch Hospital, Christchurch, New Zealand

Nour Al Jalbout Department of Emergency Medicine, Massachusetts General Hospital, Harvard Medical School, Boston, MA, USA

Eduardo R. Argaiz Tecnológico de Monterrey, Escuela de Medicina y Ciencias de la Salud, Mexico City, Mexico
Departamento de Nefrología y Metabolismo Mineral, Instituto Nacional de Ciencias Médicas y Nutrición, Salvador Zubirán, Mexico City, Mexico

Jason Arthur Department of Emergency Medicine, University of Arkansas for Medical Sciences, Little Rock, AR, USA

Jailyn Avila Department of Emergency Medicine, Temecula Valley Hospital, Temecula, CA, USA

Brian Bales Department of Emergency Medicine, Vanderbilt University Medical Center, Nashville, TN, USA

William Beaubien-Souligny Division of Nephrology, Department of Medicine, Université de, QC, Canada

Keith Boniface Department of Emergency Medicine, George Washington University, Washington, DC, USA

Creagh Boulger Department of Emergency Medicine, Ohio State University, Columbus, OH, USA

Jeremy S. Boyd Department of Emergency Medicine, Vanderbilt University Medical Center, Nashville, TN, USA

Katharine Burns Department of Emergency Medicine, Advocate Christ Medical Center, Oak Lawn, IL, USA
Department of Emergency Medicine, University of Illinois-Chicago, Chicago, IL, USA

Alan Chiem Department of Emergency Medicine, David Geffen School of Medicine at UCLA, Los Angeles, CA, USA

Mikaela Chilstrom Department of Emergency Medicine, Los Angeles General Medical Center, Los Angeles, CA, USA

Almaz Dessie Department of Emergency Medicine, Warren Alpert Medicine School of Brown University, Providence, RI, USA

Dana DiRenzo Division of Rheumatology, Department of Medicine, University of Pennsylvania, Philadelphia, PA, USA

Andrea Dreyfuss Department of Emergency Medicine, Hennepin County Medical Center, Minneapolis, MN, USA

Youyou Duanmu Department of Emergency Medicine, Stanford University, Palo Alto, CA, USA

Petra Duran-Gehring Department of Emergency Medicine, University of Florida College of Medicine—Jacksonville, Jacksonville, FL, USA

Robert Farrow Department of Emergency Medicine, Mount Sinai Medical Center, Miami Beach, FL, USA

Mark Favot Department of Emergency Medicine, Wayne State University School of Medicine, Detroit, MI, USA

Robinson M. Ferre Department of Emergency Medicine, Indiana University School of Medicine, Indianapolis, IN, USA

Tiffany Fong Department of Emergency Medicine, Johns Hopkins University School of Medicine, Baltimore, MD, USA

Luna Gargani Department of Surgical, Medical and Molecular Pathology and Critical Care Medicine, University of Pisa, Pisa, Italy

Andrew Goldsmith Department of Emergency Medicine, Lahey Clinic/University of Massachusetts Burlington, Burlington, MA, USA

Michael Gottlieb Department of Emergency Medicine, Rush University Medical Center, Chicago, IL, USA

Megan Guy Department of Emergency Medicine, UC Irvine Medical Center, Orange, CA, USA

Lawrence Haines Department of Emergency Medicine, SUNY Downstate/ Maimonides Medical Center, Brooklyn, NY, USA

Meghan Herbst Department of Emergency Medicine, University of Connecticut School of Medicine, Farmington, CT, USA

Tomislav Jelic Department of Emergency Medicine, University of Manitoba, Winnipeg, Canada

Jodi Jones Department of Emergency Medicine, University of Texas Southwestern Medical Center, Dallas, TX, USA

David Killeen Neighborhood Health, Alexandria, VA, USA

Daniel J. Kim Department of Emergency Medicine, University of British Columbia, Vancouver, BC, Canada

Samantha A. King Department of Emergency Medicine, University of Texas Medical Branch, Galverston, TX, USA

Andrew W. Kirkpatrick Departments of Critical Care Medicine and Surgery, University of Calgary, Calgary, AB, Canada

Abhilash Koratala Division of Nephrology, Department of Medicine, Medical College of Wisconsin, Milwaukee, WI, USA

Michael J. Lanspa Department of Pulmonary and Critical Care, Intermountain Medical Center, Salt Lake City, UT, USA

Penelope C. Lema Department of Emergency Medicine, Columbia University Vagelos College of Physicians and Surgeons, New York, NY, USA

Megan M. Leo Boston University Chobanian & Avedisian School of Medicine, Boston, MA, USA
Department of Emergency Medicine, Boston Medical Center, Boston, MA, USA

Resa E. Lewiss Department of Emergency Medicine, University of Alabama at Birmingham Heersink School of Medicine, Birmingham, AL, USA

Maya Y. Lin Department of Emergency Medicine, NYU Langone Health, New York, NY, USA

Margaret Lin-Martore Departments of Emergency Medicine and Pediatrics, University of California, San Francisco, San Francisco, CA, USA

E. Liang Liu Department of Emergency Medicine, Emory University, Atlanta, GA, USA

Rachel B. Liu Department of Emergency Medicine, Yale School of Medicine, New Haven, CT, USA

Viveta Lobo Department of Emergency Medicine, Stanford University, Palo Alto, CA, USA

Amy Marks Department of Emergency Medicine, Rush University Medical Center, Chicago, IL, USA

Paul Mayo Division of Pulmonary, Critical Care, and Sleep Medicine, Northwell Health LIJ/NSUH Medical Center, Manhasset, NY, USA
Donald and Barbara Zucker School of Medicine at Hofstra/Northwell, Hempstead, NY, USA

Carlos Mikell Department of Emergency Medicine, UC Davis Medical Center, Davis, CA, USA

Tim Montrief Division of Critical Care Medicine, DeWitt-Daughtry Family Department of Surgery, University of Miami Miller School of Medicine, Miami, FL, USA

Christy Moore Department of Emergency Medicine, University of Pennsylvania, Perelman School of Medicine, Philadelphia, PA, USA

Arun Nagdev Department of Emergency Medicine, Alameda Health System/University of California, San Francisco, CA, USA

Jason T. Nomura Department of Emergency Medicine, Christiana Care Health System, Newark, DE, USA

Laura Oh Department of Emergency Medicine, Emory University, Atlanta, GA, USA

Paul Olszynski Department of Emergency Medicine, University of Saskatchewan, Saskatoon, SK, Canada

Olusegun Olusanya Department of Critical Care, Barts Heart Centre, London, UK

Adi Osman Emergency and Trauma Department, Hospital Raja Permaisuri Bainun, Ipoh, Perak, Malaysia

Nova Panebianco Department of Emergency Medicine, University of Pennsylvania, Philadelphia, PA, USA

Stuart Prenner Department of Medicine, Division of Cardiovascular Medicine, Hospital of University of Pennsylvania, Philadelphia, PA, USA

Alexis Salerno Department of Emergency Medicine, University of Maryland School of Medicine, Baltimore, MD, USA

Aarti Sarwal Department of Neurology, Virginia Commonwealth University, Richmond, VA, USA

Monica R. Saxena Department of Emergency Medicine, Stanford University, Palo Alto, CA, USA

Jessica Schmidt Department of Emergency Medicine, University of Wisconsin, Madison, WI, USA

Christine M. Schutzer Oregon Health & Science University, Portland, OR, USA

Gillian Sheppard Discipline of Emergency Medicine, Memorial University of Newfoundland, St. John's, NL, Canada

Hamid Shokoohi Department of Emergency Medicine, Massachusetts General Hospital, Harvard Medical School, Boston, MA, USA

Manpreet Singh Department of Emergency Medicine, Harbor-UCLA Medical Center, Torrance, CA, USA

Ben C. Smith Department of Emergency Medicine, Erlanger Baroness Hospital, Chattanooga, TN, USA

Joseph Stegeman Department of Emergency Medicine, Highland Hospital/Alameda Hospital System, San Francisco, CA, USA

Robert Strony Department of Emergency Medicine, University of Pittsburgh Medical Center, North Central Region, Pittsburgh, PA, USA

Ee Tein Tay Ronald O. Perelman Department of Emergency Medicine, New York University Grossman School of Medicine, New York, NY, USA

Lindsay Taylor Department of Emergency Medicine, Virginia Commonwealth University, Richmond, VA, USA

Felipe Teran Laboratory of Translational Resuscitation Science, Department of Emergency Medicine, Weill Cornell Medicine, New York, NY, USA

Rajiv Thavanathan Department of Emergency Medicine, University of Ottawa, Ottawa, ON, Canada

Melissa Villa Department of Emergency Medicine, University of Pennsylvania, Philadelphia, PA, USA

Vietvuong Vo Department of Emergency Medicine, University of Texas Southwestern, Dallas, TX, USA

Eileen Y. Wang Department of Obstetrics and Gynecology, University of Pennsylvania, Philadelphia, PA, USA

Anthony J. Weekes Department of Emergency Medicine, Atrium Health's Carolinas Medical Center, Wake Forest School of Medicine, Charlotte, NC, USA

Amie Hall Woods Department of Emergency Medicine, UVA School of Medicine, Inova Campus - Inova Fairfax Hospital, Annandale, VA, USA

Michael D. Zwank Department of Emergency Medicine, Regions Hospital, Saint Paul, MN, USA
University of Minnesota Medical School, Minneapolis, MN, USA

An Introduction to Point-of-Care Ultrasound

1

Michael Gottlieb and Nova Panebianco

Background

Point-of-care ultrasound (POCUS) has become an integral aspect of patient care, evolving from a large machine producing static images to complex, handheld devices that can fit in a pocket. Alongside the technology, the training and applications have evolved, resulting in a wider range of clinicians across a variety of specialties adopting this practice. Importantly, as this has evolved, so has the nomenclature. As POCUS has grown simultaneously across multiple specialties, there is a need to disambiguate some key terms [1]. Table 1.1 provides a summary of common terms and definitions used in POCUS to facilitate this understanding. It is only with an understanding of how POCUS has developed

Table 1.1 Common terms and definitions used in point-of-care ultrasound

Term	Definition
Advanced emergency medicine ultrasonography	Ultrasound by emergency physicians with advanced training. This term is used by the American Board of Emergency Medicine, Focused Practice Designation
Focused practice designation	A pathway created by the American Board of Medicine Specialties to recognize advanced training. The pathway is specialty-specific and applies to advanced knowledge in an area. The American Board of Emergency Medicine offers an FPD in AEMUS
Point-of-care ultrasound	Ultrasound performed by clinicians directly caring for the patient that answers a specific clinical question. It is not defined by the location where the exam is performed, the capabilities of the machine, or the complexity of the exam. This may also be referred to as clinical ultrasound
Educational ultrasound	Ultrasound performed on a patient, volunteer, or in simulation for the educational benefit of the operator. It t is not intended to provide information to further the clinical care of that individual
Consultative ultrasound	Ultrasound performed by consultant service (e.g., radiology, cardiology) at the request of another clinician.
Resuscitative ultrasound	Ultrasound use that is directly related to cardiac resuscitation, general medical resuscitation (e.g., sepsis), or resuscitation from unknown causes
Diagnostic ultrasound	Ultrasound used in a purely diagnostic capacity
Sign- or symptom-based ultrasound	Ultrasound used in a clinical pathway based upon the patient's symptoms or signs (e.g., chest pain, shortness of breath)
Therapeutic ultrasound	Ultrasound used as a part of therapy for patient care
Ultrasound-guided procedure	Ultrasound used to guide a procedure in real time
Ultrasound-assisted procedure	Ultrasound used to assist with a procedure that is not performed in real time (e.g., pre-procedural identification)
Limited ultrasound	Ultrasound imaging of an organ or organ system that is not comprehensive. This term is used to represent a level of ultrasound for coding and billing

This table was adapted from the American College of Emergency Physicians 2023 Policy Statement [17]

M. Gottlieb (✉)
Department of Emergency Medicine, Rush University Medical Center, Chicago, IL, USA
e-mail: michaelgottliebmd@gmail.com

N. Panebianco
Department of Emergency Medicine, University of Pennsylvania, Philadelphia, PA, USA
e-mail: nova.panebianco@pennmedicine.upenn.edu

M. Gottlieb, N. Panebianco (eds.), *Advanced Point-of-Care Ultrasound*, https://doi.org/10.1007/978-3-031-85308-1_1

and evolved that we can understand where it will go next. In this chapter, we will review the history of POCUS, the current state, and future directions.

A Brief History of Point-of-Care Ultrasound

The exploration of ultrasound for medical diagnostics began in the late 1940s [2, 3]. In 1949, Dr. Douglas Howry and colleagues built an ultrasound device using surplus radio and Air Force radar parts, which they subsequently combined with a 35-mm camera to record the first cross-sectional image with ultrasound [2]. In 1951, Dr. Howry and a team of engineers developed a two-dimensional compound ultrasound scanner [2]. This eventually led to one of the earliest medical ultrasound devices, the "pan-scanner" [2, 3]. This device included a single transducer that would rotate around a patient who was seated in a chair submerged in saline and produced static images. Recognizing some of the inherent issues with this device, Dr. Howry and team collaborated with two engineers (William Wright and Edward Meyer) to create a direct contact ultrasound scanner, which included a mounted scanning head which could be positioned by the operator [2]. In 1961, Wright and Meyer later formed Physionic Engineering, Inc., where they developed the first, commercially available handheld scanning device (Figs. 1.1, 1.2, 1.3 and 1.4) [2].

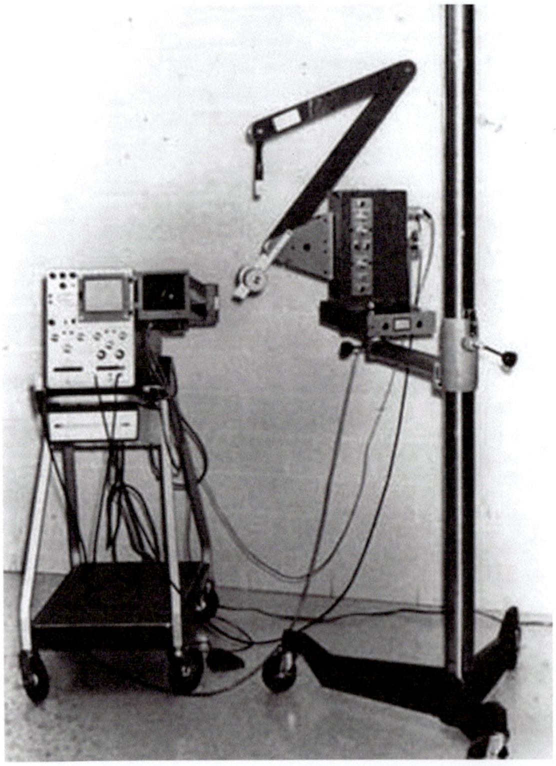

Fig. 1.1 The first commercial model of a portable ultrasound machine, the Porta-arm Scanner by Physionic Engineering, Inc. (*Image courtesy of The American Institute of Ultrasound in Medicine*)

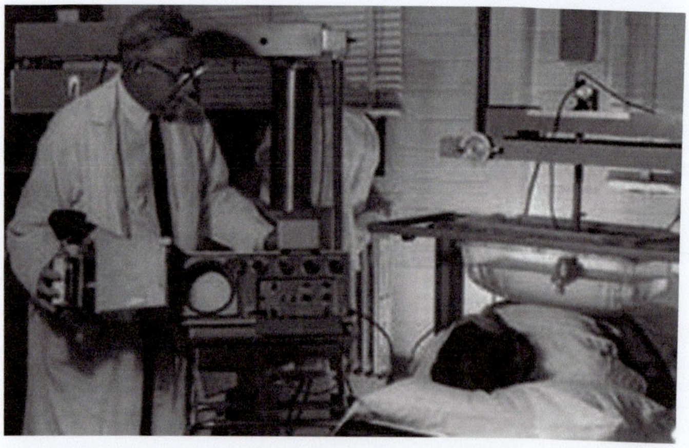

Fig. 1.2 Early use of portable ultrasound machines at the patient's bedside in the early 1960s. (*Image courtesy of The American Institute of Ultrasound in Medicine*)

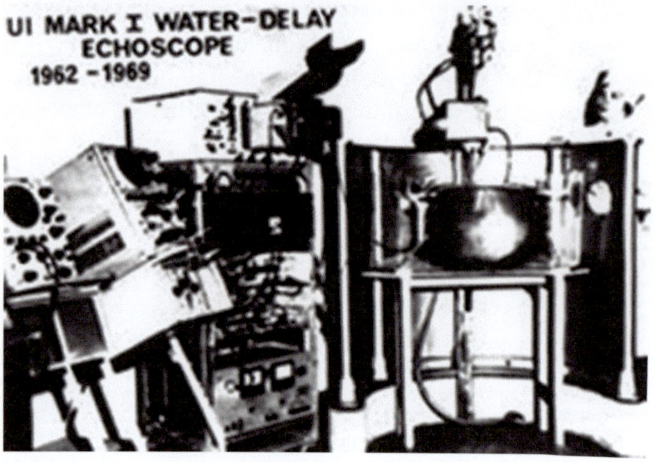

Fig. 1.3 The "UI Mark I" created by Dr. George Kossoff and his coworkers at the Australian Department of Health in the 1960s. (*Image courtesy of The American Institute of Ultrasound in Medicine*)

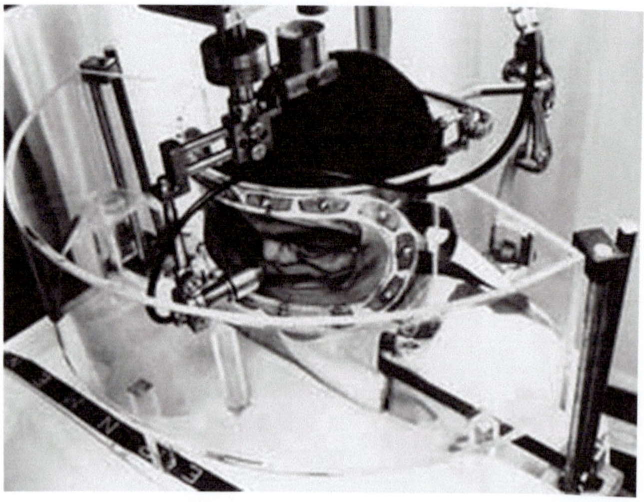

Fig. 1.4 "Second generation" B-mode scanners provided more resolution to detect tumors, cysts, and other lesions. Ultrasonic coupling was performed using a water bath and goggles. (*Image courtesy of The American Institute of Ultrasound in Medicine*)

While the field continued to evolve, the use of ultrasound in the United States remained primarily limited to radiologists, cardiologists, and obstetricians, with little adoption beyond these specialties until the 1980s [4]. In 1984, Dr. Alexander Trott published an editorial stating that with proper training in POCUS, "the emergency physician can add markedly to his or her diagnostic capabilities." [5] Some of the earliest research in POCUS published by emergency physicians occurred in 1987. Dr. Michael Heller and team assessed the feasibility of POCUS by emergency physicians [4]. Dr. Ray Mayron and colleagues published on the use of single-view cardiac ultrasound to diagnose pericardial effusions and pulseless electrical activity [6]. Dr. Dietrich Jehle and collaborators studied the ability of emergency physicians to diagnose pericardial effusion, pulseless electrical activity, intrauterine pregnancy, intrauterine device location, biliary disease, and abdominal aortic aneurysms [7]. The literature evolved and was fueled by the focused use of ultrasound in trauma in the early 1990s [8–12]. This led to the creation of the Focused Abdominal Sonography in Trauma (FAST) examination, which was later renamed to the "Focused Assessment with Sonography in Trauma" to reflect inclusion of cardiac and thoracic elements [13].

As the field expanded, there was a surge of interest. Some of the earliest courses within emergency medicine were conducted in 1991 [4]. The University of Buffalo created a 14-day "mini ultrasound fellowship" shortly after [4]. This was later incorporated into residency training across multiple specialties, and the first official clinical ultrasound fellowship was launched by Dr. James Mateer at the Medical College of Wisconsin in 1993 [4]. Some of the first graduates from emergency ultrasound fellowship at the Medical College of Wisconsin included Drs. Thomas, Valley, and Phelan.

Development and Evolution of POCUS Guidelines and Policies

Over time numerous specialties have developed POCUS guidelines. In 1990, the American College of Emergency Physicians (ACEP) released a position statement supporting the use of POCUS by properly trained emergency physicians [14]. Since then, other specialty groups issued position statements. In 1999, the American Medical Association passed House Resolution 802, which defined ultrasound as within the scope of appropriately trained physicians, regardless of specialty (Fig. 1.5) [15]. This provided critical support and further validation to support the use of POCUS by a wider range of users.

In 2001, ACEP developed the first emergency ultrasound guidelines, which established recommendations for documentation, quality assurance, and hospital credentialing for POCUS examinations [16]. These initial guidelines focused on seven core applications: trauma, pregnancy, cardiac, abdominal aortic aneurysm, biliary, renal, and procedural [16]. As time has passed, these guidelines have evolved to include a much broader range of applications, with many of the previously advanced topics now deemed core applications in the current iteration [17].

Other specialties have also adopted guidelines over these ensuing years. In 2015, Society of Critical Care Medicine released their guidelines for POCUS in the critically ill patient [18]. In 2015, the American Academy of Pediatrics also released guidelines on POCUS use by pediatric emergency physicians [19]. The American Medical Society for Sports Medicine released a position statement on interventional musculoskeletal ultrasound in sports medicine in the same year [20]. This was followed by the American Academy of Family Physicians' "Recommended Curriculum Guidelines for Family Medicine Residents Point-of-Care Ultrasound" in 2016 [21]. In 2019, the Society of Hospital Medicine issued a position statement on POCUS for hospitalists [22]. These provide just a few select examples of the rapidity of spread throughout a wide range of specialties, wherein POCUS was adopted as among core skills of the practicing clinician.

Looking internationally, POCUS has also seen substantial growth. The World Interactive Network Focused on Critical UltraSound (WINFOCUS) is one of the largest international organizations with representation from over 120 countries. WINFOCUS has hosted thousands of courses, and has been the entity for numerous consensus statements including medical student education, lung ultrasound, and cardiac imaging [23–25].

Fig. 1.5 American Medical Association House Resolution 802 [15]. (*AMA* American Medical Association)

1. AMA affirms that ultrasound imaging is within the scope of practice of appropriately trained physicians;
2. AMA policy on ultrasound acknowledges that broad and diverse use and application of ultrasound imaging technologies exist in medical practice;
3. AMA policy on ultrasound imaging affirms that privileging of the physician to perform ultrasound imaging procedures in a hospital setting should be a function of hospital medical staffs and should be specifically delineated on the Department's Delineation of Privileges form; and
4. AMA policy on ultrasound imaging states that each hospital medical staff should review and approve criteria for granting ultrasound privileges based upon background and taining for the use of ultrasound technology and strongly recommends that these criteria are in accordance with recommended training and education standards developed by each physician's respective specialty.

Current State of POCUS

As POCUS has expanded, the breadth and depth of applications have followed. Applications such as thoracic ultrasound for undifferentiated dyspnea have gathered increasingly widespread support, including via the American College of Physicians in their 2022 Clinical Guidelines statement [26]. Other applications, such as ocular and musculoskeletal ultrasound, have also experienced rapid rises in use [27]. Within POCUS examinations, there has been growth in their application including more sophisticated measurements and protocols [28–30].

There have also been advances in education. While in the early stages, this focused on hands-on teaching sessions at select conferences, modern uses have included tele-ultrasound, simulation, and even artificial intelligence (AI) to enhance learning [31–33]. Training and assessment have also evolved to include more robust and evidence-informed measures, such as competency-based medical education over pure numerical assessments [34–37]. With the expansion of training, there has also been a concomitant rise in clinical ultrasound fellowships across multiple specialties [38–40].

More recently, the American Board of Medicine Specialties approved a focused practice designation (FPD) in Advanced Emergency Medicine Ultrasonography (AEMUS). This demonstrates a deeper and more robust understanding of POCUS, including the administrative, educational, clinical, and research components. To be eligible for FPD certification, ultrasound fellows must complete training in a fellowship program accredited by the Emergency Ultrasound Fellowship Accreditation Council and pass the FPD examination [41, 42].

Importantly, at times, POCUS has led to conflict across groups. This may reflect variations in definitions and understanding of the clinical use of POCUS, which has led to the development of POCUS practice in silos and contributed to the diverse nomenclature around the imaging modality. Therefore, going forward, it will be critical to ensure greater collaboration across specialties and groups to advance the practice at-large.

Future Directions

Over time, there has been remarkable progress in ultrasound technology. Newer devices have become more compact, extending to handheld devices that can be easily transported throughout the clinical environment. Transducers have evolved from traditional piezoelectric crystals to microarray computer chips [43]. Advances in imaging technology and processing features can enhance image quality. Notably, while this can allow for improved visualization, this must be balanced by the risk of potential false positives [44].

While contrast has been used in consultative echocardiography since the 1960s (with the first published use in 1968) [45, 46], it was only more recently expanded to POCUS. Contrast-enhanced ultrasound is particularly well-suited for POCUS, where physical limitations may preclude the optimized environment seen in echocardiography suites. While this is well-suited for and often considered in the context of cardiac and vascular assessment, contrast-enhanced ultrasound can be utilized for a wider array of applications, including assessing solid organ injury in trauma, gastrointestinal pathology, or even muscle perfusion in suspected compartment syndrome [47].

AI has also experienced a rapid expansion. While early AI focused primarily on diagnostic assessment across a limited number of applications, this has expanded broadly and now includes measures such as systolic and diastolic dysfunction [48], - B-lines for pulmonary edema [49, 50], inferior vena cava assessments for volume status [51, 52], pericardial effusion [53], and hemopericardium in trauma [54], among others. Other advances include auto-labeling and auto-measuring structures, sorting and classifying images, and even automated measures of image quality for quality improvement and education [33, 55, 56].

There is precedent for patients to self-generate medical data for independent and clinician-supervised health care. Examples include home blood pressure monitoring, glycemic regulation with glucometers and insulin pumps, and point-of-care testing for acute SARS-CoV-2 infection. Early data of patients self-performing POCUS suggest that this may be a viable technology for home use in the future [57].

Conclusion

In the last 30 years, POCUS has rapidly evolved to allow advanced imaging via a mobile cart or handheld probe. The number of examinations and breadth of specialties using POCUS, coupled with expansion of clinical ultrasound fellowships and educational advances, has positioned POCUS to be a key tool in the skillset of every practicing clinician. As the field continues to evolve at a nearly exponential rate, many of the novel applications and newer advances will become standard across machines and commonplace in training. The skill of the operator remains the greatest barrier in POCUS imaging. Therefore, it is critical to establish a robust foundation to ensure that our patients receive the highest quality care.

References

1. Kirkpatrick JN, Panebianco N, Díaz-Gómez JL, et al. Recommendations for cardiac point-of-care ultrasound nomenclature. J Am Soc Echocardiogr. Published online July 11. 2024;S0894-7317(24):00222. https://doi.org/10.1016/j.echo.2024.05.001.
2. Goldberg BB, Gramiak R, Freimanis AK. Early history of diagnostic ultrasound: the role of American radiologists. Am J Roentgenol. 1993;160(1):189–94. https://doi.org/10.2214/ajr.160.1.8416623.
3. Salerno A, Gottlieb M. Point-of-care ultrasound in the emergency department: past, present, and future. Emerg Med Clin North Am. Published online June. 2024;42:S0733862724000737. https://doi.org/10.1016/j.emc.2024.05.016.
4. Von Kuenssberg JD, Wilson C. Some recollections of early work with bedside ultrasound in emergency medicine: the first 10 years. JACEP Open. 2020;1(5):871–5. https://doi.org/10.1002/emp2.12115.
5. Trott A. Ultrasonography in emergency medicine. J Emerg Med. 1984;1(6):549. https://doi.org/10.1016/0736-4679(84)90011-8.
6. Mayron R, Gaudio FE, Plummer D, Asinger R, Elsperger J. Echocardiography performed by emergency physicians: impact on diagnosis and therapy. Ann Emerg Med. 1988;17(2):150–4. https://doi.org/10.1016/s0196-0644(88)80301-9.
7. Jehle D, Davis E, Evans T, et al. Emergency department sonography by emergency physicians. Am J Emerg Med. 1989;7(6):605–11. https://doi.org/10.1016/0735-6757(89)90283-0.
8. Kimura A, Otsuka T. Emergency center ultrasonography in the evaluation of hemoperitoneum: a prospective study. J Trauma. 1991;31(1):20–3. https://doi.org/10.1097/00005373-199101000-00004.
9. Tso P, Rodriguez A, Cooper C, et al. Sonography in blunt abdominal trauma: a preliminary progress report. J Trauma. 1992;33(1):39–43.; discussion 43–44. https://doi.org/10.1097/00005373-199207000-00009.
10. Plummer D, Brunette D, Asinger R, Ruiz E. Emergency department echocardiography improves outcome in penetrating cardiac injury. Ann Emerg Med. 1992;21(6):709–12. https://doi.org/10.1016/s0196-0644(05)82784-2.
11. Jehle D, Guarino J, Karamanoukian H. Emergency department ultrasound in the evaluation of blunt abdominal trauma. Am J Emerg Med. 1993;11(4):342–6. https://doi.org/10.1016/0735-6757(93)90164-7.
12. Ma OJ, Kefer MP, Mateer JR, Thoma B. Evaluation of hemoperitoneum using a single- vs multiple-view ultrasonographic examination. Acad Emerg Med. 1995;2(7):581–6. https://doi.org/10.1111/j.1553-2712.1995.tb03593.x.
13. Scalea TM, Rodriguez A, Chiu WC, et al. Focused assessment with sonography for trauma (FAST): results from an international consensus conference. J Trauma. 1999;46(3):466–72. https://doi.org/10.1097/00005373-199903000-00022.
14. American College of Emergency Physicians. Council resolution on ultrasound. ACEP News. 1990;9:11.
15. American Medical Association. Privileging for Ultrasound Imaging H-230.960. 2020. Accessed 13 May 2024. https://policysearch.ama-assn.org/policyfinder/detail/Ultrasoundimaging?uri=%2FAMADoc%2FHOD.xml-0-1591.xml
16. American College of Emergency Physicians. American College of Emergency Physicians. ACEP emergency ultrasound guidelines-2001. Ann Emerg Med. 2001;38(4):470–81.
17. American College of Emergency Physicians. Ultrasound guidelines: emergency, point-of-care, and clinical ultrasound guidelines in medicine. Ann Emerg Med. 2023;82(3):e115–55. https://doi.org/10.1016/j.annemergmed.2023.06.005.
18. Frankel HL, Kirkpatrick AW, Elbarbary M, et al. Guidelines for the appropriate use of bedside general and cardiac ultrasonography in the evaluation of critically ill patients-part I: general ultrasonography. Crit Care Med. 2015;43(11):2479–502. https://doi.org/10.1097/CCM.0000000000001216.
19. Marin JR, Lewiss RE. American Academy of Pediatrics, Committee on Pediatric Emergency Medicine, Society for Academic Emergency Medicine, Academy of Emergency Ultrasound, American College of Emergency Physicians, Pediatric Emergency Medicine Committee, World Interactive Network Focused on Critical Ultrasound. Point-of-care ultrasonography by pediatric emergency medicine physicians. Pediatrics. 2015;135(4):e1113–22. https://doi.org/10.1542/peds.2015-0343.
20. Finnoff JT, Hall MM, Adams E, et al. American Medical Society for Sports Medicine (AMSSM) position statement: interventional musculoskeletal ultrasound in sports medicine. PM R. 2015;7(2):151–168.e12. https://doi.org/10.1016/j.pmrj.2015.01.003.
21. American Academy of Family Physicians. Recommended Curriculum Guidelines for Family Medicine Residents: Point-of-Care Ultrasound. Accessed 6 Oct 2024. https://www.aafp.org/dam/AAFP/documents/medical_education_residency/program_directors/Reprint290D_POCUS.pdf
22. Soni NJ, Schnobrich D, Mathews BK, et al. Point-of-care ultrasound for hospitalists: a position statement of the Society of Hospital Medicine. J Hosp Med. 2019;14:E1–6. https://doi.org/10.12788/jhm.3079.
23. Hoppmann RA, Mladenovic J, Melniker L, et al. International consensus conference recommendations on ultrasound education for undergraduate medical students. Ultrasound J. 2022;14(1):31. https://doi.org/10.1186/s13089-022-00279-1.
24. International Liaison Committee on Lung Ultrasound (ILC-LUS) for the International Consensus Conference on Lung Ultrasound (ICC-LUS), Volpicelli G, Elbarbary M, et al. International evidence-based recommendations for point-of-care lung ultrasound. Intensive Care Med. 2012;38(4):577–91. https://doi.org/10.1007/s00134-012-2513-4.
25. Via G, Hussain A, Wells M, et al. International evidence-based recommendations for focused cardiac ultrasound. J Am Soc Echocardiogr. 2014;27(7):683.e1–683.e33. https://doi.org/10.1016/j.echo.2014.05.001.
26. Qaseem A, Etxeandia-Ikobaltzeta I, Mustafa RA, et al. Appropriate use of point-of-care ultrasonography in patients with acute dyspnea in emergency department or inpatient settings: a clinical guideline from the American College of Physicians. Ann Intern Med. 2021;174(7):985–93. https://doi.org/10.7326/M20-7844.
27. Gottlieb M, Cooney R, King A, et al. Trends in point-of-care ultrasound use among emergency medicine residency programs over a 10-year period. AEM Educ Train. 2023;7(2):e10853. https://doi.org/10.1002/aet2.10853.
28. Alerhand S, Sundaram T, Gottlieb M. What are the echocardiographic findings of acute right ventricular strain that suggest pulmonary embolism? Anaesth Crit Care Pain Med. 2021;40(2):100852. https://doi.org/10.1016/j.accpm.2021.100852.
29. Alerhand S, Adrian RJ, Taylor LA. Cardiac point-of-care ultrasound: an emergency medicine review. Emerg Med Clin North Am. 2024;42(4):731–54. https://doi.org/10.1016/j.emc.2024.05.004.
30. Lin J, Rosario J, Saltarelli N. Resuscitative ultrasound and protocols. Emerg Med Clin North Am. 2024;42(4):947–66. https://doi.org/10.1016/j.emc.2024.05.014.
31. Soni NJ, Boyd JS, Mints G, et al. Comparison of in-person versus tele-ultrasound point-of-care ultrasound training during the COVID-19 pandemic. Ultrasound J. 2021;13(1):39. https://doi.org/10.1186/s13089-021-00242-6.
32. Zavitz J, Sarwal A, Schoeneck J, et al. Virtual multispecialty point-of-care ultrasound rotation for fourth-year medical students during COVID-19: innovative teaching techniques improve ultra-

sound knowledge and image interpretation. AEM Educ Train. 2021;5(4):e10632. https://doi.org/10.1002/aet2.10632.

33. Kayarian F, Patel D, O'Brien JR, Schraft EK, Gottlieb M. Artificial intelligence and point-of-care ultrasound: benefits, limitations, and implications for the future. Am J Emerg Med. 2024;80:119–22. https://doi.org/10.1016/j.ajem.2024.03.023.
34. Damewood SC, Leo M, Bailitz J, et al. Tools for measuring clinical ultrasound competency: recommendations from the ultrasound competency work group. AEM Educ Train. 2020;4(Suppl 1):S106–12. https://doi.org/10.1002/aet2.10368.
35. Rider AC, Miller DT, Ashenburg N, et al. Using a simulated model and mastery learning approach to teach the ultrasound-guided serratus anterior plane block to emergency medicine residents: a pilot study. AEM Educ Train. 2021;5(3):e10525. https://doi.org/10.1002/aet2.10525.
36. Bailitz J, O'Brien J, McCauley M, et al. Development of an expert consensus checklist for emergency ultrasound. AEM Educ Train. 2022;6(4):e10783. https://doi.org/10.1002/aet2.10783.
37. Gottlieb M, Duanmu Y. Beyond the numbers: assessing competency in point-of-care ultrasound. Ann Emerg Med. 2023;81(4):427–8. https://doi.org/10.1016/j.annemergmed.2023.01.020.
38. Adhikari S, Leo M, Liu R, et al. The 2023 Core content of advanced emergency medicine ultrasonography. J Am Coll Emerg Physicians Open. 2023;4(4):e13015. https://doi.org/10.1002/emp2.13015.
39. Cramer N, Cantwell L, Ong H, et al. Pediatric emergency medicine fellowship point-of-care ultrasound training in 2020. AEM Educ Train. 2021;5(4):e10643. https://doi.org/10.1002/aet2.10643.
40. Baston CM, Wallace P, Chan W, Dean AJ, Panebianco N. Innovation through collaboration: creation of a combined emergency and internal medicine point-of-care ultrasound fellowship. J Ultrasound Med. 2019;38(8):2209–15. https://doi.org/10.1002/jum.14908.
41. American Board of Emergency Medicine. Advanced EM Ultrasonography. Accessed 13 May 2024. https://www.abem.org/public/become-certified/focused-practice-designation/advanced-em-ultrasonography
42. Gottlieb M, Duran-Gehring P, Coneybeare D, Lema P. Creation of a novel course for the advanced emergency medicine ultrasound focused practice designation examination. AEM Educ Train. 2022;6(5):e10810. https://doi.org/10.1002/aet2.10810.
43. Baribeau Y, Sharkey A, Chaudhary O, et al. Handheld point-of-care ultrasound probes: the new generation of POCUS. J Cardiothorac Vasc Anesth. 2020;34(11):3139–45. https://doi.org/10.1053/j.jvca.2020.07.004.
44. Parker MA, Hicks BG, Kaili M, et al. The lipliner sign: potential cause of a false positive Focused Assessment with Sonography in Trauma (FAST) Examination. J Emerg Med. Published online June 28, 2024:S0736-4679(24)00212-9. https://doi.org/10.1016/j.jemermed.2024.06.013.
45. Gramiak R, Shah PM. Echocardiography of the aortic root. Investig Radiol. 1968;3(5):356–66. https://doi.org/10.1097/00004424-196809000-00011.
46. Frinking P, Segers T, Luan Y, Tranquart F. Three decades of ultrasound contrast agents: a review of the past, present and future improvements. Ultrasound Med Biol. 2020;46(4):892–908. https://doi.org/10.1016/j.ultrasmedbio.2019.12.008.
47. Kummer T, Oh L, Phelan MB, Huang RD, Nomura JT, Adhikari S. Emergency and critical care applications for contrast-enhanced ultrasound. Am J Emerg Med. 2018;36(7):1287–94. https://doi.org/10.1016/j.ajem.2018.04.044.
48. Gottlieb M, Schraft E, O'Brien J, Patel D. Diagnostic accuracy of artificial intelligence for identifying systolic and diastolic cardiac dysfunction in the emergency department. Am J Emerg Med. 2024;86:115–9. https://doi.org/10.1016/j.ajem.2024.10.019.
49. Gottlieb M, Patel D, Viars M, Tsintolas J, Peksa GD, Bailitz J. Comparison of artificial intelligence versus real-time physician assessment of pulmonary edema with lung ultrasound. Am J Emerg Med. 2023;70:109–12. https://doi.org/10.1016/j.ajem.2023.05.029.
50. Russell FM, Ehrman RR, Barton A, Sarmiento E, Ottenhoff JE, Nti BK. B-line quantification: comparing learners novice to lung ultrasound assisted by machine artificial intelligence technology to expert review. Ultrasound J. 2021;13(1):33. https://doi.org/10.1186/s13089-021-00234-6.
51. Blaivas M, Adhikari S, Savitsky EA, Blaivas LN, Liu YT. Artificial intelligence versus expert: a comparison of rapid visual inferior vena cava collapsibility assessment between POCUS experts and a deep learning algorithm. J Am Coll Emerg Physicians Open. 2020;1(5):857–64. https://doi.org/10.1002/emp2.12206.
52. Blaivas M, Blaivas L, Philips G, et al. Development of a deep learning network to classify inferior vena cava collapse to predict fluid responsiveness. J Ultrasound Med. 2021;40(8):1495–504. https://doi.org/10.1002/jum.15527.
53. Yıldız Potter İ, Leo MM, Vaziri A, Feldman JA. Automated detection and localization of pericardial effusion from point-of-care cardiac ultrasound examination. Med Biol Eng Comput. 2023;61(8):1947–59. https://doi.org/10.1007/s11517-023-02855-6.
54. Leo MM, Potter IY, Zahiri M, Vaziri A, Jung CF, Feldman JA. Using deep learning to detect the presence and location of Hemoperitoneum on the focused assessment with sonography in trauma (FAST) examination in adults. J Digit Imaging. 2023;36(5):2035–50. https://doi.org/10.1007/s10278-023-00845-6.
55. Blaivas M, Arntfield R, White M. Creation and testing of a deep learning algorithm to automatically identify and label vessels, nerves, tendons, and bones on cross-sectional point-of-care ultrasound scans for peripheral intravenous catheter placement by novices. J of Ultrasound Medicine. 2020;39(9):1721–7. https://doi.org/10.1002/jum.15270.
56. Blaivas M, Arntfield R, White M. DIY AI, deep learning network development for automated image classification in a point-of-care ultrasound quality assurance program. JACEP Open. 2020;1(2):124–31. https://doi.org/10.1002/emp2.12018.
57. Chiem AT, Lim GW, Tabibnia AP, Takemoto AS, Weingrow DM, Shibata JE. Feasibility of patient-performed lung ultrasound self-exams (patient-PLUS) as a potential approach to telemedicine in heart failure. ESC Heart Fail. 2021;8(5):3997–4006. https://doi.org/10.1002/ehf2.13493.

Ultrasound Physics, Knobology, and Safety

2

Hamid Shokoohi and Nour Al Jalbout

Introduction

Ultrasound in medicine utilizes sound waves for image generation, while using frequencies above the range of human hearing. While audible sound is measured in hertz (Hz), diagnostic ultrasound is measured in megahertz (MHz). The technology has evolved tremendously in the last decade, including the development of more compact ultrasound systems and handheld ultrasound devices. The sound waves emitted from these devices have their own physical properties and interact uniquely with different tissue media thus creating images of different resolutions. A comprehensive understanding of the physics of ultrasound waves allows clinicians to better acquire and interpret images, accurately differentiate pathology from artifact, and adjust the ultrasound machine processing to optimize image quality.

The concepts and principles of producing high-quality images and safe ultrasound practice are emphasized by the American Institute of Ultrasound in Medicine (AIUM) Curriculum for Fundamentals of Ultrasound Physics and Instrumentation [1]. In this chapter, we will explore the principles of ultrasound physics, including sound wave properties, imaging planes, modes of ultrasound, image artifacts, and safety of ultrasound imaging. As more clinicians are integrating point-of-care ultrasound (POCUS) in medical decision-making, a thorough understanding of these foundational principles can lead to improved image acquisition, interpretation, and patient care outcomes.

H. Shokoohi (✉) · N. Al Jalbout
Department of Emergency Medicine, Massachusetts General Hospital, Harvard Medical School, Boston, MA, USA
e-mail: hshokoohi@mgh.harvard.edu; naljalbout@mgh.harvard.edu

Knobology

Understanding how to operate the ultrasound machine is the first step towards mastering the skill and art of POCUS. The majority of ultrasound machines share basic controls for power, probe selection, measurement, and the functions of image optimization including depth, gain, focus, and time gain compensation (TGC).

Depth corresponds to the distance the ultrasound beam travels into the body and is reflected back. Depth can be increased or decreased depending on the area of interest. The greater the depth of the area of interest, the longer the ultrasound beam has to travel from the deeper structures. This can result in a loss of image resolution and a lower frame rate(number of images displayed per second). The focus button on the machine can compensate by creating a "focal zone" where the image has the best resolution at the depth of interest [2].

Gain is the uniform amplification of the ultrasound beam returning from the imaged tissue, allowing the images to appear bright (hyperechoic), dark (hypoechoic), or black (anechoic). By increasing the gain of an image, operators are amplifying the returning ultrasound signals, which increases the brightness of the image [2]. TGC is an additional ultrasound feature that allows clinicians to adjust the strength of returning ultrasound beams at various depths by the factor of time required for the echos to return. This compensates for the attenuation of energy as the beam travels deeper into the body. TGC can be adjusted at different levels of the imaged organ, from the near field closest to the probe to the far field away from the probe to improve and balance the brightness of the image.

Multibeam imaging is another feature of ultrasound transducers that sends out signals at multiple angles across the probe. This results in multiple angles of incidence and reflection back to the probe. This technique enhances image quality, especially for surrounding structures susceptible to refraction artifacts.

M. Gottlieb, N. Panebianco (eds.), *Advanced Point-of-Care Ultrasound*, https://doi.org/10.1007/978-3-031-85308-1_2

Tissue harmonics is an ultrasound imaging technique that uses a tissue's resonance at multiples of the incident frequency transmitted by the probe to produce an image of higher resolution with fewer artifacts. For example, if the incident frequency from the probe is 4 MHz, the imaged tissue has the tendency to resonate at 4 MHz, 8 MHz, and 12 MHz. Transducers can be set to receive both the incident and harmonic frequencies, combining them to create an image with higher resolution. This feature is especially useful in patients with a large body habitus to improve image quality. Additionally, using tissue harmonic settings helps reduce artifacts by listening at multiple frequencies thus producing a clearer image [3, 4].

Transducers and Sonographic Techniques

Transducer Physics

The principles of ultrasound imaging depend on sending sound waves to the tissues and receiving the reflected waves to create images. These sound waves are generated by using piezoelectric crystals. Piezoelectric crystals have unique properties, vibrating when receiving an electric current and converting this energy into mechanical ultrasound waves. They are also capable of doing the opposite thus producing images from reflected waves. During the majority of the time, the transducer is waiting for reflected waves, spending only 1% of the time generating ultrasound waves [2, 4, 5].

Ultrasound waves are produced in pulses, with each pulse consisting of 2–3 cycles of the same frequency. The time between two pulses is the pulse repetition period (PRP) and the number of pulses generated in one second is the pulse repetition frequency (PRF), making PRP = 1/PRF. In other words, PRF is the number of pulses in a given period of time.

Imaging deeper structures requires a longer PRP to extend the listening time and allow sound waves to return from longer distances before the next pulse. Conversely, a higher PRF means there are more pulses in a second and shorter listening times resulting in an improved image resolution at shallow depths.

The ultrasound probe has other components around the piezoelectric crystals that ensure safe and proper imaging (Fig. 2.1). The backing layer situated behind the crystals suppresses the crystal vibrations so sound waves can be sent in shorter pulses, producing better resolution. The matching layer in front of the crystal layer reduces the impedance difference with the imaged tissue, allowing more sound waves to penetrate the tissue. The most anterior layer in front of the matching layer is the acoustic lens which focuses the ultrasound waves, leading to less scatter and enhanced resolution. Coating the transducer is the acoustic insulation layer which ensures that no other sound waves affect the transducer [2, 5].

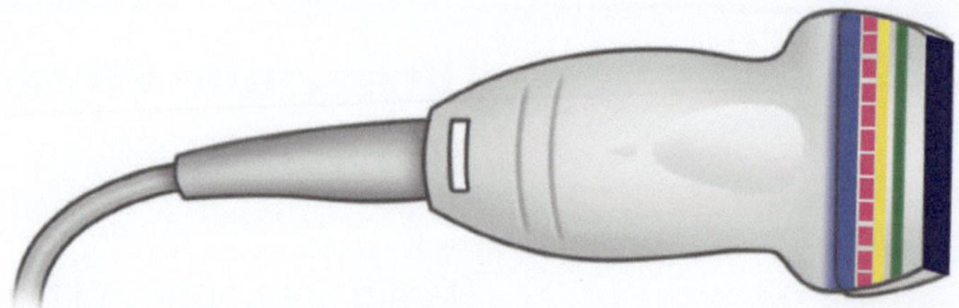

Fig. 2.1 Ultrasound probe components. In the accompanying diagram, the backing layer is blue, the crystals are pink, the matching layer is yellow, and the acoustic lens is green

Types of Probes

When performing POCUS, one must choose the appropriate probe based on the area of interest. Each probe has a different bandwidth or a range of possible frequencies depending on the backing material used. The most common types of probes are:

Linear array probes (5–15 MHz): high-frequency probes with a linear flat footprint containing crystals arranged in a line. These probes have high resolution but low penetration capabilities, and thus are used to evaluate superficial structures.

Curvilinear or convex array probes (1–6 MHz): low-frequency probes with a large footprint containing crystals arranged in a curvilinear fashion. These probes are best suited for deeper imaging of the abdominal organs due to their ability to deep penetrationpenetrate deeper, at the expense of proximal image resolution.

Phased array or sector probes (1–5 MHz): low-frequency probes with a flat footprint containing crystals arranged into a cluster producing a pie-shaped image. These probes are ideal for cardiac imaging given their high temporal resolution and smaller footprint to navigate narrow intercostal spaces. Similar to curvilinear probes, they allow better imaging of deeper structures, with reduced proximal resolution.

Endocavitary probe (4–13 MHz): higher-frequency probes with a curvilinear footprint and wide field of view up to 180 degrees, leading to an optimal tissue resolution. The most common applications are in pelvic, prostatic, or intraoral imaging.

Silicon Chip Probes

Recent advancements in handheld ultrasound devices have introduced silicon chip probes that use microelectromechanical systems (MEMS). The two main types of MEMS systems are capacitive micromachined ultrasonic transducers (CMUTs) and piezoelectric micromachined ultrasonic transducers (PMUTs) [6, 7].

CMUTs work by placing a thin membrane over a cavity, creating a capacitor. When voltage is applied, the membrane vibrates like a drum, generating ultrasound waves. Adjusting the voltage changes the wave frequency, and when echoes return, the membrane moves, altering the capacitance and producing an electrical signal to create an image (Fig. 2.2).

PMUTs, on the other hand, use piezoelectric crystals combined with silicon. Thousands of micromachines cause the piezoelectric material to expand and contract, bending the structure and producing ultrasound waves. By adjusting the voltage, PMUTs can generate a broad range of frequencies [6–8].

These chip-based transducers are small, housing 4000–9000 transducers on a 2-by-3-centimeter silicon chip. They can handle a wide range of frequencies, making them versatile, cost-effective, and capable of delivering high-quality images across various frequencies with just one transducer.

Ultrasound Probe Movement

Mastering the sonographic technique starts by understanding the six cardinal movements of the ultrasound probe: slide, sweep, rock, fan, rotate, and compress [9]. (Fig. 2.3).

Slide: moving along the long axis of the probe while being 90 degrees to the imaged structure in order to identify the best window for imaging.

Sweep: moving along the short axis of the probe while being 90 degrees to the imaged structure in order to identify the best window for imaging.

Rock: rocking the probe toward or away from the probe indicator along its long axis while maintaining the imaged structure in plane at a fixed point.

Fan: pivot the probe from side to side along the short axis at a fixed point on the body allowing the visualization of multiple cross sectional images of the structure.

Rotate: turning the probe along its central axis in clockwise or counterclockwise fashion to switch between transverse and longitudinal planes.

Compress: applying pressure on the probe while keeping the footprint at a fixed position, causing the probe to move into the body and displace structures in the way (e.g., bowel loops, air).

When performing these movements, one should be optimizing the angle of the beam emitted from the probe relative to the organ of interest, which is often aligning the beam with a non-parallel structure. This angle is known as the angle of insonation (Fig. 2.4). The strongest echo signal is produced by adjusting the angle of insonation to 90 degrees thus having the angle of incidence (angle of engagement of the beam with the structure) on the tissue equal to the angle of reflection. When rocking or fanning, the angle of insonation is changed away from or toward 90 degrees whereas the angle remains fixed when sliding or sweeping the probe relative to the underlying structure.

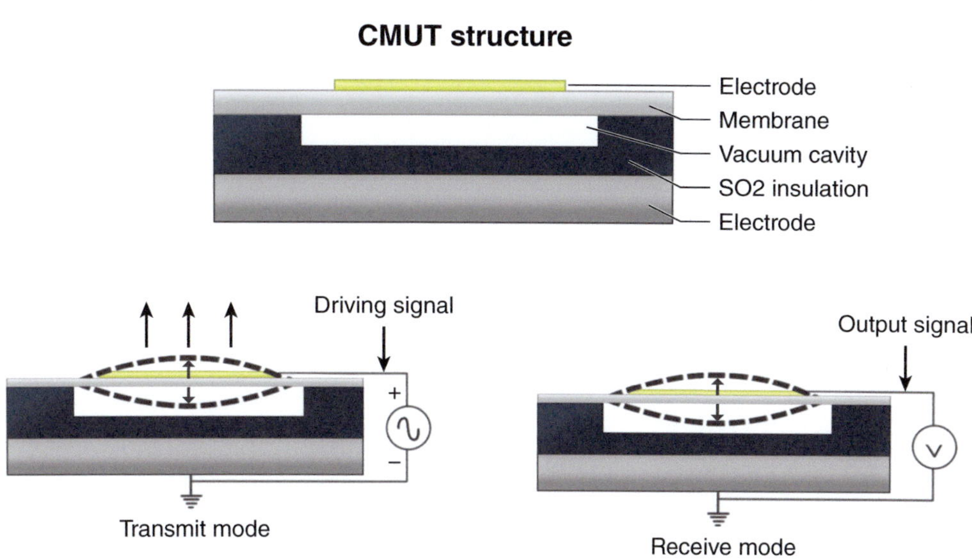

Fig. 2.2 Schematic illustration of Capacitive Micromachined Ultrasonic Transducer (CMUT)

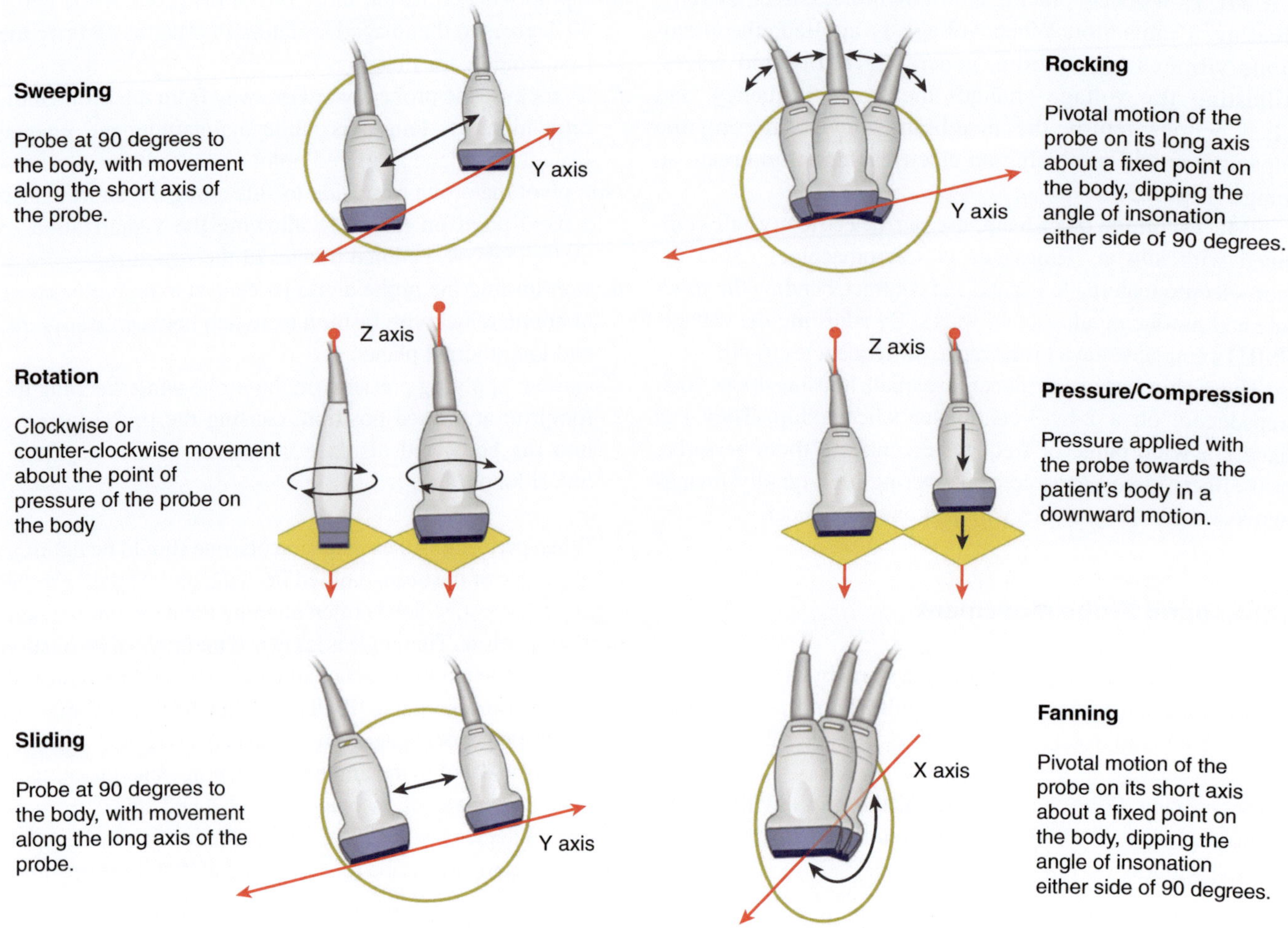

Fig. 2.3 Six cardinal probe movements

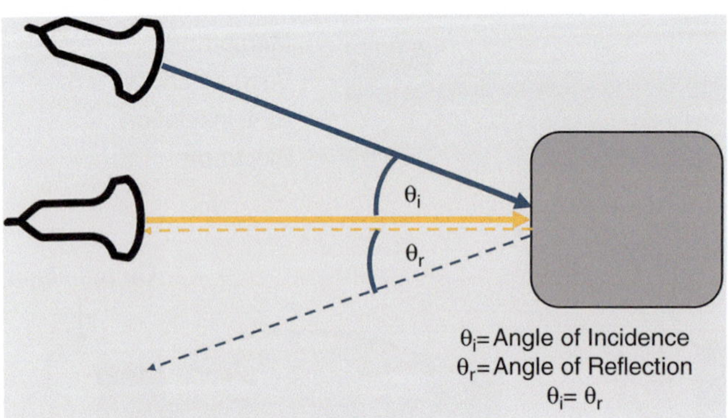

Fig. 2.4 Ultrasound beam reflection and angle of incidence. An ultrasound beam strikes an interface at an angle (θ_i) and reflects at the same angle (θ_i), following $\theta_i = \theta_i$. Aligning the angle of insonation to 90 degrees to the structure of interest produces the strongest echoes

Anatomical Planes

The imaged structure can be evaluated in multiple planes when performing POCUS. These are often divided into two main types: body planes and structure planes. Body planes refer to external anatomic reference planes, while structure planes are specific to the orientation of the structure being examined.

The body is divided into three main planes (Fig. 2.5):

1. Sagittal Plane: the plane dividing the body into right and left sections, parallel to the long axis of the body.
2. Transverse (or Axial) Plane: the plane dividing the body into superior and inferior sections, perpendicular to the long axis of the body.

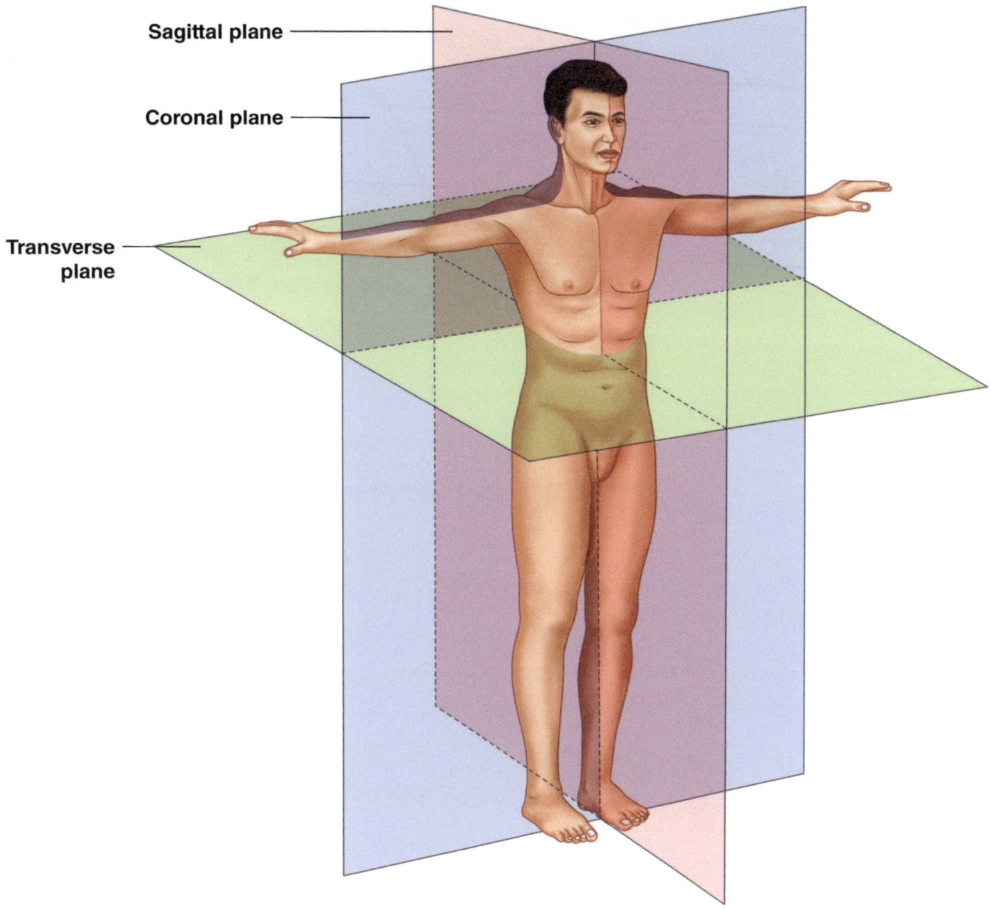

Fig. 2.5 Illustration of the three main imaging planes of the body

3. Coronal Plane: the plane dividing the body into anterior and posterior sections, also parallel to the long axis of the body.

Commonly in ultrasound, specific structures do not perfectly align with the conventional anatomic planes (e.g., long bones, gallbladder, heart). In these instances, a structure-based system is used, with imaging conventions of short-axis and long-axis, which refer to the axis in relation to the specific structure rather than the external anatomic plane. In a structure-based system, the long axis is the plane parallel to the longest dimension of the structure, while the short axis is perpendicular to the long axis. Images between these two planes are often termed oblique.

Properties of Sound Waves

The most common type of ultrasound waves used in medical imaging are compression waves, also known as longitudinal waves. These waves displace the medium parallel to the direction of the propagating source wave to create the ultrasound image. Key components of ultrasound waves are presented in Table 2.1 and Fig. 2.6. Common propagation speeds for various structures are presented in Table 2.2.

Table 2.1 Characteristics of ultrasound waves

Frequency (MHz)	The number of cycles emitted per one second, ranging from 1 to 20 MHz
Period (msec)	Time required to complete a wave cycle; reciprocal of frequency
Wavelength (mm)	Distance between two troughs or crests on the wave; inversely related to frequency
Amplitude (dB)	The strength of the sound wave signal
Power (Watts)	The amount of energy (joules) generated per unit of time
Intensity (Watts/cm^2 or milliWatts/cm^2)	The power delivered over a specific area
Propagation speed (m/s)	The rate at which ultrasound waves pass through a medium
Bulk modulus (Pa)	The measure of the ability to withstand changes in volume under compression (incompressibility)

Image Quality

The displayed image on the ultrasound machine is influenced by multiple factors. Intrinsic factors related to the probe include the number of piezoelectric crystals, aperture diameter, or frequency used. Other factors depend on the property of the medium through which the ultrasound beam travels.

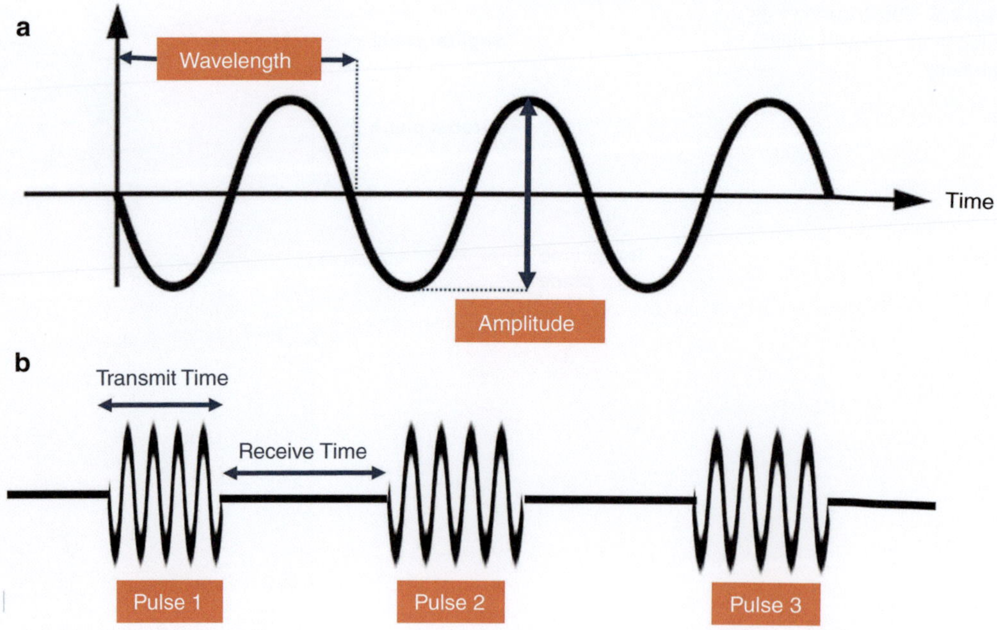

Fig. 2.6 The ultrasound wave and its properties. (**a**) Shows the wavelength (distance between peaks) and amplitude (height from baseline to peak) of a wave over time. (**b**) Depicts ultrasound pulses (Pulse 1, Pulse 2, Pulse 3) with intervals of transmit time (when pulse is sent) and receive time (when echo is received)

Table 2.2 Propagation speeds for common structures in the body

Structure	Propagation speed
Air	331 m/s
Fat	1430 m/s
Soft tissue	1540 m/s
Blood	1570 m/s
Muscle	1575 m/s
Liver	1580 m/s
Bone	3000–5000 m/s

In discussing the image quality, it is important to distinguish between the different types of resolution, defined as the ability to differentiate echoes in terms of space, time, and strength.

There are three types of resolution:

- Spatial resolution: This is the ability of the beam to distinguish two structures close to each other in space and is divided into two types:
  - *Axial resolution*: The ability to display two objects as separate when they are parallel to the axis of the beam, displaying them as two separate objects in depth. Axial resolution highly depends on the length of the pulse used to form the beam or the spatial pulse length. The shorter the spatial pulse length, the better the axial resolution. Thus, higher frequency probes produce shorter pulses leading to better axial resolution.
  - *Lateral resolution*: The ability to display objects as separate when perpendicular to the axis of the beam, displaying them next to each other as two separate objects, at the same distance from the probe. This highly depends on the width of the ultrasound beam. The lateral resolution is best at the narrowest area of the beam.
- Temporal resolution: This is the ability of the beam to distinguish changes in the imaged structure across time, most importantly in cardiac imaging. It is mainly determined by the image frame rate of the system. Higher frame rates increase the likelihood of visualizing rapidly moving structures like valves.
- Contrast resolution: This is the ability of the beam to differentiate between tissues with different image intensities (e.g., kidney and liver).

A single image produced on an ultrasound machine screen is known as a frame. Multiple frames produced in rapid sequence form the moving image we see on the screen. Frame rate, or the number of frames produced in one second, is typically around 15 frames per second allowing sonographers to achieve a smooth, real-time image while scanning. Frame rates depend on the depth of the field, with shallower structures requiring shorter pulse travel distances, thus enhancing the frame rate. Increased propagation speed through the tissue, selecting the appropriate probe frequency, decreasing the width of the ultrasound beam, and reducing the number of focal points also improve the frame rate.

Beam Profile

The shape of the ultrasound beam coming out of the probe is important for image quality. As the ultrasound beam exits the probe, it travels as a parallel bundle for a certain distance and then disperses away from the center. The parallel component is known as the near field (or Fresnel zone), the divergent component is known as the far field (or Fraunhofer zone),

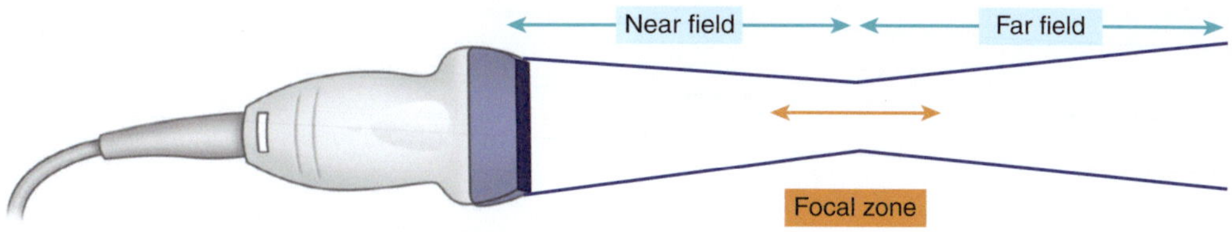

Fig. 2.7 Ultrasound beam profile: The probe sends out sound waves, forming the near field or Fresnel zone (closer to the probe) and the far field or Fraunhofer zone (further away). The focal zone (orange arrow) is where the beam narrows, providing the highest image resolution

and the point separating both is the transition zone (or focal point) where resolution is highest (Fig. 2.7).

Dynamic Range

One factor essential in determining the image quality is the dynamic range. The dynamic range is defined as the difference between the strongest and the weakest signal of echoes available for display, which affects the contrast of the image on the screen. Broad dynamic ranges produce more shades of gray, enhancing spatial resolution by increasing contrast levels and improving image detail and clarity. A narrow dynamic range increases the contrast of the image by having fewer shades of gray and more black and white. This is beneficial when imaging blood vessels and fluid-filled cavities.

Attenuation

As a sound wave travels through a medium, its intensity and amplitude decreases, weakening its energy as it travels farther distances and when emitted at higher frequencies. Therefore, the highest resolution images are produced when imaging superficial structures. This concept is referred to as attenuation [4, 10].

There are three main modes of attenuation:

(i) *Absorption*: Absorption refers to the conversion of acoustic energy into heat. Scattered ultrasound waves can be absorbed by the imaged tissues, generating heat in small amounts without significant measurable temperature changes. Absorption tends to increase with high-frequency probes and with deeper imaging.
(ii) *Refraction*: Refraction refers to the diversion of the ultrasound beam from its original straight path as it crosses the boundary between two media having different propagation speeds. The amount of beam deflection is proportional to the difference in stiffness or elasticity between the two media and increases if the angle of incidence of the original beam is not perpendicular.
(iii) *Scatter*: Scatter refers to the redirection of the sound waves in different directions when meeting a structure with a different acoustic impedance compared to the surrounding tissue. This is particularly common when the tissue interface is smaller than the wavelength of the sound wave, and is encountered more with high-frequency compared to low-frequency probes. This property allows the visualization of different echogenic structures within a particular tissue.

Reflection

The image quality produced is greatly influenced by the degree of reflection of the sound waves off a tissue surface. The main properties influencing reflection include:

(i) *The angle of incidence*: This is the angle at which ultrasound waves engage with any structure. Ideally, a perpendicular angle of incidence helps reflected waves return in their greatest concentration thus producing the best image.
(ii) *Tissue Density*: High-density tissues (e.g., bone) reflect more sound, resulting in hyperechoic images while low-density tissues (e.g., water) allow sound waves to penetrate resulting in anechoic ultrasound images.
(iii) *Interface Type*: A higher proportion of waves return to the probe when meeting large smooth flat interfaces like the diaphragm. Sound waves scatter away from the probe in higher concentrations when meeting irregular interfaces thus reducing the image quality.
(iv) *Acoustic Impedance*: This is an intrinsic property of different tissue types and a product of tissue density and speed of sound in the medium. The difference in acoustic impedance between two media determines the amount of transmitted energy compared to reflected energy. Sound waves are completely reflected when the acoustic impedance difference between the two interfaces is large. Using ultrasound gel in imaging is one example of decreasing the acoustic impedance between the probe and the imaged structures to improve the transmission of sound beams and thus decrease reflection.

Ultrasound Modes

Ultrasound images can be shown in different modes, which include B-mode, M-mode, color Doppler, and spectral Doppler. Brightness mode (B-mode), also known as 2D mode, creates a two-dimensional grayscale image. It is the

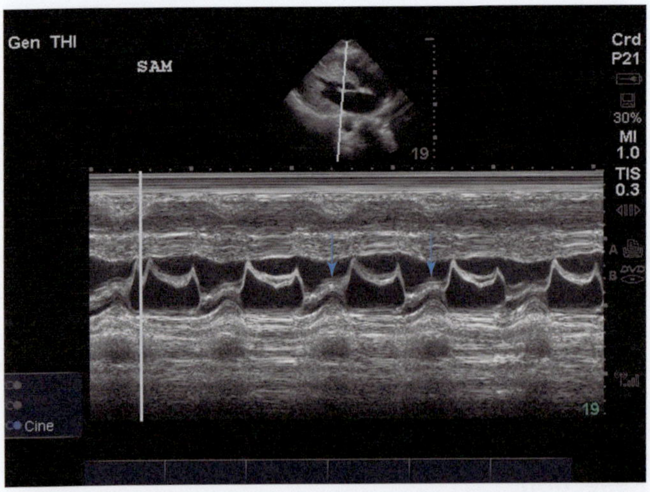

Fig. 2.8 M-mode display at the level of the mitral valve in a patient with hypertrophic cardiomyopathy illustrating systolic anterior motion (SAM) of the mitral valve

most fundamental mode in ultrasound imaging, and all other imaging modes rely on having a good B-mode image as a foundation. Motion mode (M-mode) displays the movement of a structure over time along a specific line of interest. The y-axis shows the motion, while the x-axis represents time. M-mode is commonly used in cardiac imaging to assess functions like ejection fraction or right ventricular dysfunction. (Fig. 2.8).

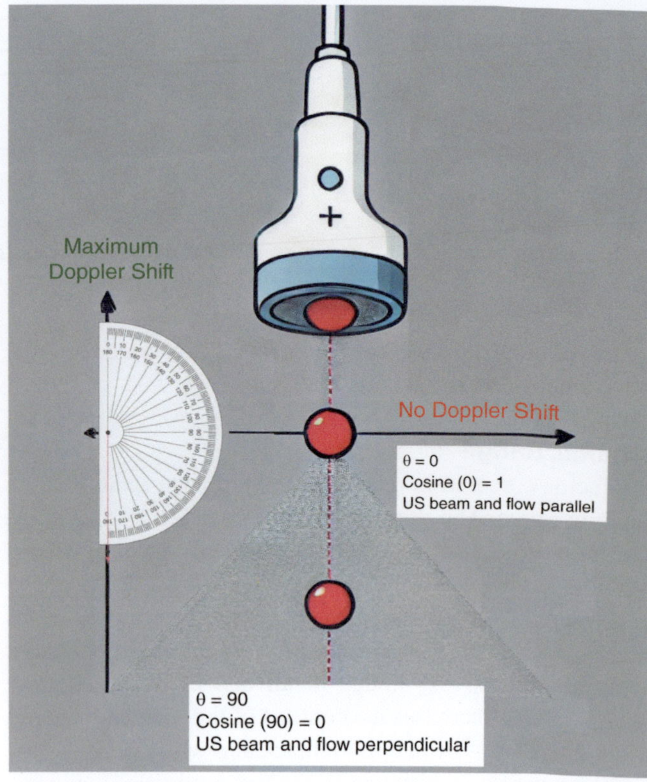

Fig. 2.9 Doppler shift. Velocity is proportional to the cos θ, such that the Doppler shift is maximized the closer the angle is to 0 degrees and is minimized the closer the angle is to 90 degrees

Doppler Ultrasound

Doppler ultrasound is a technique used to measure the movement and speed of blood flow through the heart and blood vessels. It works based on the Doppler effect, which refers to changes in the frequency of sound waves as they bounce off moving objects, like red blood cells. This frequency change is called the Doppler shift [4, 10, 11].

Doppler Shift

The Doppler shift refers to the change in sound wave frequency as it reflects off moving blood or tissue, allowing the measurement of flow direction and speed (i.e., velocity). This is useful for diagnosing and monitoring various conditions, including cardiac and vascular pathologies. When blood flows toward the ultrasound probe, the returning sound frequency increases, and when it flows away, the frequency decreases. The more aligned the blood flow is with the ultrasound beam, the greater the Doppler shift [10–12].

Doppler Equation

The Doppler equation links the frequency of ultrasound waves to the velocity of blood flow. The Doppler shift, or change in frequency, depends on the original frequency emitted by the probe and the velocity of the moving blood. This shift is highly affected by the angle between the ultrasound beam and the blood flow. A 0-degree angle (parallel to the flow) provides the most accurate velocity measurement, while a 90-degree angle (perpendicular to the flow) does not detect movement at all (Fig. 2.9). In practice, an angle under 20 degrees is generally considered acceptable for accurate measurements. Many ultrasound machines also offer angle correction, which adjusts for the beam's angle and is particularly effective in uniform flow situations, such as in major blood vessels. While it is not perfect, angle correction can be useful when achieving a parallel beam is difficult [4, 12].

A common use of the Doppler shift is in cardiac Doppler ultrasound to assess valvular function. To accurately measure peak blood flow velocities, it is important to align the ultrasound beam as parallel as possible to the blood flow. This maximizes the reflection of Doppler signals, providing clearer and more accurate data on how the blood is moving through the heart valves.

This is why most valvular assessments are done using the apical 4-chamber view of the heart. In this view, the ultrasound beam is directed from the apex of the heart, aligning with the blood flow through the mitral, aortic, and tricuspid valves. This alignment ensures more accurate measurements of blood velocities and better reflection of

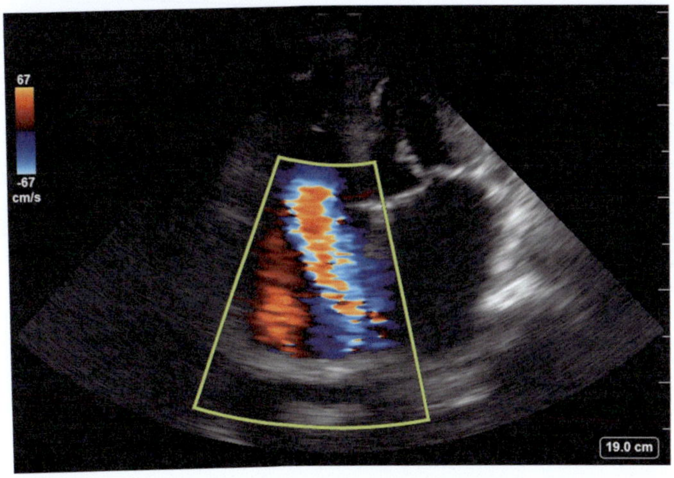

Fig. 2.10 Apical 4-chamber view representing severe tricuspid regurgitation as the retrograde jet reaches the posterior wall of the right atrium

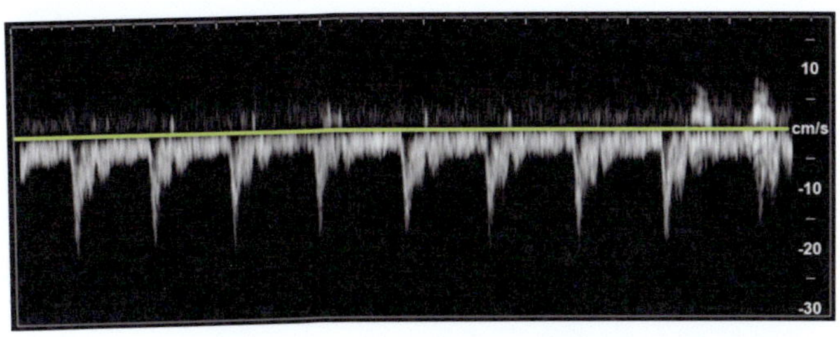

Fig. 2.11 Spectral Doppler tracing of the internal carotid artery

Doppler signals, optimizing the assessment of valve function (Fig. 2.10).

Doppler Display

In Doppler ultrasound, blood cell movement is analyzed through spectral analysis (Fig. 2.11). This process captures the Doppler shifts, which are displayed on a graph: upward shifts represent blood moving toward the probe, and downward shifts show blood moving away. The vertical axis of the graph represents the velocity of the blood or tissue, while the horizontal axis shows time. This provides a clear visual of both the speed and rhythm of blood flow over a given period.

Doppler Types

Doppler ultrasound utilizes three primary forms: color flow Doppler, pulsed-wave Doppler, and continuous-wave Doppler.

1. Color Flow Doppler

Color flow Doppler visualizes blood movement and flow velocities across multiple points by using colors to represent both direction and speed. Blue indicates flow moving away from the probe, while red shows flow toward it, easily remembered by the mnemonic BART (blue away, red toward) (Fig. 2.12). This color data is layered over regular

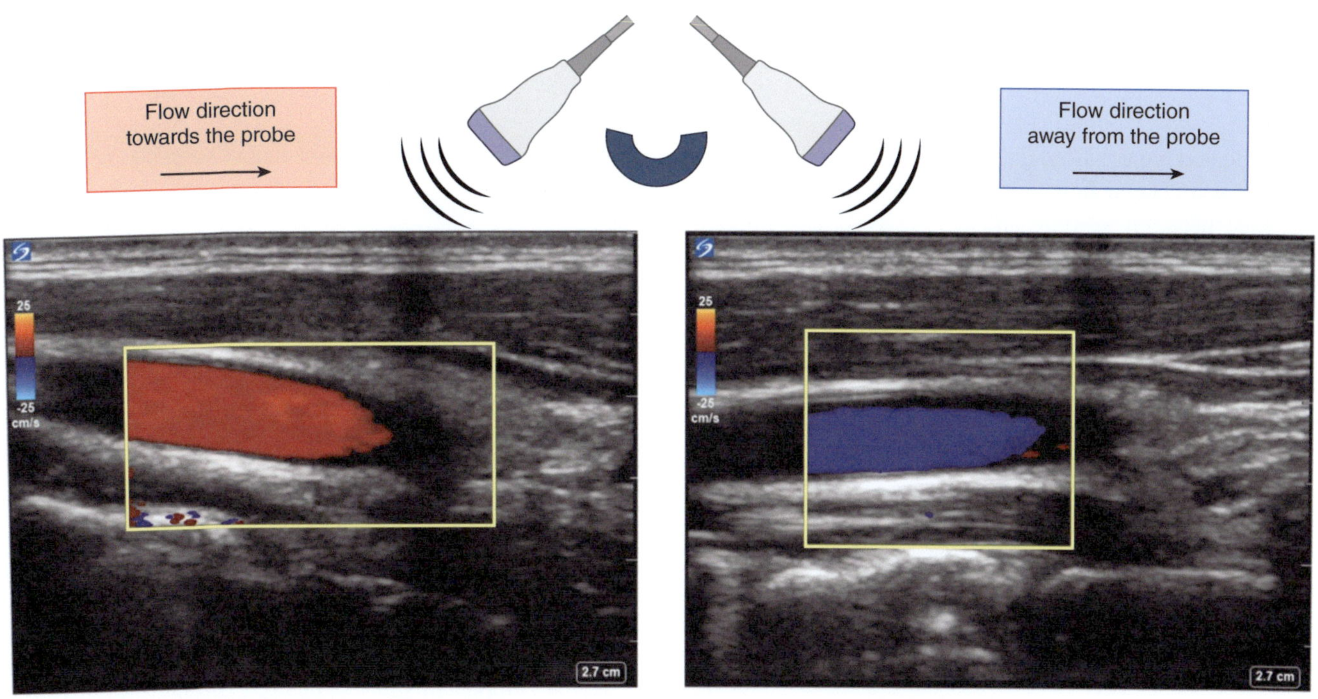

Fig. 2.12 Changing the angle of the ultrasound probe in carotid artery ultrasound results in the blood flow appearing either red (toward the probe) or blue (away from the probe). These colors only represent direction, not arterial or venous blood flow

B-mode images, helping to better assess flow patterns, their locations, and how different heart chambers or vessels are functioning.

To optimize color Doppler imaging, start by choosing the proper angle and aligning the ultrasound beam correctly with the blood vessel. Then, adjust the color gain by increasing it fully and gradually lowering it until areas around the vessels that should be free of echoes appear anechoic. Reducing the size of the color Doppler box can improve the frame rate, which helps enhance the image quality and allows for a more accurate assessment of valvular diseases. Color Doppler is also commonly used to assess tissue perfusion in cases of testicular torsion, soft tissue masses, and peripheral blood vessels (Fig. 2.13) [13].

Color Doppler imaging can encounter aliasing, which happens when blood flow speeds are higher than what the system can accurately measure. This leads to errors in the Doppler display (Fig. 2.14). The system's ability to measure these velocities depends on the PRF. Faster blood flow requires a higher PRF to correctly capture the Doppler shifts. PRF plays a key role in determining the maximum blood flow speed the system can measure without errors. To reduce aliasing, the PRF scale can be adjusted, or, in some cases, the transmission frequency can be lowered.

Power Doppler is a variation of color Doppler that highlights the intensity of blood flow signals but does not account for the direction of flow (Fig. 2.15). This makes it particularly useful for detecting very low blood flow, such as in conditions like testicular torsion.

2. Pulsed-wave Doppler

Pulsed-wave Doppler (PWD) uses a single transducer to send and receive ultrasound signals in short bursts, allowing it to measure blood flow at specific locations. By adjusting the time between sending and receiving signals, sonographers can target a particular area to assess blood flow (Fig. 2.16). This makes PWD especially helpful for obtaining spatial information about blood flow in cardiac exams, like checking for diastolic dysfunction by measuring mitral inflow velocities. However, like color Doppler, it can also experience aliasing.

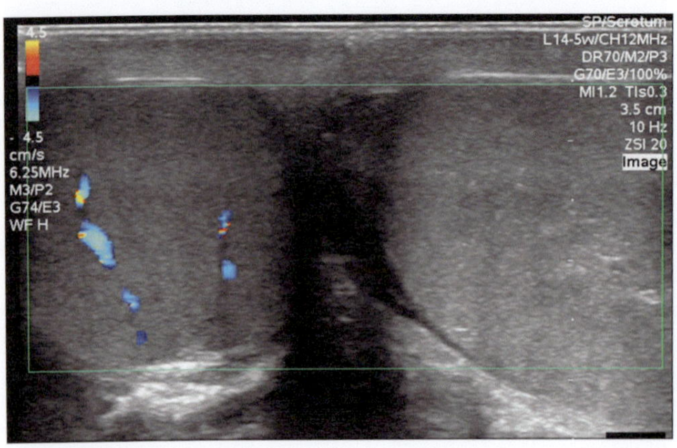

Fig. 2.13 Color Doppler shows flow to the patient's right testicle (left side of the image) but an absence of flow in the patient's left testicle (right side of the image), indicating testicular torsion

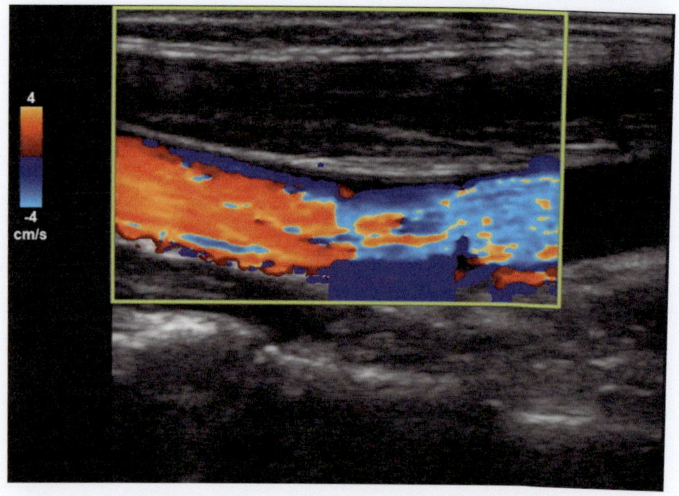

Fig. 2.14 Aliasing in a color Doppler image of a right carotid artery, where the velocity exceeds the threshold. The resulting Doppler signals appear as if they are moving in the opposite direction (Red)

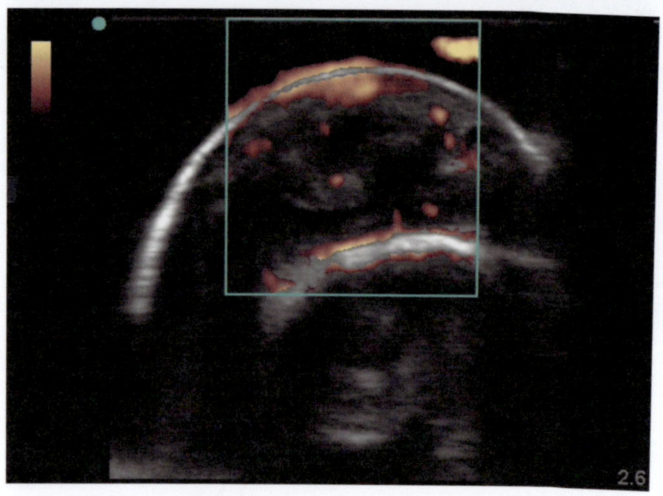

Fig. 2.15 Power Doppler used to assess inflammation at the fingertip in a patient with suspected felon

To get the best signal, start by using color Doppler to locate the desired area for measuring flow. Then, align the ultrasound beam as parallel as possible to the blood vessel or structure, and keep the sample volume size (often referred to as the "gate") between 3 and 5 mm for better accuracy.

Tissue Doppler Imaging (TDI) is a special form of PWD to assess tissue movement velocity, most commonly used to evaluate myocardial function. Instead of detecting blood cell movement, TDI captures the low-speed, high-intensity sig-

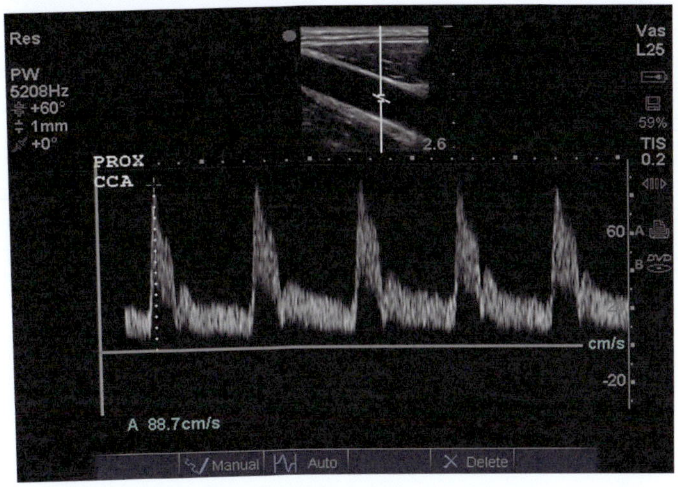

Fig. 2.16 Using pulsed-wave Doppler to measure the peak flow velocity of the proximal common carotid artery

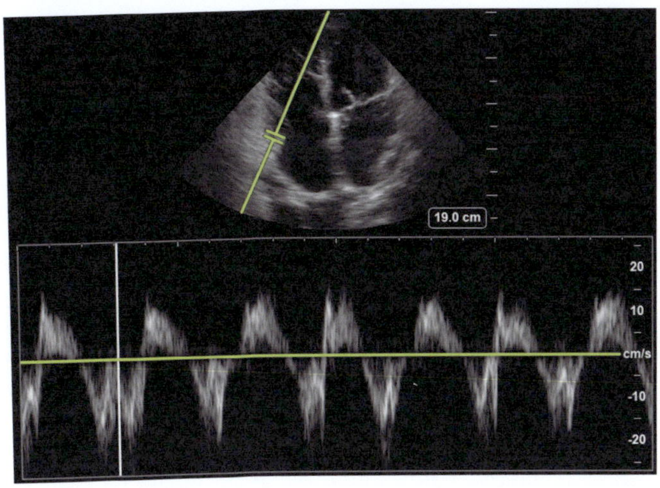

Fig. 2.17 Using Tissue Doppler Imaging to measure the velocity of the lateral tricuspid valve annulus (S′) movement to evaluate right ventricular dysfunction

nals from heart tissue. It measures the velocity of myocardial movement throughout the cardiac cycle, helping to understand regional cardiac function and diagnose conditions like diastolic dysfunction. With its high temporal resolution, TDI is great for tracking any part of myocardial wall movement during the cardiac cycle. It is often used to measure early diastolic relaxation velocity (e′) at the mitral valve annulus to assess diastolic dysfunction. TDI can also evaluate the right ventricular dysfunction by measuring systolic contraction velocity (S′) at the lateral tricuspid valve annulus (Fig. 2.17).

3. Continuous-wave Doppler

Continuous-wave Doppler (CWD) constantly transmits and receives ultrasound signals, using two separate crystals, one for sending and one for receiving. This method is great for measuring high blood flow velocities, which is key in diagnosing conditions like valvular or congenital heart diseases. However, CWD is unable to differentiate depth, meaning it picks up data from all the cells along the beam's path, making it harder to interpret when multiple structures, like the mitral and aortic valves, are in close proximity. It is particularly useful for assessing conditions like aortic stenosis or estimating pulmonary artery pressure through tricuspid regurgitation, where detecting high-velocity flow is important (Fig. 2.18).

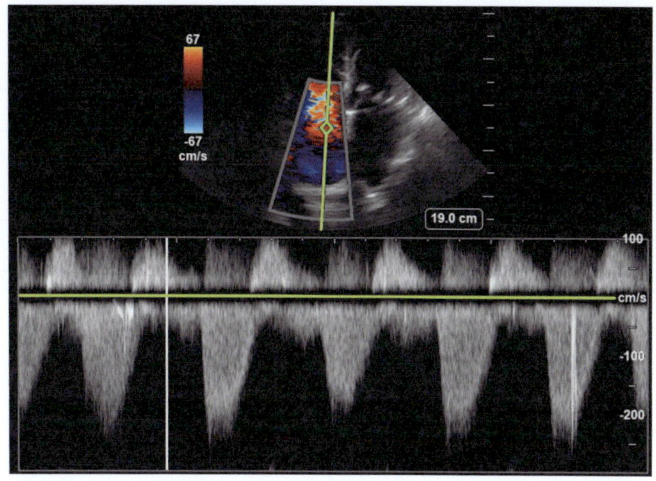

Fig. 2.18 Using continuous-wave Doppler to measure the tricuspid regurgitation in a patient with a pulmonary embolism

To perform CWD, first use color Doppler to identify the area of interest. Then, align the ultrasound beam with the direction of flow. Unlike PWD, CWD captures flow along the entire beam path without a sample gate or specific location and it is not affected by aliasing.

Image Artifacts in Clinical Scenarios

Ultrasound imaging relies on the clinician's skill to recognize and manage artifacts. Correct interpretation of these artifacts is crucial for accurate diagnosis, as they can either obscure real findings or reveal critical information when understood within the physics of ultrasound.

Shadowing

Shadowing happens when a dense object absorbs or reflects ultrasound waves more than the surrounding tissues, resulting in a dark, anechoic "shadow" behind it. This effect is often seen behind dense structures such as bone, metal, or calcium stones, where the sound waves are either fully reflected or absorbed (Fig. 2.19). Additionally,

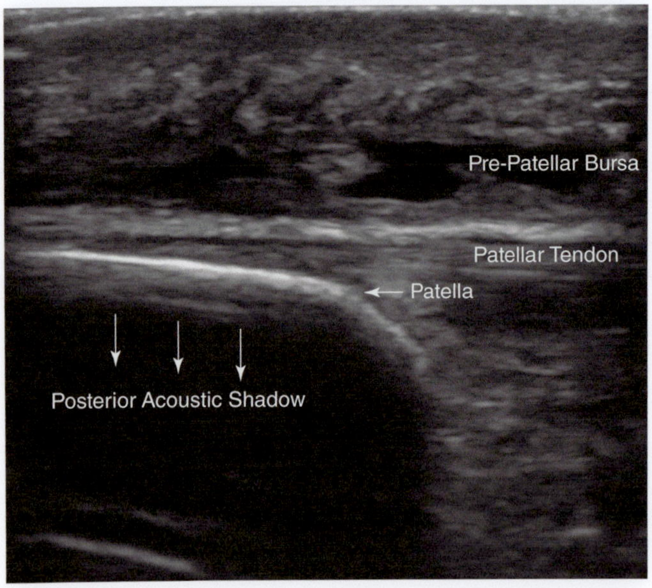

Fig. 2.19 Posterior acoustic shadow of the lower pole of the patella with the proximal insertion of the patellar tendon

"dirty" shadowing can occur when sound waves are scattered or refracted at air interfaces, like in the lungs or bowel, causing a more disorganized shadowing pattern [4, 14]. In contrast to anechoic shadowing from a dense object, dirty shadowing will create a gray and hazy appearance deep to the structure, resulting from the scattered ultrasound beams.

Posterior Acoustic Enhancement

Posterior acoustic enhancement occurs when a fluid-filled structure, such as a cyst, allows more sound waves to pass through at a faster speed (due to a higher propagation rate and less attenuation) than the tissue. This causes the area behind it to appear brighter (hyperechoic) than the surrounding tissues. These effects are influenced by the frequency used, with higher frequencies enhancing this artifact. While shadowing often points to gas or solid materials, posterior enhancement typically indicates a fluid-filled space (Fig. 2.20) [4, 14].

Reverberation Artifact

Reverberation artifact, also called "ringdown" or "comet tail" artifact, happens when sound waves bounce back and forth between two reflective surfaces before returning to the ultrasound probe. This creates bright, evenly spaced lines on the image, corresponding to the distance or frequency of the reverberation. While the first reflections accurately represent anatomy, the later echoes are artifacts and do not correspond to real structures. Clinically, these artifacts can be seen as A-lines in lung ultrasound or when visualizing metallic foreign bodies (Fig. 2.21) [15, 16].

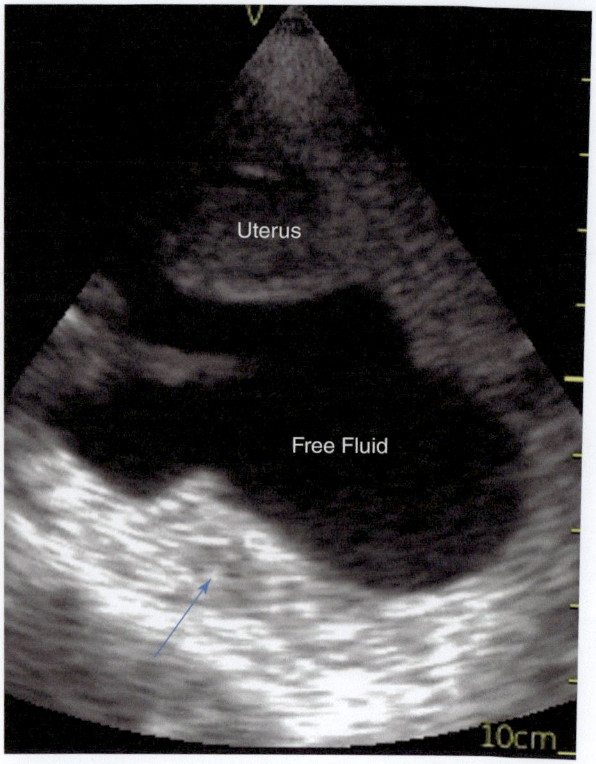

Fig. 2.20 Posterior acoustic enhancement behind pelvic free fluid (arrow)

Side Lobe Artifact

Ultrasound image reconstruction is based on the assumption that echoes return from structures directly in the path of the ultrasound beam. However, artifacts occur when echoes come from multiple reflections or from side lobes of the beam. Side lobes are weaker, off-axis emissions that can pick up reflections from nearby reflective objects and misplace them in the image, often showing up as bright (hyperechoic) lines within fluid-filled (anechoic) areas (Fig. 2.22). This is commonly seen in the heart's cavities and the bladder. To differentiate between real pathology and artifacts,

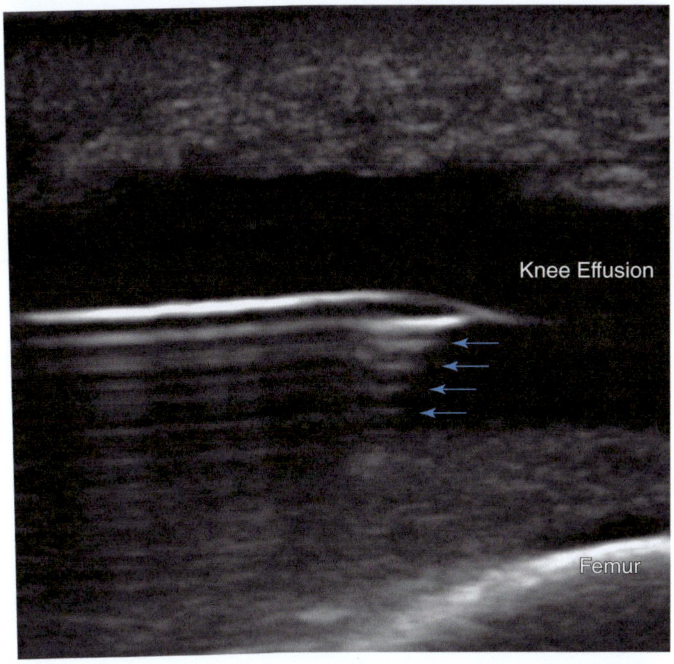

Fig. 2.21 Reverberation artifact finding (arrows) behind a needle during a knee arthrocentesis

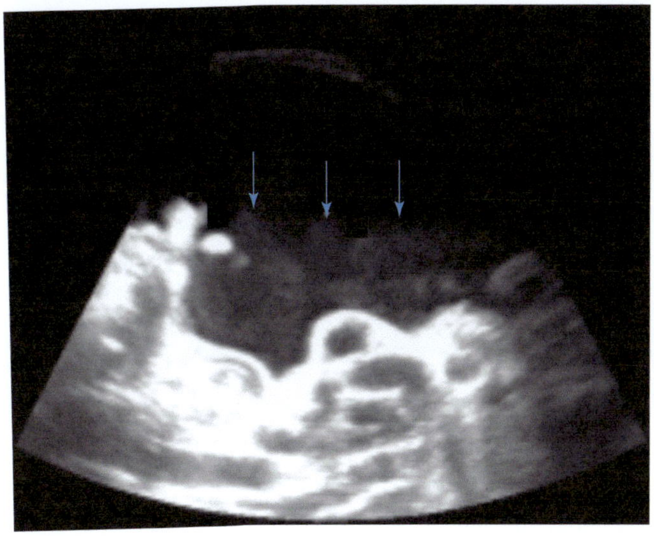

Fig. 2.22 Side lobe artifact (arrows) seen during an abdominal ultrasound in a patient with ascites

clinicians can adjust the probe angle or rotate it to get multiple views, helping to avoid misdiagnosis [14–16].

Edge Artifact

Edge artifact, a type of refraction artifact, occurs when ultrasound waves hit the curved edges of structures like the

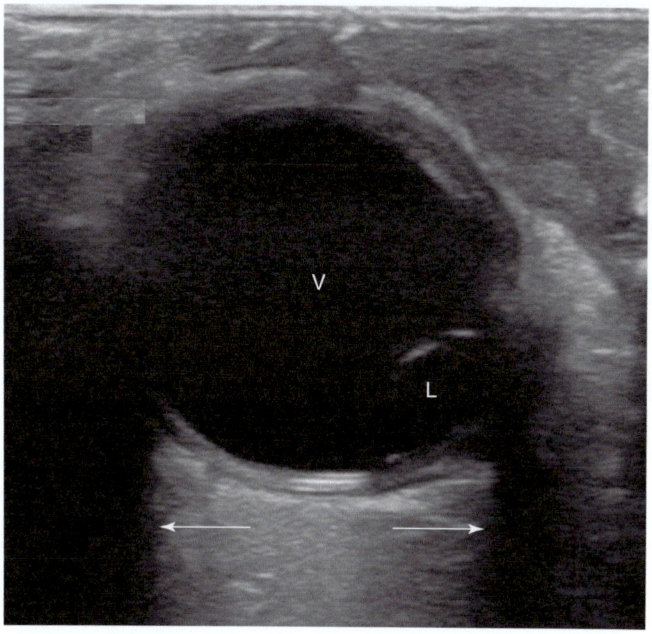

Fig. 2.23 Edge artifact (arrows) in an ocular ultrasound of a patient with a dislocated lens. *V = vitreous, L = lens*

gallbladder or bladder, or when the waves cross between tissues with different speeds of sound (Fig. 2.23). When the ultrasound waves strike a structure at an oblique angle, they bend away from their original path and send fewer echoes back to the probe. This results in a hypoechoic zone, where the ultrasound beam's intensity is reduced after bending around the curved edge. This thin acoustic shadow can sometimes be mistaken for pathology, such as the shadow behind a calcified gallstone. To differentiate an edge artifact from true pathology, the sonographer can trace the shadow to its origin. If there is a bright, echogenic structure at the start of the shadow, it is likely a gallstone. Another approach is to image the structure from a different angle; if the shadow disappears, it is likely an edge artifact [15, 16].

Mirror Image Artifact

Mirroring is an ultrasound artifact where a false or duplicate image appears on the opposite side of a strong reflector, often deeper than the real structure. This commonly occurs at the diaphragm, which is a strong reflector. Sound waves bounce off the diaphragm, reflect off another structure like the liver, and then return to the diaphragm before finally heading back to the probe. This extra travel time causes the ultrasound system to misinterpret the reflected signals as coming from a deeper structure, creating the illusion of a structure that is not actually there.

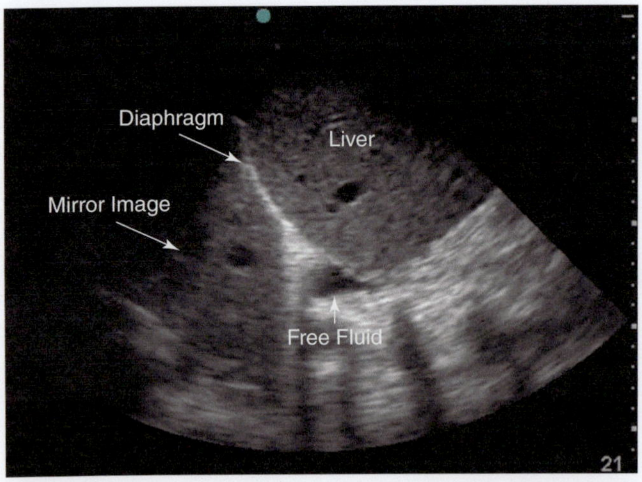

Fig. 2.24 Mirror image artifact during a FAST ultrasound. The diaphragm acts as a strong reflector, causing a mirror image of the liver tissue to be seen superior to the diaphragm with a trace of fluid in the thoracic cavity. *FF* free fluid

While this can be misleading during diagnosis, true anatomical structures usually produce stronger echoes, which can help minimize the mirroring effect. Mirrored images might also appear distorted due to the curvature of reflective surfaces, like the pericardium, complicating interpretation. Although commonly seen at the diaphragm, this artifact can occur at any strong reflective interface in the body. Clinically, it can be useful for ruling out free fluid above the diaphragm, as the mirror artifact disappears if fluid is present behind the reflecting surface (Fig. 2.24) [14, 16].

Anisotropy

Anisotropy is a common artifact in musculoskeletal ultrasound, particularly affecting tendons and nerves due to their fibrous structure. It occurs because sound waves behave differently depending on the angle they strike the fibers. When the waves hit the fibers at a perpendicular angle, attenuation increases, making tendons appear more hypoechoic, which can be mistaken for tendinitis or fluid-filled spaces (Figs. 2.25 and 2.26) [14].

To get a clear image of tendons, the ultrasound beam needs to be aligned perpendicularly to the tendon's axis; otherwise, anisotropy can distort the image. This artifact can be corrected by adjusting the probe angle to be parallel to the tendon or by having the patient contract the muscle to straighten the tendon. Anisotropy affects both long- and short-axis imaging planes, so careful probe manipulation is necessary for accurate orientation. It can also help differentiate between tendons and nerves, as tendons are more anisotropic, experiencing changes with as little as 2 degrees of angulation, whereas nerves require at least a 10-degree change to show similar effects [17].

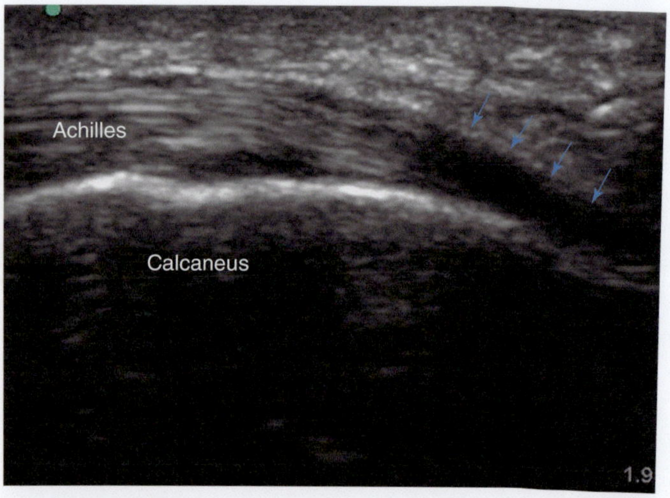

Fig. 2.25 Anisotropy (arrows) at the insertion of Achilles tendon due the anatomical curve

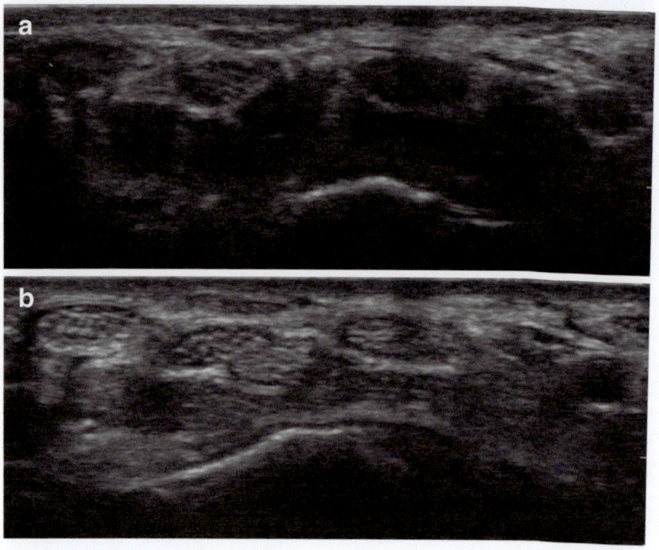

Fig. 2.26 Anisotropy causes a wrist flexor tendons to shift between hypoechoic (**a**) and echogenic (**b**) with slight fanning of the ultrasound probe

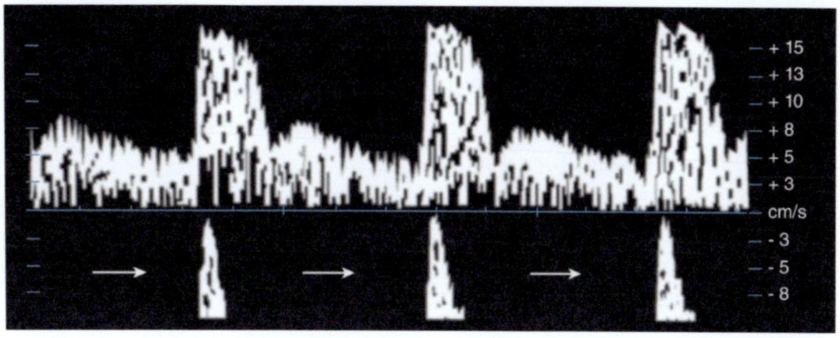

Fig. 2.27 Example of aliasing

Table 2.3 Technical modifications to manage or prevent aliasing

Shifting the baseline	Broadens the range of displayed velocities without aliasing
Shallower sample volume	Reduces time delay between pulse emission and return; allows for higher PRF and a higher Nyquist limit
Increasing velocity scale	Accommodates higher velocities
Increasing angle of insonation	Impacts the Doppler frequency shift; helps manage aliasing
Switching to CW Doppler	No Nyquist limit; measures higher velocities without aliasing

Aliasing

Aliasing occurs when blood flow velocities exceed the Nyquist limit, which is defined as half of the PRF. The Nyquist limit represents the maximum velocity that can be accurately measured without distortion. When the velocity surpasses this limit, the Doppler signals are misrepresented, making the flow appear as if it is moving in the opposite direction (referred to as aliasing). This is commonly seen in high-speed blood flow, such as in aortic insufficiency. To prevent or manage aliasing, several strategies can be applied, such as increasing the PRF, lowering the Doppler frequency, or using CWD for high velocities (Fig. 2.27, Table 2.3) [10, 18].

Biological Effects and Safety

Increasing ultrasound intensity can increase the risk of potential tissue damage. While this is often discussed as a theoretical risk, there remains no evidence to date confirming a clinically significant impact on tissue, including fetal tissues. Nonetheless, the "as low as reasonably achievable" (ALARA) principle in ultrasound should be followed. The ALARA principle advises using the minimum power output for safe imaging (especially in obstetric and ocular exams) and is consistent with the United States Food & Drug Administration (FDA) guidelines that recommend keeping power output low [1, 19–21]. Selecting the obstetrics or ocular examination presets should maintain the power output below the levels approved by the FDA for these tissue types. AIUM has stated there are no confirmed bioeffects from current diagnostic equipment, and views the benefits as outweighing any risks, recommending informing participants about exposure levels akin to normal diagnostic use [20, 21].

There are two main proxy measures of the ultrasound beam's biological effects:

1. The thermal index (TI) which is a measure of the ultrasound beam's thermal bioeffects as absorption of ultrasound waves by tissue can cause heating. At a given condition, TI reflects the power needed to raise the temperature by 1 °C. Absorption of heat is directly proportional to the frequency, so superficial structures are at higher theoretical risk. TI is most relevant in ocular and obstetric imaging. Intraocular structures are considered to be particularly at risk because their minimal blood flow cannot dissipate the heat generated. In fetal tissue, there is increased theoretical risk due to the small size and early embryological state. When using color or spectral Doppler, ultrasound output power increases, in turn increasing the TI. This is why the use of these modes is discouraged when imaging an embryo to avoid crossing a theoretical TI threshold. The International Society of Ultrasound in Obstetrics and Gynecology currently recommends a TI <1.0 for first trimester screening, limiting exposure time to Doppler imaging to preferably less than 5–10 min. The same is true for ocular imaging as recommended by the FDA [22, 23].
2. The mechanical index (MI) which is a measure of the ultrasound beam's micromechanical damage defined by its ability to cause cavitation-related bioeffects or mechanical stress. MI is inversely proportional to the ultrasound frequency and can be decreased by setting the focal zone away from the probe surface or by decreasing the beam output. Clinically, MI is relevant in contrast-enhanced ultrasound where cavitation of bubbles is needed, with smaller bubbles requiring higher pressure and higher frequency for cavitation. Lungs and intestines are the most sensitive to these cavitation effects because they are gas-filled organs. The FDA recommends keeping the MI <1.9 when imaging [4, 24].

In keeping with the principle of ALARA, the operator of the ultrasound machine should closely monitor the TI and MI to ensure that these values remain as low as possible, while maintaining appropriate settings to obtain adequate high-resolution images for patient care.

Key Ultrasound Findings

Term	Definition
Anechoic	Completely dark appearance, indicating no internal echoes Commonly seen in fluid-filled structures like cysts or the bladder
Hypoechoic	Appears darker than surrounding tissues, indicating fewer internal echoes
Hyperechoic	Appears brighter than surrounding tissues, indicating more internal echoes like calcified areas and fatty tissue
Isoechoic	Similar brightness to surrounding tissues, making it hard to distinguish from its surroundings
B-mode (brightness mode)	Two-dimensional image showing varying intensities of echoes, providing structural information about tissues and organs
M-mode (motion mode)	Single-dimensional representation of motion over time, typically used to assess the movement of structures like heart valves or the diaphragm
Gain	Adjusts amplification of returning echoes, affecting overall image brightness
Time Gain Compensation (TGC)	Adjusts gain at different depths to compensate for attenuation, ensuring a uniform image from near to far field
Tissue Harmonic Imaging (THI)	Utilizes the nonlinear propagation of ultrasound waves through tissue, enhancing image quality by reducing artifacts and improving resolution
Dynamic range	The range of echo intensities that an ultrasound system can process and display affecting image contrast
Spatial resolution	The ability of an ultrasound system to distinguish between two closely spaced objects, determining image detail and clarity
Temporal resolution	The ability to accurately track moving objects over time, related to the frame rate of the ultrasound system
Multibeam imaging	Uses multiple simultaneous beams to acquire data, increasing frame rates and improving temporal resolution
Doppler effect	Change in frequency of sound waves as they reflect off moving objects. It is used to measure blood flow velocity and direction
Color Doppler	Displays blood flow velocity and direction in color on a B-mode image
Power Doppler	Detects presence of blood flow without providing velocity or direction. More useful for detecting low flow
Spectral Doppler	Graphical display of blood flow velocities over time. Used to measure peak velocities and flow patterns in vessels and around the heart valves. Pulsed-wave Doppler has range specificity, but can have aliasing. Continuous-wave Doppler has no range specificity and no aliasing
Acoustic shadowing	Dark area behind a solid or calcified object where sound waves are blocked. Seen behind bones or stones
Posterior acoustic enhancement	Increased brightness behind a fluid-filled structure due to lower sound wave attenuation. It is typically seen behind cysts or the bladder
Reverberation	Multiple, equally spaced echoes caused by repeated reflection between two strong reflectors. B-lines in lung ultrasound or reverberation behind a needle
Edge shadowing	Dark bands on either side of a round structure like cyst or bladder due to bending (refraction) and scattering of sound waves
Aliasing	An artifact in Doppler ultrasound where high-velocity blood flow appears to reverse direction due to limitations in sampling frequency
Attenuation	Reduction in sound wave intensity as they pass through tissue, due to absorption, scattering, and reflection
Thermal index	A measure of the potential for tissue heating due to ultrasound exposure, important for assessing the safety of the examination
Mechanical index	A measure of the potential for mechanical bioeffects, such as cavitation, from ultrasound exposure

Pearls and Pitfalls

- Adjust the depth to keep the organ centered on the screen for clearer images and better diagnosis. Avoid setting the depth too deep, as it slows down returning echoes, reducing image quality and slowing frame rate.
- Fine-tune gain and TGC settings to improve brightness and contrast at different depths. Too much gain can make the image overly bright, hiding important details.
- Use multibeam imaging and tissue harmonics to sharpen images and reduce artifacts, especially in larger patients.
- Choose the right transducer based on how deep the organ is; high-frequency probes work best for shallow structures like blood vessels and soft tissues.

(continued)

- Keep the angle of insonation as close to 90 degrees as possible to improve image quality and avoid unnecessary artifacts.
- For cardiac and vascular Doppler exams, adjust the frame rate and depth settings to optimize spatial and temporal resolution. Properly sizing the color box and adjusting image depth are key for improving resolution.
- Learn to spot common artifacts (like shadowing, side lobe, edge artifact, or reverberation) to avoid misinterpreting images.
- Follow the ALARA principle to limit patient exposure to ultrasound energy, especially in ocular and obstetric ultrasound.

References

1. AIUM curriculum for fundamentals of ultrasound physics and instrumentation. J Ultrasound Med. 2019;38(8):1933–5.
2. Lawrence JP. Physics and instrumentation of ultrasound. Critic Care Med. 2007;35(Suppl):S314–22.
3. Uppal T. Tissue harmonic imaging. Australas J Ultrasound Med. 2010;13(2):29–31.
4. Aldrich JE. Basic physics of ultrasound imaging. Crit Care Med. 2007;35(5 Suppl):S131–7.
5. Rathod VT. A review of acoustic impedance matching techniques for piezoelectric sensors and transducers. Sensors. 2020;20(14):4051.
6. Rothberg JM, Ralston TS, Rothberg AG, et al. Ultrasound-on-chip platform for medical imaging, analysis, and collective intelligence. Proc Natl Acad Sci USA. 2021;118(27):e2019339118. https://doi.org/10.1073/pnas.2019339118. PMID: 34210796; PMCID: PMC8271708
7. He Y, Wan H, Jiang X, Peng C. Piezoelectric micromachined ultrasound transducer technology: recent advances and applications. Biosensors (Basel). 2022;13(1):55. https://doi.org/10.3390/bios13010055. PMID: 36671890; PMCID: PMC9856188
8. Ergun AS, Oralkan O, Yarahoglu GG, et al. Capacitive micromachined ultrasonic transducers: fabrication technology. IEEE Trans Ultrason Ferroelectris Freq Control. 2005;52(12):2242–58.
9. Bahner DP, Blickendorf JM, Bockbrader M, et al. Language of transducer manipulation: codifying terms for effective teaching. J of Ultrasound Medicine. 2016;35(1):183–8.
10. Shokoohi H, Chu D, Al Jalbout N. Ultrasound physics. Emerg Med Clinic. 2024;42:711. https://doi.org/10.1016/j.emc.2024.05.002.
11. Edler I, Lindström K. The history of echocardiography. Ultrasound Med Biol. 2004;30(12):1565–644.
12. Kruskal JB, Newman PA, Sammons LG, Kane RA. Optimizing doppler and color flow US: application to hepatic sonography. Radiographics. 2004;24(3):657–75. https://doi.org/10.1148/rg.243035139.
13. Yagil Y, Naroditsky I, Milhem J, et al. Role of doppler ultrasonography in the triage of acute scrotum in the emergency department. J Ultrasound Med. 2010;29(1):11–21.
14. Quien MM, Saric M. Ultrasound imaging artifacts: how to recognize them and how to avoid them. Echocardiography. 2018;35(9):1388–401.
15. Prabhu SJ, Kanal K, Bhargava P, Vaidya S, Dighe MK. Ultrasound artifacts: classification, applied physics with illustrations, and imaging appearances. Ultrasound Q. 2014;30(2):145–57.
16. Feldman M, Katyal S, Blackwood M. US artifacts, vol. 29(4). Radiographics: a review publication of the Radiological Society of North America, Inc; 2009. p. 1179–89.
17. Jamadar DA, Robertson BL, Jacobson JA, Girish G, Sabb BJ, Jiang Y, Morag Y. Musculoskeletal sonography: important imaging pitfalls. AJR Am J Roentgenol. 2010;194(1):216–25. https://doi.org/10.2214/AJR.09.2712. PMID: 20028926
18. Rubens DJ, Bhatt S, Nedelka S, Cullinan J. Doppler artifacts and pitfalls. Radiol Clin North Am. 2006;44(6):805–35. https://doi.org/10.1016/j.rcl.2006.10.014. PMID: 17147988
19. Abramowicz JS, Adhikari S, Dickman E, et al. Ocular ultrasound: review of bioeffects and safety, including fetal and point-of-care perspective. J of Ultrasound Medicine. 2022;41(7):1609–22.
20. American Institute of Ultrasound in Medicine. Recommended maximum scanning times for displayed thermal index (TI) values. American Institute of Ultrasound in Medicine website. https://www.aium.org/resources/official-statements. Approved October 30, 2016
21. https://www.fda.gov/radiation-emitting-products/medical-imaging/ultrasound-imaging
22. Bigelow TA, Church CC, Sandstrom K, et al. The thermal index: its strengths, weaknesses, and proposed improvements. J Ultrasound Med. 2011;30(5):714–34.
23. Harris GR. Safety considerations for diagnostic ultrasound in the eye. J Ultrasound Med. 2019;38(5):11.
24. Sen T, Tufekcioglu O, Koza Y. Mechanical index. Anatol J Cardiol. 2015;15(4):334–6.

3 Ultrasound for Trauma Evaluation

Jailyn Avila, Ben C. Smith, and Megan Guy

Background

Trauma is the leading cause of death in persons under 45 years of age [1]. Rapid identification of the etiology of traumatic shock is essential to expedite appropriately tailored treatment. While the history and physical examination are important in the evaluation of a trauma patient, diagnostic imaging is helpful for planning management and disposition. Computed tomography (CT) is often considered the gold standard for trauma imaging. However, it requires transportation of a potentially unstable patient out of the acute care area, where resuscitation efforts can be more challenging. Point-of-care ultrasound (POCUS) performed at the bedside can thereby be used as the initial (and in some instances, only) diagnostic assessment. The Focused Assessment with Sonography in Trauma (FAST) examination was first described in 1995 as a bedside assessment for hemoperitoneum and hemopericardium [2]. The extended FAST (EFAST) built upon this to incorporate evaluation for a pneumothorax and was coined in 2004 [3].

A meta-analysis consisting of 34 studies with 8,635 adult and pediatric patients who suffered blunt abdominal trauma found that the FAST examination was 74% sensitive and 96% specific for hemoperitoneum [4]. Aside from its accuracy, the use of POCUS in the evaluation of these patients carries other benefits. One randomized controlled trial of trauma patients found that those who received a FAST examination demonstrated a shorter time to operative care, lower rate of CT scans, shorter admission length of stay, fewer number of complications, and reduced cost of care compared to those who did not receive a FAST examination [5]. Other studies have demonstrated decreased use of diagnostic peritoneal lavage and CT when POCUS was introduced into the diagnostic algorithm [6–10], changes in management upon performing the POCUS examination [6, 11–13], and decreased cost to the patient [14].

Indications

Indications
- Hemodynamically unstable patients with abdominal or thoracic trauma
- Hemodynamically stable patients with abdominal or thoracic trauma

Diagnoses
- Hemopericardium and tamponade
- Solid organ injury (e.g., liver, spleen, kidney)
- Hemoperitoneum
- Hemothorax
- Pneumothorax

Supplementary Information The online version contains supplementary material available at https://doi.org/10.1007/978-3-031-85308-1_3.

J. Avila (✉)
Department of Emergency Medicine, Temecula Valley Hospital, Temecula, CA, USA

B. C. Smith
Department of Emergency Medicine, Erlanger Baroness Hospital, Chattanooga, TN, USA

M. Guy
Department of Emergency Medicine, UC Irvine Medical Center, Orange, CA, USA

M. Gottlieb, N. Panebianco (eds.), *Advanced Point-of-Care Ultrasound*, https://doi.org/10.1007/978-3-031-85308-1_3

Core Views

View	Image	Approach
Right Upper Quadrant (RUQ)	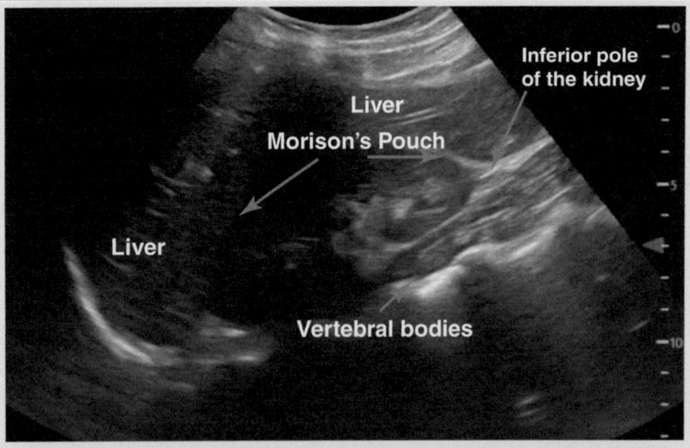 Core View 1. Right upper quadrant view demonstrating Morison's pouch Core Video 1. Right upper quadrant view	Technique: Place a low-frequency probe in the coronal plane at the mid-axillary line between T5 and T7. Fan from an anterior to posterior plane (or vice versa). Structures visualized (from highest to lowest sensitivity for free fluid): Right paracolic gutter (interface between caudal tip of the liver and inferior pole of the kidney) Morison's pouch (hepatorenal fossa) Subdiaphragmatic recess
Pelvis	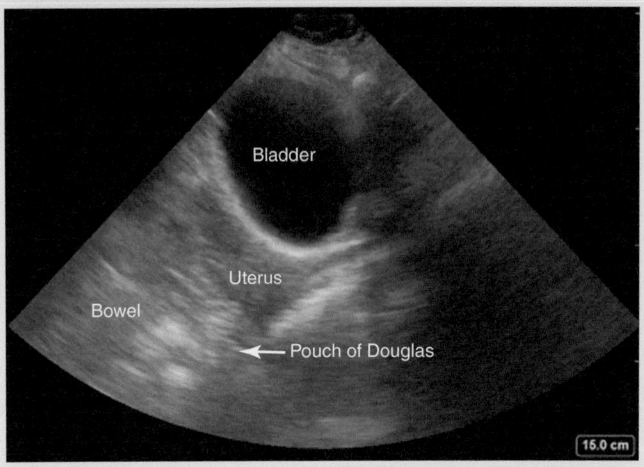 Core View 2. Pelvic view demonstrating the pouch of Douglas in a patient with a uterus Core Video 2. Pelvic view demonstrating the pouch of Douglas in a patient with a uterus	Technique: Place probe cephalad to the pubic symphysis, using the bladder as a landmark and acoustic window. Perform a sweep of the area in the sagittal plane. Then, rotate the probe 90 degrees and perform a sweep in the transverse plane. Structures visualized: Rectovesicular pouch (patients without a uterus) Rectouterine pouch (patients with an anteverted uterus) Uterovesicular recess (patients with a retroverted uterus)
Left Upper Quadrant (LUQ)	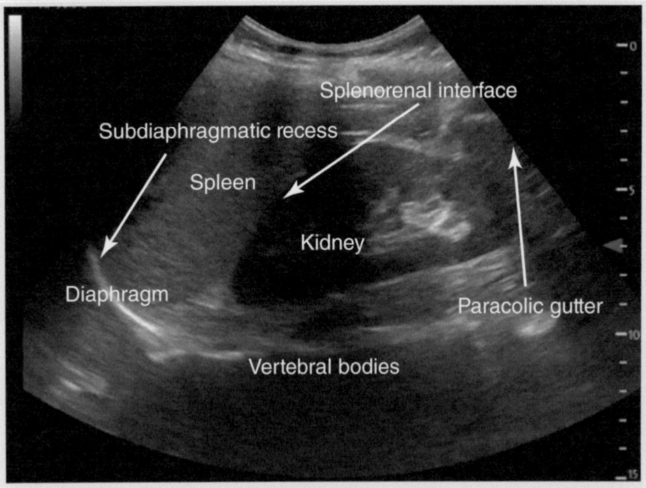 Core View 3. Left upper quadrant view Core Video 3. Left upper quadrant view	Technique: Place probe slightly more posterior and cephalad, as compared to the RUQ view. Fan from an anterior to posterior plane (or vice versa). Structures visualized (from highest to lowest sensitivity for free fluid): Subdiaphragmatic recess Splenorenal recess Left paracolic gutter (interface between inferior pole of the kidney and caudal tip of the spleen)

View	Image	Approach
Cardiac	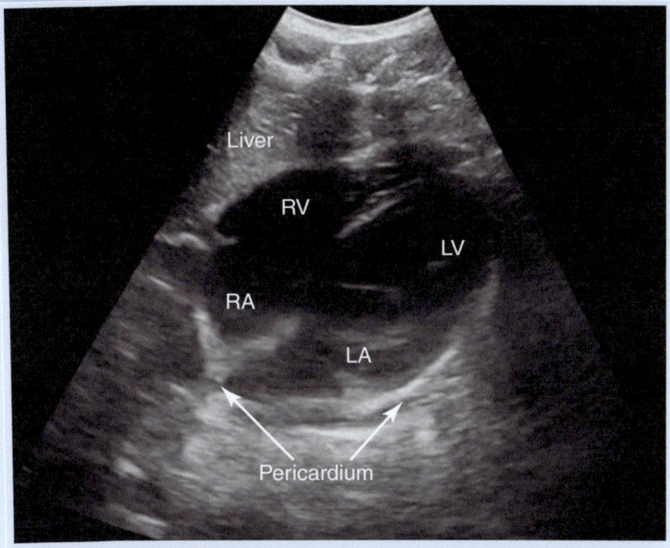 Core View 4. Subxiphoid cardiac view Core Video 4. Subxiphoid cardiac view	Technique For the subcostal window, place the probe in the subxiphoid region with the marker aligning with its location on the screen. The tail of the probe should be flattened against the abdomen in order to direct the ultrasound beam up toward the heart. For the parasternal long-axis view, place the probe to the left of the sternum, at around the level of T4 with the probe marker toward the right shoulder. Structures visualized Right and left ventricles Right and left atria Pericardial lining
Thoracic view for pneumothorax	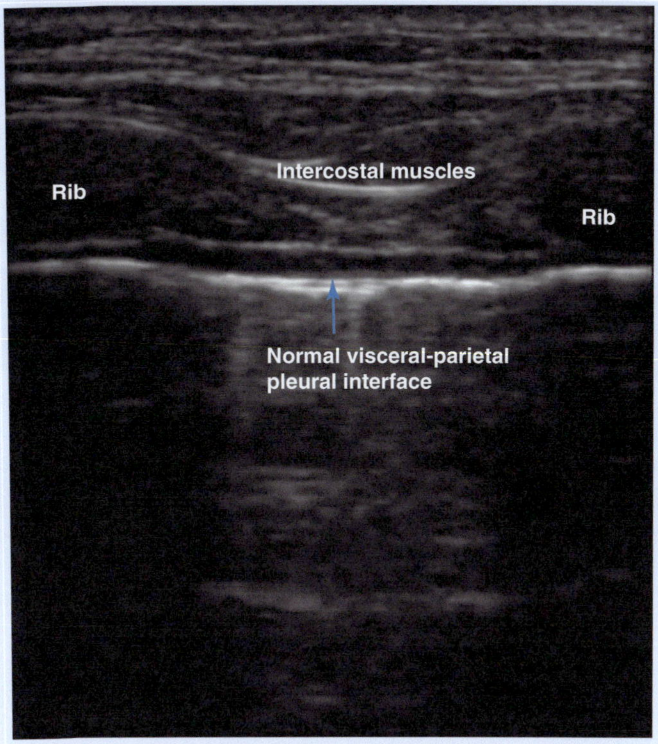 Core View 5. Thoracic pleural view for pneumothorax Core Video 5. Thoracic pleural view for pneumothorax	Technique Place a high-frequency probe in the sagittal orientation with the marker facing cephalad, focusing on the intercostal recess in the anterior and lateral regions of each hemithorax. Structures visualized (from superficial to deep) Ribs Intercostal muscles Pleural line

View	Image	Approach
Thoracic view for hemothorax	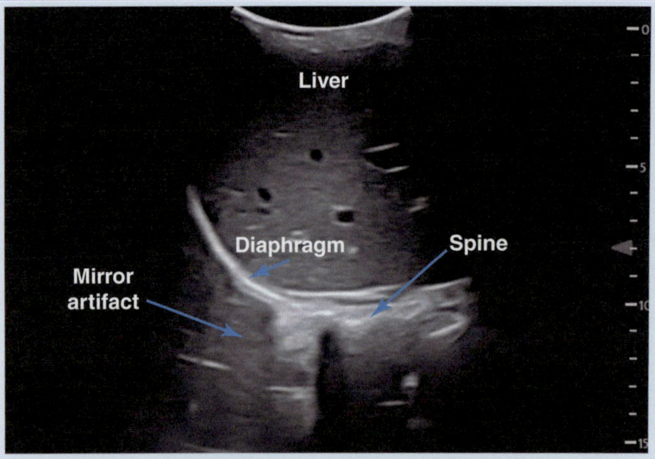 Core View 6. Thoracic view at the lung base for hemothorax Core Video 6. Thoracic view at the lung base for hemothorax	Technique Place a low-frequency probe in the coronal plane at the mid-axillary or posterior axillary line in the most dependent region of each hemithorax. Structures visualized Liver or spleen Lumbar and lower thoracic vertebral bodies Diaphragm

Clinical Applications

EFAST Examination

General Considerations

With regard to the specific probe to use, the curvilinear probe has the widest footprint and often has a higher frequency compared to the phased array probe, which supplies an image with a higher resolution. This makes the curvilinear probe the preferred one for the FAST examination, especially for the abdominal component. The phased array probe may be utilized as well, but suffers from a lower resolution relative to the curvilinear probe. One advantage of the phased array probe would be for visualizing the heart (especially in the parasternal long-axis view), as the smaller footprint is less likely to be obscured by ribs. As with any ultrasound examination, the depth should be decreased to only contain the structures of interest in order to maximize the resolution and increase the frame rate. Operators should also be careful to avoid excess gain, which could lead to missing free fluid.

Free fluid will appear as a hypoechoic area not contained within a cystic structure, such as the bladder. It is best identified by performing thorough sweeps in each region. The order in which the abdominal FAST examination components are performed should be based on where the gravitationally dependent free fluid is most likely to be present. For example, in most blunt trauma patients, the right upper quadrant (RUQ) should be performed first as this is the area most likely to be positive [15]. This should be followed by the pelvic and left upper quadrant (LUQ) views. Some have proposed a cranial to caudal approach where the RUQ is performed first, followed by the LUQ and then the pelvis. However, the LUQ is typically the least likely to have isolated blood when hemoperitoneum is present [15] and is the most common of the three abdominal windows to be inadequately visualized[16]. Therefore, we recommend progressing from RUQ to pelvis followed by LUQ.

The FAST examination is primarily utilized as a binary examination (either positive or negative). A positive RUQ view (i.e., free fluid present) does not necessarily need the additional pelvic or LUQ view to diagnose hemoperitoneum. Additionally, when there is thoracic or combined trauma, it may be preferable to begin with the cardiac and thoracic components prior to the abdominal components, particularly when there is a clinical concern for hemopericardium, pneumothorax, or hemothorax. Regardless of the specific order, it is important that this examination be performed quickly and thoroughly.

Importantly, the FAST examination does not necessarily identify the source or composition of abdominal free fluid. For example, RUQ fluid may be the only sign of a splenic injury, even when the LUQ view is negative [17]. Additionally, while free fluid after trauma is most likely hemoperitoneum, it could alternatively be ascites, urine, bile, or bowel contents in the appropriate clinical context. In patients who have a delayed presentation to the ED after trauma, or who have a slow bleed, the blood can clot and become isoechoic relative to surrounding structures and may be missed.

Right Upper Quadrant View

In the RUQ view, the areas most likely to demonstrate free fluid (in order of frequency) are: the interface between the caudal tip of the liver and inferior pole of the kidney, hepatorenal recess (i.e., Morison's pouch), and subdiaphrag-

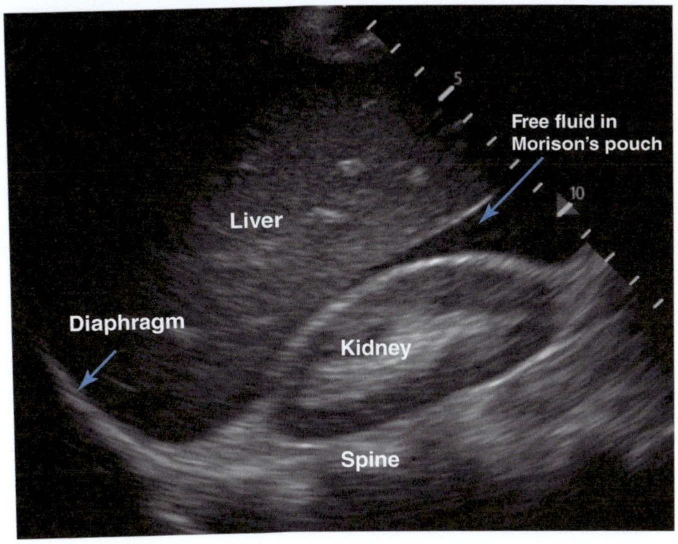

Fig. 3.1 Free fluid in the right upper quadrant view. In this image, there is a wedge of hypoechoic free fluid visible in Morison's pouch, which in the setting of trauma may be indicative of blood

matic recess (also known as the suprahepatic recess) [15] (Fig. 3.1, Video 1). Accuracy of the RUQ view can be increased by placing the patient in 30 degrees Trendelenberg positioning [18].

Pelvic View

In a person with a uterus, fluid will be preferentially located in the rectouterine recess (i.e., pouch of Douglas) (Fig. 3.2, Video 2) or rectovesicular recess. If the uterus is retroverted, fluid may preferentially accumulate first between the bladder and the uterus (i.e., the uterovesicular recess). In a person with a prostate, fluid will more likely be found in the rectovesicular recess (Fig. 3.3, Video 3). Importantly, in persons with a prostate, the seminal vesicles are often seen posterior to the bladder and should not be mistaken as free fluid within the peritoneum (Fig. 3.4, Video 4). Differentiating between free fluid and the seminal vesicles can be accomplished by turning the transducer in the sagittal orientation and observing the paired seminal vessels attached to the prostate with or without free fluid visualized cephalad to the tips of the seminal vesicles.

Because a distended bladder can create posterior acoustic enhancement, it is possible to miss small amounts of fluid (particularly if it contains heterogeneous components such as clotted blood). To avoid this, consider reducing the time gain compensation deep to the bladder to maintain a consistent echogenicity throughout the image.

Differentiating between physiologic free fluid and pathologic free fluid should be accomplished via careful consideration of preexisting risk factors, the patient's current symptoms, serial examinations, and complimentary medical tests and imaging. Some references state that physiologic

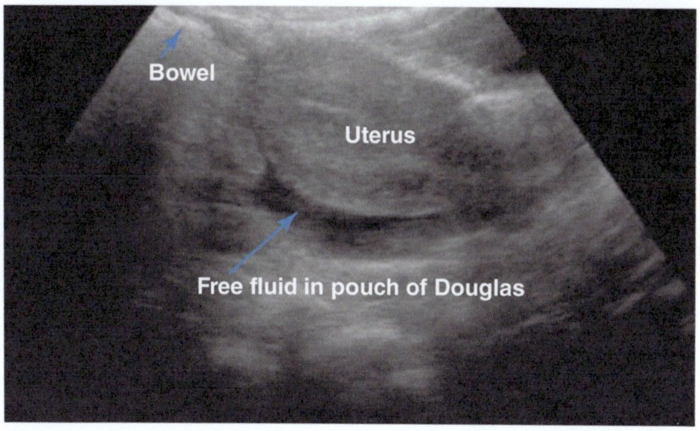

Fig. 3.2 Sagittal suprapubic view in a patient with a uterus demonstrating hypoechoic blood posterior to the uterus in the pouch of Douglas

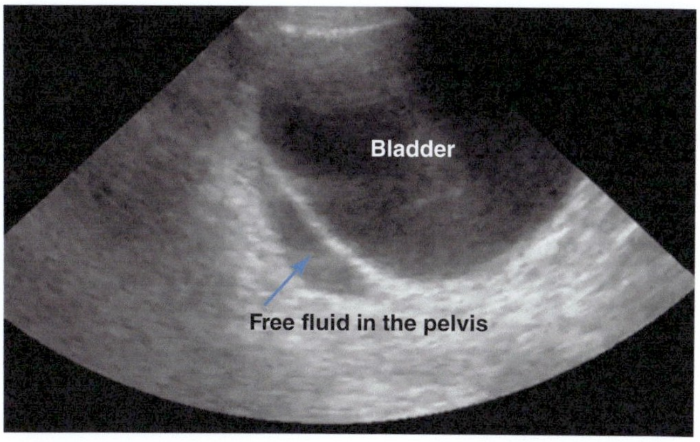

Fig. 3.3 Transverse suprapubic view of a patient without a uterus. The bladder has anechoic urine contained within it. Posterolateral to the bladder, hypoechoic blood is visualized

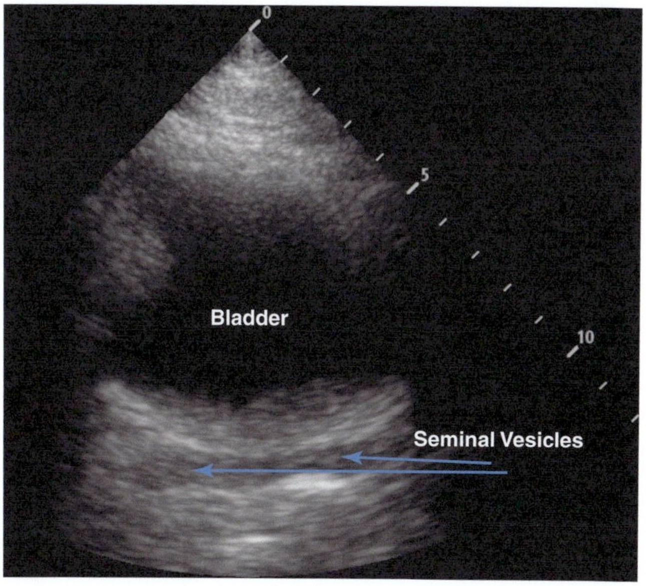

Fig. 3.4 Seminal vesicles are fluid-filled hypoechoic tubular structures posterior to the bladder in the male pelvis that can be mistaken for free fluid

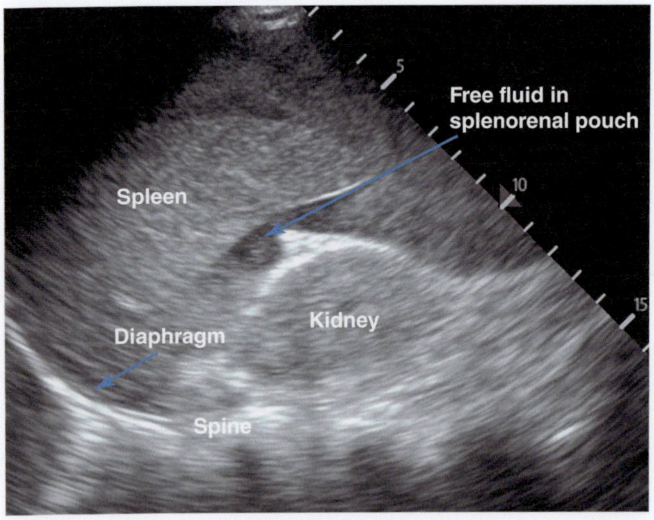

Fig. 3.5 Free fluid in the left upper quadrant view. This image contains hypoechoic free fluid between the spleen and the kidney concerning for blood in the setting of trauma

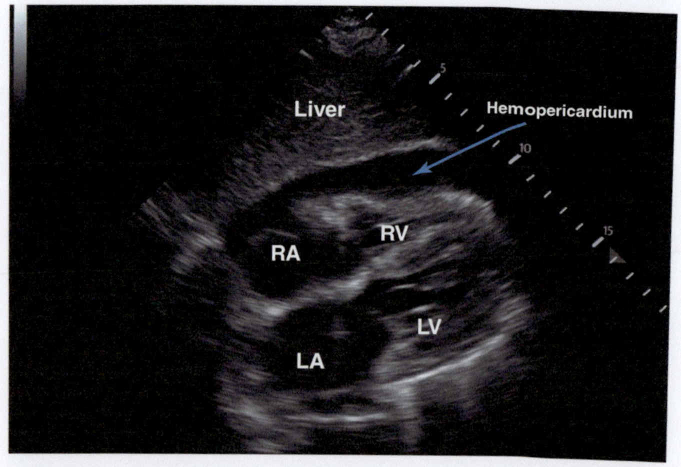

Fig. 3.6 Hemopericardium. In this image, blood surrounds the heart within the pericardium. The blood is anechoic in the setting of an acute bleed prior to coagulation. *LA* left atrium, *RA* right atrium, *LV* left ventricle, *RV* right ventricle

free fluid may be a relatively common finding in patients with a uterus. However, subsequent data has shown this idea to potentially be a cause of catastrophic oversight. In a large study of 2319 patients with a uterus who presented with blunt abdominal trauma, 2% of nonpregnant patients and 3% of pregnant patients had isolated free fluid to the pelvis. Among these patients, 30% of pregnant and 40% of nonpregnant patients were ultimately found to have traumatic injuries as the cause of their isolated pelvic free fluid [19].

Left Upper Quadrant View

Care should be taken to remember that the LUQ is not a mirror image of the RUQ and that fluid preferentially accumulates in different locations relative to the RUQ. The most common regions for free fluid to accumulate in the LUQ are (in order): the subdiaphragmatic recess, the left paracolic region, and splenorenal recess (Fig. 3.5, Video 5) [15, 16, 20]. Another important consideration is that the LUQ view is typically the most difficult view to obtain [16]. One study reported that over half of 405 reviewed FAST examinations had inadequate LUQ views, mostly due to poor subdiaphragmatic views [16].

Pericardial Effusion and Tamponade

The evaluation of the heart for the presence of hemopericardium and tamponade can be performed using the curvilinear or phased array probe. Traditionally, it has been taught that a subxiphoid view is the preferred view for the EFAST; however, any acoustic window that can visualize the heart is sufficient. A pericardial effusion will appear as a rim of fluid surrounding the heart (Fig. 3.6, Video 6). While there is normally 15–30 mL of physiologic fluid in the pericardial sac, this fluid is rarely seen with ultrasound [21]. Therefore, a non-trace pericardial effusion is generally considered abnormal. Importantly, one study found that up to 2% of cardiac POCUS examinations had an incidental pericardial effusion, so this must be correlated with the patient's symptoms and examination [22].

Epicardial fat pads may be mistaken for hemopericardium. Differentiation involves careful inspection of the suspected fat pad. If the pericardial structure is seen to be completely adhered to the myocardium, it is more likely to be an epicardial fat pad rather than a clot in the pericardium. Additionally, in patients with significant abdominal trauma, the subcostal view may be difficult to adequately obtain due to abdominal pain. A parasternal or apical view of the heart is acceptable for the evaluation of hemopericardium in these cases.

In the context of trauma, the primary focus is identifying early tamponade that would require prompt decompression. The echocardiographic findings suggestive of tamponade include systolic right atrial collapse (sensitive), diastolic right ventricular collapse (specific), and a dilated and noncollapsible inferior vena cava (sensitive) [23–25]. If hemopericardium is identified but tamponade is not suspected, one must keep in mind that rapid collection of pericardial fluid within a noncompliant pericardium is poorly tolerated and may quickly progress to tamponade. Therefore, serial cardiac examinations may be useful, particularly in patients with hemopericardium without initial tamponade physiology, especially if there is a decline in hemodynamics. Of note, the diagnosis of tamponade should preferentially be made based on the sonographic identification of obstruction to cardiac outflow (i.e., right ventricular diastolic collapse) rather than the presence of hypotension. This is due to the fact that most patients in early tamponade are normotensive or hypertensive, or they may be hypotensive for reasons other than the pericardial fluid [26].

Pneumothorax

While chest x-ray is commonly used to identify a traumatic pneumothorax, in supine trauma patients, it has been found to have low sensitivity, especially for smaller pneumothoraces [27]. POCUS has been found to have similar specificities to supine chest x-ray (99% POCUS vs 100% chest x-ray) but markedly improved sensitivities (91% POCUS vs 47% chest x-ray) [27].

Either the curvilinear or linear probe may be used for this assessment [28, 29]. While the linear probe is often preferred, the curvilinear probe may be advantageous if already being used as part of the remainder of the FAST examination. In order to optimize the image, the clinician should decrease the depth so that the bottom of the ultrasound window extends 2-4 cm deep to the pleura. Additionally, decreasing the gain will allow for easier visualization of pleural sliding.

The probe should be placed at the level of T5–T8 along the midclavicular line in the sagittal orientation with the probe marker facing cephalad [30]. The visceral-parietal pleural interface (i.e., pleural line) should be identified as a hyperechoic line just deep to the ribs. This white line represents the visceral and parietal pleural interface between the chest wall and the lungs. This is the primary area of focus and the focal point should be set to this location if possible.

If either lung sliding is visible or reverberation artifacts are seen, this indicates that the visceral and parietal pleura are in contact with one another, and pneumothorax has been ruled out in that area (Fig. 3.7, Video 7). Conversely, a pneumothorax is suggested when the hyperechoic line of the pleura does not slide with respiration. This absence of sliding suggests that there is air in between the parietal and visceral pleura, which obstructs sound waves from visualizing the mobile visceral pleura (Fig. 3.8, Video 8).

There are, however, other pathologies that can also abolish lung sliding such as blebs, adhesions, and apnea. Additionally, if there is subcutaneous emphysema, the air in the subcutaneous tissue will obstruct the sound waves from reaching the pleura. This would render the ultrasound unable to make any assessment of the lungs due to the inability to visualize the pleura itself [31]. Patients with previous lung surgery may not have the typical apical or anterior pneumothorax location. In these instances, pleural sliding may be lost if the visceral and parietal pleura are adherent. Similarly, small pneumothoraces close to the mediastinum may be missed because the findings can be obscured by bone.

Whereas lung sliding rules out a pneumothorax in the area that is being evaluated, the lung point has a high specificity for pneumothorax. A lung point refers to when lung sliding is visualized in one region of the pleural line and absent on another part of the pleural line (Video 9). The lung point represents the border of the pneumothorax, where the visceral pleura contacts the parietal pleura. Lung point can also be used to predict the size of the pneumothorax [32]. Data report that the specificity of a lung point for pneumothorax is 100%; however, these studies consisted predominantly of patients in the intensive care unit patients, with few traumatic pneumothoraces [33–37]. Additionally, there have been false-positives reported, including the interface between

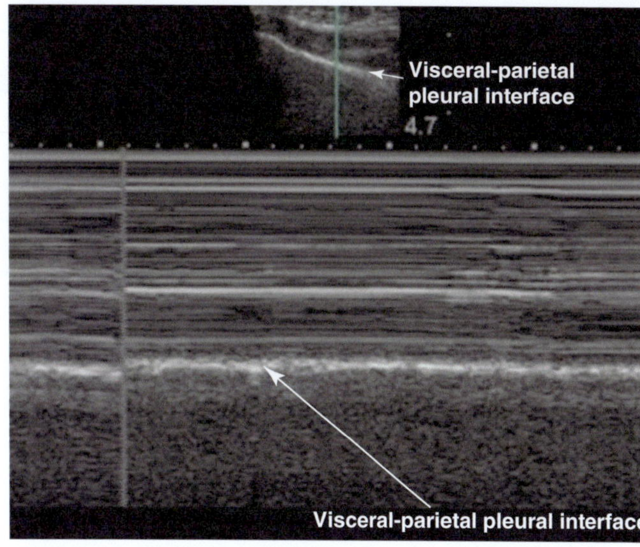

Fig. 3.7 Normal lung ultrasound. The M-mode cursor is centered over the intercostal recess with a linear probe. As represented by the "seashore sign," movement is seen at the pleural line with artifacts deep to it. This signal is indicative of lung sliding, ruling out a pneumothorax in this specific rib recess

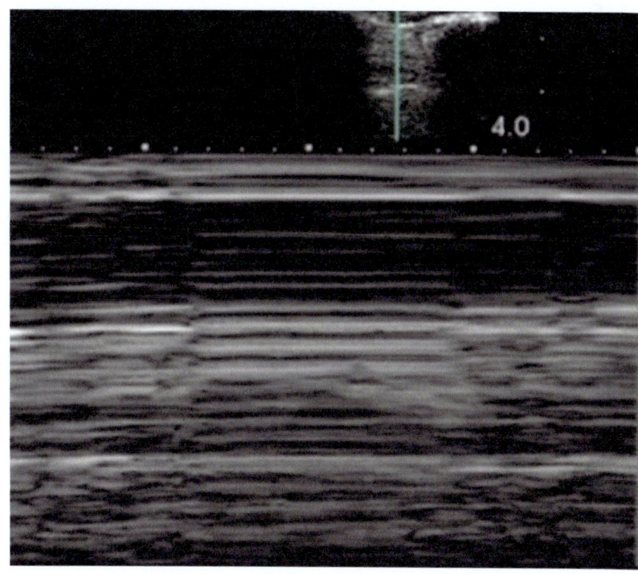

Fig. 3.8 Pneumothorax. The waveform from superficial to deep has a similar pattern on the M-mode tracing. This "Barcode" or "Stratosphere" sign indicates that the visceral pleura is not directly touching the parietal pleural. This represents the absence of lung sliding in that specific rib recess, which may be indicative of a pneumothorax in the correct clinical setting

the diaphragm and lung, the heart, and the lung, and in bullous lung disease [38].

In the scenario of apnea or right mainstem intubation, lung sliding and visceral-based reverberation artifacts may not appear. The presence of a lung pulse, horizontal rhythmic sliding that occurs at the same rate as the heart typically in the left lung adjacent to the contracting heart, can also rule out pneumothorax under these conditions [39]. This is often identified using motion mode (M-mode), but it can also be seen with brightness mode (B-mode).

Additional Applications

Hemothorax

The sonographic diagnosis of a hemothorax is not significantly different from the evaluation for a nontraumatic pleural effusion. The curvilinear probe is placed along the mid-axillary or posterior axillary line at the level of the diaphragm with the marker facing cephalad. A hemothorax is diagnosed by identifying dependent fluid within the thoracic cavity (Fig. 3.9, Video 10) [40]. The composition of the pleural effusion may range sonographically from relatively anechoic to a mixed density of hyper- and hypoechoic fluid, depending on the chronicity of the hemothorax [41]. For instance, an anechoic fluid collection is likely more consistent with an acute hemothorax, whereas a more complex effusion might suggest a subacute presentation with clotted blood [41].

Ultrasound findings that can assist in the diagnosis of a hemothorax are the "spine sign" and mirror artifact. In an air-filled thorax, the spine is generally not visualized cephalad to the diaphragm as air does not transmit sound. If there is fluid in that dependent pleural cavity, the vertebral bodies immediately cephalad to the diaphragm will be seen due to the fluid within the thoracic cavity transmitting sound to those thoracic vertebral bodies. A positive "spine sign" is when you can see the spine above the diaphragm and is generally indicative of a hemothorax, pleural effusion, or other pathology of increased density in the thorax. A mirror artifact is present when you see a mirror image of what is below the diaphragm above the diaphragm. This occurs because the diaphragm is a strong reflector and the air superior to it enhances the reflective nature, whereas fluid above the diaphragm would allow the beam to transmit above the diaphragm. The presence of a mirror artifact rules out a hemothorax because it implies that the hemithorax is air-filled and without fluid. A positive spine sign can help rule in a hemothorax, whereas a negative spine sign or the presence of mirror artifact help rule one out.

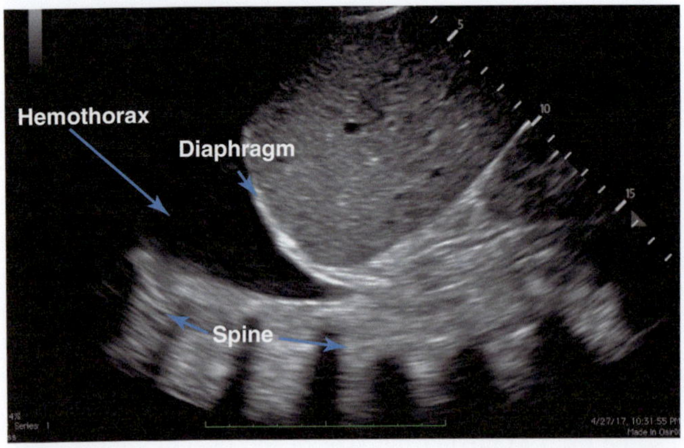

Fig. 3.9 Hemothorax. The liver is seen as a homogenous structure. Cephalad to the diaphragm, hypoechoic intrathoracic fluid is identified. In the setting of trauma, this would be indicative of a hemothorax. Hemothorax will appear as a fluid collection relatively hypoechoic to the echogenicity of the liver or spleen. Also visualized is the "spine sign" deep to the pleural effusion

Pulmonary Contusion

A chest x-ray is often used for diagnosing pulmonary contusion. However, ultrasound has been found to be significantly more sensitive at the bedside compared to chest x-ray [42]. While the gold standard diagnostic modality for the diagnosis of pulmonary contusions is CT, data suggest POCUS can accurately diagnose them with a specificity approaching 100% [43]. However, POCUS is only 58% sensitive and is, therefore, insufficient to exclude the diagnosis [44].

The curvilinear probe is preferred due to its wide field of view. The lung or thoracic preset should be used to enhance B-line identification. Start by examining the chest wall in multiple intercostal spaces, focusing on the areas of the chest where the patient has pain or bruising. A pulmonary contusion is diagnosed by identifying pleural line abnormalities (e.g., subpleural consolidations) or B-lines (Fig. 3.10, Video 11). Of note, a pulmonary contusion can also create a false-positive lung point due to the contusion creating an adhesive area of the pleura, which does not slide [45].

How to Utilize the EFAST Examination in Clinical Practice

The EFAST examination should be utilized as one of many data points in the clinical assessment of a patient who has suffered trauma. A negative EFAST examination does not have sufficient sensitivity for ruling out intra-abdominal injury in the setting of a patient with high pretest probability. This is an important consideration because not all patients with serious intra-abdominal injuries have hemoperitoneum. One retrospective study of 575 blunt abdominal trauma patients receiving CT reported that 34% of patients with abdominal visceral injuries did not have hemoperitoneum, and of those, 17% required surgical or angiographic inter-

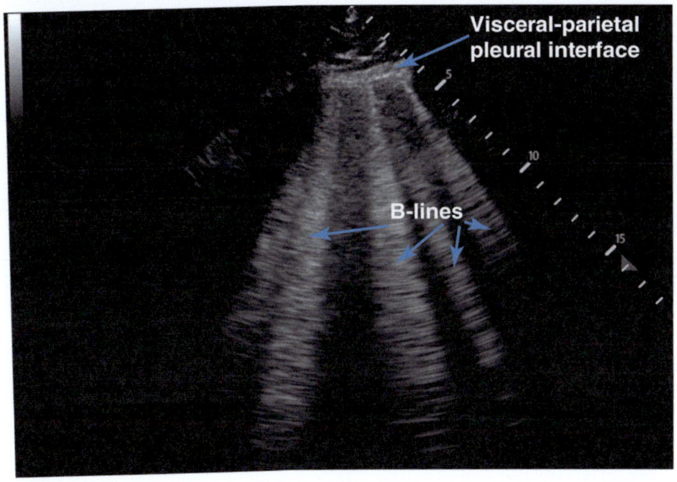

Fig. 3.10 Pulmonary contusion. This image demonstrates ≥3 B-lines in this lung field, indicative of interstitial edema, which in the setting of trauma could indicate pulmonary contusion

vention [46]. In another study of 3,392 consecutive blunt trauma admissions with CT imaging, 196 had abdominal injury and 26% did not have any detectable hemoperitoneum on admission [47].

The EFAST examination is most useful when employed in a hemodynamically unstable trauma patient. If the abdominal portion of the EFAST examination is positive for free fluid, it is likely that the patient has an underlying injury that requires immediate exploratory laparotomy. If the abdominal portion of the EFAST examination is negative in a hemodynamically unstable patient, it is unlikely that intra-abdominal hemorrhage is the etiology of hypotension, and other sources should be evaluated. The same holds true for the evaluation of pneumothorax and cardiac tamponade in a hypotensive patient. In a non-hypotensive patient, the EFAST examination still has value from a specificity standpoint. If a hemoperitoneum is identified in a non-hypotensive patient, resources can be deployed more quickly to diagnose and address the underlying etiology before hemodynamic instability in the so-called "golden hour" of the patient's trauma presentation.

The amount of fluid that needs to accumulate in the peritoneum before it is reliably identified with the FAST examination varies in the literature from 75 to 670 mL, with a mean hovering around 300-400 mL [18, 48–52]. However, studies show that the presence of larger volumes of fluid is correlated with a higher likelihood of hemodynamic instability and need for operative intervention [53–59].

Role of Serial Examinations

A limitation of the FAST examination is that a certain amount of fluid needs to accumulate before it can be detected reliably using POCUS. As noted above, the minimum amount of hemoperitoneum detectable can vary widely depending on the specific abdominal window utilized, patient positioning, and operator experience. This variability means that hemoperitoneum may not be sonographically visible earlier in the patient's hospital course [18, 48–52]. Therefore, if the initial examination is negative but there is a moderate or high suspicion for intra-abdominal injury or a change in the patient's hemodynamic status, serial FAST examinations may be beneficial, especially if an alternative imaging modality such as CT is unavailable or the patient is unsafe for transport. Two retrospective studies of patients with blunt abdominal trauma found that the sensitivity of the FAST examination increased from 38.5% to 85.2% and from 31.1% to 72.1%, respectively, after repeat scans were performed between 30 min and 24 h after the initial POCUS was performed [60, 61].

Solid Organ Injury

While the FAST examination focuses on indirect signs of injury via hemoperitoneum, free fluid may not always be present or visualized on ultrasound. Therefore, some experts have also used ultrasound to evaluate for solid organ injury. The sonographic identification of traumatic solid organ injuries of the spleen, liver, and kidney have been previously described [62–65]. Intracapsular injuries have been described as areas of hyper- and hypoechoic regions within the parenchyma (Fig. 3.11, Video 12), while lacerations have been described as thin, irregular hyper- or hypoechoic lines that traverse the affected organs (Fig. 3.12, Video 13) [62–65]. The accuracy of the sonographic diagnosis of solid organ injury detection has also been shown to improve after the administration of ultrasound contrast agents [66].

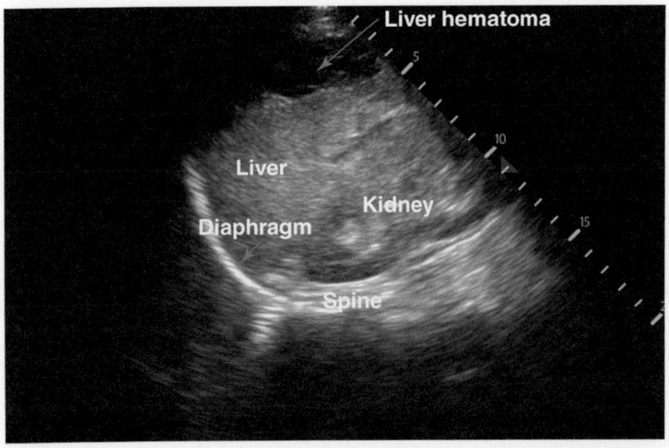

Fig. 3.11 Liver hematoma. This image demonstrates an intracapsular injury of the liver, which is seen as a hypoechoic area within the liver parenchyma

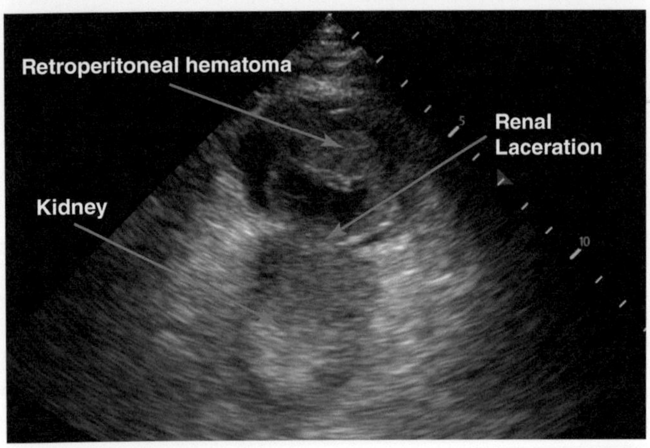

Fig. 3.12 Kidney laceration with development of a retroperitoneal hematoma

Key Ultrasound Findings

Sonographic finding	Key ultrasound findings
Hemopericardium	Anechoic or hypoechoic fluid in the pericardial space
Hemoperitoneum in Morison's pouch	Anechoic or hypoechoic fluid between the liver and the right kidney
Hemoperitoneum in the right subdiaphragmatic space	Anechoic or hypoechoic fluid under the diaphragm (above the liver)
Hemoperitoneum in the right paracolic gutter	Anechoic or hypoechoic fluid around the caudal liver tip between the lateral abdominal wall and the ascending colon The most common location to find free fluid in the RUQ
Hemoperitoneum in the pelvis (uterus present)	Anechoic or hypoechoic fluid in the rectouterine pouch, also known as the pouch of Douglas or the "cul-de-sac" (between the bladder and the uterus)
Hemoperitoneum in the pelvis (uterus absent)	Anechoic or hypoechoic fluid in the rectovesicular pouch (between the bladder and the rectum)
Hemoperitoneum in the splenorenal pouch	Anechoic or hypoechoic fluid between the spleen and the left kidney
Hemoperitoneum in the left subdiaphragmatic space	Anechoic or hypoechoic fluid under the diaphragm (above the spleen) The most common location to find free fluid in the LUQ
Hemoperitoneum in the left paracolic gutter	Anechoic or hypoechoic fluid inferior to the caudal tip of the spleen between the lateral abdominal wall and the descending colon
Pneumothorax	Absence of lung sliding seen on B-mode or seashore sign seen on M-mode A "lung point" indicates the point where a normal lung (with normal lung sliding) meets the collapsed lung (with no lung sliding)
Hemothorax	Anechoic or hypoechoic fluid in the chest above the diaphragm in the costophrenic recess "Spine sign" is when the thoracic vertebral bodies are visualized extending superior to the diaphragm in the presence of free fluid within the pleural space rather than aerated lung

Pearls and Pitfalls

- The abdominal portion of the FAST comprises three views: the RUQ, pelvis, and LUQ. Hypoechoic free fluid in any of those areas indicates a positive test.
- The caudal tip of the liver is the most sensitive area to detect free intraperitoneal fluid.
- When performing the abdominal portion of the FAST examination, false negative results can occur due to insufficient blood accumulation or too quick of a probe sweep through an area, while false positives can result from the misidentification of physiological structures as hemoperitoneum such as the bladder, gallbladder, bowel, stomach, or seminal vesicles.
- When evaluating a patient for hemopericardium, a positive examination is confirmed when a pathologic amount of fluid is seen within the pericardium. While the cardiac portion of the FAST may identify sonographic tamponade, it was created to identify pericardial fluid.
- Clotted blood has a more hyperechoic appearance on ultrasound. Careful evaluation of structures, as well as an adequate history with regards to when the trauma occurred, are essential to avoid missing this finding.

(continued)

- The presence of lung sliding rules out a pneumothorax in the intercostal recess evaluated, while the absence of lung sliding increases suspicion of a pneumothorax in that region but is not definitive. Conditions that can cause the absence of lung sliding on ultrasound without a pneumothorax include pleurodesis, pleural adhesions, contralateral mainstem intubation, severe asthma or COPD exacerbation, pulmonary fibrosis, atelectasis, large consolidations, and phrenic nerve paralysis.
- The presence of comet-tail artifacts or B-lines indicates that the visceral and parietal pleura are approximated, thereby ruling out pneumothorax.
- The epicardial fat pad can be echolucent and is, therefore, frequently mistaken for pericardial fluid; however, the fat pad is anterior, affixed to the heart and will move with the heart, whereas fluid is circumferential and will not appear fixed to the heart.

References

1. Curtin SC, Tejada-Vera B, Bastian BA. Deaths: leading causes for 2020. Natl Vital Stat Rep. 2023;72(13):1–115. PMID: 38085308
2. Rozycki GS, Ochsner MG, Schmidt JA, Frankel HL, Davis TP, Wang D, Champion HR. A prospective study of surgeon-performed ultrasound as the primary adjuvant modality for injured patient assessment. J Trauma. 1995;39(3):492–8. https://doi.org/10.1097/00005373-199509000-00016. discussion 498–500. PMID: 7473914
3. Kirkpatrick AW, Sirois M, Laupland KB, Liu D, Rowan K, Ball CG, Hameed SM, Brown R, Simons R, Dulchavsky SA, Hamiilton DR, Nicolaou S. Hand-held thoracic sonography for detecting post-traumatic pneumothoraces: the Extended Focused Assessment with Sonography for Trauma (EFAST). J Trauma. 2004;57(2):288–95. https://doi.org/10.1097/01.ta.0000133565.88871.e4. PMID: 15345974
4. Stengel D, Leisterer J, Ferrada P, Ekkernkamp A, Mutze S, Hoenning A. Point-of-care ultrasonography for diagnosing thoracoabdominal injuries in patients with blunt trauma. Cochrane Database Syst Rev. 2018;12:CD012669. https://doi.org/10.1002/14651858.CD012669.pub2. PMID: 30548249; PMCID: PMC6517180.
5. Melniker LA, Leibner E, McKenney MG, Lopez P, Briggs WM, Mancuso CA. Randomized controlled clinical trial of point-of-care, limited ultrasonography for trauma in the emergency department: the first sonography outcomes assessment program trial. Ann Emerg Med. 2006;48(3):227–35. https://doi.org/10.1016/j.annemergmed.2006.01.008. Epub 2006 Mar 24. PMID: 16934640
6. Ollerton JE, Sugrue M, Balogh Z, D'Amours SK, Giles A, Wyllie P. Prospective study to evaluate the influence of FAST on trauma patient management. J Trauma. 2006;60(4):785–91. https://doi.org/10.1097/01.ta.0000214583.21492.e8. PMID: 16612298
7. Rose JS, Levitt MA, Porter J, Hutson A, Greenholtz J, Nobay F, Hilty W. Does the presence of ultrasound really affect computed tomographic scan use? A prospective randomized trial of ultrasound in trauma. J Trauma. 2001;51(3):545–50. https://doi.org/10.1097/00005373-200109000-00022. PMID: 11535908
8. Kern SJ, Smith RS, Fry WR, Helmer SD, Reed JA, Chang FC. Sonographic examination of abdominal trauma by senior surgical residents. Am Surg. 1997;63(8):669–74. PMID: 9247431
9. Sheng AY, Dalziel P, Liteplo AS, Fagenholz P, Noble VE. Focused assessment with sonography in trauma and abdominal computed tomography utilization in adult trauma patients: trends over the last decade. Emerg Med Int. 2013;2013:678380. https://doi.org/10.1155/2013/678380. Epub 2013 Aug 29. PMID: 24073336; PMCID: PMC3773453
10. Stengel D, Rademacher G, Ekkernkamp A, Güthoff C, Mutze S. Emergency ultrasound-based algorithms for diagnosing blunt abdominal trauma. Cochrane Database Syst Rev. 2015;2015:CD004446. https://doi.org/10.1002/14651858.CD004446.pub4. PMID: 26368505; PMCID: PMC6464800.
11. Walcher F, Kortüm S, Kirschning T, Weihgold N, Marzi I. Optimierung des Traumamanagements durch präklinische Sonographie [Optimized management of polytraumatized patients by prehospital ultrasound]. Unfallchirurg. 2002;105(11):986–94. https://doi.org/10.1007/s00113-002-0517-1. German. PMID: 12402124
12. Walcher F, Weinlich M, Conrad G, Schweigkofler U, Breitkreutz R, Kirschning T, Marzi I. Prehospital ultrasound imaging improves management of abdominal trauma. Br J Surg. 2006;93(2):238–42. https://doi.org/10.1002/bjs.5213. PMID: 16329081
13. Blaivas M, Kuhn W, Reynolds B, Brannam L. Change in differential diagnosis and patient management with the use of portable ultrasound in a remote setting. Wilderness Environ Med Spring. 2005;16(1):38–41. https://doi.org/10.1580/1080-6032(2005)16[38:ciddap]2.0.co;2. PMID: 15813146
14. Boulanger BR, McLellan BA, Brenneman FD, Ochoa J, Kirkpatrick AW. Prospective evidence of the superiority of a sonography-based algorithm in the assessment of blunt abdominal injury. J Trauma. 1999;47(4):632–7. https://doi.org/10.1097/00005373-199910000-00005. PMID: 10528595
15. Lobo V, Hunter-Behrend M, Cullnan E. Caudal edge of the liver in the Right Upper Quadrant (RUQ) view is the most sensitive area for free fluid on the FAST exam. West J Emerg Med. 2017;18(2):270–80. [PMID: 28210364]
16. O'Brien KM, Stolz LA, Amini R, Gross A, Stolz U, Adhikari S. Focused assessment with sonography for trauma examination: reexamining the importance of the left upper quadrant view. J Ultrasound Med. 2015;34(8):1429–34. [pubmed]
17. Rozycki GS, Ochsner MG, Feliciano DV, Thomas B, Boulanger BR, Davis FE, Falcone RE, Schmidt JA. Early detection of hemoperitoneum by ultrasound examination of the right upper quadrant: a multicenter study. J Trauma. 1998;45(5):878–83. https://doi.org/10.1097/00005373-199811000-00006. PMID: 9820696
18. Abrams BJ, Sukumvanich P, Seibel R, Moscati R, Jehle D. Ultrasound for the detection of intraperitoneal fluid: the role of Trendelenburg positioning. Am J Emerg Med. 1999;17(2):117–20. https://doi.org/10.1016/s0735-6757(99)90040-2. PMID: 10102306
19. Ormsby EL, Geng J, McGahan JP, Richards JR. Pelvic free fluid: clinical importance for reproductive age women with blunt abdominal trauma. Ultrasound in obstetrics & gynecology: the official journal of the International Society of Ultrasound in Obstetrics and Gynecology. 2005;26(3):271–8. [PMID: 16116567]
20. Meyers MA. The spread and localization of acute intraperitoneal effusions. Radiology. 1970;95:547–54.
21. Roy CL, Minor MA, Brookhart MA, Choudhry NK. Does this patient with a pericardial effusion have cardiac tamponade? JAMA. 2007;297(16):1810–8. https://doi.org/10.1001/jama.297.16.1810. PMID: 17456823
22. Stolz LA, Stolz U, Fields JM, Saul T, Secko M, Flannigan MJ, Sheele JM, Rifenburg RP, Weekes AJ, Josephson EB, Bedolla J, Resop DM, Dela Cruz J, Boysen-Osborn M, Caffery T, Derr C, Bengiamin R, Chiricolo G, Backlund B, Heer J, Hyde RJ, Adhikari

S. Emergency medicine resident assessment of the emergency ultrasound milestones and current training recommendations. Acad Emerg Med. 2017;24:353.
23. Alerhand S, Adrian RJ, Long B, Avila J. Pericardial tamponade: a comprehensive emergency medicine and echocardiography review. Am J Emerg Med. 2022;58:159–74. https://doi.org/10.1016/j.ajem.2022.05.001. Epub 2022 May 6. PMID: 35696801
24. Alerhand S, Carter JM. What echocardiographic findings suggest a pericardial effusion is causing tamponade? Am J Emerg Med. 2019;37(2):321–6. https://doi.org/10.1016/j.ajem.2018.11.004. Epub 2018 Nov 17. PMID: 30471929
25. Pérez-Casares A, Cesar S, Brunet-Garcia L, Sanchez-de-Toledo J. Echocardiographic evaluation of pericardial effusion and cardiac tamponade. Front Pediatr. 2017;5:79. https://doi.org/10.3389/fped.2017.00079. PMID: 28484689; PMCID: PMC5401877
26. Argulian E, Messerli F. Misconceptions and facts about pericardial effusion and tamponade. Am J Med. 2013;126(10):858–61. https://doi.org/10.1016/j.amjmed.2013.03.022. Epub 2013 Jul 24. PMID: 23891285
27. Chan KK, Joo DA, McRae AD, Takwoingi Y, Premji ZA, Lang E, Wakai A. Chest ultrasonography versus supine chest radiography for diagnosis of pneumothorax in trauma patients in the emergency department. Cochrane Database Syst Rev. 2020;7:CD013031. https://doi.org/10.1002/14651858.CD013031.pub2. PMID: 32702777; PMCID: PMC7390330.
28. Ketelaars R, Gülpinar E, Roes T, Kuut M, van Geffen GJ. Which ultrasound transducer type is best for diagnosing pneumothorax? Crit Ultrasound J. 2018;10(1):27. Published 2018 Oct 22. https://doi.org/10.1186/s13089-018-0109-0.
29. Walsh MH, Smyth LM, Desy JR, Fischer EA, Goffi A, Li N, Lee M, St-Pierre J, Ma IWY. Lung ultrasound: A comparison of image interpretation accuracy between curvilinear and phased array transducers. Australas J Ultrasound Med. 2023;26(3):150–6. https://doi.org/10.1002/ajum.12347. PMID: 37701767; PMCID: PMC10493348
30. Mennicke M, Gulati K, Oliva I, Goldflam K, Skali H, Ledbetter S, Platz E. Anatomical distribution of traumatic pneumothoraces on chest computed tomography: implications for ultrasound screening in the ED. Am J Emerg Med. 2012;30(7):1025–31. https://doi.org/10.1016/j.ajem.2011.06.020. Epub 2011 Sep 9. PMID: 21908143
31. Rovida S, Orso D, Naeem S, Vetrugno L, Volpicelli G. Lung ultrasound in blunt chest trauma: a clinical review. Ultrasound. 2022;30(1):72–9. https://doi.org/10.1177/1742271X21994604. Epub 2021 Mar 17. PMID: 35173781; PMCID: PMC8841950
32. Volpicelli G, Boero E, Sverzellati N, Cardinale L, Busso M, Boccuzzi F, Tullio M, Lamorte A, Stefanone V, Ferrari G, Veltri A, Frascisco MF. Semi-quantification of pneumothorax volume by lung ultrasound. Intensive Care Med. 2014;40(10):1460–7. https://doi.org/10.1007/s00134-014-3402-9. Epub 2014 Jul 24. PMID: 25056671
33. Lichtenstein D, Mezière G, Biderman P, Gepner A. The "lung point": an ultrasound sign specific to pneumothorax. Intensive Care Med. 2000;26(10):1434–40. https://doi.org/10.1007/s001340000627. PMID: 11126253
34. Lichtenstein DA, Mezière G, Lascols N, Biderman P, Courret JP, Gepner A, Goldstein I, Tenoudji-Cohen M. Ultrasound diagnosis of occult pneumothorax. Crit Care Med. 2005;33(6):1231–8. https://doi.org/10.1097/01.ccm.0000164542.86954.b4. PMID: 15942336
35. Lichtenstein DA, Mezière GA. Relevance of lung ultrasound in the diagnosis of acute respiratory failure: the BLUE protocol. Chest. 2008;134(1):117–25. https://doi.org/10.1378/chest.07-2800. Epub 2008 Apr 10. Erratum in: Chest. 2013;144(2):721. PMID: 18403664; PMCID: PMC3734893
36. Soldati G, Testa A, Sher S, Pignataro G, La Sala M, Silveri NG. Occult traumatic pneumothorax: diagnostic accuracy of lung ultrasonography in the emergency department. Chest. 2008;133(1):204–11. https://doi.org/10.1378/chest.07-1595. Epub 2007 Oct 9. PMID: 17925411
37. Bataille B, Riu B, Ferre F, Moussot PE, Mari A, Brunel E, Ruiz J, Mora M, Fourcade O, Genestal M, Silva S. Integrated use of bedside lung ultrasound and echocardiography in acute respiratory failure: a prospective observational study in ICU. Chest. 2014;146(6):1586–93. https://doi.org/10.1378/chest.14-0681. PMID: 25144893
38. Skulec R, Parizek T, David M, Matousek V, Cerny V. Lung point sign in ultrasound diagnostics of pneumothorax: imitations and variants. Emerg Med Int. 2021;2021:6897946. Published 2021 May 28. https://doi.org/10.1155/2021/6897946.
39. Alerhand S, Tsung JW. Unmasking the lung pulse for detection of endobronchial intubation. J Ultrasound Med. 2020;39(11):2105–9. https://doi.org/10.1002/jum.15318. Epub 2020 May 1. PMID: 32356589
40. Staub LJ, Biscaro RRM, Kaszubowski E, Maurici R. Chest ultrasonography for the emergency diagnosis of traumatic pneumothorax and haemothorax: a systematic review and meta-analysis. Injury. 2018;49(3):457–66. https://doi.org/10.1016/j.injury.2018.01.033. Epub 2018 Feb 8. PMID: 29433802
41. Brogi E, Gargani L, Bignami E, Barbariol F, Marra A, Forfori F, Vetrugno L. Thoracic ultrasound for pleural effusion in the intensive care unit: a narrative review from diagnosis to treatment. Crit Care. 2017;21(1):325. https://doi.org/10.1186/s13054-017-1897-5. PMID: 29282107; PMCID: PMC5745967
42. Hosseini M, Ghelichkhani P, Baikpour M, Tafakhori A, Asady H, Haji Ghanbari MJ, Yousefifard M, Safari S. Diagnostic accuracy of ultrasonography and radiography in detection of pulmonary contusion; a systematic review and meta-analysis. Emerg (Tehran). 2015;3(4):127–36. PMID: 26495401; PMCID: PMC4608349
43. Dallagnol C, Alcala JMF, de Vargas RM, Escuissato DL. Imaging findings of pulmonary contusions on multidetector CT: a retrospective study comparing adults and children. Medicine (Baltimore). 2022;101(36):e30498. https://doi.org/10.1097/MD.0000000000030498. PMID: 36086733
44. Jahanshir A, Moghari SM, Ahmadi A, Moghadam PZ, Bahreini M. Value of point-of-care ultrasonography compared with computed tomography scan in detecting potential life-threatening conditions in blunt chest trauma patients. Ultrasound J. 2020;12(1):36. https://doi.org/10.1186/s13089-020-00183-6. PMID: 32747992; PMCID: PMC7399008
45. Gillman LM, Alkadi A, Kirkpatrick AW. The "pseudo-lung point" sign: all focal respiratory coupled alternating pleural patterns are not diagnostic of a pneumothorax. J Trauma. 2009;67(3):672.
46. Shanmuganathan K, Mirvis SE, Sherbourne CD, Chiu WC, Rodriguez A. Hemoperitoneum as the sole indicator of abdominal visceral injuries: a potential limitation of screening abdominal US for trauma. Radiology. 1999;212(2):423–30. https://doi.org/10.1148/radiology.212.2.r99au18423. PMID: 10429699
47. Chiu WC, Cushing BM, Rodriguez A, Ho SM, Mirvis SE, Shanmuganathan K, Stein M. Abdominal injuries without hemoperitoneum: a potential limitation of focused abdominal sonography for trauma (FAST). J Trauma. 1997;42(4):617–23. https://doi.org/10.1097/00005373-199704000-00006. discussion 623–625. PMID: 9137247
48. Branney SW, Wolfe RE, Moore EE, Albert NP, Heinig M, Mestek M, Eule J. Quantitative sensitivity of ultrasound in detecting free intraperitoneal fluid. J Trauma. 1995;39(2):375–80. https://doi.org/10.1097/00005373-199508000-00032. PMID: 7674411
49. Paajanen H, Lahti P, Nordback I. Sensitivity of transabdominal ultrasonography in detection of intraperitoneal fluid in humans. Eur Radiol. 1999;9(7):1423–5. https://doi.org/10.1007/s003300050861. PMID: 10460387

50. Rose JS. Ultrasound in abdominal trauma. Emerg Med Clin North Am. 2004;22(3):581–99., vii. https://doi.org/10.1016/j.emc.2004.04.007. PMID: 15301840
51. Miller MT, Pasquale MD, Bromberg WJ, Wasser TE, Cox J. Not so FAST. J Trauma. 2003;54(1):52–9. discussion 59–60. [PMID: 12544899]
52. Von Kuenssberg JD, Stiller G, Wagner D. Sensitivity in detecting free intraperitoneal fluid with the pelvic views of the FAST exam. Am J Emerg Med. 2003;21(6):476–8. https://doi.org/10.1016/s0735-6757(03)00162-1. PMID: 14574655
53. Ma OJ, Kefer MP, Stevison KF, Mateer JR. Operative versus nonoperative management of blunt abdominal trauma: role of ultrasound-measured intraperitoneal fluid levels. Am J Emerg Med. 2001;19(4):284–6. https://doi.org/10.1053/ajem.2001.24476. PMID: 11447513
54. McKenney KL, McKenney MG, Cohn SM, Compton R, Nunez DB, Dolich M, Namias N. Hemoperitoneum score helps determine need for therapeutic laparotomy. J Trauma. 2001;50(4):650–4. https://doi.org/10.1097/00005373-200104000-00009. discussion 654–656. PMID: 11303159
55. Porter RS, Nester BA, Dalsey WC, O'Mara M, Gleeson T, Pennell R, Beyer FC. Use of ultrasound to determine need for laparotomy in trauma patients. Ann Emerg Med. 1997;29(3):323–30. https://doi.org/10.1016/s0196-0644(97)70343-3. PMID: 9055770
56. Bode PJ, Niezen RA, van Vugt AB, Schipper J. Abdominal ultrasound as a reliable indicator for conclusive laparotomy in blunt abdominal trauma. J Trauma. 1993;34(1):27–31. https://doi.org/10.1097/00005373-199301000-00005. PMID: 8437192
57. Lee BC, Ormsby EL, McGahan JP, Melendres GM, Richards JR. The utility of sonography for the triage of blunt abdominal trauma patients to exploratory laparotomy. AJR Am J Roentgenol. 2007;188(2):415–21. https://doi.org/10.2214/AJR.05.2100. PMID: 17242250
58. Rose JS, Richards JR, Battistella F, Bair AE, McGahan JP, Kuppermann N. The fast is positive, now what? Derivation of a clinical decision rule to determine the need for therapeutic laparotomy in adults with blunt torso trauma and a positive trauma ultrasound. J Emerg Med. 2005;29(1):15–21. https://doi.org/10.1016/j.jemermed.2005.01.004. PMID: 15961002
59. Dolich MO, McKenney MG, Varela JE, Compton RP, McKenney KL, Cohn SM. 2,576 ultrasounds for blunt abdominal trauma. J Trauma. 2001;50(1):108–12. https://doi.org/10.1097/00005373-200101000-00019. PMID: 11231679
60. Mohammadi A, Ghasemi-Rad M. Evaluation of gastrointestinal injury in blunt abdominal trauma "FAST is not reliable": the role of repeated ultrasonography. World J Emerg Surg. 2012;7(1):2. https://doi.org/10.1186/1749-7922-7-2. PMID: 22264345; PMCID: PMC3287959
61. Blackbourne LH, Soffer D, McKenney M, Amortegui J, Schulman CI, Crookes B, Habib F, Benjamin R, Lopez PP, Namias N, Lynn M, Cohn SM. Secondary ultrasound examination increases the sensitivity of the FAST exam in blunt trauma. J Trauma. 2004;57(5):934–8. https://doi.org/10.1097/01.ta.0000149494.40478.e4. PMID: 15580013
62. Richards JR, McGahan JP, Jones CD, Zhan S, Gerscovich EO. Ultrasound detection of blunt splenic injury. Injury. 2001;32(2):95–103. https://doi.org/10.1016/s0020-1383(00)00147-9. PMID: 11223039
63. Alswaimil NF, Alzahrani SA, Alfuraih MA, Alfaraj D, Alshahrani A. Splenic heterogeneity in focused Assessment with Sonography for Trauma (FAST) scan led to the diagnosis of Grade 2 splenic injury in a pediatric blunt abdominal trauma. Cureus. 2022;14(12):e33128. https://doi.org/10.7759/cureus.33128. PMID: 36601219; PMCID: PMC9801666
64. Iacobellis F, Schillirò ML, Di Serafino M, Borzelli A, Grimaldi D, Verde F, Caruso M, Dell'Aversano Orabona G, Rinaldo C, Sabatino V, Cantisani V, Vallone G, Romano L. Multimodality ultrasound assessment of the spleen: Normal appearances and emergency abnormalities. J Clin Ultrasound. 2023;51(3):543–59. https://doi.org/10.1002/jcu.23414. Epub 2022 Dec 14. PMID: 36515988
65. Catalano O, Lobianco R, Raso MM, Siani A. Blunt hepatic trauma: evaluation with contrast-enhanced sonography: sonographic findings and clinical application. J Ultrasound Med. 2005;24(3):299–310. https://doi.org/10.7863/jum.2005.24.3.299. PMID: 15723842
66. Sutarjono B, Kessel M, Alexander D, Grewal E. Is it time to re-think FAST? A systematic review and meta-analysis of Contrast-Enhanced Ultrasound (CEUS) and conventional ultrasound for initial assessment of abdominal trauma. BMC Emerg Med. 2023;23(1):8. https://doi.org/10.1186/s12873-023-00771-4. PMID: 36703099; PMCID: PMC9881326

Core Cardiac Ultrasound

4

Petra Duran-Gehring, Jason Arthur, and Stuart Prenner

Background

Echocardiography was initially developed by cardiologists in the 1970s and performed primarily by dedicated technicians [1]. By the early 1990s, other specialties, such as emergency medicine, began to use this tool at the bedside to diagnose pericardial effusion and tamponade, improving both time to diagnosis and survival in penetrating trauma [2, 3]. By 1997, the American College of Emergency Physicians (ACEP) released its first policy statement in regards to point-of-care ultrasound (POCUS), advocating for its use in the evaluation of pericardial effusion [4]. During the early 2000s, the use of ultrasound to evaluate cardiac pathology broadened to include nontraumatic etiologies of pericardial effusion, the evaluation of left ventricular function, and several protocols to address cardiac function in shock and sepsis. [5–9] Cardiac POCUS has been considered a core application of clinical ultrasound since the initial ACEP Emergency Ultrasound Imaging Criteria Compendium in 2006, with the most recent 2021 iteration now including pericardial effusion and cardiac tamponade, gross cardiac function during cardiac arrest, left ventricular systolic function, right heart dysfunction, aortic root, and inferior vena cava evaluations [10]. In this chapter, we will review the basic echocardiography views and relevant anatomy identified in each view. This chapter will also discuss the evaluation of left ventricular function, pericardial effusion and tamponade, and the inferior vena cava.

While there are different conventions for cardiac scanning, this chapter will assume that the machine screen indicator is on the right (cardiology convention). If one chooses to scan with the screen indicator on the left, the probe will need to be rotated 180 degrees to make the same conventional image. When describing probe movements, it will be relative to the beam of the probe (like a flashlight), not the tail of the probe.

Supplementary Information The online version contains supplementary material available at https://doi.org/10.1007/978-3-031-85308-1_4.

P. Duran-Gehring (✉)
Department of Emergency Medicine, University of Florida College of Medicine—Jacksonville, Jacksonville, FL, USA
e-mail: petra.duran@jax.ufl.edu

J. Arthur
Department of Emergency Medicine, University of Arkansas for Medical Sciences, Little Rock, AR, USA
e-mail: jarthur@uams.edu

S. Prenner
Department of Medicine, Division of Cardiovascular Medicine, Hospital of University of Pennsylvania, Philadelphia, PA, USA
e-mail: Stuart.Prenner@pennmedicine.upenn.edu

Indications

Indications
- Chest pain
- Dyspnea
- Lower extremity edema
- Tachycardia
- Hypotension
- Tachypnea
- Hypoxia
- Abnormal laboratory values (e.g., brain-type natriuretic peptide, troponin)

Diagnoses
- Left ventricular systolic dysfunction
- Pericardial effusion
- Cardiac tamponade
- Plethoric inferior vena cava

M. Gottlieb, N. Panebianco (eds.), *Advanced Point-of-Care Ultrasound*, https://doi.org/10.1007/978-3-031-85308-1_4

Core Views

View	Image	Approach
Parasternal Long-Axis (PLAX) 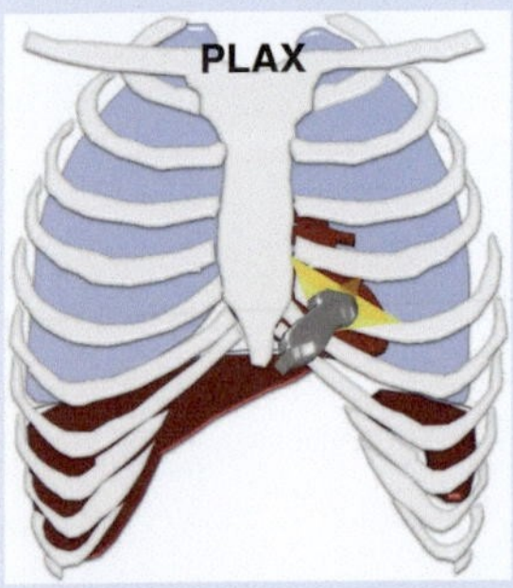	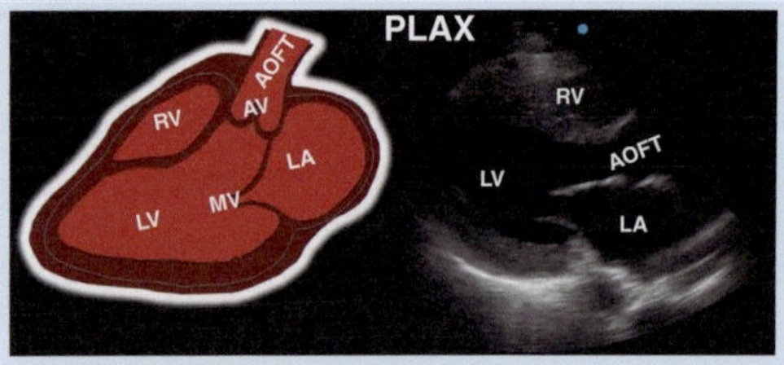 Core view 1. PLAX view	*Technique* Use the cardiac preset with the probe indicator to the right side of the screen. The probe marker should point toward the patient's right shoulder. This view is best visualized left of the sternum at the third or fourth intercostal space. *Anatomy visualized* Right ventricle (RV) Left atrium (LA) Mitral valve (MV) Left ventricle (LV) Aortic valve (AV) Aortic outflow tract (AOFT)
Right ventricular inflow (RVI) 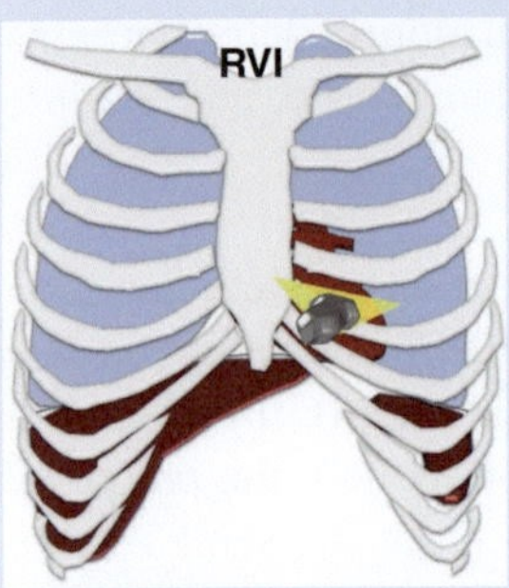	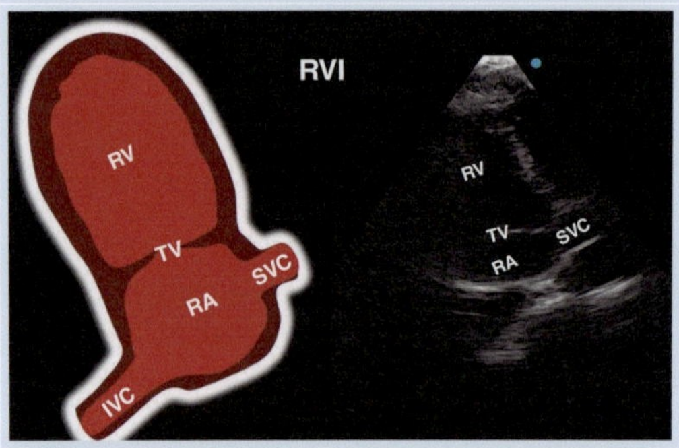 Core view 2. RVI view	*Technique* From the PLAX view, fan the probe toward the patient's right hip. *Anatomy visualized* Inferior vena cava (IVC) Superior vena cava (SVC) Right atrium (RA) Tricuspid valve (TV) Right ventricle (RV)
Parasternal short-Axis (PSAX) 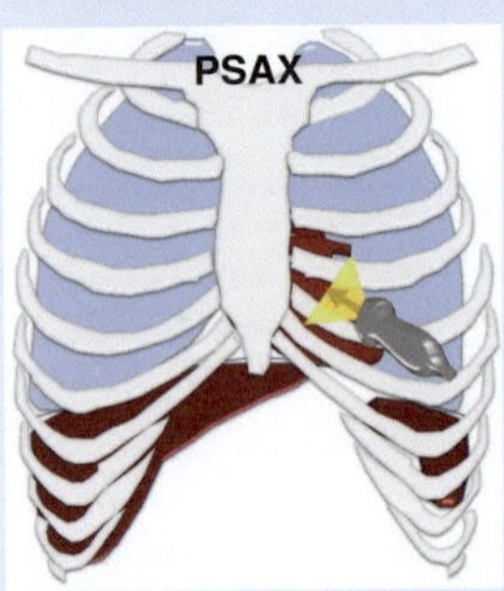	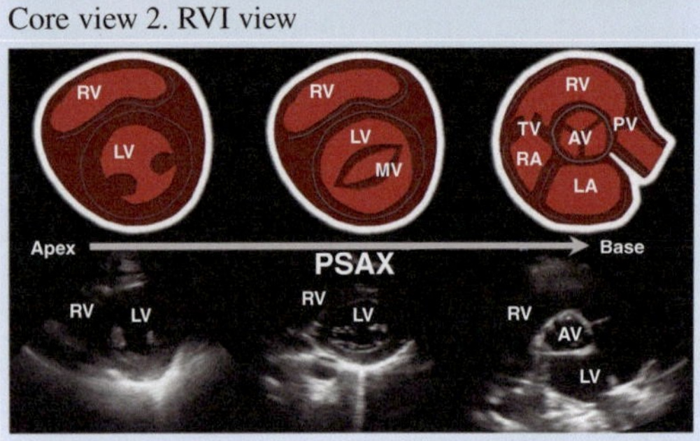 Core view 3. PSAX	*Technique* From the PLAX view, rotate the probe 90°, so that the probe marker points toward the patient's left shoulder. Fan the probe through this window from inferior to superior in order to visualize the different cuts of the short-axis view. The left ventricle is visualized deep to the right ventricle with papillary muscles visible at the apex. As the probe is fanned to the base of the heart superiorly, the papillary muscles give way to the mitral valve leaflets. Fanning the ultrasound beam further toward the base of the heart will demonstrate the tri-leaflet aortic valve in the center of the screen, often described as the "Mercedes-Benz sign." *Anatomy visualized* Apical: Right ventricle (RV) RV papillary muscles Left ventricle (LV) Mid: Right ventricle (RV) Mitral valve (MV) Left ventricle (LV) Basal: Right atrium (RA) Tricuspid valve (TV) Right ventricle (RV) Pulmonic valve (PV) Left atrium (LA) Aortic valve (AV)

View	Image	Approach
Apical 4-chamber (A4C) 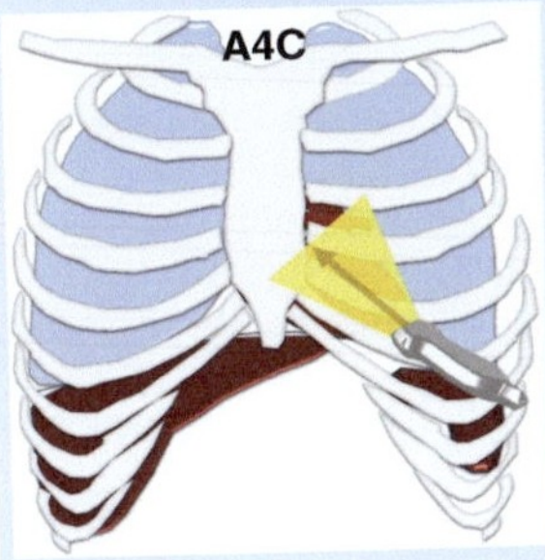	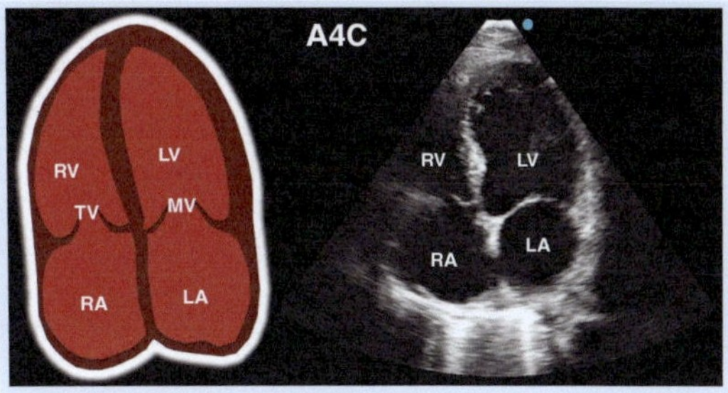 Core view 4. A4C view	*Technique* Place the probe at the point of maximal impulse (PMI) with the probe marker aiming toward the patient's left. Flatten the probe so that the angle of insonation is directed toward the patient's right shoulder. Rotate the probe until the interventricular septum is oriented vertically. Another way to acquire this view is to slide the probe inferiorly and laterally from the PSAX view to the PMI, while flattening the probe until the A4C is visualized. In order to avoid foreshortening of the chambers, the probe should be placed at the most inferior rib space possible where the heart is visualized. This helps to ensure the angle of insonation is directed through the long-axis of the heart. *Anatomy visualized* Right atrium (RA) Tricuspid valve (TV) Right ventricle (RV) Left atrium (LA) Mitral valve (MV) Left ventricle (LV)
Apical 5-chamber (A5C)	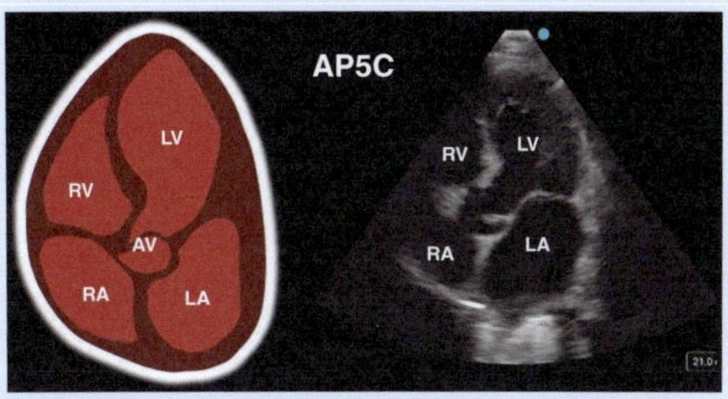 Core view 5. A5C view	*Technique* From the A4C view, flatten the probe and angle the beam of insonation more superiorly until the LVOT appears. *Anatomy visualized* Right atrium (RA) Tricuspid valve (TV) Right ventricle (RV) Left atrium (LA) Mitral valve (MV) Left ventricle (LV) Aortic valve (AV) Left ventricular outflow tract (LVOT)
Apical 2-chamber (A2C)	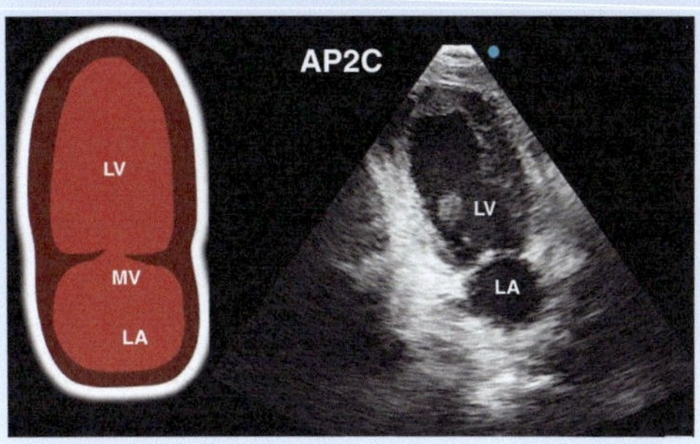 Core view 6. A2C view	*Technique* Rotate the probe 90° clockwise from the A4C view and the heart will be visualized along the left side with the left atrium and left ventricle in view. The inferior wall is now on screen left and the anterior wall is on screen right. *Anatomy visualized* Left ventricle (LV) Mitral valve (MV) Left atrium (LA)

View	Image	Approach
Subxiphoid Long-Axis (SXLA) 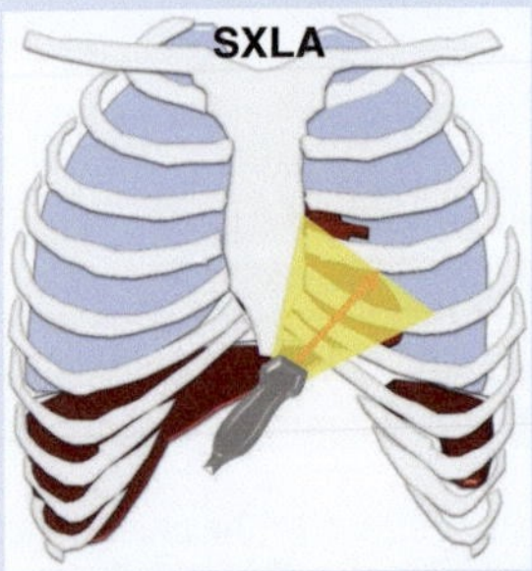 	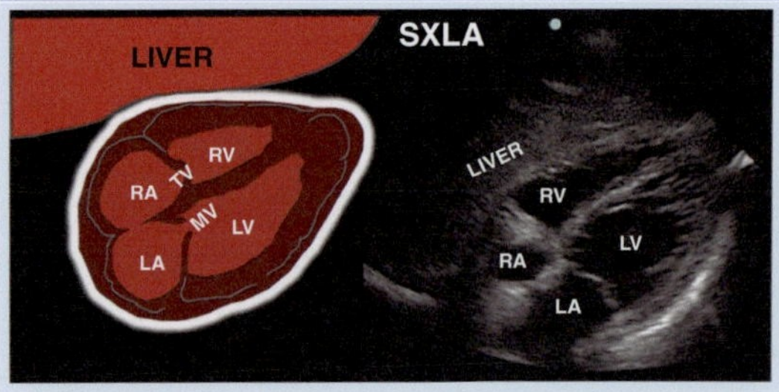 Core view 7. SXLA view	*Technique* Gripping the probe from the top face using an overhand grip, place it in the subxiphoid region with the probe marker facing toward the patient's left. The probe should be placed nearly flat against the patient, with the angle of insonation pointing toward the patient's left shoulder. This allows the beam to penetrate through the liver and diaphragm into the chest cavity. Since the probe is now farther away from the heart itself, increase the depth for a deeper field of view. *Anatomy visualized* Right atrium (RA) Tricuspid valve (TV) Right ventricle (RV) Left atrium (LA) Mitral valve (MV) Left ventricle (LV) Aortic valve (AV)
Subxiphoid short-Axis (SXSA) 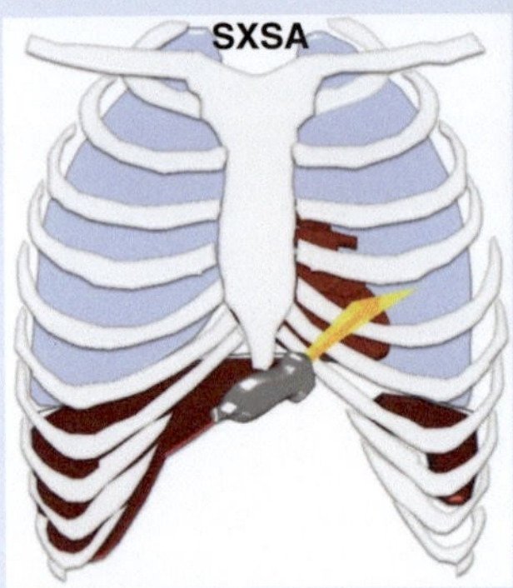 	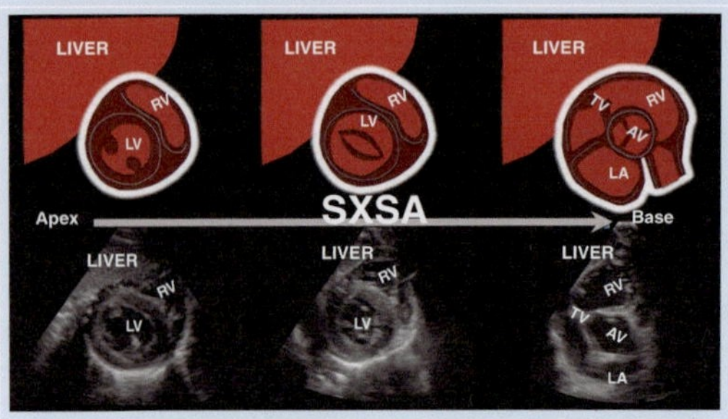 Core view 8. SXSA view	*Technique* From the SXLA view, rotate the probe so that the marker is pointed inferiorly. As with the different cuts of the PSAX view, fan the probe in order to visualize the apical, mid, and basal planes. *Anatomy visualized* Right ventricle (RV) Liver Right atrium (RA) Tricuspid valve (TV) Right ventricle (RV) Left atrium (LA) Mitral valve (MV) Aortic valve (AV)
Inferior vena cava (IVC) 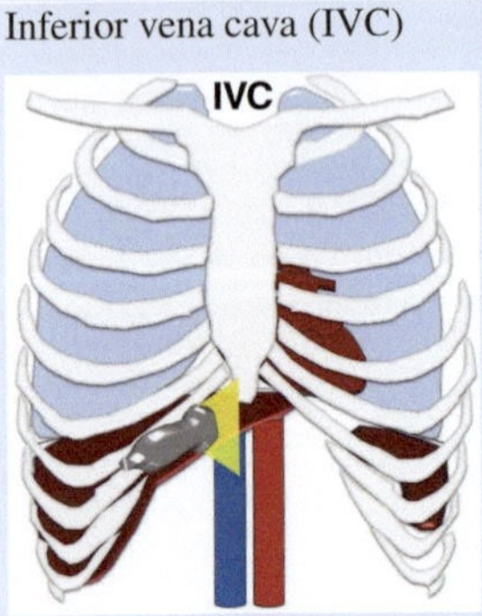 	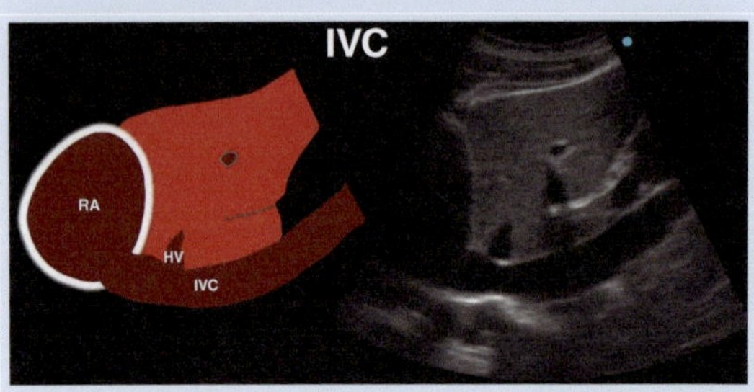 Core view 9. IVC view	*Technique* Place the probe in the subxiphoid region with the marker facing inferiorly, such that the heart appears on the left of the screen, with a horizontal longitudinal view of the IVC on the right. If the probe is located too medially, the aorta will be visualized instead. The IVC is thin-walled, converges with hepatic veins just prior to crossing the diaphragm, and drains directly into the RA. The aorta is thicker-walled, pulsatile, and branches into the celiac trunk at this location. Alternatively, from the SXLA view, identify the RA and rotate the probe 90° to visualize the IVC as it drains into the RA. *Anatomy visualized* Inferior vena cava (IVC) Right atrium (RA) Liver Hepatic vein (HV)

Clinical Applications

Left Ventricular Systolic Function

Cardiac POCUS can be used to evaluate whether left ventricular (LV) systolic function is normal or impaired, as well assess the severity of impairment if present. There are several methods that can be used to assess LV function. These include the global qualitative assessment, E-point septal separation, fractional shortening, and Simpson biplane methods of discs.

Global Qualitative Assessment

With proper training and experience, the simplest method to estimate LV ejection fraction (EF) is by visual estimation, which can be particularly beneficial in the acute care setting when more detailed quantitative assessment is not immediately needed. Grossly normal LV function refers to normal systolic contraction and inward excursion of the endocardial walls with thickening of those walls (Video 1A). Grossly abnormal function refers to when contraction and wall thickening are decreased (Video 1B). Diagnostic accuracy of visual estimation is increased by imaging the LV in multiple views. Global LV systolic function can be assessed qualitatively with strong accuracy. [11–14]

E-Point Septal Separation

E-point septal separation (EPSS) is a quantitative tool that can differentiate patients with normal and abnormal left ventricular EF. EPSS refers to the distance in diastole between the tip of the open anterior mitral valve leaflet and the interventricular septum in the PLAX view. To acquire this measurement, the motion mode (M-mode) beam is placed perpendicularly over the interventricular septum and the tip of the anterior mitral valve leaflet (Fig. 4.1) [15]. Therefore, it is critical that the heart is oriented such that the interventricular septum is horizontal (perpendicular to the ultrasound probe), as a more vertical (i.e., oblique) septum can lead to artificially inflated EPSS values.

A normal, healthy anterior mitral valve leaflet may come in contact with the septum to produce an EPSS of 0 mm. In patients with decreased LV contractility, a lesser volume of blood flows down the pressure gradient through the mitral valve in diastole, so the anterior leaflet of the mitral valve does not open as widely. Moreover, the LV cavity increases in size as a compensatory mechanism to maintain stroke volume. These factors lead to an increase in EPSS values [16–18]. When EPSS is >7 mm, LV systolic dysfunction is likely present (Fig. 4.2). In one study, an EPSS >7 mm was 87% sensitive and 75% specific for identifying an EF < 50% [16]. Another study demonstrated that an EPSS >7 mm was 100% sensitive and 52% specific for an EF < 30% [19]. Correlation data between EPSS and visually estimated or calculated EF has ranged between $r = 0.68–0.87$ [16, 17, 19, 20]. An elevated EPSS may occur despite a normal EF when the opening of the anterior mitral valve leaflet toward the septum is restricted for other reasons (e.g., mitral stenosis, aortic regurgitation) [16, 17]. EPSS may be of limited utility in atrial fibrillation when there is beat-to-beat variability due to changes in LV filling.

Fractional Shortening

Fractional shortening entails comparing the LV cavity diameter in systole and diastole between the interventricular septum and the posterior left ventricular wall. In the PLAX view, linear measurements in M-mode or brightness mode (B-mode) are taken from the LV cavity perpendicular (at either the endocardium or midwall) to the long axis to obtain the left ventricular end-diastolic diameter (LVEDD) and left ventricular end-systolic diameter (LVESD) in cm (Fig. 4.3).

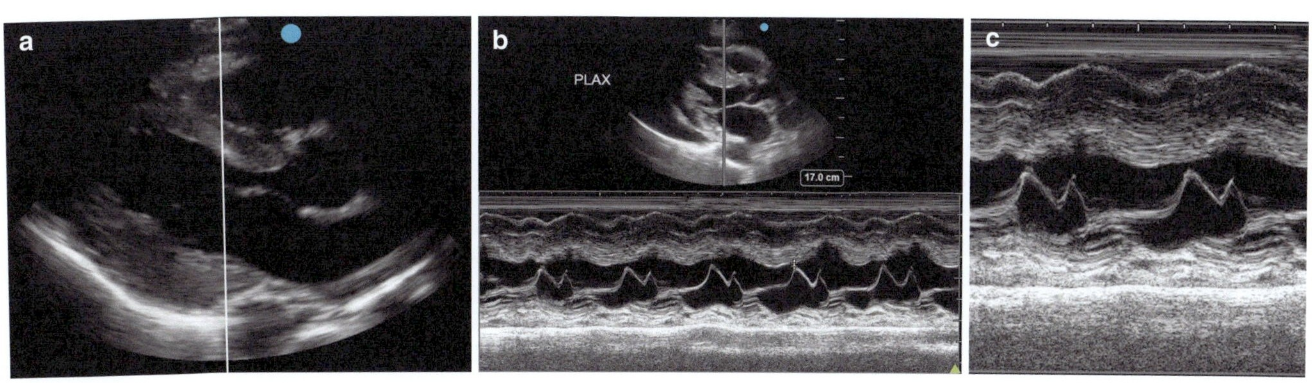

Fig. 4.1 E-Point septal separation. (**a**) M-mode cursor placement over the anterior leaflet of the mitral valve in the PLAX view through the interventricular septum. (**b**) M-mode tracing demonstrating the mitral valve excursion. (**c**) M-mode tracing of the mitral valve, with the first peak representing the maximal mitral valve opening in early LV diastole (E-wave) followed by the second peak of the atrial contraction later in LV diastole (A-wave). Distance is measured between the E-wave (E) and the interventricular septum (S)

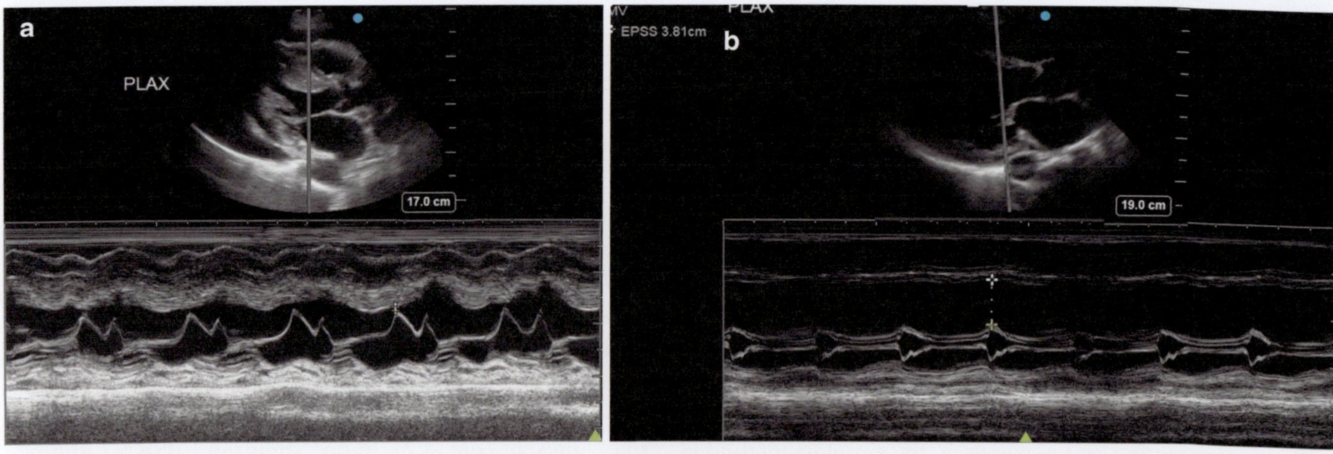

Fig. 4.2 E-Point septal separation. (**a**) Normal EPSS <7 mm. (**b**) An elevated EPSS signifying decreased ejection fraction

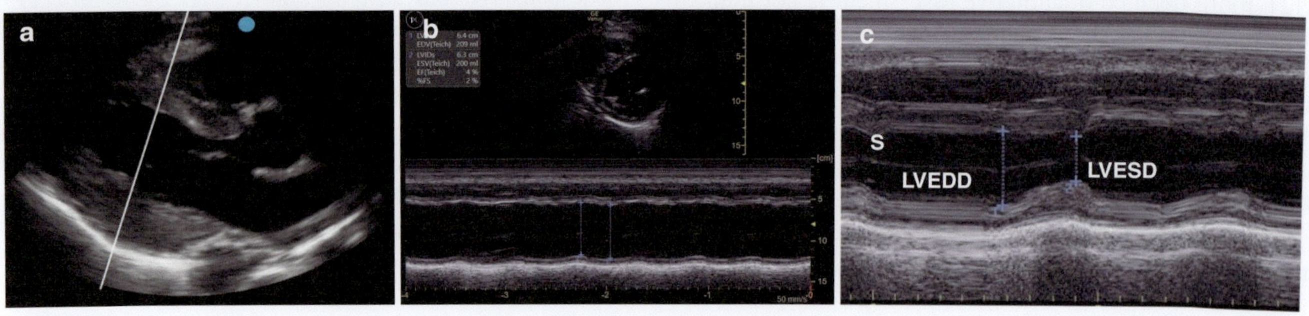

Fig. 4.3 Fractional shortening. (**a**) M-mode cursor placement in the PLAX view through the mid LV, not to include the papillary muscles or mitral valve. (**b**) M-mode tracing demonstrating the LV contraction. (**c**) M-mode tracing of the LV contraction, measuring the maximum diameter (LVEDD) and the minimum diameter (LVESD) between the interventricular septum (S) and the LV posterior wall (LV)

$$\text{The equation for fractional shortening is}: \left(\left[\text{LVEDD} - \text{LVESD}\right] / \text{LVEDD}\right) \times 100$$

Fractional shortening is expressed as a percentage that reflects the change in the LV cavity in one dimension, and, thus, these percentages should not be confused with the EF [20]. When LV systolic dysfunction is present, there is a lesser change in the LV cavity diameter from diastole (when the diameter is longest) to systole (when the diameter is shortest) (Fig. 4.4). Normal values of endocardial fractional shortening are 27–45% for women and 25–43% for men, with severely abnormal denoted as ≤16% and ≤14% for women and men, respectively [20].

Of note, this technique for evaluating LV dysfunction is inaccurate in the presence of regional wall motion abnormalities. Additionally, the operator needs to ensure that measurements are taken perpendicular to the LV cavity long axis in order to avoid overestimation, similar to EPSS [21].

Simpson Biplane Method of Discs

The most accurate method of determining LV systolic function is the Simpson biplane method of discs [21]. This method entails tracing the LV cavity in both the A2C and A4C views, in systole and diastole. Using these tracings, the LV cavity is divided into a series of disks, and the cumulative volume is used to estimate the LV volume (Fig. 4.5). This method is the most time-consuming and may not be realistic or necessary in emergent situations. As this approach relies on the calculation of LV volume, it is dependent on accurately tracing the LV cavity and distinguishing the endocardium from the blood pool. Another limitation includes beat-to-beat variation of volumes in patients who are in atrial fibrillation [21].

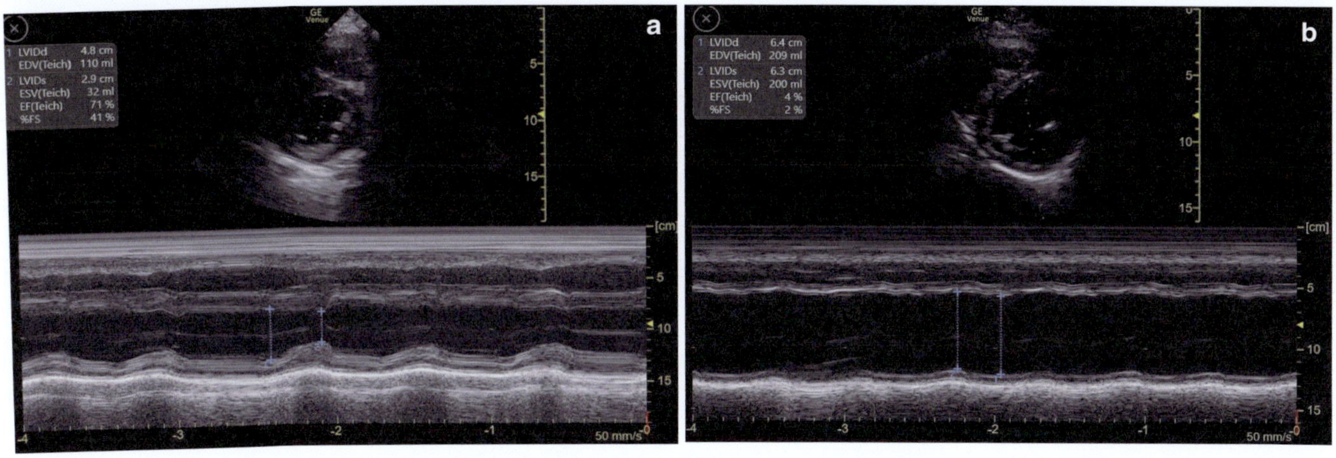

Fig. 4.4 Fractional Shortening. (**a**) Normal fractional shortening. (**b**) Abnormal fractional shortening

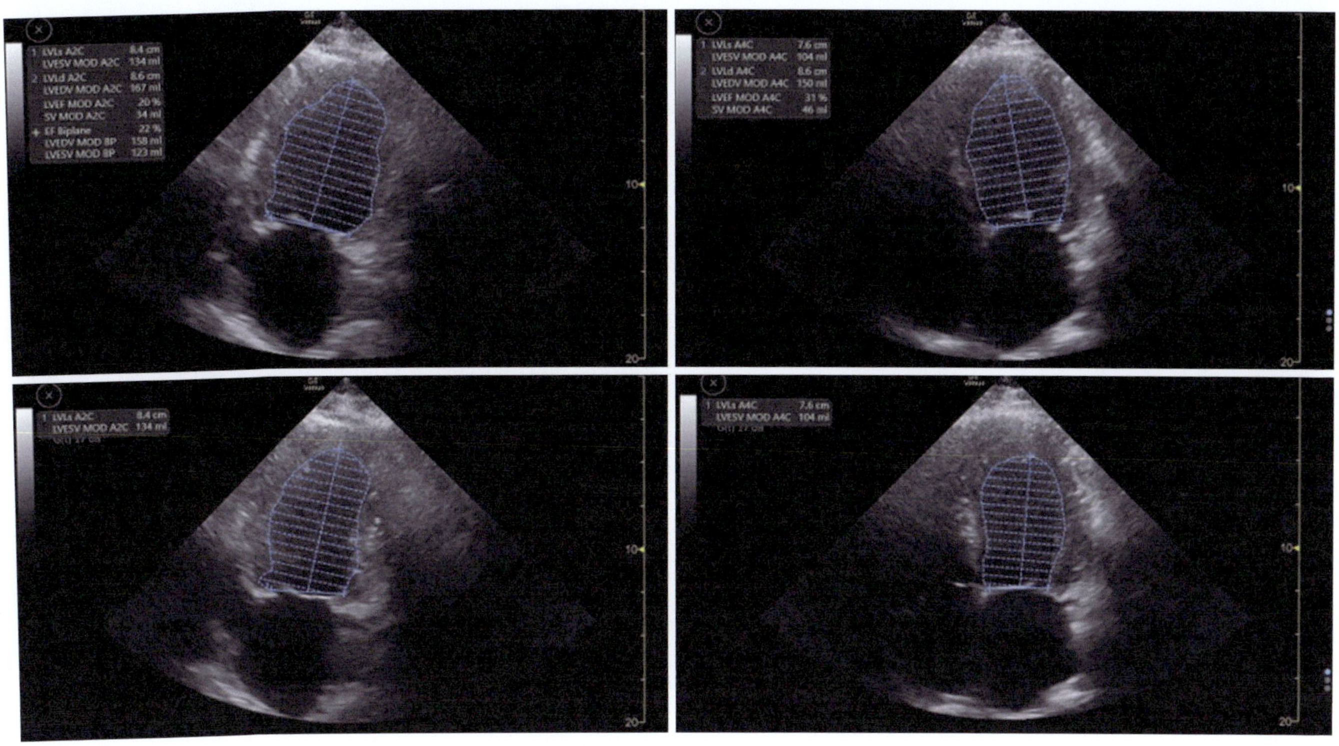

Fig. 4.5 Simpson biplane method of discs showing an abnormal left ventricular ejection fraction

Left Ventricular Regional Wall Motion Abnormalities

Assessment of regional wall motion abnormalities (RWMA) during echocardiography may be a useful tool in the diagnosis of acute coronary syndrome, especially in patients with a concerning history and nondiagnostic electrocardiogram (ECG) or biomarkers, as echocardiography has been demonstrated to be more sensitive in the detection of cardiac ischemia [22–25]. Emergency physicians have accurately identified RWMA using multiple echocardiographic views to visualize segmental wall thickening and endocardial motion [21, 24–27]. Coronary artery distributions on ECG may be correlated to specific wall segments (e.g., anterior, posterior, inferior, lateral); however, multiple echocardiographic views should be used to determine the likely vascular distribution as there is some overlap of segments (Fig. 4.6, Video 2) [26]. The presence of a new RWMA in patients presenting with acute chest pain can indicate an increased risk for acute coronary syndrome and the subsequent need for intervention [28, 29].

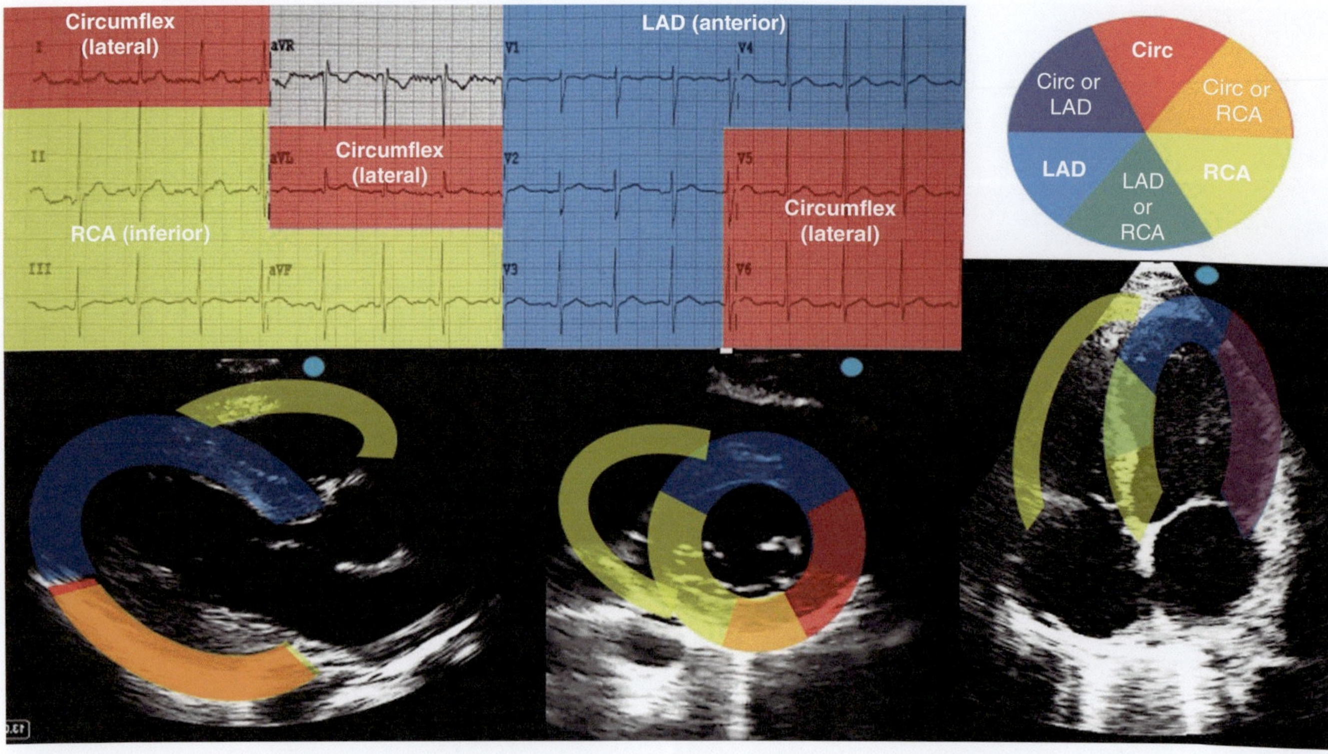

Fig. 4.6 Regional wall motion abnormality vascular territories and the corresponding ECG distribution. Each color reflects the corresponding vascular territories. *LAD* left anterior descending artery, *Circ* left circumflex artery, *RCA* right coronary artery

Cardiac Output

Cardiac output (CO) can be measured in a variety of ways: using the Fick principle, thermodilution, pulse contour analysis, and echocardiography. The Fick principle calculates CO based on oxygen consumption divided by arteriovenous oxygen difference. Thermodilution requires invasive pulmonary artery catheters. Pulse contour analysis requires dedicated devices. Echocardiography offers a rapid, noninvasive method of measuring CO using assessment of stroke volume (SV) and heart rate (HR) with the equation: CO = SV x HR. Stroke volume can be measured by subtracting end-systolic volume from end-diastolic volume, measures which can be obtained with echocardiography. More commonly, SV is calculated using the Left Ventricular Outflow Tract (LVOT) Velocity Time Integral (VTI) multiplied by the LVOT cross-sectional area [28, 30].

$$\text{SV} = \text{LVOT VTI} \times \text{Cross-sectional area of the LVOT}$$

$$\text{LVOT Cross-sectional area} = 3.14 * (\text{LVOT diameter} / 2)^2$$

In the A4C view, LVOT VTI is determined by placing the pulsed-wave Doppler sampling gate in the LVOT proximal to the aortic valve and recording the velocity (cm/s). The velocity signal is integrated with respect to time by measuring the area within the envelope (Fig. 4.7) [29]. The VTI is obtained by outlining the velocity curve and multiplying the value by the LVOT cross-sectional area. A normal LVOT diameter is 20 mm. Normal stroke volume is 74.3 ± 17.2 mL for men and 62.5 ± 14.3 mL for women [28]. LVOT VTI has been shown to correlate with invasive measurements of cardiac output. [31, 32] Extremely low LVOT VTI < 10 cm is predictive of both short- and long-term mortality and risk of decompensation in several populations, including post-myocardial infarction [33–35] (Fig. 4.8).

Inferior Vena Cava

The inferior vena cava (IVC) lies proximal to the right atrium, and, thus, assessment of the IVC can be helpful to determine whether right atrial filling pressure is low, normal, or elevated. IVC diameter and respirophasic collapsibility can be integrated into the resuscitation of critically ill patients. In a spontaneously breathing patient, the IVC collapses in inspiration due to an increase in negative intrathoracic pressures and increased return to the right atrium. On expiration, the IVC distends due to a decrease in the negative intrathoracic pressures and decreased return to the right atrium. The IVC is typically imaged in the subcostal view in the longitudinal plane in B-mode, approximately 2 cm distal to the right atrial junction. (Fig. 4.9). However, some have advocated for measuring this in the short axis to avoid mismeasurement due to lateral movement during respiration, creating a cylindrical tangential effect. (Fig. 4.10,

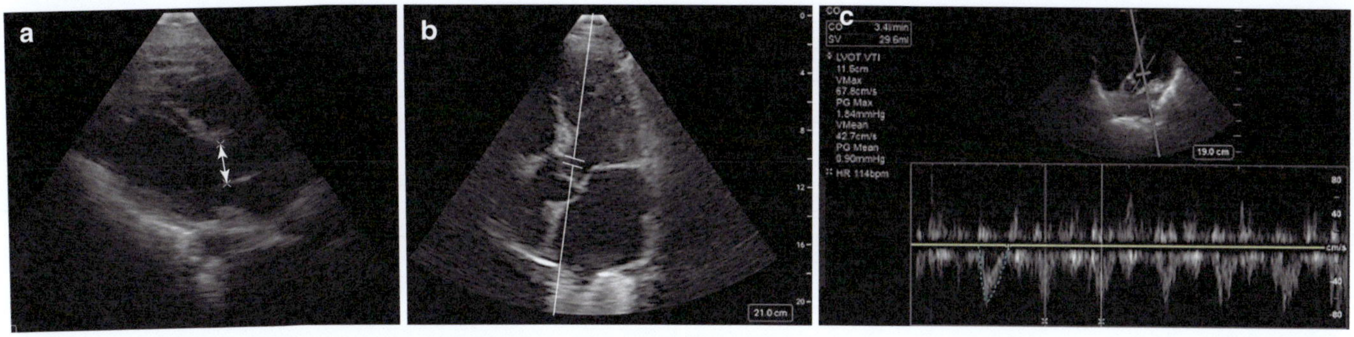

Fig. 4.7 Cardiac output utilizing left ventricular outflow tract (LVOT) velocity time integral (VTI). (**a**) LVOT diameter measured in the PLAX view during mid-systole. (**b**) Pulsed-wave Doppler gates are placed in the LVOT proximal to the aortic valve. (**c**) Doppler tracing of the flow through LVOT as a downward deflection is noted and outlined utilizing auto trace or manual trace function on the ultrasound machine to get a VTI measurement

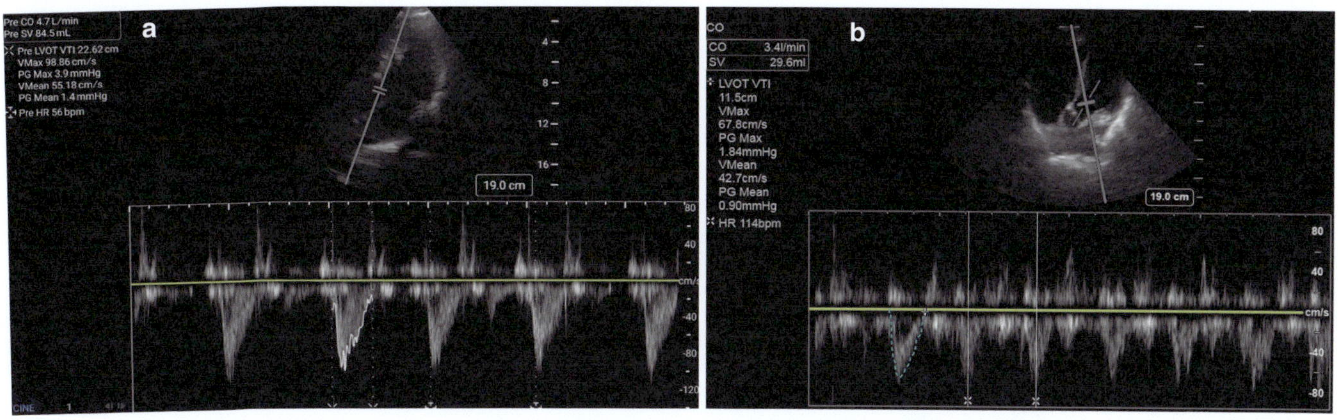

Fig. 4.8 Cardiac output measures using left ventricular outflow tract velocity time integral (LVOT VTI). (**a**) Normal cardiac output using LVOT VTI. (**b**) Abnormal cardiac output using LVOT VTI. (*Image B courtesy of Henrique Puls, MD*)

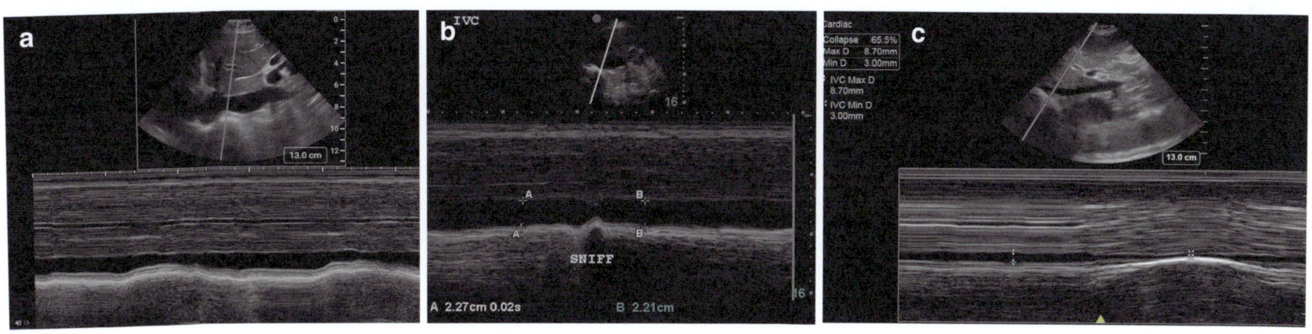

Fig. 4.9 IVC B-mode image with M-mode tracing of respiratory variation. (**a**) Normal IVC, (**b**) Plethoric IVC, (**c**) Volume depleted IVC

Fig. 4.11). Measurement of the IVC diameter is obtained at rest and during a quick forced inhalation maneuver (e.g., sniff). The normal IVC diameter is <2.1 cm, with >50% collapse during inspiration (Table 4.1) [36]. Right atrial pressure is estimated as normal when the IVC is <2.1 cm and collapses >50%, while the right atrial pressure is considered elevated when the IVC > 2.1 cm and does not collapse with respiration [37] (Video 3). These estimates only apply to spontaneously breathing patients who are not on mechanical ventilation.

The caval index is defined as the ratio between the end-expiratory (maximum) IVC diameter and the inspiratory (minimum) IVC diameter. Caval index >50% is associated with lower right atrial pressures [39]. When compared to

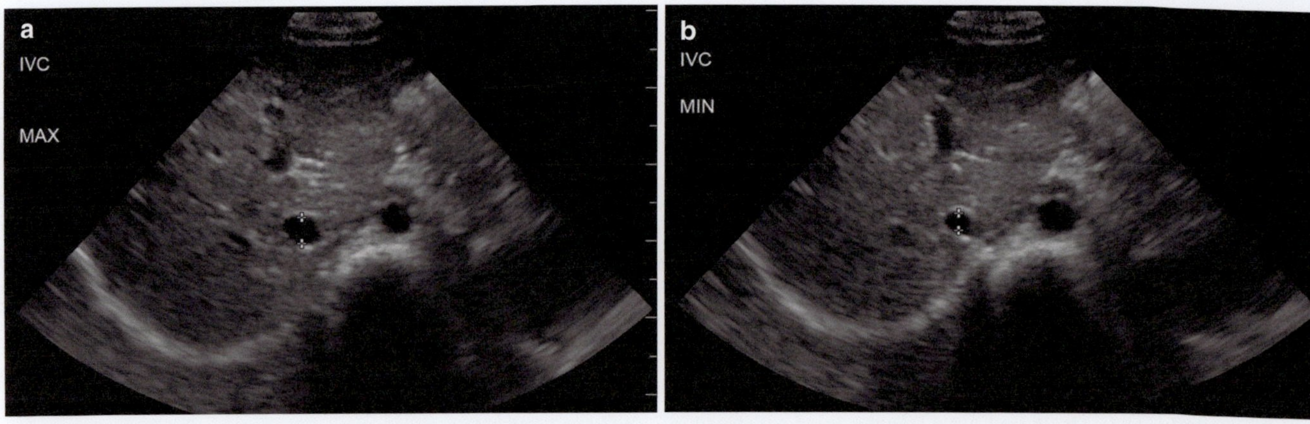

Fig. 4.10 IVC B-mode image in the short-axis demonstrating respiratory variation. (**a**) IVC maximum diameter (**b**) IVC minimum diameter

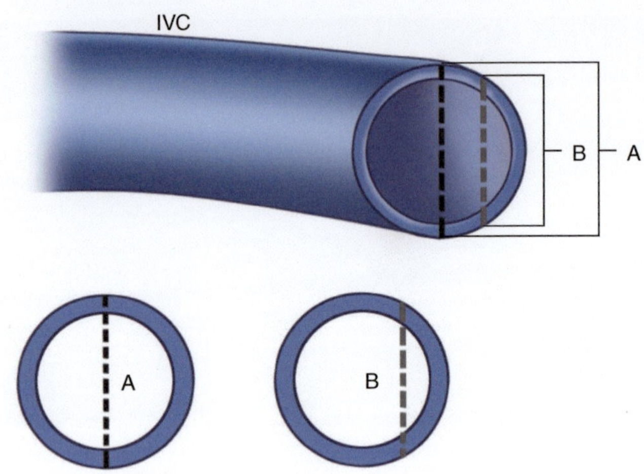

Fig. 4.11 IVC cylinder tangential effect. Measurement at midpoint (**a**) vs measurement along outer edge (**b**) may lead to inaccurate measurement in the long-axis plane

Table 4.1 Inferior vena cava diameter measurement, collapsibility, and estimated right atrial pressure range

Inferior vena cava diameter	Collapsibility	Estimated right atrial pressure range
<2.1 cm	> 50%	0–5 mmHg
<2.1 cm	< 50%	5–10 mmHg[a]
>2.1 cm	> 50%	5–10 mmHg[a]
>2.1 cm	< 50%	10–20 mmHg

[a]The following indices can be used to upgrade the right atrial pressures in indeterminate cases: dilated right atrium, an interatrial septum bowing right to left throughout the cardiac cycle, restrictive right-sided diastolic filling pattern, tricuspid E/e' > 6, and hepatic vein diastolic flow predominant. [38]

right atrial pressure measured with a central line, caval index ≥50% predicted a central venous pressure < 8 mm Hg with 91% sensitivity and 94% specificity [36].

In patients who are mechanically ventilated, the mechanical ventilation causes positive intrathoracic pressures during inspiration, the opposite of spontaneous respiration. Thus, the IVC is at maximum diameter at inspiration and at minimum diameter during expiration in patients on mechanical ventilation. The distensibility index has been used in mechanically ventilated patients and is calculated as ([maximum diameter on inspiration — minimum diameter on expiration]/minimum diameter on expiration)*100. Distensibility index values >18% have been associated with volume depletion and favor volume resuscitation in septic patients [40]. However, there remains no clear consensus on the ideal cut-off, as values vary across studies [41].

Pericardial Effusion

The size and location of a pericardial effusion are important to document due to the implications for hemodynamics and potential intervention. Because the pericardium is fibrous with relatively little capacity for distension, small volume pericardial effusions may influence hemodynamics if accumulation occurs rapidly. Alternatively, effusions that develop slowly over time allow for the pericardium to stretch and may grow to very large volumes before leading to tamponade physiology (Fig. 4.12) [42].

Effusions may be global or collect in a specific region of the pericardium, such as anterior, posterior, or apical region. Recognition and documentation of the distribution of effusion is important for comparison on repeat imaging and for procedural planning.

There has been limited research into which specific echocardiographic view is superior for evaluating pericardial effusion. The subcostal view is commonly taught as part of the Focused Assessment with Sonography in Trauma and in penetrating cardiac trauma has robust data suggesting 100% sensitivity and 100% specificity [43]. The PLAX view may be of most value in assessing for posterior effusions. The PSAX and A4C views are useful to assess the distribution of the effusion relative to the heart.

Effusion size is determined by measurement of the distance from the visceral pericardium to the parietal pericardium at the deepest pocket during end-diastole [38, 44] (Fig. 4.13, Video 4). Effusions visible only during systole are considered trace effusions and do not convey an increased risk for tamponade. Guidelines from the American Society of Echocardiography and the European Society of Cardiology recommend estimating size of effusion using this method as either small (< 10 mm), moderate (10–20 mm), or large (> 20 mm) (Table 4.2) [38, 44].

Pericardial effusions may be anechoic or have internal echoes. Acute hemorrhage into the pericardium is often anechoic, though as blood coagulates it may develop into a discrete clot or create layers. Uremic effusions are often anechoic. Increased echoes within an effusion, including loculations or fibrin deposition along the visceral and parietal pericardium, should be noted as these may have implications for procedures such as pericardiocentesis. To date, little research exists on the ability of ultrasound to distinguish exudative from transudative pericardial effusions. A notable exception to this is the rare finding of air within the pericardium, which when found suggests either trauma, recent intervention, or the presence of a gas-forming organism within the pericardium [45].

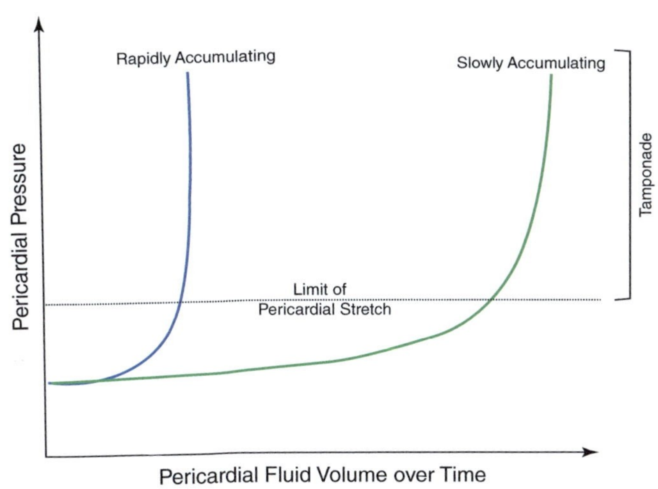

Fig. 4.12 Comparison of pericardial fluid volume and pericardial pressure for short versus long periods of fluid accumulation

Anterior epicardial adipose tissue (commonly referred to as an epicardial fat pad) is a normal anatomic finding and a common cause of a false-positive isolated anterior pericardial effusion. There are several strategies to differentiate epicardial adipose tissue from pericardial effusion. The epicardial adipose typically has mixed echogenicity while most effusions are anechoic. Increasing gain can also be helpful in identifying the internal echoes. Additionally, isolated anterior pericardial effusions are uncommon, as liquid is gravitationally dependent. Occasionally, a clot in the anterior epicardium can also mimic epicardial adipose. Careful evaluation of the movement of the myocardium will show that the epicardial adipose, because it is adhered to the heart, moves simultaneously with the myocardium while the clot will move in response to the motion of the heart in slightly delayed fashion (Fig. 4.14, Video 5). In these cases, it can be helpful to decrease the sector width to produce a higher frame rate and increase lateral resolution. It may also be helpful to play cine clips back at half or quarter speed.

Other common causes of a false positive pericardial effusion include left-sided pleural effusions and ascites. Pericardial effusions can be distinguished from left pleural effusions by using the descending thoracic aorta as a refer-

Table 4.2 Quantification of effusion size

Effusion size	Effusion depth during diastole
Trace	Present only during systole
Small	< 10 mm
Moderate	10–20 mm
Large	> 20 mm

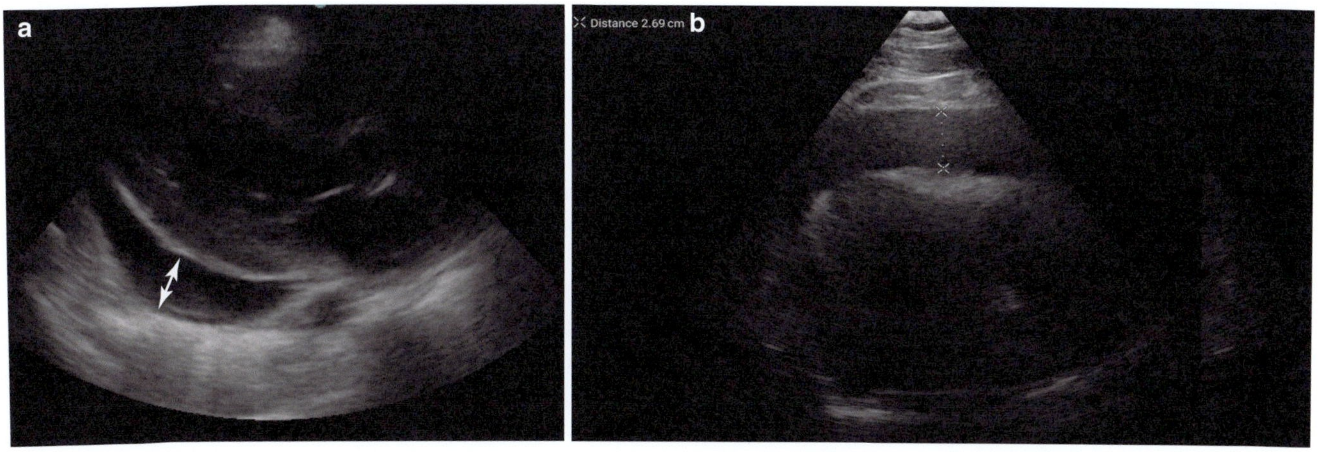

Fig. 4.13 Pericardial effusion measurement in end-diastole. (**a**) Measured in the posterior pericardial space via PLAX view. (**b**) Measured in the inferior pericardial space via subxiphoid view

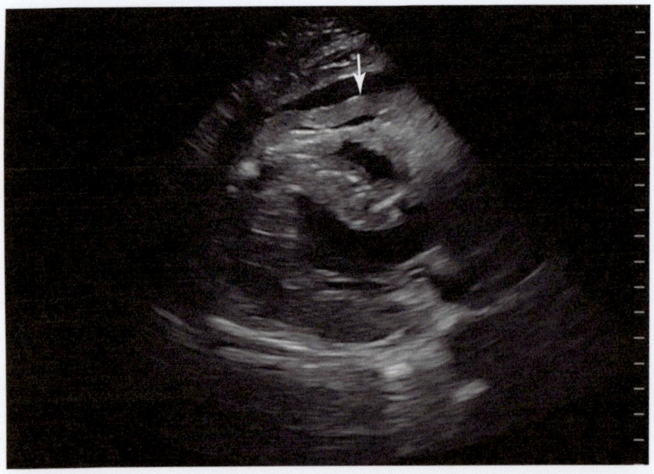

Fig. 4.14 Pericardial effusion with clot (arrow). (*Image courtesy of Michael Gottlieb, MD*)

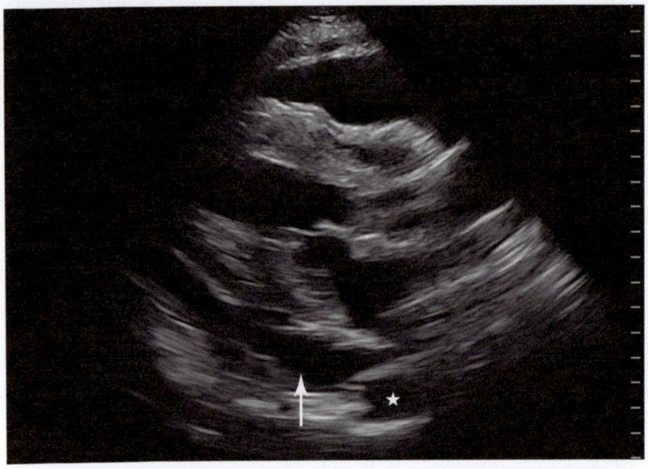

Fig. 4.15 Pericardial effusion (arrow) with extension anterior to the descending aorta (star). (*Image courtesy of Michael Gottlieb, MD*)

ence. Pleural effusions should remain posterior to the descending thoracic aorta, whereas dependent pericardial effusions typically course anterior to the descending thoracic aorta (Fig. 4.15). Ascites is another common false positive for pericardial effusion in the subxiphoid space. Identification of the falciform ligament within a fluid collection distinguishes a pericardial effusion from ascitic fluid in the subxiphoid space [46].

Cardiac Tamponade

Cardiac tamponade is defined as compression of the cardiac chambers by a pericardial effusion, which inhibits normal filling [38]. Tamponade occurs when the compliance of the fluid-filled pericardium is exhausted and can no longer stretch to accommodate a greater volume. With the volume of the pericardium fixed, a trade-off between filling of the right and left heart occurs. Inspiration increases the right heart filling at the expense of left heart filling. This reverses during expiration, when the right heart filling is reduced for the benefit of the left heart and cardiac output. This reflects the principle of ventricular interdependence (i.e., what happens with one ventricle affects the other) and is the physiology responsible for *pulsus paradoxus* (i.e., exaggerated decreases in systolic blood pressure during inspiration). Tamponade most commonly occurs due to increased pressure within the pericardial space, termed high-pressure tamponade. Low-pressure tamponade, where the pressure within the pericardium is minimally elevated, may occur in the setting of pericardial effusion and hypovolemia resulting from a decrease in preload [47].

Effusions may cause tamponade without typical echographic findings as a result of their location. This is especially true for loculated effusions in circumstances such as trauma and following procedures when a clot can exert localized mass effect on the adjacent cardiac chamber. These effusions located adjacent to the left ventricle or atrium may exert physiologic effects of tamponade but without right-sided diastolic collapse [46, 48, 49]. Similarly, extra-cardiac compression can result in tamponade and has been reported from pleural effusions compressing the left atrium in isolation [50]. For this reason, it is important to carefully evaluate the pericardium in multiple orthogonal views to assess for effusion and evaluate all chambers of the heart for diastolic collapse if tamponade is high on the list of differential diagnoses.

Systolic Right Atrial Collapse

Collapse of the right atrium as it is filling during ventricular systole is the earliest echocardiographic indicator of tamponade with a sensitivity of up to 100% (Fig. 4.16). However, it suffers from wide specificity ranging from 33% to 82% [51–54]. Increasing duration of right atrial collapse is associated with a greater probability of tamponade physiology. In cases where the right atrium is collapsed during greater than one-third of the cardiac cycle, sensitivity and specificity for tamponade increase [51]. It is important to differentiate right atrial collapse during systole from right atrial collapse during diastole, which is a normal finding. The echographic window that most easily allows for assessment of the right atrium for the purposes of assessing tamponade is the A4C and SXLA views because of the ability to assess for right atrial collapse during ventricular systole when the right atria should be filling. Alternative views, including PSAX and the right ventricular inflow view, may be helpful for viewing the right atrium but may make assessment of the timing of the cardiac cycle difficult in the absence of ECG leads.

Diastolic Right Ventricular Collapse

Collapse of the right ventricular free wall during ventricular diastole is a finding highly concerning for tamponade (Fig. 4.17, Video 6). Studies have reported this finding to be 40–75% sensitive and 75–90% specific for tamponade [52, 55]. It can be difficult to differentiate whether collapse of the right ventricular free wall is occurring during systole or diastole due to tachycardia. Right ventricular systolic collapse during systole may instead suggest an underfilled right ventricle. M-mode may be particularly useful in these cases by aligning the M-mode tracing over the area of right ventricular collapse and the anterior leaflet of the mitral valve in the PLAX view (Fig. 4.18). Because the mitral valve E and A waves represent diastole, collapse of the right ventricular free wall during diastole can be readily determined.

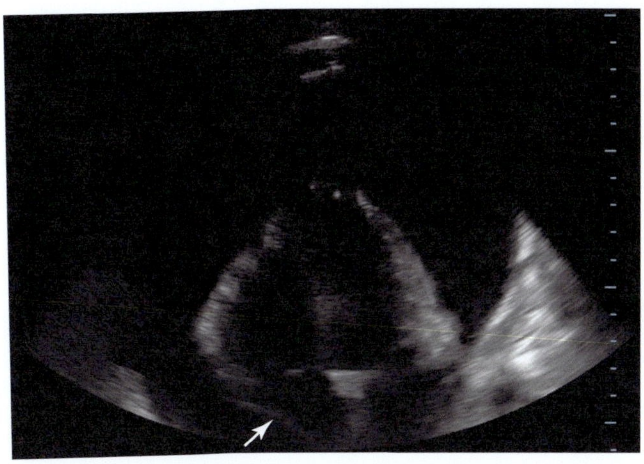

Fig. 4.16 Right atrial collapse (arrow) in early tamponade physiology. *(Image courtesy of Michael Gottlieb, MD)*

Plethoric IVC

A dilated and plethoric IVC has been described as 95–97% sensitive for cardiac tamponade [55, 56]. Physiologically, this is attributed to impaired right atrial filling causing venous return pooling in the IVC resulting in dilation. However, IVC plethora can result from a variety of etiologies, which may limit its use in isolation. Dilation of the IVC is well-described in multiple pathologic states and as a result is not specific for tamponade [56–58]. IVC diameter may be falsely reduced by factors including intra-abdominal hypertension and the presence of extracorporeal membrane oxygenation (ECMO) catheters within the IVC [59]. Additionally, the influence of positive-pressure ventilation on the relation to IVC plethora and pericardial effusions has not been well described.

Respirophasic Variability

Another sign of cardiac tamponade is increased respiratory variation of inflow velocity across the valves on spectral Doppler, a finding known as *sonographic pulsus paradoxus*. Doppler patterns typically show a diastolic restrictive filling pattern with high E-wave velocities, short deceleration times, increased E/A ratio, and reduced A-waves [38]. The tricuspid and pulmonary valves have increased inflow velocities with inspiration due to increased preload. Consensus guidelines from the American Society of Echocardiography and European Society of Cardiology support using >30% of mitral inflow variation and > 60% across the tricuspid valve as concerning for tamponade which is different from previous recommendations of >25% across the MV and >$0% across the TV [38, 44]. In clinical practice, respiratory variation across the tricuspid and mitral valves are the most commonly assessed (Table 4.3). Evaluation of inflow velocities to assess for increased respiratory variation should be performed from A4C view using pulsed-wave Doppler (Fig. 4.19). Doppler gates should be placed between the tips

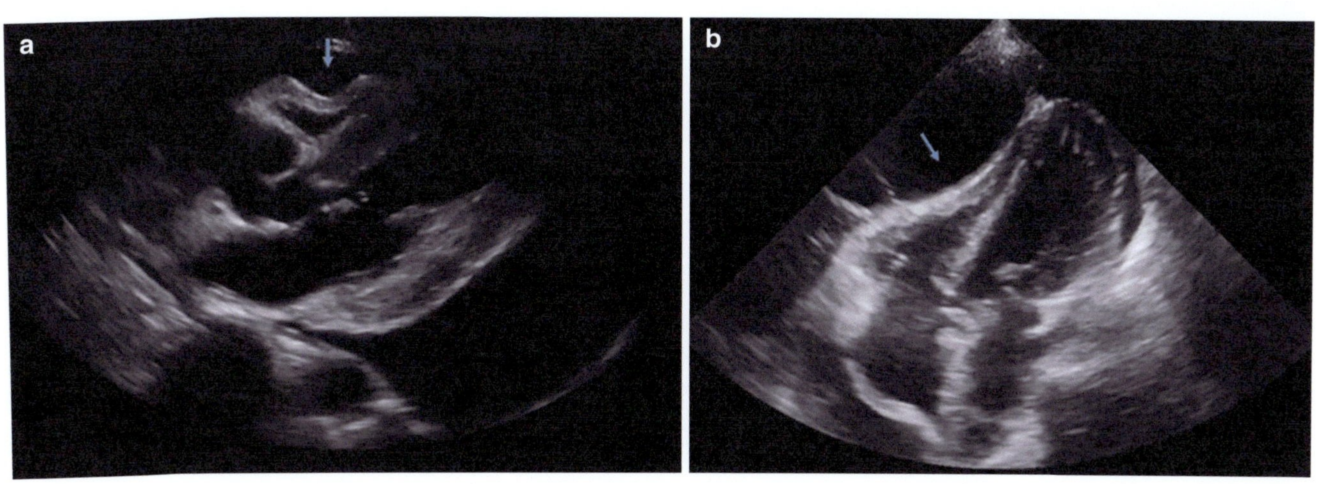

Fig. 4.17 Right ventricular collapse in diastole consistent with cardiac tamponade physiology. (**a**) PLAX view of the right ventricle with collapse (arrow). (**b**) Apical 4-chamber view showing right ventricular collapse (arrow)

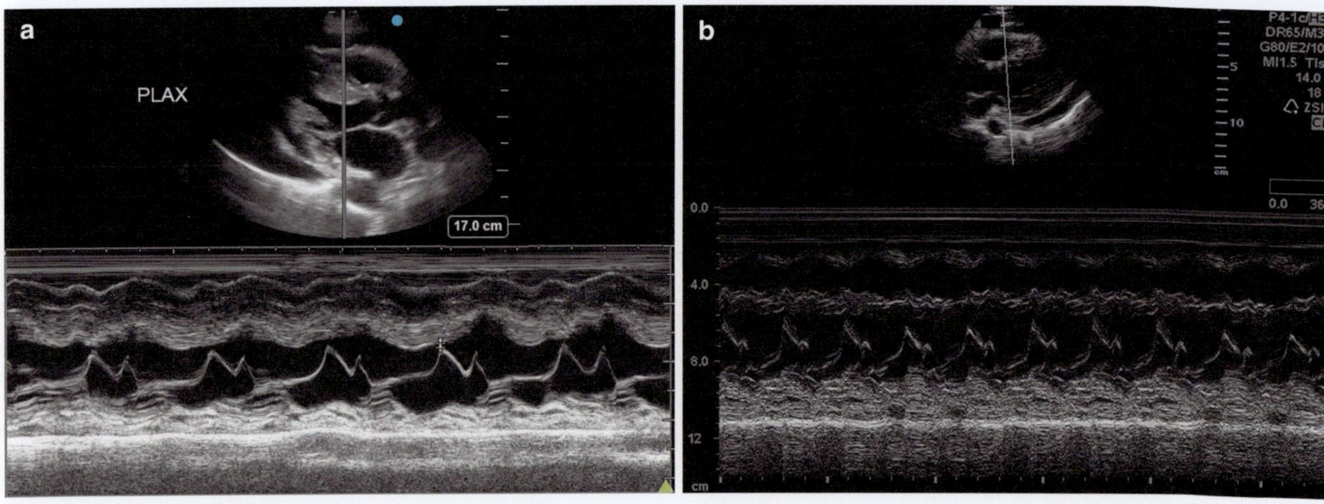

Fig. 4.18 M-mode tracing of the right ventricle and mitral valve. (**a**) Normal (**b**) Right ventricular collapse seen during diastole

Table 4.3 Sensitivity and specificity of increased respiratory variation across cardiac valves for cardiac tamponade. Of note, expert consensus guidelines in 2013 suggested values of 30% across the mitral valve, and 60% across the tricuspid valve [38], and should be taken into consideration with other sonographic and clinical findings when making the diagnosis of cardiac tamponade

Valve	Cutoff	Sensitivity	Specificity
Tricuspid	>30%	50%	69%
Pulmonary	>25%	87%	85%
Mitral	>22%	77%	80%
Aortic	>20%	75%	89%

Table adapted from Materazzo et al. [52]

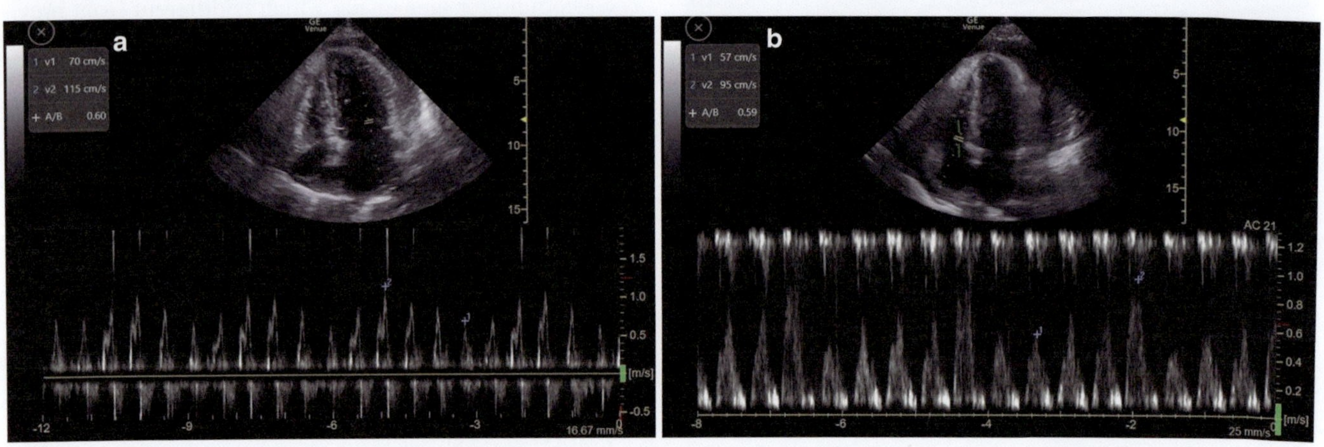

Fig. 4.19 (**a**) Pulsed-wave Doppler tracing of respiratory variation across the mitral valve. (**b**) Pulsed-wave Doppler tracing of respiratory variation across the tricuspid valve

of the open mitral and tricuspid valves. The probe should be oriented such that the flow of blood is perpendicular to the probe face. Depending on the duration of the respiratory cycle, it may be necessary to decrease sweep speed from 100 mm/second to 25–50 mm/second to allow comparison between peak and trough inflow velocities. Care should be taken to measure the E-wave, as this is the wave which reflects diastolic filling without atrial kick and is the lowest pressure point of ventricular diastole.

Cardiac Tamponade in the Context of Pulmonary Hypertension

Diagnosis and management of tamponade is challenging in the setting of pulmonary hypertension. Due to increased right-sided cardiac pressures and right ventricular hypertrophy, it may be more difficult for the ventricle to collapse during diastole. One systematic review and meta-analysis found that right atrial or right ventricular collapse was present in only 10% of cases of cardiac tamponade in those with pulmonary hypertension [60]. Studies have shown that the diagnostic accuracy of right atrial collapse, right ventricle diastolic collapse, trans-mitral respiratory variation, and IVC plethora is lower compared to those without pulmonary hypertension [48]. Interestingly, the predictive value of IVC plethora has been shown to persist even in pulmonary hypertension, in whom IVC plethora has predictive accuracy of 83% [48]. An important consideration is the value of pericardiocentesis among patients with pulmonary hypertension. A fluid-filled pericardium is relatively noncompliant and may buttress a failing right ventricle, preventing the ventricle from becoming distended. Removal of fluid in the pericardium may result in a pressure differential which may lead to sudden right ventricular dilation and right ventricular failure. Previous studies have shown that patients with pulmonary hypertension who undergo pericardiocentesis suffer a higher rate of post-procedure cardiogenic shock and a higher mortality rate [46].

Key Ultrasound Findings

Diagnosis	Key ultrasound findings
Left ventricular systolic function	Gross qualitative estimation E-point septal separation Fractional shortening Simpson biplane method of discs
Pericardial effusion	Effusions are categorized as trace (present only during systole), small (<10 mm), moderate (10–20 mm), or large (>20 mm) False-positives for a pericardial effusion include a pericardial fat pad, left-sided pleural effusion, and ascites
Cardiac tamponade	The echocardiographic findings suggestive of tamponade are: Systolic right atrial collapse (sensitive) Diastolic right ventricular collapse (specific) Dilated, non-collapsible IVC (sensitive) Sonographic pulsus paradoxus
Inferior vena cava	Thin and collapsible—RAP 0–5 mmHg In-between—RAP 5–10 mmHg Plethoric and non-collapsible—RAP 10–20 mmHg

RAP right atrial pressure

Pearls and Pitfalls

- Consider rolling the patient into the left lateral decubitus position to bring the heart closer to the chest wall and obtain clearer cardiac POCUS windows.
- Left lateral decubitus positioning ranges from 0 to 130 degrees. Evaluate differences in visualization with small movements along the range, rather than limiting to only 90 degrees.
- To identify the ideal parasternal window, start with the probe as superior as possible and slide inferiorly until the first adequate cardiac window appears.
- To locate the apical view, start in the parasternal short-axis and slide apically until the heart is just out of view and then flatten the probe. This should be the point of maximal impulse and the ideal view for apical imaging.
- In contrast to the left ventricle, the right ventricle should generally be smaller, have a thinner free wall, more apical atrioventricular valve, and have a moderator band. The surest distinguishing characteristic is that the LV ejects into the LVOT and aortic outflow tract.
- Findings that suggest an oblique cut in the parasternal short-axis include: asymmetric papillary muscle sizes in the mid-chamber view, an oval-shaped left ventricle, and visualization of the left ventricle and tricuspid valve simultaneously.
- The typical echocardiographic findings of tamponade are less likely in patients with pulmonary hypertension, as the elevated right-sided filling pressures would only collapse with higher pericardial pressures from the effusion.

References

1. Moore C. Current issues with emergency cardiac ultrasound probe and image conventions. Acad Emerg Med Off J Soc Acad Emerg Med. 2008;15(3):278–84.
2. Mazurek B, Jehle D, Martin M. Emergency department echocardiography in the diagnosis and therapy of cardiac tamponade. J Emerg Med. 1991;9(1–2):27–31.
3. Plummer D, Brunette D, Asinger R, Ruiz E. Emergency department echocardiography improves outcome in penetrating cardiac injury. Ann Emerg Med. 1992;21(6):709–12.
4. Use of ultrasound imaging by emergency physicians. American College of Emergency Physicians. Ann Emerg Med. 1997;30(3):364–5.
5. Bahner DP. Trinity: a hypotensive ultrasound protocol. J Diagn Med Sonogr. 2002;18(4):193–8.

6. Rose JS, Bair AE, Mandavia D, Kinser DJ. The UHP ultrasound protocol: a novel ultrasound approach to the empiric evaluation of the undifferentiated hypotensive patient. Am J Emerg Med. 2001;19(4):299–302.
7. Breitkreutz R, Walcher F, Seeger FH. Focused echocardiographic evaluation in resuscitation management: concept of an advanced life support-conformed algorithm. Crit Care Med. 2007;35(5 Suppl):S150–61.
8. Atkinson PRT, McAuley DJ, Kendall RJ, Abeyakoon O, Reid CG, Connolly J, et al. Abdominal and cardiac evaluation with sonography in shock (ACES): an approach by emergency physicians for the use of ultrasound in patients with undifferentiated hypotension. Emerg Med J EMJ. 2009;26(2):87–91.
9. Hernandez C, Shuler K, Hannan H, Sonyika C, Likourezos A, Marshall J. C.A.U.S.E.: Cardiac arrest ultra-sound exam—a better approach to managing patients in primary non-arrhythmogenic cardiac arrest. Resuscitation. 2008;76(2):198–206.
10. Emergency Ultrasound Imaging Criteria Compendium. Ann Emerg Med. 2016;68(1):e11–48.
11. Moore CL, Rose GA, Tayal VS, Sullivan DM, Arrowood JA, Kline JA. Determination of left ventricular function by emergency physician echocardiography of hypotensive patients. Acad Emerg Med Off J Soc Acad Emerg Med. 2002;9(3):186–93.
12. Unlüer EE, Karagöz A, Akoğlu H, Bayata S. Visual estimation of bedside echocardiographic ejection fraction by emergency physicians. West J Emerg Med. 2014;15(2):221–6.
13. Adhikari S, Fiorello A, Stolz L, Jones T, Amini R, Gross A, et al. Ability of emergency physicians with advanced echocardiographic experience at a single center to identify complex echocardiographic abnormalities. Am J Emerg Med. 2014;32(4):363–6.
14. Randazzo MR, Snoey ER, Levitt MA, Binder K. Accuracy of emergency physician assessment of left ventricular ejection fraction and central venous pressure using echocardiography. Acad Emerg Med Off J Soc Acad Emerg Med. 2003;10(9):973–7.
15. Prada G, Vieillard-Baron A, Martin AK, Hernandez A, Mookadam F, Ramakrishna H, et al. Echocardiographic applications of M-mode ultrasonography in anesthesiology and critical care. J Cardiothorac Vasc Anesth. 2019;33(6):1559–83.
16. Ahmadpour H, Shah AA, Allen JW, Edmiston WA, Kim SJ, Haywood LJ. Mitral E point septal separation: a reliable index of left ventricular performance in coronary artery disease. Am Heart J. 1983;106(1 Pt 1):21–8.
17. Massie BM, Schiller NB, Ratshin RA, Parmley WW. Mitral-septal separation: new echocardiographic index of left ventricular function. Am J Cardiol. 1977;39(7):1008–16.
18. Strunk BL, Guss SB, Hicks RE, Kotler MN. Echocardiographic recognition of the mitral valve-posterior aortic wall relationship. Circulation. 1975;51(4):594–8.
19. McKaigney CJ, Krantz MJ, La Rocque CL, Hurst ND, Buchanan MS, Kendall JL. E-point septal separation: a bedside tool for emergency physician assessment of left ventricular ejection fraction. Am J Emerg Med. 2014;32(6):493–7.
20. Lang RM, Bierig M, Devereux RB, Flachskampf FA, Foster E, Pellikka PA, et al. Recommendations for chamber quantification: a report from the American Society of Echocardiography's Guidelines and Standards Committee and the Chamber Quantification Writing Group, developed in conjunction with the European Association of Echocardiography, a branch of the European Society of Cardiology. J Am Soc Echocardiogr Off Publ Am Soc Echocardiogr. 2005;18(12):1440–63.
21. Lang RM, Badano LP, Mor-Avi V, Afilalo J, Armstrong A, Ernande L, et al. Recommendations for cardiac chamber quantification by echocardiography in adults: an update from the American Society of Echocardiography and the European Association of Cardiovascular Imaging. J Am Soc Echocardiogr Off Publ Am Soc Echocardiogr. 2015;28(1):1–39.e14.
22. Kontos MC. Role of echocardiography in the emergency department for identifying patients with myocardial infarction and ischemia. Echocardiogr Mt Kisco N. 1999;16(2):193–205.
23. Peels CH, Visser CA, Kupper AJ, Visser FC, Roos JP. Usefulness of two-dimensional echocardiography for immediate detection of myocardial ischemia in the emergency room. Am J Cardiol. 1990;65(11):687–91.
24. Bracey A, Massey L, Pellet AC, Thode HC, Holman TR, Singer AJ, et al. FOCUS may detect wall motion abnormalities in patients with ACS. Am J Emerg Med. 2023;69:17–22.
25. Sağlam C, Ünlüer EE, Yamanoğlu NGÇ, Kara PH, Ediboğlu E, Bektaşlı R, et al. Accuracy of emergency physicians for detection of regional wall motion abnormalities in patients with chest pain without ST-elevation myocardial infarction. J Ultrasound Med Off J Am Inst Ultrasound Med. 2021;40(7):1335–42.
26. Kerwin C, Tommaso L, Kulstad E. A brief training module improves recognition of echocardiographic wall-motion abnormalities by emergency medicine physicians. Emerg Med Int. 2011;2011:483242.
27. Croft PE, Strout TD, Kring RM, Director L, Vasaiwala SC, Mackenzie DC. WAMAMI: emergency physicians can accurately identify wall motion abnormalities in acute myocardial infarction. Am J Emerg Med. 2019;37(12):2224–8.
28. Patel HN, Miyoshi T, Addetia K, Henry MP, Citro R, Daimon M, et al. Normal values of cardiac output and stroke volume according to measurement technique, age, sex, and ethnicity: results of the world Alliance of societies of echocardiography study. J Am Soc Echocardiogr Off Publ Am Soc Echocardiogr. 2021;34(10):1077–1085.e1.
29. Huntsman LL, Stewart DK, Barnes SR, Franklin SB, Colocousis JS, Hessel EA. Noninvasive Doppler determination of cardiac output in man. Clinical validation. Circulation. 1983;67(3):593–602.
30. Baumgartner H, Hung J, Bermejo J, Chambers JB, Edvardsen T, Goldstein S, et al. Recommendations on the echocardiographic assessment of aortic valve stenosis: a focused update from the European Association of Cardiovascular Imaging and the American Society of Echocardiography. J Am Soc Echocardiogr. 2017 Apr;30(4):372–92.
31. Gola A, Pozzoli M, Capomolla S, Traversi E, Sanarico M, Cobelli F, et al. Comparison of Doppler echocardiography with thermodilution for assessing cardiac output in advanced congestive heart failure. Am J Cardiol. 1996;78(6):708–12.
32. Pozzoli M, Capomolla S, Cobelli F, Tavazzi L. Reproducibility of Doppler indices of left ventricular systolic and diastolic function in patients with severe chronic heart failure. Eur Heart J. 1995;16(2):194–200.
33. Tan C, Rubenson D, Srivastava A, Mohan R, Smith MR, Billick K, et al. Left ventricular outflow tract velocity time integral outperforms ejection fraction and Doppler-derived cardiac output for predicting outcomes in a select advanced heart failure cohort. Cardiovasc Ultrasound. 2017;15(1):18.
34. Trent RJ, Rawles JM. Risk stratification after acute myocardial infarction by Doppler stroke distance measurement. Heart Br Card Soc. 1999;82(2):187–91.
35. Ristow B, Na B, Ali S, Whooley MA, Schiller NB. Left ventricular outflow tract and pulmonary artery stroke distances independently predict heart failure hospitalization and mortality: the heart and soul study. J Am Soc Echocardiogr Off Publ Am Soc Echocardiogr. 2011;24(5):565–72.
36. Rudski LG, Lai WW, Afilalo J, Hua L, Handschumacher MD, Chandrasekaran K, et al. Guidelines for the echocardiographic assessment of the right heart in adults: a report from the American Society of Echocardiography endorsed by the European Association of Echocardiography, a registered branch of the European Society of Cardiology, and the Canadian Society of Echocardiography.

J Am Soc Echocardiogr Off Publ Am Soc Echocardiogr. 2010;23(7):685–713. quiz 786–8

37. Porter TR, Shillcutt SK, Adams MS, Desjardins G, Glas KE, Olson JJ, et al. Guidelines for the use of echocardiography as a monitor for therapeutic intervention in adults: a report from the American Society of Echocardiography. J Am Soc Echocardiogr Off Publ Am Soc Echocardiogr. 2015;28(1):40–56.
38. Klein AL, Abbara S, Agler DA, Appleton CP, Asher CR, Hoit B, et al. American Society of Echocardiography clinical recommendations for multimodality cardiovascular imaging of patients with pericardial disease: endorsed by the Society for Cardiovascular Magnetic Resonance and Society of cardiovascular computed tomography. J Am Soc Echocardiogr Off Publ Am Soc Echocardiogr. 2013;26(9):965–1012.e15.
39. Kircher BJ, Himelman RB, Schiller NB. Noninvasive estimation of right atrial pressure from the inspiratory collapse of the inferior vena cava. Am J Cardiol. 1990;66(4):493–6.
40. Nagdev AD, Merchant RC, Tirado-Gonzalez A, Sisson CA, Murphy MC. Emergency department bedside ultrasonographic measurement of the caval index for noninvasive determination of low central venous pressure. Ann Emerg Med. 2010;55(3):290–5.
41. Barbier C, Loubières Y, Schmit C, Hayon J, Ricôme JL, Jardin F, et al. Respiratory changes in inferior vena cava diameter are helpful in predicting fluid responsiveness in ventilated septic patients. Intensive Care Med. 2004;30(9):1740–6.
42. Pérez-Casares A, Cesar S, Brunet-Garcia L, Sanchez-de-Toledo J. Echocardiographic evaluation of pericardial effusion and cardiac tamponade. Front Pediatr. 2017;5:79.
43. Ashoobi MA, Homaie Rad E, Rahimi R. Diagnostic performance of sonography in penetrating torso trauma: a systematic review and meta-analysis. Eur J Trauma Emerg Surg Off Publ Eur Trauma Soc. 2024;50:1347.
44. Adler Y, Charron P, Imazio M, Badano L, Barón-Esquivias G, Bogaert J, et al. 2015 ESC guidelines for the diagnosis and management of pericardial diseases: the task force for the diagnosis and management of pericardial diseases of the European Society of Cardiology (ESC) endorsed by: the European Association for Cardio-Thoracic Surgery (EACTS). Eur Heart J. 2015;36(42):2921–64.
45. Imazio M, Adler Y. Management of pericardial effusion. Eur Heart J. 2013;34(16):1186–97.
46. Vasquez MA, Iskander M, Mustafa M, Quintero-Martinez JA, Luna A, Mintz J, et al. Pericardiocentesis outcomes in patients with pulmonary hypertension: a Nationwide analysis from the United States. Am J Cardiol. 2024;210:232–40.
47. Sagristà-Sauleda J, Angel J, Sambola A, Alguersuari J, Permanyer-Miralda G, Soler-Soler J. Low-pressure cardiac tamponade: clinical and hemodynamic profile. Circulation. 2006;114(9):945–52.
48. Plotnick GD, Rubin DC, Feliciano Z, Ziskind AA. Pulmonary hypertension decreases the predictive accuracy of echocardiographic clues for cardiac tamponade. Chest. 1995;107(4):919–24.
49. Chuttani K, Pandian NG, Mohanty PK, Rosenfield K, Schwartz SL, Udelson JE, et al. Left ventricular diastolic collapse. An echocardiographic sign of regional cardiac tamponade. Circulation. 1991;83(6):1999–2006.
50. Khaja M, Santana Y, Rodriguez Guerra MA, Rehmani A, Perez Lara JL. Isolated left atrial cardiac tamponade caused by pleural effusion. Cureus. 2020;12(11):e11578.
51. Gillam LD, Guyer DE, Gibson TC, King ME, Marshall JE, Weyman AE. Hydrodynamic compression of the right atrium: a new echocardiographic sign of cardiac tamponade. Circulation. 1983;68(2):294–301.
52. Materazzo C, Piotti P, Meazza R, Pellegrini MP, Viggiano V, Biasi S. Respiratory changes in transvalvular flow velocities versus two-dimensional echocardiographic findings in the diagnosis of cardiac tamponade. Ital Heart J Off J Ital Fed Cardiol. 2003;4(3):186–92.
53. Kronzon I, Cohen ML, Winer HE. Diastolic atrial compression: a sensitive echocardiographic sign of cardiac tamponade. J Am Coll Cardiol. 1983;2(4):770–5.
54. Guntheroth WG. Sensitivity and specificity of echocardiographic evidence of tamponade: implications for ventricular interdependence and pulsus paradoxus. Pediatr Cardiol. 2007;28(5):358–62.
55. Alerhand S, Adrian RJ, Long B, Avila J. Pericardial tamponade: a comprehensive emergency medicine and echocardiography review. Am J Emerg Med. 2022;58:159–74.
56. Himelman RB, Kircher B, Rockey DC, Schiller NB. Inferior vena cava plethora with blunted respiratory response: a sensitive echocardiographic sign of cardiac tamponade. J Am Coll Cardiol. 1988;12(6):1470–7.
57. Kawata T, Daimon M, Nakanishi K, Kimura K, Sawada N, Nakao T, et al. Factors influencing inferior vena cava diameter and its respiratory variation: simultaneous comparison with hemodynamic data. J Cardiol. 2022;79(5):642–7.
58. Stone MB, Huang JV. Inferior vena cava assessment: correlation with CVP and plethora in tamponade. Glob Heart. 2013;8(4):323–7.
59. Via G, Tavazzi G, Price S. Ten situations where inferior vena cava ultrasound may fail to accurately predict fluid responsiveness: a physiologically based point of view. Intensive Care Med. 2016;42(7):1164–7.
60. Adrian RJ, Alerhand S, Liteplo A, Shokoohi H. Is pulmonary hypertension protective against cardiac tamponade? A systematic review. Intern Emerg Med. 2024;19:1987.

Advanced Cardiac Ultrasound

5

Alan Chiem, Mark Favot, and Lindsay Taylor

Introduction

This chapter will focus on advanced components of cardiac ultrasound. Many of the advanced applications in this chapter will build upon elements in Chap. 4, so readers are advised to review that chapter as a foundation before beginning this advanced cardiac chapter. The chapter will sequentially cover three main applications: diastolic dysfunction, right ventricular function, and valvular pathology. After this chapter, the reader will have a strong foundation in these advanced uses of cardiac ultrasound.

Diastology

Background

The definition of diastology is simply the study of filling of the left ventricle (LV) during diastole. Assessment of LV diastolic function provides valuable information in patients with all variants of heart failure, as well as changes in volume status and responses to heart failure management therapies. Changes in diastolic function precede findings on serology, radiography, as well as on physical examination.

Supplementary Information The online version contains supplementary material available at https://doi.org/10.1007/978-3-031-85308-1_5.

A. Chiem
Department of Emergency Medicine, David Geffen School of Medicine at UCLA, Los Angeles, CA, USA
e-mail: achiem@mednet.ucla.edu

M. Favot
Department of Emergency Medicine, Wayne State University School of Medicine, Detroit, MI, USA
e-mail: mfavot@med.wayne.edu

L. Taylor (✉)
Department of Emergency Medicine, Virginia Commonwealth University, Richmond, VA, USA
e-mail: Lindsay.Taylor@vcuhealth.org

An understanding of diastolic dysfunction can also be valuable for diagnosing new heart failure, differentiating acute from chronic heart failure, and assessing for ischemia-related impaired relaxation in early acute coronary syndrome (which often precedes regional wall motion abnormalities or systolic dysfunction) [1, 2]. Diastology can also assist with differentiating restrictive cardiomyopathies from pericardial disease processes such as cardiac tamponade or constrictive pericarditis [3, 4]. Diastology has tremendous potential in terms of recent telemedicine approaches that use portable, implantable left atrial pressure and pulmonary artery pressure monitoring devices to detect early, pre-symptomatic acute heart failure [5, 6]. Lastly, diastology serves as the foundation for emerging POCUS applications such as Venous Excess Ultrasound (VExUS) [7].

LV diastolic function is determined by two normal forces in two distinct phases in diastole—LV relaxation and left atrial (LA) contraction. In pathological states, these normal forces are supplanted by a positive pressure gradient between the LA and LV due to pathological left atrial pressure (LAP) elevation.

Assessment of diastolic function is performed by: (1) measurement of maximal filling velocities during early and late diastole using pulsed-wave Doppler (PWD) and (2) measurement of LV relaxation velocities through Tissue Doppler Imaging (TDI). Diastolic dysfunction severity is determined by the severity of LAP elevation, which can be reduced or normalized via administration of diuretics and blood pressure control.

Indications

Indications
- Chest pain
- Dyspnea
- Fatigue
- Lower extremity swelling
- Rales

Diagnoses
- Diastolic dysfunction

M. Gottlieb, N. Panebianco (eds.), *Advanced Point-of-Care Ultrasound*, https://doi.org/10.1007/978-3-031-85308-1_5

Core Views

View	Image	Approach
Mitral Valve Inflow Velocity	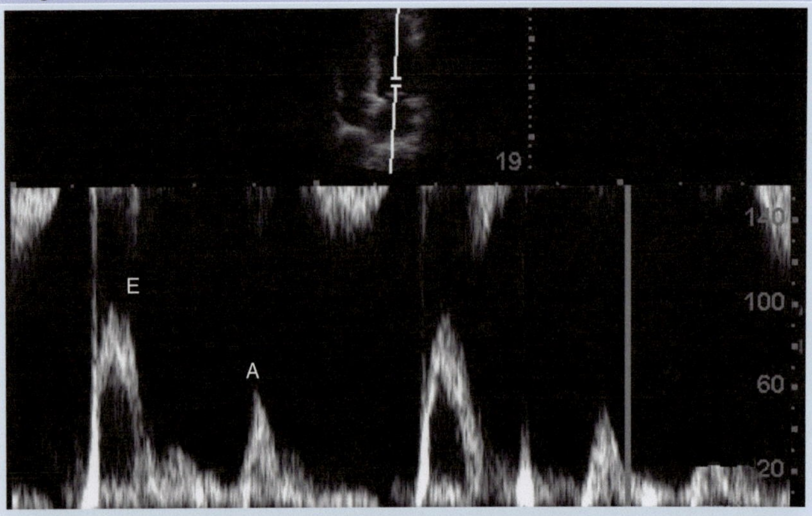 Core View 1. Apical 4-chamber view with pulsed-wave Doppler over the mitral inflow	After obtaining an apical 4-chamber view, place the pulsed-wave Doppler gate over the area of maximal mitral inflow, just below the mitral valve within the left ventricle. Ensure the Doppler gate is sufficiently distal to avoid accidentally capturing the mitral valve leaflet. Adjust the scale and baseline as needed to maximize visualization of the waveform and avoid aliasing. E wave, early filling; A wave, atrial contraction.
Tissue Doppler Imaging of LV Wall	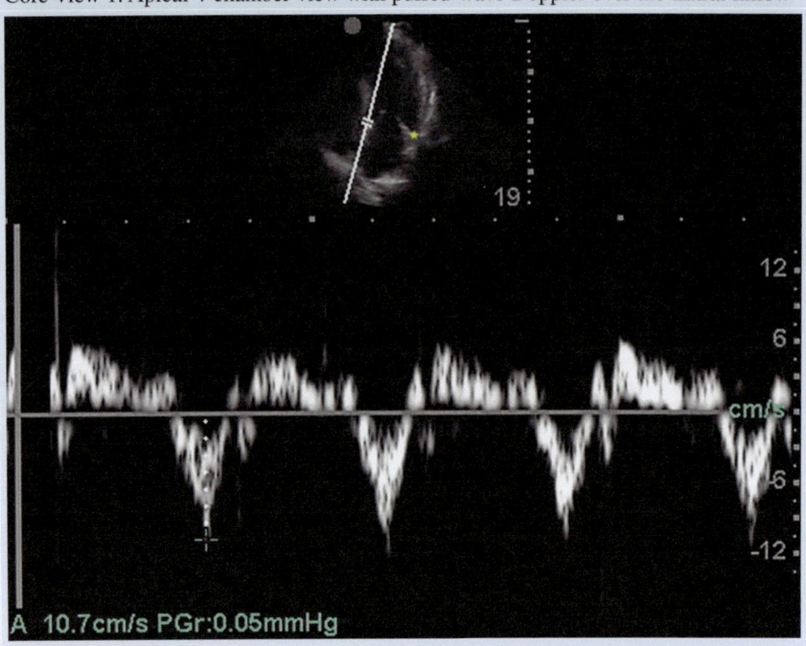 *Lateral annulus Core View 2. Apical 4-chamber view and TDI of lateral and septal mitral annulus	From the apical 4-chamber view, use tissue Doppler imaging (TDI) and place the gait over the septal edge of the mitral valve annulus. Ensure that the Doppler is as parallel to the wall as possible. This can then be repeated on the lateral edge of the mitral valve annulus (asterisk).

View	Image	Approach
Left Atrial Size (Qualitative)	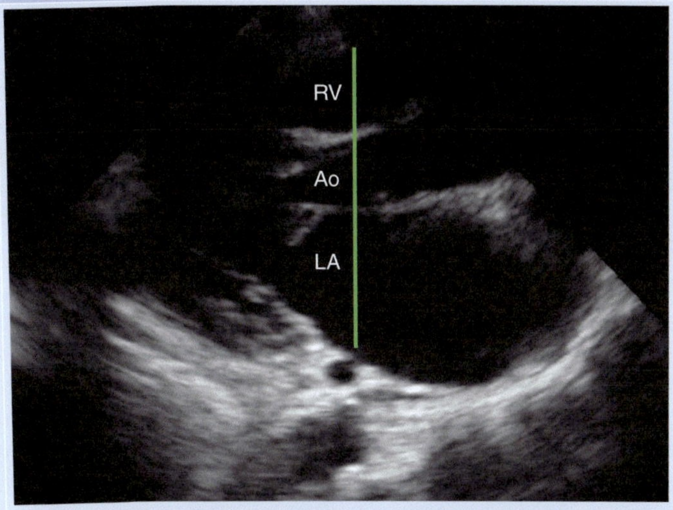 Core View 3. Left atrial assessment using qualitative criteria	Using the parasternal long-axis view, the left atrium can be qualitatively assessed using the rule of thirds. The anterior-posterior dimension of the right ventricle (RV), aortic root (Ao), and left atrium (LA) should be approximately the same size normally. When enlarged (as in this image), the left atrium will be >1/3 of the total diameter.
Left Atrial Size (Quantitative)	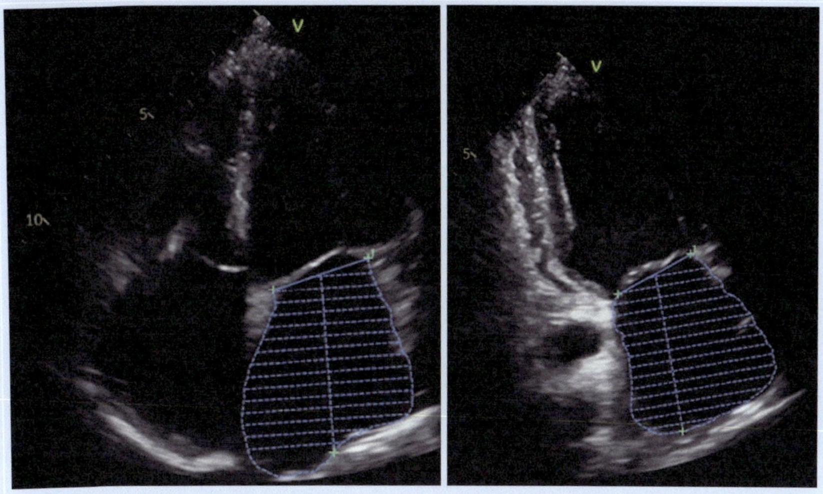 Core View 4. Left atrial assessment using quantitative measurements	Quantitative assessment of left atrial volume index is performed using the apical 4-chamber and the apical 2-chamber views with the Simpson's biplane method of discs. Begin by obtaining an end-systolic atrial view (with the mitral valve closed), as this reflects when the atria is maximally dilated. Simpson's biplane is calculated by tracing the diameter of the inner wall and then calculated by the ultrasound machine. This volume is then divided by the patient's total body surface to determine the left atrial volume index (normal ≤34 mL/m^2). This is repeated in the atrial 2-chamber view and the two values are averaged.

There are two primary mechanisms or forces responsible for filling, each occurring in two separate phases of diastole. These two forces affect the pressure gradient between the LA and LV.

The first force is the relaxation of the LV during early diastole, sometimes termed isovolumetric relaxation or lusitropy. Due to the inverse relationship between pressure and volume in a chamber, as the LV expands in early diastole, its chamber pressure drops. This leads to a negative pressure gradient between the LV and LA, leading to suctioning of blood from the LA to the LV. Fluid flows into the LV as a result of this negative pressure gradient and only stops when the pressure in the LA and the LV are equal. This pressure equalization between the LA and LV is also affected by LV compliance. A more compliant LV will continue to expand with increasing blood volume filling the LV before the LV pressure starts to increase and equilibrates with the LA, leading to cessation of filling during this early phase of diastole.

The maximal velocity of the fluid that fills the chamber is directly proportional to the volume of filling that occurs. Likewise, the velocity of expansion of the LV (as measured at standardized points of the mitral annulus) is proportional to the amount of the negative pressure gradient generated, which itself determines the amount of filling. The filling velocity is denoted as the E wave, while the velocity of LV tissue relaxation is denoted as the e′ wave. After early diastolic filling, there is no flow between LA and LV because the pressures are equalized. This point during diastole is called diastasis.

The second stage of diastole follows diastasis. It occurs when the LA contracts, leading to a positive pressure gradient between LA and LV. There is a brief resultant filling of the LV. This velocity profile is called the A wave. Filling of the LV due to atrial contraction also leads to LV expansion, and this is seen in the mitral annular movement known as the a′ wave. Of note, a′ is largely passive, whereas e′ is due to energy-dependent relaxation of the LV. Normal LV relaxation and expansion lead to approximately 70–80% of chamber filling, while atrial contraction is responsible for the remaining 20–30% of filling.

Echocardiographic Assessment of Diastolic Function

The standard approach to diastolic assessment is performed using an apical 4-chamber (A4C) view. First, mitral inflow velocities are assessed using PWD, with the sampling gate placed in between and just distal to the mitral leaflet tips. The sampling gate should be 1–2 mm apart, and the sampling line should be inline with the LA to LV direction (i.e., the vector of diastolic filling) [8]. Applying color Doppler before PWD can assist in identifying the course of blood flow into the LV. A normal mitral inflow profile will show a characteristic repeating pattern of a taller and usually wider E wave coupled with a smaller and narrower A wave, with a typical height ratio of roughly 1–1.5, reflecting the relative greater importance of LV relaxation in normal diastolic function [8].

Second, TDI of both the medial (septal) and lateral mitral annulus are assessed to evaluate left ventricular myocardial relaxation. TDI is a modified form of PWD, where the gain is severely reduced to prevent imaging of less dense blood inflow, while still preserving the visualization of the denser movement of the mitral annuli. The scale in TDI is also reduced to 0–20 cm/s, which is the normal velocity range of the annuli, as opposed to blood inflow, which travels 5–10 times faster. TDI assessment is performed at the septal and lateral mitral annulus. Normal TDI waveforms of either annuli show a profile similar to the E and A wave pattern but are negative in direction. This is due to the mitral annulus moving toward the base of the heart (i.e., away from the probe) during each phase of diastole. The lateral e′ is normally ≥10 cm/s while the septal e′ is normally ≥7 cm/s [8]. The septal annulus is tethered to the interatrial and interventricular septum, accounting for its lower tissue velocity. Both the medial and lateral measurements should be measured and then averaged.

Clinical Applications

Diastolic Dysfunction

Impaired relaxation may occur due to decreased lusitropy, which, similar to inotropy and chronotropy, is very energy-dependent and mediated by adrenergic pathways. This is why diastolic dysfunction occurs before systolic dysfunction in the ischemic cascade associated with acute coronary syndrome [9], as well as in restrictive cardiomyopathies [10]. Impaired relaxation is also associated with decreased compliance, which typically occurs in patients with longstanding uncontrolled hypertension and left ventricular hypertrophy [11]. Atrial contraction can be described by a Frank-Starling curve in which increased preload of the atria leads to increased atrial contraction and stroke volume [12]. As a result of decreased filling of the LV during early diastole (E wave) in impaired relaxation, the atrial volume is greater during the late diastolic phase. This increased atrial preload leads to both a higher inflow pattern (A wave) and greater annular velocity (a′) during late diastole.

As a result, the impaired relaxation profile shows a smaller E wave compared to a taller A wave, as well as a smaller e′ (due to impaired relaxation) and larger a′. During impaired relaxation, the increased atrial contraction and stroke volume compensates for reduced filling during early diastole. This is important to note since patients with impaired relaxation often do not have symptoms of acute heart failure, such as pulmonary or systemic congestion.

Atrial compensation in impaired relaxation is a tenuous state, as increases in LV afterload, LV end-diastolic pressure, or systemic congestion, can lead to further decompensation. This leads to a rise in LAP, which results in pulmonary edema, elevated right heart pressures, decreased venous return, and peripheral edema. This increase in LAP is the crucial transition point between asymptomatic and symptomatic patients. The severity and duration of LAP elevation are associated with the severity of pulmonary and systemic congestion [13]. For example, flash pulmonary edema results from acute increases in systemic blood pressure and LV afterload, leading to increased pulmonary congestion but little to no systemic congestion. This is why patients with flash pulmonary edema dramatically improve within hours of anti-hypertensive therapy and can often be discharged within 24 h of admission [14]. In contrast, patients who experience slowly worsening pulmonary and systemic congestion due to steady increases in fluid retention can have a more prolonged recovery.

Regardless of etiology, the common result in symptomatic diastolic and systolic dysfunction is an elevation in LAP. The severity of this LAP increase can be described by the relative amplitudes of the E and A waves, as well as e′ and a′. When LAP is elevated in early diastole, the normal mechanism of relaxation-mediated filling of the LV is subsequently replaced by a positive pressure gradient between LA and LV. When the mitral valve opens in early diastole, this pressure gradient forces blood from the LA to the LV. This leads to an increase in the E wave such that the E:A ratio is now roughly 1–1.5, similar to a heart without diastolic dysfunction. However, the e′ and a′ are still depressed since the mechanism of this LV filling is not lusitropic but rather due to the positive pressure gradient from elevated LAP. This pattern is referred to as "pseudonormalization" since the E:A filling profile is indistinguishable from the normal diastolic filling profile. TDI must be used to differentiate this pseudonormal or Grade II diastolic dysfunction from normal diastolic function.

With worsening LAP, this positive pressure gradient between LA and LV leads to further increases in passive filling of the LV, with a higher E wave and declining A wave. The A wave declines slightly because atrial preload is severely elevated, and atrial contraction, according to the Frank-Starling curve, is impaired due to excessive atrial stretch. The E:A ratio is >2 in this Grade III diastolic dysfunction, which is termed restrictive. TDI assessment also shows diminishing e′ and a′, indicating the increasing dominance of the positive LA:LV pressure gradient in LV filling and the much diminished role of lusitropy.

Grades II–III of diastolic dysfunction are often reversible at the initial assessment with a Valsalva maneuver or after heart failure therapy, which reduces or normalizes LAP. The Valsalva maneuver temporarily decreases venous return, which will also temporarily reduce LAP so that the influence of the positive LA-LV gradient on LV filling is reduced in comparison to the negative gradient generated by LV relaxation. This temporarily decreases the E wave velocity as well as possibly increasing the e′, allowing for a reduction in diastolic dysfunction severity. For example, patients with Grade III diastolic dysfunction can revert back to Grade II temporarily with a Valsalva maneuver [15].

Traditional classification of diastolic dysfunction includes a Grade IV, which is similar to Grade III, except that it is considered irreversible, either with Valsalva or traditional heart failure therapies. This is owing to the negligible effect of the Valsalva maneuver on LAP reduction in relation to the dramatically elevated LAP. A summary of the grades and sonographic findings is included in Fig. 5.1.

Estimating LAP with E/e′

Left atrial pressure can be assessed by myriad calculations [16]. However, the most applicable for point-of-care ultrasound (POCUS) are E/e′, isovolumic relaxation time (IVRT), and deceleration time (DT) (Fig. 5.2). IVRT is the time between closure of the aortic valve to onset of filling with the E wave. Deceleration time is the interval from the peak of the E wave to the projected E wave baseline or where it meets 0 cm/s. IVRT and DT both have an upside-down parabolic relationship with diastolic function. For example, normal IVRT is between 60 and 80 ms, while >90 ms indicates impaired relaxation, and <60 ms indicates restrictive filling physiology. Normal DT is between 150 and 240 ms, whereas impaired relaxation is associated with DT >240 ms, and restrictive filling is associated with DT <150 ms [17].

E/e′ can be calculated based on the mitral E wave and the average of the septal and lateral annular e′, as described above. An E/e′ <13 is associated with normal LAP, while values ≥13 are associated with elevated LAP. Furthermore, LAP can be estimated using the formula E/e′ + 4. However, severe mitral regurgitation (MR) or aortic regurgitation (AR) can limit the reliability of E wave assessment. In addition, tachycardia may lead to fusion of the E and A waves. In such cases, decreasing the sweep speed may help to delineate the E and A velocities. The e′ may be influenced by the presence of any pathologies that further restrict movement of the mitral annulus, such as in calcific mitral stenosis or mitral valve replacement. In general, E/e′ is considered one of the most reliable and reproducible measures of LAP [18].

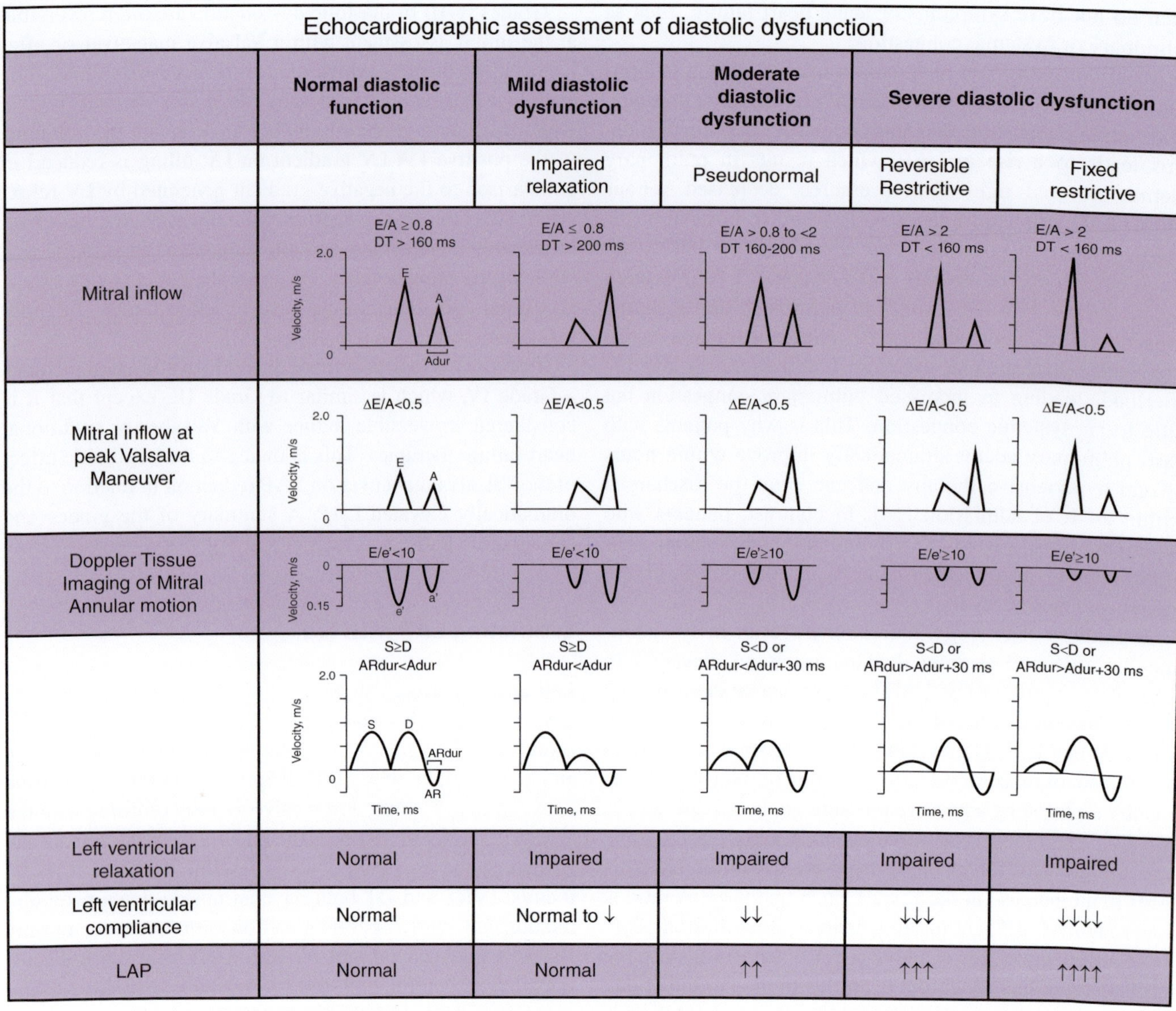

Fig. 5.1 Grades of diastolic dysfunction. Grade I is characterized by impaired relaxation and normal left atrial pressure (LAP). Grade II is characterized by a pseudonormal E/A profile but diminished e′ velocities. Grade III is characterized by severely elevated LAP that drives the high E velocity passively, with minimal contribution from lusitropy, as seen by severely diminished e′ velocities *Adur* atrial contraction duration, *ARdur* atrial reversal duration, *DT* deceleration time, *LAP* left atrial pressure

Evaluation of Acute Decompensated Heart Failure

One common misconception is that diastolic dysfunction is a steady-state diagnosis that does not change. In fact, aside from patients with severely depressed LV ejection fractions and heart failure symptoms at rest, the majority of patients with heart failure can have improvement or resolution of their diastolic function as well as their congestion with appropriate management.

In patients with known heart failure, LAP assessment is a powerful tool in both diagnosing acute decompensated heart failure (ADHF) and helping to guide treatment. This has been supported by recent telemedicine studies with invasive LAP and pulmonary artery pressure (PAP) devices, such as V-LAPS and CardioMEMS, that have led to significant reductions in hospitalizations and mortality [19, 20]. PAP devices function similarly to LAP devices, but in a downstream fashion as elevated LAP leads to pulmonary congestion which will increase PAP. In addition, small recent studies of the use of E/e′ to guide management of ADHF have shown strong associations between E/e′ and pulmonary congestion as well as reductions in length of stay [21, 22].

If the diagnosis of ADHF is uncertain due to mixed findings from pulmonary and inferior vena cava (IVC) ultrasound, E/e′ >13 may be used to increase the likelihood of

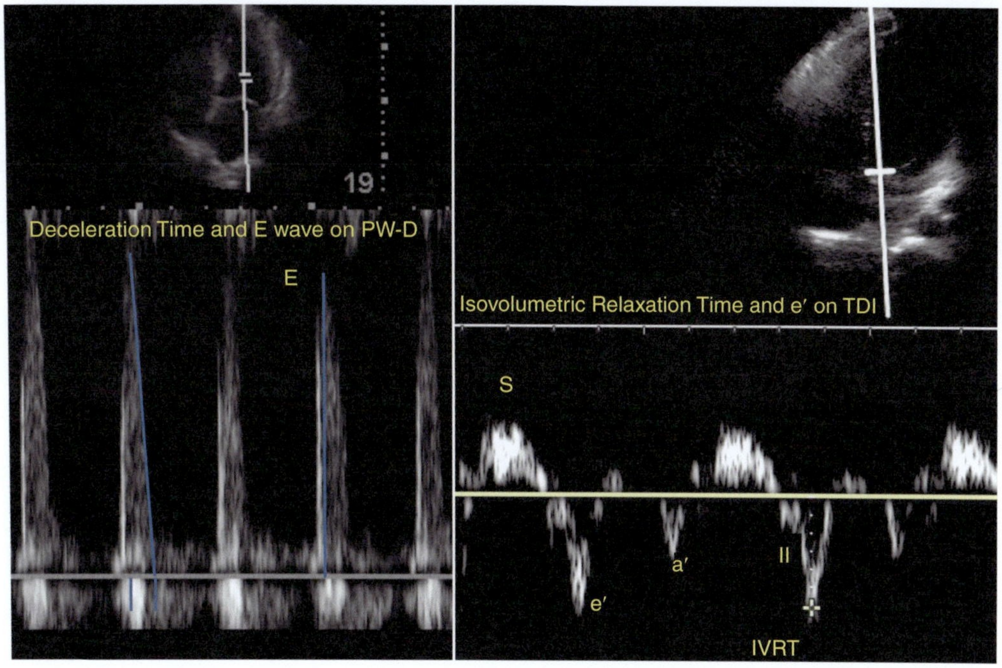

Fig. 5.2 Deceleration time (DT) is measured as the time from peak to baseline for the E wave. Isovolumetric relaxation time (IVRT) is measured as the time from closure of the aortic valve to onset of filling for the E wave

ADHF. Once the diagnosis is made, serial E/e′ may be performed, similar to serial point-of-care glucose assessments for the treatment of patients with hyperglycemia or serial heart rates in the management of tachycardia. If the E/e′ is reduced significantly after treatment-associated diuresis or blood pressure reduction, these patients may be identified as responders that may be suitable for discharge [23]. There is a tremendous need to identify these responders who may benefit from rapid and focused management to avoid unnecessary hospital admissions.

Evaluation of New Isolated Diastolic Heart Failure

While the diagnosis of systolic dysfunction is based primarily on the ejection fraction, diagnosing diastolic dysfunction requires several criteria to be present and combined with the clinical presentation. The most widely used criteria, and those recommended by the American Society of Echocardiography, assesses four main criteria [8]:

- E/e′ > 14
- Left atrial volume index >34 mL/m^2 (performed using Simpson's biplane method of discs)
- Septal e′ <7 m/s or lateral e′ <10 m/s
- Tricuspid regurgitation jet >2.8 m/s

If ≥3 criteria are met, the patient is diagnosed with diastolic heart failure, while two criteria suggest an indeterminate diagnosis, and <2 criteria indicate no diastolic dysfunction. This approach leads to a high specificity, though sensitivity may be as low as 35% [24].

Table 5.1 H2FPEF criteria

Clinical variables	Definition	Points
Heavy	BMI > 30 kg/m^2	2
Hypertensive	On ≥2 antihypertensive medications	1
Atrial fibrillation	Paroxysmal or permanent	3
Pulmonary hypertension	PASP >35 mm Hg	1
Elderly	Age >60 years	1
Filling pressure	E/e′ >9	1

BMI body mass index, *PASP* pulmonary artery systolic pressure

A newer decision instrument that can be used in the acute care setting by advanced POCUS practitioners is the H2FPEF score (Table 5.1). It uses four historical and clinical variables as well as E/e′ >9 and pulmonary artery systolic pressure (PASP) >35 mm Hg, with a total assigned number of 9 points. A score ≤1 is associated with a ≤25% likelihood of diastolic heart failure, while a score ≥6 is associated with a ≥90% likelihood of diastolic heart failure. This model has been validated with high sensitivity and moderate specificity, with an area under the curve (AUC) of >0.85 [25].

Assessing Diastolic Dysfunction When Atrial Fibrillation Is Present

Patients with atrial fibrillation depend solely on early diastolic LV relaxation for LV filling as they lack an organized atrial contraction during late diastole. Therefore, Doppler analysis reveals only E and e′ waves but no A or a′ wave (Fig. 5.3). DT of the mitral inflow <170 ms or IVRT <65 ms indicates elevated LAP. E/e′ can also be used, with a ratio

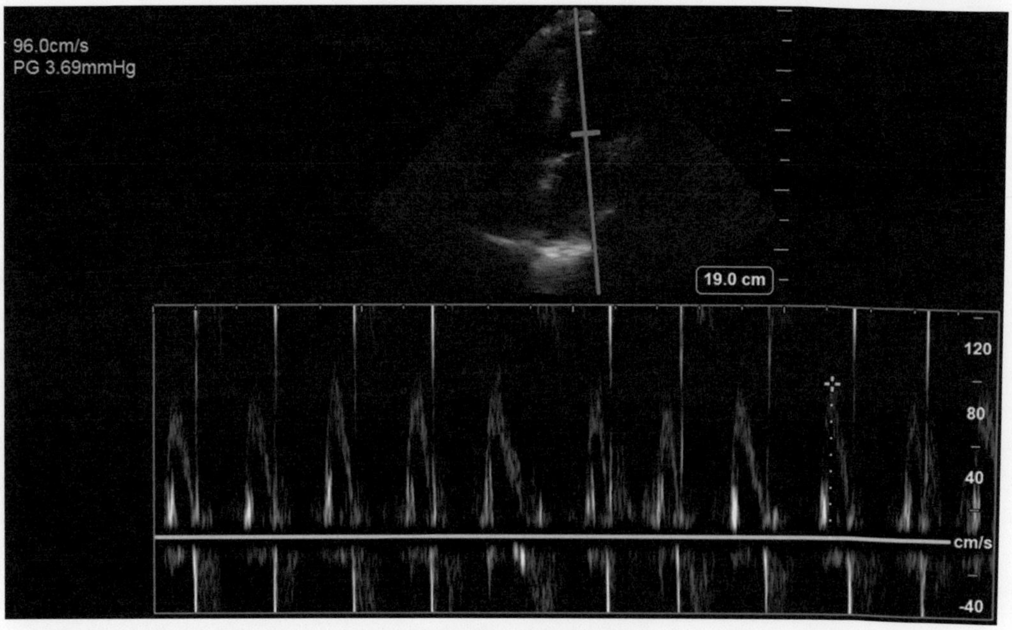

Fig. 5.3 Pulsed-wave Doppler in atrial fibrillation. Note the absence of A waves and the irregular intervals between the E waves

>11 indicating elevated LAP [8]. However, the average value of at least three E/e′ measurements from three nonconsecutive beats should be used. This will account for the variability in the ventricular rate, which affects LV filling, stroke volume ejected, as well as remaining LV volume after systole. As a corollary, if there is little E wave variability between beats, that is usually a sign that LV filling pressures are elevated [25].

Assessing Diastolic Dysfunction When Mitral Valve Pathology Is Present

According to the continuity equation, mass or blood volume must be preserved as it travels through a valvular area. So when blood travels through a stenotic orifice, it will accelerate to preserve this blood volume. Its velocity will be inversely proportional to the stenotic orifice area. In mitral stenosis (MS), both the E and A wave velocities increase in an inverse relationship to the mitral valve area. While the E wave is not reliable, an A wave >1.5 m/s is correlated with elevated LAP. In addition, the e′ and a′ wave velocities may be reduced and delayed compared to the E and A wave, especially if the mitral annulus is heavily calcified. As a result, E/e′ is not useful when there is MS. IVRT <60 ms is still helpful in diagnosing elevated LAP. Another more technically challenging measurement is the IVRT/Te-e′ ratio. If this value is <4.2, this indicates elevated LAP. The Te-e′ is the time interval between the onset of systole and the onset of either the E wave or the e′ wave (Fig. 5.4) [8].

Mitral regurgitation is commonly due to elevated LV filling pressures or failure of the mitral leaflets to coapt in patients with a dilated LV. In these cases, it is considered functional MR, and common diastolic assessments can still be applied, including the E/e′. In patients with valvular MR, IVRT <60 ms and IVRT/Te-e′ <5.2 can be used to predict elevated LAP.

While mitral valve disease may limit application of the above assessments, the increase in LAP can still be seen as a diminished inflow pattern into the LA from the pulmonary veins. There are three distinct phases of pulmonary vein inflow (Fig. 5.5). The first is the S wave, which corresponds to atrial filling during systole. This flow is due to the expansion of the LA, which (similar to LV relaxation in diastole) causes a suction effect of blood from the pulmonary vein to the LA. The D wave is flow during early diastole, when the mitral valve opens and the LV relaxation actually occurs. Flow into the LA continues as blood flows from LA to LV. Lastly, there is an atrial reversal wave (A_R), which is negatively deflected and occurs as a result of atrial contraction during late diastole. This contraction forces a temporary retrograde flow back into the pulmonary veins that is seen as the A_R wave.

In normal LAP, the S wave is bigger than the D wave, owing to the significance of the suction effect due to LA expansion in systole. When LAP is elevated, the S wave is diminished since an elevated LAP reduces the amount of filling from the pulmonary veins. Additionally, just as an elevated LAP causes a tall E wave, the D wave also increases above the amplitude of the S wave. An S/D ratio <1 signifies elevated LAP. Likewise, the A wave in diastolic dysfunction with elevated LAP is diminished, as the pressure generated by LA contraction is insufficient in the face of elevated LV filling pressures. The blood in the LA during LA contraction has to be ejected retrograde to the pulmonary veins. Therefore, in elevated LAP, the A wave diminishes while the

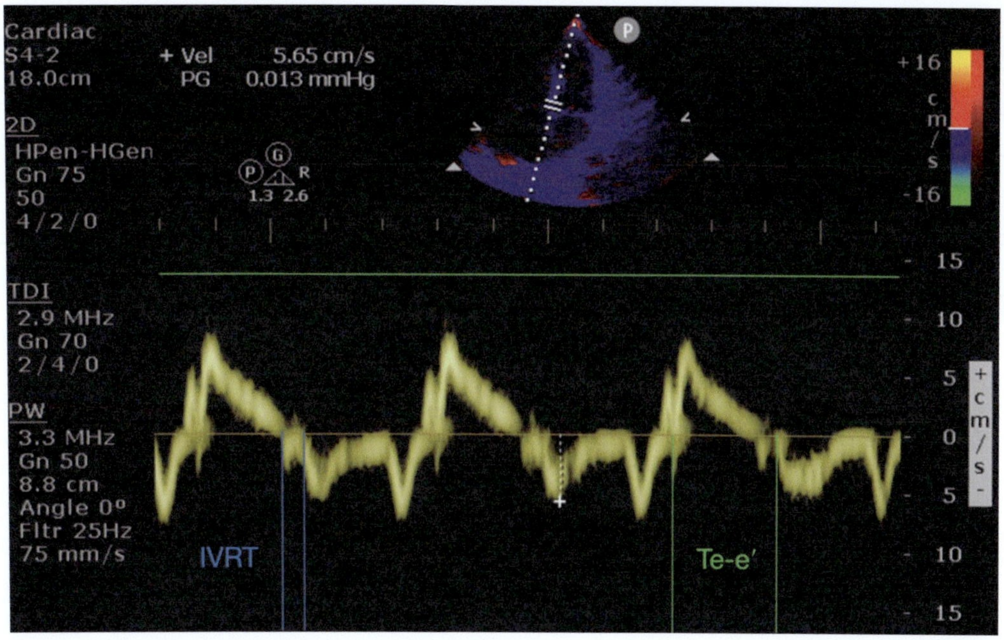

Fig. 5.4 Te-e′ and isovolumetric relaxation time (IVRT) in mitral stenosis

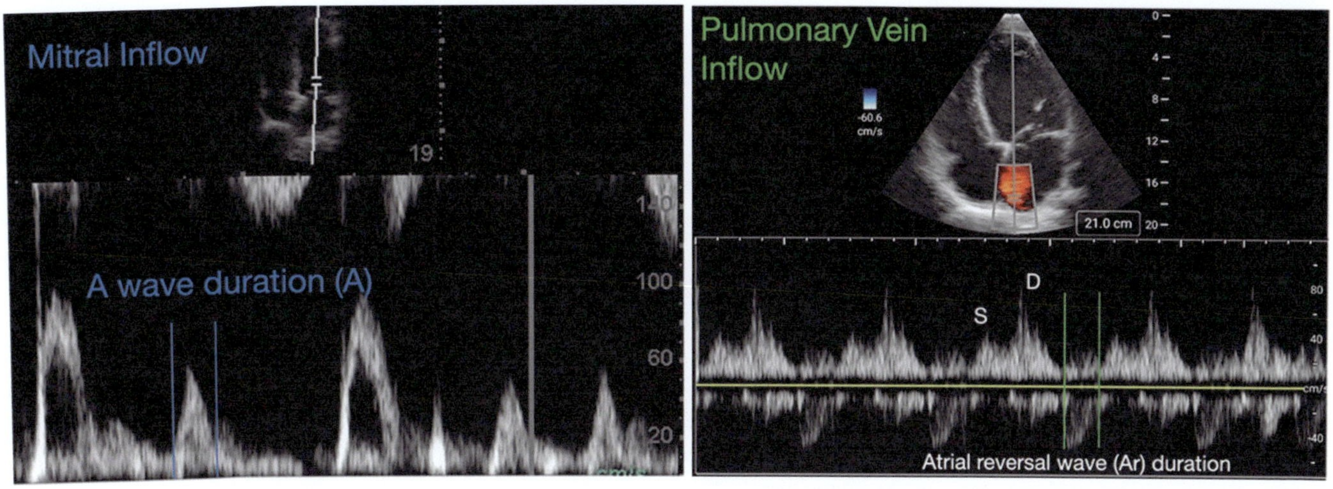

Fig. 5.5 Pulmonary vein flow analysis for assessing diastolic function. The left image demonstrates mitral valve inflow assessment. The right image demonstrates the pulmonary vein inflow patterns, characterized by S, D, and A_R waves. A_R duration and A wave duration (on mitral inflow) can be calculated, and the difference can help to detect elevated LAP. In addition, an S/D amplitude <1 also signifies elevated LAP

A_R wave increases. An A_R-A wave duration of >30 ms signifies elevated LAP [8].

Note that this profile can be assessed and is consistent in more distal structures, such as the hepatic vein and portal vein. The difference is the directionality of flow; for example, the hepatic vein flows posteriorly toward the IVC, so the deflection of the S and D peaks are negative. These distal structures are assessed in the VExUS protocol, which is essentially an extension of diastology to peripheral vessels that are organ-specific. With increasing diastolic dysfunction and congestion, more and more peripheral organs and vessels are affected, from the IVC to the liver (i.e., hepatic vein), gastrointestinal tract (i.e., portal vein), and kidneys (i.e., renal veins). This underscores the importance of central congestion and diastolic assessment in predicting the degree of organ-specific congestion [7]. A summary of the key diastolic measures discussed is presented in Table 5.2.

Table 5.2 Summary of key diastolic findings

Assessing diastolic function in the context of common associated pathologies	Normal	Impaired relaxation	Elevated left atrial pressure/restrictive filling
Heart failure with reduced ejection fraction	E/A < 0.8 and E < 50 (impaired relaxation is the baseline)		E/A > 2 OR E/A 0.8–2 plus ≥2 of the following: 1. E/e′ > 14 2. TR jet >2.8 cm/s 3. LA volume >34 ml/m^2
Preserved systolic function with no prior diagnosis of heart failure	≤2 of the criteria to the right.	>2 of the following criteria: E/e′ > 14 TR jet >2.8 cm/s LA volume > 34 ml/m^2 Septal e′ < 7 cm/s or lateral e′ < 10 cm/s	
Heart failure with preserved ejection fraction	E/A < 0.8 (impaired relaxation is the baseline)		E/A > 0.8 and e′ diminished E/e′ > 14
Atrial fibrillation	E/e′ ≤ 14 (no A or a′ seen in atrial fibrillation)		E/e′ > 11 using septal e′ DT < 170 ms IVRT < 65 ms
Moderate-severe mitral stenosis	None of the criteria to the right. (E/e′ not reliable in moderate-severe stenosis)		A > 1.5 m/s IVRT < 65 ms IVRT/Te-e′ < 4.2
Moderate-severe mitral regurgitation	None of the criteria to the right.		E/e′ > 14 if LVEF reduced IVRT < 60 ms IVRT/Te-e′ < 5.6 Ar-A > 30 ms

Ar atrial reversal wave, *DT* deceleration time, *IVRT* isovolumetric relaxation time, *LA* left atrium, *LVEF* left ventricular ejection fraction, *TR* tricuspid regurgitation

Adapted from Nagueh et al. [8]

Right Ventricular Dysfunction

Background

The right ventricle (RV) can present unique challenges to the sonographer compared to the more well-studied LV. The retrosternal location of the RV can make attaining optimal images more challenging, and its unique shape limits the determination of volumes through mathematical equations as is commonly done with the LV. Additionally, the standard echocardiographic views are oriented relative to the LV, which can make the RV appear abnormal or misshapen in an oblique plane. Nevertheless, the RV has an important role in the hemodynamic assessment of critically ill patients and in patients undergoing evaluation for pulmonary embolism (PE) and pulmonary hypertension.

Indications

Indications
- Chest pain
- Dyspnea
- Hypoxia
- Hypotension

Diagnoses
- Pulmonary embolism
- Pulmonary hypertension
- Right ventricular regional wall motion abnormality in myocardial infarction
- Shock

Core Views

View[a]	Image	Approach
PLAX RV Inflow (RVI)	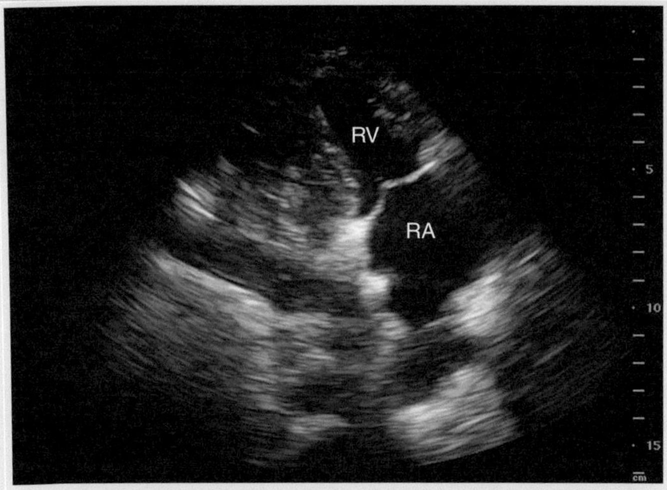 Core View 6. PLAX RVI. RA, right atrium; RV, right ventricle Core View Video 5.1. PLAX RVI	Begin by obtaining the standard PLAX view. Then, fan the probe toward the right iliac crest until the RA and RV are visible.
PLAX RV Outflow (RVOT)	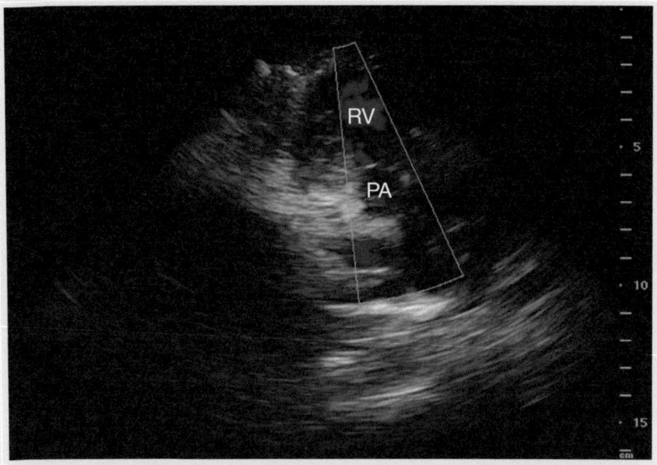 Core View 7. PLAX RVOT. RV, right ventricle; PA, pulmonary artery Core View Video 5.2. PLAX RVOT	Begin by obtaining the standard PLAX view. Then, fan the probe toward the left shoulder until the pulmonic valve and main pulmonary artery (PA) are visible.
RV-Focused A4C	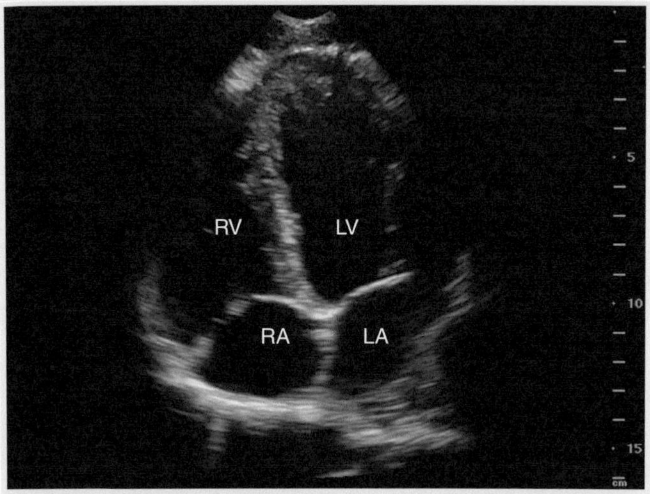 Core View 8. RV-Focused A4C. LA, left atrium; LV, left ventricle; RA, right atrium; RV, right ventricle Core View Video 5.3. RV-Focused A4C	Begin by obtaining the standard A4C view. Then, fan the probe medially toward the right shoulder and gently rotate the probe counterclockwise as needed to obtain the RV at its maximal length (major axis).

View[a]	Image	Approach
RV-Modified A4C	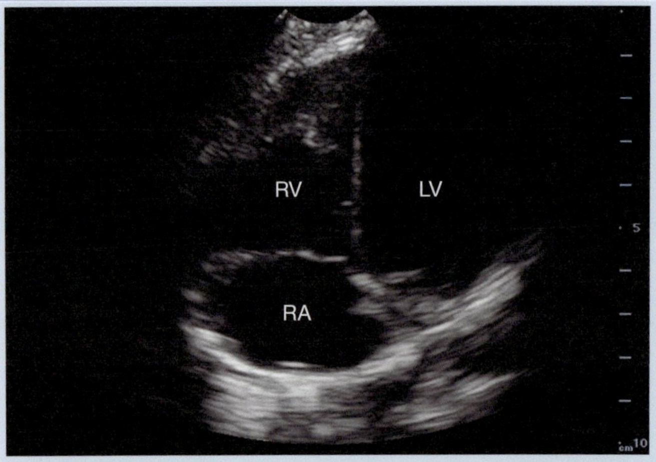 Core View 8. RV Modified A4C. LV, left ventricle; RA, right atrium; RV, right ventricle Core View Video 5.4. RV Modified A4C	Begin by obtaining the standard A4C view. Then, fan the probe laterally toward the left shoulder. It may be necessary to slide the probe medially (toward the sternum) as well. Gently rotate counterclockwise as needed to obtain maximum RV length (major axis). This view focuses more on the apex of the RV.

[a]Note: This section focuses on advanced RV views. Please review Chap. 4 for additional views; *A4C* apical 4-chamber, *PLAX* parasternal long-axis

Clinical Applications

Right Ventricular Size Assessment

Due to the complex shape and orientation of the RV, there is no simple geometric shape that approximates this chamber well. Therefore, making RV volumetric calculations is challenging using echocardiography. The RV is a thin-walled, compliant chamber that is essentially wrapped around the LV in a U-shaped (or crescent-shaped) fashion [26]. The A4C and subxiphoid windows typically give a more consistent appearance to the RV as compared to the parasternal windows. The parasternal long-axis (PLAX) window will often underestimate RV size; however, the parasternal short-axis (PSAX) view at the base of the heart can give a more reliable measurement of the right ventricular outflow tract (RVOT) [26].

A qualitative approach can be used by more experienced users. The qualitative approach compares the maximal diameter of the LV to the RV using the A4C view (Table 5.3, Figs. 5.6, 5.7, 5.8, and 5.9). Quantitative measurements of the RV are taken at end-diastole from multiple imaging windows. The basal annular dimension is obtained from the A4C window and should measure <4.2 cm. The RV free wall thickness is measured using the subxiphoid long-axis view with the zoom feature, and right ventricular hypertrophy is suggested by a thickness >5 mm [27]. The RVOT proximal diameter measurement is performed using a standard PLAX window and should measure <3.3 cm, while the distal RVOT diameter measurement is taken using the PSAX window at the base of the LV and should measure <2.7 cm [27].

Dilation is the normal response of the RV to both volume overload (e.g., atrial septal defect, pulmonic valve regurgitation, tricuspid valve regurgitation) or acute pressure overload (e.g., PE, pulmonary hypertension). It is also the first marker of increased pulmonary vascular resistance

Table 5.3 Qualitative assessment of right ventricular size [27]

RV size classification	RV:LV size ratio
Normal	< 0.67:1
Mild dilation	0.67–1:1
Moderate dilation	1–1.5:1
Severe dilation	> 1.5: 1

LV left ventricle, *RV* right ventricle

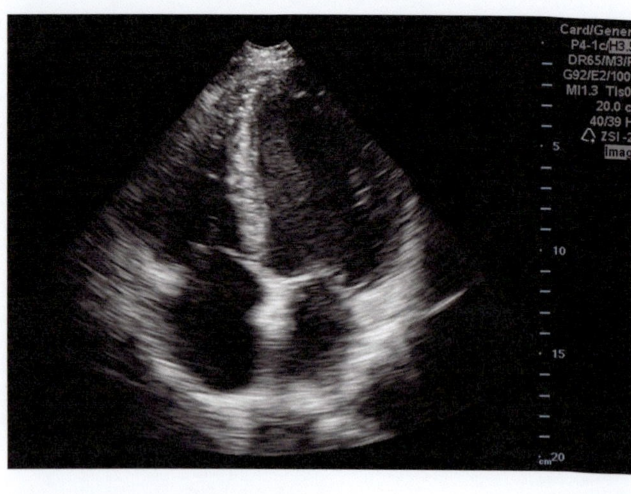

Fig. 5.6 Apical 4-chamber image showing a normal right ventricle size

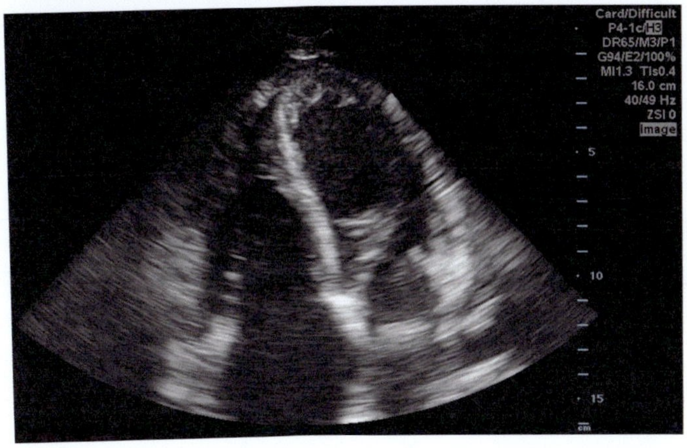

Fig. 5.7 Apical 4-chamber image showing a mildly enlarged right ventricle

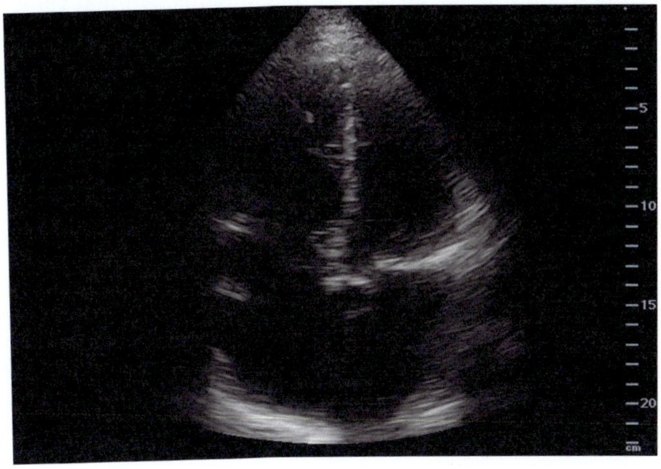

Fig. 5.8 Apical 4-chamber image showing a moderately enlarged right ventricle. (*Image courtesy of Michael Gottlieb, MD*)

[28]. RV hypertrophy is indicative of a sustained increase in pressure over time (e.g., chronic pulmonary hypertension, pulmonic stenosis), though it can also be seen in infiltrative diseases of the heart (e.g., amyloidosis) and hypertrophic cardiomyopathy. Care must be taken when measuring the RV free wall thickness to exclude epicardial fat or RV trabeculations. Measurements >5 mm are considered abnormally high and indicative of chronic RV pressure overload [29].

Septal Dyskinesia

The interventricular septum functions as part of the LV and in the normal heart it bows into the RV in diastole due to the higher pressure of the LV. At the onset of systole, the interventricular septum thickens and the endocardium moves toward the center of the LV such that at the end of systole, the PSAX window shows a circular-shaped LV chamber. When there is RV dilation or hypertrophy, interventricular septal motion is altered. When the RV and LV masses are equal (as occurs in RV dysfunction), septal motion will be "flat." When RV mass exceeds LV mass, the interventricular septum will move paradoxically anterior in systole and reverse in curvature in diastole [30]. Eventually, as RV mass increases, the LV will take on a characteristic D-shape (i.e., "D sign") in the PSAX view in early diastole due to rapid, high-pressure filling of the RV (Fig. 5.10).

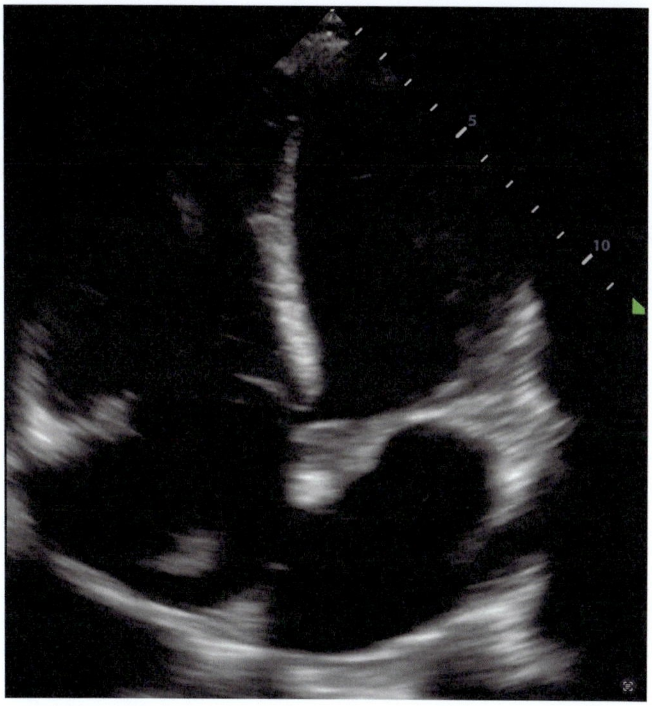

Fig. 5.9 Apical 4-chamber image showing a severely enlarged right ventricle. (*Image courtesy of Nova Panebianco, MD*)

RV pressure overload manifests as a leftward shift of the interventricular septum throughout the entire cardiac cycle, with a maximum reversed curvature at end-systole (Video 5.1). In RV volume overload, the maximum reversed curvature is seen in mid-diastole with normalization of the curvature in systole (Video 5.2) [31]. Importantly, several conditions can mimic septal dyskinesia. These conditions include impaired conduction (particularly left bundle branch block) altering the sequence of RV and LV contraction, valvular disease affecting the timing of RV and LV diastolic filling, and tamponade or constriction. Additionally, oblique views (including a probe placed too far lateral) can lead to a false "D sign."

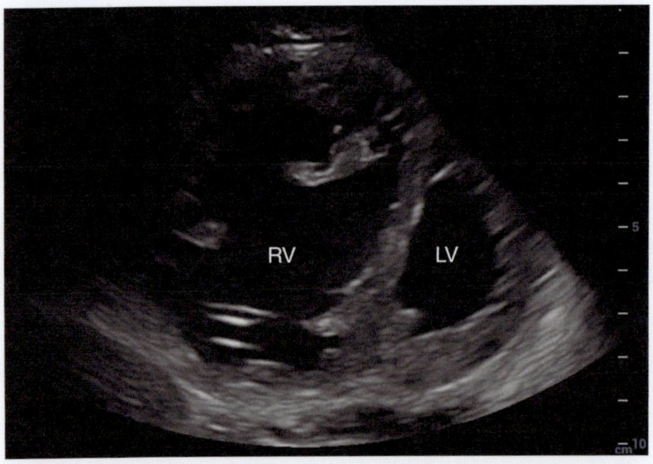

Fig. 5.10 Characteristic "D sign" with right ventricular (RV) dilation leading to flattening of the septal wall, creating a D-shaped left ventricle (LV). (*Image courtesy of Michael Gottlieb, MD*)

Right Ventricular Systolic Function

Given the inherent difficulties in measuring RV volumes, indices of systolic function such as RV ejection fraction have no practical role in echocardiography and should be reserved for three-dimensional echocardiography or cardiac magnetic resonance imaging (MRI). Compared with the LV, the base-to-apex longitudinal shortening of the RV is the primary determinant of RV systolic function. The most widely accepted and commonly employed method to assess RV systolic function is tricuspid annular plane systolic excursion (TAPSE) [32]. TAPSE takes advantage of this important base-to-apex longitudinal contraction and uses motion mode (M-mode) to measure the linear distance that the lateral tricuspid annulus moves toward the RV apex in systole. While TAPSE is primarily measuring the degree of free wall longitudinal contraction, it assumes that this is representative of the systolic function of the entire RV thus rendering it less useful when there are regional wall motion abnormalities such as in acute myocardial infarction. A TAPSE measurement <17 mm is the American Society of Echocardiography-defined threshold for abnormal (Fig. 5.11) [26]. TAPSE has demonstrated a strong association with predicting 30-day mortality in PE, though thresholds have varied across studies (Table 5.4) [33–37]. Care must be taken to align the M-mode cursor to be as close as possible to being parallel with the free wall, and also ensure that the same point on the M-mode tracing is being marked for both systole (the peak) and diastole (the trough).

While TAPSE measures the distance that the tricuspid annulus moves during the cardiac cycle, S′ TDI of the RV measures the tissue velocity of that same movement [29]. Using the spectral Doppler tracing, the echocardiographer measures the highest systolic velocity by placing the TDI sampling gate at the lateral tricuspid annulus. Normal values are 14.1 cm/s (±2.3 cm/s), whereas values below 9.5 cm/s are considered abnormal (Fig. 5.12) [29].

Table 5.4 Thresholds for tricuspid annular plane systolic excursion used in the literature.

First author	Outcome measure	TAPSE lower cutoff (mm)	TAPSE upper cutoff (mm)
Lobo 2014 [33]	All-cause and PE-related 30-day mortality	<16	>18
Schmid 2015 [34]	Intraoperative CPR and death while undergoing emergent embolectomy	<18	–
Paczyńska 2016 [35]	PE-related 30-day mortality	<15	>18
Ciurzyński 2018 [36]	PE-related mortality or need for rescue thrombolysis at 30 days	–	>20
Pruszczyk 2020 [37]	PE-related 30-day mortality	<15	>20

PE Pulmonary Embolism, *CPR* Cardiopulmonary Resuscitation

A third method of RV systolic function assessment is fractional area change (FAC). FAC is calculated using the formula:

$$\text{RVFAC} = \left(\left[\text{RVEDA} - \text{RVESA}\right] / \text{RVEDA}\right) \times 100$$

$$RV\,FAC = right\ ventricular\ fractional\ area\ change$$
$$RVEDA = right\ ventricular\ end\text{-}diastolic\ area$$
$$RVESA = right\ ventricular\ end\text{-}systolic\ area$$

RV FAC <35% correlates with RV ejection fraction by cardiac MRI, and is an independent predictor of heart failure, sudden death, stroke, and mortality after myocardial infarction [29, 38]. FAC is obtained by tracing the RV endocardium in both systole and diastole in an RV-focused A4C view from the tricuspid valve annulus, along the free wall to the apex, then back to the annulus along the interventricular septum. The leaflets of the tricuspid valve, chords of the tricuspid valve, and RV trabeculations are also included in the chamber.

Pulmonary Artery Pressure Measurements

Tricuspid Regurgitation Pressure Gradient

Among the more useful tools of Doppler echocardiography is the estimation of pulmonary artery and other right heart pressures. The key measurement to facilitate the calculation of right-sided pressures is the tricuspid regurgitation pressure gradient (TRPG). Dilation and ballooning of the normally thin and compliant RV free wall leads to pulling of the anterior leaflet of the tricuspid valve outward. The chordae tendineae also get displaced apically which leads to poor coaptation of the tricuspid valve leaflets and resul-

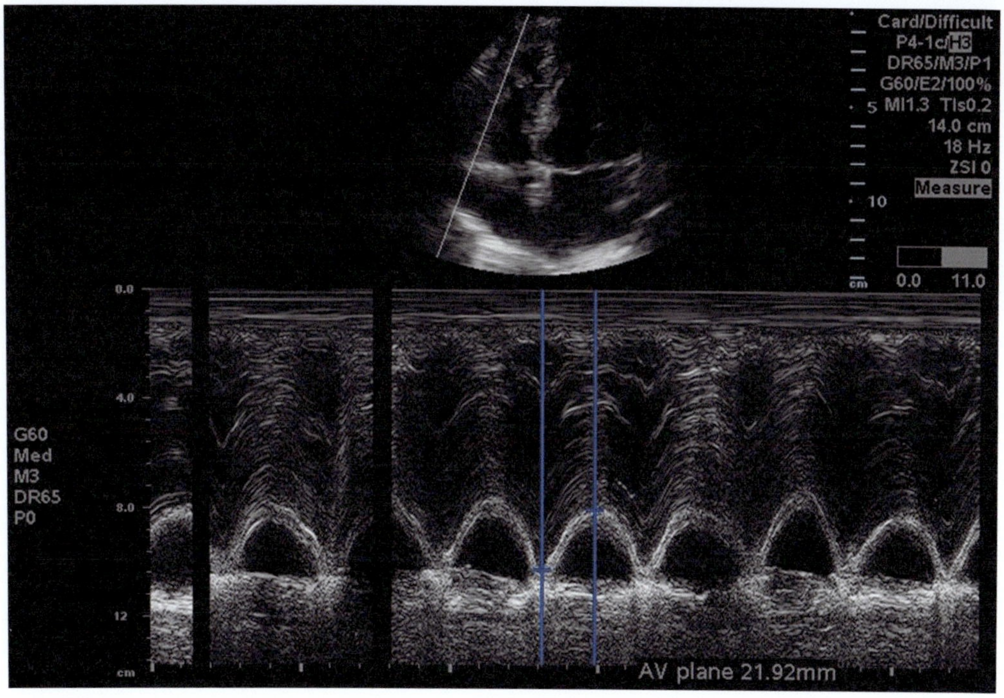

Fig. 5.11 Apical 4-chamber image with M-mode with a normal tricuspid annular plane systolic excursion

tant tricuspid regurgitation. The greater the rise in the RV pressure in response to the various pathophysiologic insults that it faces, the greater the velocity of tricuspid regurgitation (TR).

To estimate the TRPG, begin by applying color Doppler over the tricuspid valve and RA. If there is no regurgitant jet, the gradient cannot be measured. Estimation of the TRPG can be performed from the A4C view, PSAX view at the level of aortic valve, PLAX RV inflow view, and subxiphoid short-axis views at the level of the RVOT. It is best to obtain measurements from as many views as possible and to utilize the measure that gives the highest maximum TR velocity. The highest velocity is used rather than the average of the different peak velocities, as it is easy to underestimate if the Doppler angle is too high (i.e., more perpendicular to the direction of flow). A Doppler angle less than 20 degrees is recommended for TRPG measurement [29].

Utilizing continuous-wave Doppler (CWD), align the gate with the center of the TR jet and place the marker at the peak of the envelope. Include only the dense, well-defined spectral envelope and avoid the grainy, noisy signals at the periphery of the envelope. Normal resting values for TR velocity are <2.9 m/s [29]. From the peak velocity, the simplified Bernoulli equation is used to estimate the TRPG:

$$\mathrm{TRPG} = 4 * \left(\mathrm{TRV}_{\max}\right)^2$$

$$TRPG = tricuspid\ regurgitation\ pressure\ gradient$$

$$TRV_{\max} = maximal\ tricuspid\ regurgitant\ velocity$$

The TRPG is the difference in pressure between the RV and the RA. The RV systolic pressure (RVSP) is calculated by adding the TRPG to the estimated RAP (Fig. 5.13). RAP is estimated by evaluating size and collapsibility of the IVC from the subxiphoid window. An IVC diameter <2.1 cm with >50% decrease in diameter during inspiration corresponds with RAP 0–5 mm Hg. An IVC diameter >2.1 cm with >50% decrease in diameter during inspiration corresponds with RAP 5–10 mm Hg. An IVC diameter >2.1 cm with <50% decrease in diameter during inspiration corresponds with RAP 10–20 mm Hg [29]. Given that these measurements are ranges, it is recommended to use values of 3 mm Hg, 8 mm Hg, and 15 mm Hg in any equations involving RAP. Assuming there is no tricuspid stenosis, RVSP is calculated by the following equation:

$$\mathrm{RVSP} = \mathrm{TRPG} + \mathrm{RAP}$$

$$RVSP = right\ ventricular\ systolic\ pressure$$

$$TRPG = tricuspid\ regurgitant\ pressure\ gradient$$

$$RAP = right\ atrial\ pressure$$

If there is tricuspid stenosis, the pressure gradient across the tricuspid valve is subtracted from the TRPG and this value is added to the RA. Tricuspid stenosis is fortunately rare. The normal TR velocity correlates to RVSP <36 mm Hg [29]. In a dyspneic patient with RVSP >40 mm Hg, the American College of Cardiology and American Heart Association recommend further evaluation because of increased risk of RV dysfunction and mortality [39]. In patients with very severe TR, the Doppler spectral envelope may be cut off because of an early equalization of RV and RA pressures through a wide tricuspid valve orifice. With severe TR, the RV and RA essen-

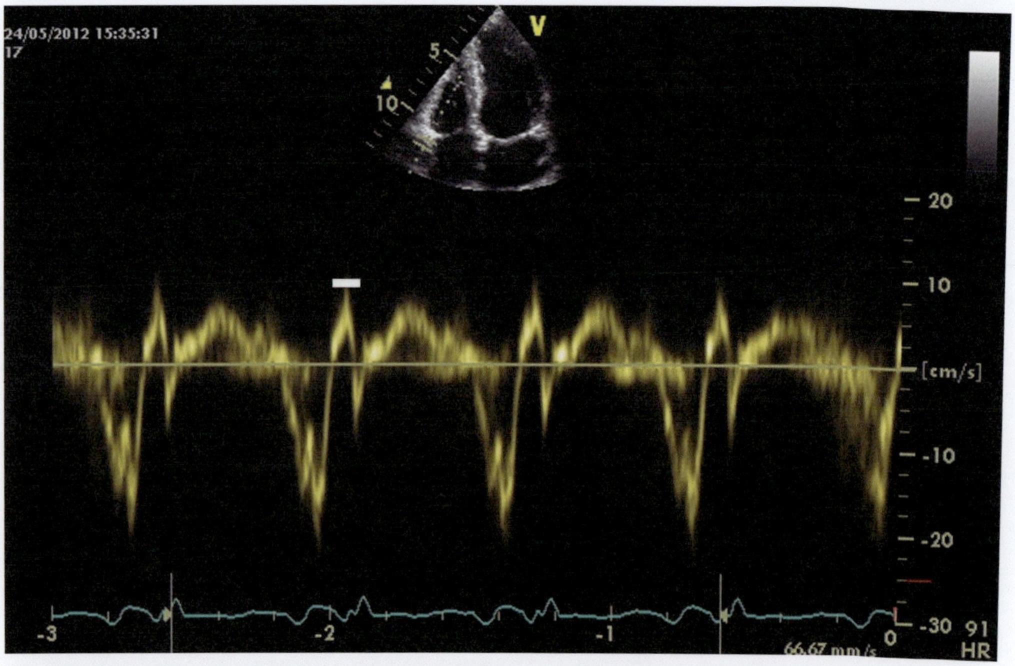

Fig. 5.12 Apical 4-chamber image using tissue Doppler imaging at the tricuspid annulus to calculate right ventricle S′ which is reduced in this patient

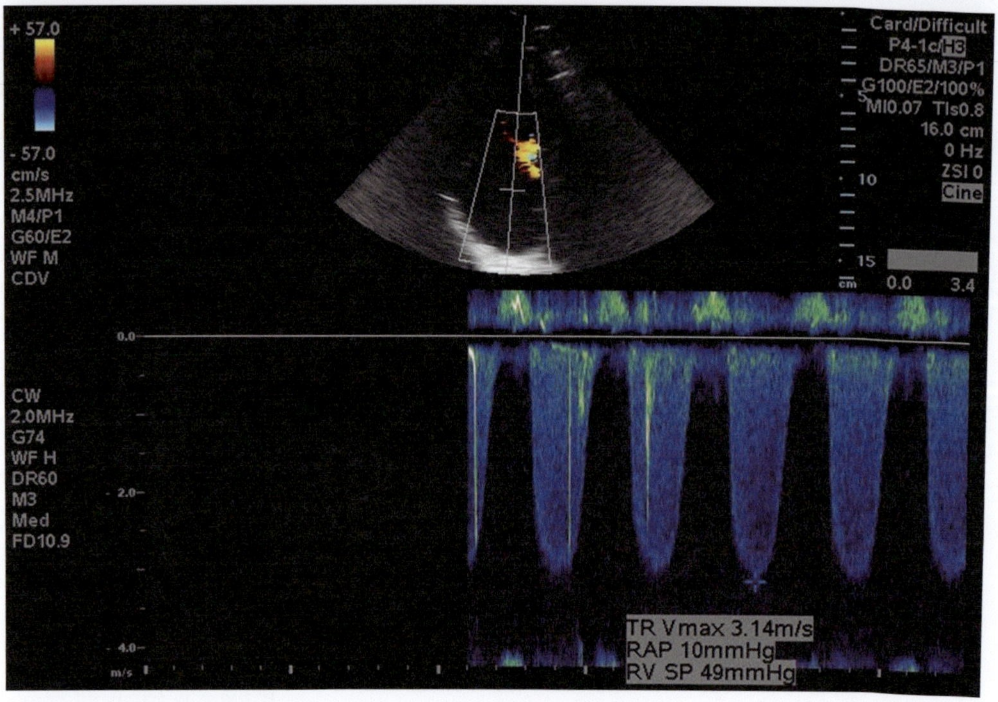

Fig. 5.13 Apical 4-chamber image showing the method used to calculate right ventricular systolic pressure (RVSP) through determination of the tricuspid regurgitation pressure gradient (TRPG). In this patient, the RVSP is estimated to be 49 mm Hg after adding the TRPG, which is calculated by squaring the maximum velocity of the tricuspid regurgitation jet (3.14 m/s in this patient) and multiplying by 4 [TRPG = 4 * $(TRV_{max})^2$]

tially act as a single chamber during systole, resulting in rapid deceleration of the spectral waveform leading to underestimation of TRPG by the modified Bernoulli equation. The RVSP is equal to PASP in the absence of pulmonic stenosis.

When pulmonic stenosis is present:

$$\mathrm{PASP} = \mathrm{RVSP} - \mathrm{PVPG}$$

$$PASP = pulmonary\ artery\ systolic\ pressure$$

$$RVSP = right\ ventricular\ systolic\ pressure$$

$$PVPG = pulmonary\ valve\ pressure\ gradient$$

Pulmonary artery diastolic pressure (PADP) is estimated using the end-diastolic velocity of the pulmonary valve regurgitation gradient with the equation (Fig. 5.14):

$$\mathrm{PADP} = 4 * (\mathrm{PR\,end\text{-}diastolic\ velocity})^2 + \mathrm{RAP}$$

$$PADP = pulmonary\ artery\ diastolic\ pressure$$

$$PR = pulmonary\ regurgitation$$

$$RAP = right\ atrial\ pressure$$

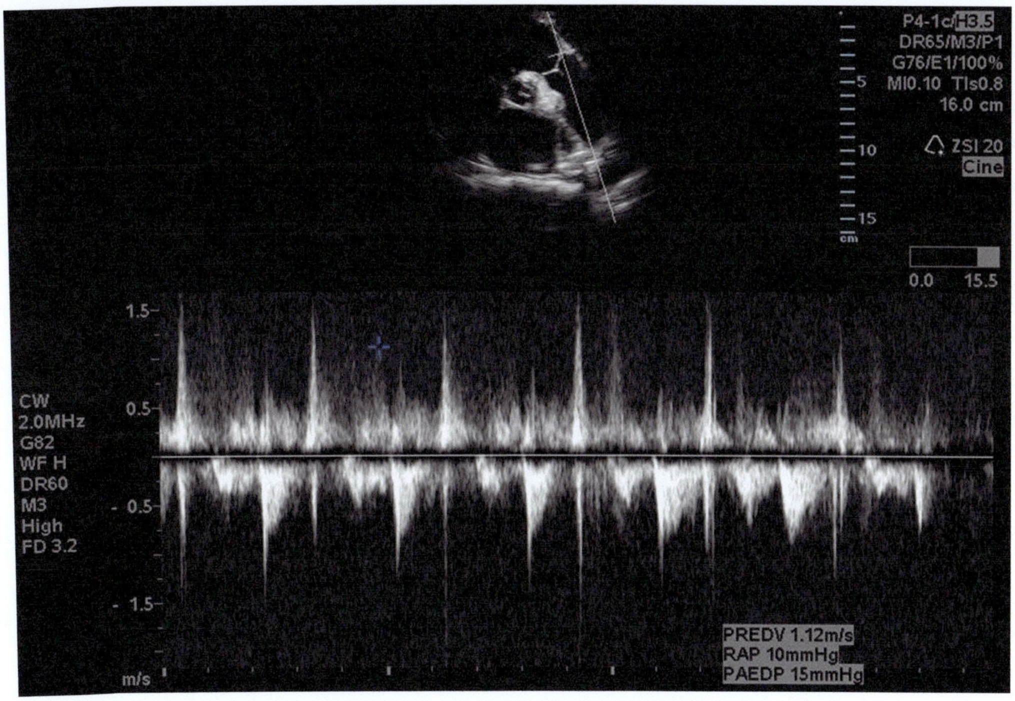

Fig. 5.14 Parasternal short-axis image at the basal level demonstrating the pulmonary regurgitation end-diastolic velocity (PREDV) to calculate the pulmonary artery diastolic pressure (PADP) using the equation: PADP = 4 * $(\text{PREDV})^2$ + RAP

The pulmonary regurgitation gradient is calculated using CWD over the pulmonary valve from either the PSAX view at the level of the AV, the PLAX RV outflow view, or if these two windows prove inadequate it can be obtained from the subxiphoid short-axis window at the RVOT.

Mean pulmonary artery pressure (mPAP) can be determined using a variety of methods. The simplest method is using the equation:

$$\text{mPAP} = \frac{1}{3} * \text{PASP} + \frac{2}{3} * \text{PADP}$$

Alternatively, the Chemla formula can be used. It is derived from the linear regression of the reasonably consistent relationship between PASP and mPAP using the formula [40]:

$$\text{mPAP} = 0.61 * \text{PASP} + 2\,\text{mmHg}$$

It can also be derived using the pulmonary acceleration time (AT) by the equation:

$$\text{mPAP} = 79 - (0.45 * \text{pulmonary AT})$$

Lastly, one can use the velocity time integral (VTI) of the PR jet and add the RAP.

According to the American Society of Echocardiography, the cutoff values of 2.1 cm diameter and 50% collapsibility are used to classify the IVC. IVC assessment tends to be more accurate at the low and the high end of the RAP continuum and less so for mid-range values [41]. It also tends to be less reliable for patients undergoing mechanical ventilation. While 50% collapsibility provides optimal sensitivity and specificity for detecting RAP greater or less than 10 mm Hg, it can lead to underestimation in patients with RAP exceeding 15 mm Hg (Video 5.3) [31].

Pulmonary Artery Systolic Ejection Waveform

The normal PA systolic ejection waveform shows a gradual acceleration to the peak velocity (which occurs in mid-systole), followed by a gradual symmetric deceleration. It is obtained using PWD with the sampling gate placed approximately 0.5 cm proximal to the pulmonary valve leaflets in either the PLAX RV inflow view or the PSAX view at the level of the aortic valve. In a pooled analysis of 1479 healthy patients, mean pulmonary artery acceleration time (PAAT) was 138.7 ± 17.5 ms [42]. A very precise Doppler angle is not required for PAAT because it is a time-based measurement along the x-axis of the spectral tracing. Even if the peak velocity is underestimated because of a large Doppler angle, the time-to-peak velocity will remain the same. Increasing the sweep speed will cause each spectral envelope to broaden out and make it easier for the sonographer to find the precise peak velocity time, particularly with faster heart rates. As RV afterload (pulmonary vascular resistance) increases acutely, the PWD waveform will show a steeper acceleration and an earlier peak velocity (shorter PAAT), as well as a steeper deceleration due to earlier pressure equilibration between the RVOT and PA. PAAT values less than 60–80 ms are strongly suggestive of acute RV dysfunction, whereas values between 80 and 105 ms are more likely associated with chronic RV dysfunction such as pulmonary hypertension (Figs. 5.15 and 5.16) [43]. Guidelines and studies denote a PAAT <105 ms as a cutoff for elevated pulmonary artery pressures [42].

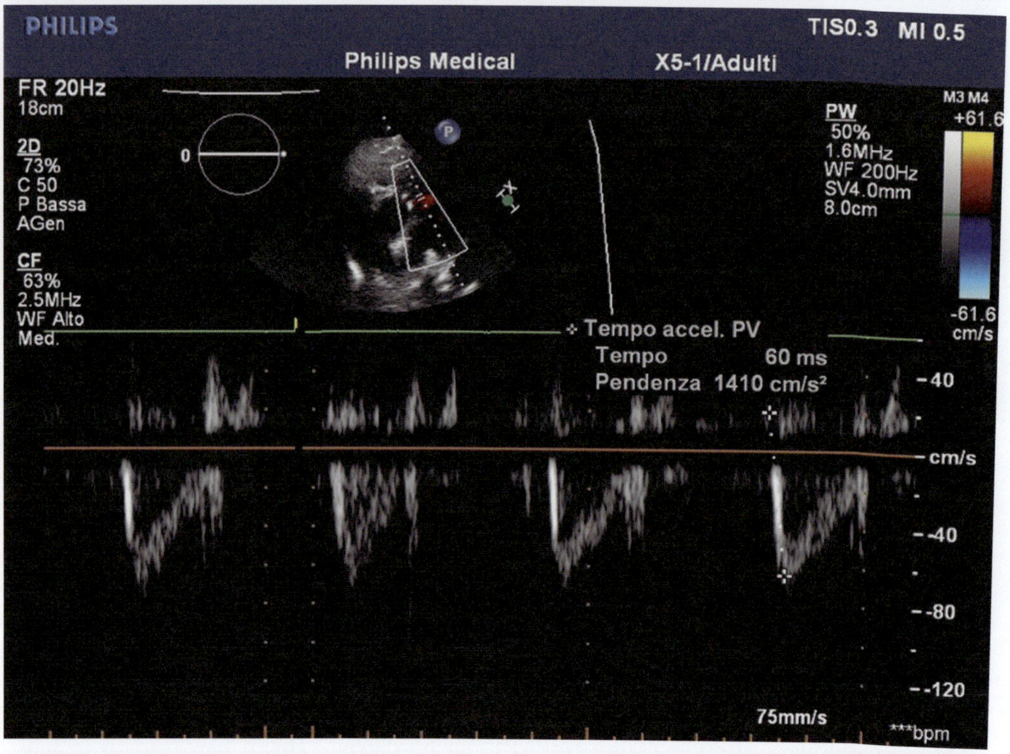

Fig. 5.15 Pulmonary artery acceleration time measured at 60 ms, suggesting an acute rise in pulmonary vascular resistance in a patient with an acute pulmonary embolism

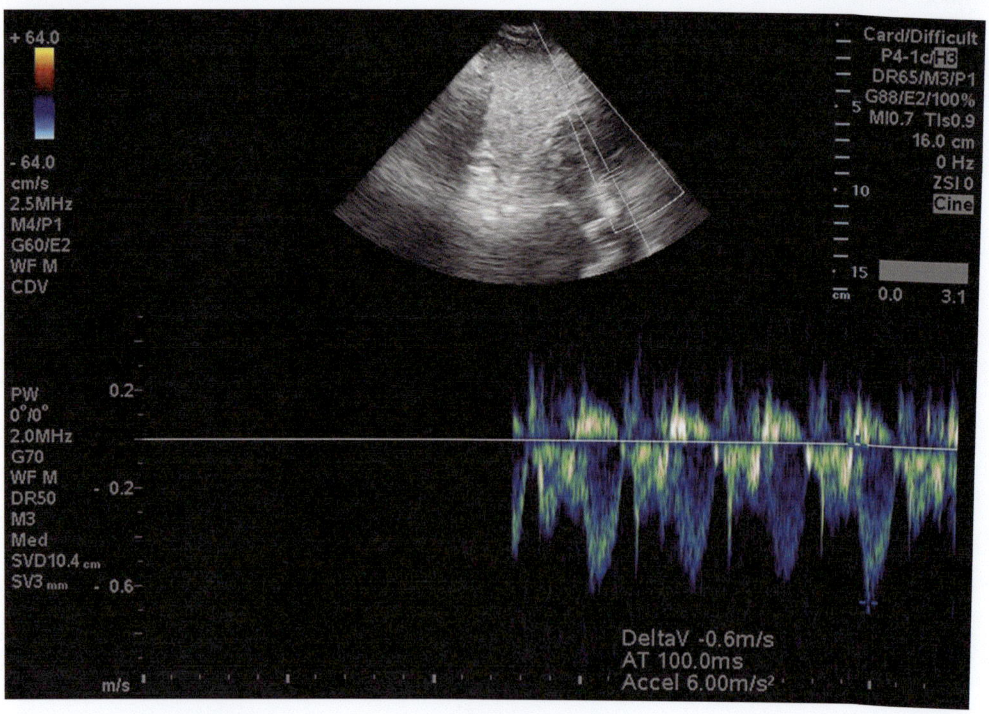

Fig. 5.16 Pulmonary artery acceleration time measured at 100 ms, indicative of chronic pulmonary hypertension

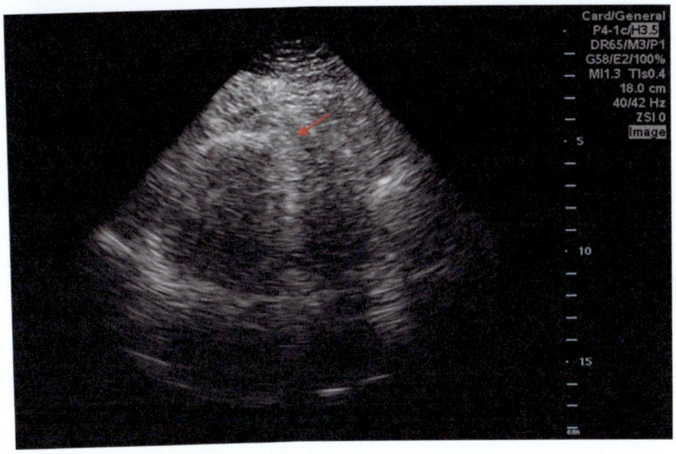

Fig. 5.17 McConnell's sign. The arrow is pointing toward the apex of the right ventricle which has preserved contractility, while the rest of the right ventricle is dilated and hypokinetic

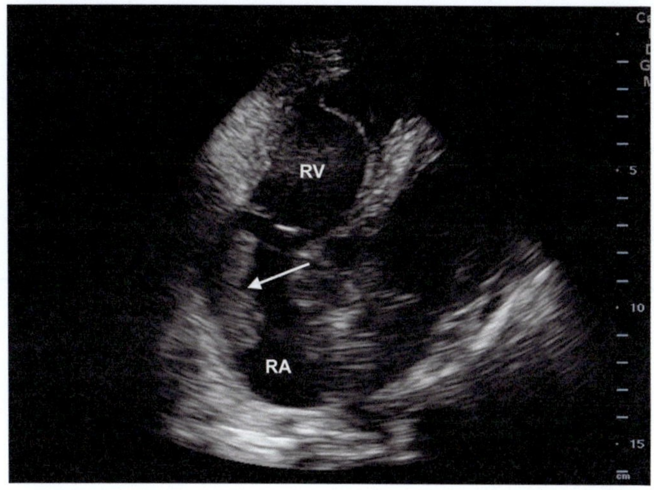

Fig. 5.18 Right heart thrombus (arrow). RA right atrium, RV right ventricle

McConnell's Sign

McConnell's sign is a characteristic pattern of disturbed RV systolic function that was once felt to be highly specific for acute PE. Findings of McConnell's sign include that the mid-portion (and to a lesser extent the basal portion) of the RV free wall becomes hypokinetic, with preservation of normal apical contraction (Fig. 5.17 and Video 5.4) [44, 45]. Several mechanisms have been postulated to explain this regional RV dysfunction pattern. One proposed rationale is the tethering of the RV apex to the LV apex, causing the thin RV apex to get pulled inward by a contracting and often hyperdynamic LV apex. Another potential mechanism is that, as the RV dilates abruptly in PE, it takes on a more spherical shape to distribute wall stress more equally. This leads to a greater outward bulging of the mid-cavity of the RV compared to the apex, which only gives the appearance of RV mid-wall hypokinesis. A third potential explanation is increased wall tension from an acutely increased RV pressure load and subsequent RV chamber dilation increasing the RV free wall's oxygen demand with a simultaneous reduction in right coronary artery perfusion. The apex is spared from dysfunction because it has a dual blood supply from both the right coronary artery and left anterior descending artery [27]. The finding of McConnell's sign maintains relatively high specificity for acute PE (as high as 97%) while it suffers from poor sensitivity (as low as 22%) [46]. Any condition that can lead to RV ischemia can potentially be associated with McConnell's sign [47].

Right Heart Thrombus

Visualizing a right heart thrombus (RHT) is essentially a pathognomonic finding for acute PE [27, 46]. Sensitivity of RHT is poor (<10%), while specificity is quite high (approximately 99%) [46]. Prevalence increases in a sicker patient population, such as in the intensive care unit [48]. Also known as a "clot in transit," an RHT is seen on echocardiography when the clot lingers temporarily or lodges in the RA or RV (Fig. 5.18 and Video 5.5). Although there can be some variability in size and shape of the RHT, the typical appearance is an oblong or worm-like, echogenic, mobile mass in the RA or RV chamber [29]. It may be seen floating back and forth through the tricuspid valve and pulmonary valve. An RHT can be seen in the PLAX RV inflow view, PSAX at the basal level, A4C, or the subxiphoid long-axis view.

It is important to recognize mimics of RHT which include a prominent eustachian valve remnant, a Chiari network, valvular vegetations, and cardiac tumors. A prominent eustachian valve remnant can be seen arising from the cavo-atrial junction (often best seen on the subcostal long-axis IVC window) and will have a thin, hyperechoic, mobile appearance (Video 5.6). Transesophageal echocardiography may be required in some cases to determine the origin of this mass, but most often, it can be easily distinguished from an RHT. A Chiari network is a network of thin fibers connected to the eustachian valve and is the embryological remnant of the right valve of the sinus venosus. It is seen on echocardiography as a series of very thin, highly mobile strands near the opening of the IVC and coronary sinus (Video 5.7). The extremely thin and long appearance makes it quite easy to differentiate it from an RHT.

Valvular vegetations from endocarditis can have a highly variable appearance, ranging in size from barely detectable with conventional imaging to greater than 3 cm in length (Video 5.8). A vegetation will be attached to the low-pressure flow side of the valve and can attach anywhere on that side of the valve, although the coaptation line of the valve is the most common point of attachment. Mobility of the vegetation will be independent of the movement of the valve itself. When there is valvular regurgitation in the setting of a valvular mass, the likelihood of endocarditis is increased. Primary cardiac tumors are fortunately rare but can be seen when using POCUS to evaluate for right ventricular dysfunction. The most likely cardiac tumor that will be encountered is an atrial myxoma, which will arise from the fossa ovalis of the interatrial septum. As it increases in size, the myxoma will become more mobile and may even be seen "plopping" through the tricuspid valve.

Differentiating Between Acute Pulmonary Embolism and Chronic Pulmonary Hypertension

As many of the aforementioned findings can be seen in both acute PE and chronic pulmonary hypertension, it can be challenging to delineate the ultimate etiology. However, there are several echocardiographic findings that can help to distinguish the chronicity of the findings [49]. One useful parameter that is fairly specific to an acute etiology like PE is the 60/60 sign [50]. The 60/60 sign is a combination of two previously described findings, the TRPG and the PAAT. A positive 60/60 sign is when a patient has both a TRPG between 36 and 60 mmHg and PAAT <60 ms. Sensitivity of the 60/60 sign for acute PE is 25%, whereas the specificity for acute PE is much greater at 94% [43].

Another discriminatory finding is pulmonary artery early-systolic notching (ESN). PWD is used to interrogate the RVOT just as one would to calculate PAAT. The ESN pattern can be detected by visual assessment. It appears as a "spike and dome" morphology where the spectral envelope exhibits a narrow peaked initial wave (spike) with early deceleration of the envelope producing a sharp notch within the first half of systole, followed by a second Doppler wave (dome) that is more rounded in appearance. ESN was observed in 92% of patients with massive or submassive PE, 2% of those with subsegmental PE, and in no patients without PE [51]. The mechanism underlying this finding is related to the reflection distance from the RVOT to the reflection site and the markedly elevated pulmonary vascular resistance. The closer the source of the arterial wave reflection to the clot-associated vasoconstriction, the earlier the systolic notching is seen on the spectral tracing (Fig. 5.19) [51].

On the subxiphoid view, a thickened RV free wall (>5mm) (Video 5.9) and an enlarged RA (Video 5.10) (major dimension >5.3 cm or end-systolic area >18 cm^2) would favor a diagnosis of chronic pulmonary hypertension [29]; however, a patient with pulmonary hypertension can develop an acute PE. In assessing chronic pulmonary hypertension versus an acute process in a patient with pulmonary hypertension, additional data such as a positive deep venous thrombosis study, or recent echocardiogram with quantitative data are useful. Table 5.5 provides a summary of key findings for distinguishing acute PE from chronic pulmonary hypertension

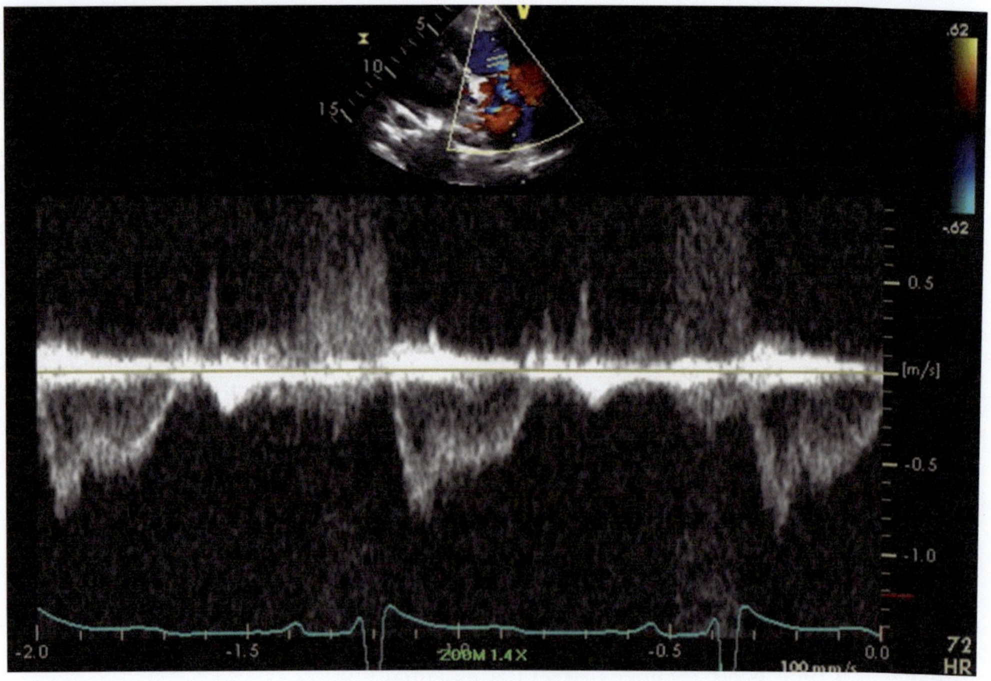

Fig. 5.19 Early systolic notching with a "spike and dome" pattern

Table 5.5 Findings to distinguish acute pulmonary embolism vs. chronic pulmonary hypertension [27, 46, 52, 53]

Finding	Acute PE	Chronic PH	Diagnostic accuracy
RV: LV size: > 1:1.5	X	X	For acute PE: Sensitivity: 55% Specificity: 86%
RA enlargement		X	For chronic RV dysfunction: RA area: 18.0–41.9 cm^2
Septal dyskinesia	X	X	For acute PE: Sensitivity: 26% Specificity: 95%
McConnell's sign	X		For acute PE: Sensitivity: 22% Specificity: 97%
Right heart thrombus	X		For acute PE: Sensitivity: 5% Specificity: 99%
TAPSE <18 mm	X	X	For acute PE: Sensitivity: 64% Specificity: 61%
RV free wall thickness > 5 mm		X	For RV Hypertrophy: Sensitivity: 90–93% Specificity: 94–95%
Reduced RV S′ (<11–12 cm/s)	X	X	For RV ejection fraction <45–50% Sensitivity: 74–90% Specificity: 68–85%
PAAT	<60–80 ms	81–105	For chronic PH: Sensitivity: 84% Specificity: 84%
Early systolic notching	X		For acute PE: Sensitivity: 34% Specificity: 97%
60/60 sign	X		For acute PE: Sensitivity: 24% Specificity: 84%

LV left ventricle, *PAAT* pulmonary artery acceleration time, *PE* pulmonary embolism, *RA* right atrium, *RV* right ventricle, *TAPSE* tricuspid annular plane systolic excursion, *PH* pulmonary hypertension

Valvular Assessment

Background

Valvular heart disease is a common cardiovascular disease that accounts for 10–20% of all cardiac surgical procedures in the United States [54]. In the acute care setting, it is important to quickly identify causes of life-threatening valvulopathy. Cardiac POCUS can rapidly identify the etiology and severity of valvular pathology [55].

Indications

Indications
- Hemodynamic instability
- Dyspnea
- Hypoxia
- Acute onset of heart failure
- Sepsis with suspected endocarditis
- Syncope

Diagnoses
- Tricuspid regurgitation
- Pulmonic regurgitation
- Mitral regurgitation
- Aortic regurgitation
- Aortic stenosis

Clinical Applications

Valvular Regurgitation Assessment

Acute valvular regurgitation will cause a rapid increase in preload without significant remodeling of the heart chambers. In chronic regurgitation, the myocardium has time to compensate due to the slower increases in pressure and volume over time. After long-term volume and pressure overload, overall function will decrease [56, 57].

Brightness mode (B-mode) imaging is the first process in the assessment of valvular pathology. This entails close examination of the leaflets (e.g., prolapse, flail, calcifications, abnormal thickening, or vegetations), as well as their attachments and supporting structures. Evaluating the surrounding chambers for enlargement provides information to assess severity and chronicity [57].

Doppler examination is the next step in assessing the severity of regurgitation [57]. In clinical ultrasound, some of the most utilized methods include: color jet area to estimate severity of regurgitation (TR, MR), color jet width at origin relative to left ventricular outflow tract (LVOT) in AR, vena contracta width (AR, MR), and flow convergence (AR, MR).

Color jet area allows the visual estimation of the jet profile in MR and TR and is a simple way of assessing severity. The regurgitant jet can be central or eccentric (i.e., directed toward the atrium's medial or lateral wall). In the latter case, the jet will demonstrate a smaller jet area than a centrally directed jet of equal or lower severity [58–61]. This hydrodynamic phenomenon, known as the Coanda effect, occurs due to the loss of the jet's kinetic energy as it gets absorbed by the atrial wall. The associated friction, thermal, and viscous losses between moving blood and stationary vessel wall are not accounted for by the simplified Bernoulli equation, leading to underestimation of the Doppler shift [61, 62].

Color jet width in LVOT is a ratio of the width of the AR jet in comparison to the diameter of the LVOT. The best view to obtain this measurement is in the PLAX view, just proximal to the aortic valve [57].

The vena contracta (VC) is the narrowest diameter of the regurgitant jet just past the regurgitant orifice. It directly correlates with the diameter of the effective regurgitant orifice area (EROA) independent of volume flow rate and driving pressure [56, 57]. The orientation of the ultrasound beam should be perpendicular to flow in order to achieve the best spatial resolution and therefore the most accurate measurement. The VC is a small measurement (typically <1 cm); therefore, a small error in measurement will lead to a large error in quantifying the severity of regurgitation. This measurement is valid for central and eccentric regurgitant jets and is a true parameter of the severity of the lesion [57].

Flow convergence is another method used to measure the severity of regurgitation. In AR and MR, the flow of blood is reversed and converges at the site of the closed valve leaflets. The area where blood flow convergence occurs is proximal to the regurgitant orifice and can identify the location and magnitude of the lesion causing the regurgitation [63]. As the flow of blood merges, it accelerates toward the narrow opening resulting in concentric proximal isovelocity surface areas (PISA). PISA is a quantitative echocardiographic method utilizing both color and spectral Doppler to calculate an orifice area and flow volumes through that orifice. As the flow is moving toward the valve, it forms concentric rings of increasing velocities with decreasing surface area and takes the shape of a hemisphere [58]. Table 5.6 provides a summary of echocardiographic parameters in a limited evaluation of valvular regurgitation.

Color flow offers the ability to image the hemisphere that corresponds to the aliasing velocity as one moves out from the regurgitant orifice. The radius (r) of the hemisphere is measured from the point of color Doppler aliasing (Nyquist limit 50–70 cm/s) to the VC. The r is then used to calculate the surface area ($2\pi r^2$). The regurgitant flow rate (R_{FR}) is the product of the surface area and the color Doppler aliasing velocity (V_a) [58].

$$R_{FR} = 2\pi r^2 * V_a$$

The regurgitant orifice area (ROA) is estimated by dividing the R_{FR} by the maximum velocity of the regurgitant jet (V_{RJ}) using PWD or CWD.

$$ROA = R_{FR} / V_{RJ}$$

Table 5.6 Summary of echocardiographic parameters in evaluation of valvular regurgitation

Parameters	
B-Mode	Motion of the leaflets: coaptation, prolapse, flail, restriction
	Annulus dilation
Color Doppler	Origin of the site of regurgitation and the direction
	Components of the jet: Color jet area (MR, TR) Color jet width at origin relative to left ventricular outflow tract (LVOT) in AR Vena contracta (AR, MR) Flow convergence (AR, MR)
	Flow reversal in pulmonary/hepatic veins (MR/TR)
Spectral Doppler	Density of the velocity jet, continuous-wave Doppler
Quantitative	Valvular annular diameter
	PISA optimization for calculating R_{Vol} and EROA

AR aortic regurgitation, *EROA* effective regurgitant orifice area, *LVOT* left ventricular outflow tract, *MR* mitral regurgitation, *PISA* proximal isovelocity surface areas, R_{Vol} regurgitant volume, *TR* tricuspid regurgitation

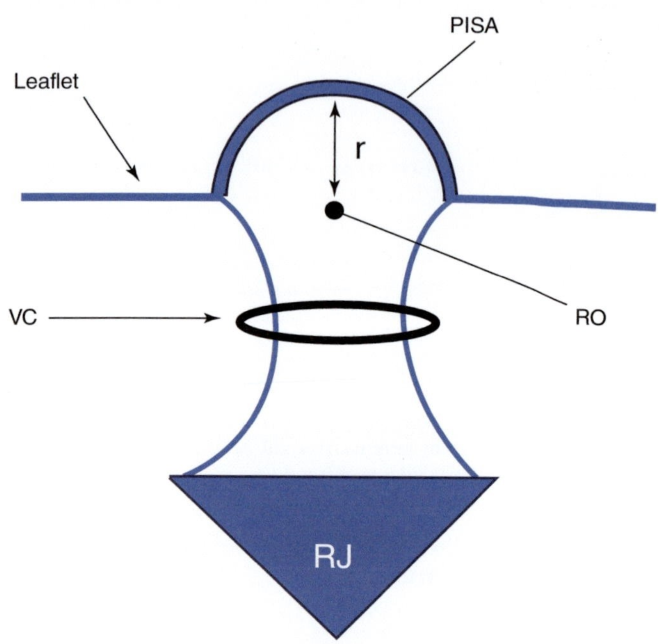

Fig. 5.20 Proximal flow convergence. PISA proximal isovelocity surface area, r radius, RO, regurgitant oriface, VC vena contracta, RJ regurgitant jet. (*Adapted from Otto* [56])

Regurgitant volume (R_{Vol}) is then calculated by multiplying ROA by the velocity time integral (VTI) of the regurgitant jet (Fig. 5.20).

$$R_{Vol} = ROA * VTI$$

Specific Valvular Regurgitation Lesions

Mitral Valve Regurgitation

The etiology of MR is divided into two distinct categories: primary and secondary. An intrinsic abnormality of the leaflets is considered primary. Some examples include myxomatous changes (e.g., mitral valve prolapse), degenerative changes, infectious (e.g., endocarditis), inflammatory, or congenital. MR that results from distortion of the mitral valve apparatus due to LV or LA remodeling is considered secondary. Some examples include remodeling from ischemia, nonischemic cardiomyopathy, or annular dilation (e.g., atrial fibrillation). Patients with acute MR may present clinically with acute pulmonary edema. To thoroughly assess the severity of MR, the color flow jet area should be considered in conjunction with the origin of the jet, the VC, and its flow convergence (Fig. 5.21 and Video 5.11) [56, 57]. Table 5.7 summarizes qualitative measures for MR severity.

Aortic Valve Regurgitation

AR results from disease of either the aortic leaflets or the aortic root that results in an abnormality in the valve coaptation [64]. The disease processes that cause aortic stenosis (e.g., congenital bicuspid valve, calcification, rheumatic disease) can also cause AR because of alterations in leaflet shape causing inadequate diastolic coaptation of the leaflets [56]. Patients with acute AR present clinically in shock with or without pulmonary edema. AR originates from the aortic valve during diastole. Three important components to consider when assessing the origin, direction, and severity of AR include (1) jet width in the LVOT, (2) VC, and (3) flow convergence (Fig. 5.22 and Video 5.12). Table 5.8 summarizes qualitative measures for AR severity.

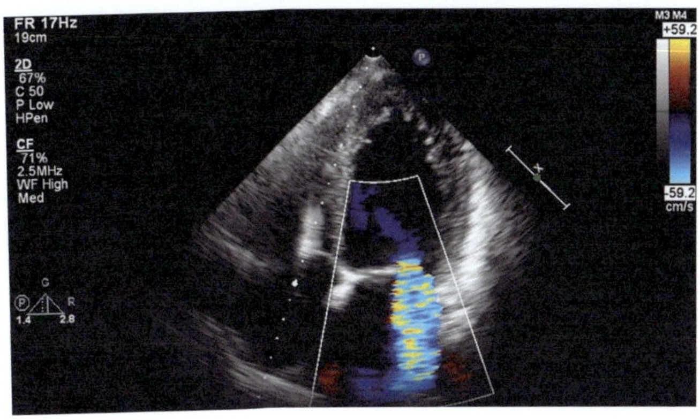

Fig. 5.21 Color jet area allows the visual estimation of the jet profile in mitral regurgitation and is a simple way of assessing severity. This is an example of an eccentric regurgitant jet directed toward the lateral wall of the left atrium

Tricuspid Valve Regurgitation

The etiology of TR is divided into two distinct categories: primary and secondary. An intrinsic abnormality of the leaflets is considered primary and an abnormality that affects the supporting structures (e.g., tricuspid annulus, right ventricle) is considered secondary [56]. There are several ways to assess the severity of TR; however, color jet area is a simple visual estimation of the jet profile in TR (Fig. 5.23 and Video 5.13). Table 5.9 summarizes qualitative measures for TR severity.

Valvular Stenosis Assessment

Valvular stenosis causes remodeling of the chamber proximal to the stenotic valve. This occurs due to an increase in pressure proximal to the lesion, which results in an increase in afterload. The chamber will enlarge or hypertrophy in response to this increase in pressure, which will eventually lead to a decrease in function when it fails [56].

Aortic Stenosis

The most common causes of aortic stenosis (AS) are calcification of the trileaflets, congenital bicuspid valve, or rheumatic valve disease. Using B-mode, a stenotic valve may appear as a hyperechoic, calcified valve with reduced leaflet excursion and a small valve orifice [65].

Doppler measurements can be applied to quantify the severity of AS [65, 66]. The three most important parameters needed to classify aortic valve stenosis include:

1. *Peak Velocity* (V_{max}) is the systolic velocity across the aortic valve. It is performed using CWD because of the high velocities of AS. Align the Doppler gate parallel to the aortic jet for the most accurate measurement (Fig. 5.24) [65].

Table 5.7 Qualitative assessment of mitral regurgitation

Mitral regurgitation	Structural parameters	Color flow jet area	VC width	ROA	R_{Vol} (mL/beat)
Mild	Normal LA/LV Size	<20%	<0.3 cm	<0.20 cm^2	<30 mL
Moderate		20–40%	0.3–0.7 cm	0.20–0.39 cm^2	30–59 mL
Severe	Enlarged LA, Flail Leaflet, Papillary Muscle Rupture	>40% or Eccentric Pulmonary vein flow reversal during systole	>0.7 cm	≥0.4 cm^2	≥60 mL

LA left atrium, *LV* left ventricle, *ROA* regurgitant orifice area, *VC* vena contracta, R_{Vol} regurgitant volume

2. *Mean Pressure Gradient (Δp)* is the gradient between the LV and the aorta during systole. In clinical practice, the gradient is calculated using the simplified Bernoulli equation, using the peak systolic velocity (V_{max}) and applying it to the equation [65].

$$\Delta p = 4 \times V_{max}{}^2$$

3. *Aortic Valve Area (AVA)* is measured using the continuity equation. To calculate the AVA, three measurements are needed: The diameter of the LVOT ($LVOT_{diameter}$), the velocity-time integral (VTI) of the LVOT (VTI_{LVOT}), and the aortic jet VTI (VTI_{Ao}). The LVOT should be measured in the PLAX view in mid-systole, the VTI_{LVOT} is measured with PWD in the apical 5-chamber view with the Doppler gate on ventricular side of the aortic valve, and the VTI_{Ao} is measured with CWD to obtain the highest velocity signal. The $LVOT_{diameter}$ is used to calculate the cross-sectional area (CSA) of the blood flow (cm²) [65].

$$CSA_{LVOT} = \frac{\pi \left(LVOT_{diameter}\right)^2}{2}$$

The CSA_{LVOT} is then used to calculate the AVA.

$$AVA = CSA_{LVOT} \times \left(VTI_{LVOT} / VTI_{Ao}\right)$$

The dimensionless index (DI) is another method to evaluate the severity of AS that reduces the measurement errors caused when calculating the CSA of the LVOT. The DI measures the effective valvular area as a proportion of the cross-sectional area of the LVOT [67]. Table 5.10 summarizes qualitative measures for AS severity.

$$\text{Dimensionless Index} = \left(VTI_{LVOT} / VTI_{Ao}\right)$$

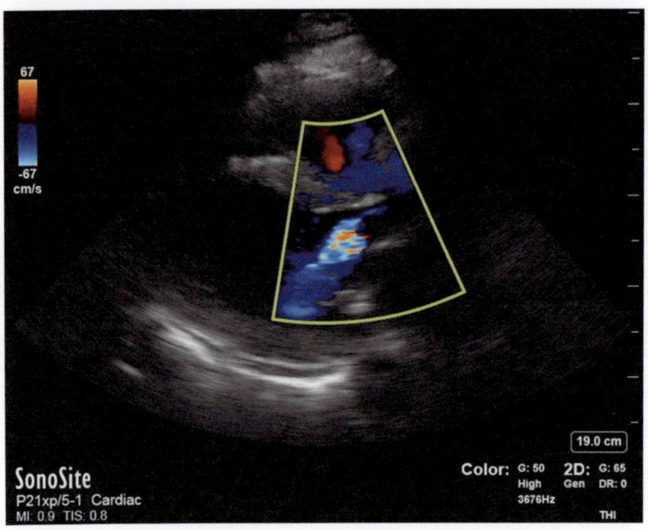

Fig. 5.22 Color jet width in the left ventricular outflow tract (LVOT) is a ratio of the width of the aortic regurgitant jet in comparison to the diameter of the LVOT. The best view to obtain this measurement is in the parasternal long-axis view, just proximal to the aortic valve

Mitral Stenosis

Rheumatic disease remains to be a common cause of MS followed by mitral annular calcification typically as a result of aging. On B-mode, rheumatic valvular disease causes commissural fusion resulting in an immobile posterior mitral valve leaflet and bowing of the anterior mitral valve leaflet in diastole [68]. The bowing of the anterior mitral valve leaflet is colloquially described as having a "hockey stick" appearance (Fig. 5.25 and Video 5.14) [68]. Other common findings in rheumatic valvular disease include thickening of the leaflet tips, as well as scarring and calcification of the chordae tendineae. Mitral annular calcification does not affect the leaflets, and there is no commissural fusion, which is a way to distinguish it from rheumatic valvular disease on B-mode [65].

Doppler measurements can be applied to quantify the severity of MS. The recommended parameters needed to classify the severity of MS include the mean pressure gradient and mitral valve area.

Mean Pressure Gradient (Δp) is the gradient between the LA and the LV during diastole. In clinical practice, the gradient is calculated using the simplified Bernoulli equation, using the peak diastolic velocity (V_{max}) across the mitral valve and applying it to the equation [65].

$$\Delta p = 4 \times V_{max}{}^2$$

Table 5.8 Qualitative assessment of aortic regurgitation

Aortic regurgitation	Structural parameters	Color flow Jet width: LVOT width	VC width	ROA	R_{Vol} (mL/beat)	Aortic color flow reversal
Mild	Normal Leaflets Normal LV size	<25% LVOT	<0.3 cm	<0.10 cm²	<30 mL	
Moderate	Normal or Abnormal Leaflets Normal or Dilated LV	25–65%	0.3–0.6 cm	10–30 cm²	30–60 mL	
Severe	Flail Leaflet or Coaptation Defect Dilated LV	>65% LVOT	> 0.6 cm	≥0.30 cm²	>60 mL	Color flow reversal in the proximal abdominal aorta

LV left ventricle, *LVOT* left ventricular outflow tract, *ROA* regurgitant orifice area, *VC* vena contracta, R_{Vol} regurgitant volume

Mitral Valve Area (MVA) is the most specific measurement in the assessment of mitral stenosis. Two common ways to measure MVA are planimetry and the continuity equation.

The most direct technique is planimetry. Scan through the LV in the PSAX view until the smallest orifice of the leaflet tips is identified in mid-diastole. Trace the orifice and the planimeter result is quantified within the ultrasound system [65].

The continuity equation is similar to AVA, $LVOT_{diameter}$ is used again (applying the law of conservation of mass) because the stroke volume of the mitral valve is equal to the stroke volume through the LVOT [65]. Table 5.11 summarizes qualitative measures for MS severity.

$$LVOT_{area} = \frac{\pi\left(LVOT_{diameter}\right)^2}{2}$$

$$MVA = LVOT_{area} \times \left(VTI_{LVOT} / VTI_{MV}\right)$$

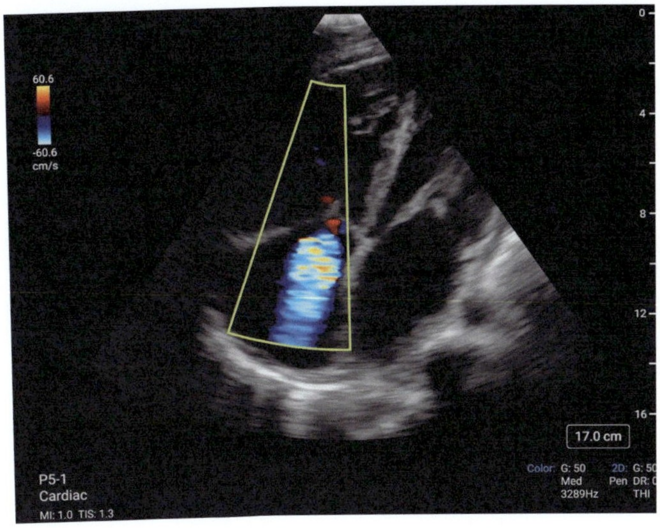

Fig. 5.23 Color jet area allows the visual estimation of the jet profile in tricuspid regurgitation and is a simple way of assessing severity

Endocarditis

Endocarditis on echocardiography appears as an echogenic mass (vegetation) that moves independently of the valve motion (Fig. 5.26 and Video 5.15). The vegetations often form on the leading edge of the valve at the coaptation line on the lower pressure side (Fig. 5.27). In prosthetic valves, they are commonly located at the junction between the sewing ring and the valvular annulus [69]. Vegetations range in size from small (<5 mm) to large (≥10 mm), with evidence suggesting those ≥10 mm on the left side and >20 mm on the right side are at increased risk for embolic events and an increase in mortality risk [70]. In addition to identifying a vegetation, evaluate the leaflet for thickening, abnormal coaptation, chordal rupture, or prolapse. Severe valvular destruction or chordal rupture may result in a flail leaflet (Fig. 5.28 and Video 5.16).

Other complications of infective endocarditis include paravalvular abscess, pericardial effusion, and dehiscence of a prosthetic valve. A paravalvular abscess (most commonly associated with the aortic valve) may be echolucent or echodense and can occur at the valve annulus adjacent to the infected leaflet. Purulent pericarditis can result in a large pericardial effusion due to direct extension from a paravalvular abscess [71–73]. Infective endocarditis causes the affected valve to prolapse and results in valvular regurgitation on Doppler examination [74].

High-risk populations include patients with a prosthetic valve, intracardiac device, congenital disease, previous endocarditis, heart failure, new atrioventricular block, or have community-acquired Staphylococcus bacteremia [56]. Transthoracic echocardiography (TTE) has a relatively low sensitivity of 61% (95% CI, 45–75%) but has a high specificity of 94% (95% CI, 85–98%) [75]. In any population where endocarditis is suspected, a transesophageal echocardiogram (TEE) should be performed, especially in high-risk patients and when the TTE is nondiagnostic [56].

Table 5.9 Qualitative assessment of tricuspid regurgitation

Tricuspid regurgitation	Structural parameters	Color flow jet area	VC width	ROA	R_{Vol} (mL/beat)	Color flow reversal
Mild	Normal Leaflets Normal RV/RA	Thin, Small, Central	<0.3 cm	<0.20 cm^2	<30 mL	
Moderate	–	–	0.3–0.69 cm	0.2–0.4 cm^2	30–44 mL	
Severe	Flail Leaflet or Coaptation Defect End-diastolic diameter ≥ 40 mm Dilated RA/RV, IVC Dilation	>50% of RA	≥0.7 cm	>0.40 cm^2	≥45 mL	Systolic flow reversal into the hepatic veins

IVC inferior vena cava, *RA* right atrium, *RV* right ventricle, *ROA* regurgitant orifice area, *VC* vena contracta, R_{Vol} regurgitant volume

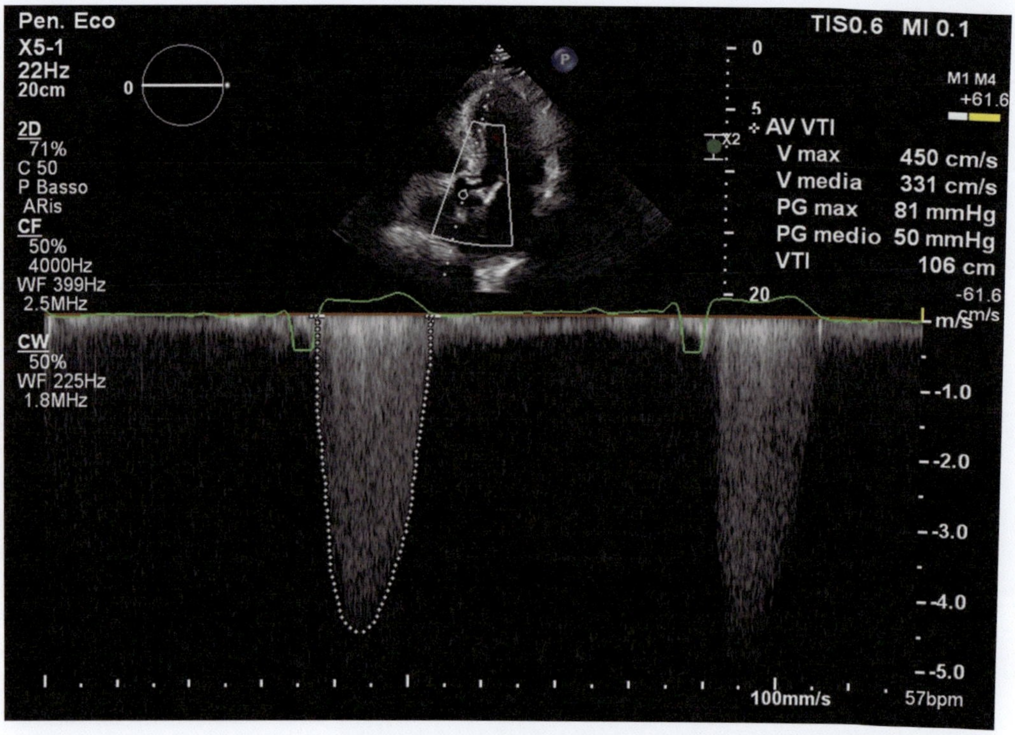

Fig. 5.24 Continuous-wave Doppler through the aortic valve for assessing the severity of aortic stenosis. (*Image courtesy of Luna Gargani, MD*)

Table 5.10 Qualitative assessment of aortic stenosis

Aortic stenosis	AVA (cm^2)	Mean gradient (mmHg)	Peak velocity (m/s)	Dimensionless index
Normal	–	–	<2.5	–
Mild	>1.5	<20	2.6–2.9	>0.50
Moderate	1.0–1.5	20–40	3–4	0.25–0.50
Severe	<1.0	>40	>4	<0.25

AVA aortic valve area

Table 5.11 Qualitative assessment of mitral stenosis

Mitral stenosis	Structural findings	MVA	Mean gradient	Peak velocity
Mild	Mild LA enlargement	>1.5 cm^2	<5 mm Hg	2.6–2.9 m/s
Moderate	Moderate LA enlargement	1.0–1.5 cm^2	5–10 mm Hg	3–4 m/s
Severe	Moderate-Severe LA enlargement	<1.0 cm^2	>10 mm Hg	>4 m/s

LA left atrium, *MVA* mitral valve area

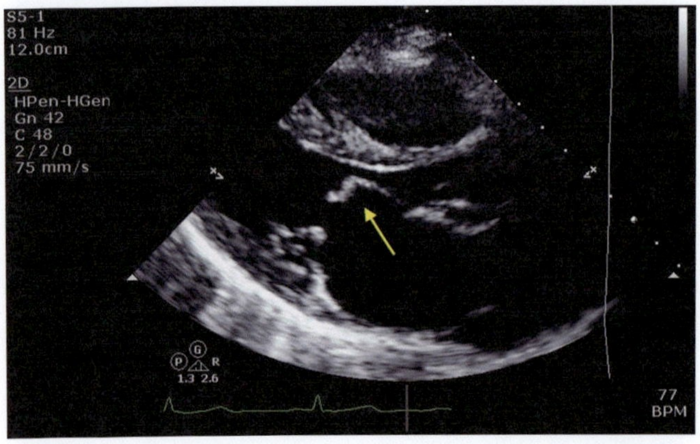

Fig. 5.25 Yellow arrow pointing to the "hockey stick" appearance of the anterior mitral valve leaflet in rheumatic heart disease. (*Image courtesy of Muhamed Saric, MD*)

Prosthetic Valves

The two general types of prosthetic valves are bioprosthetic (tissue) or mechanical. When compared to a native valve, prosthetic valves have different fluid dynamics, flow velocities, and acoustic shadowing from the prosthesis that can make it difficult to interpret [76].

In general, bioprosthetic valve leaflets are made of natural tissue (xenograft or homograft), supported by a stent or a strut, and attached to the annulus via a sewing ring. The sewing ring and framework of the bioprosthetic valve can cause acoustic shadowing or reverberation artifacts which can affect the ability to obtain accurate measurements and evaluate for pathology [76].

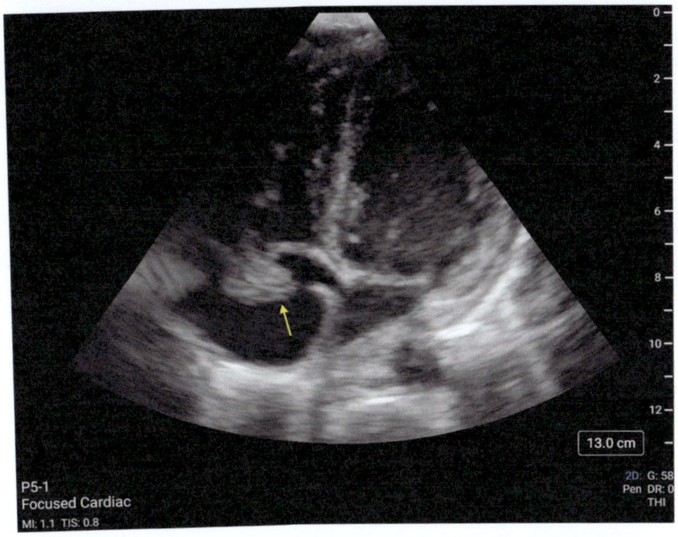

Fig. 5.26 Endocarditis. The yellow arrow points to vegetation on the tricuspid valve

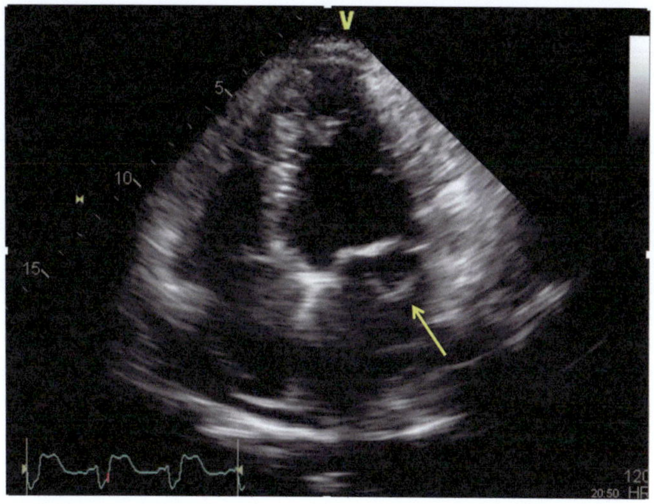

Fig. 5.28 Flail posterior mitral valve leaflet indicated by the yellow arrow in diastole

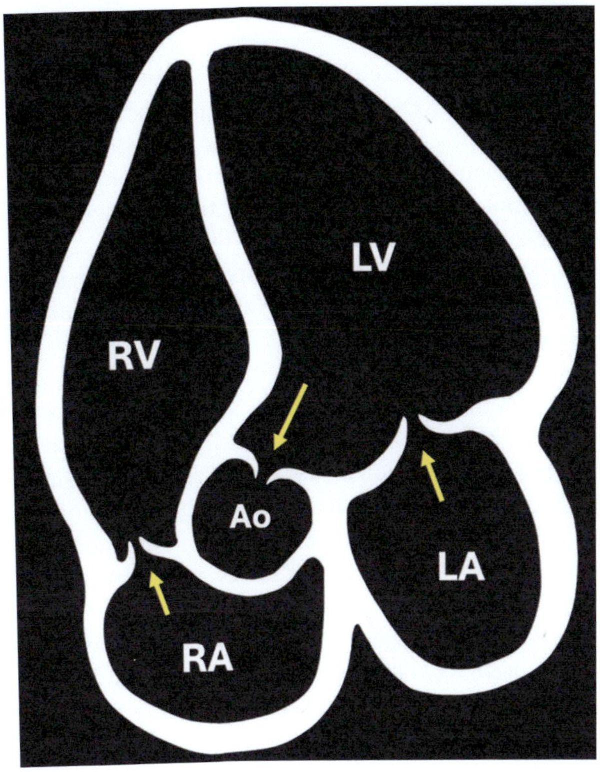

Fig. 5.27 Vegetations attach on the leading edge of the valves. The yellow arrows point to the side of the valves that the echogenic mass would be most likely to adhere to. On the aortic valve (AV), the leaflet will prolapse into the outflow tract during diastole, the mitral valve will prolapse into the LA during systole and the tricuspid valve will prolapse into the RA during systole

Table 5.12 Common types of prosthetic valves

Types of prosthetic valves	Bioprosthetic	Mechanical
Most Common	Stented Xenograft (porcine or bovine)	Bileaflet tilting disc
Less Common	Homografts (cadaver)	Single tilting disc Ball-in-cage[a]

[a]No longer implanted but may be seen in clinical practice

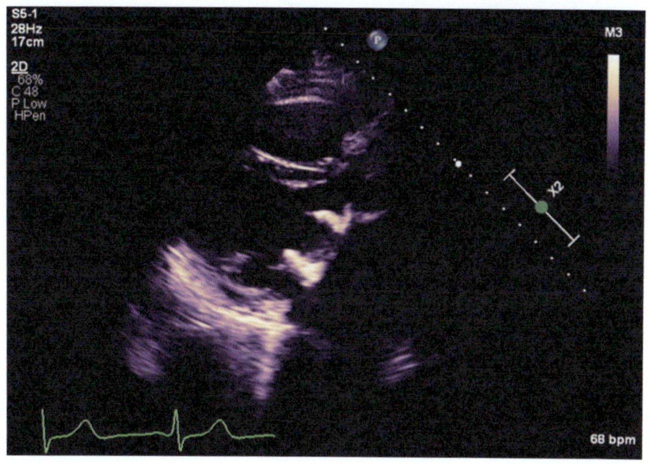

Fig. 5.29 Stented xenograft prosthetic valve. (*Image courtesy of Muhamed Saric, MD*)

There are several types of mechanical valves that have varying patterns of acoustic shadowing (Table 5.12, Figs. 5.29, 5.30, 5.31, and 5.32, Videos 5.17, 5.18, 5.19, and 5.20). These artifacts can help delineate the type but also make it difficult to assess for dysfunction, thrombosis, or endocarditis posteriorly [56]. Advanced imaging such as TEE, cardiac MRI, or cardiac computed tomography are becoming more useful in assessing prosthetic valve dysfunction [76].

Prosthetic valve dysfunction can occur intrinsically from wear and tear, calcification of the leaflets, or struc-

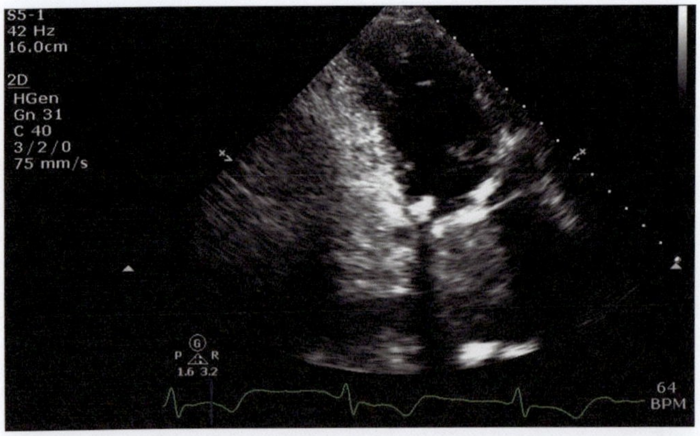

Fig. 5.30 Bileaflet tilting disc prosthetic valve. (*Image courtesy of Muhamed Saric, MD*)

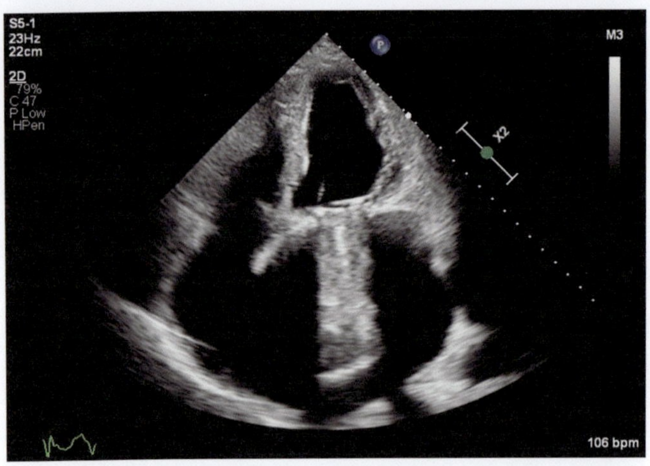

Fig. 5.31 Single tilting disc prosthetic valve. (*Image courtesy of Muhamed Saric, MD*)

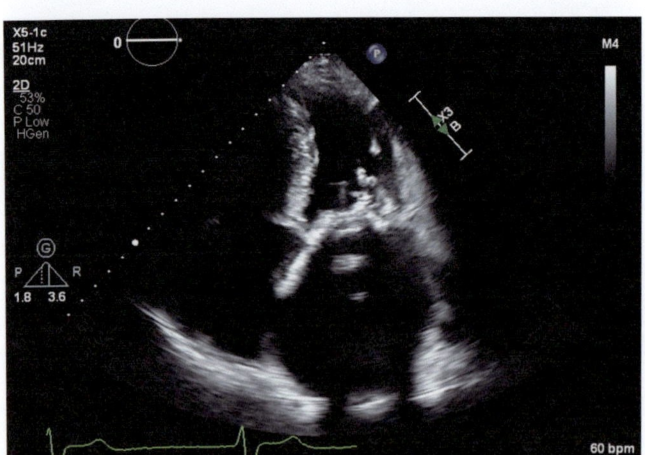

Fig. 5.32 Ball-in-cage prosthetic valve. (*Image courtesy of Muhamed Saric, MD*)

Table 5.13 Qualitative assessment of prosthetic valves

Prosthetic valve doppler parameters	PrAV (DVI)	PrMV (DVI)
Normal	≥0.30	<2.2
Possible Stenosis	0.29–0.25	2.2–2.5
Suggests Significant Stenosis	<0.25	>2.5

DVI Doppler velocity index, *PrAV* prosthetic aortic valve, *PrMV* prosthetic mitral valve

tural damage such as a fracture in the supportive frame. Prosthetic valve dysfunction can also be nonstructural from a size mismatch (prosthesis-patient mismatch), paravalvular leak, or dilation of the surrounding chambers after implantation. Other extrinsic factors of prosthetic valve dysfunction include endocarditis or thrombus formation [77].

When compared to the hemodynamics of native valves, the prosthetic valves have a smaller orifice area and therefore in a normally functioning prosthetic valve, the velocity of blood flow will be higher than that of a normal native valve. The velocity of blood flow through a normal functioning prosthetic valve may be akin to a native valve having mild-to-moderate stenosis [76].

Measuring the effective orifice area can be technically difficult because of the artifact from the prosthesis. Therefore, instead of using Doppler velocities and gradients, the Doppler velocity index (DVI) can be implemented. DVI provides a simple way to evaluate prosthetic valve hemodynamics using a simplified continuity equation. In prosthetic aortic valves (PrAV), the velocity of blood flow proximal to the valve (using PWD) is divided by the velocity distal to the valve (using CWD) [77].

For prosthetic mitral valve (PrMV) evaluation, dividing the VTI of the mitral valve by the VTI of the LVOT is the method of choice to assess severity of PrMV stenosis. The reason this method is used for PrMV is because the transmitral velocities can be elevated in stenosis and regurgitation. If the DVI is elevated, this indicates PrMV dysfunction [77]. The DVI for PrMV is the inverse of the DVI for PrAV.

Prosthetic valve regurgitation is evaluated using the same methods used for native valvular regurgitation. It may be normal to have trivial-to-mild central valvular regurgitation due to leaflet retraction that occurs during implantation [76]. Table 5.13 summarizes qualitative measures for prosthetic valve stenosis severity.

Key Ultrasound Findings

Diagnosis	Key ultrasound findings
RV Enlargement	Normal: < 0.67:1 Mild Dilation: 0.67–1:1 Moderate Dilation: 1–1.5:1 Severe Dilation: > 1.5: 1
Septal Dyskinesia	Paradoxical movement of the interventricular septum, creating a "D sign"
TAPSE	Measurement of tricuspid annular movement during systole Abnormal <17 mm
RV FAC	RV FAC = ([RVEDA − RVESA]/RVEDA) × 100
PASP	PASP = RVSP = TRPG + RAP TRPG = 4 * $(TRV_{max})^2$
PAAT	Measurement from start to peak of pulmonary artery flow Acute RV dysfunction: 60–80 ms Chronic RV dysfunction: 80–105 ms Normal: >105 ms
McConnell's sign	Hypokinetic mid-RV with normal apical contraction
Right heart thrombus	Visualization of an echogenic thrombus within the RA or RV
60/60 sign	60/60 sign is abnormal if TRPG is between 36 and 60 mmHg and PAAT <60 ms
PA ESN	"Spike and dome" morphology of the pulmonary artery
Chronic pulmonary hypertension	Chronic pulmonary hypertension is more likely with a thickened RV free wall >5 mm or an enlarged RA
Color jet area/width	Visual estimation of regurgitation
Vena contracta width	Narrowest diameter of the regurgitant jet just past the regurgitant orifice
Flow convergence	Convergence of blood flow reversal at the side of closed valve leaflets
Endocarditis	An echogenic mass (vegetation) that moves independently of the valve motion Most commonly on the leading edge of the valve

PA ESN pulmonary artery early systolic notching, *PAAT* pulmonary artery acceleration time, *PASP* pulmonary artery systolic pressure, *RA* right atrium, *RAP* right atrial pressure, *RV* right ventricle, *RVEDA* right ventricular end-diastolic area, *RVESA* right ventricular end-systolic area, *RV FAC* right ventricular fractional area change, *RVSP* right ventricular systolic pressure, *TAPSE* tricuspid annular plane systolic excursion, *TRPG* tricuspid regurgitation pressure gradient, TRV_{max} maximal tricuspid regurgitant velocity

Pearls and Pitfalls

- An impaired relaxation profile is seen in patients with chronic heart failure, and not in patients with acute heart failure.
- Elevated LAP is the common pathway leading to pulmonary and systemic congestion.
- E/e′ is a powerful real-time measurement of elevated LAP, and can be used to trend the efficacy of acute heart failure therapies.
- Adjunct measurements of diastolic function should be used if patients have severe mitral stenosis, mitral regurgitation, or atrial fibrillation.
- Owing to the Doppler equation, it is very easy to underestimate TRPG. Carefully choose the best spectral envelope and measure the maximum velocity using the dense portion of the waveform. Evaluate TRPG from multiple windows. The window where the angle of insonation can be kept closest to 0 degrees will give the most accurate data. Use color Doppler findings to guide where to place the spectral Doppler.
- Always consider valvular disease (especially mitral valve) when patients have a very enlarged left atrium combined with findings of chronic pulmonary hypertension.
- All right ventricular size measurements must be interpreted in the context of the left ventricular size measurements.
- Septal dyskinesia can be seen in pericardial disease (tamponade and constriction) as well as restrictive cardiomyopathies.
- Color jet width in LVOT is not a valid tool for evaluating eccentric jets.
- The mitral regurgitation color jet area can be underestimated when LA pressure is elevated, it prevents the regurgitation from displacing into the pulmonary veins.
- Valvular endocarditis can be misinterpreted as or falsely identified as other anomalies such as thrombi, degenerative or myxomatous valve disease, or marantic vegetations.
- There is significant variability in normally functioning prosthetic valves because of the different manufacturer types and sizes. Refer to the manufacturer guide of each prosthetic valve for these parameters.

References

1. Nesto RW, Kowalchuk GJ. The ischemic cascade: temporal sequence of hemodynamic, electrocardiographic and symptomatic expressions of ischemia. Am J Cardiol. 1987;59:C23–30.
2. Gottlieb M, Schraft E, O'Brien J, Patel D, Peksa GD. Prevalence of undiagnosed stage B heart failure among emergency department patients. Am J Emerg Med. 2024;85:153–7.
3. Alerhand S, Adrian RJ, Long B, Avila J. Pericardial tamponade: a comprehensive emergency medicine and echocardiography review. Am J Emerg Med. 2022;58:159–74.
4. Reuss CS, Wilansky SM, Lester SJ, Lusk JL, Grill DE, Oh JK, Tajik AJ. Using mitral "annulus reversus" to diagnose constrictive pericarditis. Eur J Echocardiogr. 2009;10:372–5.
5. Clephas PRD, Radhoe SP, Boersma E, Gregson J, Jhund PS, Abraham WT, McMurray JJV, De Boer RA, Brugts JJ. Efficacy of

pulmonary artery pressure monitoring in patients with chronic heart failure: a meta-analysis of three randomized controlled trials. Eur Heart J. 2023;44:3658–68.
6. D'Amario D, Meerkin D, Restivo A, et al. Safety, usability, and performance of a wireless left atrial pressure monitoring system in patients with heart failure: the VECTOR-HF trial. Eur J Heart Fail. 2023;25:902–11.
7. Beaubien-Souligny W, Rola P, Haycock K, Bouchard J, Lamarche Y, Spiegel R, Denault AY. Quantifying systemic congestion with Point-Of-Care ultrasound: development of the venous excess ultrasound grading system. Ultrasound J. 2020;12:16.
8. Nagueh SF, Smiseth OA, Appleton CP, et al. Recommendations for the evaluation of left ventricular diastolic function by echocardiography: an update from the American Society of Echocardiography and the European Association of Cardiovascular Imaging. Eur Heart J Cardiovasc Imaging. 2016;17:1321–60.
9. Stillman AE, Oudkerk M, Bluemke DA, et al. Imaging the myocardial ischemic cascade. Int J Cardiovasc Imaging. 2018;34:1249–63.
10. Rapezzi C, Aimo A, Barison A, Emdin M, Porcari A, Linhart A, Keren A, Merlo M, Sinagra G. Restrictive cardiomyopathy: definition and diagnosis. Eur Heart J. 2022;43:4679–93.
11. Slivnick J, Lampert BC. Hypertension and heart failure. Heart Fail Clin. 2019;15:531–41.
12. Anwar AM, Geleijnse ML, Soliman OII, Nemes A, ten Cate FJ. Left atrial Frank-Starling law assessed by real-time, three-dimensional echocardiographic left atrial volume changes. Heart. 2007;93:1393–7.
13. Bowcock EM, Mclean A. Bedside assessment of left atrial pressure in critical care: a multifaceted gem. Crit Care. 2022;26:247.
14. Gheorghiade M, Pang PS. Acute heart failure syndromes. J Am Coll Cardiol. 2009;53:557–73.
15. Wierzbowska-Drabik K, Drożdż J, Plewka M, Kurpesa M, Krzemińska-Pakuła M, Kasprzak JD. Assessment of mitral inflow during standardized valsalva maneuver in stratification of diastolic function. Echocardiography. 2007;24:464–71.
16. Nagueh SF. Left ventricular diastolic function. JACC Cardiovasc Imaging. 2020;13:228–44.
17. Jeong E-M, Dudley SC Jr. Diastolic dysfunction:—potential new diagnostics and therapies. Circ J. 2015;79:470–7.
18. Park J-H, Marwick TH. Use and limitations of E/e' to assess left ventricular filling pressure by echocardiography. J Cardiovasc Ultrasound. 2011;19:169.
19. Perl L, Meerkin D, D'amario D, et al. The V-LAP system for remote left atrial pressure monitoring of patients with heart failure. J Card Fail. 2022;28:963–72.
20. Radhoe SP, Brugts JJ. CardioMEMS™: a tool for remote hemodynamic monitoring of chronic heart failure patients. Futur Cardiol. 2022;18:173–83.
21. Öhman J, Harjola V-P, Karjalainen P, Lassus J. Assessment of early treatment response by rapid cardiothoracic ultrasound in acute heart failure: cardiac filling pressures, pulmonary congestion and mortality. Eur Heart J Acute Cardiovasc Care. 2018;7:311–20.
22. Öhman J, Harjola V, Karjalainen P, Lassus J. Focused echocardiography and lung ultrasound protocol for guiding treatment in acute heart failure. ESC Heart Failure. 2018;5:120–8.
23. Akiyama E, Cinotti R, Čerlinskaitė K, et al. Improved cardiac and venous pressures during hospital stay in patients with acute heart failure: an echocardiography and biomarkers study. ESC Heart Failure. 2020;7:996–1006.
24. MacNamara JP, Sarma S. Faltering under pressure: limitations to noninvasive diastolic function assessments. JAHA. 2021;10:e023189.
25. Reddy YNV, Carter RE, Obokata M, Redfield MM, Borlaug BA. A simple, evidence-based approach to help guide diagnosis of heart failure with preserved ejection fraction. Circulation. 2018;138:861–70.
26. Lang RM, Badano LP, Mor-Avi V, et al. Recommendations for cardiac chamber quantification by echocardiography in adults: an update from the American Society of Echocardiography and the European Association of Cardiovascular Imaging. J Am Soc Echocardiogr. 2015;28:1–39.e14.
27. Alerhand S, Sundaram T, Gottlieb M. What are the echocardiographic findings of acute right ventricular strain that suggest pulmonary embolism? Anaesth Crit Care Pain Med. 2021;40:100852.
28. Ventetuolo CE, Klinger JR. Management of acute right ventricular failure in the intensive care unit. Ann Am Thorac Soc. 2014;11:811–22.
29. Rudski LG, Lai WW, Afilalo J, Hua L, Handschumacher MD, Chandrasekaran K, Solomon SD, Louie EK, Schiller NB. Guidelines for the echocardiographic assessment of the right heart in adults: a report from the American Society of Echocardiography endorsed by the European Association of Echocardiography, a registered branch of the European Society of Cardiology, and the Canadian Society of Echocardiography. J Am Soc Echocardiogr. 2010;23:685–713. quiz 786–788
30. Clancy DJ, Mclean A, Slama M, Orde SR. Paradoxical septal motion: a diagnostic approach and clinical relevance. Aust J Ultrasound Med. 2018;21:79–86.
31. La Gereche A, Wright L. Pulmonary hypertension. In: Solomon SD, Wu JC, Gillam LD, editors. Essential echocardiography: a companion to Braunwald's Heart disease. Philadelphia, PA: Elsevier; 2019. p. 376–84.
32. Mitchell C, Rahko PS, Blauwet LA, Canaday B, Finstuen JA, Foster MC, Horton K, Ogunyankin KO, Palma RA, Velazquez EJ. Guidelines for performing a comprehensive transthoracic echocardiographic examination in adults: recommendations from the American Society of Echocardiography. J Am Soc Echocardiogr. 2019;32:1–64.
33. Lobo JL, Holley A, Tapson V, et al. Prognostic significance of tricuspid annular displacement in normotensive patients with acute symptomatic pulmonary embolism. J Thromb Haemost. 2014;12:1020–7.
34. Schmid E, Hilberath JN, Blumenstock G, Shekar PS, Kling S, Shernan SK, Rosenberger P, Nowak-Machen M. Tricuspid annular plane systolic excursion (TAPSE) predicts poor outcome in patients undergoing acute pulmonary embolectomy. Heart Lung Vessel. 2015;7:151–8.
35. Paczyńska M, Sobieraj P, Burzyński Ł, Kostrubiec M, Wiśniewska M, Bienias P, Kurnicka K, Lichodziejewska B, Pruszczyk P, Ciurzyński M. Tricuspid annulus plane systolic excursion (TAPSE) has superior predictive value compared to right ventricular to left ventricular ratio in normotensive patients with acute pulmonary embolism. Arch Med Sci. 2016;12:1008–14.
36. Ciurzyński M, Kurnicka K, Lichodziejewska B, et al. Tricuspid regurgitation peak gradient (TRPG)/tricuspid annulus plane systolic excursion (TAPSE) – a novel parameter for stepwise echocardiographic risk stratification in normotensive patients with acute pulmonary embolism. Circ J. 2018;82:1179–85.
37. Pruszczyk P, Kurnicka K, Ciurzyński M, et al. Defining right ventricular dysfunction by echocardiography in normotensive patients with pulmonary embolism. Pol Arch Intern Med. 2020;130:741–7.
38. Anavekar NS, Skali H, Bourgoun M, et al. Usefulness of right ventricular fractional area change to predict death, heart failure, and stroke following myocardial infarction (from the VALIANT ECHO Study). Am J Cardiol. 2008;101:607–12.
39. Huston JH, Maron BA, French J, Huang S, Thayer T, Farber-Eger EH, Wells QS, Choudhary G, Hemnes AR, Brittain

EL. Association of mild echocardiographic pulmonary hypertension with mortality and right ventricular function. JAMA Cardiol. 2019;4:1112–21.
40. Chemla D, Castelain V, Humbert M, Hébert J-L, Simonneau G, Lecarpentier Y, Hervé P. New formula for predicting mean pulmonary artery pressure using systolic pulmonary artery pressure. Chest. 2004;126:1313–7.
41. Nagueh SF, Bhatt R, Vivo RP, Krim SR, Sarvari SI, Russell K, Edvardsen T, Smiseth OA, Estep JD. Echocardiographic evaluation of hemodynamics in patients with decompensated systolic heart failure. Circ Cardiovasc Imaging. 2011;4:220–7.
42. Marra AM, Benjamin N, Ferrara F, et al. Reference ranges and determinants of right ventricle outflow tract acceleration time in healthy adults by two-dimensional echocardiography. Int J Cardiovasc Imaging. 2017;33:219–26.
43. Kurzyna M, Torbicki A, Pruszczyk P, et al. Disturbed right ventricular ejection pattern as a new Doppler echocardiographic sign of acute pulmonary embolism. Am J Cardiol. 2002;90:507–11.
44. McConnell MV, Solomon SD, Rayan ME, Come PC, Goldhaber SZ, Lee RT. Regional right ventricular dysfunction detected by echocardiography in acute pulmonary embolism. Am J Cardiol. 1996;78:469–73.
45. Platz E, Hassanein AH, Shah A, Goldhaber SZ, Solomon SD. Regional right ventricular strain pattern in patients with acute pulmonary embolism. Echocardiography. 2012;29:464–70.
46. Fields JM, Davis J, Girson L, Au A, Potts J, Morgan CJ, Vetter I, Riesenberg LA. Transthoracic echocardiography for diagnosing pulmonary embolism: a systematic review and meta-analysis. J Am Soc Echocardiogr. 2017;30:714–723.e4.
47. Shah P, Schleifer JW, Mookadam F, Chandrasekaran K. Right ventricular myocardial infarction: an underrecognized aetiology of McConnell's sign. Eur Heart J Cardiovasc Imaging. 2015;16:225.
48. Kurnicka K, Lichodziejewska B, Goliszek S, et al. Echocardiographic pattern of acute pulmonary embolism: analysis of 511 consecutive patients. J Am Soc Echocardiogr. 2016;29:907–13.
49. Alerhand S, Adrian RJ. What echocardiographic findings differentiate acute pulmonary embolism and chronic pulmonary hypertension? Am J Emerg Med. 2023;72:72–84.
50. Shah BR, Velamakanni SM, Patel A, Khadkikar G, Patel TM, Shah SC. Analysis of the 60/60 sign and other right ventricular parameters by 2D transthoracic echocardiography as adjuncts to diagnosis of acute pulmonary embolism. Cureus. 2021;13:e13800.
51. Afonso L, Sood A, Akintoye E, et al. A Doppler echocardiographic pulmonary flow marker of massive or submassive acute pulmonary embolus. J Am Soc Echocardiogr. 2019;32:799–806.
52. Wang Y-C, Huang C-H, Tu Y-K. Pulmonary hypertension and pulmonary artery acceleration time: a systematic review and meta-analysis. J Am Soc Echocardiogr. 2018;31:201–210.e3.
53. Aslaner MA, Karbek Akarca F, Aksu ŞH, et al. Diagnostic accuracy of early systolic notching in pulmonary embolism. J Ultrasound Med. 2022;41:637–44.
54. Maganti K, Rigolin VH, Sarano ME, Bonow RO. Valvular heart disease: diagnosis and management. Mayo Clin Proc. 2010;85:483–500.
55. Maheshwari V, Barr B, Srivastava M. Acute valvular heart disease. Cardiol Clin. 2018;36:115–27.
56. Otto CM. Textbook of clinical echocardiography. 5th ed. Philadelphia, PA: Elsevier; 2013.
57. Zoghbi WA, Enriquez-Sarano M, Foster E, et al. Recommendations for evaluation of the severity of native valvular regurgitation with two-dimensional and Doppler echocardiography. J Am Soc Echocardiogr. 2003;16:777–802.
58. Zoghbi WA, Adams D, Bonow RO, et al. Recommendations for noninvasive evaluation of native valvular regurgitation. J Am Soc Echocardiogr. 2017;30:303–71.
59. Lancellotti P, Moura L, Pierard LA, et al. European Association of Echocardiography recommendations for the assessment of valvular regurgitation. Part 2: mitral and tricuspid regurgitation (native valve disease). Eur J Echocardiogr. 2010;11:307–32.
60. Chao K, Moises VA, Shandas R, Elkadi T, Sahn DJ, Weintraub R. Influence of the Coanda effect on color Doppler jet area and color encoding. In vitro studies using color Doppler flow mapping. Circulation. 1992;85:333–41.
61. Giardini A, Tacy TA. Non-invasive estimation of pressure gradients in regurgitant jets: an overdue consideration. Eur J Echocardiogr. 2008;9:578–84.
62. Akins CW, Travis B, Yoganathan AP. Energy loss for evaluating heart valve performance. J Thorac Cardiovasc Surg. 2008;136:820–33.
63. Bargiggia GS, Tronconi L, Sahn DJ, Recusani F, Raisaro A, De Servi S, Valdes-Cruz LM, Montemartini C. A new method for quantitation of mitral regurgitation based on color flow Doppler imaging of flow convergence proximal to regurgitant orifice. Circulation. 1991;84:1481–9.
64. Bekeredjian R, Grayburn PA. Valvular heart disease: aortic regurgitation. Circulation. 2005;112:125–34.
65. Baumgartner H, Hung J, Bermejo J, et al. Echocardiographic assessment of valve stenosis: EAE/ASE recommendations for clinical practice. Eur J Echocardiogr. 2009;10:1–25.
66. Rana M. Aortic valve stenosis: diagnostic approaches and recommendations of the 2021 ESC/EACTS guidelines for the management of valvular heart disease – a review of the literature. Cardiol Cardiovasc Med. 2022;6:315–24.
67. Altes A, Thellier N, Rusinaru D, et al. Dimensionless index in patients with low-gradient severe aortic stenosis and preserved ejection fraction. Circ Cardiovasc Imaging. 2020;13:e010925.
68. Omran AS, Arifi AA, Mohamed AA. Echocardiography in mitral stenosis. J Saudi Heart Assoc. 2011;23:51–8.
69. Rasalingam R, Makan M, Pérez JE. Washington manual of echocardiography. Philadelphia: Wolters Kluwer Health; 2012.
70. Okonta KE, Adamu YB. What size of vegetation is an indication for surgery in endocarditis? Interact Cardiovasc Thorac Surg. 2012;15:1052–6.
71. Habib G, Hoen B, Tornos P, et al. Guidelines on the prevention, diagnosis, and treatment of infective endocarditis (new version 2009): the Task Force on the Prevention, Diagnosis, and Treatment of Infective Endocarditis of the European Society of Cardiology (ESC). Endorsed by the European Society of Clinical Microbiology and Infectious Diseases (ESCMID) and the International Society of Chemotherapy (ISC) for Infection and Cancer. Eur Heart J. 2009;30:2369–413.
72. Habib G, Badano L, Tribouilloy C, et al. Recommendations for the practice of echocardiography in infective endocarditis. Eur J Echocardiogr. 2010;11:202–19.
73. Mügge A, Daniel WG, Frank G, Lichtlen PR. Echocardiography in infective endocarditis: reassessment of prognostic implications of vegetation size determined by the transthoracic and the transesophageal approach. J Am Coll Cardiol. 1989;14:631–8.
74. Habib G, Lancellotti P, Antunes MJ, et al. 2015 ESC Guidelines for the management of infective endocarditis: the Task Force for the Management of Infective Endocarditis of the European Society of Cardiology (ESC) Endorsed by: European Association for Cardio-Thoracic Surgery (EACTS), the European Association of Nuclear Medicine (EANM). Eur Heart J. 2015;36:3075–128.
75. Bai AD, Steinberg M, Showler A, Burry L, Bhatia RS, Tomlinson GA, Bell CM, Morris AM. Diagnostic accuracy of transthoracic echocardiography for infective endocarditis findings using transesophageal echocardiography as the reference standard: a meta-analysis. J Am Soc Echocardiogr. 2017;30:639–646.e8.
76. Zoghbi WA, Chambers JB, Dumesnil JG, et al. Recommendations for evaluation of prosthetic valves with echocardiography and

doppler ultrasound: a report From the American Society of Echocardiography's Guidelines and Standards Committee and the Task Force on Prosthetic Valves, developed in conjunction with the American College of Cardiology Cardiovascular Imaging Committee, Cardiac Imaging Committee of the American Heart Association, the European Association of Echocardiography, a registered branch of the European Society of Cardiology, the Japanese Society of Echocardiography and the Canadian Society of Echocardiography, endorsed by the American College of Cardiology Foundation, American Heart Association, European Association of Echocardiography, a registered branch of the European Society of Cardiology, the Japanese Society of Echocardiography, and Canadian Society of Echocardiography. J Am Soc Echocardiogr. 2009;22:975–1014; quiz 1082–1084

77. Fernandes V, Olmos L, Nagueh SF, Quiñones MA, Zoghbi WA. Peak early diastolic velocity rather than pressure half-time is the best index of mechanical prosthetic mitral valve function. Am J Cardiol. 2002;89:704–10.

Transesophageal Echocardiography

6

Katharine Burns, Paul Mayo, and Felipe Teran

Background

Transesophageal echocardiography (TEE) was previously only used in cardiac surgery and comprehensive cardiology applications. Over time, TEE has rapidly become a modality of choice in the evaluation of patients with acute hemodynamic decompensation, undifferentiated shock, and cardiac arrest, mainly when transthoracic echocardiography (TTE) is inadequate [1]. In contrast to comprehensive TEE, focused TEE is employed with a goal-directed approach to provide immediate and actionable information at the point of care. As such, focused TEE represents an additional imaging approach to the already well-established scope of point-of-care ultrasound (POCUS). While TTE can be limited by the interference of lung pathology (e.g., chronic obstructive pulmonary disease), excess subcutaneous tissue, or other obstacles to adequate views, TEE can reliably obtain high-quality images of the heart due to its retrocardiac position in the esophagus.

Over the last three decades, multiple studies have demonstrated focused TEE's feasibility and clinical impact to help establish the etiology of cardiac arrest and circulatory failure in emergency, critical care, and operative settings [2–6]. Building on this experience, emergency physician and intensivist-performed TEE programs using focused protocols have been demonstrated to be feasible, safe, and clinically impactful in the management of critically ill patients [7–10].

As an extension of POCUS, TEE can be used to obtain data across several clinical scenarios, syndromes, and specific pathologies affecting critically ill patients. In some cases, focused TEE represents a helpful alternative when TTE images are insufficient or unobtainable. Other scenarios may include patients in cardiac arrest or undergoing cannulation for extracorporeal membrane oxygenation (ECMO).

Supplementary Information The online version contains supplementary material available at https://doi.org/10.1007/978-3-031-85308-1_6.

K. Burns (✉)
Department of Emergency Medicine, Advocate Christ Medical Center, Oak Lawn, IL, USA

Department of Emergency Medicine, University of Illinois-Chicago, Chicago, IL, USA

P. Mayo
Division of Pulmonary, Critical Care, and Sleep Medicine, Northwell Health LIJ/NSUH Medical Center, Manhasset, NY, USA

Donald and Barbara Zucker School of Medicine at Hofstra/Northwell, Hempstead, NY, USA

F. Teran
Laboratory of Translational Resuscitation Science, Department of Emergency Medicine, Weill Cornell Medicine, New York, NY, USA

Indications

Indications
Cardiac arrest
Intra-arrest
Evaluation of potentially reversible pathologies
Optimization of chest compression location and depth
Assist in the characterization of type of myocardial activity and identification of ventricular arrhythmias
After the return of spontaneous circulation
Monitor the response to interventions
Shock
Refractory hypoxemia
Dyspnea
Respiratory failure
Hemodynamic monitoring
Procedural guidance
Trauma
Diagnoses
Cardiac tamponade
Pulmonary embolism
Right heart thrombus and saddle embolism
Hypovolemia
Cardiogenic shock
Left ventricular outflow obstruction
Severe valvular disease causing hemodynamic compromise
Atrial septal defect causing left to right shunt

(continued)

M. Gottlieb, N. Panebianco (eds.), *Advanced Point-of-Care Ultrasound*, https://doi.org/10.1007/978-3-031-85308-1_6

Hemothorax
Pleural effusion
Acute thoracic aortic aneurysms and dissection
Traumatic aortic hematomas and dissection

Probe Mechanics

In place of the hand movements when performing TTE (e.g., fanning, sliding, rotating), the TEE probe uses a combination of mechanical and digital components to achieve the requisite imaging planes and produce the desired images (Fig. 6.1). The endoscopic shaft can be advanced, withdrawn, and turned left or right in the esophagus or stomach. Two wheels on the handle provide mechanical flexion of the probe's tip. The main wheel (usually larger) bends the tip forward (anteflexion) or backward (retroflexion), while a secondary wheel (generally smaller) bends it laterally (right or left flexion).

In addition to mechanical controls and probe movements, digital components allow for rotation of the imaging plane (i.e., the ultrasound beam) with a range of 180°. This is referred to as the omniplane and is displayed by a half-circle

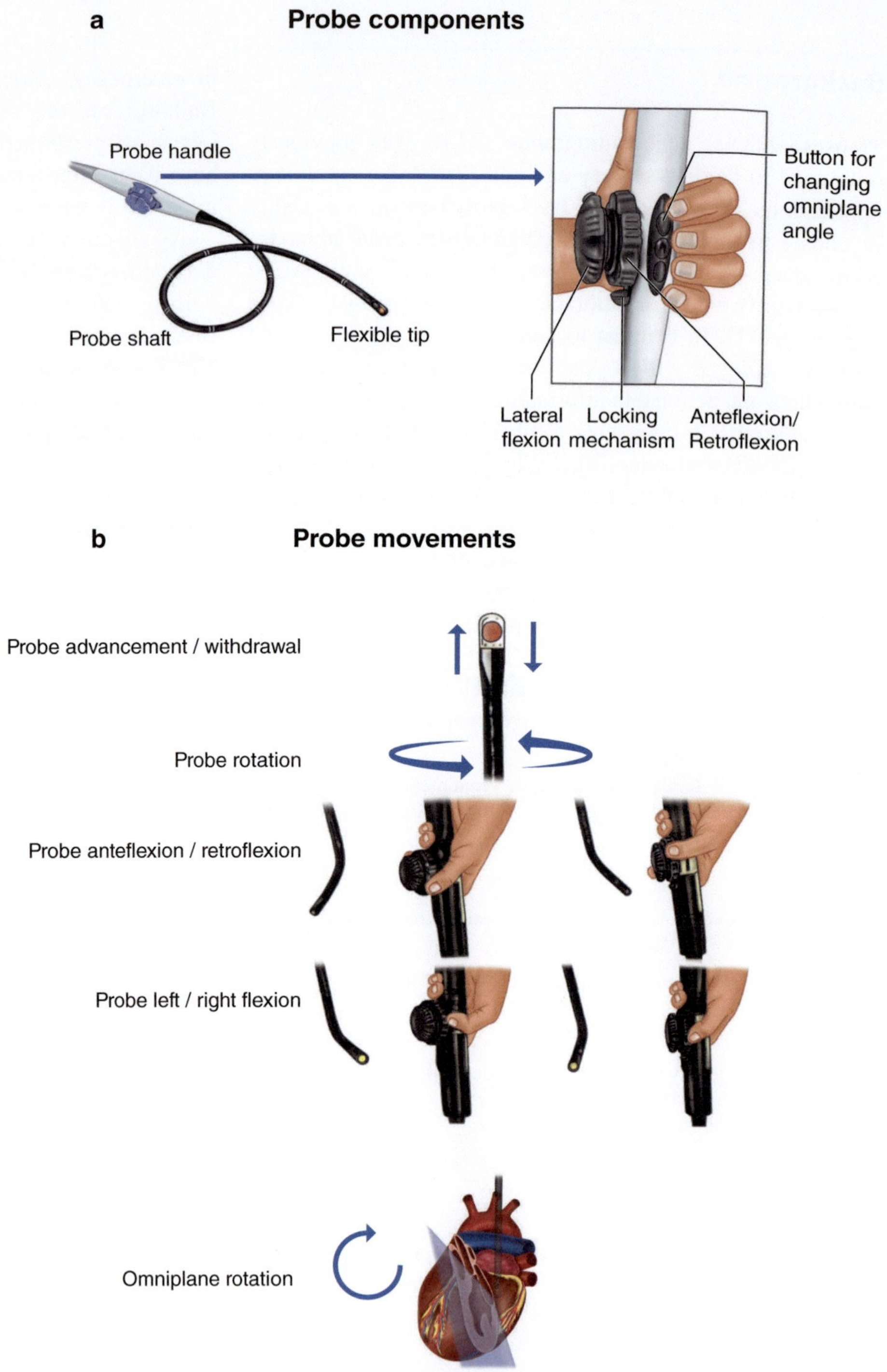

Fig. 6.1 (**a**) Transesophageal probe components. (**b**) Transesophageal probe movements

with a range of 0–180° located at one of the top corners of the screen. The rotation of the omniplane provides a broad range of imaging planes, including transverse, sagittal, and oblique planes of the heart and other cardiopulmonary structures.

Safety of Transesophageal Echocardiography

The safety of TEE in cardiology practice and perioperative settings has been well documented, with several large studies consistently reporting a very low risk of serious mechanical injury to the gastrointestinal tract or procedure-related complications. Rates of iatrogenic perforation of the esophagus when performing TEE are extremely low, ranging from 0.03% to 0.09% of all procedures [11–13]. In a retrospective review of 2508 TEE cases occurring in the intensive care unit (ICU), no procedure-related deaths or serious mechanical injuries were reported [14]. A recent multicenter study of 1045 prospectively enrolled focused TEE studies in the emergency, critical care, and operating room settings reported no esophageal perforations or oropharyngeal injuries [10].

As focused TEE is performed only in patients with a definitive airway, any complications related to aspiration or respiratory depression do not apply to this modality. Additionally, sedative and paralytic medications are often used during focused TEE procedures, which can reduce complications related to patient movement or changes in intrathoracic pressure [15].

There are only a few absolute contraindications to performing focused TEE (Table 6.1) [16]. Relative contraindications include Barrett's esophagus, recent gastrointestinal surgery, mediastinal radiation, esophageal varices, and symptomatic hiatal hernia. However, the emergent nature of focused TEE examinations usually prevents adequate screening for these contraindications. In the case of cardiac arrest, clinicians may have no access to a patient's medical history and will not know if the patient has any adverse conditions. The opportunity to acquire potentially lifesaving clinical information from TEE at the point of care outweighs the potential risk of these rare complications.

Table 6.1 Absolute contraindications to performing focused transesophageal echocardiography

Absolute contraindications
Ongoing esophageal hemorrhage
Esophageal tumor
Esophageal perforation or laceration
Known esophageal stricture or tracheoesophageal fistula

Probe Insertion

Focused TEE examinations are performed only in intubated patients. The placement of the TEE probe is performed similarly to the placement of an oral gastric tube. Before insertion, the flexion wheels must be placed in the unlocked position to allow for unrestricted movement of the probe tip. With the transducer facing anteriorly, the probe is advanced into the mouth and pharynx under direct visualization and manual guidance to maintain midline position. The arytenoid cartilage and piriform fossa are the most common anatomic sites obstructing the TEE probe during insertion. Therefore, to access the esophagus and avoid pharyngeal injuries, it is critical to maintain the midline position while advancing the probe in the hypopharynx. This can be performed by digitally guiding the probe over the base of the tongue or under direct visualization using a video laryngoscope. To aid in the passage of the probe tip past the upper esophageal sphincter, the mandible may be pulled forward gently, and the patient's neck partially flexed. While advancing the probe, it is important to be mindful of the endotracheal tube placement to avoid its dislodgement. If resistance is encountered, gently retract the TEE probe and proceed again, ensuring the tip is not flexed. Using a bite block can prevent damage to the probe from the patient's teeth during ongoing chest compressions or defibrillation. For ease of use, it is recommended to place the bite block onto the probe and secure it high near the handle before probe insertion. Once the probe is inserted into the esophagus, slide the bite block down the probe shaft and affix it inside the patient's mouth.

Focused Transesophageal Echocardiography Views

While a comprehensive TEE examination includes 28 views [17], focused TEE examinations involve fewer views (usually 4–12 views) [10, 18–20], with an emphasis on obtaining essential clinical information in a maximally efficient manner [1]. Consequently, what defines focused TEE is the scope of the examination and the goal-directed nature of the examination rather than a specific number of views. Furthermore, the complexity and sophistication of focused TEE examinations can vary depending on the clinical environment, the diagnostic question or procedure for which TEE is being used, and the background training level of the physician.

Our suggested core imaging planes for a focused TEE examination include the mid-esophageal 4-chamber (ME 4C; Video 6.1), mid-esophageal long-axis (ME LAX; Video 6.2), trans-gastric short-axis (TG SAX; Video 6.3), mid-esophageal bicaval (ME bicaval; Video 6.4), mid-esophageal descending thoracic aorta short-axis (ME DTA SAX; Video 6.5), and mid-esophageal descending thoracic aorta long-axis (ME DTA LAX; Video 6.6) views. These views allow the evaluation of right and left heart function, volume status, presence of a pericardial effusion, thoracic aorta dissection, aneurysm, or rupture, and guidance for endovascular procedures such as transvenous pacemaker placement and ECMO. The ME 4C, ME LAX, and TG SAX are analogous to basic views in TTE (Table 6.2), whereas the additional views of ME DTA SAX, ME DTA LAX, and ME bicaval are unique to TEE. These core views provide the necessary diagnostic and procedural information to guide management in most emergent clinical scenarios (Table 6.3).

Supplementary Views

In certain clinical scenarios, such as when specific pathology is suspected (e.g., pulmonary embolism, dissection of the ascending thoracic aorta, regional wall motion abnormality), additional information may be obtained in a similar goal-directed manner by expanding beyond the core views described above. Some of these include the mid-esophageal 2-chamber (ME 2C; Video 6.7), mid-esophageal aortic valve short-axis (ME AV SAX; Video 6.8), mid-esophageal ascending aorta in short-axis (ME Asc Aorta SAX; Video 6.9) and long-axis (ME Asc Aorta LAX; Video 6.10), mid-esophageal right ventricular inflow–outflow (ME RV I-O; Video 6.11), and deep trans-gastric 5-chamber (Deep TG 5C; Video 6.12) views (Table 6.4).

Generally used on a case-by-case basis, these views can provide additional diagnostic and therapeutic information on the same core elements of the abovementioned resuscitative examination. However, they can also provide supplemental information about the presence of proximal aortic pathology, fluid tolerance, stroke volume estimation, heart–lung interactions, enhanced right ventricular assessment, and a cardiac source of embolism. Additionally, they can assist with select procedural guidance and device evaluation (e.g., intravenous pacemaker, veno-arterial and veno-venous ECMO, ventricular assist devices, intra-aortic balloon pump).

Transesophageal Lung Ultrasound

The TEE probe can also examine the lung and pleural space. Examination of the thoracic space with transesophageal lung ultrasound (TELUS) is particularly valuable in the supine critically ill patient where the posterolateral thorax is challenging to examine with transthoracic lung ultrasound due to patient-related factors that degrade the image or life support devices restricting access to the chest [21].

Once the operator has obtained the necessary cardiac views, TELUS is performed in conjunction with an examination of the descending aorta. The probe is withdrawn from the transgastric position back to the mid-esophageal position and turned counterclockwise toward the patient's left to obtain the posterior cross-sectional view of the descending aorta. Immediately adjacent to the aorta is the left posterior thoracic space. This allows for visualization of the left lower lobe of the lung and characterization of its aeration pattern, which will be familiar to the clinician with knowledge of transthoracic lung ultrasonography (e.g., A lines, B lines, consolidations). Pleural fluid is also readily identified and characterized with TELUS. The omniplane is increased to 90°, and the operator rotates the probe clockwise, sweeping through the pleural space in the tomographic plane and obtaining a longitudinal view of the left thoracic space. The diaphragm and underlying spleen are best identified in the longitudinal scanning plane, which can help to identify a pleural effusion overlying the diaphragm or ascites within the abdominal cavity.

In contrast to the left side, where the thoracic aorta serves as a guiding landmark, the right hemithorax is more difficult to scan with TELUS due to the lack of an identifying landmark structure. To scan the right hemithorax, we recommend advancing the probe into the transgastric position and then rotating right to locate the liver and, within it, the inferior vena cava. The omniplane is then increased to 90°. Withdrawal of the probe allows identification of the diaphragm and the lung and pleural space above it. Figures 6.2, 6.3, 6.4, and 6.5 and Videos 6.13, 6.14,6.15, 6.16,6.17 and 6.18 depict pathology seen on TELUS exam.

Table 6.2 Comparison of analogous views between transesophageal and transthoracic echocardiography

Transesophageal Echo (TEE)	Transthoracic Echo (TEE)
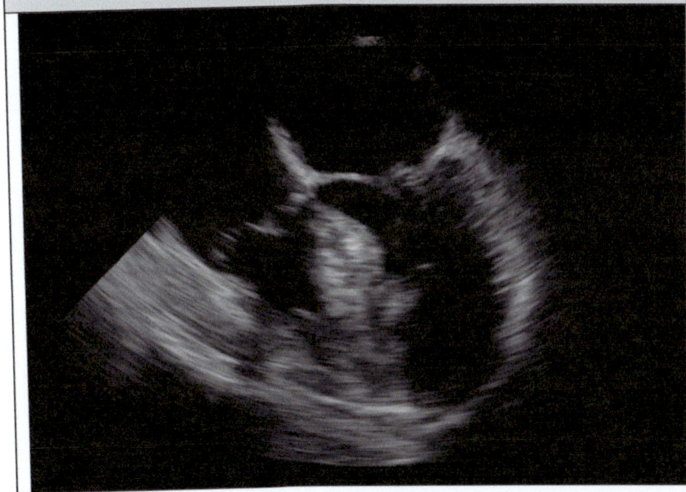	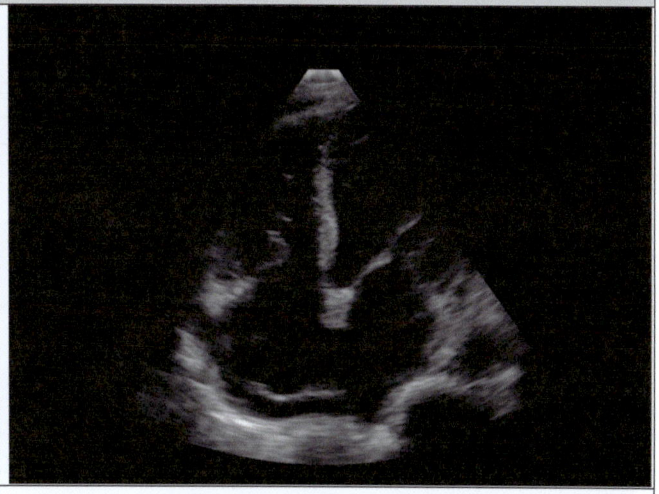
Mid-esophageal 4 Chamber (ME 4C)	Apical 4-Chamber (A4CH)
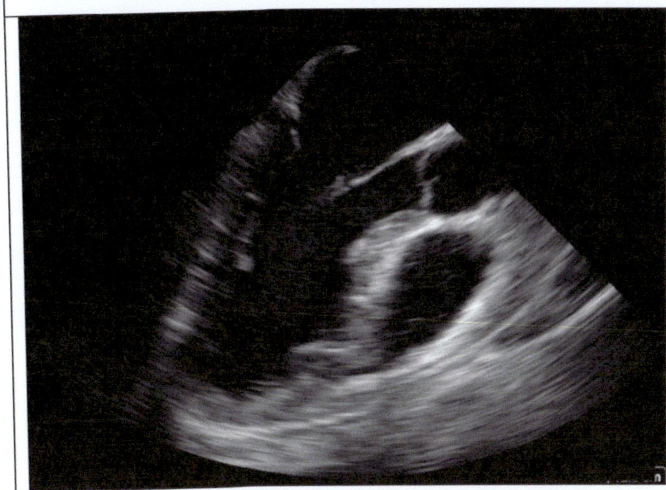	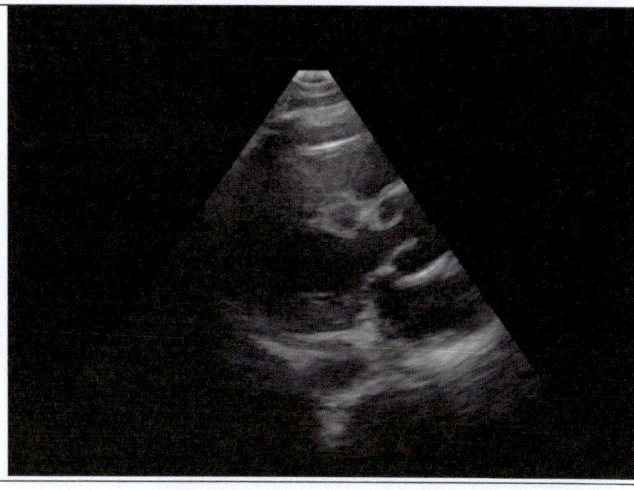
Mid-esophageal Long-Axis (ME LAX)	Parasternal Long-Axis (PLAX)
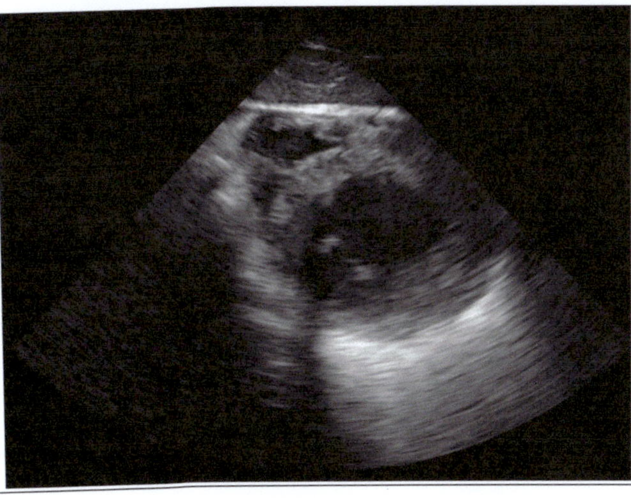	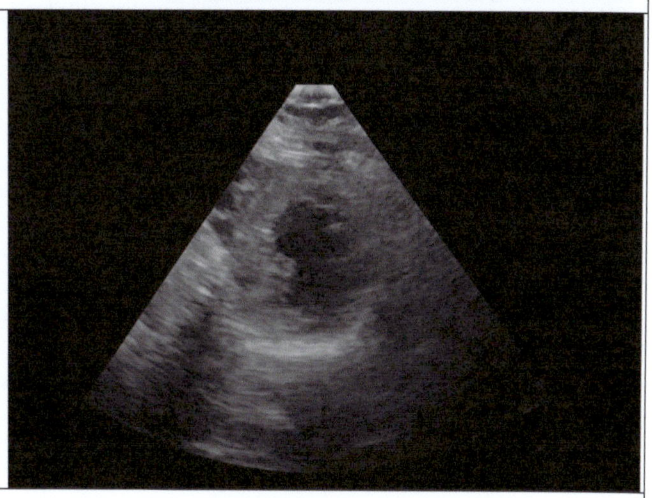
Trans-Gastric Short-Axis (TG SAX)	Parasternal Short-Axis (PSAX)

Table 6.3 Core TEE views

Image	View	Acquisition	Application
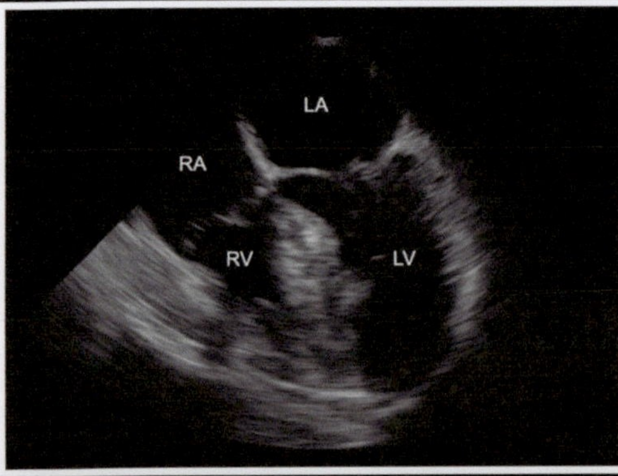	**Mid-esophageal 4-Chamber (ME 4C)**	Omniplane: 0° *Retroflexion to optimize LV apex* Location: Mid-esophagus Anatomy: RA, RV, LA, LV, MV, TV	Clinical Applications: -RV and LV size and function -RWMA -Valvular pathology -Pericardial pathology
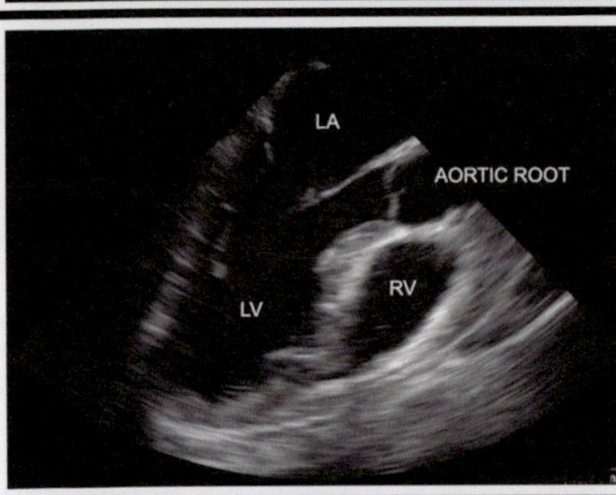	**Mid-esophageal Long-Axis (ME LAX)**	Omniplane: 120-140° Location: Mid-esophagus Anatomy: LA, LV, MV, LVOT, AV, RV	Clinical Applications: -LV function -RWMA -Valvular pathology -Pericardial pathology -Chest compression quality and location of the area of maximal compression
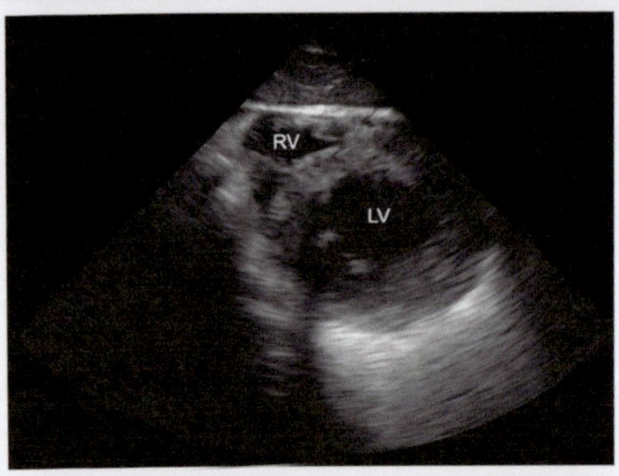	**Trans-Gastric Short Axis at Mid-Papillary (TG SAX)**	Omniplane: 0° *Anteflex to make contact with the stomach wall and displace gastric air* Location: Stomach Anatomy: RV, LV	Clinical Applications: -LV function -RWMA -Pericardial pathology
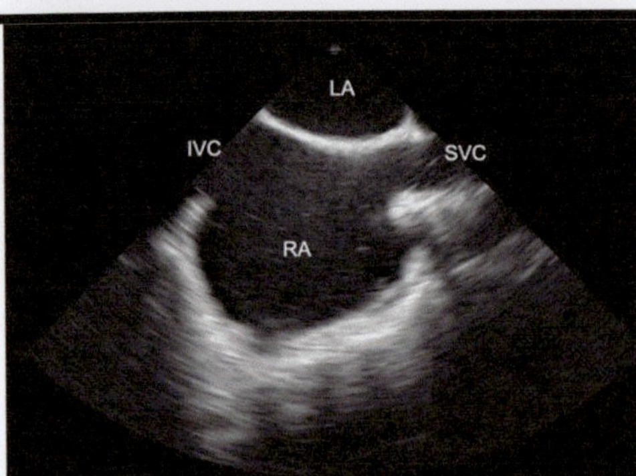	**Mid-esophageal Bicaval (ME Bicaval)**	Omniplane: 90° Location: Mid-esophagus Anatomy: LA, RA, IVC, SVC, IAS	Clinical Applications: -Procedural guidance (venous guidewire ECMO, transvenous pacemaker) -Significant interatrial septal pathology -Volume responsiveness

Table 6.3 (continued)

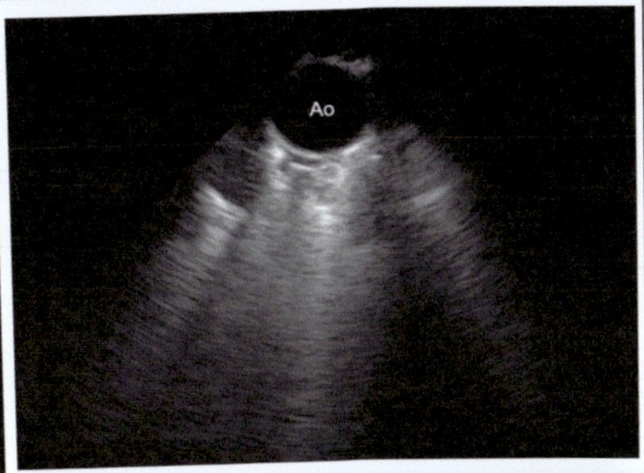

Mid-esophageal Descending Thoracic Aorta Short-Axis (ME DTA SAX)	
Acquisition	**Application**
Omniplane: 0° *Advance and withdraw probe to scan entire length of aorta* Location: Mid-esophagus Anatomy: DTA	Clinical Applications: -Procedural guidance (arterial guidewire ECMO, confirm placement of intra-aortic balloon pump) -Aortic pathology

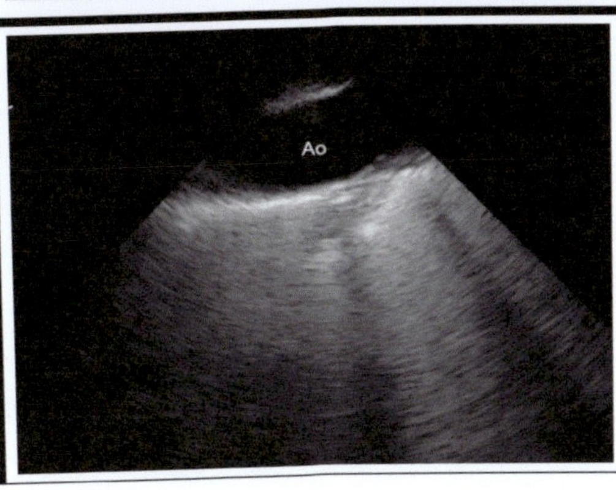

Mid-esophageal Descending Thoracic Aorta Long-Axis (ME DTA LAX)	
Acquisition	**Application**
Omniplane: 90° *Advance and withdraw probe to scan entire length of aorta* Location: Mid-esophagus Anatomy: DTA	Clinical Applications: -Procedural guidance (arterial guidewire ECMO, confirm placement of intra-aortic balloon pump) -Aortic pathology

RA right atrium, *RV* right ventricle, *LA* left atrium, *LV* left ventricle, *MV* mitral valve, *TV* tricuspid valve, *RWMA* regional wall motion abnormality, *LVOT* left ventricular outflow tract, *AV* aortic valve, *IVC* inferior vena cava, *SVC* superior vena cava, *ECMO* extracorporeal membrane oxygenation, *Ao* aorta, *DTA* descending thoracic aorta

Table 6.4 Additional focused TEE views

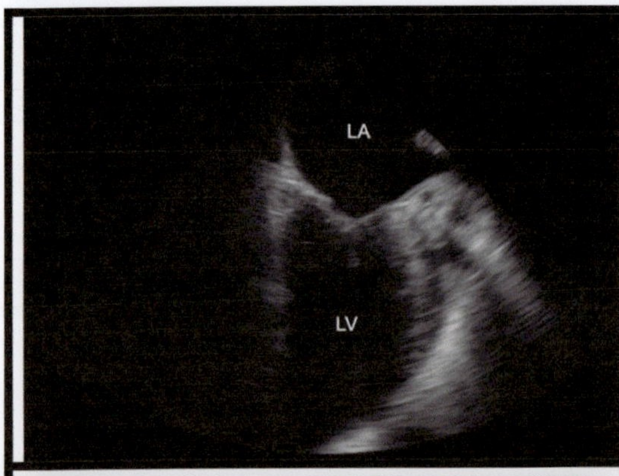

Mid-esophageal 2-Chamber (ME 2C)

Acquisition	Application
Omniplane: 90° Location: Mid-esophageal Anatomy: LA, LV including posteromedial papillary muscle, MV, LAA	Clinical Applications: -LV size and function -RWMA: anterior and inferior walls of LV -Valvular pathology -Pericardial pathology -Thrombus in LAA

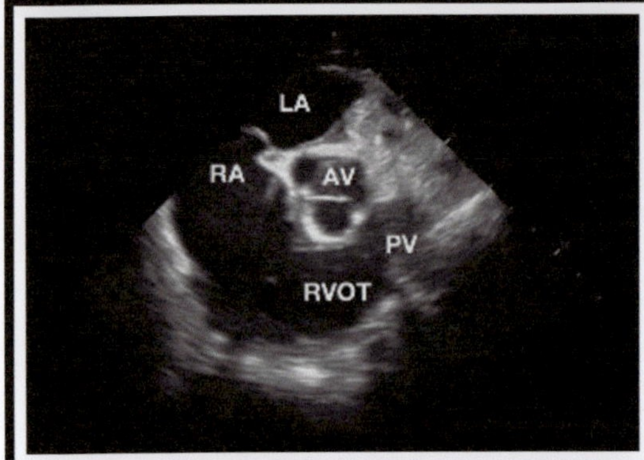

Mid-esophageal Aortic Valve (ME AV SAX)

Acquisition	Application
Omniplane: 30-45° *From ME 4C, withdraw to ME 5C view to see the AV. Center image on AV then rotate omniplane* Location: Mid-esophageal Anatomy: AV, LA, RA, RV, PV	Clinical Applications: -Aortic stenosis -ASD -Pathology at RVOT -Doppler at RCA and LMCA

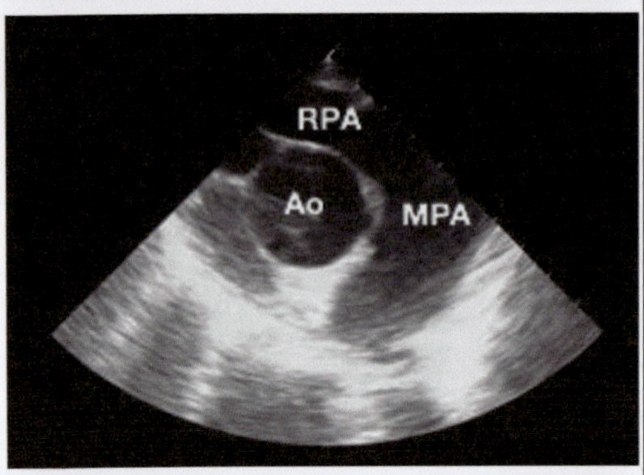

Mid-esophageal Ascending Aorta Short-Axis (ME Asc Ao SAX)

Acquisition	Application
Omniplane: 0° Location: Mid-esophageal Anatomy: Asc Ao, Main PA, RPA *Anatomy may be obstructed by air-filled trachea and airways*	Clinical Applications: -Pulmonary embolism (saddle clot) -Aortic pathology (dissection, aneurysm) -RVOT VTI -Pathology of PA

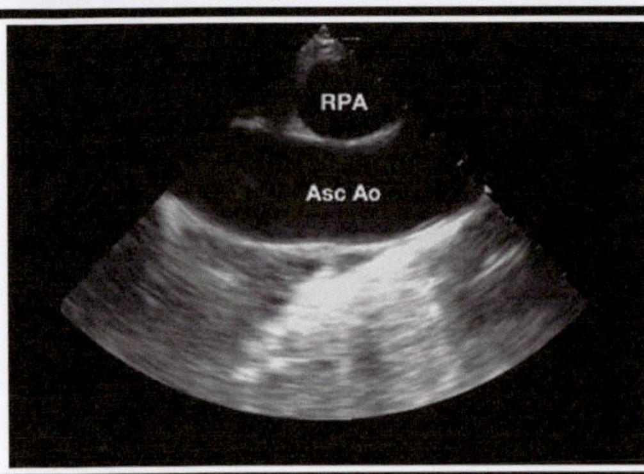

Mid-esophageal Ascending Aorta Long-Axis (ME Asc Ao LAX)

Acquisition	Application
Omniplane: 90-110° Location: Mid-esophageal Anatomy: Asc Ao, RPA *Anatomy may be obstructed by air-filled trachea and airways*	Clinical Applications: -Aortic pathology (dissection, aneurysm) -Pulmonary embolism -Pathology PA -Outflow cannula in LVAD patients -IABP

Table 6.4 (continued)

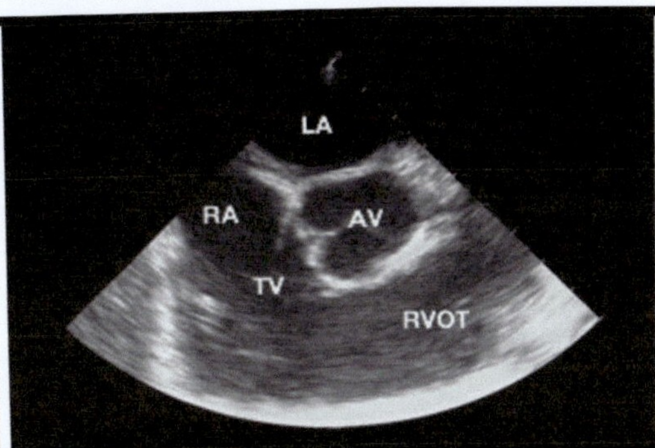

Mid-esophageal Right Ventricular Inflow-Outflow (ME RV I-O)	
Acquisition	**Application**
Omniplane: 60-75° Location: Mid-esophageal Anatomy: LA, RA, RV, TV, PV, AV	Clinical Applications: -Pathology of TV, RVOT -Doppler TV, PV -Transvenous pacemaker

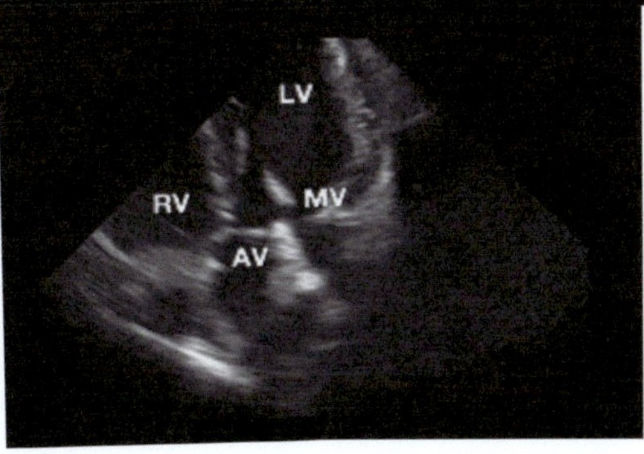

Deep Trans-Gastric 5-Chamber (Deep TG 5C)	
Acquisition	**Application**
Omniplane: 0° *From TG SAX, increase anteflexion and advance distally into stomach* Location: Deep trans-gastric; 45-50 cm from incisors Anatomy: LA, LV, RA, RV, MV, TV, AV, LVOT	Clinical Applications: -Doppler LVOT (VTI), AV -TAPSE/MAPSE (prior modification to visualize TV)

LA left atrium, *LV* left ventricle, *MV* mitral valve, *LAA* left atrial appendage, *RWMA* regional wall motion abnormality, *ME 4C* mid-esophageal four-chamber view, *ME 5C* mid-esophageal five-chamber view, *AV* aortic valve, *RA* right atrium, *RV* right ventricle, *PV* pulmonic valve, *ASD* atrial septal defect, *RVOT* right ventricular outflow tract, *RCA* right coronary artery, *LMCA* left main coronary artery, *Asc* Ao ascending aorta, *PA* pulmonary artery, *RPA* right pulmonary artery, *Ao* aorta, *MPA* main pulmonary artery, *VTI* velocity time interval, *LVAD* left ventricular assist device, *IABP* intra-aortic balloon pump, *TV* tricuspid valve, *TG SAX* trans-gastric short axis view, *LVOT* left ventricular outflow tract, *TAPSE* tricuspid annular plane systolic excursion, *MAPSE* mitral annular plane systolic excursion

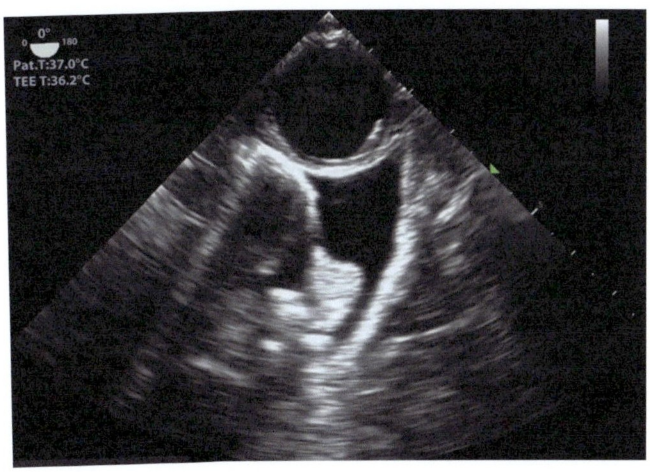

Fig. 6.2 This image was obtained at the mid-esophageal level at 0° omniplane, with the tomographic plane oriented through the descending aorta and the posterior left hemithorax. There is an anechoic pleural effusion with associated atelectatic lung

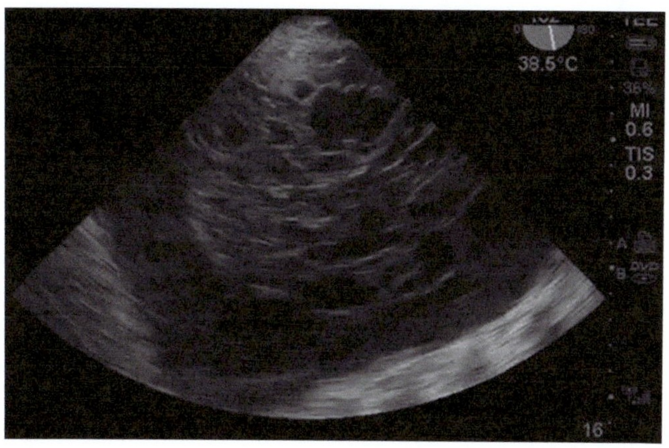

Fig. 6.3 This image was obtained at the mid-esophageal level at 100° omniplane with the tomographic plane oriented to scan through the right posterior hemithorax. A large multiseptated pleural effusion was present

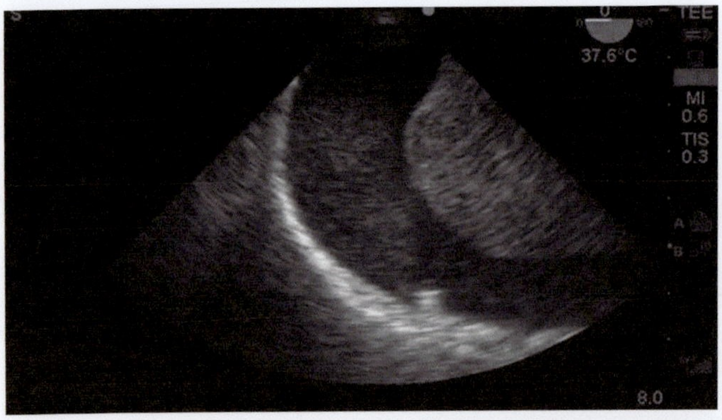

Fig. 6.4 This image was obtained at the mid-esophageal level at 0° omniplane with the tomographic plane oriented to scan through the right hemithorax. There is a large homogeneously echogenic pleural effusion associated with the atelectatic lung. There is partitioning of echogenicity in the effusion with an interface suggesting the distribution of cellular material into the dependent portion of the pleural effusion. The circular echogenic element in the dependent thorax is a chest tube placed for the management of this hemothorax

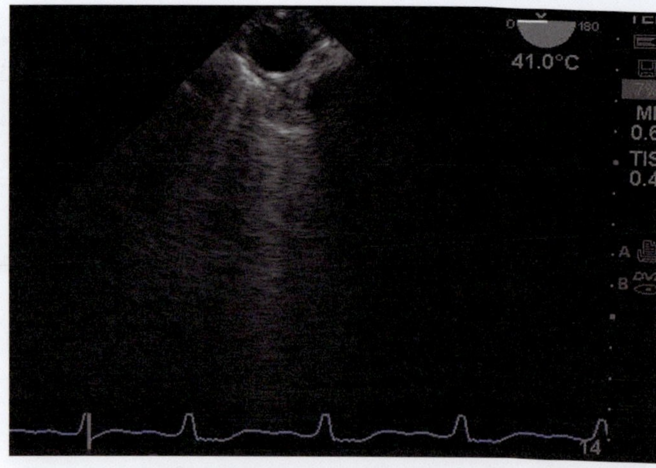

Fig. 6.5 This image was obtained at the mid-esophageal level at 0° with the tomographic plane oriented through the descending aorta and the posterior left hemithorax. There is a subsegmental consolidation of the left lower lobe with associated comet tail artifacts

Clinical Applications

Cardiac Arrest

The goal of cardiopulmonary resuscitation (CPR) is to provide high-quality chest compressions with minimal interruptions to promote cerebral and coronary perfusion during cardiac arrest [22, 23]. Unique to this modality, TEE offers the ability to visualize the ideal location of chest compressions in real-time. Performing TEE intra-arrest allows for continuous cardiac visualization, with one retrospective study suggesting TEE was associated with shortened pulse check duration compared to TTE [24].

For adequate circulation during CPR, the area of maximal compression should overlie the left ventricle while maintaining patency of the left ventricular outflow tract (LVOT) and aortic root. This is best visualized in the ME LAX view (Fig. 6.6; Videos 6.19 and 6.20). Current American Heart Association guidelines posit that hands should be positioned in the middle of the patient's chest at the lower half of the sternum when performing CPR [23]. However, studies evaluating chest computed tomography (CTs) and cardiac magnetic resonance imaging (MRIs) have revealed that, in many patients, the left ventricle (LV) is not located directly beneath the sternum. Instead, the LVOT and aortic root were positioned beneath the sternum in 50–80% of patients [25, 26]. Similar anatomy has been seen in intra-arrest TEE examinations where the area of maximal compression has been positioned over the LVOT or aortic root, causing significant narrowing of the LVOT, thereby impeding optimal circulation (Fig. 6.7; Videos 6.21 and 6.22) [27, 28]. TEE can guide a change in hand position to direct forces over the LV and reduce obstruction of the LVOT and aortic valve, which may lead to improved hemodynamics during CPR [29, 30]. When used intra-arrest, TEE may thus offer an individualized approach to enhance the quality of chest compressions, with the potential to positively affect resuscitation outcomes.

The American Heart Association and the American Society of Echocardiography support using focused echocardiography to investigate reversible causes of cardiac arrest [23, 31]. The 2023 American College of Emergency Physicians policy statement on the use of TEE details the diagnostic capability of TEE in cardiac arrest, including identification of cardiac tamponade, intra-arrest evaluation of cardiac activity, and post-arrest function of the left and right heart [1].

TEE use during cardiac arrest in the emergency department (ED) was first described in 2008 [32]. The superior-quality images of the heart obtained with TEE intra-arrest can reveal fine ventricular fibrillation, pseudo-PEA, and cardiac standstill, which can impact ongoing resuscitation and treatment [10]. Studies in the ED and ICU report TEE as integral in diagnosing potentially treatable causes, including cardiac tamponade, aortic dissection, intracardiac thrombus, pulmonary embolism, hypovolemia, and myocardial infarction, among others (Fig. 6.8; Videos 6.23, 6.24, 6.25, and 6.26) [9, 10, 33–35]. TEE has similar diagnostic capability in cardiac arrests in the perioperative setting and can likewise impact the management of these critically ill patients [4]. A prospective observational study of cardiac arrest patients in the ED showed that information obtained from TEE examinations contributed to changes in management in 97% of cases [18]. Additional studies of TEE in critically ill patients in the ICU setting found similar rates [9, 35]. Described management changes include defibrillation of shockable rhythms, thrombolysis, adjusted location of chest compressions, pericardiocentesis, initiation of pressors or inotropes, and commencement of ECMO.

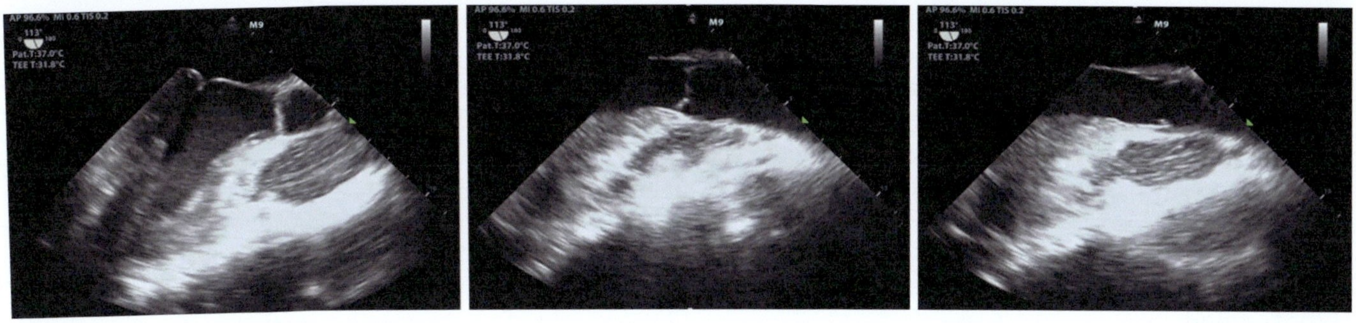

Fig. 6.6 Mid-esophageal long-axis view during ongoing chest compressions. The left ventricle is compressed while the left ventricular outflow tract and aortic root remain patent

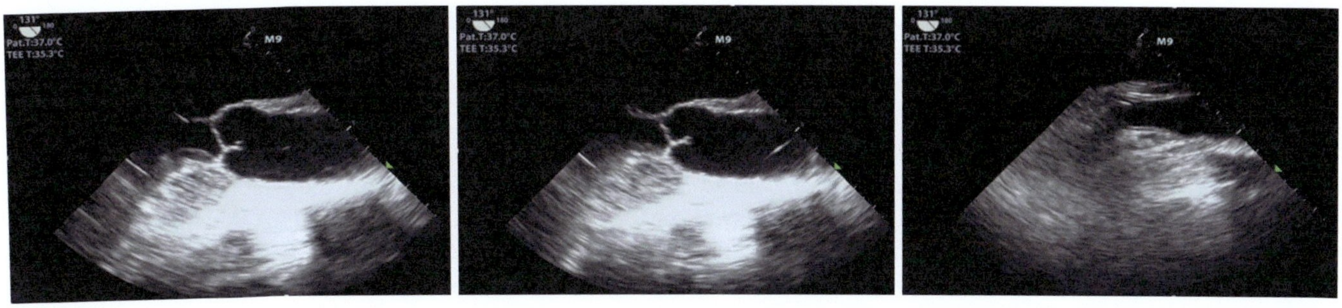

Fig. 6.7 Mid-esophageal long-axis view during inadequate compressions where the aortic root is compressed, thereby impeding optimal circulation

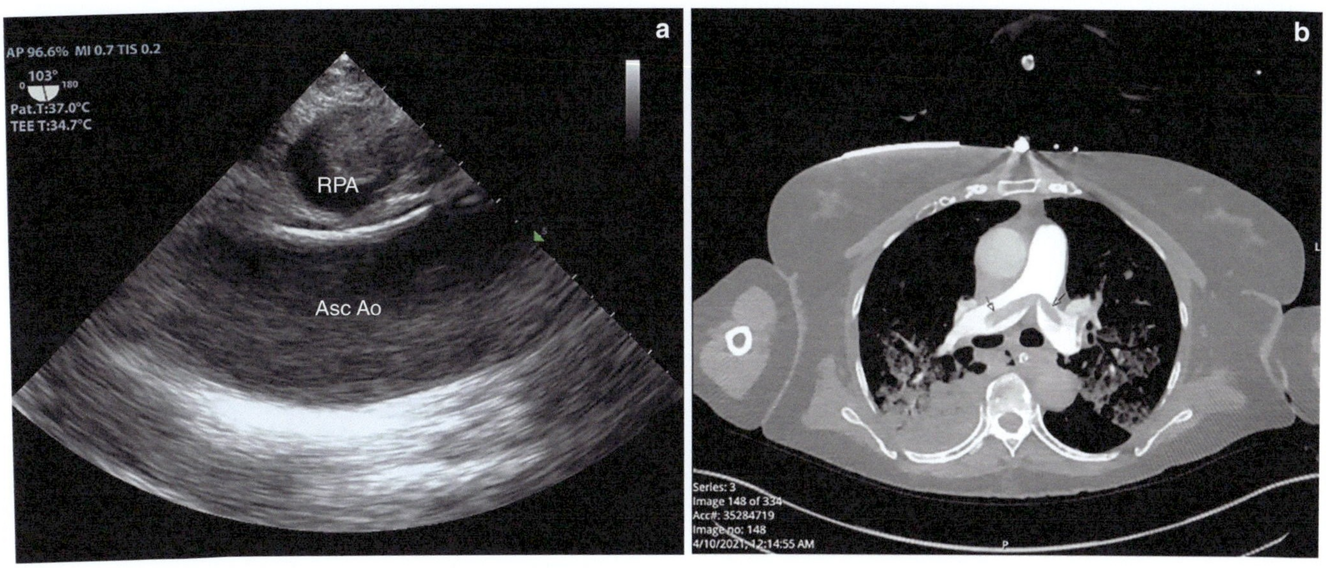

Fig. 6.8 (**a**) TEE image of ascending aorta long-axis view. In the near-field of the image there is a partially obstructive thrombus in the right pulmonary artery. *RPA right pulmonary artery, Asc Ao ascending aorta.* (**b**) Computed tomography image at the level of the pulmonary trunk shows the same saddle embolism visualized previously in TEE

Prognosis after an arrest event and the likelihood of neurologically intact survival are often dependent on identifying and treating a reversible cause. However, intra-arrest TEE findings of prolonged cardiac standstill or irreversible cardiac damage may suggest the futility of further interventions and support the decision to terminate resuscitation [9, 18, 35].

Evaluation of Shock and Undifferentiated Hypotension

While transthoracic cardiac ultrasound remains the first-line point-of-care imaging modality for assessing patients in shock in the ED, TEE is a powerful alternative for intubated patients in whom TTE windows are inadequate or unavailable. Once placed, TEE can help to establish the etiology or predominant mechanism of shock, perform serial hemodynamic assessments estimating stroke volume and stroke volume variation (Fig. 6.9), determine preload sensitivity using respirophasic variation of superior vena cava (SVC) diameter (Fig. 6.10 and Video 6.27), and monitor the response to hemodynamic interventions (e.g., initiating or titrating vasopressor therapy) [9, 36, 37]. One study using TEE to evaluate the SVC collapsibility index as a tool for evaluating intravascular volume in critically ill patients showed that a higher SVC collapsibility (greater than 35%) was associated with lower intravascular volume, indicating that these patients were more likely to be hypovolemic and could benefit from fluid resuscitation [37].

Cardiac function can be assessed with the core views ME 4C, ME LAX, and TG SAX. In most cases, these views are sufficient to evaluate global left and right ventricular function (Video 6.28), cardiac filling status, presence of pericardial effusion (Video 6.29), and regional wall motion abnormalities.

An underfilled LV showing "kissing" papillary muscles in the TG SAX view (Video 6.30) and small LV chamber size in the ME 4C and ME LAX views can qualitatively indicate hypovolemia. Systolic anterior motion of the mitral valve physiology, seen in the context of hypertrophic cardiomyopathy or in the setting of hypovolemia, can be visualized at the ME LAX as well as the Deep TG 5C. Preload assessment of IVC and SVC at the ME bicaval view can provide information on volume status and responsiveness. Evaluation of the pericardium and diagnosis of tamponade and obstructive shock can be accomplished with multiple views, including core views ME 4C, ME LAX, TG SAX and advanced views ME 2C, RV I/O, and Deep TG 5C. When evaluating the patient for aortic dissection, views including ME AV SAX, ME Asc Ao SAX, ME Asc Ao LAX, Upper Esophageal Aortic Arch SAX and LAX, and ME DTA SAX and LAX are recommended (Figs. 6.11 and 6.12; Videos 6.31 and 6.32). However, one limitation of TEE is the difficulty in imaging the distal ascending aorta and arch due to air artifacts from the trachea. Imaging with CT or MRI should be used if there is concern for injury to this area.

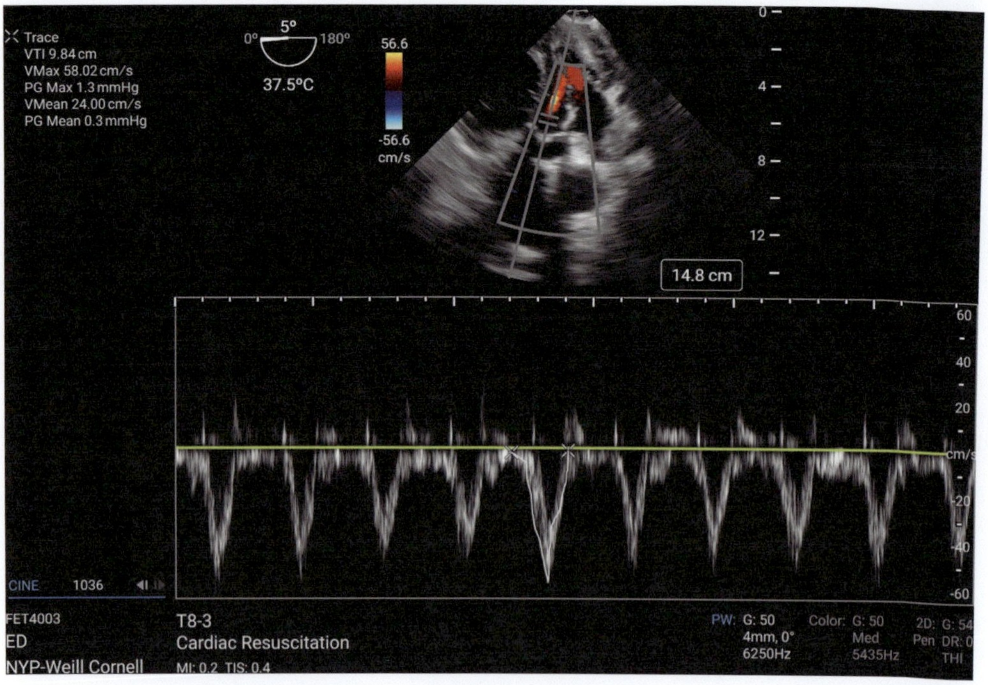

Fig. 6.9 Deep transgastric 5-chamber view using pulsed-wave Doppler to generate the velocity-time integral (VTI). The VTI, as a surrogate of stroke volume, can be used to monitor hemodynamic interventions and to estimate cardiac output. In this case, the VTI is 9.8 cm, consistent with low stroke volume

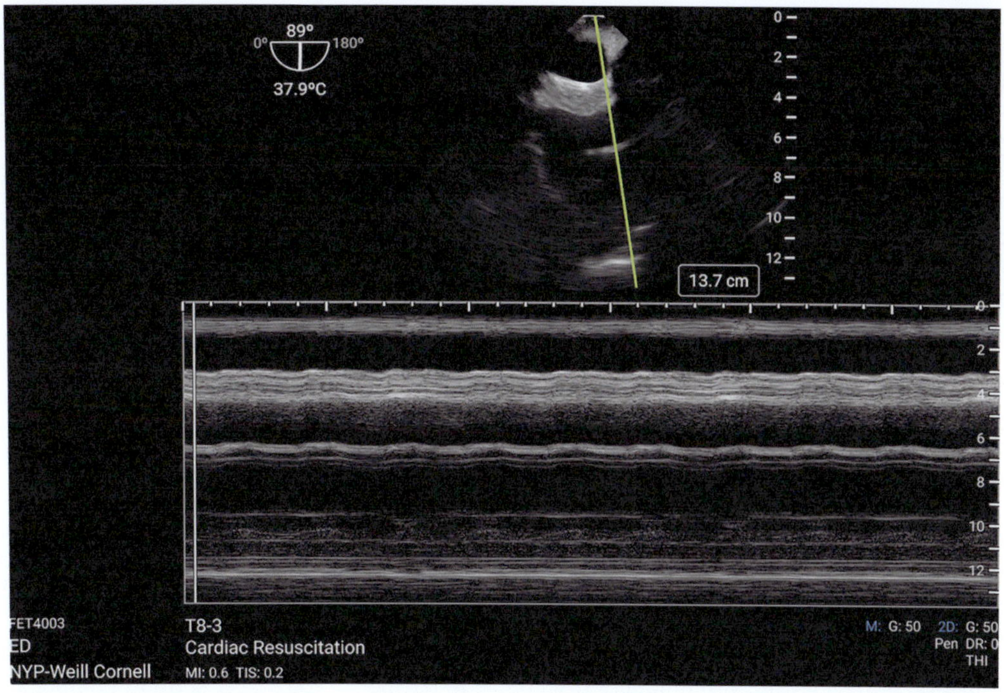

Fig. 6.10 Mid-esophageal bicaval view with M-mode tracing through the superior vena cava (SVC). The unidimensional tracing of the SVC allows the clinician to measure the respiratory variation of the diameter of this vessel as an indicator of central venous pressure and preload responsiveness. In this example, the lack of SVC diameter variation suggests elevated central venous pressure and low likelihood of stroke volume responsiveness to fluid administration

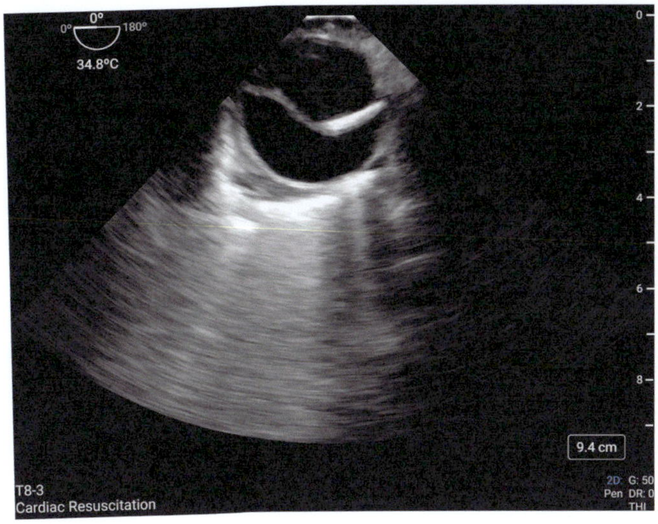

Fig. 6.11 Mid-esophageal descending thoracic aorta in the short axis with the presence of aortic dissection

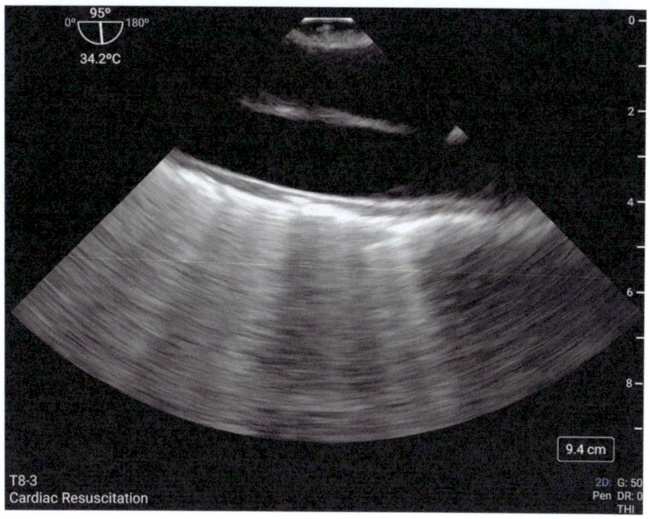

Fig. 6.12 Mid-esophageal descending thoracic aorta in the long axis with presence of aortic dissection

Trauma

The immediate identification of acute hemorrhage and cardiac tamponade can lead to life-saving interventions in the trauma patient. Unfortunately, transthoracic and transabdominal approaches may be limited by trauma-specific factors such as subcutaneous emphysema, positive-pressure ventilation, and ongoing sterile surgical procedures restricting access to the chest and abdomen. Beyond the heart, TEE also allows for visualization of the ascending aorta, arch, and descending aorta to evaluate for blunt traumatic aortic injuries, which, while rare, are one of the leading causes of mortality in trauma patients [38, 39]. While focused TEE is a relatively novel application in trauma resuscitation, it has been shown to provide additional diagnostic yield and may lead to changes in management [40].

Patients who survive transport to the ED with blunt traumatic aortic injury are often critically ill with unstable vital signs, preventing them from obtaining the necessary CT or MRI for diagnosis. TEE has been shown to compare reliably with CT and MRI for accuracy and diagnosis of aortic injury [41]. It may even be more sensitive in detecting injury to the intimal and medial layers of the aorta [42]. Chest injuries causing traumatic aortic dissection, mediastinal hematoma, aortic tear and pseudoaneurysm, intramural hematoma, and aortic rupture have been seen on TEE evaluation and can be diagnosed in minutes thus expediting the acute management of these patients [43–45].

Patients with penetrating and blunt traumatic injuries commonly suffer hemorrhagic shock, which is essential to recognize early. In TEE examinations performed during acute resuscitation of trauma in the ED, ICU, and operating room, evidence of hypovolemia and decreased preload were the most common findings [40, 46, 47]. A recent retrospective review described multiple patients with dynamic LVOT and systolic anterior motion of the mitral valve, recognizing that trauma patients are particularly susceptible to this physiology because of their hypovolemia and vasoplegia (Video 6.32) [40]. TEE can also provide hemodynamic monitoring in patients with burn injuries who require careful management of volume status. These patients can experience massive fluid shifts in the acute phase that can affect myocardial function [48]. They are also uniquely susceptible to bacteremia and distributive shock [49].

However, there are also precautions within this population. Penetrating trauma to the neck with concern for esophageal injury is an absolute contraindication to TEE. Thermal burns to the oropharynx can cause the potential for bleeding or perforation of edematous tissue, so TEE should be performed only after weighing the risks and benefits of the procedure [48]. TEE should also be performed with caution in patients with suspected unstable cervical spine injuries, with care taken to minimize head and neck movement during probe insertion and manipulation [16].

Procedural Guidance

Focused TEE also has a unique role in guiding several emergency procedures, such as initiation and monitoring of ECMO, assistance in placement of pulmonary artery catheters, placement of intravenous pacemaker wires, or placement of an intra-aortic balloon pump [50–55]. Utilizing existing acute care resources, critically unstable patients can effortlessly move from a diagnostic TEE examination to a TEE-guided procedure.

The insertion of a transvenous pacemaker (TVP) is a time-critical procedure with potentially severe complications. Traditionally, TVP insertion has been performed using a landmark-based technique with external telemetry monitoring for cardiac capture or with fluoroscopic guidance. Although fluoroscopy can theoretically be used at the bedside, issues with bed compatibility, workflow, and logistics often make this impractical. Given that blind insertion, though common, can result in misplacement, failure to capture, and serious complications, TEE-guided insertion of TVP has the potential to reduce time to procedure completion and reduce complications [53].

During ECMO cannulation, TEE offers advantages comparable to those of TEE-guided TVP insertion (Fig. 6.13; Videos 6.33 and 6.34). Regardless of the configuration (e.g., veno-venous or veno-arterial ECMO), TEE provides real-time structural details, along with important functional information such as left ventricular filling status, identification of contraindications to the procedure (e.g., aortic dissection, severe aortic regurgitation), and optimal cannula positioning. Moreover, TEE allows for the immediate detection of complications and improves cardiac monitoring for patient progress and recovery.

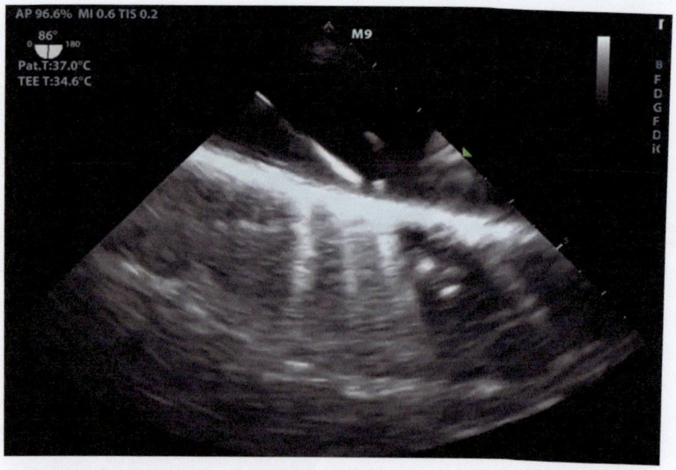

Fig. 6.13 Descending thoracic aorta in long-axis view showing the tip of an arterial guidewire during cannulation for veno-arterial ECMO. The guidewire is seen on the left side of the image and corresponds to the direction of the patient's femoral artery where the wire was inserted

Implementation of a Focused TEE Program

An essential first step for implementation of a TEE program is establishing an institution-specific protocol that describes indications, patient selection criteria, probe processing workflow, and physician requirements. To this end, it is key to establish clearly the indications and scope for focused TEE, in order to distinguish it from comprehensive or consultative TEE.

When choosing a TEE system and probe, the most common choice is a reusable probe, available from most POCUS system providers, which can be connected to existing machines. Once a system and probe have been acquired, a workflow to process the TEE probe must be established. As with any other endoscopic device, TEE probes require high-level disinfection rather than sterilization [56]. The cleaning process includes the following steps: (1) decontamination, (2) high-level disinfection, and (3) a leak test. A leak test checks for damage to the TEE probe's external components and structural integrity. It is performed with a special device that places the probe in a fluid bath to detect the presence of electrical discharge. Leak testing is mandated by the Intersocietal Accreditation Commission (IAC), an international accreditation body supported by many surgical and procedural specialties, including the American Society of Echocardiography and the American Institute of Ultrasound in Medicine [57]. There are two methods for cleaning TEE probes: using the hospital's central processing department or cleaning the probe in the ED, similar to an endocavitary probe. Central processing by the hospital allows for process logging and performance of the leak test. Once cleaned, the probe should be stored fully extended to prevent damage (Fig. 6.14).

Another important aspect to consider during implementation is clinician training. Due to the relatively low frequency of use, high-fidelity simulation is essential for acquiring and maintaining competency. Currently, there are several TEE simulator systems which can provide training with varying degrees of fidelity. Beyond simulation, training in the operating room with a cardiothoracic anesthesiologist provides invaluable experience. The perioperative setting is ideal because patients are intubated, offering a controlled environment suitable for practicing probe insertion and image acquisition. Additionally, the dynamic nature of intraoperative management, with its changing physiological states, allows trainees to conduct serial examinations and observe a high incidence of pathological findings, such as in patients undergoing thrombectomy for pulmonary embolism.

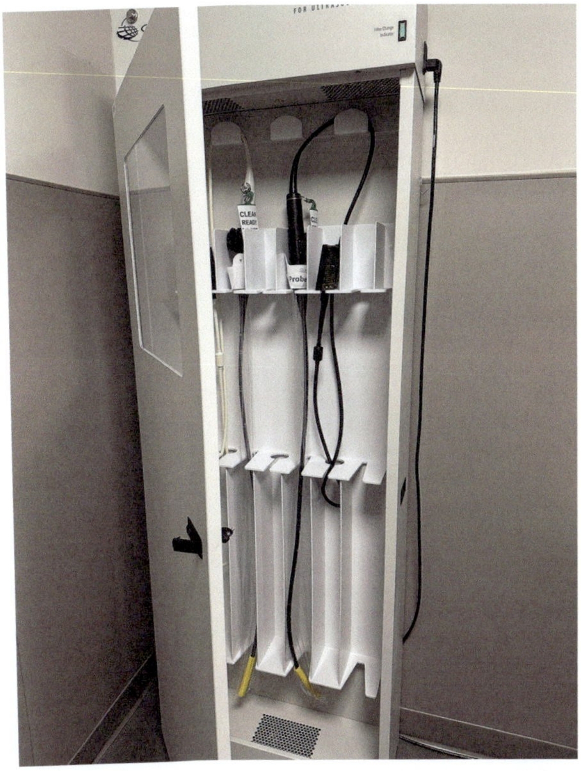

Fig. 6.14 TEE probes stored vertically in a specially designated storage cabinet

According to current guidelines from the American College of Emergency Physicians, clinicians with prior TTE experience should have at least 4–6 h of structured TEE-specific training (e.g., continuing medical education course, workshop, didactics), conduct 10 proctored TEE examinations, and complete a standardized assessment supervised by a TEE-credentialed physician [1]. In addition, we recommend establishing credentialing guidelines and privileges in collaboration with hospital leadership to ensure the protocol is accepted in the ED and throughout the hospital. In our experience, implementing a TEE program is most successful with multidisciplinary collaboration, involving anesthesiology, critical care, and cardiology. Since other specialties may use focused TEE across the hospital, we suggest aligning credentialing and guidelines to ensure consistency across locations.

Key Ultrasound Findings

Diagnosis	Key ultrasound findings
Optimal hand position during compressions in cardiac arrest	The area of maximal compression should be over the left ventricle, with the left ventricular outflow tract and aortic root remaining patent in the mid-esophageal long-axis view.
Ventricular fibrillation	Fine fibrillatory movement of the myocardium.
Anterior wall myocardial infarction	The anterior wall of the left ventricle can be isolated and assessed for regional wall motion abnormality in the mid-esophageal 2-chamber view.
Saddle pulmonary embolism	A saddle pulmonary embolism can be viewed extending between the right and left pulmonary arteries off of the main pulmonary artery in the mid-esophageal ascending aorta short-axis view.
Cardiac tamponade	Early diastolic collapse of the right ventricle in tamponade can be seen in core views, including mid-esophageal 4-chamber and transgastric short-axis views.
Thrombus in transit	A thrombus in transit can be visualized along the path of the right heart inflow and outflow, including the mid-esophageal 4-chamber view, mid-esophageal right ventricular inflow–outflow view, and mid-esophageal ascending aorta short-axis view, in which the main pulmonary artery is visualized.
Hypovolemia	"Kissing" papillary muscles in the transgastric short-axis view. Small left ventricular chamber size in the mid-esophageal 4-chamber view and mid-esophageal long-axis view.

Pearls and Pitfalls

- If the aortic root, aortic valve, and left ventricular outflow tract are seen on a ME 4C view, this would be considered a mid-esophageal 5-chamber view. Advance the probe further to reach the ME 4C and provide slight retroflexion to extend the imaging plane through the apex of the left ventricle so as not to foreshorten the apex.
- The quality and location of chest compressions can be assessed from the ME LAX view. Be wary of chest compressions that obstruct the LVOT. During ongoing CPR, the area of maximal compression should be at the left ventricle while the LVOT remains open.
- In the TG SAX view, anteflex the transducer to make contact with the anterior stomach wall to visualize the heart behind it. This will help displace any gastric air that may interfere with the image.
- When assessing for regional wall motion abnormalities, the physician should make sure the SAX view of the LV is adequately perpendicular to the heart's long axis. Both anterolateral and posteromedial papillary muscles should appear symmetric in size.
- The presence of prosthetic valves can impede visualization of the ventricles, particularly in mid-esophageal views. Trans-gastric views (e.g., Deep TG 5C view) can provide a better image of the ventricles in these cases.

References

1. American College of Emergency Physicians. Use of transesophageal echocardiography (TEE) in the ED for shock, cardiac arrest, and procedural guidance. Accessed October 26, 2024. https://www.acep.org/patient-care/policy-statements/use-of-transesophageal-echocardiography-tee-in-the-ed-for-shock-cardiac-arrest-and-procedural-guidance
2. van der Wouw PA, Koster RW, Delemarre BJ, de Vos R, Lampe-Schoenmaeckers AJ, Lie KI. Diagnostic accuracy of transesophageal echocardiography during cardiopulmonary resuscitation. J Am Coll Cardiol. 1997;30(3):780–3. https://doi.org/10.1016/s0735-1097(97)00218-0.
3. Comess KA, DeRook FA, Russell ML, Tognazzi-Evans TA, Beach KW. The incidence of pulmonary embolism in unexplained sudden cardiac arrest with pulseless electrical activity. Am J Med. 2000;109(5):351–6. https://doi.org/10.1016/s0002-9343(00)00511-8.
4. Memtsoudis SG, Rosenberger P, Loffler M, et al. The usefulness of transesophageal echocardiography during intraoperative cardiac arrest in noncardiac surgery. Anesth Analg. 2006;102(6):1653–7. https://doi.org/10.1213/01.ane.0000216412.83790.29.
5. Shillcutt SK, Markin NW, Montzingo CR, Brakke TR. Use of rapid "rescue" perioperative echocardiography to improve outcomes after hemodynamic instability in noncardiac surgical patients. J Cardiothorac Vasc Anesth. 2012;26(3):362–70. https://doi.org/10.1053/j.jvca.2011.09.029.
6. Hilberath JN, Burrage PS, Shernan SK, et al. Rescue transoesophageal echocardiography for refractory haemodynamic instability during transvenous lead extraction. Eur Heart J Cardiovasc Imaging. 2014;15(8):926–32. https://doi.org/10.1093/ehjci/jeu043.
7. Mayo PH, Narasimhan M, Koenig S. Critical care transesophageal echocardiography. Chest. 2015;148(5):1323–32. https://doi.org/10.1378/chest.15-0260.
8. Arntfield R, Pace J, Hewak M, Thompson D. Focused transesophageal echocardiography by emergency physicians is feasible and clinically influential: observational results from a novel ultrasound program. J Emerg Med. 2016;50(2):286–94. https://doi.org/10.1016/j.jemermed.2015.09.018.
9. Arntfield R, Lau V, Landry Y, Priestap F, Ball I. Impact of critical care transesophageal echocardiography in medical-surgical ICU patients: characteristics and results from 274 consecutive examinations. J Intensive Care Med. 2020;35(9):896–902. https://doi.org/10.1177/0885066618797271.
10. Teran F, Owyang CG, Wray TC, et al. Development and implementation of a multicenter registry for resuscitation-focused transesophageal echocardiography. Ann Emerg Med. 2024:147. https://doi.org/10.1016/j.annemergmed.2024.08.004.
11. Min JK, Spencer KT, Furlong KT, et al. Clinical features of complications from transesophageal echocardiography: a single-center case series of 10,000 consecutive examinations. J Am Soc Echocardiogr. 2005;18(9):925–9. https://doi.org/10.1016/j.echo.2005.01.034.
12. Ramalingam G, Choi SW, Agarwal S, et al. Complications related to peri-operative transoesophageal echocardiography – a one-year prospective national audit by the Association of Cardiothoracic Anaesthesia and Critical Care. Anaesthesia. 2020;75(1):21–6. https://doi.org/10.1111/anae.14734.
13. Sainathan S, Andaz S. A systematic review of transesophageal echocardiography-induced esophageal perforation. Echocardiography. 2013;30(8):977–83. https://doi.org/10.1111/echo.12290.
14. Hüttemann E, Schelenz C, Kara F, Chatzinikolaou K, Reinhart K. The use and safety of transoesophageal echocardiography in the general ICU – a minireview. Acta Anaesthesiol Scand. 2004;48(7):827–36. https://doi.org/10.1111/j.0001-5172.2004.00423.x.
15. Teran F, Prats MI, Nelson BP, et al. Focused transesophageal echocardiography during cardiac arrest resuscitation: JACC review topic of the week. J Am Coll Cardiol. 2020;76(6):745–54. https://doi.org/10.1016/j.jacc.2020.05.074.
16. Hilberath JN, Oakes DA, Shernan SK, Bulwer BE, D'Ambra MN, Eltzschig HK. Safety of transesophageal echocardiography. J Am Soc Echocardiogr. 2010;23(11):1115–221. https://doi.org/10.1016/j.echo.2010.08.013.
17. Hahn RT, Abraham T, Adams MS, et al. Guidelines for performing a comprehensive transesophageal echocardiographic examination: recommendations from the American Society of Echocardiography and the Society of Cardiovascular Anesthesiologists. J Am Soc Echocardiogr. 2013;26(9):921–64. https://doi.org/10.1016/j.echo.2013.07.009.
18. Teran F, Dean AJ, Centeno C, et al. Evaluation of out-of-hospital cardiac arrest using transesophageal echocardiography in the emergency department. Resuscitation. 2019;137:140–7. https://doi.org/10.1016/j.resuscitation.2019.02.013.
19. Teran F, West FM, Jelic T, et al. Resuscitative transesophageal echocardiography in emergency departments in the United States and Canada: a cross-sectional survey. Am J Emerg Med. 2024;76:164–72. https://doi.org/10.1016/j.ajem.2023.11.041.
20. Arntfield R, Pace J, McLeod S, Granton J, Hegazy A, Lingard L. Focused transesophageal echocardiography for emergency physicians-description and results from simulation training of a

structured four-view examination. Crit Ultrasound J. 2015;7(1):27. https://doi.org/10.1186/s13089-015-0027-3.
21. Weber AG, Mastroianni F, Koenig S, Mayo PH. Transesophageal lung ultrasonography as part of the critical care transesophageal echocardiography examination. Chest. 2022;161(6):e335–6. https://doi.org/10.1016/j.chest.2022.01.025.
22. Kleinman ME, Perkins GD, Bhanji F, et al. ILCOR scientific knowledge gaps and clinical research priorities for cardiopulmonary resuscitation and emergency cardiovascular care: a consensus statement [published correction appears in Circulation. 2018 Jul 31;138(5):e77. doi: 10.1161/CIR.0000000000000592]. Circulation. 2018;137(22):e802–19. https://doi.org/10.1161/CIR.0000000000000561.
23. Panchal AR, Bartos JA, Cabañas JG, et al. Part 3: Adult Basic and Advanced Life Support: 2020 American Heart Association Guidelines for Cardiopulmonary Resuscitation and Emergency Cardiovascular Care. Circulation. 2020;142(16_suppl_2):S366–468. https://doi.org/10.1161/CIR.0000000000000916.
24. Fair J 3rd, Mallin MP, Adler A, et al. Transesophageal echocardiography during cardiopulmonary resuscitation is associated with shorter compression pauses compared with transthoracic echocardiography. Ann Emerg Med. 2019;73(6):610–6. https://doi.org/10.1016/j.annemergmed.2019.01.018.
25. Nestaas S, Stensæth KH, Rosseland V, Kramer-Johansen J. Radiological assessment of chest compression point and achievable compression depth in cardiac patients. Scand J Trauma Resusc Emerg Med. 2016;24:54. https://doi.org/10.1186/s13049-016-0245-0.
26. Shin J, Rhee JE, Kim K. Is the inter-nipple line the correct hand position for effective chest compression in adult cardiopulmonary resuscitation? Resuscitation. 2007;75(2):305–10. https://doi.org/10.1016/j.resuscitation.2007.05.003.
27. Hwang SO, Zhao PG, Choi HJ, et al. Compression of the left ventricular outflow tract during cardiopulmonary resuscitation. Acad Emerg Med. 2009;16(10):928–33. https://doi.org/10.1111/j.1553-2712.2009.00497.x.
28. Teran F, Sands N, Wray T, on behalf of the Resuscitative TEE Collaborative Registry Investigators. Abstract 200: Left-ventricular outflow compression during cardiopulmonary resuscitation is associated with lower return of spontaneous circulation in out-of-hospital cardiac arrest. Circulation. 2022;146(Suppl 1) Accessed at: https://www.ahajournals.org/doi/10.1161/circ.146.suppl_1.200
29. Chu SE, Huang CY, Cheng CY, et al. Cardiopulmonary resuscitation without aortic valve compression increases the chances of return of spontaneous circulation in out-of-hospital cardiac arrest: a prospective observational cohort study. Crit Care Med. 2024;52(9):1367–79. https://doi.org/10.1097/CCM.0000000000006336.
30. Catena E, Colombo R, Volontè A, et al. Transesophageal echocardiography in patients with cardiac arrest: from high-quality chest compression to effective resuscitation. J Echocardiogr. 2021;19(1):28–36. https://doi.org/10.1007/s12574-020-00492-8.
31. Labovitz AJ, Noble VE, Bierig M, et al. Focused cardiac ultrasound in the emergent setting: a consensus statement of the American Society of Echocardiography and American College of Emergency Physicians. J Am Soc Echocardiogr. 2010;23(12):1225–30. https://doi.org/10.1016/j.echo.2010.10.005.
32. Blaivas M. Transesophageal echocardiography during cardiopulmonary arrest in the emergency department. Resuscitation. 2008;78(2):135–40. https://doi.org/10.1016/j.resuscitation.2008.02.021.
33. Jung WJ, Cha KC, Kim YW, et al. Intra-arrest transoesophageal echocardiographic findings and resuscitation outcomes. Resuscitation. 2020;154:31–7. https://doi.org/10.1016/j.resuscitation.2020.06.035.
34. Kim YW, Jung WJ, Cha KC, et al. Diagnosis of aortic dissection by transesophageal echocardiography during cardiopulmonary resuscitation. Am J Emerg Med. 2021;39:92–5. https://doi.org/10.1016/j.ajem.2020.01.026.
35. Wray TC, Johnson M, Cluff S, et al. Transesophageal echocardiography performed by intensivist and emergency physicians-a 5-year, single-center experience. J Intensive Care Med. 2022;37(7):917–24. https://doi.org/10.1177/08850666211042522.
36. Vignon P, Mentec H, Terré S, Gastinne H, Guéret P, Lemaire F. Diagnostic accuracy and therapeutic impact of transthoracic and transesophageal echocardiography in mechanically ventilated patients in the ICU. Chest. 1994;106(6):1829–34. https://doi.org/10.1378/chest.106.6.1829.
37. Vieillard-Baron A, Chergui K, Rabiller A, et al. Superior vena caval collapsibility as a gauge of volume status in ventilated septic patients. Intensive Care Med. 2004;30(9):1734–9. https://doi.org/10.1007/s00134-004-2361-y.
38. Akhmerov A, DuBose J, Azizzadeh A. Blunt thoracic aortic injury: current therapies, outcomes, and challenges. Ann Vasc Dis. 2019;12(1):1–5. https://doi.org/10.3400/avd.ra.18-00139.
39. Arthurs ZM, Starnes BW, Sohn VY, Singh N, Martin MJ, Andersen CA. Functional and survival outcomes in traumatic blunt thoracic aortic injuries: an analysis of the National Trauma Databank. J Vasc Surg. 2009;49(4):988–94. https://doi.org/10.1016/j.jvs.2008.11.052.
40. Prager R, Walser E, Balta KY, et al. Resuscitative transesophageal echocardiography during the acute resuscitation of trauma: a retrospective observational study. J Crit Care. 2024;79:154426. https://doi.org/10.1016/j.jcrc.2023.154426.
41. Shiga T, Wajima Z, Apfel CC, Inoue T, Ohe Y. Diagnostic accuracy of transesophageal echocardiography, helical computed tomography, and magnetic resonance imaging for suspected thoracic aortic dissection: systematic review and meta-analysis. Arch Intern Med. 2006;166(13):1350–6. https://doi.org/10.1001/archinte.166.13.1350.
42. Vignon P, Boncoeur MP, François B, Rambaud G, Maubon A, Gastinne H. Comparison of multiplane transesophageal echocardiography and contrast-enhanced helical CT in the diagnosis of blunt traumatic cardiovascular injuries. Anesthesiology. 2001;94(4):615–5A. https://doi.org/10.1097/00000542-200104000-00015.
43. Mollod M, Felner JM. Transesophageal echocardiography in the evaluation of cardiothoracic trauma. Am Heart J. 1996;132(4):841–9. https://doi.org/10.1016/s0002-8703(96)90320-8.
44. Smith MD, Cassidy JM, Souther S, et al. Transesophageal echocardiography in the diagnosis of traumatic rupture of the aorta. N Engl J Med. 1995;332(6):356–62. https://doi.org/10.1056/NEJM199502093320603.
45. Osman A, Fong CP, Wahab SFA, Panebianco N, Teran F. Transesophageal echocardiography at the golden hour: identification of blunt traumatic aortic injuries in the emergency department. J Emerg Med. 2020;59(3):418–23. https://doi.org/10.1016/j.jemermed.2020.05.003.
46. Burns JM, Sing RF, Mostafa G, et al. The role of transesophageal echocardiography in optimizing resuscitation in acutely injured patients. J Trauma. 2005;59(1):36–42. https://doi.org/10.1097/01.ta.0000171460.56972.42.
47. Griffee MJ, Singleton A, Zimmerman JM, Morgan DE, Nirula R. The effect of perioperative rescue transesophageal echocardiography on the management of trauma patients. A A Case Rep. 2016;6(12):387–90. https://doi.org/10.1213/XAA.0000000000000320.

48. Maybauer MO, Asmussen S, Platts DG, Fraser JF, Sanfilippo F, Maybauer DM. Transesophageal echocardiography in the management of burn patients. Burns. 2014;40(4):630–5. https://doi.org/10.1016/j.burns.2013.08.032.
49. Etherington L, Saffle J, Cochran A. Use of transesophageal echocardiography in burns: a retrospective review. J Burn Care Res. 2010;31(1):36–9. https://doi.org/10.1097/BCR.0b013e3181cb8ebc.
50. Fair J, Tonna J, Ockerse P, et al. Emergency physician-performed transesophageal echocardiography for extracorporeal life support vascular cannula placement. Am J Emerg Med. 2016;34(8):1637–9. https://doi.org/10.1016/j.ajem.2016.06.038.
51. Douflé G, Roscoe A, Billia F, Fan E. Echocardiography for adult patients supported with extracorporeal membrane oxygenation [published correction appears in Crit Care. 2016 Feb 08;20:34. doi: 10.1186/s13054-016-1214-8]. Crit Care. 2015;19:326. https://doi.org/10.1186/s13054-015-1042-2.
52. Cronin B, Robbins R, Maus T. Pulmonary artery catheter placement using transesophageal echocardiography. J Cardiothorac Vasc Anesth. 2017;31(1):178–83. https://doi.org/10.1053/j.jvca.2016.07.012.
53. Lerner RP, Haaland A, Lin J. Temporary transvenous pacer placement under transesophageal echocardiogram guidance in the Emergency Department. Am J Emerg Med. 2020;38(5):1044.e3–4. https://doi.org/10.1016/j.ajem.2019.12.027.
54. Nishioka T, Friedman A, Cercek B, et al. Usefulness of transesophageal echocardiography for positioning the intraaortic balloon pump in the operating room. Am J Cardiol. 1996;77(1):105–6. https://doi.org/10.1016/s0002-9149(97)89148-5.
55. Klopman MA, Chen EP, Sniecinski RM. Positioning an intraaortic balloon pump using intraoperative transesophageal echocardiogram guidance. Anesth Analg. 2011;113(1):40–3. https://doi.org/10.1213/ANE.0b013e3182140b9a.
56. AIUM Official Statement. Guidelines for cleaning and preparing external- and internal-use ultrasound transducers and equipment between patients as well as safe handling and use of ultrasound coupling gel. J Ultrasound Med. 2023;42(7):E13–22. https://doi.org/10.1002/jum.16167.
57. Intersocietal Accreditation Commission (IAC). IAC standards and guidelines for perioperative transesophageal echocardiography accreditation. Updated February 2023. Accessed October 26, 2024. https://intersocietal.org/wp-content/uploads/2023/02/IACPerioperativeTEEStandards2023.pdf

Thoracic and Lung Ultrasound

7

Olusegun Olusanya, Luna Gargani, and Michael J. Lanspa

Background

Ultrasonographic evaluation of the pleural space was first described more than 60 years ago; however, assessment of the lung parenchyma has been a more recent development [1]. Historically, the fact that air-filled lung scatters sound waves resulted in the belief that lung ultrasonography had no clinical utility. This led to delayed recognition of the clinical value of lung ultrasound. This was followed by a rapid expansion in research as clinicians increasingly recognized the role of reliably reproduced artifacts generated by insonation of the parenchyma under different clinical scenarios. The initial artifacts, A-lines and B-lines, have great potential for differentiation of pulmonary pathology. Similarly, closer evaluation of the pleural interface has revealed significantly more information than simply the presence or absence of an effusion.

The diagnostic performance of lung ultrasound for the evaluation of pneumothorax, pulmonary edema, pneumonia, acute respiratory distress syndrome (ARDS), and interstitial lung disease has been shown to be superior to chest radiography. The coronavirus disease of 2019 (COVID-19) pandemic resulted in an explosion of lung ultrasound research and application, as the ability to rapidly detect pulmonary abnormalities without chest radiograph demonstrated significant value.

In this chapter, we review a wide array of clinical applications in which lung ultrasound has been shown to add diagnostic or prognostic information beyond chest radiography. We will also review several of the structured protocols to guide scanning. Finally, we will discuss the role of lung point-of-care ultrasound (POCUS) to guide ventilator management.

Indications

Indications

- Dyspnea
- Chest Pain
- Hypoxemia
- Hypercarbia
- Respiratory Failure
- Shock
- Trauma

Diagnoses

- Pneumothorax
- Pulmonary Edema
- Pneumonia
- Acute Respiratory Distress Syndrome
- Atelectasis
- Rib Fracture
- Pulmonary Contusion
- Pleural Effusion
- SARS-CoV-2 Infection
- Respiratory Failure

Supplementary Information The online version contains supplementary material available at https://doi.org/10.1007/978-3-031-85308-1_7.

O. Olusanya (✉)
Department of Critical Care, Barts Heart Centre, London, UK
e-mail: segs@doctors.org.uk

L. Gargani
Department of Surgical, Medical and Molecular Pathology and Critical Care Medicine, University of Pisa, Pisa, Italy
e-mail: luna.gargani@unipi.it

M. J. Lanspa
Department of Pulmonary and Critical Care, Intermountain Medical Center, Salt Lake City, UT, USA
e-mail: michael.lanspa@imail.org

M. Gottlieb, N. Panebianco (eds.), *Advanced Point-of-Care Ultrasound*, https://doi.org/10.1007/978-3-031-85308-1_7

Core Views

View	Image	Approach
Pleura	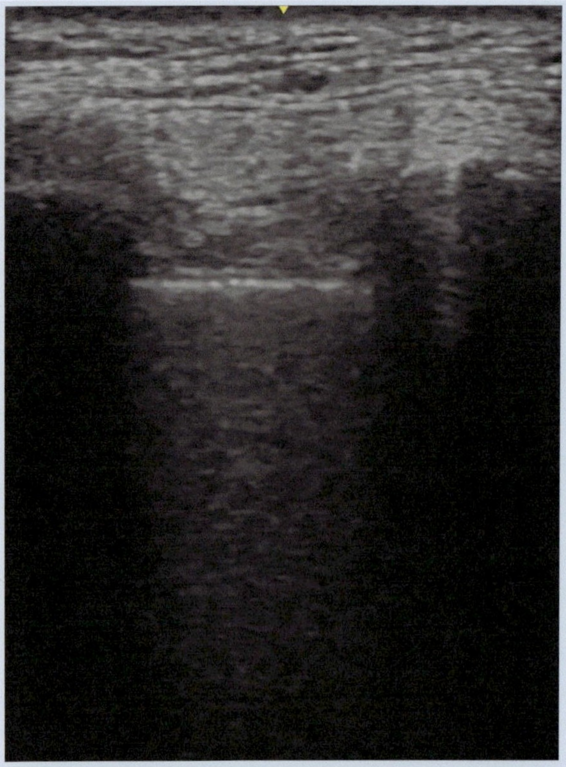 Core View 1. Evaluation of the pleura using the linear probe Core View Video 7.1. Evaluation of the pleura using the linear probe	Place the probe in the sagittal or coronal plane with the indicator superior, such that ribs superior and inferior to the zone of interest are visible in cross-section. Set the depth so that the pleural line is in the middle of the screen. Adjust the gain until the pleural artifacts are best seen. Set the focal depth at the level of the pleura. Hold the probe completely still against the skin for a full respiratory cycle. Move the probe to the next rib space of interest.
Lung parenchyma	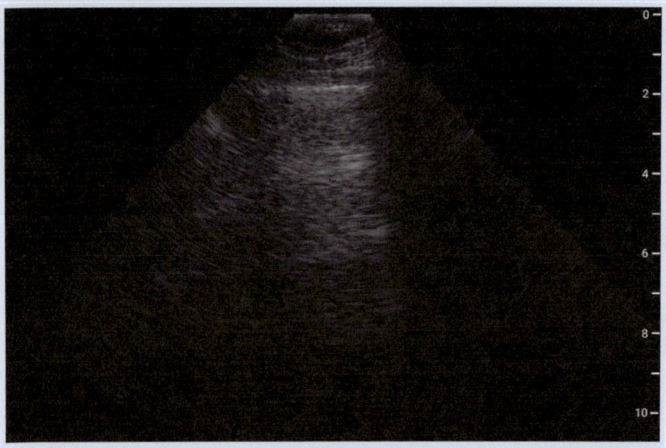 Core View 2. Evaluation of the lung parenchyma using the curvilinear probe Core View Video 7.2. Evaluation of the lung parenchyma using the curvilinear probe	Place the probe in the sagittal or coronal plane such that ribs superior and inferior to the zone of interest are visible in cross-section. Set the depth to at least three times the depth of the pleural line. While often set to 18 cm, more shallow distances can be used. Hold the probe completely still against the skin for a full respiratory cycle. Move the probe to the next rib space of interest. Substitute the phased array probe if curvilinear is not available.

View	Image	Approach
Pleural Effusions	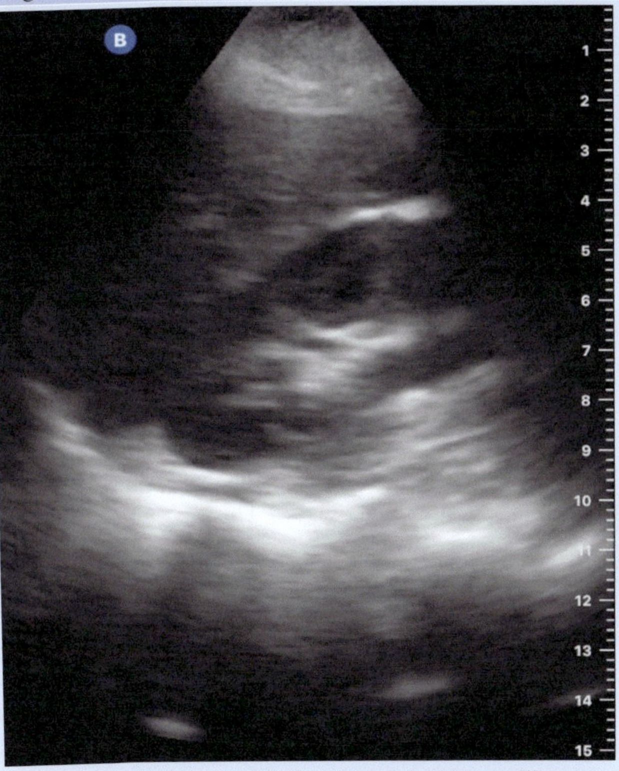 Core View 3. Evaluation of the lung base using the curvilinear probe. Core View Video 7.3. Evaluation of the lung base using the curvilinear probe.	Place the probe in the sagittal or coronal plane in the posterior or lateral inferior lung fields. Set the depth to visualize the visceral anatomy and diaphragmatic curve. Fan and rock the probe through the area of interest. Substitute the phased array probe if curvilinear is not available.

To begin the thoracic POCUS examination, the ultrasound machine should be set to the lung or thoracic examination preset if available. This lowers the ultrasound machine's mechanical index to the American Institute of Ultrasound in Medicine recommended threshold of <0.7 to decrease biological effects to the lung [2]. Additionally, this preset decreases automatic filtering of artifacts (e.g., B-lines, pleural sliding), which are clinically relevant in lung imaging.

The longitudinal approach allows confirmation of anchoring anatomy, including cross-section of the ribs. An alternate approach is the oblique approach, wherein the probe is rotated 45 degrees to lengthen the pleural space while maintaining visualization of the anatomic landmarks. The oblique approach allows visualization of a greater pleural area but carries a risk of mistaking periosteum or fascial planes for pleura. The linear probe allows much greater visualization of pleural abnormalities, but in most adult patients does not provide sufficient depth to characterize all of the important lung POCUS artifacts. B-line visualization is superior with a curvilinear probe (or phased array if curvilinear is not available) than a linear probe [3]. Clinicians should be careful to avoid undergaining images, and the ideal setting has been suggested to be a gain between 50% and 90% with the focal depth at the level of the pleura [3].

Once the space has been identified, fan from anterior to posterior is used to locate the best view. Regardless of assessing superficial or deep findings, the probe should be held completely still against the skin (ideally via anchoring of the scanning hand) for the entirety of a respiratory cycle. There is no consensus for the number of sites scanned per hemithorax, but an increased number of zones can increase the sensitivity for focal pathologies such as pneumonia. The evaluation of pleural effusions often benefits from changing to the abdominal examination preset, as it dramatically improves the visualization of liver, spleen, diaphragm, effusions, and consolidated lung.

As will be discussed in the following sections, a key component for lung ultrasound is identification of artifacts. A summary of key lung line artifacts is presented in Table 7.1.

Table 7.1 Common artifact lines on lung ultrasound

Artifact	Characteristics
A-lines	Strongly hyperechoic, long horizontal lines occurring at regular intervals, suggestive of well-aerated lung
B-lines	Strongly hyperechoic, narrow vertical lines arising from the pleura that extend at least two-thirds of the screen without fading and move with lung sliding
C-lines	Small consolidations
E-lines	Air artifact seen in the soft tissue in the presence of subcutaneous gas
M-lines	Hyperechoic artifacts arising from the margin of the rib's acoustic shadow, often fading after a short distance
R-lines	Vertical artifacts that resemble B-lines, but arise from the margin of the pericardium.
T-lines	Faint vertical artifacts occurring at a regular rate mirroring the heart rate, seen on M-mode when evaluating for lung pulse
Z-lines	Faint vertical artifacts arising from the pleura, which can help to exclude pneumothorax in that region when present

Clinical Applications

Pneumothorax

One of the earliest documented uses of lung ultrasound was for the diagnosis of pneumothorax in horses [1]. From there, this indication has spread—finally being amplified in the critically unwell by the seminal works of Lichtenstein and Volpicelli [4, 5]. Now, with nearly 40 years of experience, lung ultrasound for the identification of pneumothorax is considered a core application of the technique. POCUS has been shown to be superior to supine chest radiography, with 70–89% sensitivity and 98–99% specificity for POCUS compared with 40% sensitivity and 99% specificity for chest radiography [6, 7].

Patient positioning is crucial for diagnosing a pneumothorax. As air rises, a non-loculated pneumothorax will be seen at the most superior point of the chest. If a patient is sitting, that point may be hidden behind the trapezius and sternocleidomastoid muscles, making small pneumothoraces difficult to see. In contrast, when the patient is supine or prone, the most superior location is on the anterior or posterior thorax, respectively.

Lung sliding is a sonographic representation of the interaction between the visceral and parietal pleural interface. During normal ventilation, the parietal pleura moves over the visceral pleura, giving the appearance of lung sliding or "ants marching" on the pleural line. Normal lung should have horizontal lung sliding present throughout the respiratory cycle. This can also be supported by the presence of Z-lines, confirming the presence of lung tissue abutting the pleura.

In contrast, when a pneumothorax is present, lung sliding will not be visible at the pleural interface (Video 7.1). Additionally, as the A-line artifacts are reverberations of the pleural line, in pneumothorax, the lack of sliding and bright pleural line may cause the A-line artifacts to appear static and brighter. Lung sliding can also be enhanced by adding color or power Doppler to visualize the motion artifact associated with the sliding.

Sometimes, lung sliding may be challenging to visualize on brightness mode (B-mode). In these instances, motion mode (M-mode) can help to better delineate lung sliding, due to the greater degree of temporal resolution (Fig. 7.1). One study of emergency physicians found that the addition of M-mode increased the specificity from 89.8% to 96.0% with the largest difference seen among more novice sonographers [8].

If there is no lung sliding, this should raise suspicion for a pneumothorax in the appropriate clinical context. Once identified, the next step is to "sweep" the hemithorax from medial to lateral, to see if lung sliding can be found. If this is the case, suspicion for a pneumothorax increases, provided mimics such as bullae or pleurodesis are not present.

When time allows, the clinician should also attempt to locate the "lung point." The lung point represents the area of the lung where the accumulation of extrapleural air ends and the normal visceral and parietal pleural interface begins. This will appear as normal lung sliding intermittently entering the screen where no lung sliding was previously present (Fig. 7.2 and Video 7.2). The lung point has been previously described in the literature as 100% specific for pneumothorax [9]; however, this can be seen with other conditions, such as partial pleurodesis or severe bullous emphysema, which can create a pseudo-lung point [10]. The interface between the heart and left lingular lobe can also mimic a lung point. This is sometimes termed a "cardiac point" and needs careful understanding of probe positioning. Similarly, the interface between the lung and the diaphragm can mimic a lung point. Therefore, this finding should be interpreted with caution and consideration in the broader context (e.g., other areas with absent lung sliding, no known risk factors for mimics, proper probe positioning).

Mainstem intubation resulting in unilateral ventilation can mimic pneumothorax on the contralateral side. The "lung pulse" is a cardiophasic lung sliding that occurs with each heartbeat, resulting in rhythmic vertical artifacts from the pleura (also known as "T-lines") (Fig. 7.3) [11, 12]. Because this occurs via direct transmission of heart beats to the pleural interface, this excludes the presence of a pneumothorax on that side.

Several clinical scenarios will result in a lack of lung sliding. Therefore, it is important to consider the pretest probability and confirm this with additional lung findings as described in Table 7.2.

Pulmonary Edema

Pulmonary edema can be indirectly visualized by lung POCUS through the presence of B-lines. B-lines are hyperechoic, laser-like vertical artifacts, arising from the pleural line and extending toward the bottom of the screen, moving synchronously with respiration [13]. They are the sono-

Lung ultrasound can help to differentiate viral from bacterial pneumonia but is insufficient in isolation. A study of 200 children with clinically suspected pneumonia and abnormal chest radiographs were studied with lung ultrasound [42]. Patients with an interstitial pattern or small (0.25–0.5 cm) subpleural consolidations were classified as having viral pneumonia, while patients with an alveolar pattern (consolidation) were classified as having bacterial pneumonia. The authors found lung ultrasound was 91% sensitive and 91% specific for diagnosing bacterial pneumonia, while it was 78% sensitive and 90% specific for viral pneumonia. Another study of 85 pediatric patients found lung ultrasound was 100% sensitive and specific for bacterial pneumonia, whereas it was 77% sensitive and 80% specific for viral pneumonia [43]. While lung ultrasound is a useful tool for diagnosing pneumonia, it remains insufficient in isolation for delineating bacterial from viral etiologies. However, it may be useful in settings with high pretest probabilities for particular disease outbreaks, such as H1N1 influenza or SARS-CoV-2, or when microbial testing might otherwise be limited [44].

Atelectasis

Both atelectasis and pneumonia may manifest as consolidations on lung ultrasound. In the appropriate settings, where pneumonia is not suspected, ultrasound can be useful to identify atelectasis (B-lines and consolidation) in dependent lung areas [45]. Among patients with a consolidation, the presence of dynamic air bronchograms (hyperechoic scintillating foci present within a consolidated lung that move with respirations) has been demonstrated to be useful in differentiating pneumonia (dynamic air bronchograms) from atelectasis (static air bronchograms) with a positive predictive value of 97% (Fig. 7.10 and Video 7.9) [46]. In contrast, static air bronchograms (i.e., those that do not move with respirations) were present in both atelectasis and pneumonia, limiting the discriminatory ability of this finding (Video 7.10) [46]. Another study found that dynamic air bronchograms were only 45% sensitive but 99% specific for pneumonia [47]. In that study, the authors also assessed the pulmonary vasculature using color Doppler (small sample window with the Nyquist limit set to 25 cm/s) and found that the presence of pulsatile vascular structures was 90% sensitive and 68% specific for differentiating pneumonia from atelectasis [47].

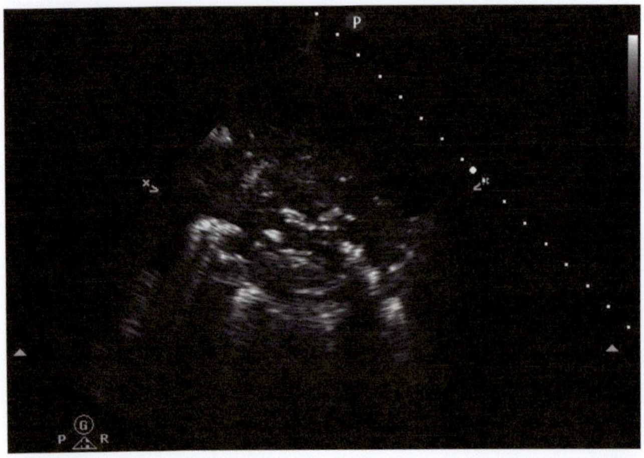

Fig. 7.10 Air bronchograms

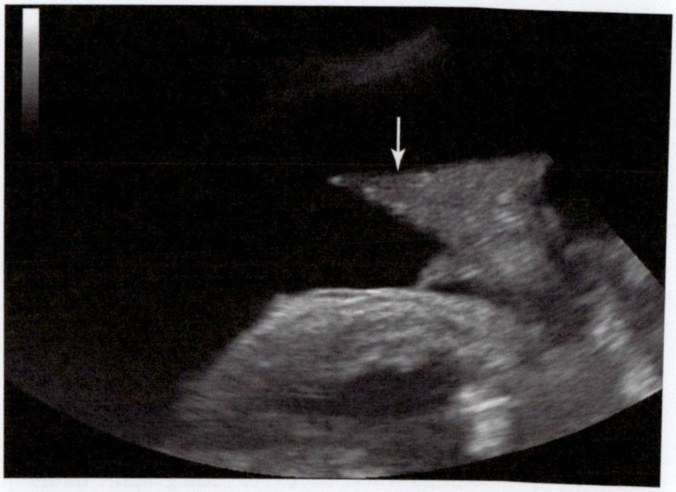

Fig. 7.11 Pleural effusion and lung with compression atelectasis (white arrow)

Compression atelectasis can also be seen in the context of pleural effusions. This will present with a similar appearance to consolidated lung but will be seen primarily in the lower lung fields in the context of a moderate or large pleural effusion (Fig. 7.11 and Video 7.11).

Pulmonary Contusion

While there are no specific signs for the diagnosis of pulmonary contusion, the presence of focal B-lines or small consolidations in a trauma patient are suggestive of the diagnosis in the absence of alternate causes (Fig. 7.12 and Video 7.12). A systematic review and meta-analysis reported lung POCUS was 92% sensitive and 89% specific for diagnosing pulmonary contusions [48]. However, as many of these findings can also be seen with other consolidative processes (e.g., atelectasis, pneumonia, pulmonary edema), it is important to consider this in the clinical context and correlate the findings with the area of trauma.

Pleural Effusion

The assessment of pleural fluid with ultrasound dates back to the 1960s where the superiority of ultrasound over chest

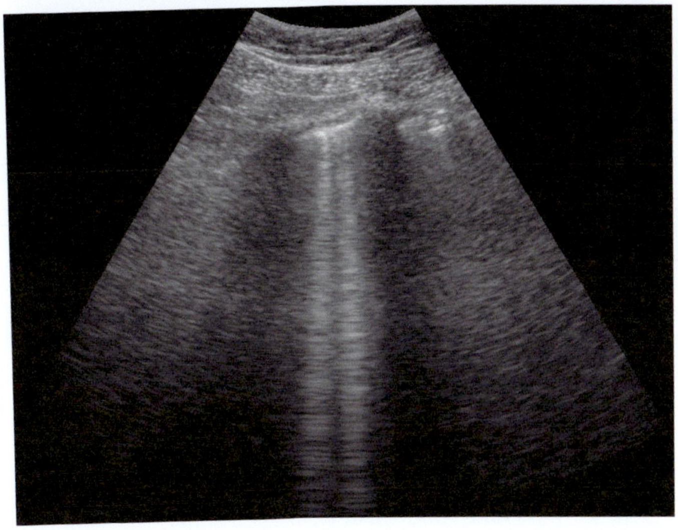

Fig. 7.12 Pulmonary contusion. (*Image courtesy of Michael Gottlieb, MD*)

radiography was clearly established [1]. Ultrasound for the assessment of pleural fluid is now a widely accepted indication for the technique, with well-established international guidelines for its use [49]. The sensitivity and specificity of ultrasound for pleural effusion approaches 100% when compared to CT. Lung ultrasound allows for the detection of small amounts of fluid (up to 5 mL), and can delineate septations and debris with a higher resolution than CT. Ultrasound is particularly useful in patients with "white out" on chest radiographs, as it can rapidly differentiate atelectasis or consolidation from effusion. Finally, the use of ultrasound dramatically increases safety when performing pleural procedures, such as thoracentesis.

A free-flowing effusion is gravity-related and will be visualized just above the diaphragm (Fig. 7.13 and Video 7.13). Thus, the preferred view to identify a pleural effusion most consistently and rapidly is via the lung base at the costophrenic angle. If the patient is supine, this will be the posterior axillary line. If the patient is sitting up, this can be the posterior axillary line extending to the patient's back. Then, the probe can be swept anteriorly to fully image the lower portion of the hemithorax.

Fluid will appear as a hypoechoic or anechoic collection above the diaphragm with posterior acoustic enhancement. If the fluid is exudative, there may be echogenic densities or septations (Figs. 7.14 and 7.15; Videos 7.14 and 7.15). While septations or loculations are useful for predicting whether fluid will be exudative, anechoic fluid does not necessarily predict transudative fluid [50].

In addition to visualization of an anechoic or hypoechoic fluid collection, operators can also visualize the spine above

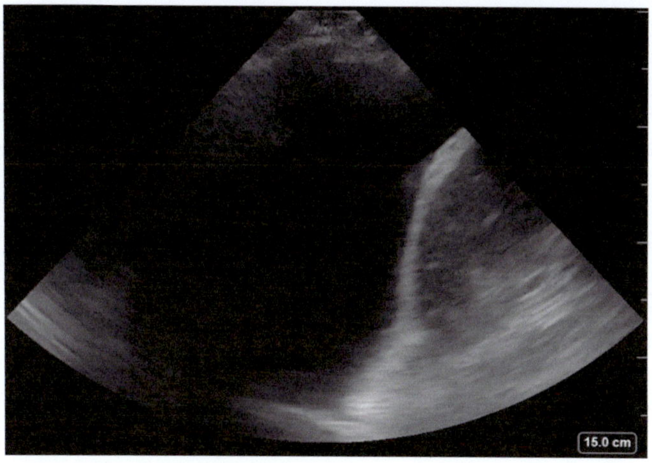

Fig. 7.13 Simple pleural effusion

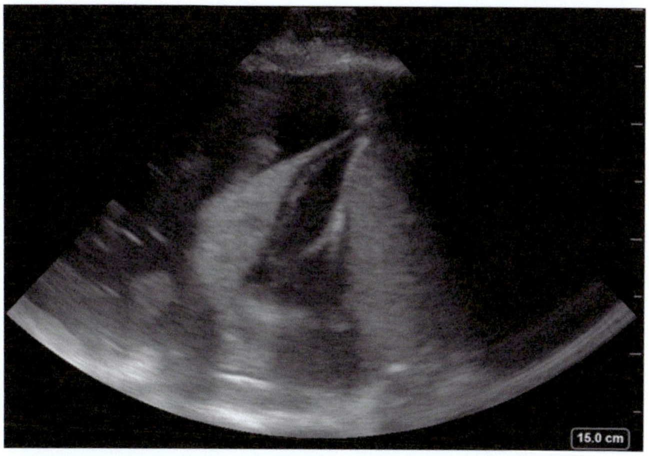

Fig. 7.14 Loculated pleural effusion

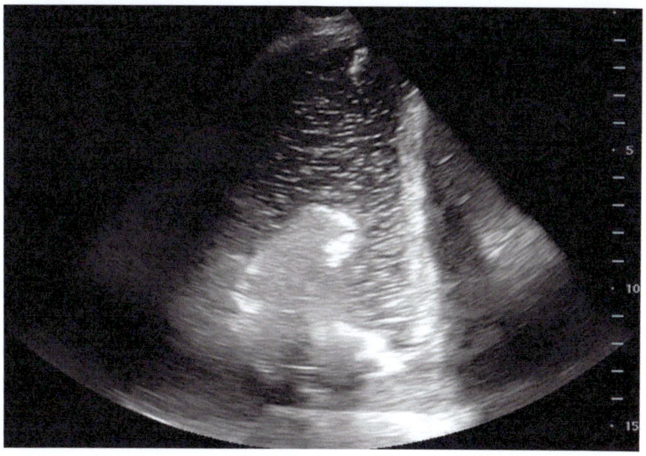

Fig. 7.15 Complex pleural effusion with air and densities within the fluid. (*Image courtesy of Michael Gottlieb, MD*)

the diaphragm, which would normally have an abrupt halt at the margin of the diaphragm due to the obscuration of the ultrasound waves from the air-filled lung. When an effusion is present, the ultrasound waves can traverse the supradiaphragmatic space, allowing visualization of the spine above the diaphragm, referred to as a positive "spine sign" (Fig. 7.16 and Video 7.16) [51].

Quantification of fluid size can be performed using a visual estimation technique (small, medium, or large). Alternatively, pleural effusion volume can be calculated using distinct measures (Table 7.4). There is a lack of consensus on which of the measurement formulas is best; therefore, decisions regarding which tool to use should be based on patient positioning and ease of calculation.

Diagnosing a pleural effusion with ultrasound requires clear visualization of the diaphragm to ensure the fluid is clearly delineated above the diaphragm. The diaphragm can be identified by tracing the spleen or liver superiorly to locate a thin muscular structure and then sliding or fanning anteriorly. Pleural effusions will appear superior to the diaphragm, while ascites will appear inferior (Fig. 7.17 and Video 7.17). The diaphragm is also important for identifying mirror image artifact. Mirror image artifact occurs because the diaphragm is a strong reflector and can create images above the diaphragm that could appear suspicious for either consolidation or effusion. However, when visualizing this finding, one will note the identical appearance of structures above and below the diaphragm (Fig. 7.18 and Video 7.18). The presence of mirror artifact effectively excludes the presence of a pleural effusion on that side. Finally, a fluid-filled distended stomach can be distinguished from pleural fluid by identifying the encapsulating walls, heterogeneous contents (often including fluid, gas, and solid matter), and absence of collapsed lung (Fig. 7.19 and Video 7.19).

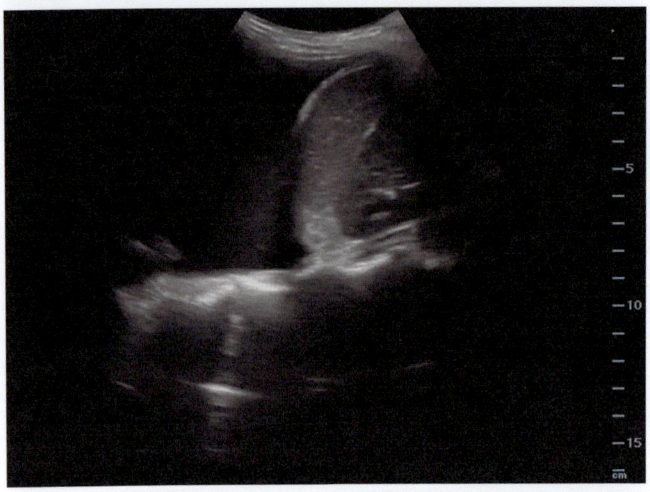

Fig. 7.16 Presence of spine sign in a patient with a pleural effusion. (*Image courtesy of Michael Gottlieb, MD*)

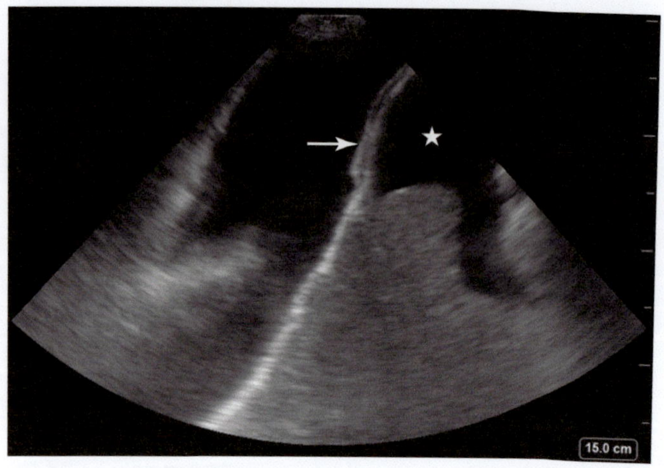

Fig. 7.17 Pleural effusion with concomitant ascites. Ascites (star) is seen inferior to the diaphragm (white arrow)

Table 7.4 Formulas for calculating pleural effusion volume

Name	Formula	Caveats
Balik [52]	LPD × 20	Patient should be supine with approximately 15° of torso elevation. Measurement is taken at end-expiration.
Eibenberger [53]	(47.6 – LPD) – 837	Patient should be supine. Measurement is taken at maximal inspiration. Cannot be used in small pleural effusions (<18 mm).
Goecke 1 [54]	CC × 90	Patient is upright. Measurement is taken at end-expiration.
Goecke 2 [54]	(CC + SPH) × 70	Patient is upright. Measurement is taken at end-expiration.

LPD Largest perpendicular distance from the chest wall to the pulmonary surface (measured in mm), *CC* Craniocaudal extent of the effusion at the dorsolateral chest wall (measured in cm), *SPH* subpulmonary height—defined as distance from the lung base to mid-diaphragm (measured in cm)

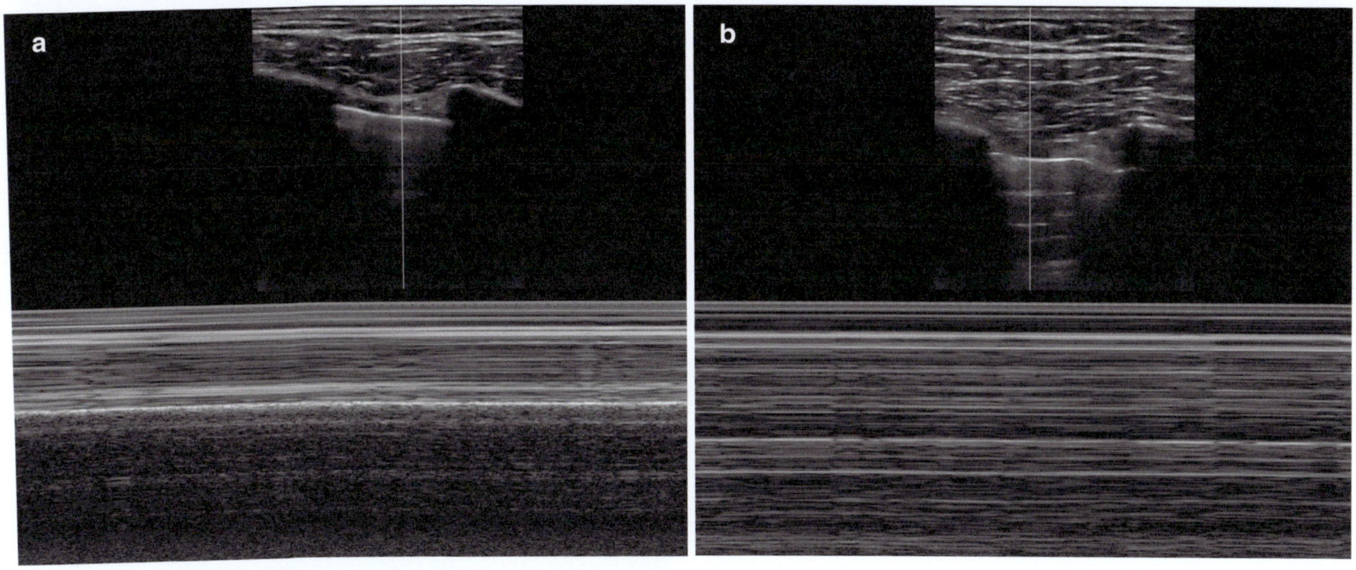

Fig. 7.1 (**a**) M-mode of normal lung demonstrating the seashore sign. (**b**) M-mode of a pneumothorax demonstrating the stratosphere or barcode sign. (*Images courtesy of Michael Gottlieb, MD*)

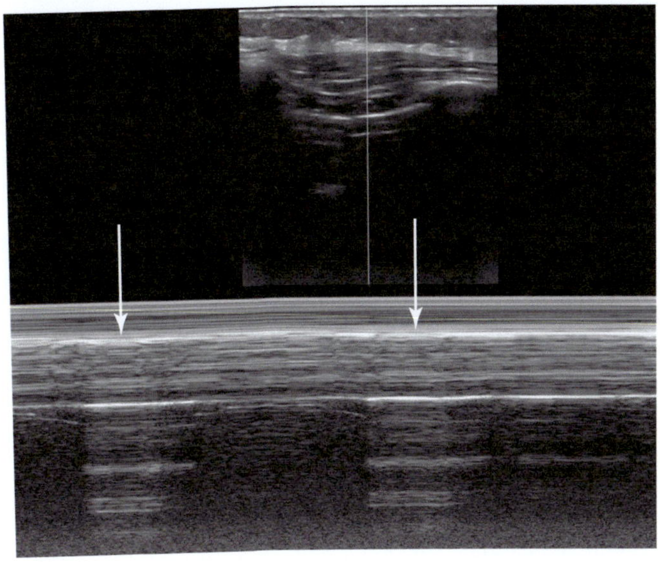

Fig. 7.2 M-mode demonstrating a lung point, with the normal lung tissue alternating with pneumothorax (white arrows). (*Image courtesy of Michael Gottlieb, MD*)

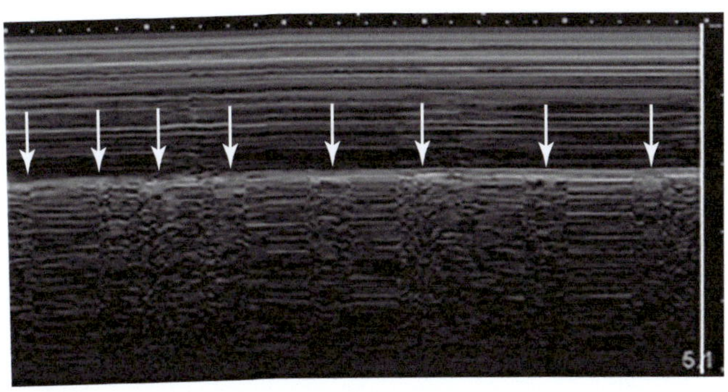

Fig. 7.3 M-mode where respirophasic lung sliding is absent, but the cardiophasic movement of the heart creates a lung pulse (arrows)

Table 7.2 Clinical causes of absent lung sliding in the absence of pneumothorax

Clinical condition	Etiology of lack of lung sliding	Mitigating factors
Endobronchial intubation	Apnea of the non-ventilated lung	Lung pulse should still be present
Bullous Emphysema	Lack of ventilation/air trapping	Lung pulse should still be present
Low tidal volume ventilation in ARDS	Limited excursion of the lung	B-lines and Z-lines rule out pneumothorax
Pleurodesis	Layers of pleura are adhered	B-lines and Z-lines rule out pneumothorax

ARDS acute respiratory distress syndrome

graphic sign of the partial deaeration of the lung and can be used for the diagnosis, monitoring, and prognosis of patients with both cardiogenic and non-cardiogenic pulmonary edema (Fig. 7.4 and Video 7.3).

Cardiogenic Pulmonary Edema

The typical lung POCUS pattern in cardiogenic pulmonary edema is the presence of multiple, diffuse B-lines present bilaterally. "Multiple" is defined as ≥3 B-lines in a single scanning zone. "Diffuse" refers to the presence of ≥3 B-lines in at least two adjacent scanning zones. "Bilateral" refers to both right and left lung involvement since cardiogenic pulmonary edema affects both lungs in almost all cases [14]. The presence of multiple diffuse bilateral B-lines is 87% sensitive and 97% specific for diagnosing acute decompensated heart failure (HF) [15–17]. Lung POCUS is more accurate than standard assessment, including chest radiography and natriuretic peptides [18], even when there is concomitant pneumonia [19]. Pleural effusion can also be present, and is

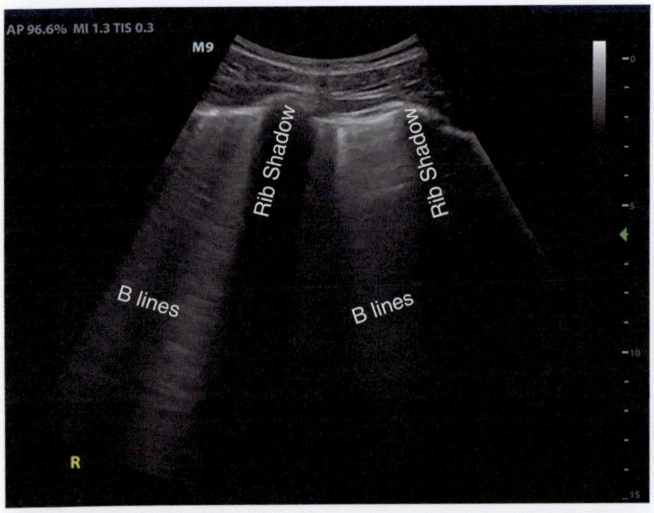

Fig. 7.4 B-mode demonstrating hyperechoic vertical artifacts known as B-lines

more frequently but not universally present on the right side more than the left [20].

In patients hospitalized for acute decompensated HF, the change in B-lines over time can help assess the degree of decongestion and are usually more dynamic than other echocardiographic signs of noninvasive hemodynamics, such as E/e′ or pulmonary artery systolic pressure. B-lines also have a strong prognostic role for predicting decompensation and readmission rates - both when assessed at admission and at discharge [21–24].

Additionally, B-lines can be used in the management of patients with chronic HF. These patients often have subclinical congestion, which may not be able to be detected by physical examination or chest x-ray but is visible through lung POCUS as B-lines [25]. Several randomized trials have shown that guiding diuretic therapy in outpatients with chronic HF using B-lines combined with standard assessment can improve their prognosis, reducing urgent HF visits and rehospitalization for HF [26–29].

Noncardiogenic Pulmonary Edema

B-lines can also be detected in patients with pulmonary congestion due to noncardiogenic causes, such as end-stage renal disease (ESRD) or ARDS [30]. When attempting to distinguish between a cardiogenic and noncardiogenic etiology for pulmonary edema, there are several features that can help predict the etiology [31]. These include the appearance of the pleural line, B-line distribution, consolidations, and spared areas (Table 7.3).

In cardiogenic pulmonary edema, the pleural line looks like a regular, thin horizontal hyperechoic line, which moves with respiration. Even when multiple diffuse B-lines are present, the pleural line usually has a normal appearance. In noncardiogenic pulmonary edema, the sonographic pleural line appears irregular and more fragmented, (Fig. 7.5 and Video 7.4). Notably, this reflects the sonographic appearance and not necessarily the anatomical pleura, which is not really "fragmented" or "thickened."

Table 7.3 Sonographic findings for distinguishing cardiogenic from noncardiogenic pulmonary edema [31]

Finding	Cardiogenic pulmonary edema	Noncardiogenic pulmonary edema
Pleural Line	Thin, normal appearance	Irregular, fragmented
Distribution of B-lines	Symmetric, gravity-related	Patchy, nongravity-related
Spared Areas	Rare	Common
Consolidations	Rare	Common

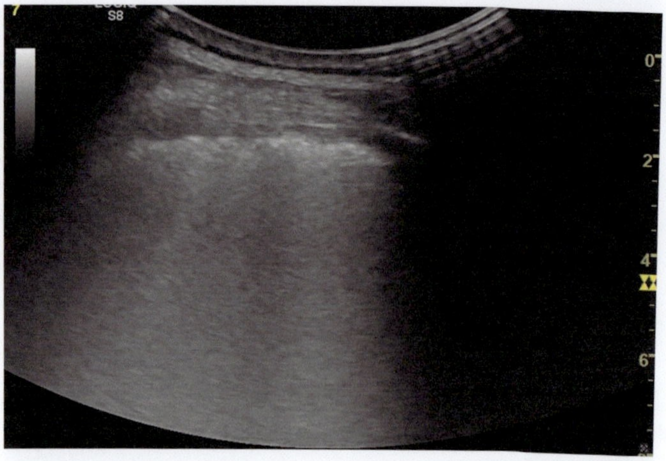

Fig. 7.5 B-lines with a fragmented pleural line suggestive of noncardiogenic pulmonary edema

In cardiogenic pulmonary edema, B-lines tend to appear first in the lower lung zones bilaterally. As the pulmonary edema worsens, they spread progressively more superior in a gravity-related distribution. In contrast, noncardiogenic pulmonary edema results in B-lines across multiple zones in a patchy and nongravity-related distribution over the chest. As such, B-lines can be seen in superior lung zones in the absence of B-lines in lower lung zones. These may also appear as "spared areas," which are areas of normal sonographic appearance surrounded by areas of multiple B-lines that are often coalescent [31, 32].

Consolidations consist of dense fluid collections resulting in a more tissue-like appearance (discussed further below). It is rare to see consolidations in the context of a cardiogenic pulmonary edema, unless there is compression atelectasis in the context of a large pleural effusion. In contrast, consolidations are common in noncardiogenic etiologies.

Data have shown that in the context of ESRD, B-lines have a prognostic role for predicting cardiovascular events [33]. Monitoring ARDS by lung POCUS is also possible and can assist with prognostic stratification. A lung POCUS score from 0 to 3 can be established for each assessed scanning zone, yielding a final "deaeration score," which can be employed for monitoring potential lung recruitment or derecruitment in case of worsening conditions [34]. A higher deaeration score correlates with increased mortality in the intensive care unit [35]. This score has been successfully applied in many conditions to monitor lung deaeration, including patients on extracorporeal membrane oxygenation, with a good correlation with signs of deaeration on computed tomography imaging in critically ill patients [34, 36, 37].

Pneumonia

Lung POCUS is 92% sensitive and 82% specific for diagnosing pneumonia [38]. When performed properly, lung POCUS is highly accurate. However, it can miss findings in the central lung parenchyma when there is interposed normally aerated peripheral parenchyma obscuring the view [39]. Lung POCUS may be particularly well-suited for patients in whom it is preferable to avoid ionizing radiation (e.g., pediatric patients), or in settings where access to radiographic imaging is limited or will be delayed.

Imaging can be performed with a high-frequency linear probe to interrogate the pleura or with a lower-frequency phased array or curvilinear probe to examine deeper structures. Ultrasound findings can include interstitial abnormalities, manifesting as B-lines, or alveolar abnormalities, appearing as a consolidation (Fig. 7.6 and Video 7.5). Interstitial patterns are sometimes graded according to the number of B-lines per intercostal space (Fig. 7.7 and Video 7.6) up to the point where the lines coalesce (Fig. 7.8 and Video 7.7). Although multiple scoring systems have been proposed, ≥3 B-lines in an intercostal space is generally considered a reasonable threshold for decreased aeration. Lung consolidation indicates near complete loss of aeration, sometimes demonstrating air bronchograms (Fig. 7.6). Because there is near-total loss of air, the consolidated lung will transmit sound better than aerated lung, allowing for deeper imaging.

Subpleural micro-consolidations may also manifest as pleural irregularities or small hypoechoic areas below the pleura (Fig. 7.9 and Video 7.8). These micro-consolidations can correlate with disease severity in pneumonia, particularly COVID-19 [40]. The detection of micro-consolidations can increase the likelihood of pneumonia in the correct clinical context [41].

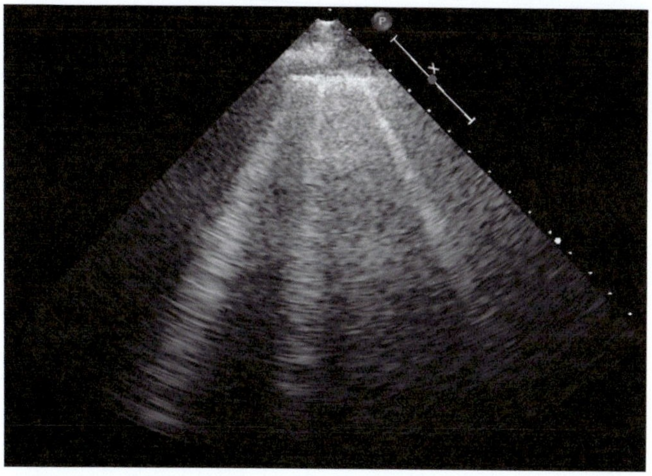

Fig. 7.7 Multiple discrete B-lines in a patient with pneumonia

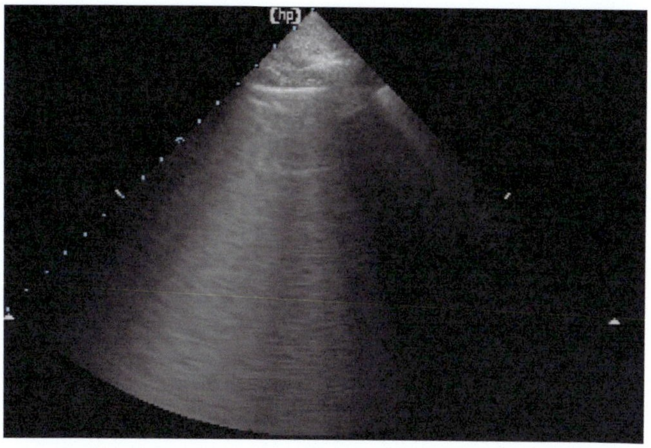

Fig. 7.8 Multiple B-lines coalescing into a single wider, dense line

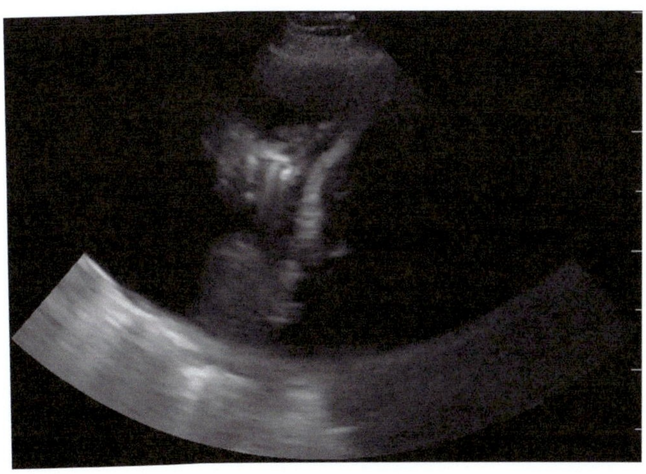

Fig. 7.6 Lung consolidation with air bronchograms

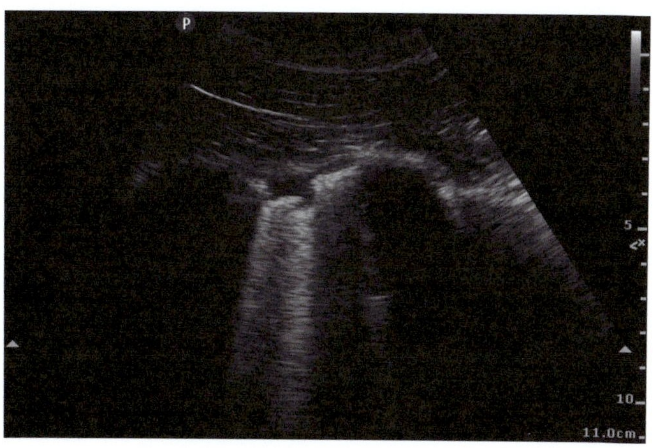

Fig. 7.9 Subpleural consolidations

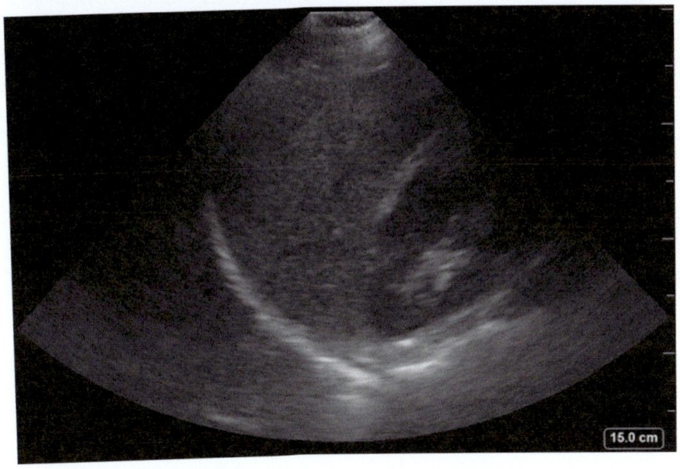

Fig. 7.18 Mirror artifact demonstrating the appearance of the liver above the diaphragm

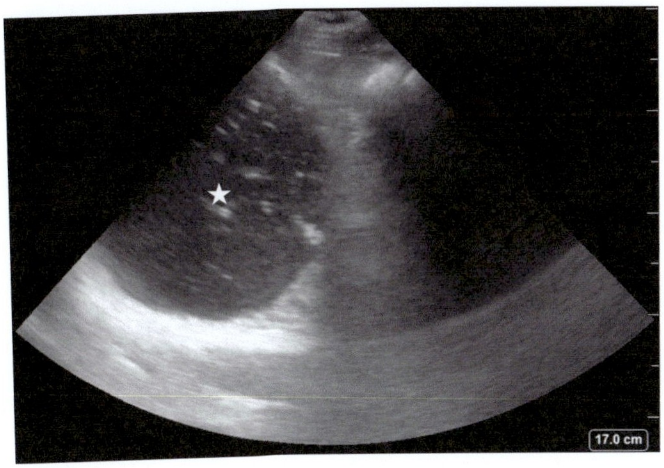

Fig. 7.19 Fluid-filled stomach (star) mimicking a pleural effusion. (*Image courtesy of Alan Chiem, MD*)

COVID-19

The use of lung POCUS as a diagnostic tool significantly expanded during the SARS-CoV-2 pandemic. Because ultrasound is portable, easily repeatable, and has a high sensitivity for detecting lung deaeration it was an excellent instrument to detect lung involvement in patients with COVID-19 [55]. Post-pandemic, this tool remains particularly beneficial for facilitating rapid diagnosis and monitoring of pulmonary conditions in critically ill patients.

Ultrasound findings in COVID-19 pneumonia can include B-lines, focal spared areas, pleural line alterations, consolidations, and pleural effusion. Both separated or coalescent B-lines can be seen in COVID-19, with separated B-lines being detected more commonly in the early phases of the disease, evolving to coalescent B-lines as a sign of worse

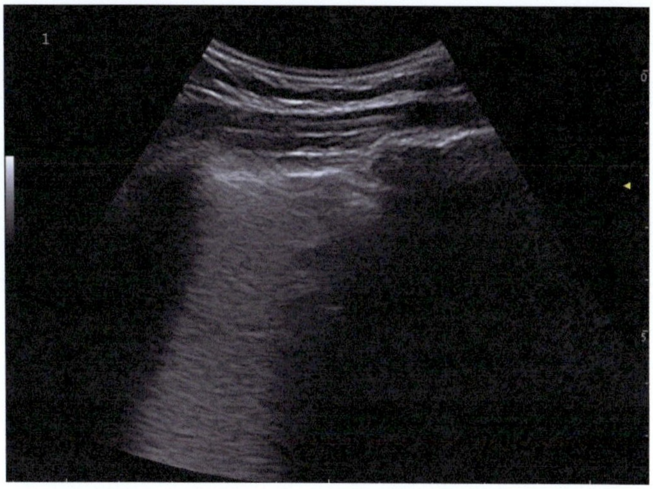

Fig. 7.20 Light beams in a patient with COVID-19

parenchymal aeration. Focal sparing of lung areas in COVID-19 pneumonia have the same appearance as in ARDS, reflecting the patchy, irregular distribution of the pulmonary involvement. In many patients with COVID-19 pneumonia, spared areas can be particularly clear with a very distinct transition between strictly coalescent B-lines. These can resemble a shining bandform, spreading down from a regular pleural line, adjacent to an area of well-aerated lung with A-lines. This sign has been defined as the "light beam," and is usually visible in the very acute phase of ground glass lesions, when limited diseased areas are in close proximity to preserved lung parenchyma (Fig. 7.20 and Video 7.20) [56].

In one large multicenter study, the authors attempted to identify patterns to assess the likelihood of COVID-19 pneumonia [57]. A high probability pattern consisted of bilateral and multifocal clusters of separated or coalescent B-lines, light beams, spared areas, small peripheral consolidations, and abnormal pleural line appearance. These findings were then combined with the pretest probability based on the symptoms and exposure to predict the likelihood of COVID-19 pneumonia. This represents one of the largest studies using lung ultrasound to assess the risk for a specific pathogen and paves the way for future diagnostic opportunities.

In addition to the diagnostic applications, lung POCUS has also been successfully employed during the pandemic for monitoring dynamic variations in parenchymal recruitment during ventilation [58, 59]. Other changes in the patterns such as the onset of a dynamic arborescent air bronchograms were shown to be very specific for the development of ventilator-associated pneumonia [60]. Lung POCUS has also demonstrated a prognostic role in patients with COVID-19 pneumonia to predict clinical progression or acute worsening of symptoms [61, 62].

Rib Fracture

Chest radiography has limited sensitivity for rib fractures, as many fractures (especially near the cartilaginous portion of the rib) are missed [63]. In contrast, ultrasound is 97% sensitive and 94% specific for this condition [64]. Ultrasound for rib fracture assessment is best performed with a high-frequency linear probe. By sliding gently in the transverse plane, the echogenic periosteum can be viewed across the entire course of the rib. Places of discontinuity are visible as anechoic breaks in the echoic periosteum and may be associated with a hematoma (Fig. 7.21 and Video 7.21). It is important to be familiar with the appearance of normal ribs and the transition at the costochondral junction to avoid a false positive diagnosis. Once a rib fracture is identified, the underlying lung parenchyma should also be evaluated for pulmonary contusion and pneumothorax, as described above.

Lung Protocols

A wide array of different protocols have been proposed for lung POCUS. Protocols are often based upon the number of views and diagnoses being evaluated for. Table 7.5 and Fig. 7.22 provide a brief review of commonly used imaging protocols.

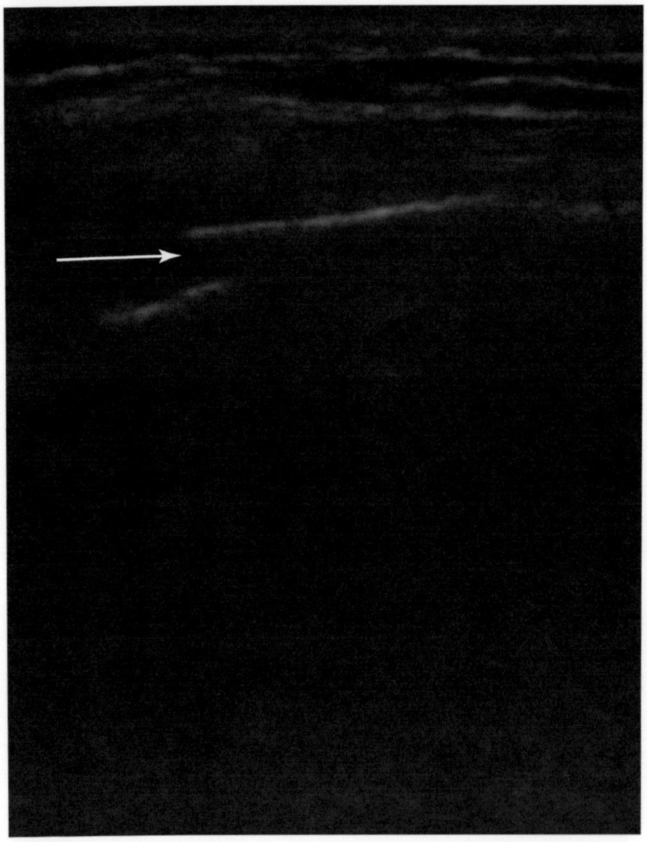

Fig. 7.21 Rib fracture with cortical step-off (white arrow)

Table 7.5 Lung ultrasound imaging protocols

Protocol	Scanning areas	Indications and Limitations
6-zone Protocol [4]	3 scanning areas per hemithorax: Anterior Lateral Postero-lateral	Able to explore the postero-lateral areas with minimal movements of the patient. Suggested for patients with acute respiratory failure in intensive care (often used for the "BLUE" protocol).
8-zone Protocol [13]	4 scanning areas per hemithorax: Antero-superior Antero-inferior Lateral-superior Lateral-inferior	Can be used in critically ill and stable patients. Requires minimal patient movement, but cannot visualize the posterior fields.
12-zone Protocol [65]	6 scanning areas per hemithorax: Antero-superior Antero-inferior Lateral-superior Lateral-inferior Postero-superior Postero-inferior	Proposed in critically ill patients, mainly for monitoring deaeration and stratifying prognosis by establishing a "LUS score" indicating the level of deaeration. To calculate the LUS score, each scanning area is assigned a score from 0 to 3.
28-zone Protocol [66, 67]	16 scanning areas on the right and 12 scanning areas on the left: Scanning from the second to the fifth ICS (on the right hemithorax) and from the second to the fourth ICS (on the left hemithorax) For each hemithorax, the following planes are used: parasternal, mid-clavicular, anterior axillary, and mid-axillary	Initially proposed to provide a standardized, comprehensive assessment for patients with heart failure. Can be more time-consuming compared with other protocols.
Interstitial Lung Disease Protocols [68, 69]	Three different approaches: Anterolateral and posterior chest Posterior chest only Postero-basal chest only	Proposed as a screening tool in connective tissue disease-associated pulmonary involvement with a cut-off value of >10 B-lines on the whole chest or >1 B-line on the postero-basal chest.
COVID-19 Protocols [70, 71]	12- and 14-zone scanning protocols: Antero-superior Antero-inferior Lateral-superior Lateral-inferior Postero-superior Postero-inferior	Different protocols (mandatory to include the posterior chest).

ICS intercostal space

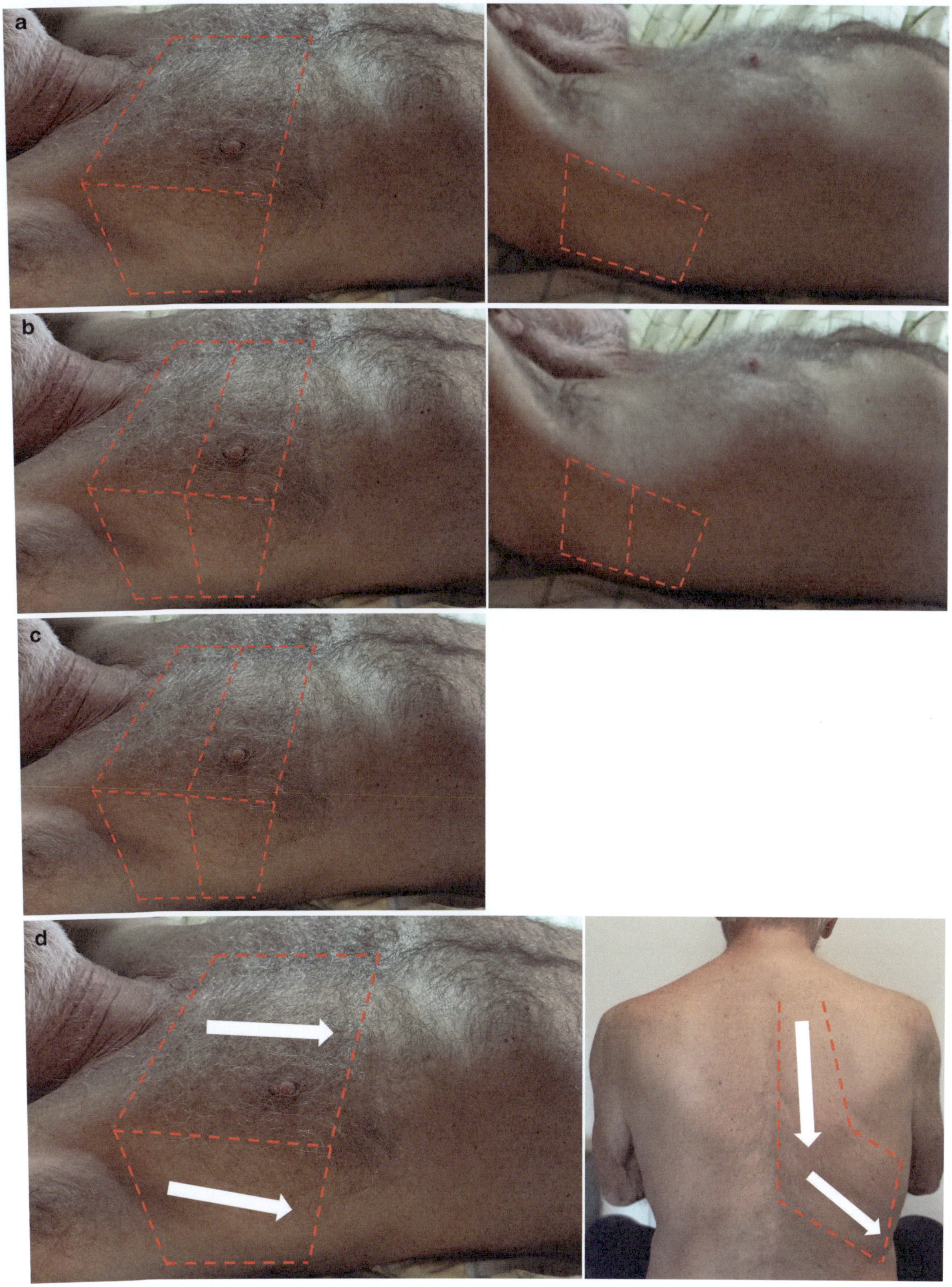

Fig. 7.22 Visualization of the scanning zones for different lung protocols. (**a**) 6-zone BLUE protocol (Three thoracic areas per side: anterior, lateral, and postero-lateral); (**b**) 12-zone protocol from the Volpicelli international consensus (Six thoracic areas per side: anterior, lateral, and postero-lateral, with upper and lower quadrants.); (**c**) 8-zone protocol from Bouhemad et al.: (Four thoracic areas per side: anterior and lateral, with upper and lower quadrants.); (**d**) COVID-19 protocol including the whole chest (scanning in all the intercostal spaces along the mid-clavicular line, midaxillary line, posterior axillary line, and then along the intercostal spaces between the spine and scapula and in the area beneath the scapula)

References

1. Joyner CR, Herman RJ, Reid JM. Reflected ultrasound in the detection and localization of pleural effusion. JAMA. 1967;200(5):399–402.
2. The Association for Medical Ultrasound. Statement and recommendations for safety assurance in lung ultrasound. Available from: https://www.aium.org/resources/official-statements/view/statement-and-recommendations-for-safety-assurance-in-lung-ultrasound. Published July 16, 2023. Accessed September 15, 2024.
3. Duggan NM, Goldsmith AJ, Saud AAA, Ma IWY, Shokoohi H, Liteplo AS. Optimizing lung ultrasound: the effect of depth, gain and focal position on sonographic B-Lines. Ultrasound Med Biol. 2022;48(8):1509–17.
4. Lichtenstein DA, Meziere GA. Relevance of lung ultrasound in the diagnosis of acute respiratory failure: the BLUE protocol. Chest. 2008;134(1):117–25.
5. Volpicelli G, Elbarbary M, Blaivas M, et al. Bedside lung ultrasound in the assessment of alveolar-interstitial syndrome. Am J Emerg Med. 2006;24(6):689–96.
6. Ding W, Shen Y, Yang J, et al. Diagnosis of pneumothorax by radiography and ultrasonography: a meta-analysis. Chest. 2011;140(4):859–66.
7. Alrajab S, Youssef AM, Akkus NI, et al. Pleural ultrasonography versus chest radiography for the diagnosis of pneumothorax: review of the literature and meta-analysis. Crit Care. 2013;17:R208.
8. Avila J, et al. Does the addition of M-mode to B-mode ultrasound increase the accuracy of identification of lung sliding in traumatic pneumothoraces? J Ultrasound Med. 2018;37(11):2681–7.
9. Lichtenstein DA, Mezière GA, Biderman P, Gepner A. The "lung point": an ultrasound sign specific to pneumothorax. Intensive Care Med. 2000;26(10):1434–40.
10. Gillman LM, Alkadi A, Kirkpatrick AW. The "pseudo-lung point" sign: all focal respiratory coupled alternating pleural patterns are not diagnostic of a pneumothorax. J Trauma. 2009;67(3):672–3.
11. Lichtenstein DA, Lascols N, Prin S, Mezière GA. The "lung pulse": an early ultrasound sign of complete atelectasis. Intensive Care Med. 2003;29(12):2187–92.
12. Alerhand S, Tsung JW. Unmasking the lung pulse for detection of endobronchial intubation. J Ultrasound Med. 2020;39(11):2105–9.
13. Volpicelli G, Elbarbary M, Blaivas M, et al. International evidence-based recommendations for point-of-care lung ultrasound. Intensive Care Med. 2012;38(4):577–91.
14. Gargani L, Girerd N, Platz E, et al. Lung ultrasound in acute and chronic heart failure: a clinical consensus statement of the European Association of Cardiovascular Imaging (EACVI). Eur Heart J Cardiovasc Imaging. 2023;24(12):1569–82.
15. Pivetta E, Tizzani M, Porrino G, et al. Lung ultrasound for diagnosis of acute cardiogenic dyspnea in the emergency department—a simeu multicenter study. Crit Ultrasound J. 2014;6:6(S2).
16. Al Deeb M, Barbic S, Featherstone R, Dankoff J, Barbic D. Point-of-care ultrasonography for the diagnosis of acute cardiogenic pulmonary edema in patients presenting with acute dyspnea: a systematic review and meta-analysis. Acad Emerg Med. 2014;21(8):843–52.
17. Anderson KL, Jenq KY, Fields JM, Panebianco NL, Dean AJ. Diagnosing heart failure among acutely dyspneic patients with cardiac, inferior vena cava, and lung ultrasonography. Am J Emerg Med. 2013;31(8):1208–14.
18. Pivetta E, Goffi A, Nazerian P, et al. Lung ultrasound integrated with clinical assessment for the diagnosis of acute decompensated heart failure in the emergency department: a randomized controlled trial. Eur J Heart Fail. 2019;21(6):754–66.
19. Mazzola M, Pugliese NR, Zavagli M, et al. Diagnostic and prognostic value of lung ultrasound B-lines in acute heart failure with concomitant pneumonia. Front Cardiovasc Med. 2021;8:693912.
20. Natanzon A, Kronzon I. Pericardial and pleural effusions in congestive heart failure-anatomical, pathophysiologic, and clinical considerations. Am J Med Sci. 2009;338(3):211–6.
21. Gargani L, Pugliese NR, Frassi F, et al. Prognostic value of lung ultrasound in patients hospitalized for heart disease irrespective of symptoms and ejection fraction. ESC Heart Fail. 2021;8(4):2660–9.
22. Gargani L, Pang PS, Frassi F, et al. Persistent pulmonary congestion before discharge predicts rehospitalization in heart failure: a lung ultrasound study. Cardiovasc Ultrasound. 2015;13(1):33.
23. Coiro S, Rossignol P, Ambrosio G, et al. Prognostic value of residual pulmonary congestion at discharge assessed by lung ultrasound imaging in heart failure. Eur J Heart Fail. 2015;17(11):1172–81.
24. Cogliati C, Casazza G, Ceriani E, et al. Lung ultrasound and short-term prognosis in heart failure patients. Int J Cardiol. 2016;218:104–8.
25. Pugliese NR, Mazzola M, Bandini G, et al. Prognostic role of sonographic decongestion in patients with acute heart failure with reduced and preserved ejection fraction: a multicentre study. J Clin Med. 2023;12(3):773.
26. Pellicori P, et al. Prevalence, pattern and clinical relevance of ultrasound indices of congestion in outpatients with heart failure. Eur J Heart Fail. 2019;21(7):904–16.
27. Rivas-Lasarte M, et al. Lung ultrasound-guided treatment in ambulatory patients with heart failure: a randomized controlled clinical trial (LUS-HF study). Eur J Heart Fail. 2019;21(12):1605–13.
28. Araiza-Garaygordobil D, et al. A randomized controlled trial of lung ultrasound-guided therapy in heart failure (CLUSTER-HF study). Am Heart J. 2020;227:31–9.
29. Marini C, et al. Lung ultrasound guided therapy reduces acute decompensation events in chronic heart failure. Heart. 2020;106(24):1934–9.
30. Reisinger N, Lohani S, Hagemeier J, Panebianco N, Baston C. Lung ultrasound to diagnose pulmonary congestion among patients on hemodialysis: comparison of full versus abbreviated scanning protocols. Am J Kidney Dis. 2022;79(2):193–201.e1.
31. Copetti R, Soldati G, Copetti P. Chest sonography: a useful tool to differentiate acute cardiogenic pulmonary edema from acute respiratory distress syndrome. Cardiovasc Ultrasound. 2008;6(1) https://doi.org/10.1186/1476-7120-6-16.
32. Baldi G, Gargani L, Abramo A, et al. Lung water assessment by lung ultrasonography in intensive care: a pilot study. Intensive Care Med. 2012;39(1):74–84. https://doi.org/10.1007/s00134-012-2694-x.
33. Zoccali C, Torino C, Tripepi R, et al. Pulmonary congestion predicts cardiac events and mortality in ESRD. J Am Soc Nephrol. 2013;24(4):639–46. https://doi.org/10.1681/asn.2012100990.
34. Bouhemad B, Liu ZH, Arbelot C, et al. Ultrasound assessment of antibiotic-induced pulmonary reaeration in ventilator-associated pneumonia. Crit Care Med. 2010;38(1):84–92. https://doi.org/10.1097/ccm.0b013e3181b08cdb.
35. Zhao Z, Jiang L, Xi X, et al. Prognostic value of extravascular lung water assessed with lung ultrasound score by chest sonography in patients with acute respiratory distress syndrome. BMC Pulm Med. 2015;15(1):98. https://doi.org/10.1186/s12890-015-0091-2.
36. Curry S, Tan A, Gargani L, et al. Lung ultrasound and the role of lung aeration score in patients with acute respiratory distress syndrome on extracorporeal membrane oxygenation. Int J Artif Organs. 2021;44(11):854–60. https://doi.org/10.1177/03913988211051395.
37. Costamagna A, Steinberg I, Pivetta E, et al. Clinical performance of lung ultrasound in predicting time-dependent changes in lung aeration in ARDS patients. J Clin Monit Comput. 2022;37(2):473–80. https://doi.org/10.1007/s10877-022-00902-5.
38. Abid I, Qureshi N, Lategan N, Williams S, Shahid S. Point-of-care lung ultrasound in detecting pneumonia: a systematic review. Can J Respir Ther. 2024;60:37–48.

39. Reissig A, et al. Lung ultrasound in the diagnosis and follow-up of community-acquired pneumonia: a prospective, multicenter, diagnostic accuracy study. Chest. 2012;142:965.
40. Bitar ZI, Shamsah M, Maadarani O, Bamasood OM, Bitar AZ, Alfoudri H. Lung ultrasound and sonographic subpleural consolidation in COVID-19 pneumonia correlate with disease severity. Crit Care Res Pract. 2021;2021:1–6. https://doi.org/10.1155/2021/6695033.
41. Nouvenne A, Zani MD, Milanese G, et al. Lung ultrasound in COVID-19 pneumonia: correlations with chest CT on hospital admission. Respiration. 2020;99(7):617–24. https://doi.org/10.1159/000509223.
42. Malla D, Rathi V, Gomber S, Upreti L. Can lung ultrasound differentiate between bacterial and viral pneumonia in children? J Clin Ultrasound. 2021;49(2):91–100. https://doi.org/10.1002/jcu.22951.
43. Stoicescu ER, Iacob R, Ilie AC, et al. Differentiating viral from bacterial pneumonia in children: the diagnostic role of lung ultrasound – a prospective observational study. Diagnostics (Basel). 2024;14(5):480.
44. Tan G, Lian X, Zhu Z, et al. Use of lung ultrasound to differentiate coronavirus disease 2019 (COVID-19) pneumonia from community-acquired pneumonia. Ultrasound Med Biol. 2020;46(10):2651–8. https://doi.org/10.1016/j.ultrasmedbio.2020.05.006.
45. Kim BR, Lee S, Bae H, Lee M, Bahk JH, Yoon S. Lung ultrasound score to determine the effect of fraction inspired oxygen during alveolar recruitment on absorption atelectasis in laparoscopic surgery: a randomized controlled trial. BMC Anesthesiol. 2020;20(1):173. https://doi.org/10.1186/s12871-020-01090-y.
46. Lichtenstein D, Mezière G, Seitz J. The dynamic air bronchogram. Chest. 2009;135(6):1421–5. https://doi.org/10.1378/chest.08-2281.
47. Haaksma ME, Smit JM, Heldeweg MLA, et al. Extended lung ultrasound to differentiate between pneumonia and atelectasis in critically ill patients: a diagnostic accuracy study. Crit Care Med. 2021;50(5):750–9. https://doi.org/10.1097/ccm.0000000000005303.
48. Hosseini M, et al. Diagnostic accuracy of ultrasonography and radiography in detection of pulmonary contusion: a systematic review and meta-analysis. Emerg (Tehran). 2015;3(4):127.
49. Laursen CB, et al. European Respiratory Society statement on thoracic ultrasound. Eur Respir J. 2021;57(3):2001519. https://doi.org/10.1183/13993003.01519-2020.
50. Shkolnik B, et al. Diagnostic accuracy of thoracic ultrasonography to differentiate transudative from exudative pleural effusion. Chest. 2020;158(2):692–7.
51. Dickman E, Terentiev V, Likourezos A, Derman A, Haines L. Extension of the thoracic spine sign: a new sonographic marker of pleural effusion. J Ultrasound Med. 2015;34(9):1555–61.
52. Balik M, et al. Ultrasound estimation of volume of pleural fluid in mechanically ventilated patients. Intensive Care Med. 2006;32:318–21.
53. Eibenberger KL, Dock WI, Ammann ME, Dorffner R, Hörmann MF, Grabenwöger F. Quantification of pleural effusions: sonography versus radiography. Radiology. 1994;191(3):681–4.
54. Ibitoye BO, Idowu BM, Ogunrombi AB, Afolabi BI. Ultrasonographic quantification of pleural effusion: comparison of four formulae. Ultrasonography. 2018;37(3):254–60.
55. Gargani L, Soliman-Aboumarie H, Volpicelli G, Corradi F, Pastore MC, Cameli M. Why, when, and how to use lung ultrasound during the COVID-19 pandemic: enthusiasm and caution. Eur Heart J Cardiovasc Imaging. 2020;21(9):941–8. https://doi.org/10.1093/ehjci/jeaa163.
56. Millington SJ, Koenig S, Mayo P, Volpicelli G. Lung ultrasound for patients with coronavirus disease 2019 pulmonary disease. Chest. 2021;159(1):205–11. https://doi.org/10.1016/j.chest.2020.08.205.
57. Volpicelli G, Gargani L, Perlini S, et al. Lung ultrasound to predict COVID-19 pneumonia: a multicenter descriptive study. SSRN Electron J. 2020; https://doi.org/10.2139/ssrn.3746266.
58. Barnikel M, Alig AHS, Anton S, et al. Follow-up lung ultrasound to monitor lung failure in COVID-19 ICU patients. PLoS One. 2022;17(7):e0271411. https://doi.org/10.1371/journal.pone.0271411.
59. Clofent D, Culebras M, Felipe-Montiel A, et al. Serial lung ultrasound in monitoring viral pneumonia: the lesson learned from COVID-19. ERJ Open Res. 2023;9(4):00017–2023. https://doi.org/10.1183/23120541.00017-2023.
60. Mongodi S, De Vita N, Salve G, et al. The role of lung ultrasound monitoring in early detection of ventilator-associated pneumonia in COVID-19 patients: a retrospective observational study. J Clin Med. 2022;11(11):3001. https://doi.org/10.3390/jcm11113001.
61. Lichter Y, Topilsky Y, Taieb P, et al. Lung ultrasound predicts clinical course and outcomes in COVID-19 patients. Intensive Care Med. 2020;46(10):1873–83. https://doi.org/10.1007/s00134-020-06212-1.
62. Banai A, Lupu L, Shetrit A, et al. Systematic lung ultrasound in Omicron-type vs. wild-type COVID-19. Eur Heart J Cardiovasc Imaging. 2022;24(1):59–67. https://doi.org/10.1093/ehjci/jeac212.
63. Awais M, Salam B, Nadeem N, Rehman A, Baloch NU. Diagnostic accuracy of computed tomography scout film and chest X-ray for detection of rib fractures in patients with chest trauma: a cross-sectional study. Cureus. 2019;11:e3875. https://doi.org/10.7759/cureus.3875.
64. Griffith JF, Rainer TH, Ching AS, Law KL, Cocks RA, Metreweli C. Sonography compared with radiography in revealing acute rib fracture. AJR Am J Roentgenol. 1999;173(6):1603–9. https://doi.org/10.2214/ajr.173.6.10584808.
65. Bouhemad B, Mongodi S, Via G, Rouquette I. Ultrasound for "lung monitoring" of ventilated patients. Anesthesiology. 2015;122(2):437–47. https://doi.org/10.1097/aln.0000000000000558.
66. Jambrik Z, et al. Usefulness of ultrasound lung comets as a nonradiologic sign of extravascular lung water. Am J Cardiol. 2004;93(10):1265–70.
67. Buessler A, et al. Accuracy of several lung ultrasound methods for the diagnosis of acute heart failure in the ED: a multicenter prospective study. Chest. 2020;157(1):99–110.
68. Barskova T, et al. Lung ultrasound for the screening of interstitial lung disease in very early systemic sclerosis. Ann Rheum Dis. 2013;72(3):390–5.
69. Gargani L, et al. Lung ultrasound B-lines in systemic sclerosis: cut-off values and methodological indications for interstitial lung disease screening. Rheumatology (Oxford). 2022;61(SI):SI56–64.
70. Volpicelli G, et al. Lung ultrasound for the early diagnosis of COVID-19 pneumonia: an international multicenter study. Intensive Care Med. 2021;47(4):444–54.
71. Tung-Chen Y, et al. The impact of different lung ultrasound protocols in the assessment of lung lesions in COVID-19 patients: is there an ideal lung ultrasound protocol? J Ultrasound. 2022;25(3):483–91.
72. Pellicori PP, et al. Ultrasound imaging of congestion in heart failure: examinations beyond the heart. Eur J Heart Fail. 2021;23(5):703–12.
73. Volpicelli G, et al. Decreased sensitivity of lung ultrasound limited to the anterior chest in emergency department diagnosis of cardiogenic pulmonary edema: a retrospective analysis. Crit Ultrasound J. 2010;2:47–52.
74. Qadir, et al. An update on management of adult patients with acute respiratory distress syndrome: an official American Thoracic Society clinical practice guideline. AJRCCM. 2024;

75. Bouhemad, et al. Bedside ultrasound assessment of positive end-expiratory pressure-induced lung recruitment. AJRCCM. 2011;183:341.
76. Stefanidis, et al. Lung sonography and recruitment in patients with early acute respiratory distress syndrome: a pilot study. Crit Care. 2011;15
77. Cavalcanti AB, et al. Effect of lung recruitment and titrated positive end-expiratory pressure (PEEP) vs low PEEP on mortality in patients with acute respiratory distress syndrome: a randomized clinical trial. JAMA. 2017;
78. Rode, et al. Positive end-expiratory pressure lung recruitment: comparison between lower inflection point and ultrasound assessment. Wien Klin Wochenschr. 2012;124:842.
79. Jardin F, et al. Is there a safe plateau pressure in ARDS? The right heart only knows. Intensive Care Med. 2007;33:444.
80. Gernoth C. Respiratory and haemodynamic changes during decremental open lung positive end-expiratory pressure titration in patients with acute respiratory distress syndrome. Crit Care. 2009;13:R59.
81. Monnet X, et al. The passive leg raising test to guide fluid removal in critically ill patients. Ann Intensive Care. 2016;6:46.
82. Papanikolaou J, et al. New insights into weaning from mechanical ventilation: left ventricular diastolic dysfunction is a key player. Intensive Care Med. 2011;37:1976.
83. de Meirelles Almeida CA, et al. Diastolic dysfunction as a predictor of weaning failure: a systematic review and meta-analysis. J Crit Care. 2016;34:135.
84. Allyn J, et al. Echocardiography to predict tolerance to negative fluid balance in acute respiratory distress syndrome/acute lung injury. J Crit Care. 2013;28:1006.
85. Alam MJ, Roy S, Iktidar MA, et al. Diaphragm ultrasound as a better predictor of successful extubation from mechanical ventilation than rapid shallow breathing index. Acute Crit Care. 2022;37(1):94–100. https://doi.org/10.4266/acc.2021.01354.
86. Parada-Gereda HM, Tibaduiza AL, Rico-Mendoza A, et al. Effectiveness of diaphragmatic ultrasound as a predictor of successful weaning from mechanical ventilation: a systematic review and meta-analysis. Crit Care. 2023;27:174. https://doi.org/10.1186/s13054-023-04430-9.

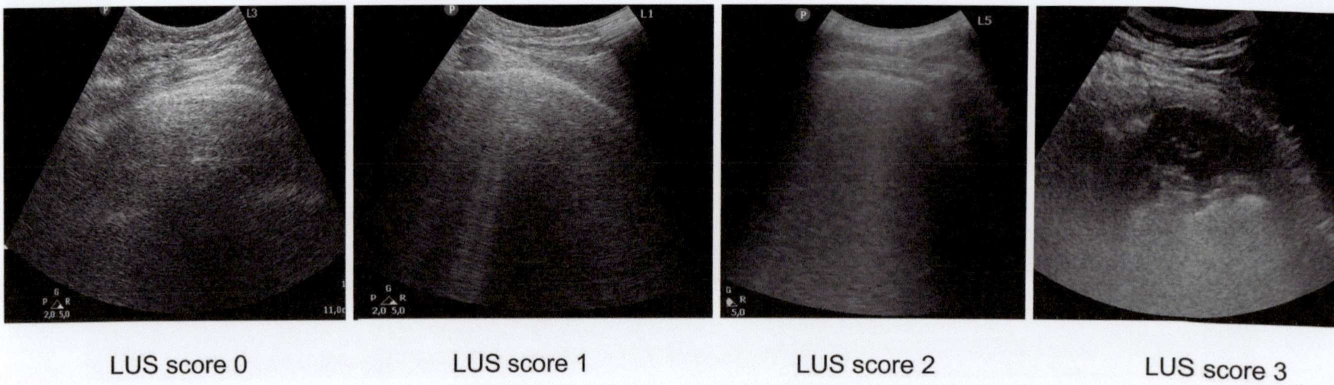

Fig. 7.23 Demonstration of the scoring system which assigns 0 points to A lines, 1 point to discrete B-lines, 2 points to coalescent B-lines, and 3 points to consolidation

Numerous scoring systems have been developed for lung ultrasound. The Lung Ultrasound (LUS) score has been used in patients with ARDS to determine the degree of lung aeration. The LUS score is calculated by assigning a number from 0 to 3 according to the different patterns (Fig. 7.23). A higher score indicates a worse degree of deaeration. This score can be used to assess changes in aeration and lung recruitment over time [65].

Quantification of B-lines can also be useful for monitoring decongestion in patients with heart failure, as well as responsiveness to intravenous diuresis or noninvasive positive pressure ventilation [72]. The number of B-lines has proved to be related to pulmonary congestion and have a clear prognostic role [14].

When B-lines can be counted one-by one as single artifacts, the total number is defined as the sum of all B-lines simultaneously present in the worst frame (i.e., when the most B-lines are simultaneously present). When B-lines become confluent, the percentage of the "white" part of the screen below the pleural line is divided by 10 (e.g., if 70% of the screen below the pleural line is composed of confluent B-lines, the number of B-lines is 7).

In addition to B-line quantification, distribution of B-lines can also be useful. In the case of cardiogenic pulmonary edema, B-lines in the upper anterior chest usually depict a more severe degree of pulmonary edema, whereas B-lines limited to the dependent zones of the chest are considered less severe [73].

Ventilator Management

At present, the use of lung POCUS to guide ventilator management is evolving and should not replace general clinical guidelines that favor low tidal volume ventilation, higher positive end-expiratory pressure (PEEP), and avoidance of large recruitment maneuvers [74]. Many of the concepts discussed in this section are provided to stimulate thought and prompt further investigation but are not yet ready for routine clinical use.

One of the more interesting applications is its use in alveolar recruitment or targeting of PEEP. Historically, ventilatory management in ARDS involved examination of the lung hysteresis curve (i.e., the pressure-volume loop). Ventilator settings were adjusted to avoid atelectasis or overdistention based on calculations of compliance. One challenge with this analysis is that it typically requires deep sedation or chemical paralysis, therapies decreasingly present in modern ARDS management that favor less sedation.

Emerging evidence suggests that ultrasound might be able to assess lung recruitment in ARDS patients. In a study of 30 patients with acute lung injury, investigators scored 12 lung areas at PEEP of 0 and 15 cm H_2O, on a scale from normal aeration, moderate aeration loss, severe loss, and consolidation [75]. They created a lung reaeration score based on how much change occurred at these lung areas. They simultaneously measured the volume of PEEP-induced lung recruitment using the ventilator pressure-volume curve method. This score was highly correlated with PEEP-induced recruitment ($\rho = 0.88$, $p < 0.0001$). A lung reaeration score $\geq +8$ was associated with recruitment ≥ 600 mL. Lung reaeration score was correlated with PEEP-induced increase in PaO_2 ($\rho = 0.63$, $P < 0.05$). Another study of 17 patients with acute lung injury were assessed using a high-frequency linear probe to measure subpleural consolidations and titrated PEEP until the consolidations reduced to nearly gone or PEEP reached 22 cm H_2O [76]. Of the 48 consolidations measured, only 4 were not recruitable.

These techniques seem promising in that lung ultrasound could be used to quantify the amount of aeration loss and potential for recruitment. However, lung ultrasound at present is not able to identify lung hyperinflation. Additionally, recruitment maneuvers have been associated with increased harm in patients with ARDS [77]. Hypotension is a common complication associated with lung recruitment, and occurred frequently in one of the PEEP titration studies using lung ultrasound [78]. A possible strategy to safeguard against this could include assessment of the right ventricle during PEEP titration [79]. The right ventricular area increases with recruitment and may indicate impending hemodynamic collapse [80]. Additionally, echocardiographic assessments of ventricular filling pressures or volume responsiveness might offer additional insights into diuresis and liberation from the ventilator [81–84].

Diaphragmatic Ultrasound for Liberation from Mechanical Ventilation

Ultrasound assessment of diaphragmatic excursion and the thickening fraction have predicted successful extubation from mechanical ventilation. In one study, these assessments were found to outperform common measures such as the Rapid Shallow Breathing Index [85]. A meta-analysis of 19 studies found that diaphragmatic excursion was 80% sensitive and 80% specific, whereas thickening fraction was 85% sensitive and 75% specific [86].

For diaphragmatic excursion, use a curvilinear probe with the patient semirecumbent at a 45-degree angle. The probe is placed between the eighth and ninth ribs at the costal margin between the midclavicular and anterior axillary lines. Measurement will occur using either the spleen or the liver as an acoustic window. Imaging should be performed in M-mode, looking for the hyperechoic diaphragm. Adjust the sweep speed to allow for at least one respiratory cycle. The threshold for diaphragmatic excursion depends on the desired sensitivity and specificity for predicting success in weaning from mechanical ventilation, with a threshold of ≤10 mm being most common (Fig. 7.24 and Video 7.22) [86].

For diaphragmatic thickness, use a linear probe with the patient semirecumbent in a 45-degree angle. The probe is placed at the zone of apposition, between the eighth and tenth intercostal spaces, at the midaxillary line or slightly ventral. The diaphragm is the hypoechoic band between the hyperechoic lines of the pleura and peritoneum. Imaging should be performed in M-mode adjusting the sweep speed for at least one respiratory cycle (Fig. 7.25 and Video 7.23). The threshold for diaphragmatic thickness similarly depends on the application, with a threshold of <20% increase at end-inspiration compared to end-expiration typically used for identification of paralysis in a spontaneously breathing patient [86].

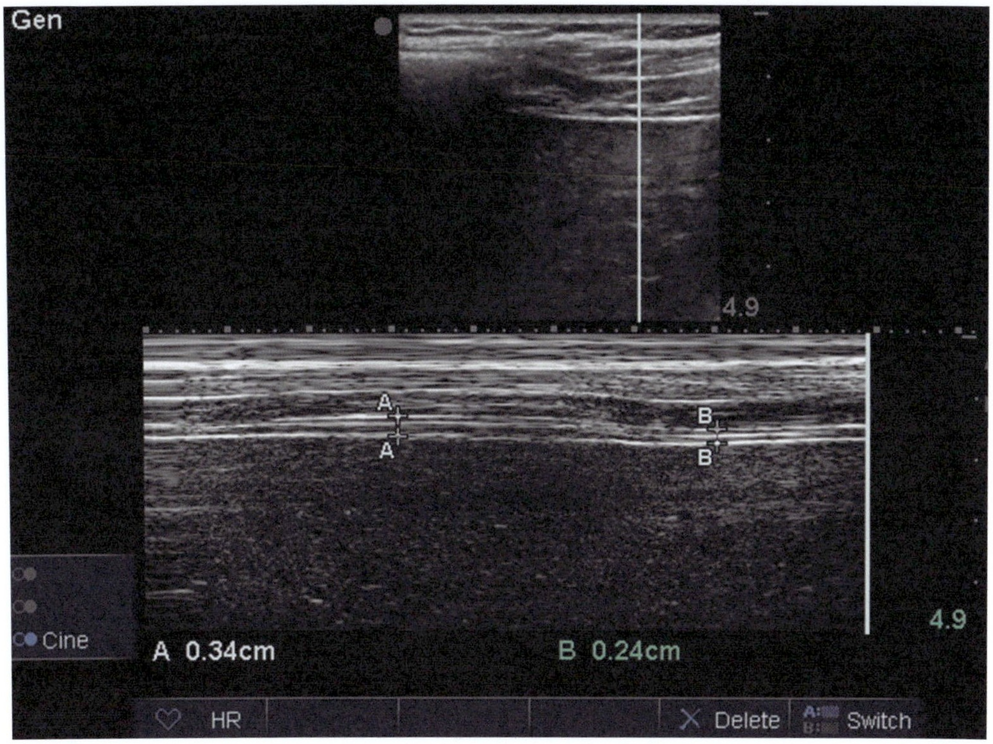

Fig. 7.24 M-mode of diaphragmatic excursion during spontaneous breathing

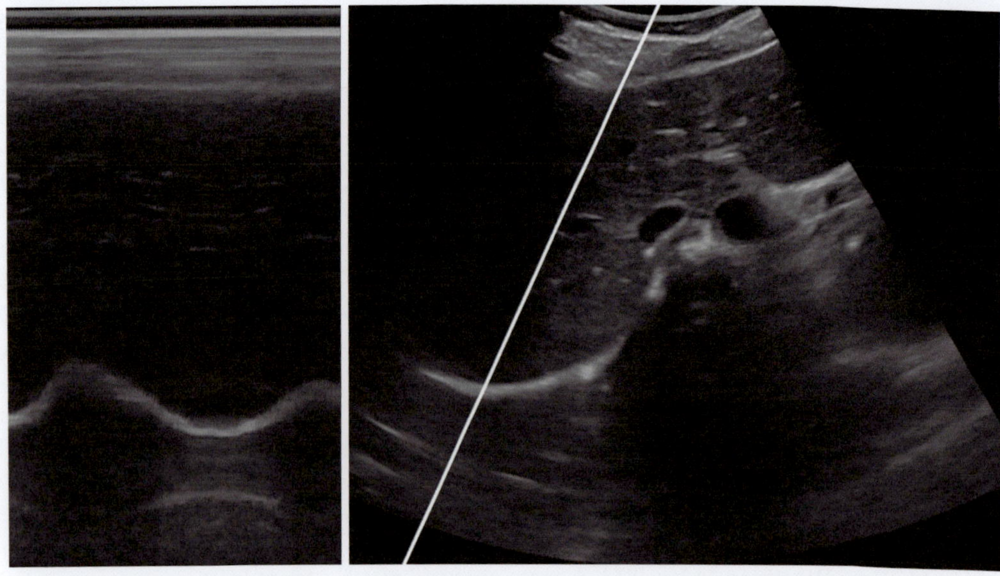

Fig. 7.25 M-Mode imaging of normal diaphragmatic thickening showing a full respiratory cycle

Key Ultrasound Findings

Diagnosis	Sonographic findings
Pneumothorax	Absence of lung sliding on B-mode or M-mode. Identification of lung point (intersection of pneumothorax and normal lung). Absence of lung pulse (rhythmic pulsations from the heart beats).
Pulmonary Edema	B-lines are vertical, hyperechoic artifacts suggestive of pulmonary edema. ≥3 B-lines is suggestive of pulmonary edema. Typically located in a gravity-related, bilateral distribution.
Pneumonia	≥3 B-lines in a single region. May have consolidations or air bronchograms.
Atelectasis	Static air bronchograms, typically located in lower lung fields. Can also present with consolidated lung in the context of a large pleural effusion.
Pulmonary Contusion	≥3 B-lines in a single region corresponding to an area of direct trauma.
Pleural Effusion	Anechoic fluid located above the diaphragm. Positive spine sign (visualization of the spine above the diaphragm). Absence of mirror artifact (visualization of abdominal structures mirrored above the diaphragm).
COVID-19 Pneumonia	B-lines with focal spared areas. Pleural line irregularity with subpleural consolidations.
Rib Fracture	Cortical irregularity in the bone best seen in the long-axis.
Diaphragmatic Excursion	Measured using M-mode with abnormal <10 mm.
Diaphragmatic Thickness	Measured using M-mode with abnormal <20% at end-inspiration compared to end-expiration.

Pearls and Pitfalls

- Ensure that the anchoring anatomy of the ribs are used to identify the pleura and avoid misidentifying other structures, such as subcutaneous emphysema.
- Beware of the pneumothorax mimics (e.g., endobronchial intubation, bullous emphysema, low tidal volume ventilation, pleurodesis) and consider this in the context of patient presentation and alternate findings (e.g., lung pulse, B-lines, Z-lines).
- Measure B-lines based on the maximal number simultaneously present in a single frame to avoid double-counting B-lines.
- Consider the distribution in addition to the number of B-lines to assess the etiology and severity of pulmonary edema.
- Multiple scanning protocols exist. Base the protocol on patient factors (e.g., positioning, body habitus) and the specific pathology (e.g., pneumonia, pulmonary edema, ARDS).
- Ensure that the diaphragm is visualized to avoid imitators of pleural effusion or basilar consolidation.

Ultrasound of the Aorta

8

Tomislav Jelic and Penelope C. Lema

Background

Diseases of the aorta can be catastrophic, yet challenging to diagnose if the clinician does not have a high suspicion. The incidence of aortic dissection in the general population is 2.6–3.5 per 100,000 person-years, and carries a mortality rate of 0.12% per hour [1–3]. At least 50% of aortic dissections originate near the sino-tubular junction [4]. Another 20–30% originate near the left subclavian artery with extension into the abdominal aorta [1]. Risk factors for the development of aortic dissection include hypertension, connective tissue disorders (e.g., Ehlers-Danlos, Marfan syndrome), aortic aneurysm, bicuspid aortic valve, trauma, or use of fluoroquinolones [1].

Aneurysms can involve any portion of the aorta. Risk factors for the development of an aortic aneurysm include smoking, hypertension, atherosclerosis, and advanced age. Abdominal aortic aneurysms (AAA) are far more common than thoracic aortic aneurysms [3]. The most common site of an AAA is the infra-renal portion of the aorta. Asymptomatic AAA often goes unnoticed until a critical size is reached. Symptomatic patients can present with abdominal or flank pain and organ or limb ischemia. In cases where AAA ruptures, patients can present in shock, with worsening abdominal pain, back pain, or cardiac arrest.

Isolated iliac artery aneurysms (IAA) are uncommon; however, the incidence is much higher if a concurrent AAA is present [2]. Clinical presentations can include abdominal, groin, or thigh pain. An expanding IAA can also cause compression of surrounding structures such as the ureter, colon, or lumbar plexus.

Point-of-care ultrasound (POCUS) allows for rapid, early assessment for aortic pathology. It is particularly helpful at the bedside in patients who are critically ill or too unstable to undergo advanced imaging, such as computed tomography (CT), or have a contraindication to contrast imaging such as a significant dye allergy. A systematic review demonstrated that POCUS has a high degree of diagnostic accuracy to identify aneurysms with 98% sensitivity and 97% specificity [4]. Patients who received POCUS compared to CT imaging had a 20–60% reduction in mortality due to rapid diagnosis and faster time to definitive management [5, 6]. Transthoracic echocardiography (TTE) carries a sensitivity ranging from 87% to 96% for type A and 60–83% for type B aortic dissection [7]. POCUS-performed assessment for aortic dissection has been shown to be 93.2% sensitive and 90.9% specific [8]. POCUS for aortic dissection also demonstrated faster time to diagnosis when compared to POCUS not being performed [9] Transesophageal echocardiography (TEE) carries a higher sensitivity of 98% and specificity of 95% for identifying aortic dissection due to its close proximity and nearly complete visualization of the thoracic aorta [10]. As TEE is already covered in Chap. 6, this chapter will focus on the noninvasive POCUS assessment of the aorta.

Indications

Indications
- Chest pain or abdominal pain, especially in the presence of back pain
- Neurologic symptoms especially if associated with chest pain
- New murmur (e.g., diastolic murmur aortic regurgitation)
- Undifferentiated hypotension
- Pulse deficit
- Syncope
- Cardiac arrest

Diagnoses
- Thoracic Aortic Aneurysm
- Abdominal Aortic Aneurysm
- Aortic Dissection

Supplementary Information The online version contains supplementary material available at https://doi.org/10.1007/978-3-031-85308-1_8.

T. Jelic (✉)
Department of Emergency Medicine, University of Manitoba, Winnipeg, Canada

P. C. Lema
Department of Emergency Medicine, Columbia University Vagelos College of Physicians and Surgeons, New York, NY, USA
e-mail: PCL2124@cumc.columbia.edu

M. Gottlieb, N. Panebianco (eds.), *Advanced Point-of-Care Ultrasound*, https://doi.org/10.1007/978-3-031-85308-1_8

Core Views

<table>
<tr><th>View</th><th>Image</th><th>Approach</th></tr>
<tr><td>Parasternal Long-axis (PLAX)</td><td>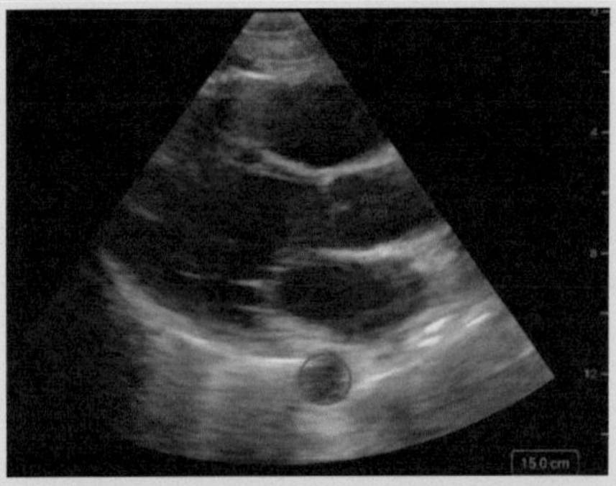

Core View 1. Parasternal long-axis demonstrating the aortic root and descending aorta</td><td>Technique
From the traditional cardiac PLAX view, slide one intercostal space superiorly or toward the sternum to image more of the ascending aorta.

Anatomy Visualized
Aortic root
Descending aorta</td></tr>
<tr><td>Parasternal Short-axis (PSAX)</td><td>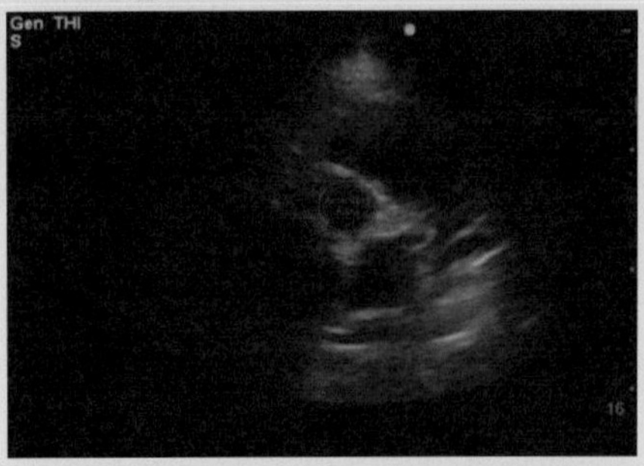

Core View 2. Parasternal short-axis demonstrating ascending aorta in cross-section</td><td>Technique
From the traditional cardiac PSAX view, slide the probe toward the sternum to visualize the aortic valve in cross-section.

Anatomy Visualized
Aortic valve
Aortic root
Ascending aorta</td></tr>
<tr><td>Apical 4-Chamber (A4C)</td><td>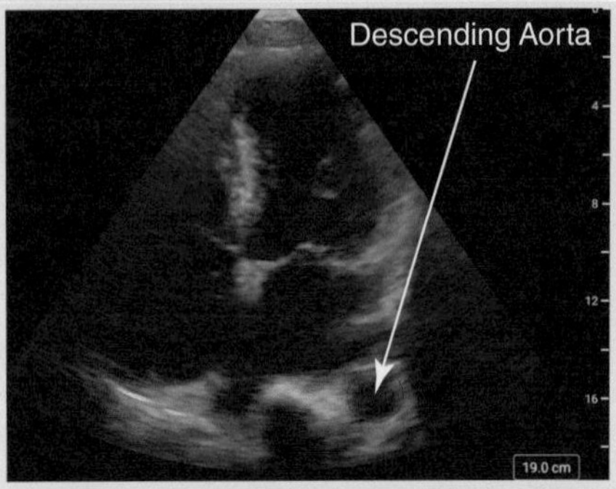

Core View 3. Apical 4-chamber demonstrating the descending aorta in short axis</td><td>Technique
Within the traditional A4C view, rock the probe to use the left atrium as a window to the descending aorta.

Anatomy Visualized
Descending aorta</td></tr>
<tr><td>Apical 5-Chamber (A5C)</td><td>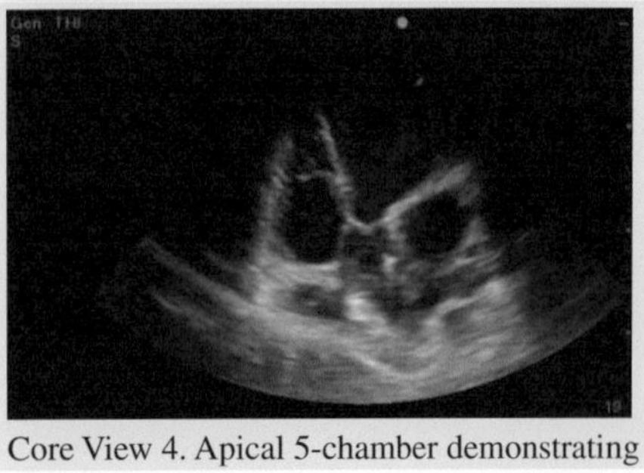
Core View 4. Apical 5-chamber demonstrating the aortic root</td><td>Technique
From the A4C view, fan the base of probe anteriorly until the left ventricular outflow tract appears in view.

Anatomy Visualized
Aortic root
Descending aorta</td></tr>
</table>

View	Image	Approach
Suprasternal Notch (SSN)	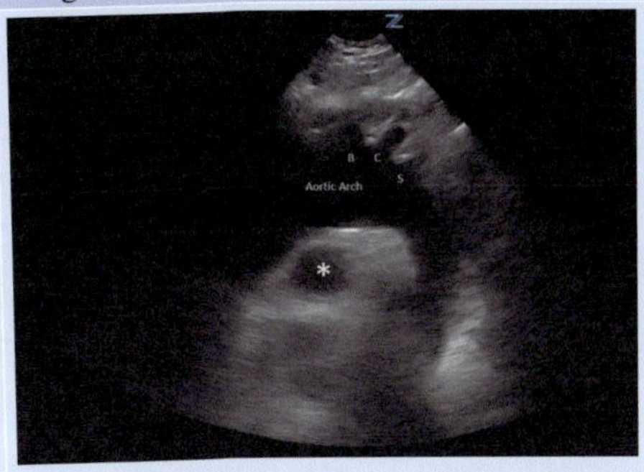 Core View 5. Suprasternal notch view demonstrating the aortic arch, brachiocephalic artery, left common carotid artery, and left subclavian artery. The right pulmonary artery is denoted with an asterisk	*Technique* Extend the patient's neck in the supine position with a pillow under the shoulders. Use a cardiac or vascular preset on the phased array probe with indicator directed toward patient's left ear or shoulder. *Anatomy Visualized* Ascending aorta Aortic arch Brachiocephalic artery Left common carotid artery Left subclavian artery Descending aorta

The Aorta

The aorta begins its course with three major branches: the innominate or brachiocephalic trunk (which divides into the right common carotid artery and right subclavian artery), left common carotid artery, and left subclavian artery. The descending (or thoracic) aorta extends from the aortic arch at the level of T4 to transition to the abdominal aorta at the level of T12. The abdominal aorta terminates at the level of L4 or umbilicus and bifurcates into the right and left iliac arteries (Fig. 8.1). The standard approach to ultrasound measurements of the diameter of the aorta is described in Table 8.1.

Thoracic Aorta

The clinical assessment should guide the segment of the aorta imaged and in which sequence. The thoracic aorta can be imaged sonographicallyin the parasternal long-axis (PLAX), parasternal short-axis (PSAX), suprasternal notch view (SSN), and apical 4-chamber (A4C) view. The thoracic aorta can be divided into three sections: the ascending aorta (which includes the aortic root and tubular ascending aorta), the aortic arch, and the descending thoracic aorta.

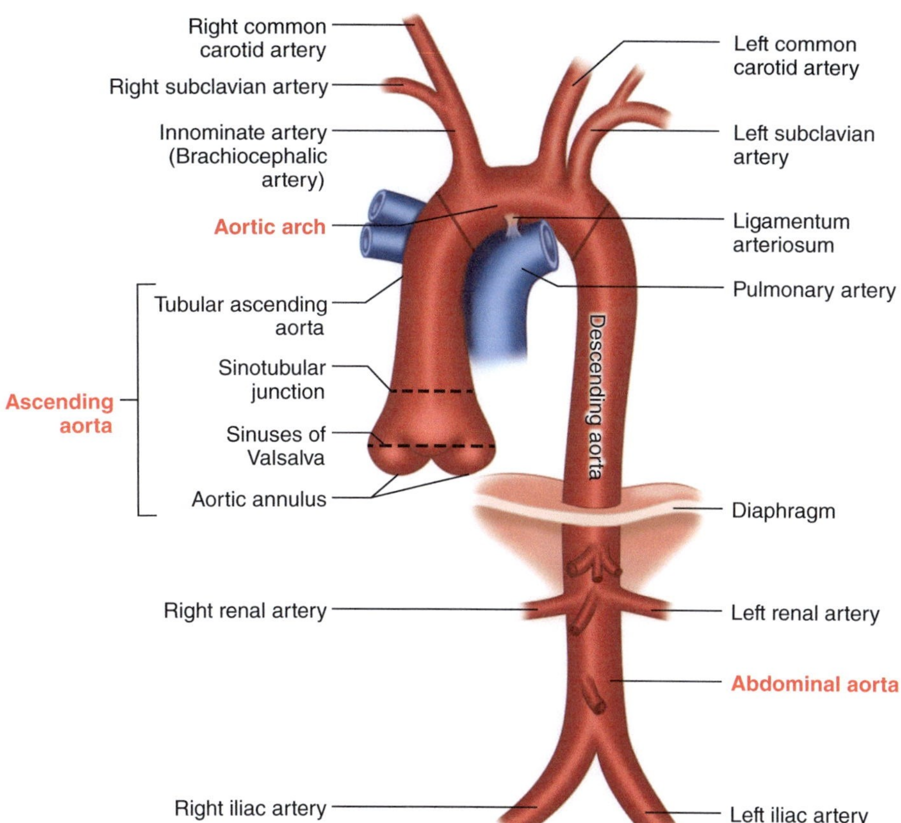

Fig. 8.1 Anatomy of the thoracic aorta

Table 8.1 Recommendations for ultrasound measurements of aorta diameter

Location	Measurement	Cardiac cycle
LVOT, Annulus	Inner wall to inner wall	Mid-systole
Sinus of Valsalva, Proximal Aorta	Leading edge to leading edge	End-diastole
Abdominal Aorta	Outer wall to outer wall	N/A

LVOT left ventricular outflow tract, *N/A* not applicable

The aortic root is a unique anatomical structure that connects the heart to the systemic circulation. The aortic root primarily consists of the annulus, the sinus of Valsalva, and the sinotubular junction. The annulus is the area where the aortic valve leaflets attach to the aortic wall and form a crown-shaped, thickened fibrous structure. The commissures are the spaces between each anchored leaflet. The three bulges of the aortic wall just distal to the aortic valve annulus are called the *sinus of Valsalva* (also known as the aortic sinuses), which is the widest cross-sectional diameter of the aortic root. The origin of the coronary arteries is located in two of the three sinuses. The left and right sinus each contain their respective coronary artery ostia, whereas the posterior sinus is referred to as the noncoronary sinus. The sinotubular junction (also called the sinotubular ridge) is where the sinuses taper off and meet the tubular ascending aorta. The aortic arch continues from the ascending aorta at the level of the second sternocostal joint and ends approximately at the level of the T4 vertebrae.

The SSN view may be helpful in evaluating the aortic arch and is obtained using a phased-array probe placed in the sternal notch (Fig. 8.2). The probe marker is pointed to the patient's left ear or shoulder, with the image or orientation marker on the right side of the screen if following the cardiology convention of image acquisition. The SSN view provides a sonographic image of the ascending, arch, and descending portions of the aorta. To improve this view, the patient can lean forward but ensure the probe is as close to the neck as possible to obtain a long-axis view of the aortic arch. Ascending and descending diameters can be variable and differ based on anatomical location and sex (Table 8.2).

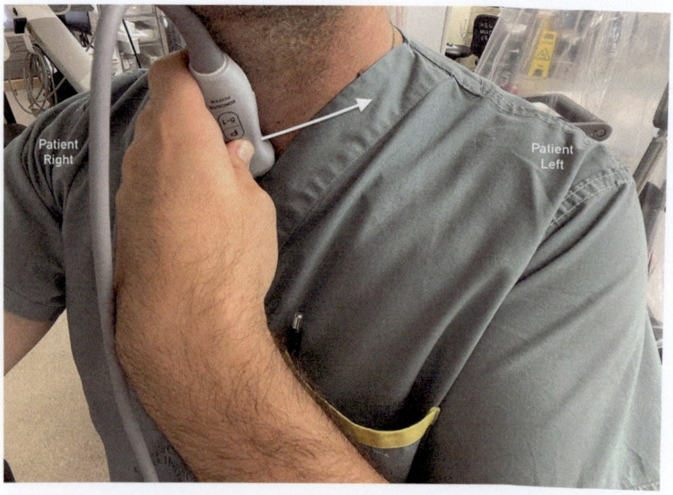

Fig. 8.2 Probe placement to obtain the suprasternal notch view. Refer to the SSN core views table to review the sonographic appearance of the suprasternal notch view

Table 8.2 Average ascending and descending aortic sizes based on sex and anatomic location [11, 12]

Anatomic location	Male	Female
Aorta Sinus	3.63–3.91 cm	3.5–3.72 cm
Ascending Aorta	2.86 cm	2.86 cm
Mid-Descending Aorta	2.39–2.98 cm	2.45–2.64 cm
At the Level of the Diaphragm	2.43–2.69 cm	2.40–2.44 cm

Abdominal Aorta

The abdominal aorta is located in the retroperitoneum and has many branches, some of which may be visualized on ultrasound (Fig. 8.3). It lies anterior and slightly to the left of the anterior part of the lumbar vertebrae, with the inferior vena cava (IVC) located to its right. Initial sonographic assessment of the abdominal aorta should begin proximally at the costal margin just beneath the subxiphoid in a transverse orientation with the indicator to the patient's right using the abdominal or aorta preset. The gain should be adjusted to allow for clear differentiation of the aortic wall from the lumen. The depth should be set such that the aorta is maximized in the field of view. Depth should be adjusted to optimize visualization as the probe moves distally toward the bifurcation. The vertebral body is a major landmark that should be localized to aid in the identification of the aorta, as the aorta is always just anterior to the spine. The sonographic appearance of the vertebral body is a very distinct hyperechoic upside down U-shaped structure with dense shadowing below it.

The abdominal aorta can be subdivided into three key areas: proximal, middle, and distal. The celiac trunk is located in the most proximal segment of the abdominal aorta and has three major branches: the left gastric artery, hepatic artery, and splenic artery. Often, only the hepatic artery and splenic artery branches may be visualized and form what is referred to as the "seagull sign." The mid-portion of the abdominal aorta is located at the level of the superior mesenteric (SMA) which is approximately 2–3 cm distal to the celiac trunk (Fig. 8.4 and Video 8.1). The distal abdominal aorta extends below the renal arteries to the level of the bifurcation (at the level of the umbilicus) into the right and left iliac arteries.

Image acquisition of the abdominal aorta should include both the short- and long-axis views with measurements obtained of the aorta diameter, typically in the short-axis

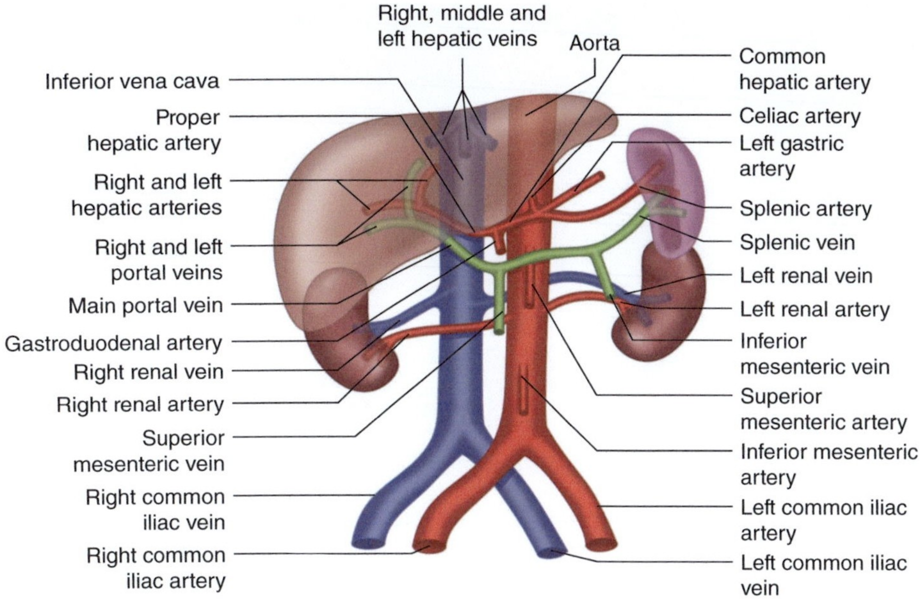

Fig. 8.3 Anatomy of the abdominal aorta

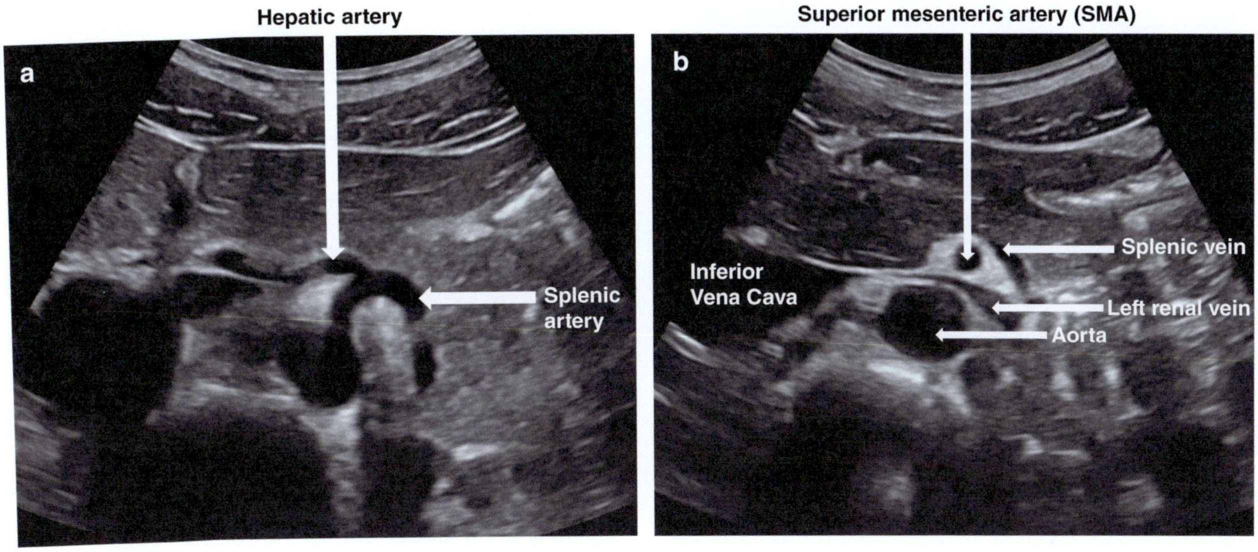

Fig. 8.4 Abdominal aorta. (**a**) Proximal abdominal aorta with the celiac trunk and hepatic and splenic artery branches visible, creating the "seagull sign." (**b**) Sonographic anatomy of the mid-abdominal aorta with the superior mesenteric artery parallel to the aorta and sandwiched between the left renal vein and splenic vein

view. This allows for a more complete assessment of the aorta and the ability to define if the AAA is fusiform or saccular. Fusiform aneurysms involve the entire circumference of the aorta, whereas saccular aneurysms tend to be isolated areas of outpouching. The abdominal aorta should always be measured from the outer-to-outer edge. This is critical to avoid underestimating the size, which can lead to a false negative assessment for AAA due to inadvertent measurement of the internal lumen of the aorta and not identifying the surrounding hematoma (Fig. 8.5). The abdominal aorta should be less than 3 cm in diameter, and each iliac artery should be less than 1.5 cm in diameter. Both common iliac arteries should be assessed for at least the first 5 cm after the bifurcation point. The right and left common iliac arteries should be measured at the same imaging level when possible.

Bowel gas can hinder the assessment of the aorta. To definitively exclude AAA, the entire abdominal aorta must be visualized. To overcome the artifacts of bowel gas, one can utilize graded compression of the abdomen with the probe to displace gas, or slide laterally away from the bowel gas and rock the probe toward the aorta to obtain a paramedian view. The patient can also flex their knees to relax the abdominal wall muscles and allow more optimal abdominal compression to displace bowel gas.

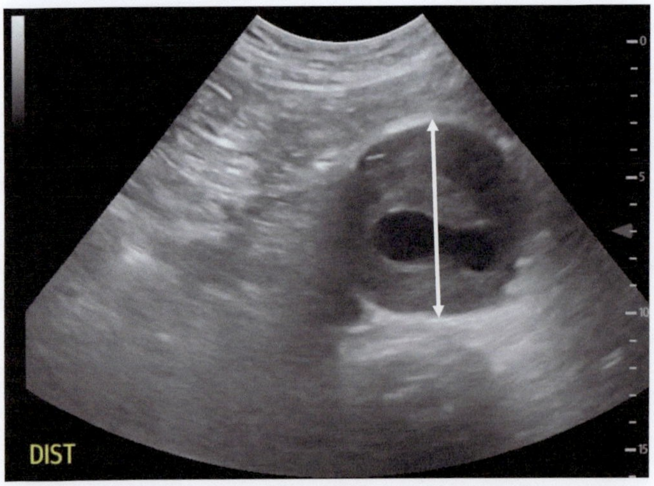

Fig. 8.5 Abdominal aortic aneurysm with a thrombus. The red line demonstrates the proper measurement of the diameter from outer wall to outer wall

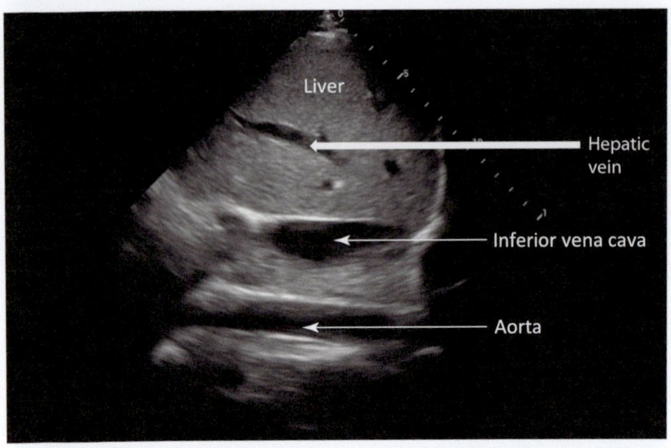

Fig. 8.6 Coronal view of the aorta obtained in the left lateral decubitus position with probe placement similar to the right upper quadrant view in the FAST examination

While a slow and methodical approach is important, the patient's clinical status may dictate otherwise. In situations of profound hemodynamic instability or cardiac arrest, we suggest a rapid slide of the probe in the short-axis orientation from the xiphoid process distally to the umbilicus to identify any visible AAA. The coronal view is an additional view of the aorta that is less commonly performed. It is obtained similar to the right upper quadrant view for the FAST examination, but the patient should be in the left lateral decubitus position. This view may be helpful if bowel gas makes ultrasound imaging impossible with the anterior abdominal views. The depth may need to be increased, and the probe may need to be positioned more posteriorly and fanned more anteriorly. The IVC will be anterior to the aorta in this view (Fig. 8.6).

Clinical Applications

Aortic Dissection

In 70–80% of cases, the primary event of an aortic dissection is a tear within the intimal layer [13]. As blood passes through a small tear in the intima, a dissection plane develops within the media, leading to a separation between the media and adventitia, creating a false lumen (Fig. 8.7). As the false lumen dilates, the true lumen collapses and there is an increase in the cross-sectional area of the aorta. The increase in the false lumen size correlates directly with blood pressure and heart rate, increasing the extent of the aorta involved. Both are related to the shear forces experienced by the aorta at these anatomic locations. Aortic dissections can be classified as Stanford Type A (any involvement proximal to the left subclavian artery) or Stanford Type B (isolated involvement distal to the left subclavian artery). This classification is important, as Type A dissection requires operative repair, whereas Type B can often be managed medically.

If there is any concern for an aortic dissection, imaging should start with the PLAX view as it allows immediate assessment of the aortic root for dilation or dissection (Fig. 8.8 and Video 8.2). To improve visualization of the aortic root, place the probe in an intercostal space higher or slide it toward the sternum, as the aorta is a cephalic structure. Type A dissection involves the ascending aorta to the proximal aspect of the left subclavian branch and can be identified using the PLAX or the SSN views.

Type B dissections will involve the aorta distal to the left subclavian branch point. The descending aorta can be difficult to visualize. Using the PLAX, PSAX, and A4C views, small portions of the aorta can be visualized and assessed for the presence of a dissection. If there is suspicion of a Type B dissection, the abdominal aorta should be assessed as well (Fig. 8.9 and Video 8.3).

If a dissection flap is encountered, color flow or pulsed-wave Doppler can be used to diagnose this and to distinguish between the true and false lumens (Fig. 8.10 and Video 8.4). The true lumen maintains brisk antegrade flow with the flap moving toward the false lumen during systole. Aliasing may be present due to the increased velocity of blood flow through a narrowed vessel lumen. The false lumen will have slow blood flow, which may demonstrate an echogenic swirling pattern of flow due to red blood cell aggregation in low-velocity blood flow on B-mode (also known as spontaneous echo contrast) and will enlarge in size during diastole. If no blood flow is visualized, a thrombosed lumen may be present. If the aorta is imaged at 90 degrees of insonation, this can produce an inadvertent false negative result as no Doppler signal will be detectable.

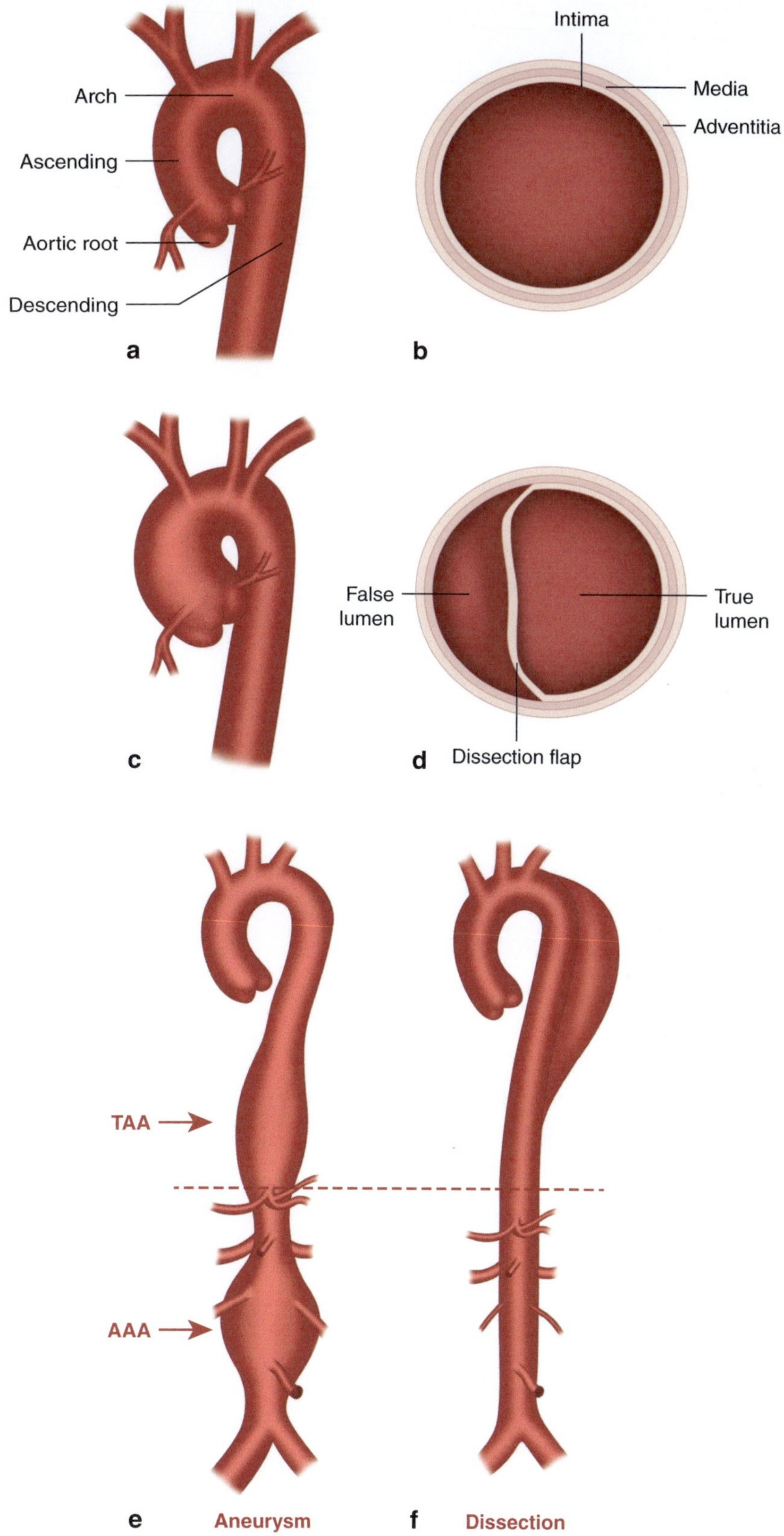

Fig. 8.7 Diagram of the aorta demonstrating normal anatomy and aortic dissection. (**a**) Normal aorta with labeled sections. (**b**) Normal aorta in cross-section. (**c**) Ascending aortic dissection. (**d**) Cross-section of aortic dissection with visualized true lumen, false lumen, and dissection flap. (**e**) Illustration of thoracic aortic aneurysm (TAA) and abdominal aortic aneurysm (AAA). (**f**) Illustration of aortic dissection

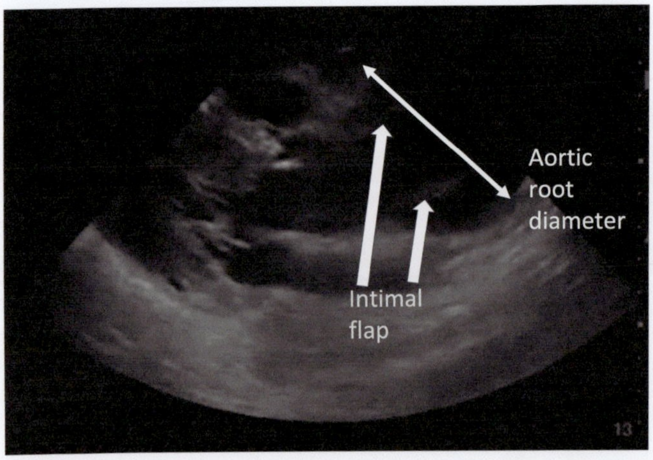

Fig. 8.8 Widened aortic root with intimal flap (in the parasternal long-axis view) in a patient with an aortic dissection

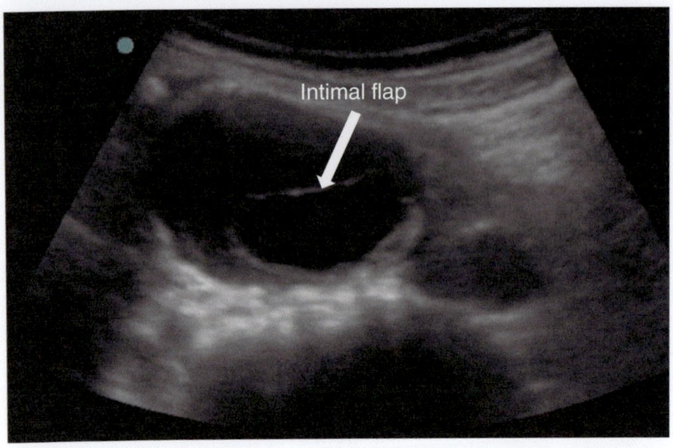

Fig. 8.9 Abdominal aortic dissection with an intimal flap

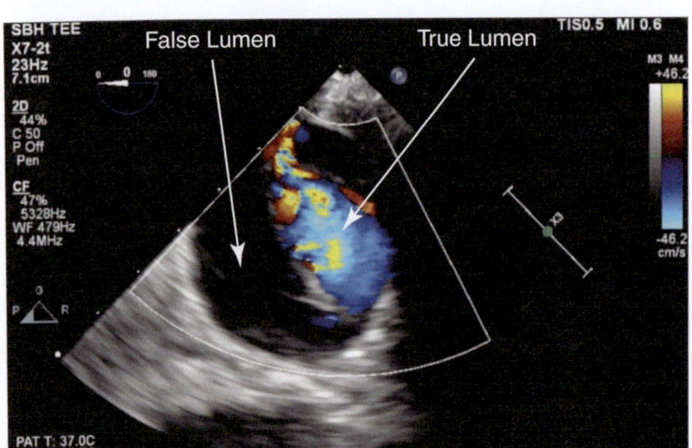

Fig. 8.10 Transesophageal echocardiogram view of an aortic dissection with color flow Doppler demonstrating a true and false lumen

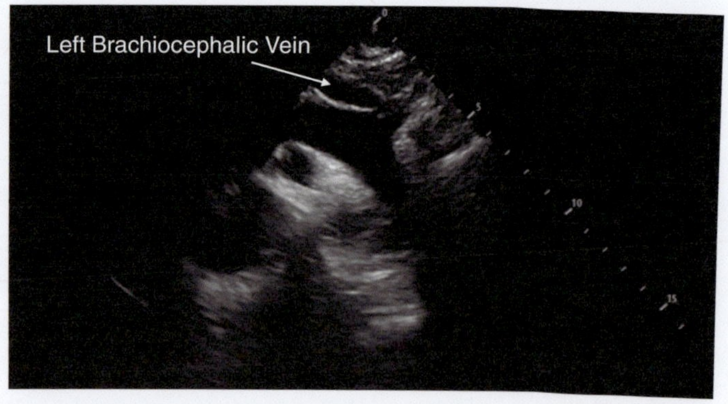

Fig. 8.11 False positive aortic dissection caused by appearance of the left brachiocephalic vein. (*Image courtesy of Michael Gottlieb, MD*)

Importantly, the left brachiocephalic vein is next to the arch of the aorta and can appear as a false positive finding of dissection on the SSN view (Fig. 8.11 and Video 8.5). Color flow and pulsed-wave Doppler can be used to identify the venous and arterial vessels. Veins should exhibit a more constant flow in both color and spectral Doppler, as opposed to the aorta, which will have a pulsatile flow. Ultrasound of the aorta can also produce reverberation artifacts, causing the appearance of a potential false dissection flap. False flaps and artifacts will have a parallel appearance to the aortic wall and will have similar blood flow velocities and color flow on both sides. False flaps and artifacts tend to be thicker (>2.5 mm) and move in perfect timing with the aortic wall itself [14]. This can be mitigated by changing the angle of insonation and Doppler gate size.

If no obvious dissection flap is identified but clinical suspicion remains high, the cardiac views should assess for findings that would raise suspicion for an aortic dissection, such as bicuspid aortic valve, new aortic regurgitation, or diastolic flow reversal within the aorta. Alternatively, complications or secondary findings of aortic dissection can be assessed even if a dissection flap is not seen. These would include findings of a unilateral hemothorax, acute regional wall motion abnormalities, aortic regurgitation, or pericardial effusion. If there is concern for an aortic dissection, CT angiography imaging of the entire aorta should ultimately be obtained when possible.

Aortic Aneurysm

There are two types of aneurysms seen in the thoracic and abdominal aorta. Fusiform aneurysms are concentric and involve the entire circumference of the wall. Saccular aneurysms are eccentric, and involve only a specific portion of the aortic wall. The presence of either does not correlate with any specific pathology. Most AAAs are saccular aneurysms [15].

Thoracic Aortic Aneurysm

Ascending and descending thoracic aortic aneurysms (TAA) account for one-third of aortic aneurysm hospital admissions, with the remainder being AAA [11]. The incidence of TAA is increasing, whereas the rates of AAA are decreasing [16]. Aneurysmal dilation is defined as a segmental dilation with at least a 50% increase in diameter compared to normal values [11]. TAA usually is asymptomatic, and it is not until complications develop (e.g., dissection, rupture) that patients become symptomatic.

Abdominal Aorta Aneurysm

The abdominal aorta is the most common part of the aorta to undergo aneurysmal dilatation and is diagnosed when the diameter is greater than 3.0 cm [17]. Due to advances in surveillance, reduction in smoking rates, and changes in operative management, the mortality rate has significantly decreased over the past several decades [18]. The most common area to find AAA is in the infrarenal portion [17]. The likelihood of rupture is significantly higher once the AAA reaches >5.5 cm or has increased in size >0.5 cm in a 6-month period [19]. Operative management is usually indicated when an AAA is >5 cm or is rapidly enlarging [19].

The evidence for the use of POCUS in the early diagnosis of AAA is compelling with a sensitivity ranging from 94% to 99% [20, 21]. Patients who received POCUS compared to CT imaging had a 20–60% reduction in mortality due to more rapid diagnosis and faster time to definitive management [5, 6]. Ruptured AAA is associated with a 81% mortality, and a one-time screening for AAA is associated with decreased AAA-related mortality and rupture rates [22]. There are limited data on physician-performed POCUS screening in the outpatient setting for AAA.

If an AAA is identified, measurements should be obtained in two orthogonal planes. It is critical that the entire aorta is measured from outer wall to outer wall as mentioned above. Care must be taken that the aorta is assessed with the probe perpendicular to the vessel, as any angulation of the probe can lead to an oblique view of the aorta and potential overestimation of its true size [23]. However, bowel gas may interfere with this approach and a paramedian view may be necessary to visualize the aorta. The aorta is a retroperitoneal structure, and while rare, free fluid in the abdomen can be found within the presence of a ruptured AAA.

After imaging the aorta, the iliac arteries should also be examined, as there is an association between IAA and AAA, with one retrospective study finding 86% of patients with IAA had an associated AAA [2]. Concern for IAA occurs when the iliac artery diameter is greater than 1.5 cm [2].

When measuring the abdominal aorta, potential sources of error can occur with misidentification of the IVC, large peri-aortic lymphadenopathy, or the spinal canal as the aorta. The aorta will be thick-walled, have monophasic pulsatility, and exhibit no respirophasic variation. It is also anterior to the spine, which should have shadowing underneath it. Longitudinally, the aorta gives off identifiable branches, such as the celiac trunk and SMA, and travels posterior to the heart more proximally.

Aortoenteric Fistula

Aortoenteric fistulas are rare and dangerous with a mortality rate of nearly 35% [23]. Primary aortoenteric fistulas result from the presence of an AAA or an inflammatory aortitis. Secondary fistulas result from the placement of an aortic graft, traumatic injury, or gastrointestinal foreign body [24]. Patients with a history of an AAA, gastrointestinal malignancy, radiation therapy involving the abdomen, or who present with a large volume gastrointestinal bleed should be evaluated for the presence of an aortoenteric fistula. POCUS can be used to identify aortic pathology and identify the communication between the aorta and gastrointestinal tract. Color Doppler may demonstrate continuous flow between the aorta and bowel (Fig. 8.12). However, evidence supporting the use of POCUS for the detection of aortoenteric fistulas is limited to case reports [25, 26].

Endovascular Leak

Endovascular aneurysm repair (EVAR) involves placement of a stent or graft at the target site of an AAA. Endovascular stents appear echogenic on ultrasound and should be found within the lumen of the AAA. Endoleak is the most common complication of this procedure and is defined as the presence of blood flow within the aneurysmal sac. Identifying an endoleak is critical as ongoing leak into the aneurysmal sac can lead to ongoing enlargement of aneurysm and eventual rupture. The visualization of spontaneous echo contrast within the vascular structure or color Doppler leaving the graft and traveling into the aneurysmal sac suggests the presence of an endoleak (Fig. 8.13 and Video 8.6). However, lack of these sonographic findings does not exclude the diagnosis.

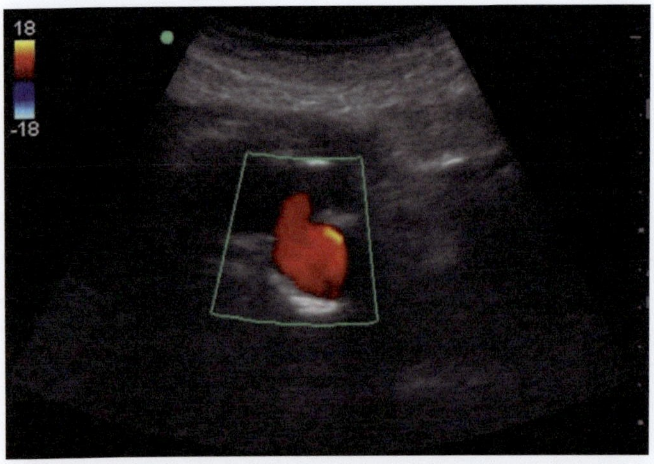

Fig. 8.12 Aortoenteric fistula. (*Image courtesy of David Mackenzie, MD*)

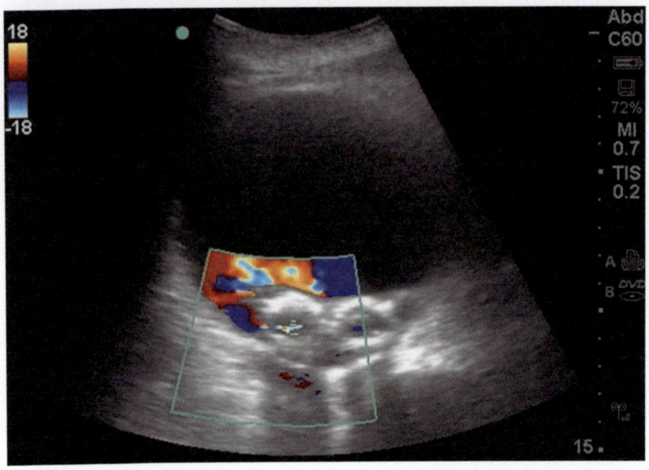

Fig. 8.13 Endovascular aneurysm repair (EVAR) leak

Key Ultrasound Findings

Aortic pathology	Anatomic location	POCUS views	POCUS findings
Dissection	Ascending aorta	PLAX, SSN	Presence of independently mobile, linear, hyperechoic structure seen in two planes
	Aortic arch	SSN	
	Descending aorta	PLAX, PSAX, A4C	
	Abdominal Aorta	Transabdominal	
Aneurysm	Ascending aorta	PLAX, SSN	Normal <4.0 cm
	Aortic arch	SSN	Normal <4.0 cm
	Descending aorta	PLAX, PSAX, A4C	Normal <3.0 cm
	Abdominal Aorta	Transabdominal	Normal <3.0 cm
	Iliac Artery	Transabdmonal	Normal <1.5 cm

PLAX parasternal long axis, *PSAX* parasternal short axis, *SSN* suprasternal notch, *A4C* apOical 4-chamber

Pearls and Pitfalls

- Bowel gas can interfere with assessments of the abdominal aorta. Compression of the bowel gas with a curvilinear probe should be performed in an effort to displace bowel gas. If the patient's abdominal wall muscles are tense, have the patient flex their knees to 90 degrees to relax the abdominal wall musculature. If necessary, the paramedian or coronal approaches can be used to image from a more lateral direction.
- The entire abdominal aorta should be scanned to evaluate for AAA.
- When measuring the aortic diameter, it is critical that the entire aortic lumen is measured from the outer wall to the outer wall, with the probe as perpendicular to the anterior abdominal wall as possible.
- False positive findings for aortic dissection can occur with reverberation artifact or by visualizing the left brachiocephalic vein. Ensure that a dissection flap is visualized in two orthogonal planes if possible and assess the movement of the potential flap. True flaps will move independently of the aortic wall.

References

1. Hagan PG, Nienaber CA, Isselbacher EM, et al. The International Registry of Acute Aortic Dissection (IRAD): new insights into an old disease. JAMA. 2000;283:897–903.
2. Huang Y, Gloviczki P, Duncan AA, Kalra M, Hoskin TL, Oderich GS, McKusick MA, Bower TC. Common iliac artery aneurysm: expansion rate and results of open surgical and endovascular repair. J Vasc Surg. 2008;47:1203–10; discussion 1210–1
3. Isselbacher EM. Thoracic and abdominal aortic aneurysms. Circulation. 2005;111:816–28.
4. Fernando SM, Tran A, Cheng W, et al. Accuracy of presenting symptoms, physical examination, and imaging for diagnosis of ruptured abdominal aortic aneurysm: systematic review and meta-analysis. Acad Emerg Med. 2022;29:486–96.
5. Hoffman M, Avellone JC, Plecha FR, Rhodes RS, Donovan DL, Beven EG, DePalma RG, Frisch JA. Operation for ruptured abdominal aortic aneurysms: a community-wide experience. Surgery. 1982;91:597–602.
6. Reed MJ, Cheung L-T. Emergency department led emergency ultrasound may improve the time to diagnosis in patients presenting with a ruptured abdominal aortic aneurysm. Eur J Emerg Med. 2014;21:272–5.
7. Erbel R, Engberding R, Daniel W, Roelandt J, Visser C, Rennollet H. Echocardiography in diagnosis of aortic dissection. Lancet. 1989;1:457–61.
8. Gibbons RC, Smith D, Feig R, Mulflur M, Costantino TG. The sonographic protocol for the emergent evaluation of aortic dissections (SPEED protocol): a multicenter, prospective, observational study. Acad Emerg Med. 2024;31:112–8.
9. Pare JR, Liu R, Moore CL, Sherban T, Kelleher MS Jr, Thomas S, Taylor RA. Emergency physician focused cardiac ultrasound

improves diagnosis of ascending aortic dissection. Am J Emerg Med. 2016;34:486–92.
10. Shiga T, Wajima Z'i, Apfel CC, Inoue T, Ohe Y. Diagnostic accuracy of transesophageal echocardiography, helical computed tomography, and magnetic resonance imaging for suspected thoracic aortic dissection: systematic review and meta-analysis. Arch Intern Med. 2006;166:1350–6.
11. Isselbacher EM, Preventza O, Hamilton Black J 3rd, et al. 2022 ACC/AHA Guideline for the Diagnosis and Management of Aortic Disease: a report of the American Heart Association/American College of Cardiology Joint Committee on Clinical Practice Guidelines. Circulation. 2022;146:e334–482.
12. Rylski B, Desjardins B, Moser W, Bavaria JE, Milewski RK. Gender-related changes in aortic geometry throughout life. Eur J Cardiothorac Surg. 2014;45:805–11.
13. Park K-H, Lim C, Choi JH, Sung K, Kim K, Lee YT, Park PW. Prevalence of aortic intimal defect in surgically treated acute type A intramural hematoma. Ann Thorac Surg. 2008;86:1494–500.
14. Vignon P, Spencer KT, Rambaud G, Preux PM, Krauss D, Balasia B, Lang RM. Differential transesophageal echocardiographic diagnosis between linear artifacts and intraluminal flap of aortic dissection or disruption. Chest. 2001;119:1778–90.
15. Ozawa H, Takahashi A, Bessho R, Hoshina K, Shukuzawa K, Ohki T. Saccular and fusiform abdominal aortic aneurysms treated with endovascular repair differ in presentation and treatment threshold: analyses using a national clinical database in Japan. J Am Heart Assoc. 2024;13:e032715.
16. Svensjö S, Björck M, Gürtelschmid M, Djavani Gidlund K, Hellberg A, Wanhainen A. Low prevalence of abdominal aortic aneurysm among 65-year-old Swedish men indicates a change in the epidemiology of the disease. Circulation. 2011;124:1118–23.
17. Chaikof EL, Brewster DC, Dalman RL, Makaroun MS, Illig KA, Sicard GA, Timaran CH, Upchurch GR Jr, Veith FJ. SVS practice guidelines for the care of patients with an abdominal aortic aneurysm: executive summary. J Vasc Surg. 2009;50:880–96.
18. Stather PW, Sidloff DA, Rhema IA, Choke E, Bown MJ, Sayers RD. A review of current reporting of abdominal aortic aneurysm mortality and prevalence in the literature. Eur J Vasc Endovasc Surg. 2014;47:240–2.
19. Brewster DC, Cronenwett JL, Hallett JW Jr, Johnston KW, Krupski WC, Matsumura JS, Joint Council of the American Association for Vascular Surgery and Society for Vascular Surgery. Guidelines for the treatment of abdominal aortic aneurysms. Report of a subcommittee of the Joint Council of the American Association for Vascular Surgery and Society for Vascular Surgery. J Vasc Surg. 2003;37:1106–17.
20. Lindholt JS, Vammen S, Juul S, Henneberg EW, Fasting H. The validity of ultrasonographic scanning as screening method for abdominal aortic aneurysm. Eur J Vasc Endovasc Surg. 1999;17:472–5.
21. Rubano E, Mehta N, Caputo W, Paladino L, Sinert R. Systematic review: emergency department bedside ultrasonography for diagnosing suspected abdominal aortic aneurysm. Acad Emerg Med. 2013;20:128–38.
22. Guirguis-Blake JM, Beil TL, Senger CA, Coppola EL. Primary care screening for abdominal aortic aneurysm: updated evidence report and systematic review for the US preventive services task force. JAMA. 2019;322(22):2219–38. https://doi.org/10.1001/jama.2019.17021.
23. Lema PC, Kim JH, St James E. Overview of common errors and pitfalls to avoid in the acquisition and interpretation of ultrasound imaging of the abdominal aorta. JVD. 2017;5:41–6.
24. Saers SJF, Scheltinga MRM. Primary aortoenteric fistula. Br J Surg. 2005;92:143–52.
25. Mackenzie DC. Aortoenteric fistula identified by clinical ultrasound. J Emerg Med. 2015;48:699–701.
26. Perrone T, Pagani C, Mossolani EE. Ultrasound detection of aortoenteric fistula in a patient with sepsis. J Ultrasound. 2017;20:157–9.

Renal and Urinary Bladder Ultrasound

9

Eduardo R. Argaiz, William Beaubien-Souligny, and Abhilash Koratala

Background

Renal ultrasound is frequently the first-line imaging modality for patients with acute kidney injury or urinary tract symptoms, being a cost-effective, radiation-free, and easily performed examination. Ultrasound can evaluate kidney anatomy and a wide range of pathologies, including hydronephrosis, renal stones, pyelonephritis, renal cysts, tumors, and vascular abnormalities. Renal ultrasound is the preferred tool for assessing renal transplants. Moreover, bladder ultrasound can estimate urine volume and common abnormalities such as enlarged prostate and urinary catheter malfunction.

Indications

Indications
- Acute kidney injury
- Flank pain
- Abdominal pain
- Urinary retention
- Suprapubic pain
- Hematuria
- Dysuria

Diagnoses
- Hydronephrosis
- Kidney and bladder stones
- Urinary catheter placement
- Prostate abnormalities
- Renal cysts
- Pyelonephritis
- Renal tumors
- Renal artery stenosis
- Congenital cardiorenal syndrome
- Renal transplant

Supplementary Information The online version contains supplementary material available at https://doi.org/10.1007/978-3-031-85308-1_9.

E. R. Argaiz (✉)
Tecnológico de Monterrey, Escuela de Medicina y Ciencias de la Salud, Mexico City, Mexico

Departamento de Nefrología y Metabolismo Mineral, Instituto Nacional de Ciencias Médicas y Nutrición, Salvador Zubirán, Mexico City, Mexico
e-mail: argaiz@tec.mx

W. Beaubien-Souligny
Division of Nephrology, Department of Medicine, Université de, QC, Canada
e-mail: William.beaubien-souligny@umontreal.ca

A. Koratala
Division of Nephrology, Department of Medicine, Medical College of Wisconsin, Milwaukee, WI, USA
e-mail: akoratala@mcw.edu

M. Gottlieb, N. Panebianco (eds.), *Advanced Point-of-Care Ultrasound*, https://doi.org/10.1007/978-3-031-85308-1_9

Core Views

View	Image	Approach
Kidneys		
Long-axis	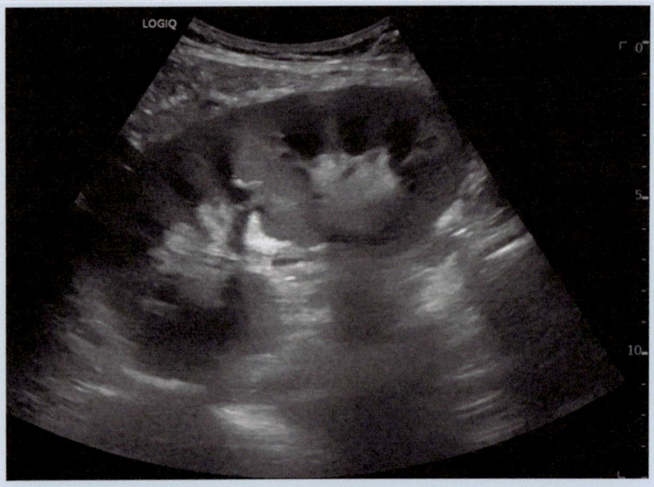 Core View 1. Long-axis view of the kidney Core Video 9.1. Long-axis view of the kidney with anteroposterior fanning	Place the probe in the mid-axillary line at the tenth rib interspace, with the marker directed superiorly with a slight posterior rotation. Fan anteroposteriorly to ensure complete imaging.
Short-axis	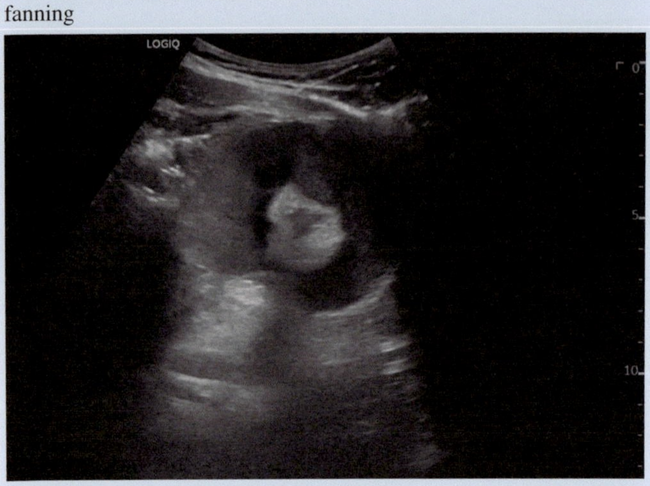 Core View 2. Short-axis view of the kidney Core Video 9.2. Short-axis view of the kidney with superoinferior fanning	Rotate the probe 90 degrees counterclockwise. Fan from the superior to inferior plane to visualize the kidney from pole to pole.
Doppler	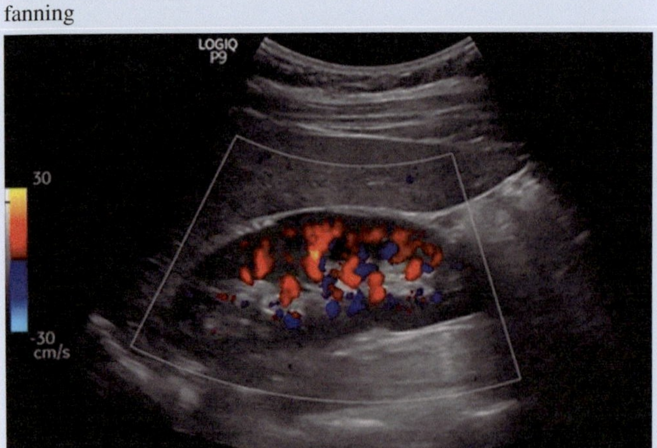 Core View 3. Long-axis view of the kidney with color Doppler	Color Doppler images offer a global assessment of renal perfusion and enable the identification of significant vascular abnormalities such as prominent vessels or arteriovenous malformations. Color Doppler can also help to delineate vessels from hydronephrosis.

View	Image	Approach
Bladder		
Transverse plane	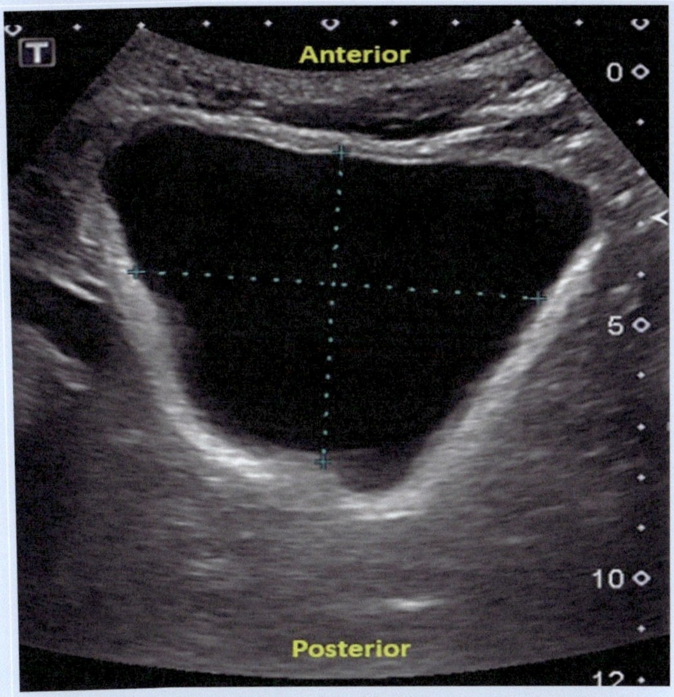 Core View 4. Transverse view of the bladder	Use a curvilinear or phased array probe just above the pubic symphysis, with the orientation marker to the right. Fan in a superoinferior direction.
Sagittal plane	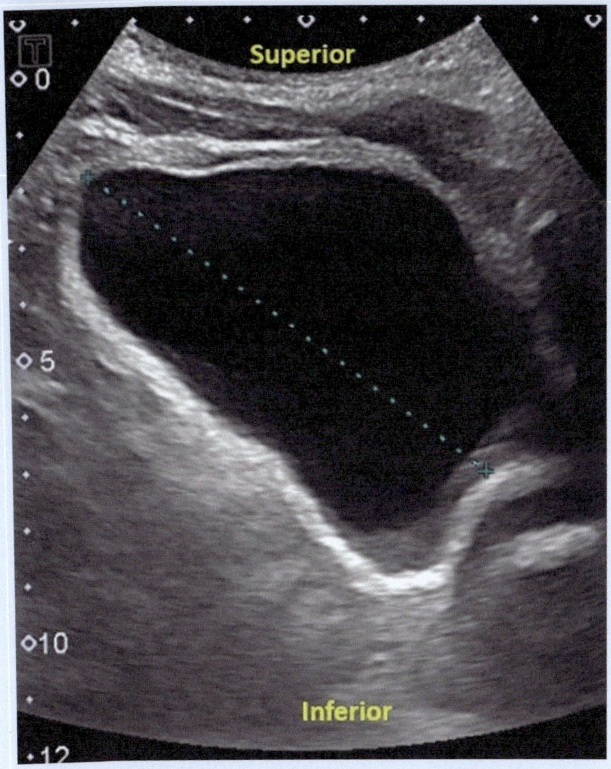 Core View 5. Sagittal view of the bladder	From the transverse plane, rotate the probe 90 degrees clockwise, with the orientation marker facing the patient's head.

View	Image	Approach
Doppler	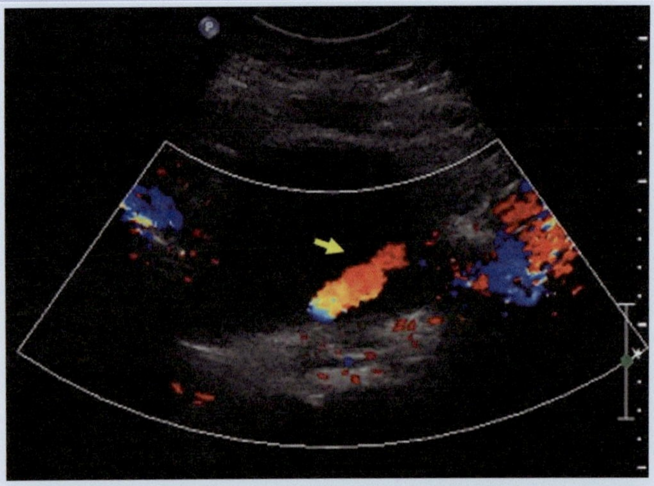 Core View 6. Ureteral jet visualized using color Doppler Core Video 9.3. Ureteral jet visualized using color Doppler	Color Doppler can identify ureteral jets, which are indicative of ureteral patency (the frequency of jets is about one every 10–15 min).

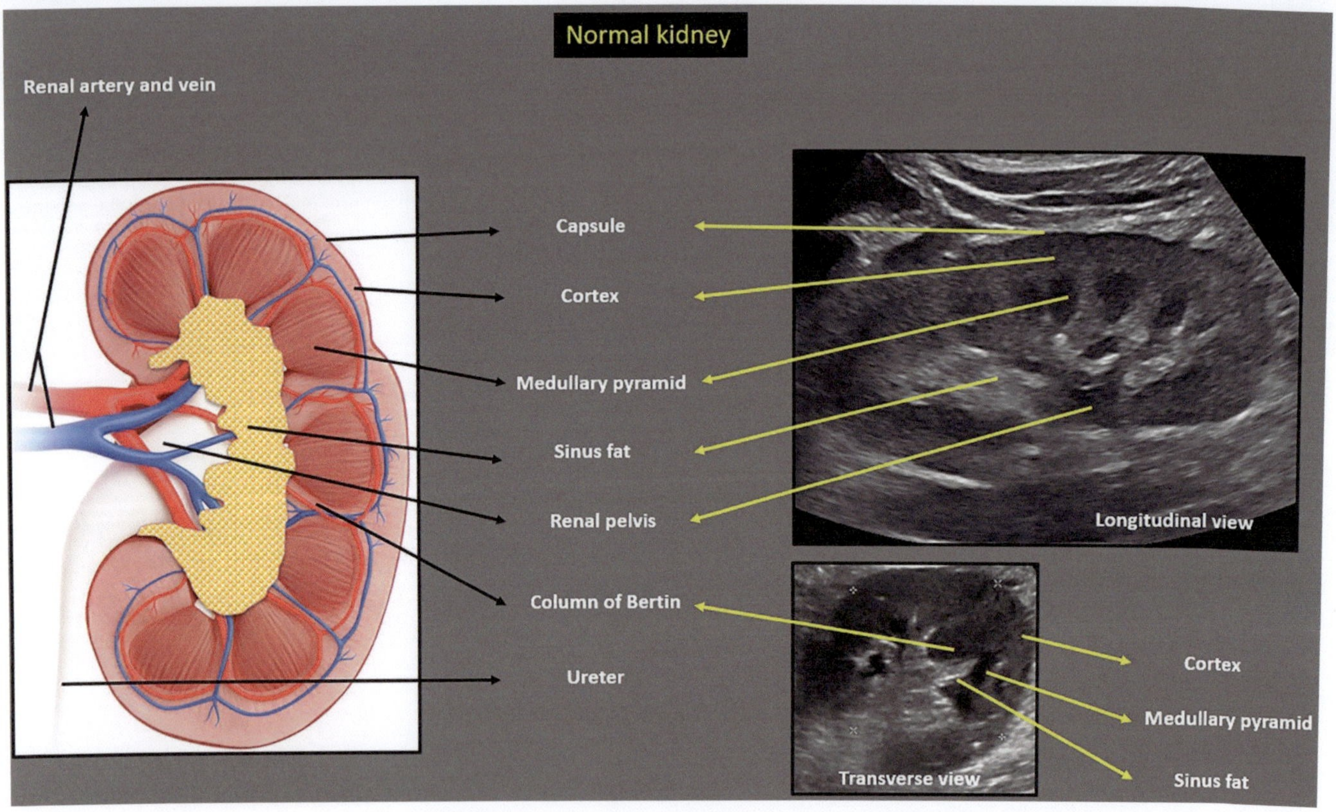

Fig. 9.1 Sonographic appearance of the kidney. (*Adapted from the Renal Fellow Network, with permission*)

Sonographically, the echogenic renal capsule makes the bean-shaped organ easily discernible (Fig. 9.1). In adults, the typical length of a kidney ranges from 10 to 12 cm and the width ranges from 3 to 5 cm, though both can vary with body size [1]. The renal parenchyma consists of an outer cortex and an inner medulla, with the latter organized into pyramids. The renal cortex is either isoechoic or hypoechoic compared to the adjacent normal liver or spleen. Medullary pyramids, in turn, are hypoechoic or anechoic compared to the cortex. Renal cortical tissue extends into the medulla, forming columns known as columns of Bertin. Hypertrophy of these columns can sometimes mimic a neoplasm. However, in contrast to a true neoplasm, the hypertrophied column of Bertin is contiguous with normal cortex, sharing a

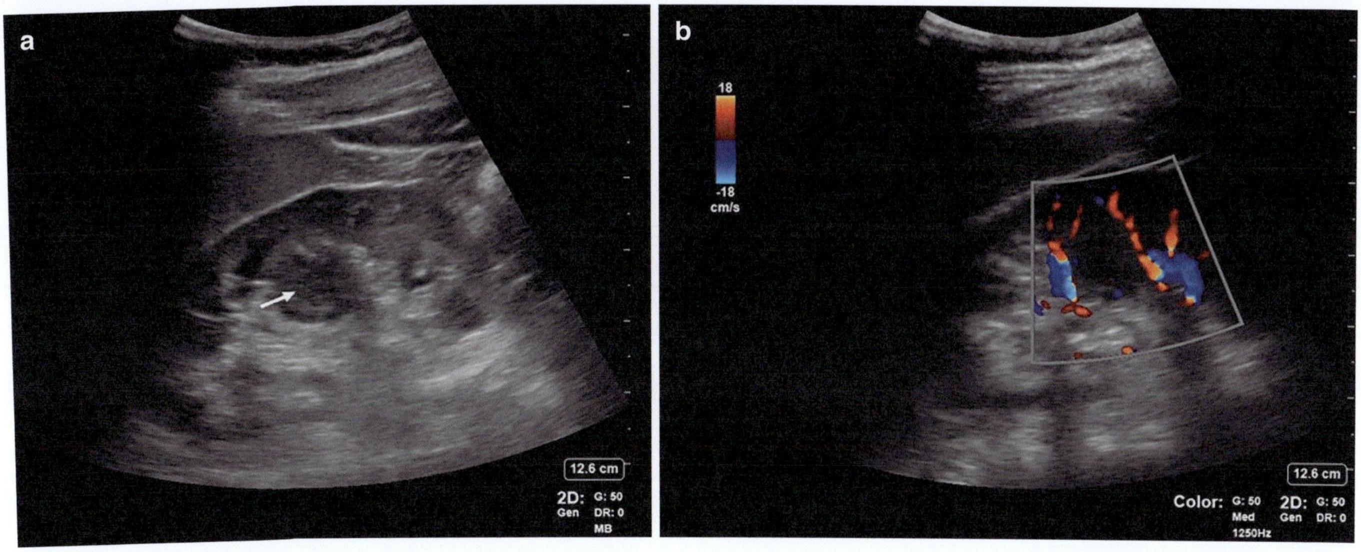

Fig. 9.2 (**a**) B-mode demonstrating a hypertrophied column of Bertin (arrow). Note that the renal outline is preserved. (**b**) Color Doppler images demonstrating preservation of normal vascular pattern (flow adjacent to medullary pyramids). (*Image courtesy of Kylie Baker, MBBS*)

similar appearance, and the renal outline is usually preserved (Fig. 9.2). The hyperechoic fat filling the renal sinus (the cavity that contains renal pelvis, calyces, and neurovascular structures) occupies a significant portion of the inner kidney. The collecting system is generally not visible due to its small caliber and the surrounding sinus fat. However, in the case of a well-functioning transplanted kidney, the collecting system may be slightly dilated. This dilation may result from an increased volume of urine production (single kidney) and the loss of the ureteric tone due to denervation.

A full bladder is optimal for proper assessment of its walls, contents, and adjacent pelvic organs. Though rarely visible unless pathologic, the ureteric orifices appear as small echogenic protuberances in the area of the trigone on the posterior aspect of the bladder. The passage of urine down the ureters occurs in pulses, detectable upon entry into the base of the bladder. These ureteral "jets" are best identified with Doppler (color or power) and are indicative of ureteral patency (Fig. 9.3 and Core Video 9.3). While the presence of ureteral jets bilaterally suggests that a complete obstruction is not present, the absence of jets does not confirm obstructive uropathy [2]. Furthermore, their practical utility is limited, and there is ongoing debate regarding their necessity and clinical relevance [2].

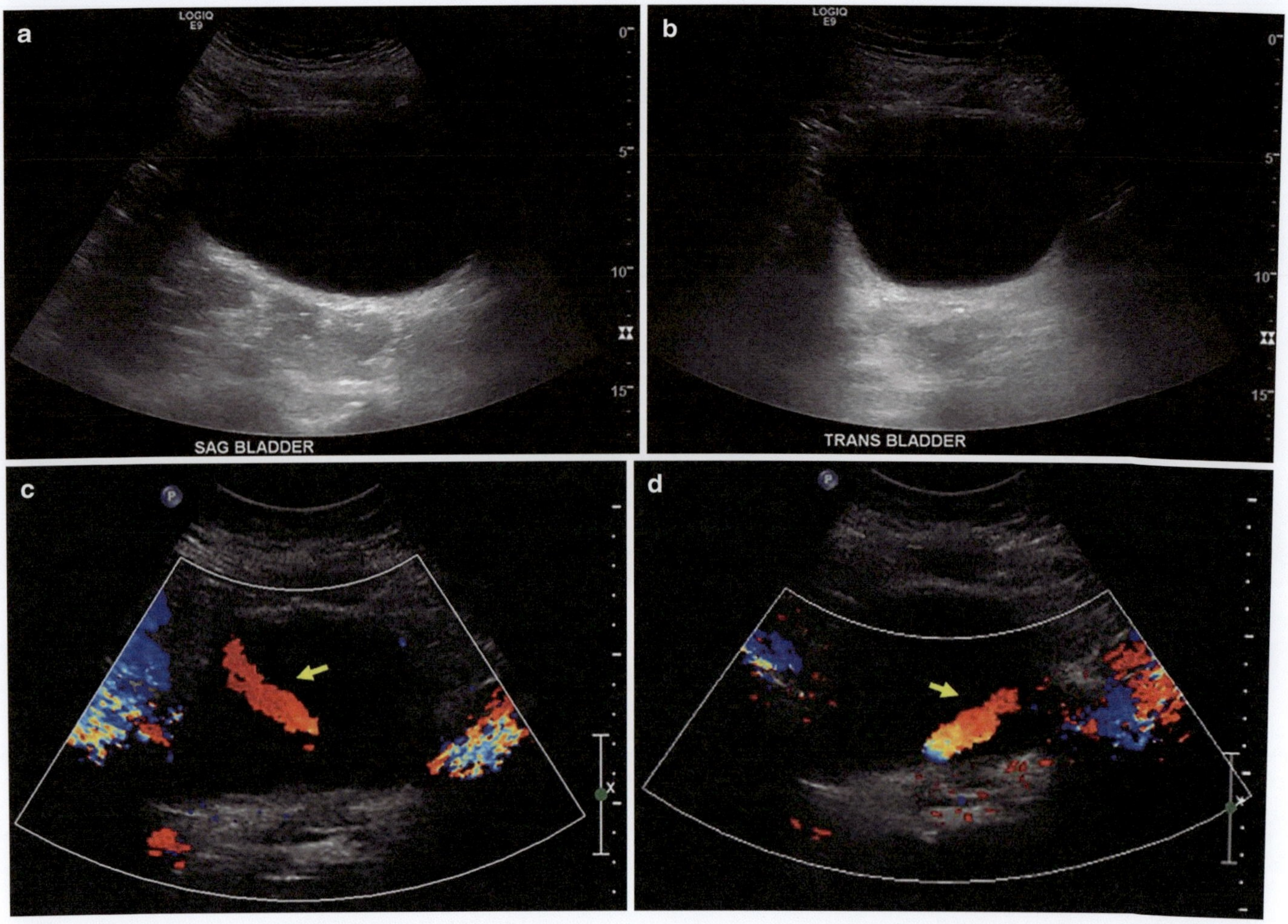

Fig. 9.3 (**a**) Sagittal view of urinary bladder on B-mode. (**b**) Transverse view of urinary bladder on B-mode. (**c**) Right ureteral jet on color Doppler. (**d**) Left ureteral jet on color Doppler

Clinical Applications

Hydronephrosis

Excluding urinary tract obstruction as a potential cause for acute pain or kidney injury is a common reason for performing renal ultrasound. Hydronephrosis appears as an anechoic branching area in the renal collecting system region, representing urine backflow. Obstruction typically originates distal to the kidney, such as when there is a stone in the ureteropelvic junction, ureter, ureterovesical junction, or when there is a bladder outlet obstruction from a stone, mass, or enlarged prostate. A gravid uterus can cause manual obstruction of the ureters and some degree of asymptomatic hydronephrosis or ureteral dilation is seen in approximately 90% of pregnancies [3]. As the severity of obstruction increases, urine moves proximally into the kidney, distorting its architecture.

Although there is no single universally accepted grading system, in routine clinical practice, hydronephrosis is qualitatively classified as mild, moderate, and severe (Fig. 9.4). Mild hydronephrosis involves slight dilation of the renal pelvis and calyces with relative preservation of the renal architecture. In moderate hydronephrosis, medullary pyramids begin to flatten due to back pressure, in addition to outpouching and confluence of the minor and major calyces, sometimes described as a "cauliflower" appearance. Severe hydronephrosis presents with a dilated renal pelvis and calyces and thinning of the renal parenchyma, which has been described as a "bear paw/claw" appearance. An alternative system has also been described using numeric grades (Table 9.1) [4].

It is important to note that the source of obstruction may not always be identified during the ultrasound examination. For instance, ureteral stones might not be visible due to the obscuration of ureters by bowel gas. For individuals suspected of having ureterolithiasis, ultrasonography remains the preferred initial imaging modality. It is associated with reduced cumulative radiation exposure compared to the initial use of computed tomography (CT) without a significant

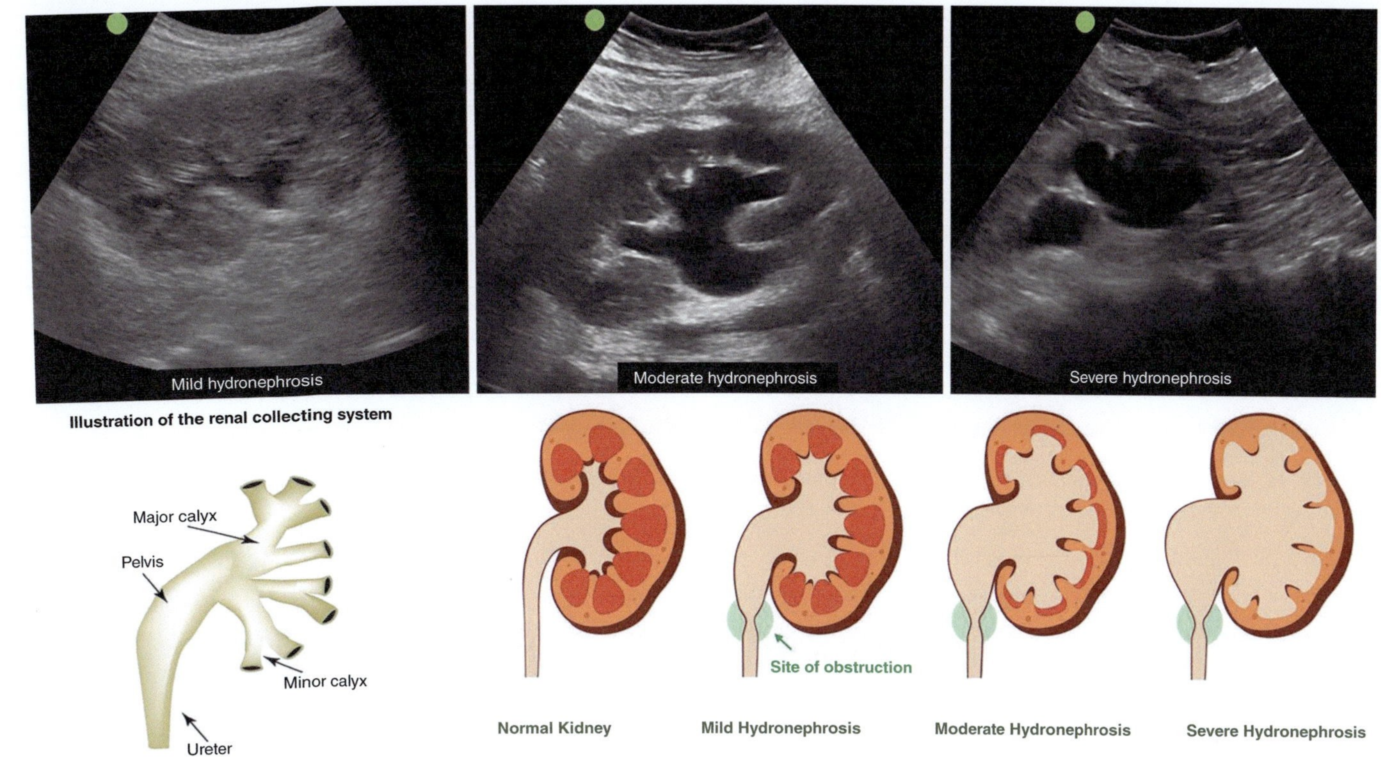

Fig. 9.4 Qualitative grading of hydronephrosis. (*Adapted from the Renal Fellow Network, with permission*)

Table 9.1 Numerical grading of hydronephrosis [4].

Grade	Description
Grade 0	No hydronephrosis
Grade 1	Isolated dilation of the renal pelvis
Grade 2	Calyceal and pelvic dilation
Grade 3	Mild-to-moderate renal parenchymal loss involving less than half of the parenchyma
Grade 4	Severe renal parenchymal loss involving more than half of the parenchyma

difference in complications [5]. Importantly, hydronephrosis can also occur in a nonobstructive context, such as during aggressive diuresis, pregnancy, papillary necrosis, or mass effect from abdominal malignancy [6].

Hydronephrosis must be differentiated from other anechoic structures such as prominent medullary pyramids (particularly in children), prominent vessels or vascular malformations, parapelvic cysts, and extrarenal pelvis [7]. Medullary pyramids are positioned external to the echogenic renal sinus fat within the parenchyma of the cortex. In contrast, hydronephrosis is in the renal pelvis area, surrounded by a rim of hyperechoic fat. Vessels can be differentiated from hydronephrosis by demonstrating flow using color or power Doppler (Fig. 9.5). Parapelvic cysts typically appear as well-circumscribed lesions without any demonstrable connection to the ureter, whereas hydronephrosis is in continuity with the ureter and branches into the kidney (Fig. 9.6). Extrarenal pelvis, an anatomical variant, presents as a cyst-like structure just outside the renal pelvis, better visualized in transverse image (Fig. 9.7a). While it is in continuity with the collecting system, it usually does not branch into the kidney. Comparison with prior imaging is beneficial when it is available. Duplicated collecting systems may or may not be apparent on ultrasound, especially when there is no hydronephrosis. Presence of two distinct moieties of sinus fat should raise the suspicion for this condition (Fig. 9.7b).

Kidney and Bladder Stones

When assessed using brightness mode (B-mode) ultrasound, stones appear as hyperechoic structures followed by an acoustic shadow, which is an area of signal void observed deep to dense structures that impede the transmission of ultrasound waves (Fig. 9.8a). However, stones may not consistently exhibit a significantly brighter appearance than the surrounding tissues. This discrepancy can be attributed to factors such as the surface curvature or the small size of a stone relative to the ultrasound wavelength, which may not scatter sound directly back to the probe [8]. Additionally, shadowing might not be evident in low-quality images or

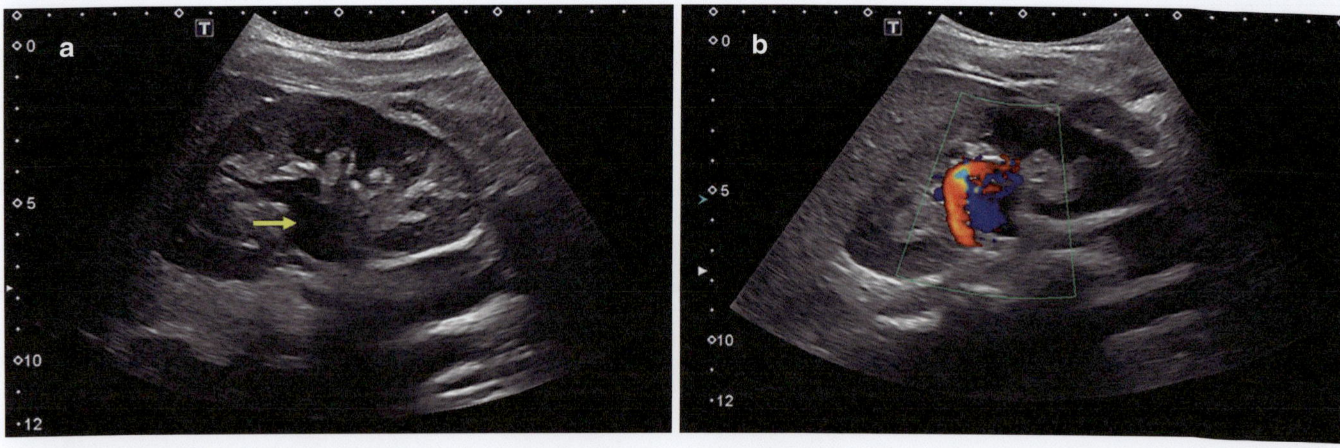

Fig. 9.5 (**a**) A vascular malformation in the hilar region mimicking mild hydronephrosis (arrow). (**b**) Color Doppler confirming the vascular malformation. (*Adapted with permission from Koratala et al.* [7])

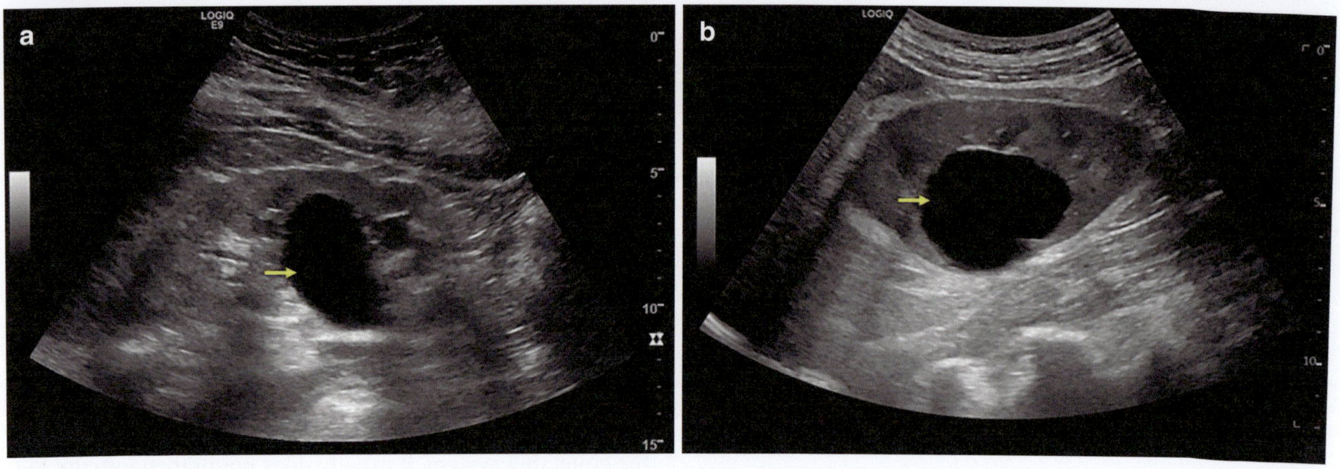

Fig. 9.6 Renal ultrasound images demonstrating two examples of parapelvic cysts obtained from different patients

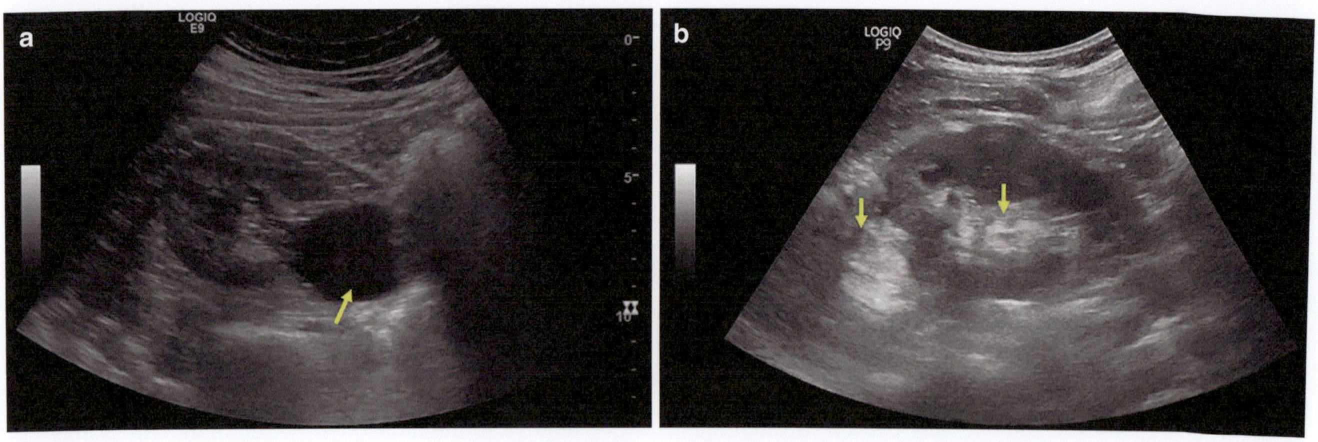

Fig. 9.7 (**a**) A distended extrarenal pelvis (arrow) in the transverse view. (**b**) A duplicated collecting system without hydronephrosis represented by two distinct sinus fat moieties (arrows)

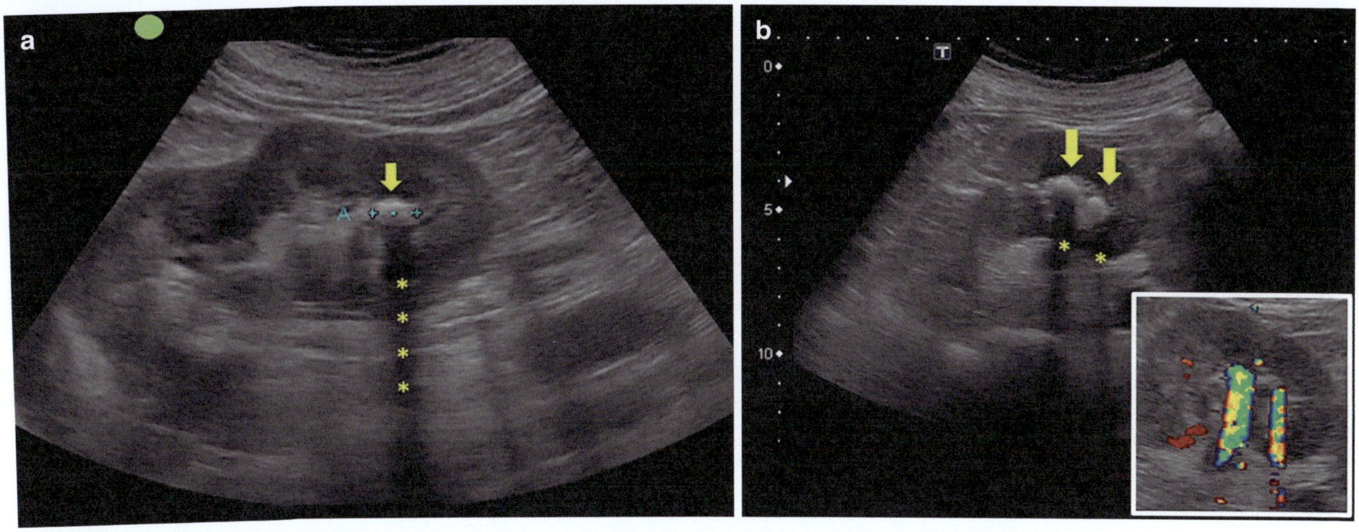

Fig. 9.8 (**a**) A renal stone (arrow) in the lower pole of the kidney with acoustic shadowing (asterisks). (**b**) Two stones (arrows) visualized on the transverse view associated with acoustic shadowing (asterisks) and twinkle artifact (inset). (*Adapted from the Renal Fellow Network, with permission*)

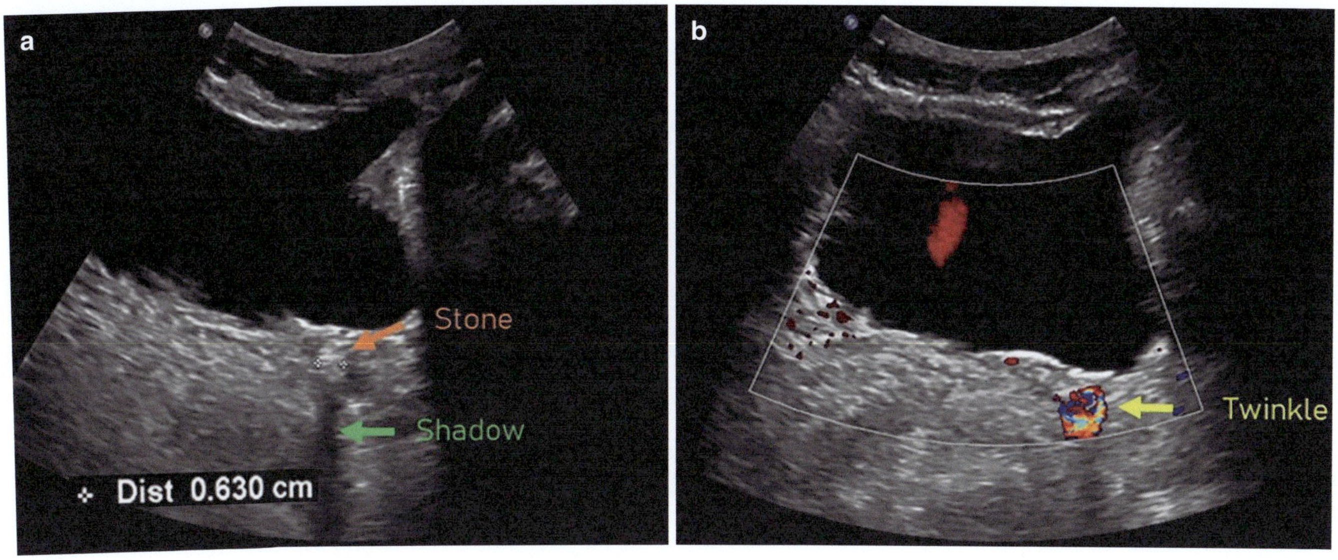

Fig. 9.9 (**a**) Bladder ultrasound images demonstrating a stone in the ureterovesical junction with acoustic shadowing. (**b**) Bladder ultrasound images demonstrating a twinkle artifact corresponding to the stone in A. (*Adapted from NephroPOCUS.com, with permission*)

those with an overall increased gain. In such instances, the "twinkling" artifact observed on color Doppler can be useful (Fig. 9.8b). It denotes a focus of swiftly alternating color Doppler signals that imitate turbulent flow and is particularly prominent with rougher stones. Of note, this sign exhibits higher sensitivity than shadowing when it comes to identifying small stones [9]. Twinkling may appear exclusively on the stone or extend as a band or tail beyond it. Adjusting the focal zone at or below the stone enhances the visibility of twinkling compared to setting it above. This artifact also aids in detecting distal ureteral stones at the ureterovesical junction [10] (Fig. 9.9).

Assessment of the Urinary Bladder Volume

Measuring bladder volume is valuable in assessing for urine retention, especially in the context of acute kidney injury (with or without hydronephrosis), postoperative states, and patients presenting with lower urinary tract symptomatology. The bladder volume is estimated through three orthogonal measurements, as illustrated in Fig. 9.10. Most point-of-care ultrasound (POCUS) machines come equipped with built-in measurement packages to compute bladder volume using these dimensions. Some machines even incorporate artificial

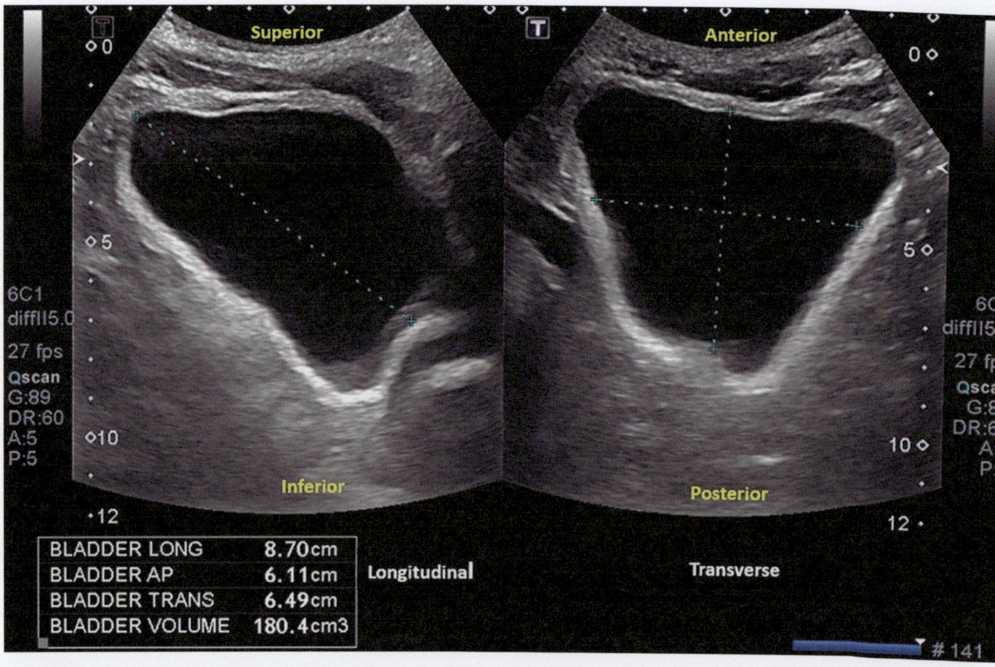

Fig. 9.10 Urinary bladder volume measurement using the ellipsoid formula. (*Adapted with permission from Koratala et al.* [7])

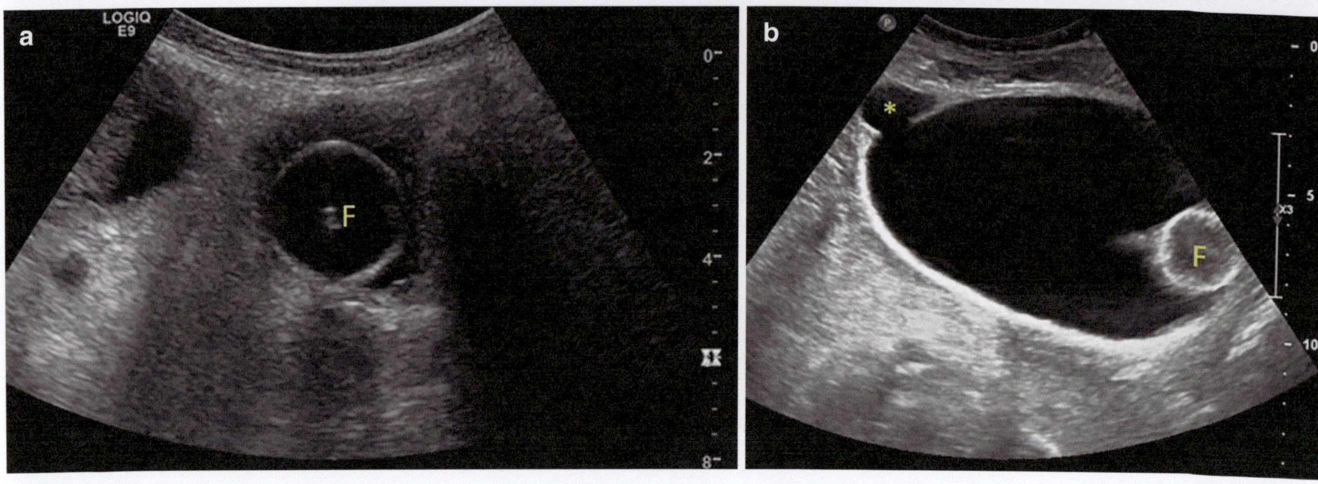

Fig. 9.11 (**a**) Bladder ultrasound demonstrating a decompressed bladder with a Foley catheter balloon (F) in place. (**b**) A distended bladder despite the presence of a Foley catheter suggestive of catheter malfunction. Asterisk indicates a small bladder diverticulum

intelligence (AI)-assisted volume estimates, eliminating the need for the operator to manually measure the dimensions. Notably, due to variations in bladder shape, several multiplication factors (ranging from 0.52 to 0.89) have been proposed beyond the traditional 0.52. In one study comparing 10 different formulas for bladder volume measurement, the most accurate one was found to be height × depth × width × 0.72, with a mean error of 17.4% ± 11.6% [11]. In general, a post-void residual volume exceeding 200 mL in adults is considered abnormal and may indicate incomplete bladder emptying, while a volume in the range of 100–200 mL falls within the indeterminate zone. Occasionally, ascitic fluid may be mistaken for a distended bladder. This can be differentiated by fanning the probe, which will reveal intestinal loops within the peritoneal fluid. However, caution must be exercised when relying on automated bladder scanners, as they are unable to distinguish between urine, fresh (unclotted) blood, and ascites [12].

Urinary Catheter Placement

Bladder ultrasound is useful for assessing the adequate placement and functioning of a urinary catheter. A well-functioning Foley catheter effectively drains the bladder, leading to bladder decompression. The Foley balloon is seen as a fluid-filled, anechoic circular structure within the decompressed bladder (Fig. 9.11a). Conversely, a bladder that remains full of urine despite the presence of a Foley catheter is indicative of catheter misplacement or malfunction (Fig. 9.11b). In some cases, visible debris responsible for the catheter obstruction may be observed.

Bladder ultrasound can be valuable in pediatric patients to determine the timing of catheter insertion when a urine sample is needed, with one study demonstrating higher success rates when ultrasound was used [13]. While urinary retention in children is rare, the formula ([age in years +2] × 30 mL) can be used to determine a greater-than-expected post-void residual volume [14].

In patients needing suprapubic catheterization, the optimal puncture site is best determined by placing the probe 2–4 cm above the pubic symphysis and excluding intervening bowel. Real-time ultrasound-guided Seldinger technique in transverse or longitudinal views can then be performed [15].

Prostate Abnormalities

In a patient with a full bladder, the enhanced acoustic window created by the fluid allows for the examination of the prostate gland, which is located deeper in the pelvis. The prostate surrounds the bladder neck and normally measures approximately 3 cm × 3 cm × 5 cm, with enlargement indicating prostatic hypertrophy, a potential underlying cause of urinary retention [16]. The assessment of echogenicity and parenchymal changes within the prostate gland is not fully achievable with transabdominal ultrasound, and additional studies such as transrectal ultrasound, CT, or magnetic resonance imaging (MRI) are often necessary. Ultrasound alone cannot be used to determine benign vs malignant causes of hyperplasia. However, transabdominal ultrasound can detect abnormalities such as an enlarged prostate causing mass effect on the bladder or a malpositioned Foley catheter with balloon inflation in the prostatic urethra (Fig. 9.12).

Renal Cysts

Renal cysts likely originate from diverticula in the distal nephron [17]. The most prevalent renal cystic lesions, simple renal cysts, are found in nearly 12% of adults, rising to more than one-third of individuals over the age of 60, and their prevalence and size tend to increase with age [18]. To diagnose a benign simple renal cyst on ultrasound, the following findings must be present: (1) a well-defined, round, and anechoic structure free of internal echoes, (2) sub-millimeter proximal wall with a thin and echogenic distal wall, and (3) increased through transmission manifested by posterior acoustic enhancement (Fig. 9.13). Simple cysts can sometimes be very large, exceeding 10–20 cm in diameter.

The presence of internal echoes, septations, calcifications, or a thickened, irregular, or nodular wall classifies the cyst as a complex one (Fig. 9.14) [19]. Internal echoes could reflect hemorrhage or infection depending on the clinical context. If infection is clinically suspected, ultrasound-guided aspiration may be considered. The presence of an irregularly thick wall, more than three septa, thick septae (greater than 2–3 mm in diameter), or any nodular elements should prompt an urgent CT or MRI to assess the potential for malignancy [7]. Of note, because commonly used classification schemes, such as the Bosniak classification system, are developed for CT and MRI use, confirmation imaging with these modalities is important [20]. Cysts situated in the renal sinus, referred to as parapelvic cysts, might resemble hydronephrosis as previously mentioned. Unlike hydronephrosis, parapelvic cysts do not have communication with the collecting system, a distinction that can be determined by fanning the probe.

Autosomal dominant polycystic kidney disease (ADPKD) is a relatively common genetic disorder that contributes significantly to chronic kidney disease. On ultrasound, kidneys with ADPKD typically exhibit enlargement and the presence

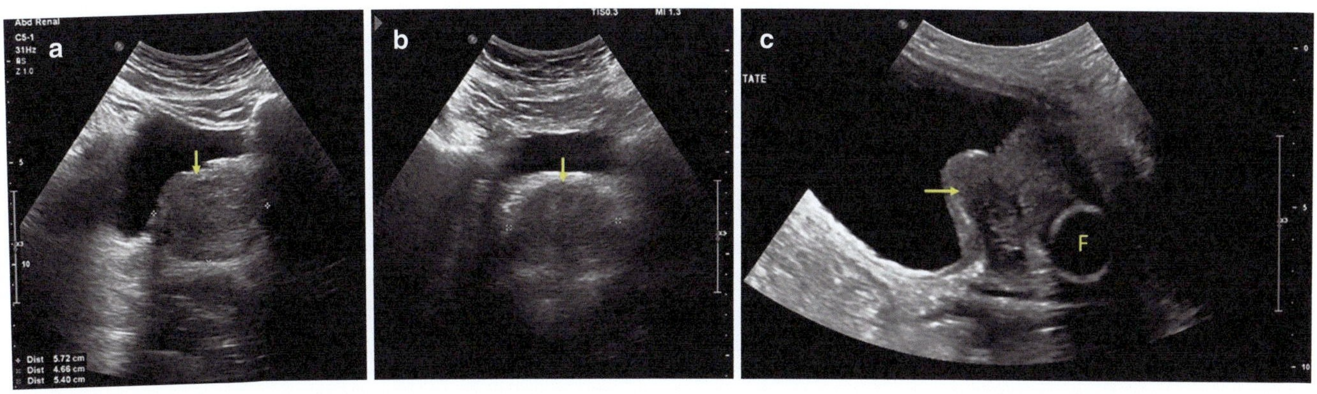

Fig. 9.12 (**a**) Sagittal view of the urinary bladder being compressed by an enlarged prostate (arrows). (**b**) Transverse view of the urinary bladder from A being compressed by an enlarged prostate (arrows). (**c**) Malpositioned Foley catheter balloon (F) within the prostate (arrow). (*Adapted from NephroPOCUS.com, with permission*)

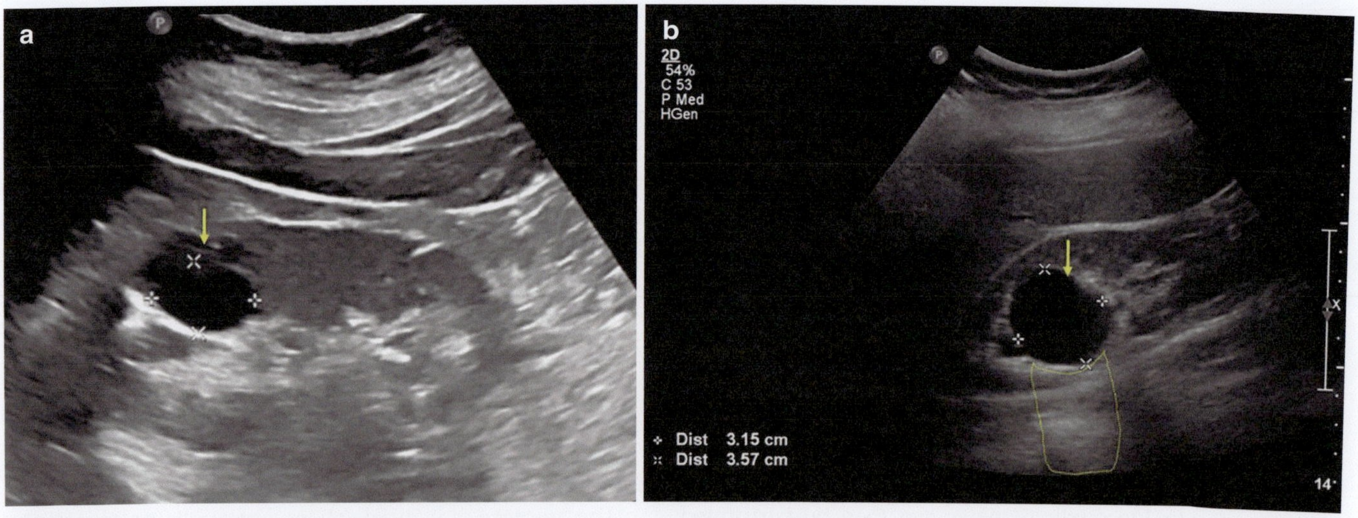

Fig. 9.13 (**a**) Renal ultrasound demonstrating a simple cysts (arrow). (**b**) Simple cyst (arrow) with a bright area deep to the cyst (dotted line) representing posterior acoustic enhancement

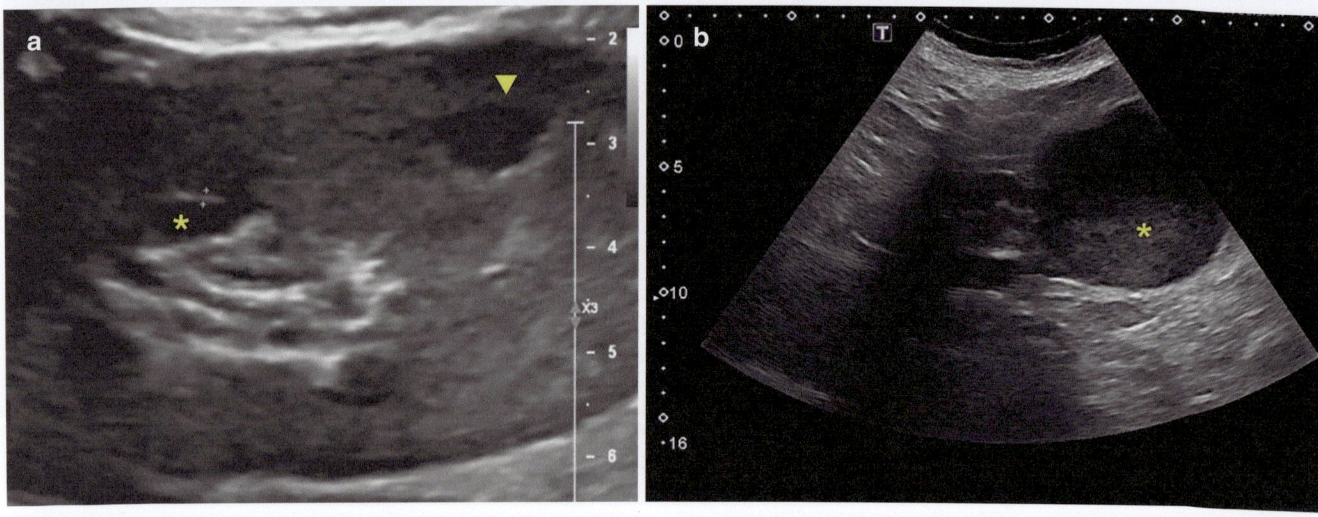

Fig. 9.14 Complex cysts. (**a**) A complex cyst with a thin septation (asterisk) and a simple cyst (arrowhead) are shown. No further imaging or follow up is needed as the septum is single, thin, and has no nodularity or solid elements. (**b**) A hemorrhagic renal cyst with layering hyperechoic material (hematocrit sign) in a patient with blunt trauma. ((**b**) was *Adapted from the Renal Fellow Network, with permission*)

of multiple cysts of varying appearance (Fig. 9.15). The diagnostic criteria vary based on the patient's age (Table 9.2) [21]. Obtaining satisfactory imaging of polycystic kidneys poses a challenge due to acoustic enhancement and reflections from numerous cysts, often requiring the use of CT or MRI. While many patients with ADPKD have a family history, the identification of more than 10 cysts per kidney on ultrasound is generally considered diagnostic, even in patients without a confirmed family history [22]. The presence of cysts in other organs (e.g., liver, spleen, and pancreas) also serves as a clue to suggest ADPKD may be present.

Patients with advanced chronic kidney disease and end-stage renal disease may present with acquired cystic disease, and its prevalence rises with the duration of renal replacement therapy [22]. Ultrasound imaging typically reveals a reduced renal size with 3–5 cysts in each kidney. In contrast to simple cysts or ADPKD, acquired cysts carry a potential for malignant transformation, necessitating periodic follow-up considerations [23].

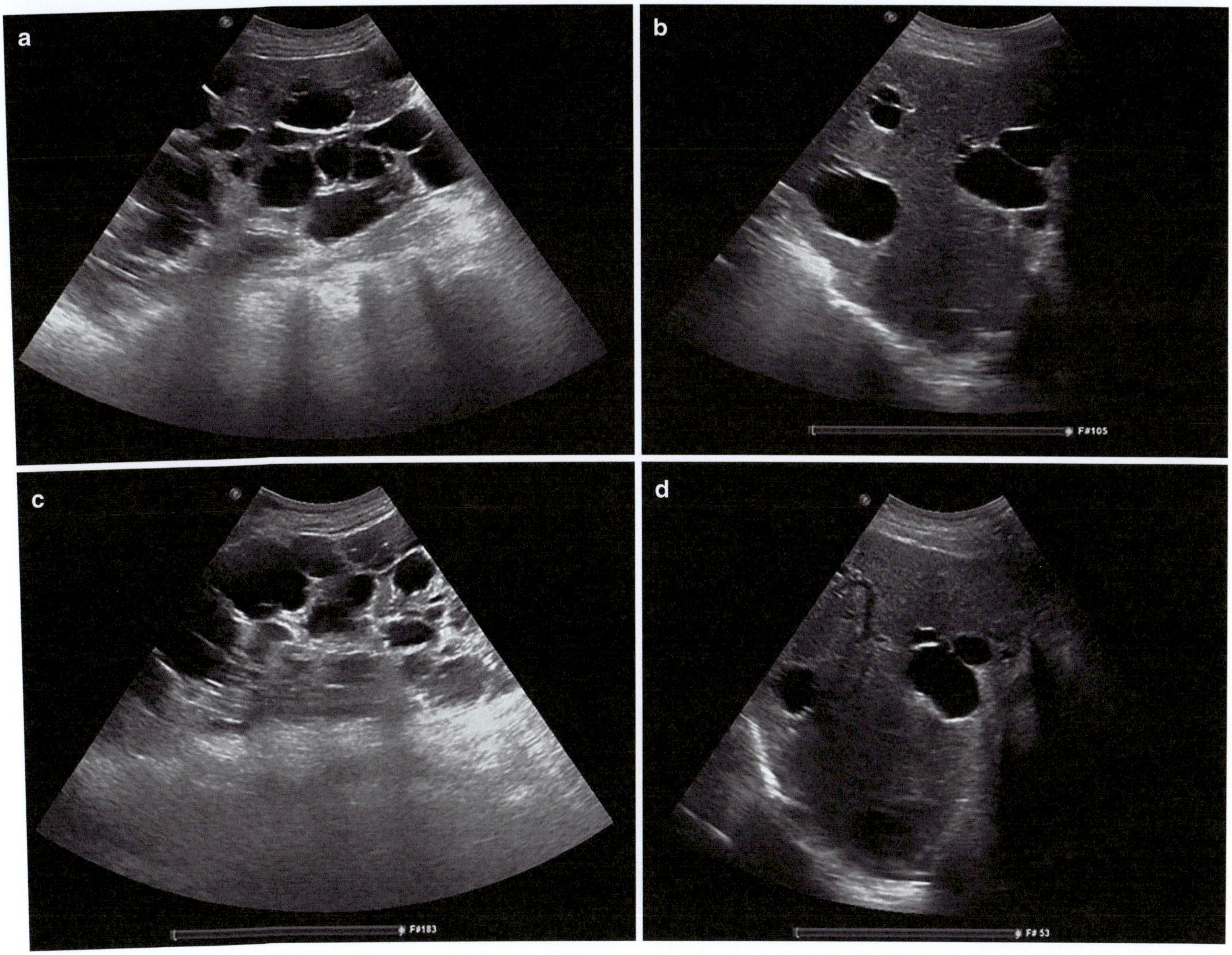

Fig. 9.15 Autosomal dominant polycystic kidney disease (ADPKD). Images (**a**) and (**c**) demonstrate innumerable renal cysts. Note that acoustic enhancement from proximal cysts may make the distal cysts appear more echogenic. Images (**b**) and (**d**) demonstrate liver cysts, which are frequently seen in patients with ADPKD. (*Adapted from the Renal Fellow Network, with permission*)

Table 9.2 Diagnostic criteria for autosomal dominant polycystic kidney disease (ADPKD) [21].

Age	Family History of ADPKD	Number of Cysts
<15 years	Positive	≥1 cysts in total
15–39 years	Positive	≥3 cysts in total
40–59 years	Positive	≥2 cysts in each kidney
>60 years	Positive	≥4 cysts in each kidney
Any age	Negative	> 10 cysts in each kidney

Pyelonephritis

Renal ultrasound is often normal in patients with uncomplicated pyelonephritis, although some nonspecific findings associated with renal inflammation may be seen, including decreased echogenicity and loss of corticomedullary differentiation. Perinephric or periureteral stranding or induration may also be seen. In severe cases, renal enlargement and loss of renal sinus signature are observed (Fig. 9.16). When involvement is focal, a hyper- or hypoechoic wedge-shaped area may be observed, potentially causing confusion with a renal mass [24]. On Doppler imaging, localized regions with either increased or decreased vascularity may indicate interstitial edema and inflammation. Another technique (referred to as sonopalpation) has been proposed, where the curvilinear probe is used to directly visualize the kidney and then pressure is applied over the area to better elucidate whether the pain localizes to the kidney versus surrounding areas [25].

Complicated pyelonephritis can encompass emphysematous pyelonephritis and the development of abscesses. In emphysematous pyelonephritis, the necrotizing infectious

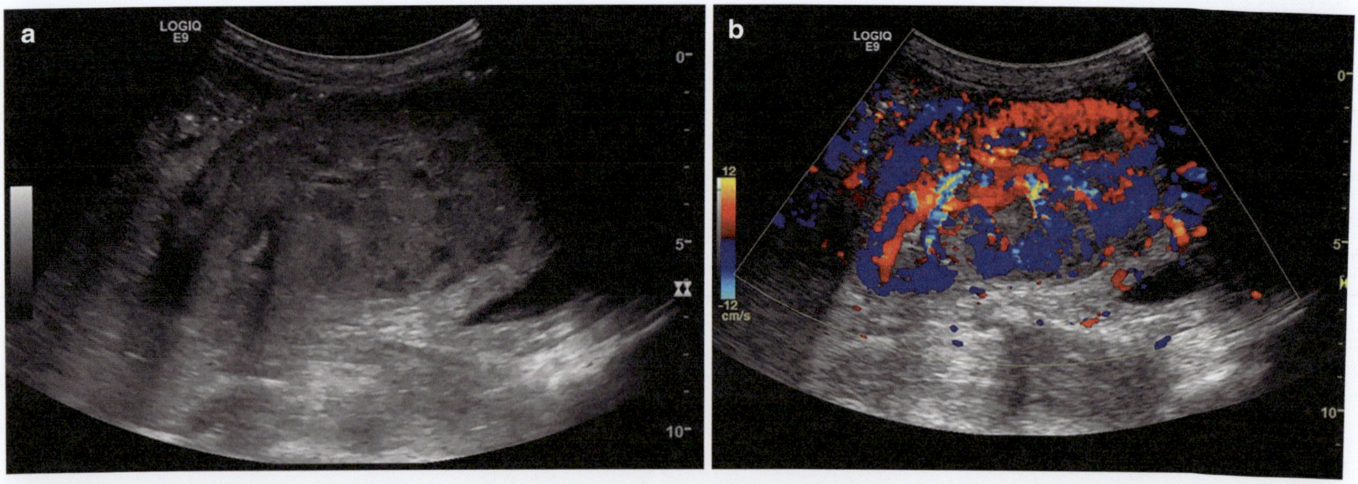

Fig. 9.16 (**a**) Renal ultrasound in a case of severe pyelonephritis demonstrating an enlarged kidney with loss of parenchymal and sinus architecture. (**b**) Color Doppler of the patient in image (a) with marked hyperemia suggestive of inflammation

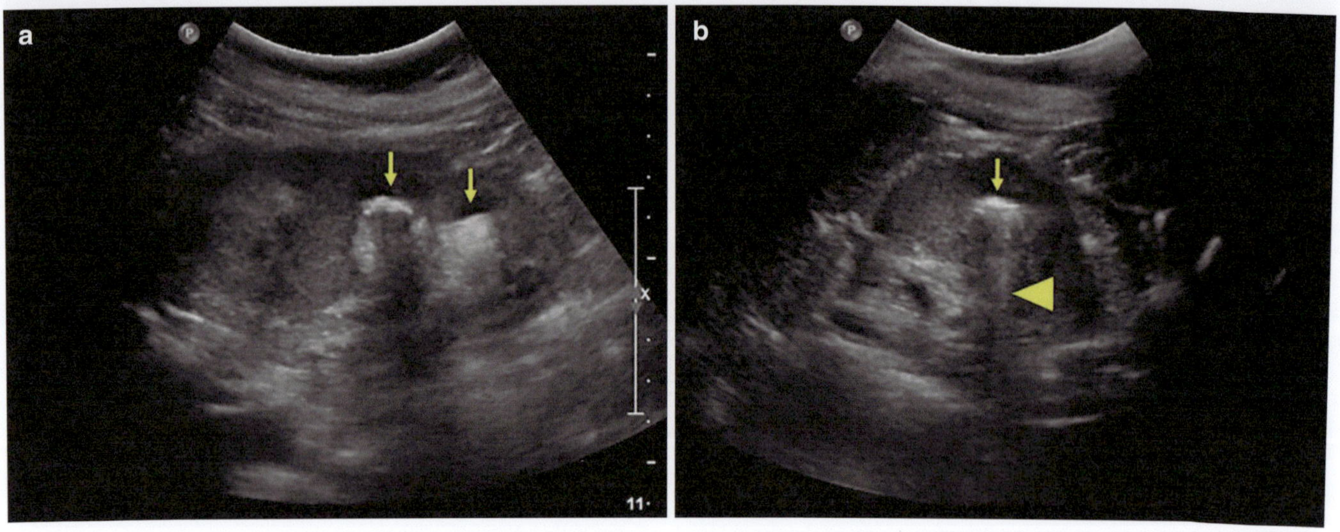

Fig. 9.17 Emphysematous pyelonephritis. (**a**) Renal ultrasound images demonstrating hyperechoic ill-defined foci with dirty shadowing suggestive of air (arrows). (**b**) Transverse view of the kidney showing air (arrows) and ringdown artifacts at the air-fluid (urine) interface (arrowhead)

process leads to gas within the renal parenchyma and surrounding structures. Gas results in bright reflective echoes, producing shadowing, usually with irregular acoustic noise (i.e., "dirty shadowing") that obscures deeper structures [26]. Moreover, the mobility of these hyperechoic foci, along with ringdown artifacts (similar to B-lines on lung ultrasound), provides clues to the presence of air within the kidney (Fig. 9.17). In emphysematous pyelitis, dirty shadowing will appear in the collecting system instead. Because the gas can interfere with visualization on ultrasound, CT is superior in determining the location and extent of gas, though ultrasound can be valuable for initial identification.

A renal abscess appears as a circular, thick-walled, hypoechoic region containing heterogeneous internal debris, which may occasionally exhibit mobility (Fig. 9.18). However, distinguishing an abscess from a hemorrhagic cyst or a cystic neoplasm can be challenging with ultrasound alone. Therefore, interpreting the findings in the appropriate clinical context and comparing them with prior imaging, when available, is essential. When an abscess ruptures into the collecting system, it results in pyonephrosis, evident on ultrasound as mobile debris within the collecting system, potentially accompanied by an associated fluid level (hydronephrosis with internal echoes) (Fig. 9.19) [27]. Although contrast-enhanced CT is sensitive for the diagnosis, revealing thickening of the renal pelvic wall and layering of contrast material around purulent fluid, it is important to note that the diagnosis might be missed on a noncontrast CT [28].

Xanthogranulomatous pyelonephritis is a chronic infection typically associated with obstructive nephrolithiasis.

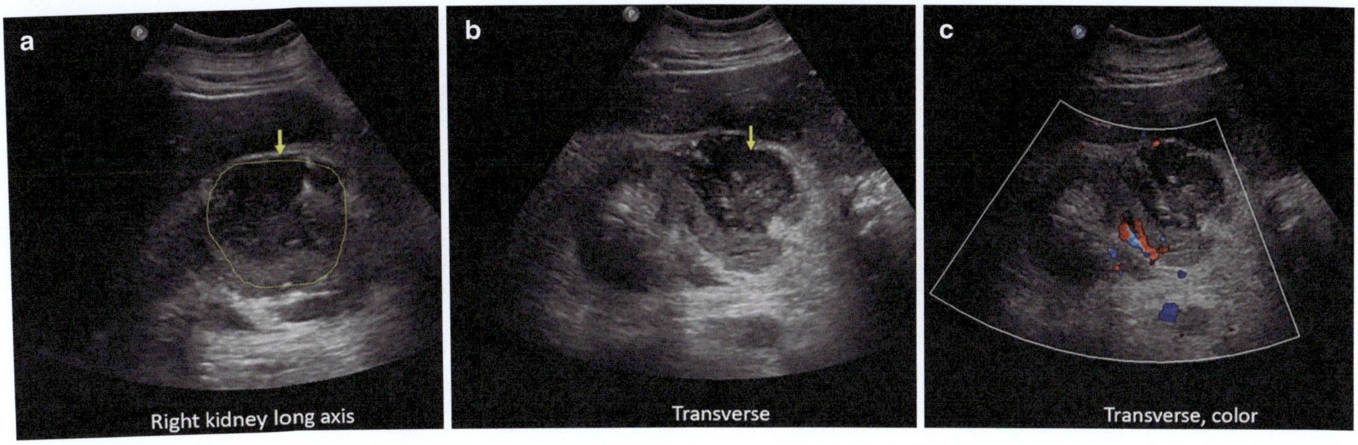

Fig. 9.18 Renal abscess. (**a**) Long-axis view of the right kidney with an abscess (arrow). (**b**) Short-axis view of the kidney with an abscess (arrow). (**c**) Color Doppler demonstrating absence of flow within the abscess in (b)

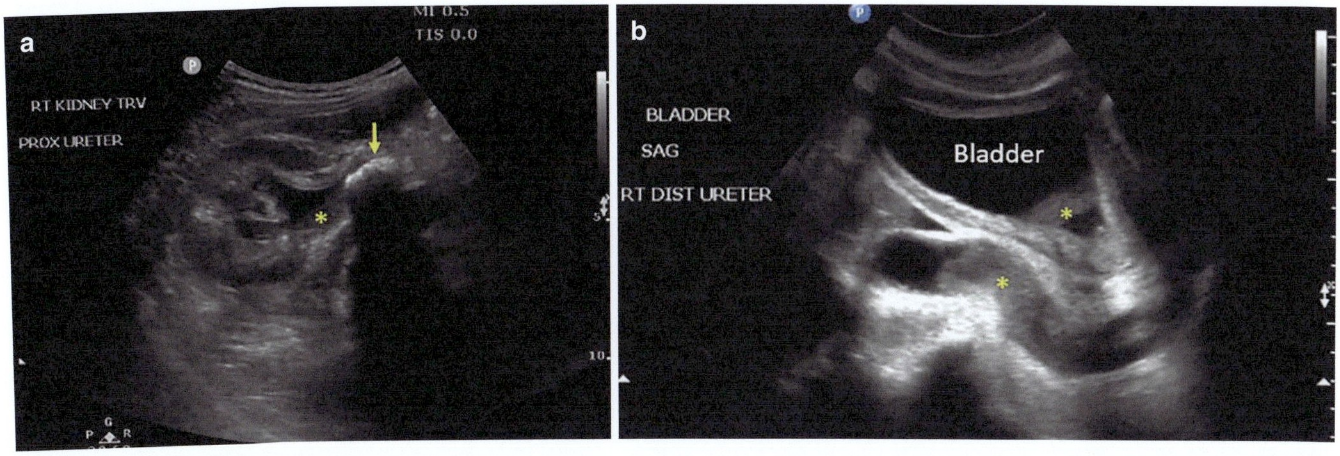

Fig. 9.19 Pyonephrosis. (**a**) Proximal ureter with debris (asterisk) and fluid-debris level. Also present is a large pelvic stone with acoustic shadowing (arrow). (**b**) Distended distal ureter and urinary bladder with visible debris (asterisk). (*Images courtesy of Robert A. Jones, DO*)

Consequently, a dilated collecting system, sometimes with internal debris, is frequently seen on ultrasound. Chronic inflammation may also cause replacement of renal parenchyma by lipid-laden macrophages, leading to multiple hypoechoic areas at the corticomedullary junction and an enlarged kidney [29]. As the imaging findings lack specificity, it is crucial to maintain a high level of suspicion in patients exhibiting chronic inflammation features, such as unintentional weight loss, poor appetite, low-grade fever, or flank pain. A tissue diagnosis is frequently necessary for a definitive diagnosis of xanthogranulomatous pyelonephritis.

Renal Tumors

Most solid renal masses are malignant, requiring thorough evaluation for accurate classification when evaluating a mass lesion. It is important to acknowledge that POCUS may not be adequate for identifying or distinguishing among different types of renal masses, and additional investigations or follow-up measures should be pursued when an incidental renal mass is detected during POCUS.

Renal cell carcinoma is the most frequent renal tumor, and it is the underlying diagnosis for more than 85% of all parenchymal malignant renal tumors [30]. The sonographic appearance can exhibit significant variability, with tumors presenting as heterogeneous hyperechoic, isoechoic, or hypoechoic masses characterized by irregular borders. Renal cell carcinomas may manifest as exophytic or be confined within the renal parenchyma, though most of them alter the renal outline (Fig. 9.20). Approximately 7% of renal cell carcinomas can manifest as cystic tumors, typically classified as complex cysts featuring thick (>2 mm) septations and nodular components [31]. Some studies suggest that microbubble contrast-enhanced ultrasound may outperform CT in diagnosing complex renal masses [32]. Although ultrasound is not ideal for evaluating lymph node or vascular extension, it may demonstrate cephalad tumor extension into the inferior

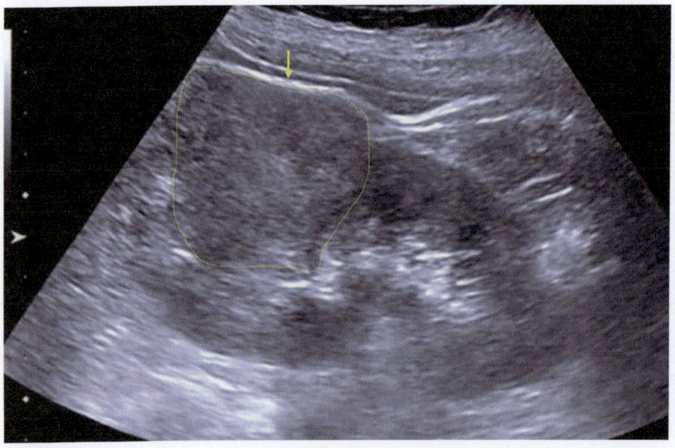

Fig. 9.20 Renal ultrasound image demonstrating a large, exophytic, heterogeneous tumor in the superior pole of the kidney (arrow). Subsequent nephrectomy confirmed renal cell carcinoma on histology.

vena cava (tumor thrombus) (Fig. 9.21). Renal cell carcinomas often display a peripheral vascular pattern on Doppler ultrasound (subject to appropriate scale and gain settings).

Renal angiomyolipomas are usually asymptomatic, although they can be associated with spontaneous retroperitoneal bleeding, a condition known as Wunderlich syndrome [33]. These tumors may manifest sporadically or can be associated with a tuberous sclerosis complex [34]. On ultrasound, they appear round and homogenous with an increased echogenicity similar to that of renal sinus fat (Fig. 9.22). However, in cases where muscular or vascular elements dominate, the tumor may appear hypoechoic. While sonographic findings are fairly sensitive to these benign hamartomatous tumors, ultrasound faces challenges in accurately distinguishing angiomyolipomas from small echogenic renal cell carcinomas. Notably, the presence of shadowing has been reported exclusively in angiomyolipomas, whereas

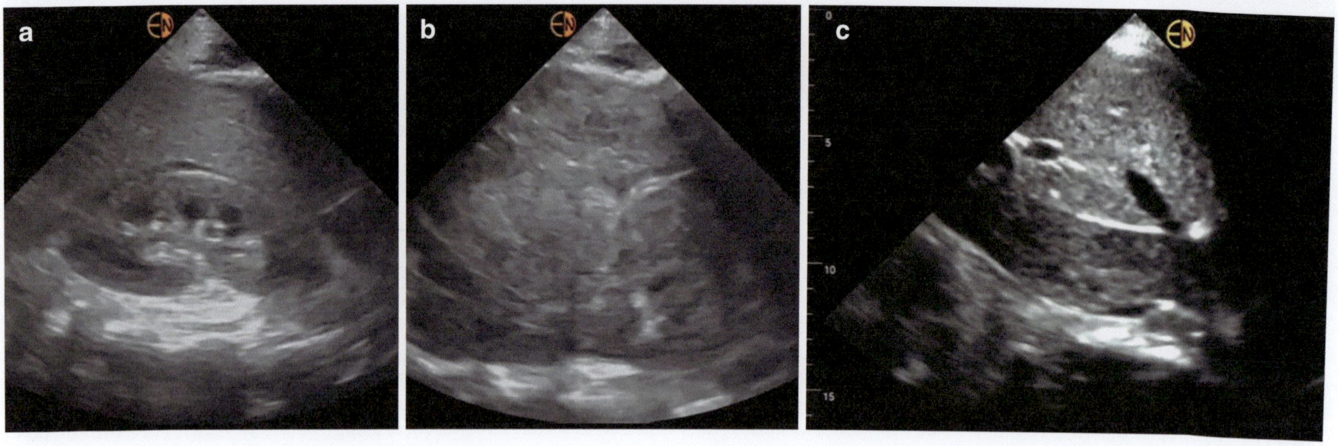

Fig. 9.21 Ultrasound findings in a patient with advanced renal cell carcinoma. (**a**) The right kidney displays a normal appearance with a surrounding rim of perirenal fluid resulting from malignant ascites. (**b**) The left kidney exhibits a loss of parenchymal architecture, replaced by a substantial heterogeneous mass. (**c**) Within the inferior vena cava, there is a presence of heterogeneous echogenic content due to a tumor thrombus. Note the hypoechoic lumen of the uninvolved hepatic vein for comparison

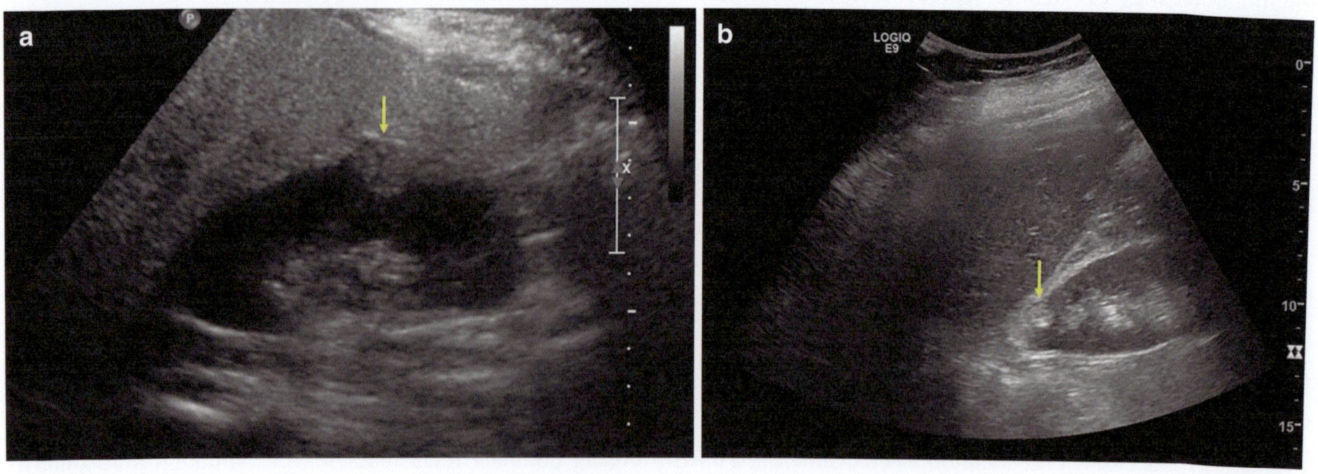

Fig. 9.22 Renal ultrasound images demonstrating solitary angiomyolipomas (arrows) in two different patients. Note the echogenicity is similar to that of adjacent sinus fat

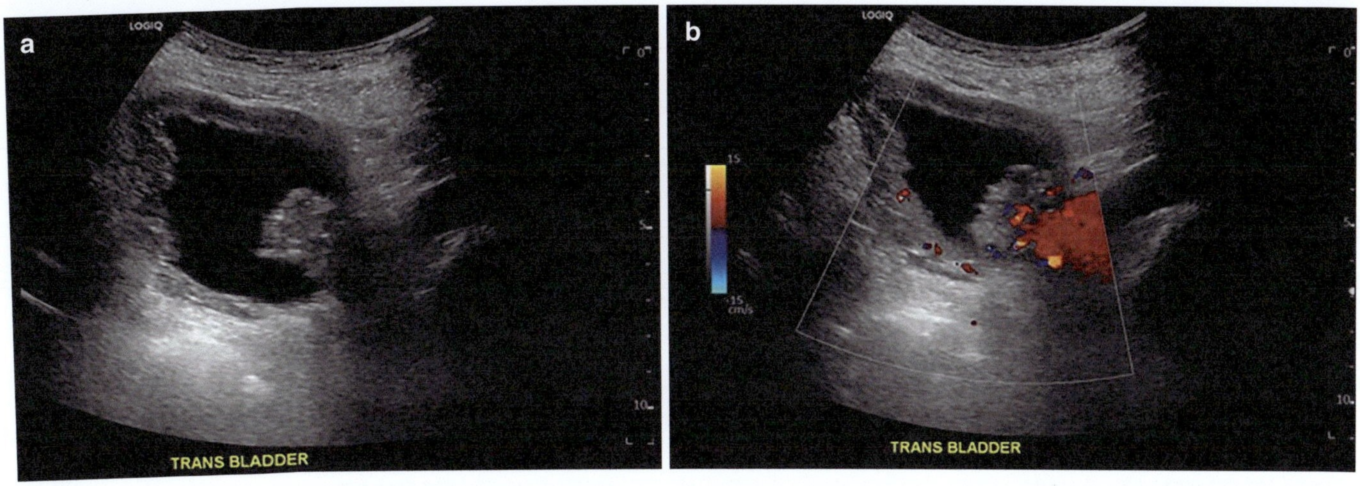

Fig. 9.23 (**a**) Bladder ultrasound images demonstrating a polypoid bladder tumor with heterogeneous echogenicity arising from the bladder wall. (**b**) Color Doppler demonstrating associated hyperemia

hypoechoic rims and intratumoral cysts have been associated with renal cell carcinoma [35]. Contrast-enhanced CT should be considered when in doubt for accurate differentiation. Other less common renal tumors include Wilms tumor, adenocarcinoma, oncocytoma, lymphoma, and metastasis.

Bladder Tumors

Urothelial carcinoma of the bladder is the most common malignant bladder tumor [36]. Approximately 70% of these tumors are superficial while the rest are invasive [36]. Ultrasound is excellent for the detection of polypoid bladder tumors with >95% sensitivity [37]. On imaging, these tumors appear as a solitary or multifocal immobile mass arising from the bladder wall or as focal wall thickening of heterogeneous echogenicity (Fig. 9.23). It is important to recognize that these findings are not specific and there is a large differential diagnosis including diffuse cystitis, extrinsic ovarian, rectal or ureterovaginal tumors, benign prostatic hypertrophy, and blood clots. Focal or asymmetric wall thickening points to bladder tumor rather than cystitis while caudal angling of the probe can usually reveal contiguity with prostate gland in benign prostatic hypertrophy. The presence of blood clots is suggested by the findings of a mobile, avascular mass [37].

Renal Artery Stenosis

During the POCUS examination of a patient with suspected secondary hypertension or progressive kidney injury, impaired arterial flow to the kidney may be evident. Parenchymal pulsed-wave Doppler at the interlobar artery level will generate the typical arterial waveform, allowing qualitative appreciation and calculation of various parameters. These include the renal resistive index (RI = [peak systolic velocity – end diastolic velocity]/peak systolic velocity), the acceleration time (which is the duration from the beginning of the systolic upstroke to the peak systolic velocity), and the acceleration index (representing the slope, in m/s^2, exhibited by the arterial Doppler signal during this period) (Fig. 9.24).

The presence of a prolonged systolic acceleration and a renal RI lower than expected are indirect indicators of a hemodynamically significant impediment to arterial flow anywhere between the heart and the kidney. The normal renal RI range is 0.5–0.7 [38]. A parenchymal absolute renal RI $\geq$ 0.05 lower than the contralateral side is considered a significant finding [39]. Additionally, an acceleration time exceeding 0.07 s or an acceleration index less than 3 m/s^2 coupled with a waveform qualitatively appearing 'dampened' (also referred to as *parvus et tardus*) serve as indirect signs of renal artery stenosis [40]. The qualitative assessment is commonly performed in point-of-care settings and has been reported to exhibit high specificity (98%) but moderate sensitivity (83%) [41]. Image acquisition is often impeded by bowel gas at the ostia and respiratory movements of the kidney. If suspicious qualitative findings are detected, it is prudent to obtain CT or MR angiography for further evaluation.

If ultrasound (typically consultative imaging) is used to confirm the diagnosis, the site of stenosis can be confirmed by identifying direct signs of stenosis including a high peak velocity at the site of the stenosis ($\geq$180 cm/s) in the renal artery, or an increased peak renal-to-aortic velocity ratio ($\geq$3.5) [41, 42]. Even after confirmation, indirect Doppler indices continue to hold clinical relevance. The presence of a high renal RI ($\geq$0.8) or kidney atrophy typically indicates a long-standing stenosis, suggesting limited potential benefits if revascularization were to be attempted [43].

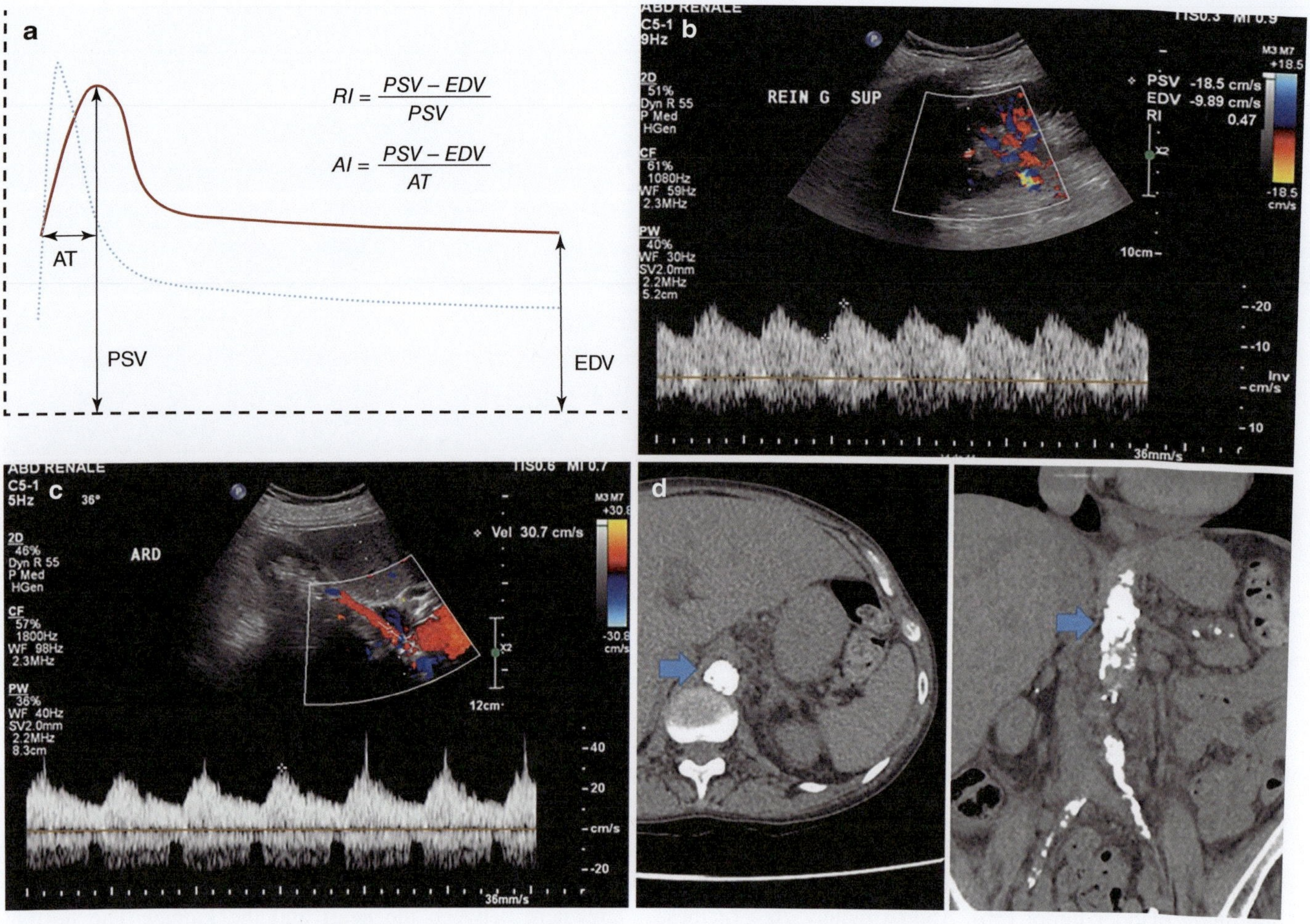

Fig. 9.24 (**a**) Quantitative measures including renal resistive index (RI), acceleration time (AT), and acceleration index (AI). Example of a blunted intrarenal arterial waveform (red) suggestive of renal artery stenosis compared to normal waveform (blue). (**b**) Renal artery Doppler of the right kidney demonstrating prolonged AT with decreased renal RI (0.47). (**c**) Similar findings to **b** were present on Doppler assessment of the right renal artery up to the ostium suggestive of a stenosis. (**d**) Abdominal CT revealed the presence of extensive calcifications resulting in the stenosis of the suprarenal abdominal aorta (arrows). *PSV* peak systolic velocity, *EDV* end-diastolic velocity

The occurrence of comparable alterations in arterial waveforms in both kidneys during Doppler assessment may suggest that the pathology is proximal to the renal arteries, such as within the abdominal aorta. This can be further validated by conducting pulsed-wave Doppler on the abdominal aorta, femoral arteries, or arteries of other abdominal organs, revealing similar waveform alterations. It is important to note that left ventricular dysfunction or aortic valve stenosis can also generate these *parvus et tardus* alterations in arterial Doppler waveforms and should be considered in the differential diagnosis when clinically relevant.

Congestive Cardiorenal Syndrome

Intra-renal Doppler can be used to assess the hemodynamic impact of venous pressure (right atrial pressure) on the kidney. Pulsed-wave Doppler at the level of the interlobar veins can identify intra-renal venous signals which are usually of a velocity between 10 and 20 cm/s [44]. The normal venous pattern is characterized by an uninterrupted signal below-the-baseline (Fig. 9.25a). As venous pressure rises, interruptions become apparent, corresponding to the absence of venous return during a portion of the cardiac cycle. Initially, these interruptions are brief, with preserved flow in both systole and diastole (i.e., a biphasic pattern) (Fig. 9.25b). However, in severe cases, they become prolonged, and venous signal is restricted to the diastole (i.e., a monophasic pattern) (Fig. 9.25c). The arterial waveform above the baseline serves as a built-in electrocardiogram aiding in the identification of different phases of the cardiac cycle. The severity of these alterations can be assessed by estimating the proportion of the cardiac cycle during which venous flow is absent, known as the renal venous stasis index (RVSI) (Fig. 9.25d). The RVSI proves useful in determining the severity of alterations within signals of the same patterns or between patterns

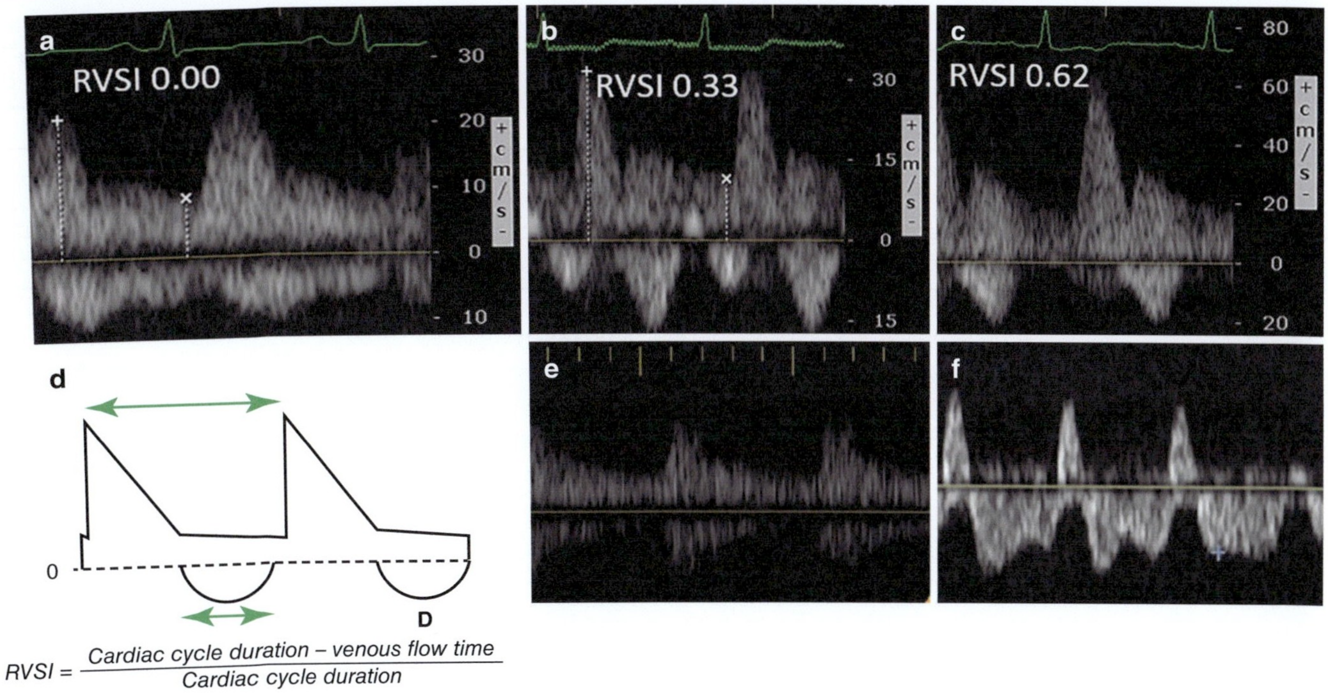

Fig. 9.25 Intra-renal venous Doppler can be classified by patterns and by the renal venous stasis index (RVSI). In the same patient, the patterns change over time from the continuous uninterrupted pattern (**a**), the pattern with short interruptions with flow in systole and diastole (**b**), and the pattern with prolonged interruptions with flow only in diastole (**c**). Calculation of the RVSI involves estimating the duration of venous flow time compared to the cardiac cycle (**d**). Common pitfalls of venous Doppler include misidentifying a mirror image of the arterial waveform (**e**) or assessing the main renal vein, which may produce a pattern similar to the hepatic vein (**f**)

with potential overlap (Fig. 9.25e). It is essential to exercise caution to avoid misinterpreting a mirror image of the arterial waveform as the venous signal or using the signal from the main renal vein, which may exhibit a higher degree of pulsatility (Fig. 9.25f).

The existence of abnormal patterns and the RVSI have both been linked to the severity of heart failure, the presence of kidney dysfunction, and the overall prognosis of patients with heart failure [45]. Intra-renal venous flow tends to show improvement during effective decongestive therapy, and such changes have been reported to correlate with concurrent improvements in kidney function [46, 47]. However, in patients with severe right heart failure or pulmonary hypertension, achieving a complete normalization of intra-renal venous flow patterns may not be attainable. The venous waveform's quality may be insufficient for interpretation or potentially misleading, particularly in critically ill patients, where the failure rate of this technique is approximately 25% [48]. In the presence of an abnormal waveform, especially if the tracing quality is suboptimal, it is advisable to verify the presence of abnormal venous waveforms at other sites, such as the portal vein or hepatic vein, as suggested by Venous Excess Ultrasound (VExUS) [47].

Evaluation of Renal Transplant

The renal allograft is typically situated in the extra-peritoneal space, either in the right or left iliac fossa, and is easily accessible for ultrasound examination. The renal arteries and veins of the allograft are anastomosed to their corresponding iliac arteries and veins. The ureters of the allograft are anastomosed to the anterolateral aspect of the bladder, and it is common to insert a temporary ureteral stent to mitigate the risk of leaks and obstruction. These factors must be considered when performing ultrasound of a renal allograft.

Ultrasound facilitates the diagnosis of common post-transplantation complications, including the timely identification of fluid collections (e.g., hematoma, urinoma, and lymphocele), obstruction, and vascular complications [49]. A mild degree of hydronephrosis is common among transplanted kidneys due to the implantation of the ureter in the bladder, even in the absence of urodynamic obstruction (Fig. 9.26). If obstruction is suspected, extrinsic obstruction from fluid collections (Figs. 9.26 and 9.27) or catheter obstruction should be considered in the immediate postoperative period, while urolithiasis or ureteral strictures should be ruled out in the late post-transplant period [50].

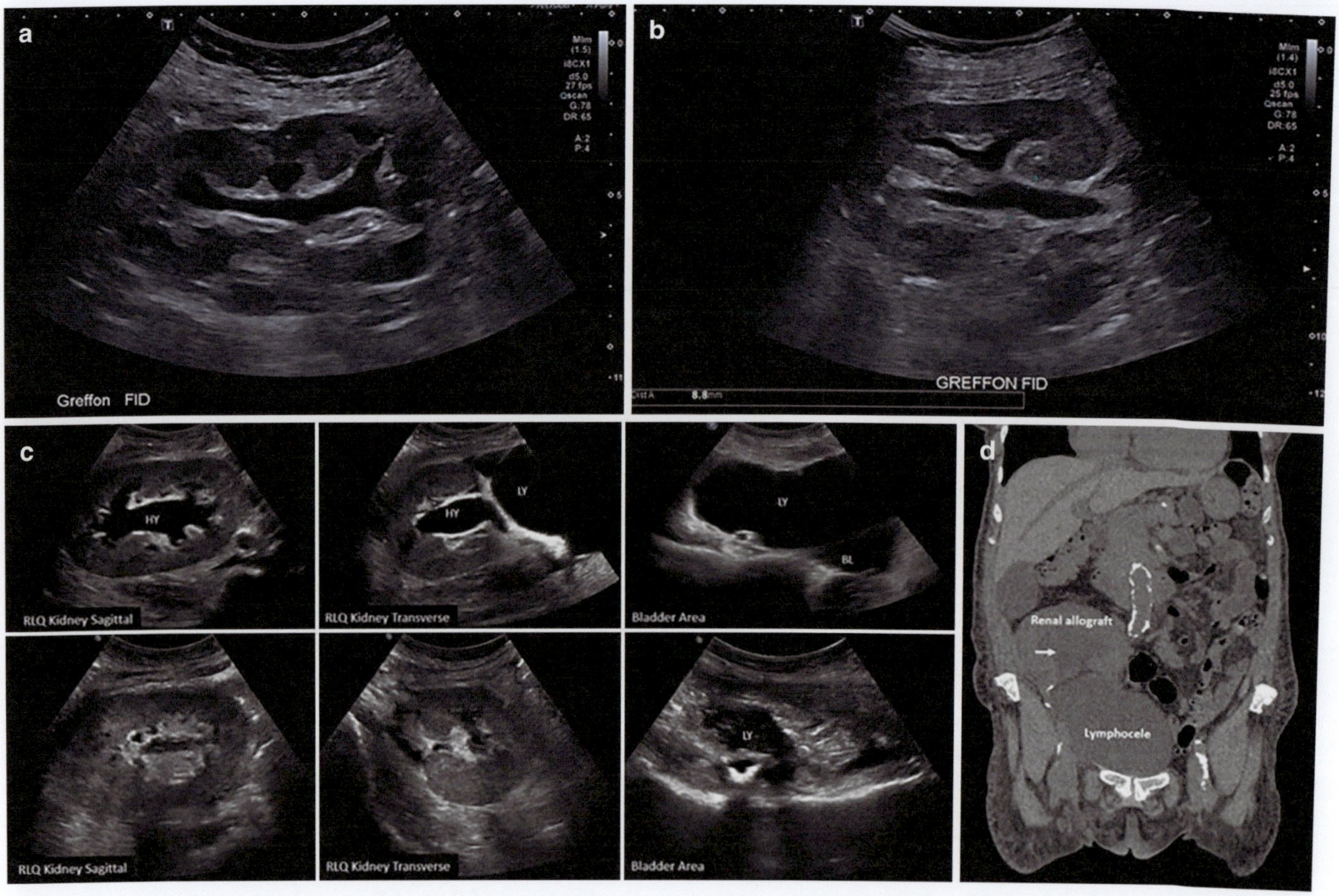

Fig. 9.26 (**a**) Mild hydronephrosis in a patient with a functioning allograft. (**b**) Mild hydroureteronephrosis in a patient with a functioning allograft. (**c**) Hydronephrosis with impaired graft function caused by a large fluid collection (*LY* lymphocele). (**d**). Abdominal CT confirming the presence of a lymphocele in the patient in image (**c**). (*Figure reused with permission from NephroPOCUS.com*)

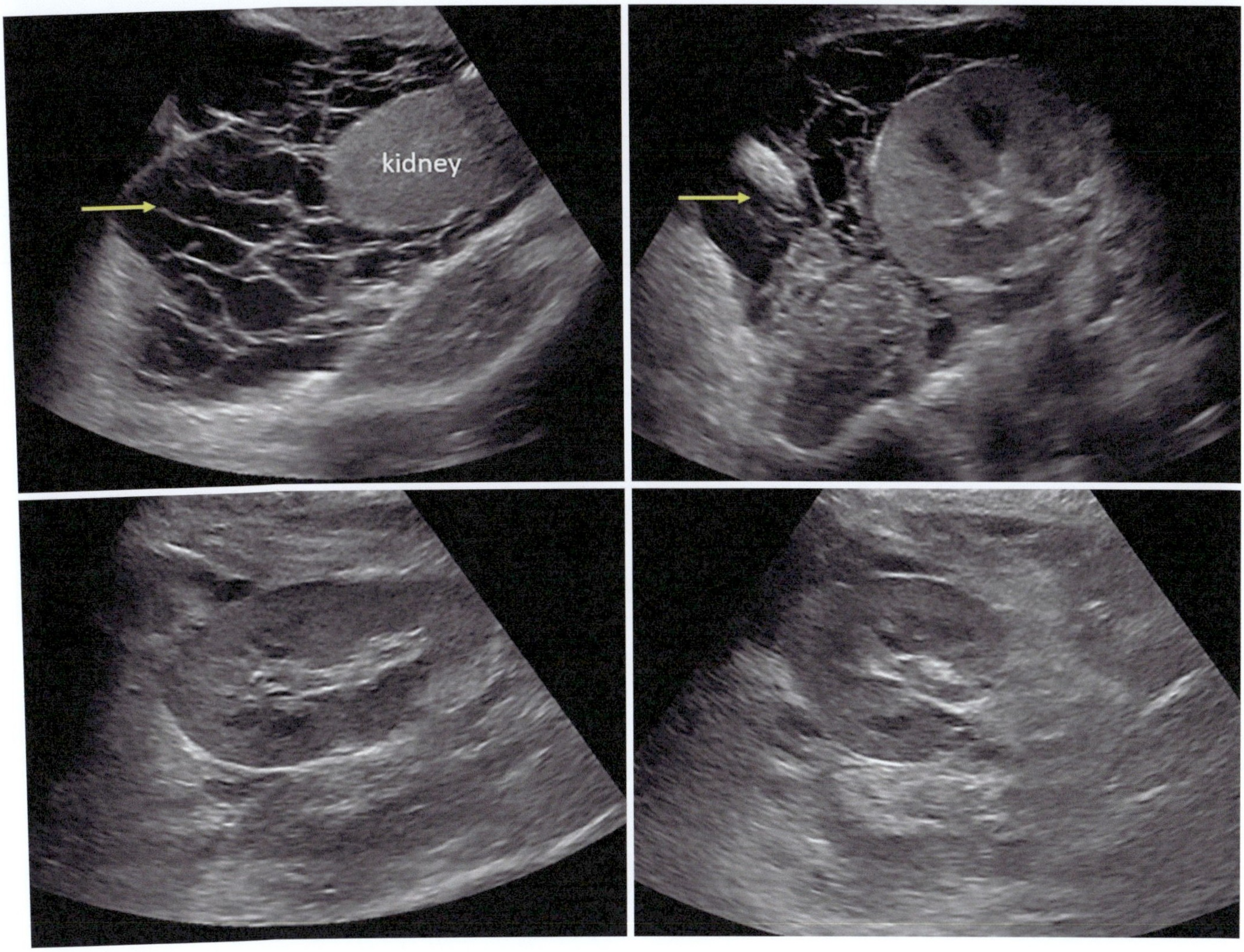

Fig. 9.27 The top ultrasound images demonstrate a transplanted kidney with a large collection of septated fluid around it (arrows). The bottom ultrasound images demonstrate substantial reduction in the perinephric collection after evacuation. Fluid analysis was consistent with a lymphocele. A hematoma can have a similar appearance, though the septations tend to be coarser.

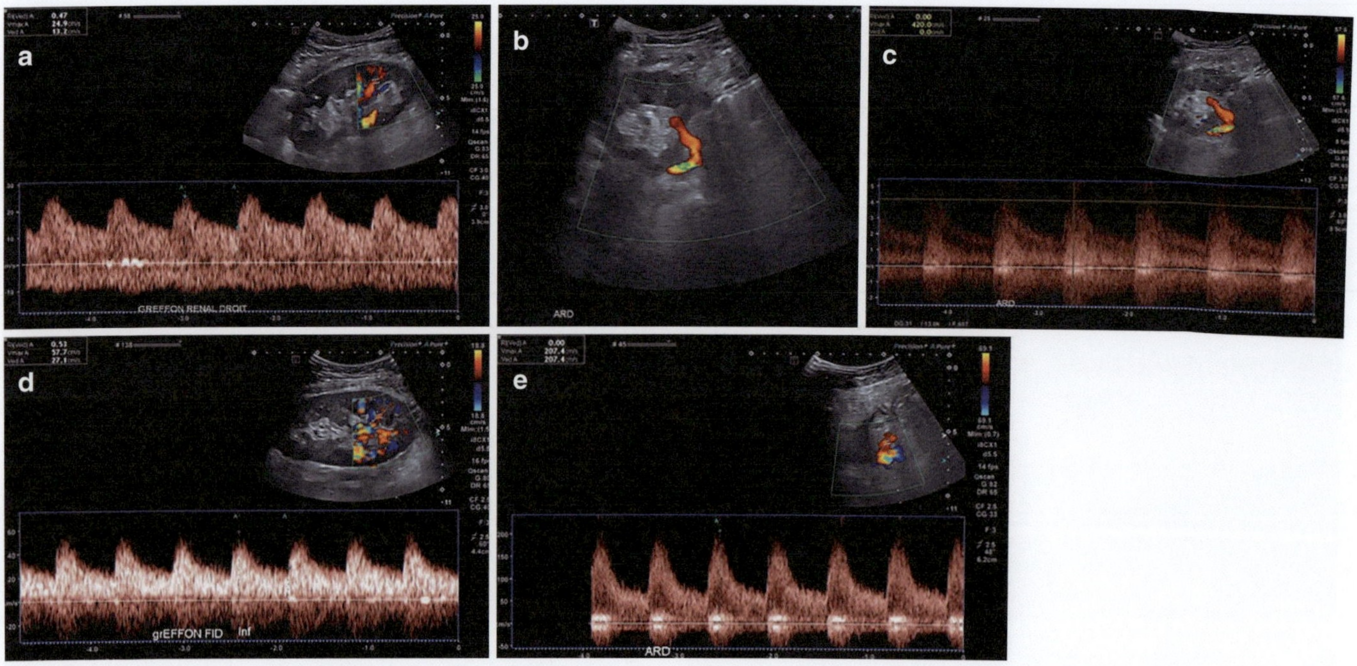

Fig. 9.28 Postoperative kidney transplant. (**a**) Blunted arterial waveform with a low renal resistive index (0.47). (**b**) Color Doppler demonstrates the kinked segment of the renal artery with flow acceleration. (**c**) Pulsed-wave Doppler evaluation of the image in B reveals accelerations up to 300–400 cm/sec in that region. (**d**) Repeat ultrasound performed 4 days later reveals improved intrarenal arterial waveform with a higher RI (0.53), suggestive of resolution of the kinked segment. (**e**) Reduced flow acceleration (207 cm/s) in the repeat ultrasound performed at 4 days

The occurrence of delayed or acute graft dysfunction should trigger an investigation into potential vascular causes. Normal renal RI in transplanted kidneys is 0.60–0.70. As mentioned earlier, a low renal RI (RI <0.60 for renal transplant), indicating slow systolic acceleration, may suggest partial occlusion of the renal transplant artery. In the immediate postoperative phase, this could be attributed to kinking of the transplanted renal artery, which may resolve spontaneously (Fig. 9.28). In the late post-transplant period, this finding could signify arterial stenosis. In contrast, an elevated renal RI (>0.70) in the context of graft dysfunction is nonspecific and can be associated with conditions such as acute or chronic transplant rejection, acute tubular necrosis causing delayed graft function, acute urinary obstruction, or be linked to extra-renal hemodynamic factors (e.g., increased pulse pressure seen with aortic regurgitation). The venous Doppler of the kidney graft should exhibit a continuous or cardiophasic pattern, as previously described. The absence of a venous Doppler signal in the presence of a high RI may suggest the presence of renal vein thrombosis.

Key Ultrasound Findings

Diagnosis	Key ultrasound findings
Hydronephrosis	Anechoic branching area in the renal collecting system region.
Ureteral stones	Hyperechoic, relatively well-defined structures followed by an acoustic shadow. Twinkling may be seen on color Doppler.
Bladder volume	Calculated as height × depth × width × 0.52.
Foley catheter placement	Foley balloon appears as a fluid-filled, anechoic circular structure within the decompressed bladder.
Simple cyst	A well-defined, round, and anechoic structure free of internal echoes and associated with acoustic enhancement.
Complex cyst	Cyst with internal echogenicities, septations, or a thick irregular wall.
Autosomal dominant polycystic kidney disease	Enlarged kidneys with multiple bilateral cysts typically in patients with a positive family history. Often associated with cysts in other organs (e.g., liver and spleen).

(continued)

Diagnosis	Key ultrasound findings
Acquired cystic kidney disease	Small kidneys with multiple cysts typically in patients with advanced chronic kidney disease.
Pyelonephritis	Ultrasound is often normal. Local changes in parenchymal echogenicity or blood flow may be present.
Emphysematous pyelonephritis	Hyperechoic, often mobile foci with dirty shadowing in the renal parenchyma and collecting system.
Pyonephrosis	Echogenic debris intermixed with hydronephrosis.
Renal tumor	A heterogeneous hyperechoic, isoechoic, or hypoechoic solid lesion characterized by irregular borders often disrupting the renal outline. May contain cystic components.
Renal artery stenosis	Indirect findings: Prolonged systolic acceleration (>0.07 s), *parvus et tardus* appearance, or lower renal resistive index than contralateral side (≥0.05). Direct findings: High peak velocity at the site of stenosis (≥190 cm/s) or increased peak renal-to-aortic ratio (≥3.5).
Venous congestion	Increased proportion of the cardiac cycle during which no venous Doppler signal is present. Severe anomalies present detectable venous signals only in diastole.

Pearls and Pitfalls

- Fanning the probe to visualize the entire kidney and bladder is essential to avoid overlooking pathologic findings.
- Parapelvic cysts may be confused with hydronephrosis. These cysts usually present as well-defined lesions in the renal pelvis area with no apparent connection to the ureter whereas hydronephrosis maintains continuity with the ureter and branches into the kidney.
- Color Doppler aids in differentiating between a dilated collecting system and prominent vessels or vascular malformations.
- A normal renal ultrasound does not exclude pyelonephritis.
- Stones are visualized as hyperechoic foci with clean shadowing, while air in the kidney parenchyma or collecting system (emphysematous pyelonephritis) manifests as mobile hyperechoic foci accompanied by dirty shadowing and ring-down artifacts.
- The presence of echogenic debris in the dilated collecting system should raise suspicion for pyonephrosis.
- The presence of a Foley catheter does not rule out bladder obstruction. Ultrasound can detect an obstructed or incorrectly placed catheter.
- Mild pelvicalyceal dilation may be a normal finding in a well-functioning renal allograft. Comparing the study with prior imaging can be helpful.
- Renal resistive index is a non-specific parameter and cannot definitively diagnose any condition.
- Renal venous congestion, often observed in the context of right heart dysfunction, is characterized by interrupted venous flow patterns. The severity of congestion correlates with the extent of venous flow interruption during each cardiac cycle.

References

1. O'Neill WC. Renal relevant radiology: use of ultrasound in kidney disease and nephrology procedures. Clin J Am Soc Nephrol. 2014;9(2):373–81. https://doi.org/10.2215/CJN.03170313.
2. Delair SM, Kurzrock EA. Clinical utility of ureteral jets: disparate opinions. J Endourol. 2006;20(2):111–4. https://doi.org/10.1089/end.2006.20.111.
3. Ferguson T, Bechtel W. Hydronephrosis of pregnancy. Am Fam Physician. 1991;43(6):2135–7.
4. Onen A. An alternative grading system to refine the criteria for severity of hydronephrosis and optimal treatment guidelines in neonates with primary UPJ-type hydronephrosis. J Pediatr Urol. 2007;3(3):200–5. https://doi.org/10.1016/j.jpurol.2006.08.002.
5. Smith-Bindman R, Aubin C, Bailitz J, Bengiamin RN, et al. Ultrasonography versus computed tomography for suspected nephrolithiasis. N Engl J Med. 2014;371(12):1100–10. https://doi.org/10.1056/NEJMoa1404446.
6. Kelahan LC, Desser TS, Troxell ML, Kamaya A. Ultrasound assessment of acute kidney injury. Ultrasound Q. 2019;35(2):173–80. https://doi.org/10.1097/RUQ.0000000000000389.
7. Koratala A, Bhattacharya D, Kazory A. Point of care renal ultrasonography for the busy nephrologist: a pictorial review. World J Nephrol. 2019;8(3):44–58. https://doi.org/10.5527/wjn.v8.i3.44.
8. Simon JC, Maxwell AD, Bailey MR. Some work on the diagnosis and management of kidney stones with ultrasound. Acoust Today. 2017;13(4):52–9.
9. Gliga ML, Chirila CN, Podeanu DM, Imola T, et al. Twinkle, twinkle little stone: an artifact improves the ultrasound performance! Med Ultrason. 2017;19(3):272–5.
10. Moesbergen TC, de Ryke RJ, Dunbar S, Wells JE, Anderson NG. Distal ureteral calculi: US follow-up. Radiology. 2011;260(2):575–80. https://doi.org/10.1148/radiol.11101077.
11. Bih LI, Ho CC, Tsai SJ, Lai YC, et al. Bladder shape impact on the accuracy of ultrasonic estimation of bladder volume. Arch Phys Med Rehabil. 1998;79(12):1553–6. https://doi.org/10.1016/s0003-9993(98)90419-1.
12. Bejjanki H, Koratala A. The TIE fighter sign on point of care ultrasonography. CEN Case Rep. 2020;9(1):91–3. https://doi.org/10.1007/s13730-019-00428-x.
13. Witt M, Baumann BM, McCans K. Bladder ultrasound increases catheterization success in pediatric patients. Acad Emerg Med. 2005;12(4):371–4.

14. Gatti JM, Perez-Brayfield M, Kirsch AJ, Smith EA, Massad HC, Broecker BH. Acute urinary retention in children. J Urol. 2001;165(3):918–21.
15. Jacob P, Rai BP, Todd AW. Suprapubic catheter insertion using an ultrasound-guided technique and literature review. BJU Int. 2012;110(6):779–84. https://doi.org/10.1111/j.1464-410X.2011.10882.x.
16. Mitterberger M, Horninger W, Aigner F, Pinggera GM, et al. Ultrasound of the prostate. Cancer Imaging. 2010;10(1):40–8. https://doi.org/10.1102/1470-7330.2010.0004.
17. Simms RJ, Ong AC. How simple are 'simple renal cysts'? Nephrol Dial Transplant. 2014;29(Suppl 4):iv106–12. https://doi.org/10.1093/ndt/gfu106.
18. Carrim ZI, Murchison JT. The prevalence of simple renal and hepatic cysts detected by spiral computed tomography. Clin Radiol. 2003;58(8):626–9. https://doi.org/10.1016/s0009-9260(03)00165-x.
19. Hélénon O, Crosnier A, Verkarre V, Merran S, et al. Simple and complex renal cysts in adults: classification system for renal cystic masses. Diagn Interv Imaging. 2018;99(4):189–218. https://doi.org/10.1016/j.diii.2017.10.005.
20. Silverman SG, Pedrosa I, Ellis JH, Hindman NM, Schieda N, Smith AD, Remer EM, Shinagare AB, Curci NE, Raman SS, Wells SA, Kaffenberger SD, Wang ZJ, Chandarana H, Davenport MS. Bosniak classification of cystic renal masses, version 2019: an update proposal and needs assessment. Radiology. 2019;292(2):475–88. https://doi.org/10.1148/radiol.2019182646.
21. Pei Y, Obaji J, Dupuis A, Paterson AD, Magistroni R, et al. Unified criteria for ultrasonographic diagnosis of ADPKD. J Am Soc Nephrol. 2009;20(1):205–12. https://doi.org/10.1681/ASN.2008050507.
22. Bergmann C, Guay-Woodford LM, Harris PC, Horie S, et al. Polycystic kidney disease. Nat Rev Dis Primers. 2018;4(1):50. https://doi.org/10.1038/s41572-018-0047-y.
23. Rahbari-Oskoui F, O'Neill WC. Diagnosis and management of acquired cystic kidney disease and renal tumors in ESRD patients. Semin Dial. 2017;30(4):373–9. https://doi.org/10.1111/sdi.12605.
24. Farmer KD, Gellett LR, Dubbins PA. The sonographic appearance of acute focal pyelonephritis 8 years' experience. Clin Radiol. 2002;57(6):483–7. https://doi.org/10.1053/crad.2002.0935.
25. Faust JS, Tsung JW. Eliciting renal tenderness by sonopalpation in diagnosing acute pyelonephritis. Crit Ultrasound J. 2017;9(1):1. https://doi.org/10.1186/s13089-016-0056-6.
26. Joseph RC, Amendola MA, Artze ME, Casillas J, et al. Genitourinary tract gas: imaging evaluation. Radiographics. 1996;16(2):295–308. https://doi.org/10.1148/radiographics.16.2.8966288.
27. Yoder IC, Pfister RC, Lindfors KK, Newhouse JH. Pyonephrosis: imaging and intervention. AJR Am J Roentgenol. 1983;141(4):735–40. https://doi.org/10.2214/ajr.141.4.735.
28. Kamboj M, Lee Loy J, Koratala A. Renal ultrasonography: a reliable diagnostic tool for pyonephrosis. Clin Case Rep. 2018;6(6):1176–8. https://doi.org/10.1002/ccr3.1512.
29. Tiu CM, Chou YH, Chiou HJ, Lo CB, et al. Sonographic features of xanthogranulomatous pyelonephritis. J Clin Ultrasound. 2001;29(5):279–85. https://doi.org/10.1002/jcu.1034.
30. Frank I, Blute ML, Cheville JC, Lohse CM, Weaver AL, Zincke H. Solid renal tumors: an analysis of pathological features related to tumor size. J Urol. 2003;170(6 Pt 1):2217–20. https://doi.org/10.1097/01.ju.0000095475.12515.5e.
31. Jhaveri K, Gupta P, Elmi A, Flor L, et al. Cystic renal cell carcinomas: do they grow, metastasize, or recur? AJR Am J Roentgenol. 2013;201(2):W292–6. https://doi.org/10.2214/AJR.12.9414.
32. Quaia E, Bertolotto M, Cioffi V, Rossi A, et al. Comparison of contrast-enhanced sonography with unenhanced sonography and contrast-enhanced CT in the diagnosis of malignancy in complex cystic renal masses. AJR Am J Roentgenol. 2008;191(4):1239–49. https://doi.org/10.2214/AJR.07.3546.
33. Shah JN, Gandhi D, Prasad SR, Sandhu PK, et al. Wunderlich syndrome: comprehensive review of diagnosis and management. Radiographics. 2023;43(6):e220172. https://doi.org/10.1148/rg.220172.
34. Nelson CP, Sanda MG. Contemporary diagnosis and management of renal angiomyolipoma. J Urol. 2002;168(4 Pt 1):1315–25. https://doi.org/10.1016/S0022-5347(05)64440-0.
35. Siegel CL, Middleton WD, Teefey SA, McClennan BL. Angiomyolipoma and renal cell carcinoma: US differentiation. Radiology. 1996;198(3):789–93. https://doi.org/10.1148/radiology.198.3.8628873.
36. Gharibvand MM, et al. The role of ultrasound in diagnosis and evaluation of bladder tumors. J Family Med Prim Care. 2017;6(4):840–3.
37. Dershaw DD, Scher HI. Sonography in evaluation of carcinoma of bladder. Urology. 1987;29(4):454e457.
38. Parolini C, Noce A, Staffolani E, Giarrizzo GF, Costanzi S, Splendiani G. Renal resistive index and long-term outcome in chronic nephropathies. Radiology. 2009;252(3):888–96.
39. Schwerk WB, Restrepo IK, Stellwaag M, Klose KJ, et al. Renal artery stenosis: grading with image-directed Doppler US evaluation of renal resistive index. Radiology. 1994;190(3):785–90. https://doi.org/10.1148/radiology.190.3.8115628.
40. Granata A, Fiorini F, Andrulli S, Logias F, et al. Doppler ultrasound and renal artery stenosis: an overview. J Ultrasound. 2009;12(4):133–43. https://doi.org/10.1016/j.jus.2009.09.006.
41. Ripollés T, Aliaga R, Morote V, Lonjedo E, et al. Utility of intrarenal Doppler ultrasound in the diagnosis of renal artery stenosis. Eur J Radiol. 2001;40(1):54–63. https://doi.org/10.1016/s0720-048x(00)00263-1.
42. Williams GJ, Macaskill P, Chan SF, Karplus TE, et al. Comparative accuracy of renal duplex sonographic parameters in the diagnosis of renal artery stenosis: paired and unpaired analysis. AJR Am J Roentgenol. 2007;188(3):798–811. https://doi.org/10.2214/AJR.06.0355.
43. Radermacher J, Chavan A, Bleck J, Vitzthum A, et al. Use of Doppler ultrasonography to predict the outcome of therapy for renal-artery stenosis. N Engl J Med. 2001;344(6):410–7. https://doi.org/10.1056/NEJM200102083440603.
44. Bateman GA, Cuganesan R. Renal vein Doppler sonography of obstructive uropathy. AJR Am J Roentgenol. 2002;178(4):921–5. https://doi.org/10.2214/ajr.178.4.1780921.
45. Deschamps J, Denault A, Galarza L, Rola P, et al. Venous Doppler to assess congestion: a comprehensive review of current evidence and nomenclature. Ultrasound Med Biol. 2023;49(1):3–17. https://doi.org/10.1016/j.ultrasmedbio.2022.07.011.
46. Husain-Syed F, Singam NSV, Viehman JK, Vaughan L, et al. Changes in Doppler-derived kidney venous flow and adverse cardiorenal outcomes in patients with heart failure. J Am Heart Assoc. 2023;12(16):e030145. https://doi.org/10.1161/JAHA.123.030145.
47. Longino A, Martin K, Leyba K, Siegel G, et al. Prospective evaluation of venous excess ultrasound (VExUS) for estimation of venous congestion. Chest. 2023;S0012-3692(23):05557–5. https://doi.org/10.1016/j.chest.2023.09.029.
48. Spiegel R, Teeter W, Sullivan S, Tupchong K, et al. The use of venous Doppler to predict adverse kidney events in a general ICU cohort. Crit Care. 2020;24(1):615. https://doi.org/10.1186/s13054-020-03330-6.
49. Leong KG, Coombs P, Kanellis J. Renal transplant ultrasound: the nephrologist's perspective. Australas J Ultrasound Med. 2015;18(4):134–42. https://doi.org/10.1002/j.2205-0140.2015.tb00220.x.
50. Kumar S, Ameli-Renani S, Hakim A, Jeon JH, et al. Ureteral obstruction following renal transplantation: causes, diagnosis and management. Br J Radiol. 2014;87(1044):20140169. https://doi.org/10.1259/bjr.20140169.

Hepatobiliary, Pancreas, and Spleen Ultrasound

10

Michael D. Zwank, Megan M. Leo, and Christine M. Schutzer

Background

Ultrasound of the upper abdominal organs can provide important information to the physician in myriad clinical scenarios. Hepatobiliary ultrasound is an effective first-line imaging modality for patients with right upper quadrant abdominal pain, ascites, hepatomegaly, or jaundice. It is commonly used to assess for gallstones and cholecystitis but also includes more advanced applications such as identifying pneumobilia, hepatomegaly, and portal vein abnormalities. Newer modalities such as contrast-enhanced ultrasound and elastography can be used to characterize cirrhosis, masses, hemorrhage, and portal vein thrombosis [1]. Hepatic vein arrival time and late phase liver enhancement level using contrast-enhanced ultrasound may help physicians diagnose and stage cirrhosis [2].

Supplementary Information The online version contains supplementary material available at https://doi.org/10.1007/978-3-031-85308-1_10.

M. D. Zwank (✉)
Department of Emergency Medicine, Regions Hospital, Saint Paul, MN, USA

University of Minnesota Medical School, Minneapolis, MN, USA

M. M. Leo
Boston University Chobanian & Avedisian School of Medicine, Boston, MA, USA

Department of Emergency Medicine, Boston Medical Center, Boston, MA, USA
e-mail: Megan.leo@bmc.org

C. M. Schutzer
Oregon Health & Science University, Portland, OR, USA
e-mail: schutzec@ohsu.edu

M. Gottlieb, N. Panebianco (eds.), *Advanced Point-of-Care Ultrasound*, https://doi.org/10.1007/978-3-031-85308-1_10

Ultrasound of the pancreas for patients with upper abdominal pain, pancreatitis, jaundice, and vomiting can provide information on pancreatic size, echogenicity, presence of lesions, and dilation of the pancreatic duct (duct of Wirsung). While the pancreas is one of the more difficult organs to visualize due to its retroperitoneal location (often obscured by air from the overlying stomach and proximal duodenum), ultrasound can provide information earlier than computed tomography (CT) or be invaluable when CT is not available.

Ultrasound of the spleen can be used to evaluate echotexture, size, and the presence of masses among patients with suspected splenomegaly, infection, or traumatic injury. While CT remains the most widely used imaging modality for many pathologies discussed in this chapter, ultrasound provides a quick, accessible alternative at the bedside without exposing patients to ionizing radiation.

Indications

Indications

- Upper abdominal pain
- Jaundice
- Vomiting
- Hepatomegaly
- Splenomegaly
- Ascites
- Sepsis without a source
- Elevated liver function tests

Diagnoses

- Steatosis or cirrhosis
- Intrahepatic ductal dilation
- Liver cysts
- Primary liver masses and metastasis
- Portal vein thrombosis
- Pneumobilia
- Portal venous air
- Abscesses or parasitic infections
- Gallstones, gallbladder sludge, or biliary colic
- Acute cholecystitis
- Biliary obstruction
- Emphysematous cholecystitis
- Gallbladder polyp or tumor
- Adenomyomatosis
- Cholesteatosis
- Pancreatic ductal dilation
- Acute pancreatitis
- Pancreatic mass
- Pancreatic pseudocyst
- Splenomegaly
- Splenic calcifications
- Splenic mass
- Splenic cyst
- Splenic infarction

Core Views

<table>
<tr><th>View</th><th>Image</th><th>Approach</th></tr>
<tr><td>Liver—Transverse View</td><td>
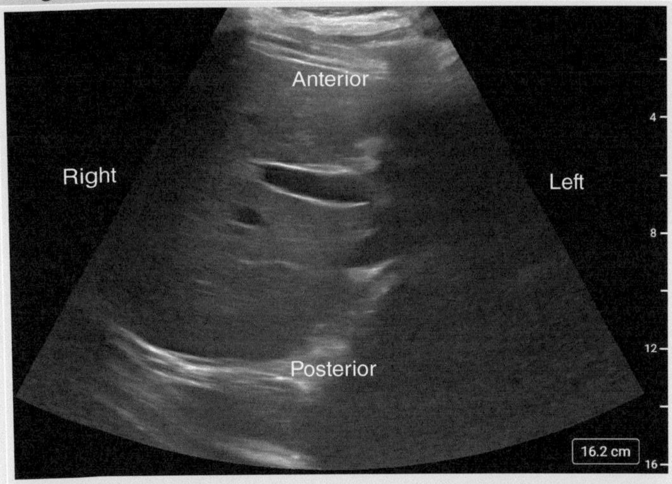

Core View 1</td><td>Place the probe at the subcostal space or right 10th intercostal space, midclavicular line, with the indicator directed to the patient's right.
Fan or slide the probe cephalad and caudad.</td></tr>
<tr><td>Liver—Sagittal View</td><td>
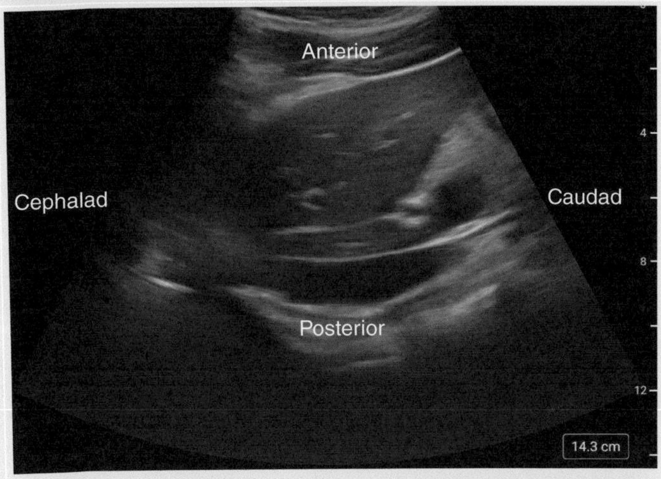

Core View 2</td><td>Place the probe at the right 10th intercostal space, midclavicular line, with the indicator directed cephalad.
Fan or slide the probe medially and laterally.</td></tr>
<tr><td>Liver—Coronal View</td><td>
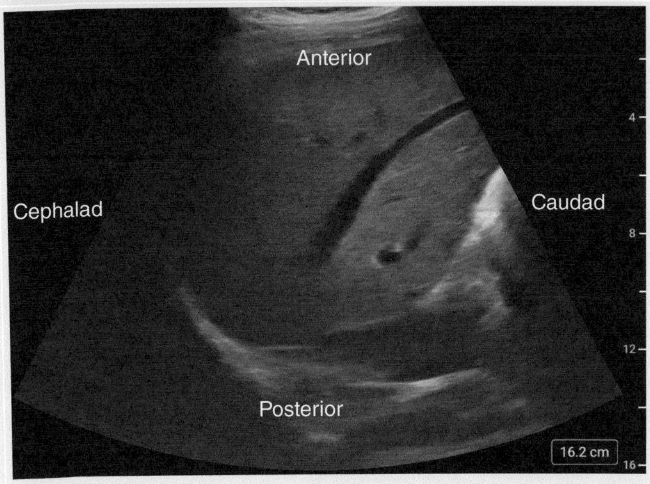

Core View 3</td><td>Place the probe at the 10th intercostal space in the right, mid-axillary line, with the indicator directed cephalad.
Fan the probe anteriorly and posteriorly.</td></tr>
</table>

View	Image	Approach
Liver—Hepatic Venous Anatomy	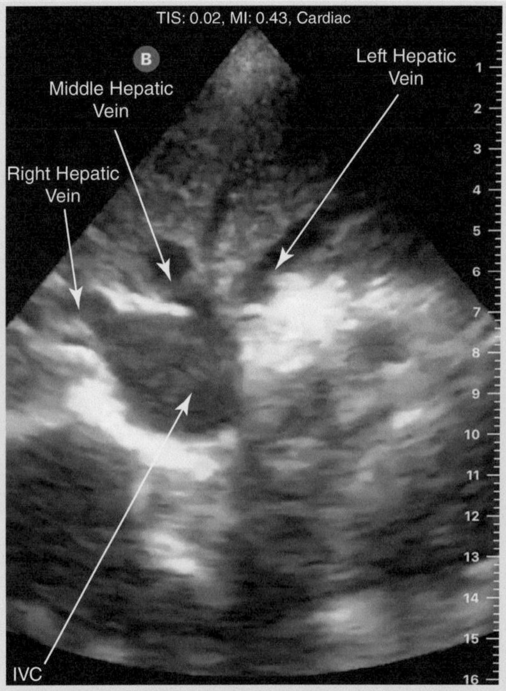 Core View 4 *Image courtesy of Meghan Herbst, MD.*	The right, middle, and left hepatic veins merge with the inferior vena cava (IVC) in the subcostal transverse view.
Liver—Portal Venous Anatomy	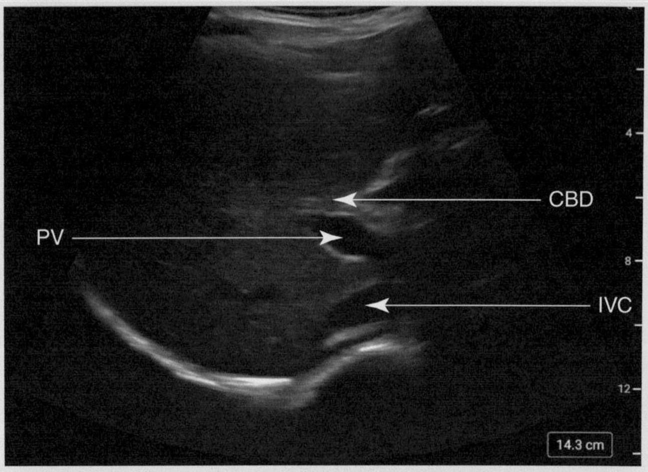 Core View 5	Place the probe at the subcostal space, midclavicular line, with the indicator directed to the patient's right. A more lateral approach or 5th intercostal space may be needed if obstructed by bowel gas. Use the IVC as a landmark to locate the portal vessels. The main portal vein is located anterior to the IVC.
Gallbladder—Long-axis View	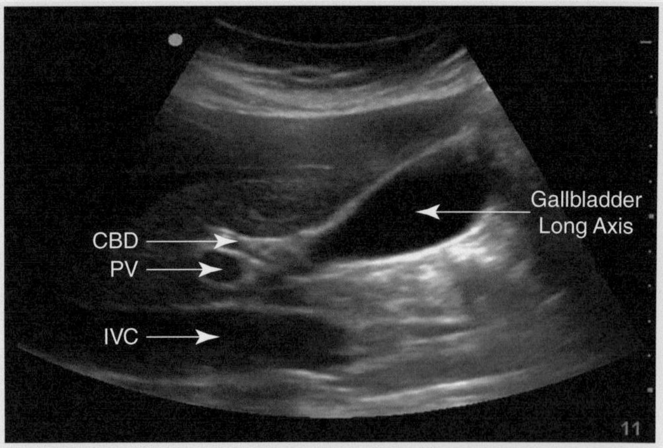 Core View 6	Place the probe inferior to the costal margin just right of midline in a sagittal plane. Slide laterally until the gallbladder is seen, then rotate clockwise to obtain a long-axis view. Fan the probe medially or laterally to visualize the entire gallbladder.

View	Image	Approach
Gallbladder—Short-axis View	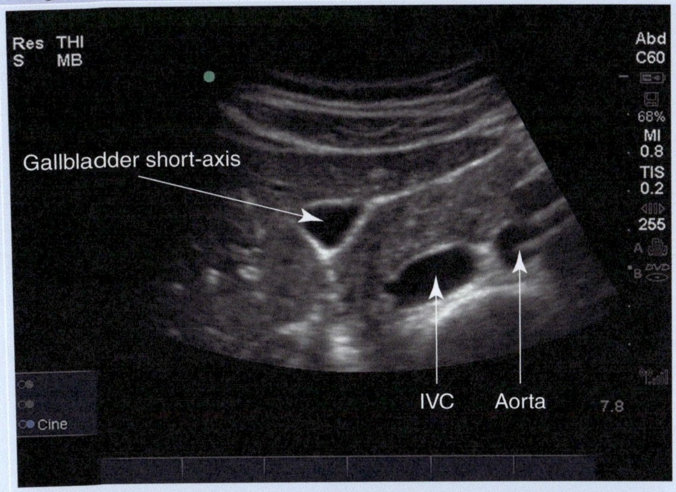 Core View 7	From the gallbladder long-axis view, rotate the probe 90° counterclockwise to obtain the short-axis view. Fan through the gallbladder from a cranial to caudal direction. Gallbladder wall thickness is best measured when viewing the gallbladder in the short axis at the thickest portion anteriorly. Avoid measuring the posterior wall as it is prone to artifactual thickening from posterior acoustic enhancement or obscuration from adjacent walls of the small intestine.
Common Bile Duct—Short-axis View	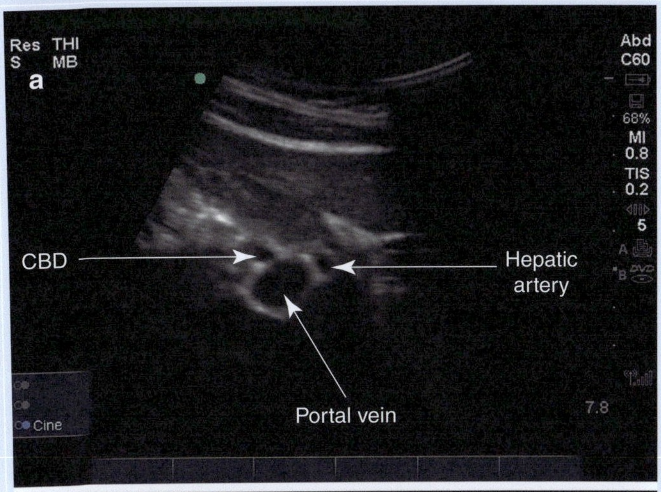	From the gallbladder long-axis view, slide laterally to locate the portal triad (common bile duct, hepatic artery, and portal vein). All three vessels will be seen next to each other (referred to as the "Mickey Mouse" sign). Use color Doppler to locate the common bile duct (the only structure in the triad that lacks flow), anterior to the portal vein and lateral to the hepatic artery.
	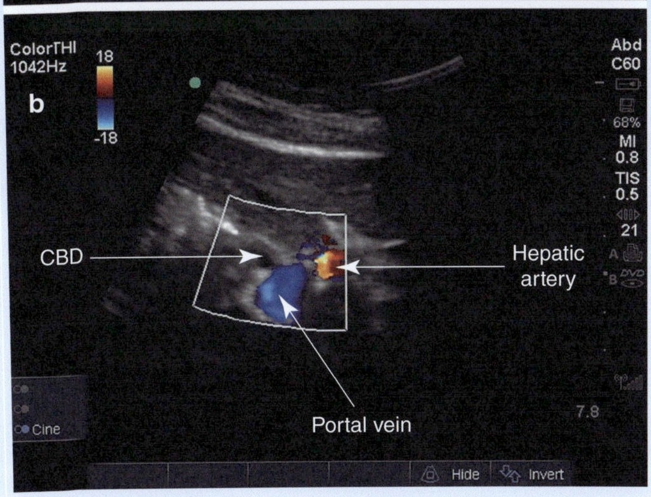 Core View 8a and 8b	

View	Image	Approach
Common Bile Duct—Long-axis View	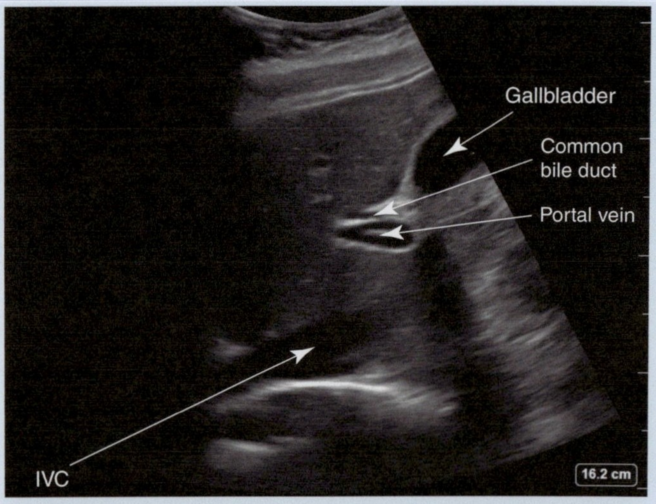 Core View 9	From the gallbladder short-axis view, slide superiorly to locate the portal vein and common bile duct in long-axis. This view can also be obtained by rotating on the common bile duct short-axis view. The portal vein and common bile duct will run parallel to each other, while the hepatic artery will remain in short-axis (referred to as the "olive sandwich" sign).
Pancreas—Long-axis View	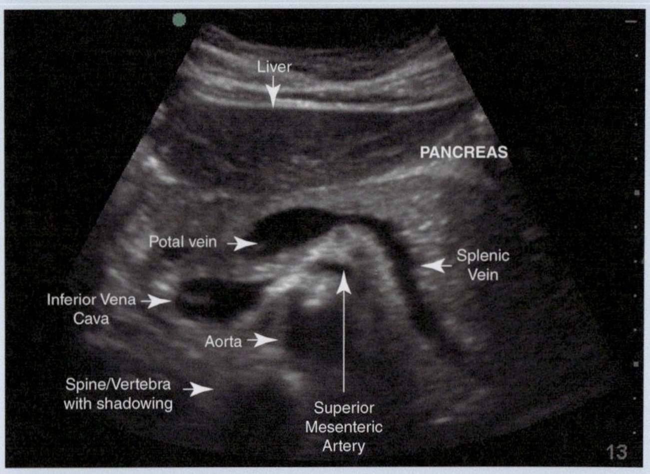 Core View 10	Place the probe at the epigastrium with the indicator directed to the patient's right. Locate the splenic vein at the level of the mid-aorta and rotate slightly counterclockwise to align the probe with the pancreas, which will be in an oblique plane.
Spleen—Long-axis View	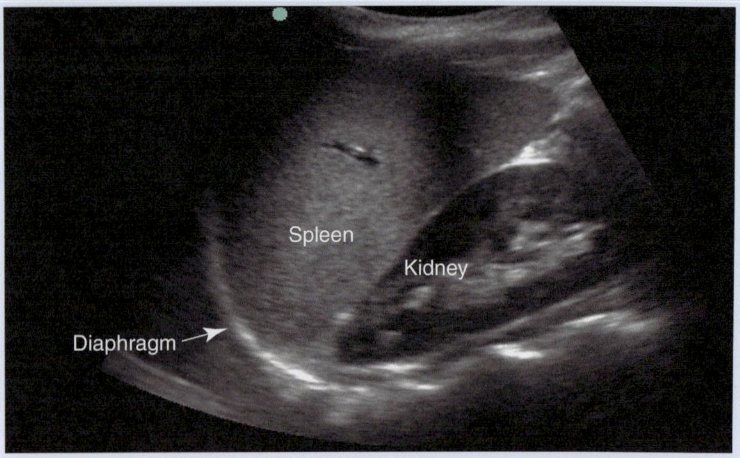 Core View 11	Place the probe between the 9th to 11th intercostal space in the left mid-axillary line with the indicator directed cephalad. Fan anterior to posterior to visualize the entire spleen.

View	Image	Approach
Spleen—Short-axis View	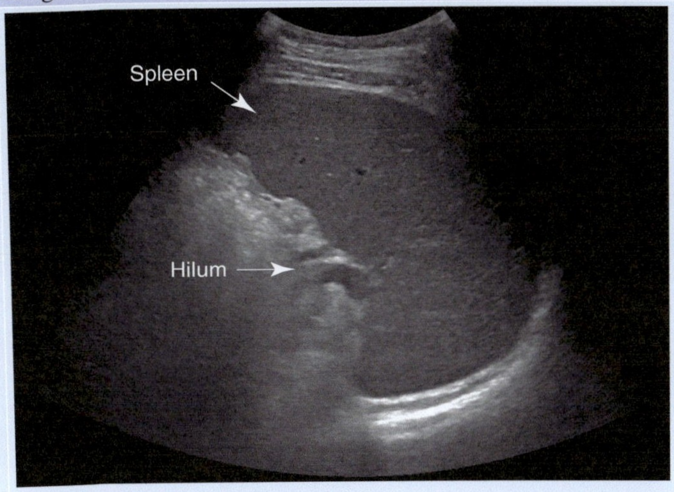 Core View 12	From the longitudinal view of the spleen, rotate the probe 90° in a counterclockwise motion. Fan cranial to caudal to visualize the entire spleen.

Clinical Applications

Liver

Normal Anatomy

The liver has four lobes: right, left, caudate, and quadrate. The right and left lobes are separated by the middle hepatic vein. The caudate lobe is situated posteriorly, bordered by the inferior vena cava (IVC) posteriorly and the ligamentum venosum anteriorly. The quadrate lobe is a small lobe located inferior to the left lobe and is bounded on the right by the gallbladder fossa and on the left by the umbilical vein. Normal liver parenchyma is uniformly hypoechoic due to the rich blood supply from both the portal venous and hepatic arterial systems. The echogenicity of the normal healthy liver should match or be slightly more echogenic than that of the renal cortex. Median liver span (as measured at the midclavicular line, sagittal plane, craniocaudal) for males is 14.5 cm and for females is 13.4 cm [3].

Hepatic Steatosis and Cirrhosis

Hepatic steatosis and cirrhosis have sonographically similar features. Steatosis is fatty infiltration of the liver that can be caused by excessive alcohol intake but also non-alcohol-related causes such as obesity, metabolic syndrome and insulin resistance, inborn errors of metabolism (e.g., Wilson's disease), infections (e.g., hepatitis C virus), and medications (e.g., tetracycline, dexamethasone) [4]. Steatosis gives the liver parenchyma a diffusely echogenic appearance that reaches deeper parts of the organ as the steatosis progresses (Fig. 10.1, Videos 10.1 and 10.2). Grading of hepatic steatosis ranges from normal (grade 0) to severe (grade 3) (Table 10.1) [5]. Subjective grading using B-mode has a sensitivity of 85–90% and specificity of 93%, and an increased accuracy toward higher grades [6, 7]. Semi-quantitative methods that compare the echogenicity between the liver and kidney (i.e., hepatorenal index) increase the sensitivity for detecting mild steatosis [5]. Quantitative measures such as backscatter coefficient and attenuation coefficient are currently outside the scope of point-of-care ultrasound (POCUS) practice but may further increase sensitivity for steatosis diagnosis.

Cirrhosis is associated with multiple conditions, including alcohol consumption, Wilson's disease, primary sclerosing cholangitis, and hemochromatosis [4]. It is defined by parenchymal necrosis, diffuse fibrosis, and regeneration that leads to disorganized lobular architecture, altered vasculature, liver cell dysfunction, and eventually portal hypertension [8]. Early stages manifest as hepatomegaly (>16 cm at the midclavicular line) with later stages leading to volume loss and a more hyperechoic appearance (similar to steatosis) and heterogeneous echotexture. [9]. The liver surface can become nodular with the presence or absence of ascites (Fig. 10.2, Video 10.3).

Regenerating nodules (new hepatocyte formation in response to cell death and fibrosis) can appear as hypoechoic components with a thin echogenic border. However, these nodules are difficult to visualize as they are often isoechoic to the surrounding parenchyma. Dysplastic nodules are premalignant and larger than regenerating nodules (typically >10 mm) [10]. The blood supply for dysplastic nodules is from the portal system, which can be confirmed using color Doppler [11]. Unlike the pulsatile Doppler characteristics of the hepatic artery that supplies hepatocellular carcinomas

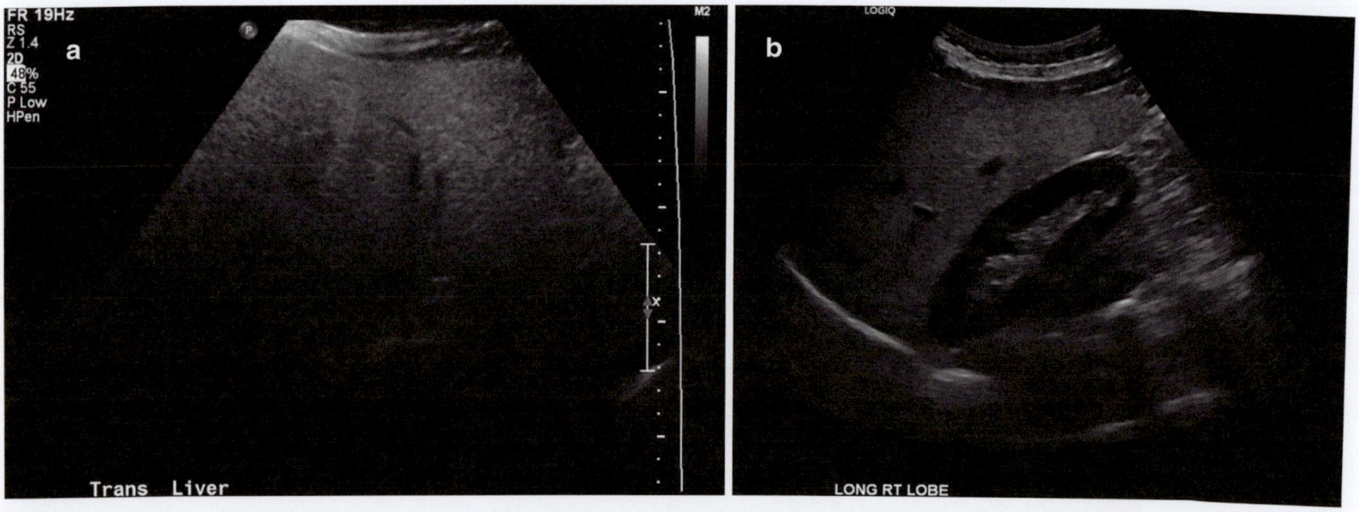

Fig. 10.1 (**a**) Diffusely echogenic appearance of steatosis. (**b**) Hepatic steatosis appears hyperechoic relative to the renal cortex

Table 10.1 Grading characteristics of hepatic steatosis [5]

Grade	Class	Sonographic Features
0	Normal	Echogenicity of the liver is normal (similar to the renal cortex) and homogeneous.
1	Mild	Echogenicity of the liver is minimally increased.
2	Moderate	Posterior beam attenuation is absent or limited to posterior segments of the right lobe of the liver (impaired diaphragm visualization) and echogenicity of the walls of the portal vessels is reduced.
3	Severe	Posterior beam attenuation impairs the visualization of anterior segments of the liver; blurring of intrahepatic vessels is observed.

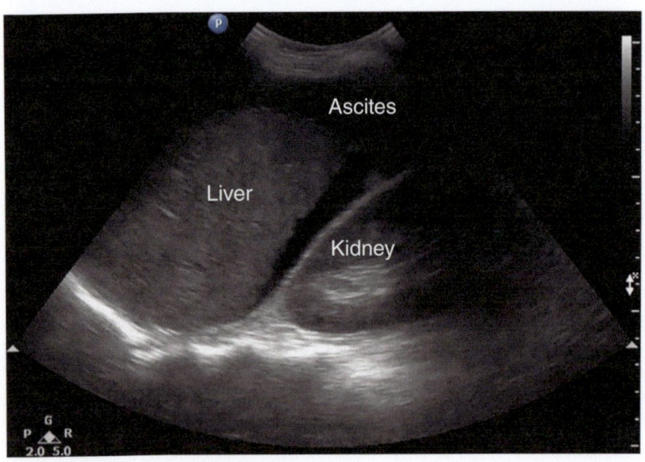

Fig. 10.2 Liver cirrhosis with ascites

(discussed later), dysplastic nodules exhibit a more static waveform.

The normal hepatic vein spectral Doppler waveform exhibits a triphasic antegrade diastolic, systolic, and smaller retrograde atrial "kick" (Fig. 10.3). Hepatic venous flow in compensated cirrhosis (before the development of portal hypertension) will change to either a decreased amplitude waveform with loss of the retrograde "kick," or a complete flattening of the waveform (Fig. 10.4) [12]. This is due to decreased compliance of the hepatic veins caused by surrounding fibrosis. Additionally, the hepatic veins narrow, resulting in higher flow velocities seen on color and spectral Doppler, often with resultant aliasing. Elastography, which assesses the stiffness of the liver tissue, can predict the presence or absence of cirrhosis but is not reliable in staging the grade of cirrhosis [13].

Contrast-enhanced ultrasound can help diagnose cirrhosis by assessing hepatic vein arrival time and liver enhancement level. Due to the hemodynamic changes of less compliant vessels and shunting that occur in cirrhosis, the contrast injected into a peripheral vein will reach the liver faster in a patient with cirrhosis than in a patient with a healthy liver. One study found that hepatic vein arrival time had a sensitivity of 100% and specificity of 96% for the diagnosis of cirrhosis [14]. Liver enhancement levels refer to the parenchyma in the late phase of contrast injection. Enhancement levels will be reduced (darker) in patients with cirrhosis due to dysfunction of the Kupffer cells compared to a normal liver [15]. Whether these techniques reliably correlate with staging is not yet clear.

Acute Hepatitis

Sonography does not play a diagnostic role in the evaluation of acute hepatitis (both infectious and noninfectious). However, sonographic findings of acute hepatitis may include hepatomegaly and decreased echogenicity of the liver parenchyma due to diffuse swelling of the hepatocytes and immune response into the portal areas. The portal

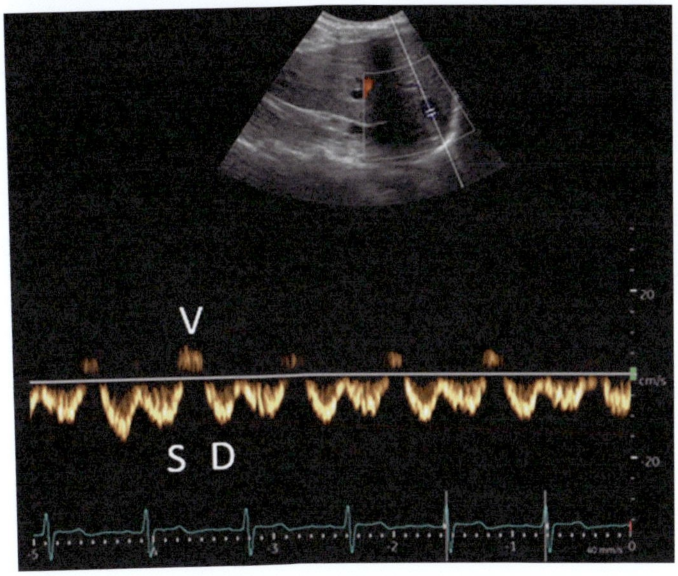

Fig. 10.3 Normal hepatic waveform demonstrating systolic (S), diastolic (D), and retrograde atrial kick (V)

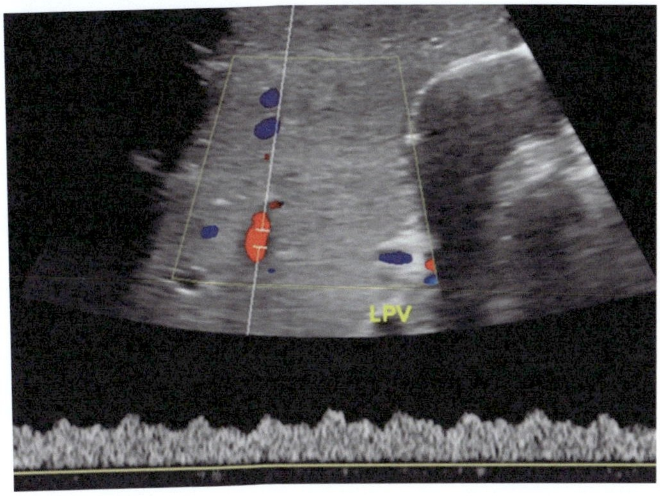

Fig. 10.4 Hepatic venous waveform with progressive portal hypertension

venous structures can also appear more echogenic with periportal cuffing, creating a "starry night" appearance (Fig. 10.5) [16].

Intrahepatic Ductal Dilation

Intrahepatic ductal dilation can be caused by intrinsic factors such as sclerosing cholangitis or extrinsic causes such as choledocholithiasis, postoperative biliary stricture, or extrinsic compression by a mass. In a normal liver, the intrahepatic ducts should not be visible. If the intrahepatic ducts are visible as multiple hyperechoic tubular channels, this is always considered pathologic (Fig. 10.6). When evaluating for intrahepatic duct dilation, color Doppler should be used to differentiate the intrahepatic ducts (flow absent) from vasculature (flow present).

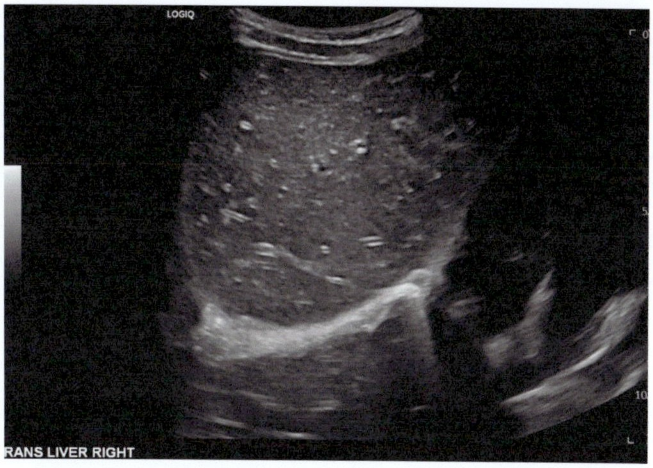

Fig. 10.5 Starry night appearance of portal venous structures seen in acute hepatitis

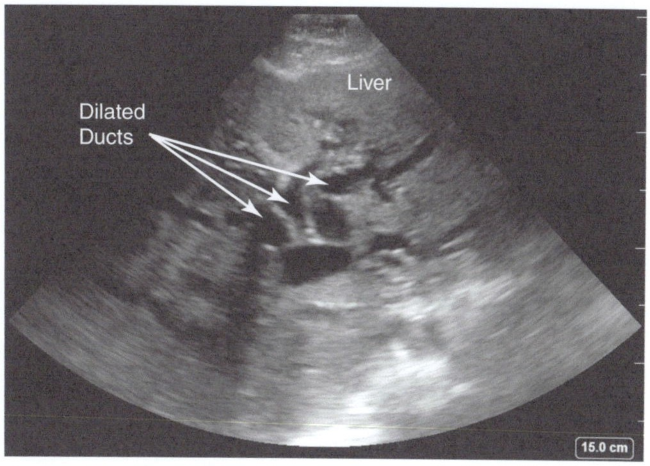

Fig. 10.6 Intrahepatic duct dilation

Liver Cysts

Cystic lesions of the liver can be categorized as infectious (discussed later) or noninfectious. Noninfectious cysts can be benign, premalignant, or malignant [17]. Benign hepatic cysts (3–5% of the general population) are typically anechoic with a well-defined circular shape [18]. They will also demonstrate posterior acoustic enhancement from the simple fluid they contain (Fig. 10.7a). Congenital cysts are simple cysts seen in females between the ages of 40–70 years, whereas acquired cysts (infectious or traumatic) tend to be more complex and are seen more commonly in males between the ages of 30–50 years [19]. Patients with polycystic kidney disease often have multiple, scattered simple cysts within the liver that can ultimately progress to liver dysfunction and failure (Fig. 10.7b, Video 10.4). No intervention is needed for simple cysts unless they are associated with pain,

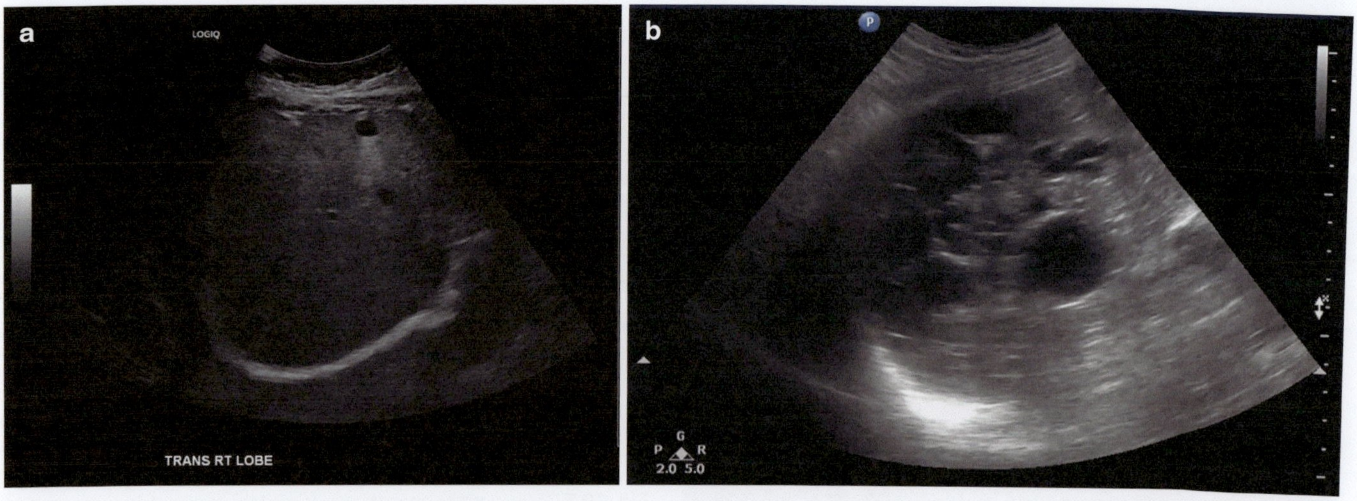

Fig. 10.7 (**a**) Simple liver cyst with posterior acoustic enhancement. (**b**) Multiple liver cysts in a patient with polycystic kidney disease

hemorrhage, or infection. Pain is experienced in approximately 15% of patients with simple cysts [20]. Ultrasound-guided aspiration can provide temporary relief of pain, but fluid reaccumulation is common. Aspiration sclerotherapy with an agent such as alcohol has longer lasting success; however, for complete resolution, surgical excision or laparoscopic fenestration is typically needed [20]. Cysts with a thick wall, heterogeneous echotexture, or septae should undergo additional imaging with CT, magnetic resonance imaging, or contrast-enhanced ultrasound to evaluate for malignancy.

Liver Masses

Liver masses can be benign or malignant. The majority of masses are benign and include hemangiomas, focal nodular hyperplasia (FNH), or adenomas. Malignant liver masses, such as hepatocellular carcinoma (HCC) and metastatic disease, are less common. B-mode can be used to assess echogenicity, size, location, cystic versus solid internal features, as well as marginal characterization. Color or spectral Doppler can differentiate a solid vascular mass from a fluid-filled cystic mass or abscess. However, Doppler is less reliable in patients with larger body habitus or with deeper lesions.

Hemangiomas are the most common benign liver tumors, with a prevalence of up to 7.3%, and are generally noted incidentally in women between 30 and 50 years old [21]. They can be solitary or multiple and appear as well-circumscribed and hyperechoic (Fig. 10.8, Video 10.5). FNH is seen in women between 20 and 50 years old [22]. They have an isoechoic appearance that blends with normal parenchyma and is only identifiable if subtle contour abnormalities or displacement of vascular structures are seen. Both hemangiomas and FNH have peripheral hypervascularity on Doppler

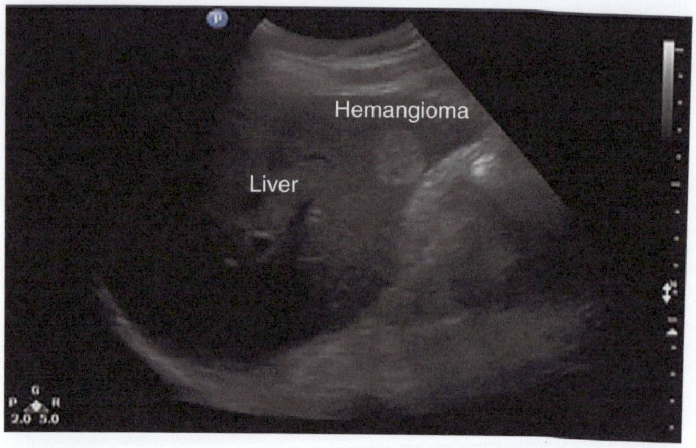

Fig. 10.8 Liver hemangioma

assessment with central sparing. Adenomas similarly occur in women of childbearing age and may be associated with oral contraception use. Although benign, adenomas can be complicated by hemorrhage (29%) or progression to malignancy (4%) [23].

Findings suggestive of a malignancy include a hypoechoic halo around the mass and heterogeneous or solid features within the mass. The presence of multiple solid masses, commonly referred to as cannonball lesions, should raise concern for metastatic disease (Fig. 10.9, Video 10.6). Identification of cannonball lesions should prompt a broad evaluation to identify the primary malignancy.

HCC is the most common primary liver malignancy. Both HCC and cholangiocarcinoma tend to manifest as a solitary liver mass. HCC tumors have variable echotextures, typically appearing hypoechoic when they are small and then converting to a heterogeneous appearance as they grow and develop internal necrosis and fibrosis. Portal vein involvement occurs in 16–30% of HCC cases, manifesting through

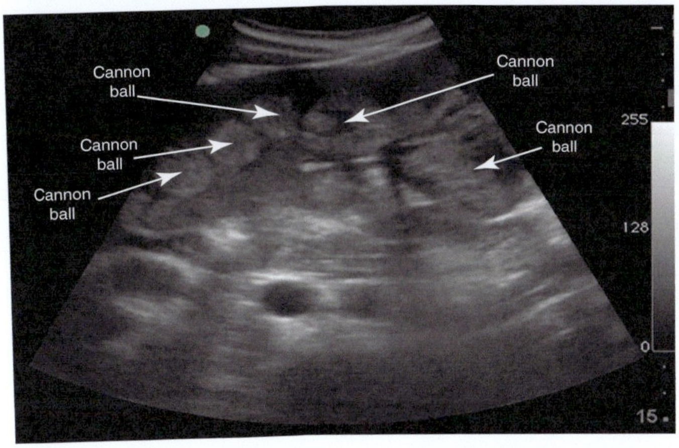

Fig. 10.9 Cannonball lesions seen with metastatic liver disease (arrows). (*Image courtesy of Meghan Herbst, MD*)

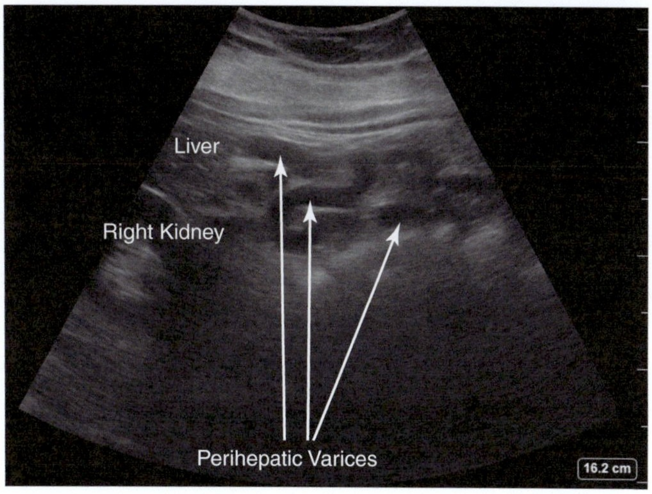

Fig. 10.10 Perihepatic varices

hemodynamic changes, tumor extension into the portal vein, and portal vein tumor thrombosis [24].

Contrast-enhanced ultrasound can evaluate liver masses in patients with both normal and cirrhotic livers. It can also differentiate focal fatty infiltration and focal fatty sparing (isovascularity) from neoplasm (hypervascularity) [25]. The vascular pattern illuminated by the contrast can predict the type of mass. For example, rim enhancement suggests a metastatic lesion, centripetal hypervascular enhancement suggests an adenoma, dysmorphic tortuous vessels with peripheral filling suggest malignant tumors, and peripheral nodular enhancement suggests hemangiomas [26].

Portal Hypertension

Portal hypertension can be extrahepatic (e.g., portal vein thrombosis) or intrahepatic (e.g., cirrhosis). Splenomegaly, ascites, and visualization of portosystemic venous collaterals suggest portal hypertension. The left gastric vein (also known as the coronary vein) and splenic hilar veins are easiest to see with ultrasound. The left gastric vein can be seen as it branches off the splenic vein in the sagittal plane. It courses into the gastroesophageal junction and varices in this region put the patient at high risk for major bleeding (Fig. 10.10). Dilated collaterals such as a left gastric vein measuring greater than 3 mm in diameter are strongly correlated with the presence of esophageal varices [27]. Tortuous varices can be seen at the splenic hilum in a coronal plane (Fig. 10.11) and occasionally in the left renal hilum [25].

Doppler analysis of the portal vein can grade the severity of the portal hypertension. Hepatic venous pressure gradient (HVPG) is now the gold standard measure of presence and severity of portal hypertension, replacing the much more invasive wedge pressure that requires catheter placement. HVPG measures the gradient between the portal vein and hepatic vein. HVPG is considered elevated when it is above 5 mmHg, but complications of portal hypertension such as varices and ascites mostly occur when HVPG rises above 10 mmHg [28]. Doppler assessment of normal portal venous flow displays undulating hepatopetal (toward the liver) flow at a velocity below 12.8 cm/s [29]. Portal hypertension is associated with monophasic portal venous flow. With increasing severity, the flow becomes biphasic and ultimately hepatofugal (away from the liver) with intrahepatic arterial-portal venous shunting (Fig. 10.12 and 10.13) [29].

Portal Vein Thrombosis

Portal vein thrombosis is typically associated with malignancy or nonmalignant hypercoagulable states such as trauma, pregnancy, inflammatory bowel disease, or pancreatitis [30]. Findings suggestive of portal vein thrombosis include visualization of an echogenic thrombus within the portal vein, portal vein diameter ≥13 mm (measured inner wall to inner wall), or cavernous transformation of the portal vein [31, 32]. Like any thrombus, the more acutely it developed, the more hypoechoic and difficult it is to see with B-mode imaging. Color Doppler may be used to display the partial or complete absence of flow in the lumen. Malignant thrombi are associated with HCC and tend to have internal arterial phases on spectral Doppler assessment [31]. Cavernous transformation appears as a wormlike collection of collaterals at the porta hepatis (Fig. 10.14).

Hepatic Vein Obstruction

Hepatic vein obstruction (historically called Budd-Chiari syndrome) is rare. It typically results from external compression of the hepatic veins with or without thrombosis due to malignancy (Fig. 10.15, Video 10.8). Hepatomegaly is an early finding and progresses to irregular regional echogenicity in the setting of infarction, followed by diffuse echogenicity with fibrosis [33]. The caudate lobe is often spared or may receive increased flow and enlarge due

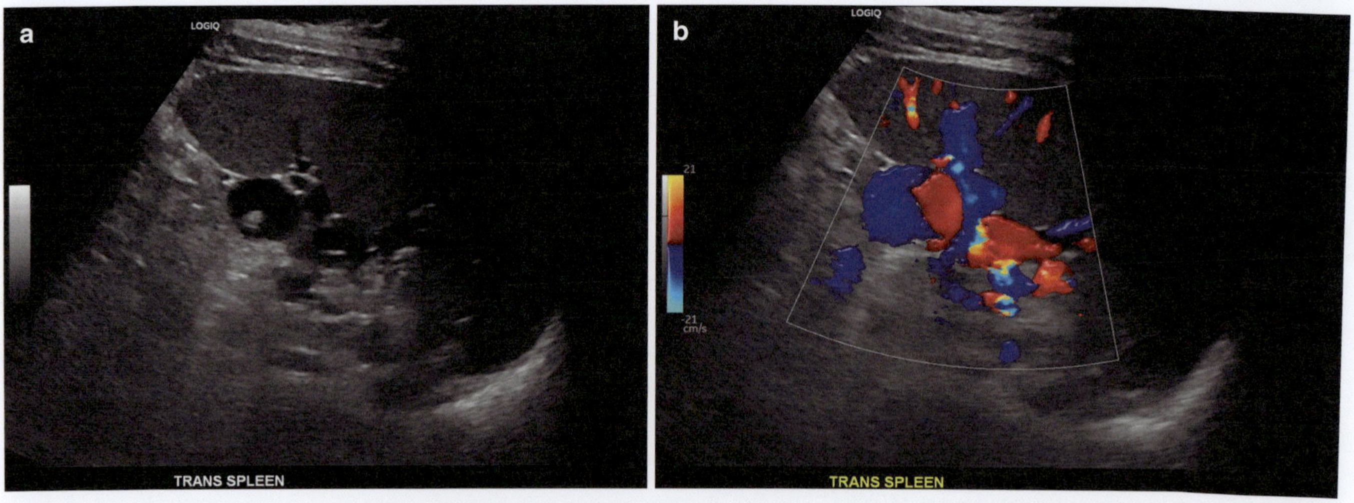

Fig. 10.11 (**a**) Perisplenic varices seen on B-mode. (**b**) Perisplenic varices with color Doppler

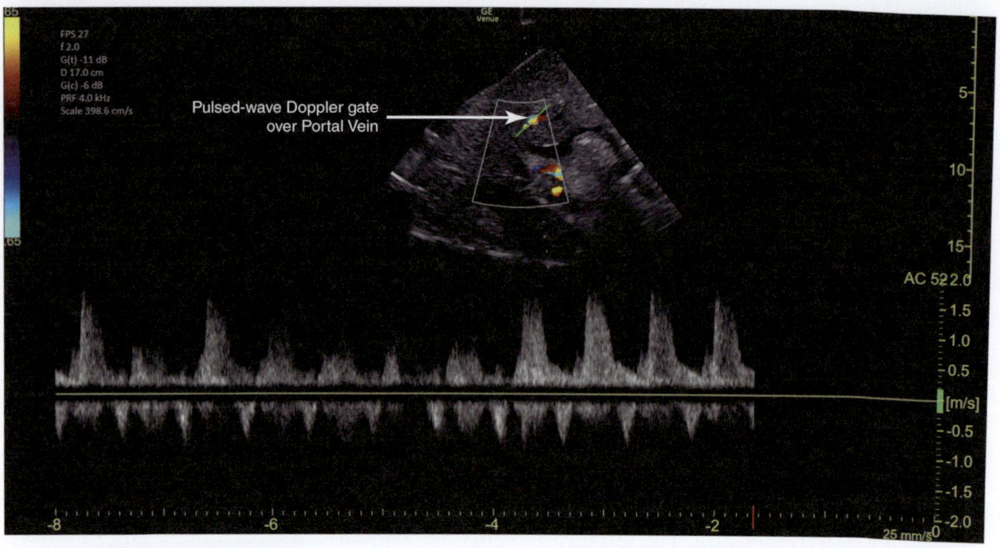

Fig. 10.12 Biphasic portal venous waveform

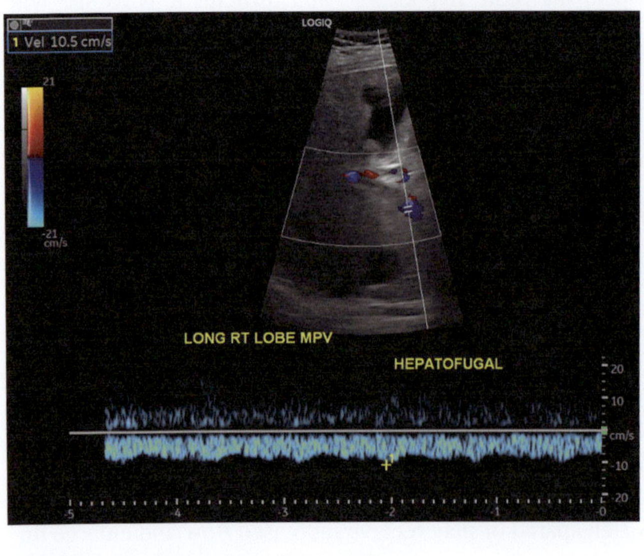

Fig. 10.13 Hepatofugal portal venous flow

to the emissary vein that drains directly into the IVC at a lower level [34]. Hepatic vein occlusion and abnormal intrahepatic collaterals can also occasionally be seen [35]. The Doppler features of hepatic vein obstruction depend on the location of the hepatic vein occlusion. The normal phasic response of the cardiac and respiratory cycle may be absent, reversed, turbulent, or continuous. The degree of hepatic occlusion or possibility of external compression by an enlarged caudate lobe may additionally affect IVC flow. Portal venous flow can slow or reverse to a hepatofugal direction [35].

Pneumobilia and Portal Venous Air

Pneumobilia is common after any procedure that involves disruption of the biliary tree, such as an esophagogastroduodenoscopy (EGD) or pancreaticoduodenectomy (Whipple procedure). Non-iatrogenic causes include trauma, sponta-

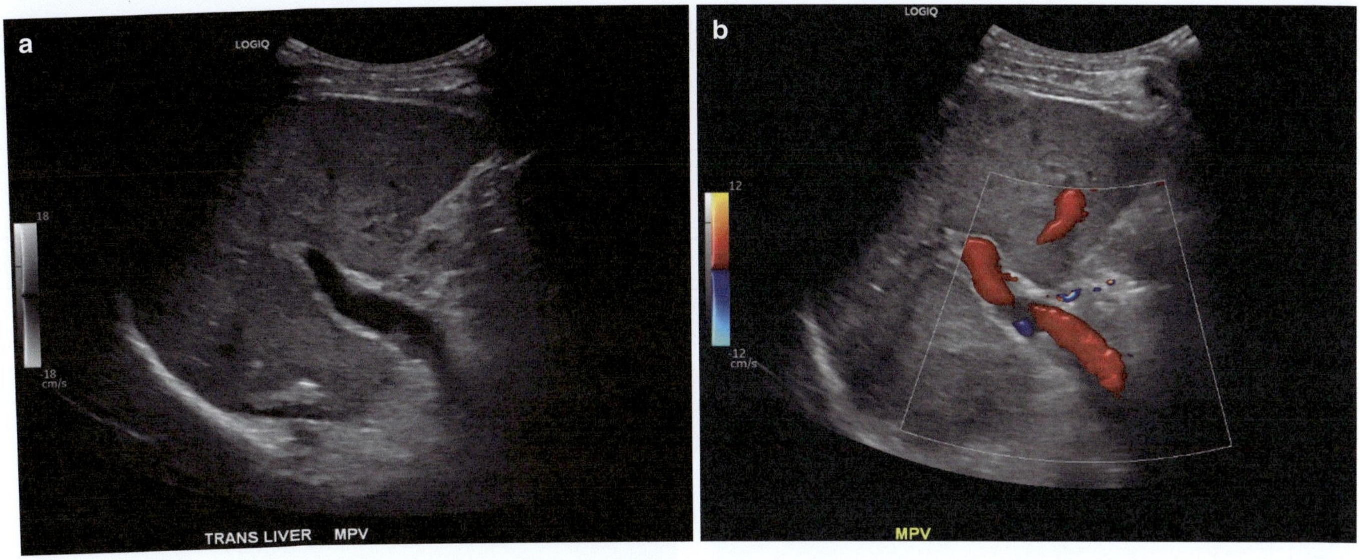

Fig. 10.14 (**a**) Main portal vein with thrombus seen on B-mode. (**b**) Main portal vein with thrombus on color Doppler

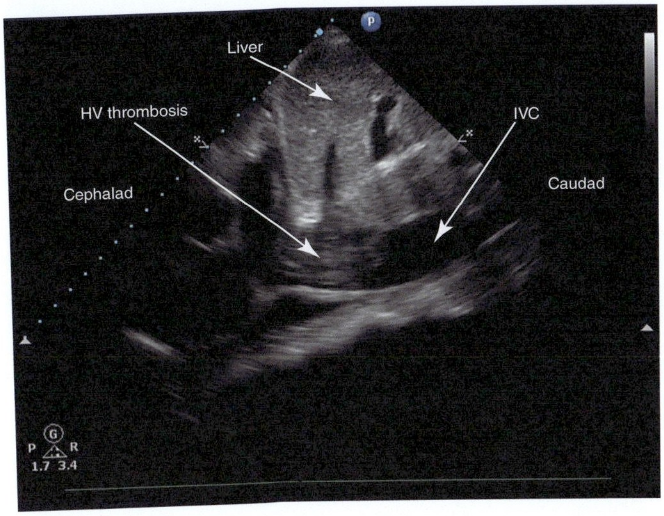

Fig. 10.15 Hepatic vein obstruction (arrow)

neous biliary-enteric fistula, choledocholithiasis, and emphysematous cholecystitis; however, these patients will generally appear more ill [36]. On ultrasound, the lumen of the biliary ducts will appear hyperechoic with posterior ring-down or reverberation artifact (Fig. 10.16).

Portal venous air is a more concerning sign that can be seen in patients with sepsis, mesenteric ischemia, or a necrotizing condition such as necrotizing enterocolitis in neonates. Pathologic air diffuses from the mesentery or spleen into their respective venous systems, which subsequently drain into the portal vein, resulting in this ominous finding. A scattering of hyperechoic air bubbles with posterior ring-down artifact can appear throughout the portal veins, extending to the periphery of the liver. The air bubbles may move centrifugally throughout the portal venous system [16]. Because the hepatic arteries and veins drain the liver parenchyma only, they are generally unaffected.

Intrahepatic Infections

Intrahepatic infections caused by a bacterial, fungal, or parasitic etiology appear as cystic lesions containing simple or complex fluid. Unlike true cysts, they lack an epithelial lining and tend to be more irregular in shape. Viral infections lead to more of a diffuse parenchymal pattern, as described earlier.

Bacterial and Fungal Abscesses

Pyogenic abscesses can arise from bacteria entering the liver through the biliary tract (e.g., from cholecystitis) or through the portal venous system (e.g., from diverticulitis). They appear as cysts with various stages of appearance (Fig. 10.17, Video 10.8). Ultrasound is 90% sensitive for detecting liver abscess [37]. Early stages of a pyogenic abscess appear like a solid isoechoic mass within the liver due to a predominance of inflammation and edema of the liver tissue without necrosis. Later stages lead to cell liquefaction and necrosis, which produce hypoechoic fluid-filled masses with posterior acoustic enhancement [38]. Timely recognition and treatment is essential. Intravenous antibiotics are the mainstay of therapy, but up to 15% of patients may require ultrasound-guided needle aspiration [39].

Hepatic fungal infections represent less than 2% of abscess contents isolated from immunocompetent patients [40]. The most common organisms are *Candida* spp., thought to be from colonization in the gastrointestinal tract and hematogenous spread through mucositis and neutropenia in immunocompromised patients such as those on chemotherapy. Other less common causes are molds and dimorphic

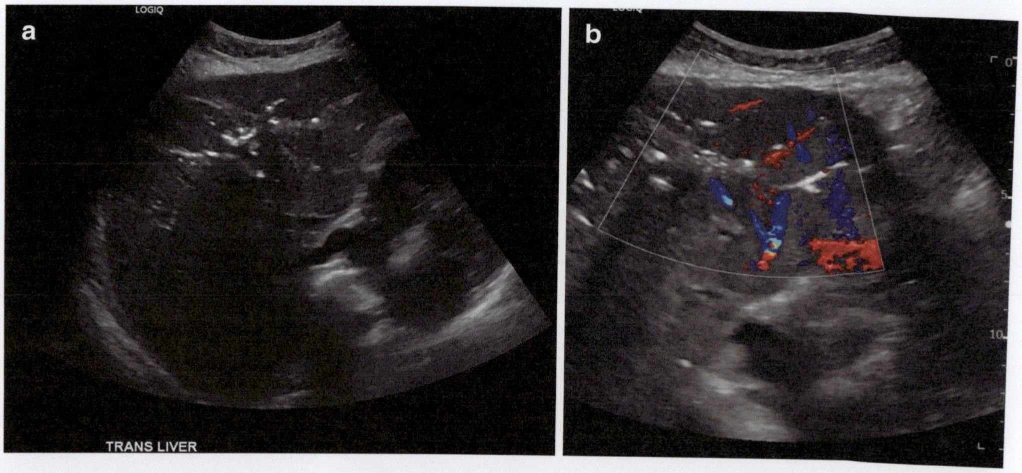

Fig. 10.16 (**a**) Pneumobilia seen on B-mode. (**b**) Pneumobilia with color Doppler to distinguish vessels from bile ducts

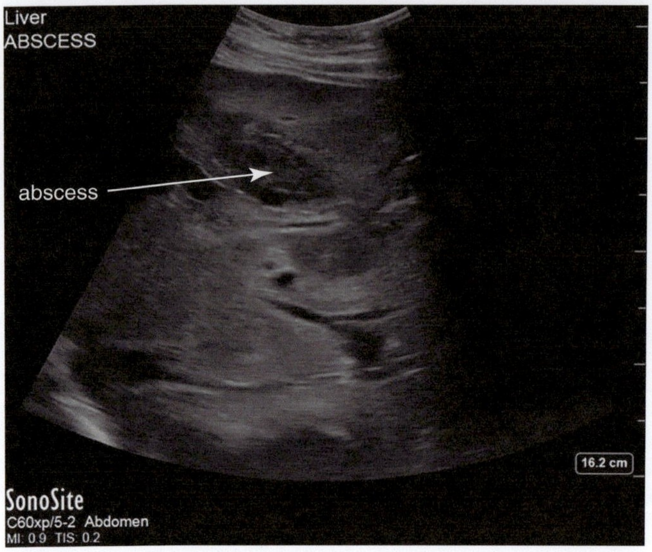

Fig. 10.17 Liver abscess (arrow)

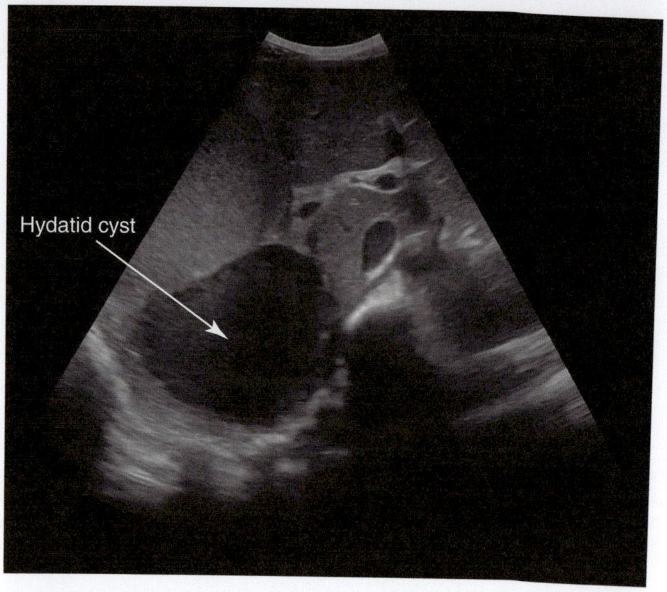

Fig. 10.18 Hydatid cyst (arrow)

fungi such as aspergillus, *Pneumocystis jirovecii*, *Rhodotorula* spp., and *Trichosporon loubieri* [40]. These abscesses have a "wheel within a wheel" appearance or a "bull's eye" pattern [41].

Parasitic Infections

Parasitic infections of the liver can be caused by a variety of organisms, including amebiasis, schistosomiasis, and echinococcus. The most common parasitic lesion of the liver is Echinococcus due to ingestion of tapeworm eggs. Patients may present with right upper quadrant or epigastric abdominal pain, hepatomegaly, or a palpable mass. Ultrasound can determine the number and location of hydatid cysts with a sensitivity of 100% and a specificity of 96% [42]. While cysts can be found in tissues such as lung and spleen, up to three-quarters of hydatid cysts develop in the liver (Fig. 10.18) [43]. These can appear as a simple cyst, a cyst with daughter cysts (matrix), a calcified cyst, or a complicated cyst (Fig. 10.19) [19].

Amebiasis, caused by *Entamoeba histolytica*, can manifest as a single liver lesion in up to 60% of cases [44]. Similar to pyogenic liver abscesses, their sonographic appearance is isoechoic with surrounding liver tissue in early stages and later becomes hypoechoic with more irregular walls and shape. For unclear reasons, these lesions tend to form in the posterior part of the right lobe of the liver [45, 46].

Gallbladder

Normal Anatomy

The gallbladder can be challenging to view due to its variable position as well as overlying bowel gas and rib shadowing. To improve visualization, the clinician can have the

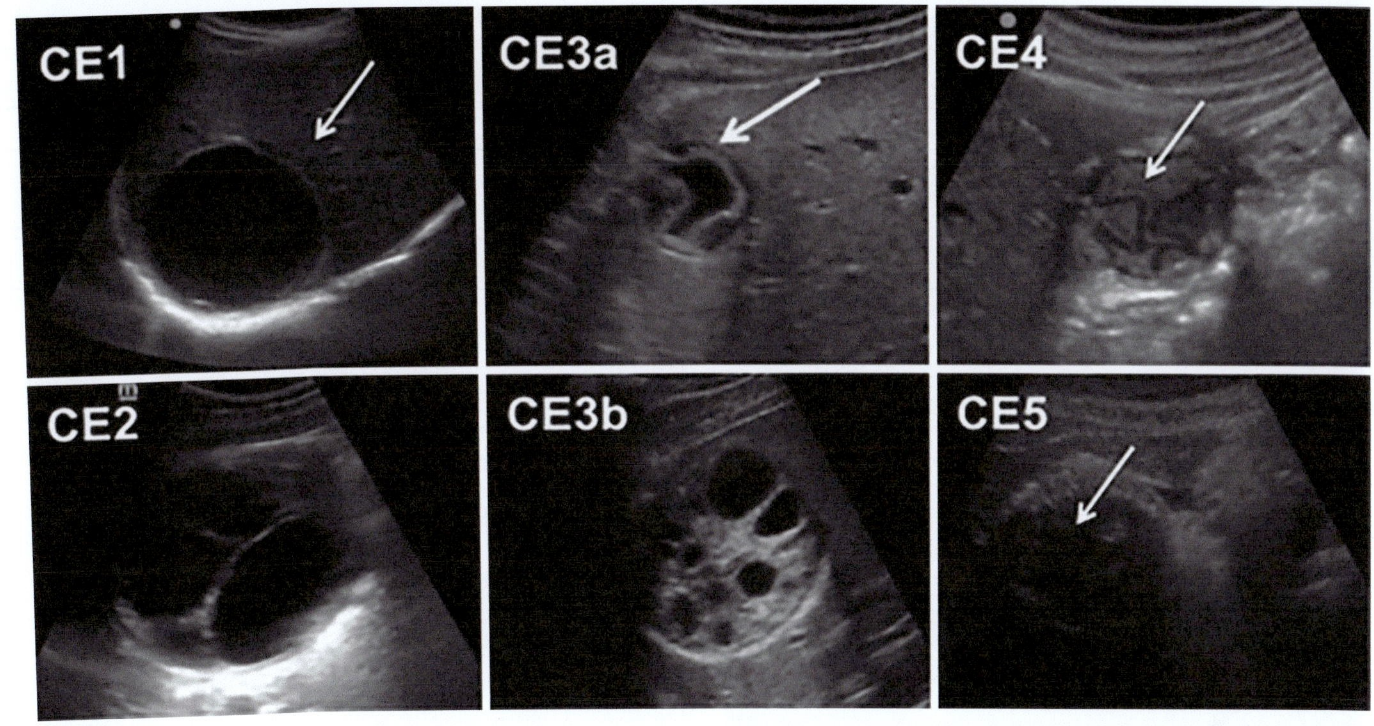

Fig. 10.19 World Health Organization Informal Working Groups on Echinococcosis (WHO-IWGE) Hydatid cyst staging. CE1: unilocular fluid-filled cyst with a double-wall (arrow); CE2: fluid-filled cysts with daughter cysts; CE3a: unilocular fluid-filled cysts with detached parasitic layers (arrow); CE3b: daughter cysts in a solid matrix with folded hypoechoic parasitic layers; CE4: solid contents with folded hypoechoic parasitic layers (arrow); CE5: egg-shell calcification with folded hypoechoic parasitic layers (arrow). (*Adapted from Tamarozzi* [106])

patient move into various positions to help improve the ultrasound window. Having the patient lie down on their left side (left lateral decubitus) will move the liver and gallbladder medially, displacing stomach and bowel gas while centering it in the more concave subxiphoid region. Adding reverse Trendelenburg positioning (supine with head up) utilizes gravity to move the liver and gallbladder inferiorly below the costal margin. Having the patient hold a deep breath can produce a similar effect by flattening the diaphragm and moving the gallbladder downward. If these maneuvers fail to provide a good imaging window, two other scanning windows can be utilized. Sliding the probe superiorly into an intercostal space allows viewing between ribs. Likewise, moving the probe laterally and utilizing a mid-axillary window (similar to the right upper quadrant FAST window) can help avoid bowel or stomach obstructing the view anteriorly. In both of these alternate windows, the probe may need to be rotated to help avoid rib shadows. A phased array or microconvex probe with a smaller footprint may also help avoid rib interference.

In addition to size, the gallbladder shape can also be variable. The gallbladder can be folded on itself creating a folded wall that can mimic an intraluminal polyp. Folds are normal variants and can be solitary or multiple. A fold in the fundus is referred to as a "phrygian cap," a floppy conical red hat with deep historical roots (Fig. 10.20). Another common anatomic variant is an outpouching of the gallbladder near the neck (termed Hartmann's pouch) where bile stasis can occur, allowing sludge and stones to form (Fig. 10.21).

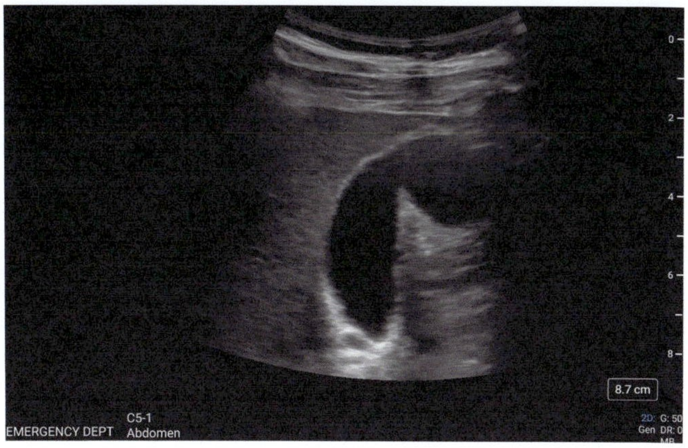

Fig. 10.20 Phrygian cap (fold in the fundus of the gallbladder)

Biliary Sludge and Gallstones

Bile is synthesized in the liver and is made of cholesterol, bile salts, and bilirubin. It is stored in the gallbladder and can form bile crystals, sludge, and stones as a result of stasis, inflammation, or genetic susceptibility. Biliary sludge is typically noted as gravity-dependent layering echoes within the gallbladder that do not shadow (Fig. 10.22). While sludge is

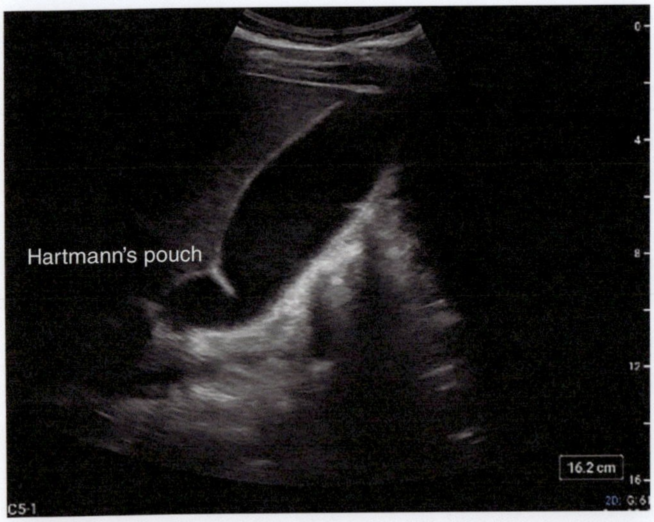

Fig. 10.21 Hartmann's pouch

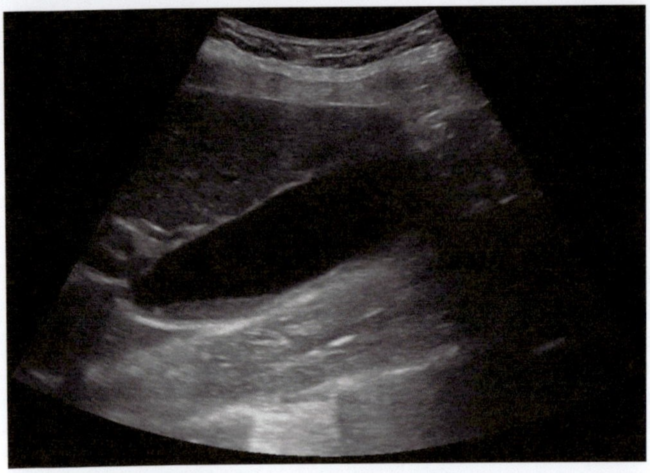

Fig. 10.22 Gallbladder with biliary sludge. (*Image courtesy of Michael Gottlieb, MD*)

typically mobile, it can become thickened (tumefactive sludge) and mimic a mass or oddly shaped stone (Fig. 10.23) [47]. Sludge can form stones, starting quite small and eventually becoming large (Fig. 10.24).

Gallstones are hyperechoic with posterior acoustic shadowing. Ultrasound has excellent test characteristics for detecting gallstones (sensitivity of 90–96%) [48]. Small stones can sometimes be challenging to detect or differentiate from sludge. Detection can be improved by assuring a perpendicular angle of ultrasound beam incidence, using a higher frequency probe, and adjusting the focal zone to the depth of the suspected stone. Color Doppler can be used as well to help define a stone as the cause of shadowing versus other causes such as overlying bowel gas. Gallstones will cause a twinkling artifact posteriorly, which appears as a multitude of "twinkling" colors [49].

Gallstones should be imaged in two different planes (long and short axis), sweeping completely through the entirety of

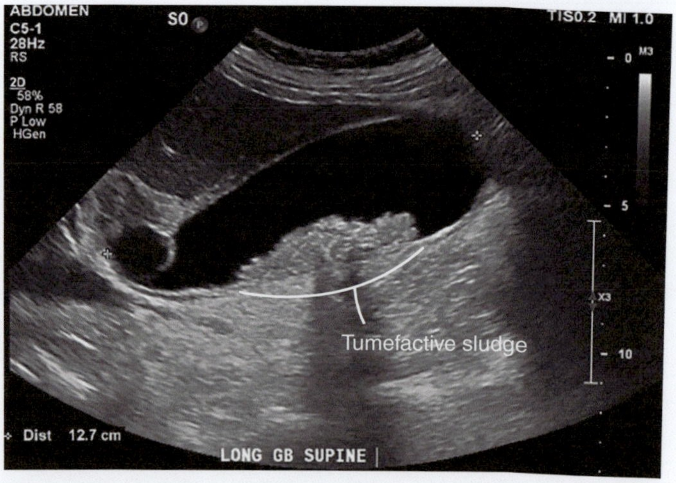

Fig. 10.23 Gallbladder with tumefactive sludge

the gallbladder, to confirm the structure is indeed a gallstone and is located intraluminally. Additionally, it is advised to image the gallbladder in more than one patient position (e.g., supine and left lateral decubitus) to potentially reveal hidden gallstones, confirm questionable stones, and indicate mobility of already identified stones. While most stones tend to be gravity-dependent, stones made primarily of cholesterol or stones containing gas can float. It is important to not confuse these rare stones with more ominous pathology such as emphysematous cholecystitis [50, 51]. Mobile stones within the gallbladder usually do not cause symptoms unless they are causing intermittent obstruction (i.e., biliary colic). However, when a stone lodges in the gallbladder neck, referred to as stone-in-neck (SIN) sign, it will become painful. A SIN can be missed if the neck is not thoroughly evaluated (Fig. 10.25). To overcome the challenges of viewing this area, the clinician can rotate the probe or slide the probe to a new angle, which may help to avoid subtle bowel gas and edge artifact.

A gallbladder completely filled with stones can be difficult to find and may resemble a gas-filled loop of bowel. This appearance is referred to as a wall-echo-shadow (WES) sign (Fig. 10.26). It represents from anterior to posterior: the anterior gallbladder wall (wall), a bright and often irregular hyperechoic line representing the surface of multiple adjacent stones (echo), and finally the anechoic posterior acoustic shadowing (shadow).

Cholecystitis

Cholecystitis is inflammation of the gallbladder typically caused by obstruction of the cystic duct with either localized or generalized inflammation as the gallbladder attempts to empty itself. The maximum dimensions of the gallbladder are 8 cm in length and 4 cm in width [52]. Its size can vary dramatically and can be contracted and difficult to see postprandially. The upper limit of normal for gallbladder wall thickness is considered to be 3 mm [53].

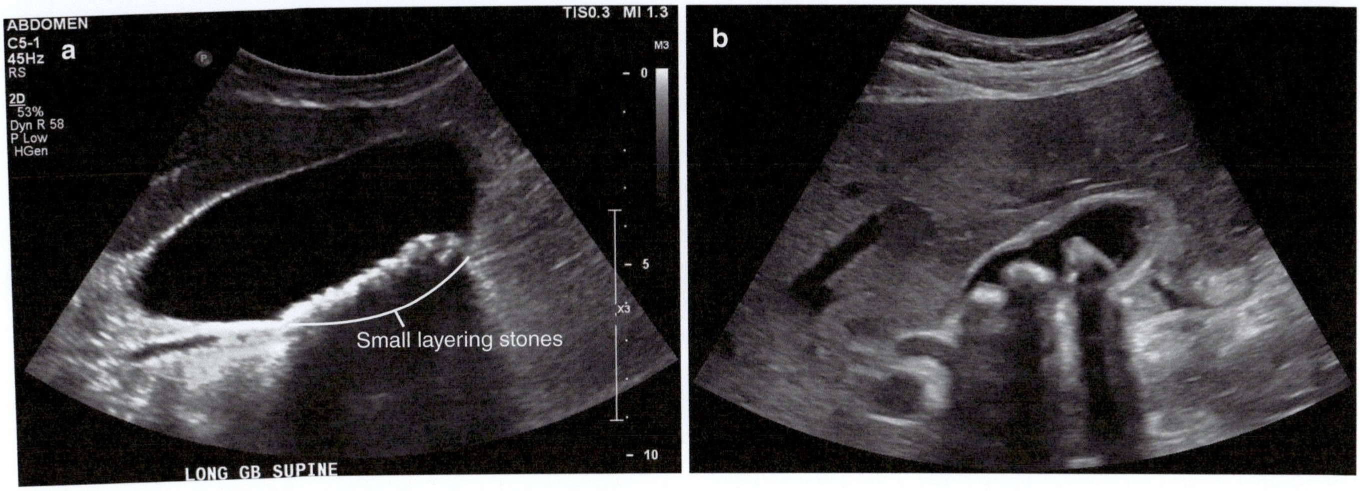

Fig. 10.24 (**a**) Gallbladder with small gallstones. (**b**) Gallbladder with three large gallstones. (*Image courtesy of Michael Gottlieb, MD*)

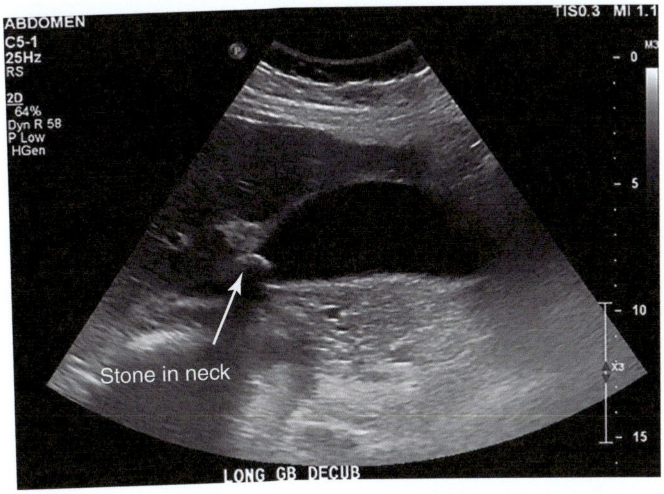

Fig. 10.25 Gallbladder with a stone in the neck

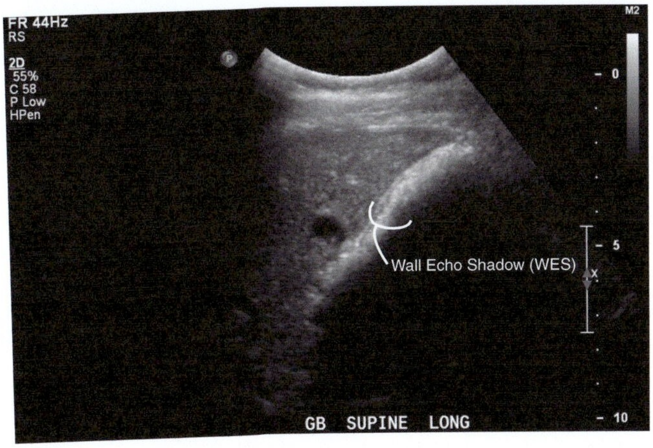

Fig. 10.26 Gallbladder with wall-echo-shadow (WES) sign

A meta-analysis demonstrated POCUS is 71% sensitive and 94% specific for the diagnosis of acute cholecystitis [54]. While diagnosis of cholecystitis is typically confirmed in the operating room under direct inspection or in the pathology lab with microscopic evaluation, making this diagnosis clinically with ultrasound can be more challenging as variable definitions are used in the medical literature when studying this. Sonographic findings that support a diagnosis of acute cholecystitis include gallbladder distention beyond normal dimensions, gallstones, wall thickening, pericholecystic fluid, and a sonographic Murphy's sign. Typically, the more findings that are noted, the more confident a clinician can be in making the diagnosis (Fig. 10.27).

Most (90–95%) acute cholecystitis cases are associated with gallstone obstruction and the absence of gallstones makes cholecystitis very unlikely [55]. The clinician should therefore focus on detecting gallstones when screening for cholecystitis, especially assessing for SIN sign, which carries a positive predictive value of 93% for cholecystitis [56]. Gallbladder distention (length greater than 10 cm) also raises concern for cholecystitis (Fig. 10.28) [57, 58].

Tenderness when the ultrasound probe compresses directly over the gallbladder (viewed below the costal margin, not through the rib cage) is called a sonographic Murphy's sign. It is important to also compress elsewhere over the liver parenchyma to assure that the tenderness is not more diffuse, in which case it is considered an indeterminate finding. The sonographic Murphy's sign is a dynamic finding with reasonable test characteristics in diagnosing cholecystitis (sensitivity 62%, specificity 96%) [59]. However, it is best used is in conjunction with other findings that support a diagnosis of cholecystitis [60].

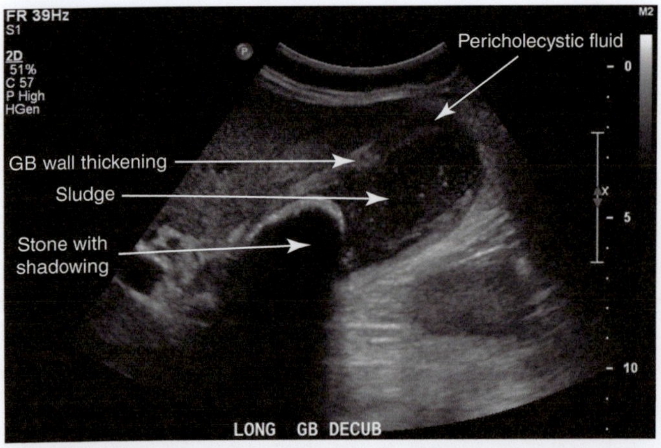

Fig. 10.27 Cholecystitis with gallstones, sludge, a thickened wall, and trace pericholecystic fluid

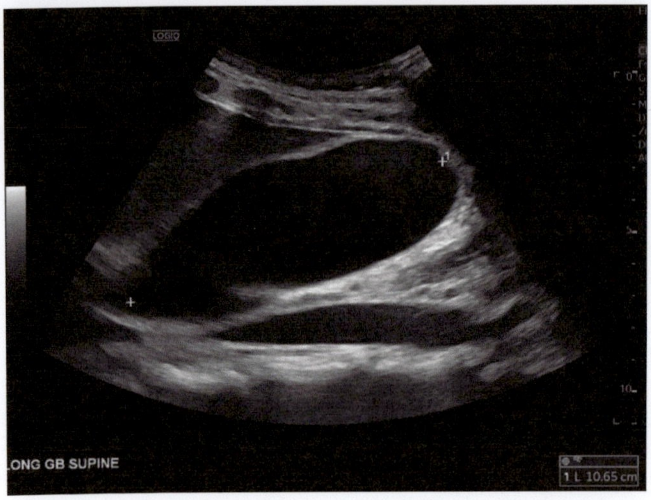

Fig. 10.28 Distended gallbladder measuring 10.65 cm in length

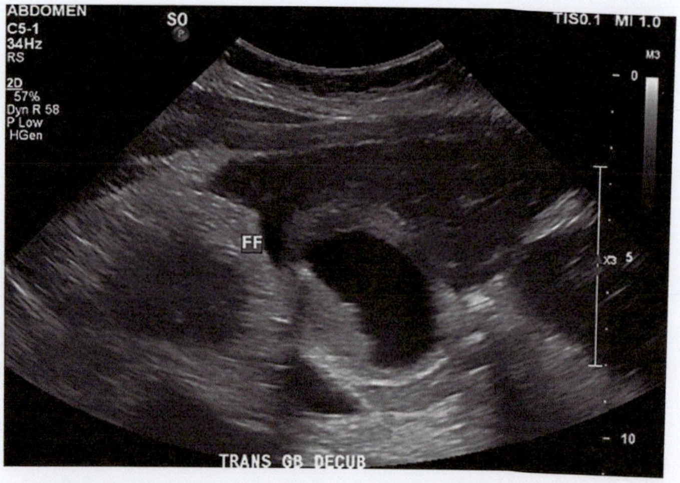

Fig. 10.29 Gallbladder with pericholecystic fluid (FF)

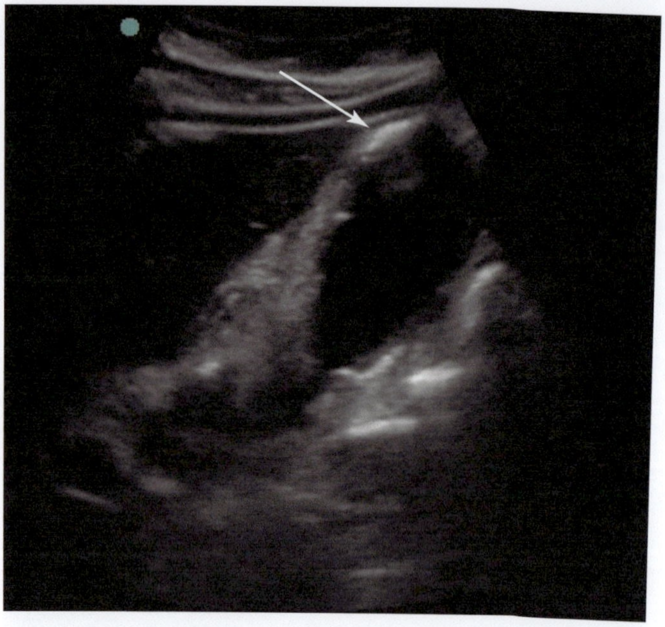

Fig. 10.30 Emphysematous cholecystitis with free air in the anterior wall (arrow). (*Image courtesy of Hamid Shokoohi, MD, MPH*)

Gallbladder wall thickening can be localized or generalized and is present when the wall thickness is >3 mm [61]. Gallbladder wall thickening is not always related to inflammation and is frequently noted in patients with a postprandial contracted gallbladder as well as in patients with extrinsic causes of edema (e.g., ascites, congestive heart failure, hypoalbuminemia). Wall changes from generalized edema typically appear as more diffuse thickening. In contrast, pus, serosal hemorrhage, and necrosis manifest as more localized wall thickening and may also demonstrate pericholecystic fluid. Pericholecystic fluid appears as a hypoechoic collection located within or adjacent to the gallbladder wall that can range from very subtle to easily discernible (Fig. 10.29).

Cholecystitis can evolve to gangrenous or emphysematous cholecystitis in which hyperechoic air with reverberation artifacts or dirty shadowing can be seen within the gallbladder and gallbladder wall (Fig. 10.30). Gangrenous and emphysematous gallbladders may be devoid of tenderness due to necrosis of the nearby nerves [62]. Gallbladder perforation and abscess are other uncommon complications of cholecystitis, noted in up to 4.8% of cases [63].

Acalculous cholecystitis is rare, lacks gallstones, and typically occurs in critically ill patients often cared for in intensive care units (Fig. 10.31). The etiology is debated but is thought to be related to biliary stasis, ascending infection, or pancreatic reflux [64]. Diagnosing acalculous cholecystitis depends heavily on the clinical context. A stable patient with diffuse wall thickening and no obvious tenderness is less likely to have acalculous cholecystitis than a febrile patient with a dilated gallbladder, wall thickening, and other signs of sepsis without an obvious source.

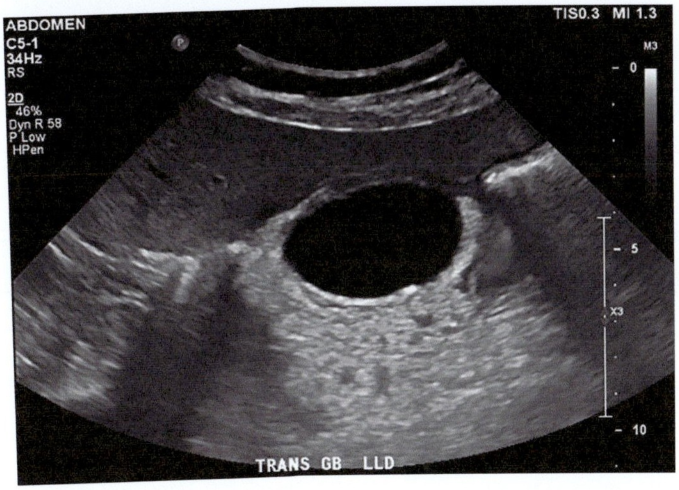

Fig. 10.31 Acalculous cholecystitis

Chronic cholecystitis is due to inflammation caused by gallstones chronically irritating the gallbladder wall. Findings are similar to acute cholecystitis with the exception of pericholecystic fluid, which is thought to be less common [65, 66]. Additionally, the clinical history of pain is more indolent.

Porcelain Gallbladder

Porcelain gallbladder is a form of chronic cholecystitis that is often an incidental finding (Fig. 10.32, Video 10.13). It occurs when there is calcification of the gallbladder wall, often thought to be related to low-grade chronic inflammation. It is rare and is associated with a small increased risk of gallbladder carcinoma (6% vs 1%) [67–69]. Risk factors are similar to other gallbladder pathologies. It is typically seen as an echogenic anterior gallbladder wall with immediate anechoic posterior acoustic shadowing.

Gallbladder Polyps

Incidental polypoid lesions of the gallbladder, including benign polyps (usually cholesterol) and benign neoplasms (usually adenoma), may be detected during gallbladder sonography. Gallbladder polyps are quite common and can be found in approximately 5% of the general population [70]. In contrast to gallstones, these masses are immobile and do not produce shadows (Fig. 10.33). Fortunately, the majority of gallbladder polyps are noncancerous. However, benign polyps can be difficult to differentiate from more serious pre-cancers and cancers of the gallbladder and therefore warrant follow-up. In general, a polyp diameter <10 mm is considered low risk for cancer [71].

Gallbladder Cancer

Gallbladder cancer is rare with approximately 5000 cases diagnosed each year [72]. Adenocarcinoma represents the vast majority of gallbladder cancers. Characteristics of a polypoid lesion that increase concern for malignancy include a solitary mass, a diameter ≥10 mm, presence of a stalk, adjacent gallbladder wall thickening, and age greater than 50 years [71]. Growths that do not meet these criteria are more likely to be benign. Metastatic disease due to direct invasion from the stomach, pancreas, and biliary tract is also possible.

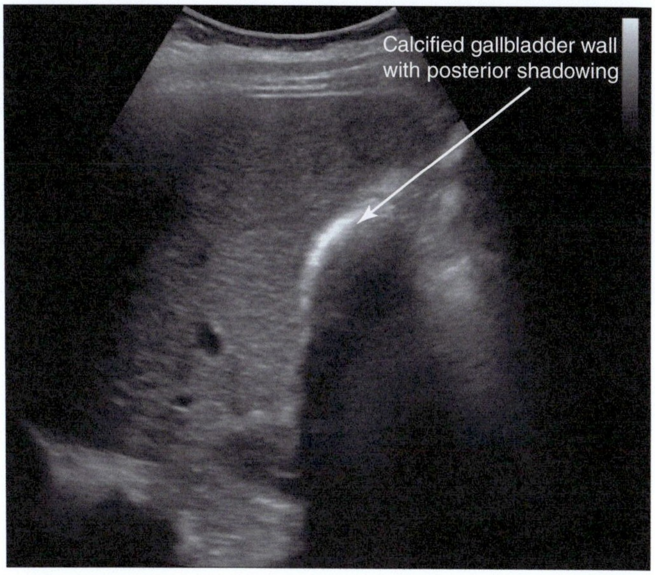

Fig. 10.32 Porcelain gallbladder. (*Image courtesy of Stephen Alerhand, MD*)

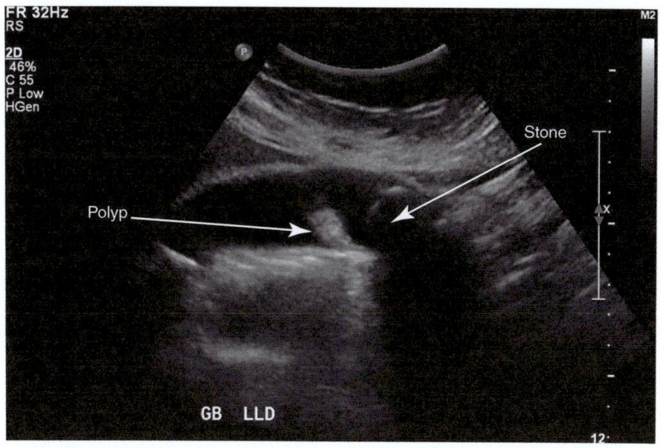

Fig. 10.33 Gallbladder polyp (arrow) and stone

Adenomyomatosis

Adenomyomatosis is proliferative growth of mucosa through the muscularis layer of the gallbladder wall, forming small intramural diverticula called Rokitansky-Aschoff sinuses (Fig. 10.34). This is often an incidental finding and can appear as wall thickening with posterior focal reverberation artifacts (comet tail artifacts), likely from cholesterol crystals within the sinuses [73, 74]. It is important to note that

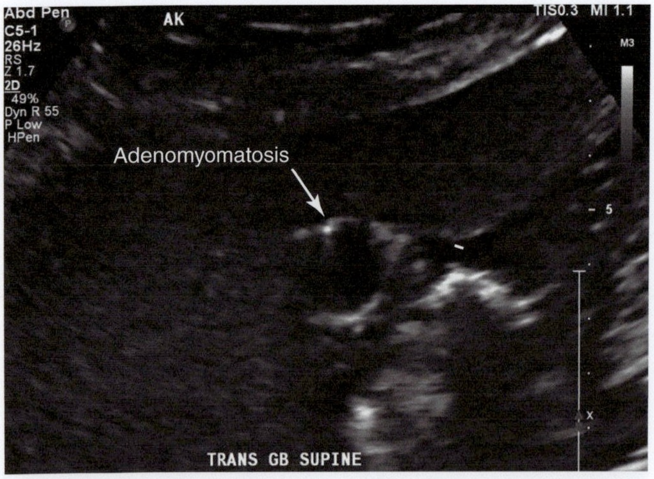

Fig. 10.34 Adenomyomatosis

differentiating adenomyomatosis, which is benign, from gallbladder cancer can be challenging. Adenomyomatosis is more likely if the wall thickening is diffuse and if pathognomonic V-shaped comet tail artifacts are present, whereas gallbladder cancer tends to be more localized [75].

Common Bile Duct Dilation

Bile ducts are elastic and able to expand with increasing intraluminal pressure. A bile duct together with a branch of a hepatic artery and a branch of a portal vein is called a portal triad. Portal veins have fatty walls that appear hyperechoic. This contrasts with hepatic veins, which have very thin walls that can be difficult to appreciate. The common hepatic duct exits the liver, connecting to the cystic duct from the neck of the gallbladder and continues further as the common bile duct (CBD) (Fig. 10.35). The CBD is usually visible anterior to the portal vein, and its diameter is normally 6 mm or less [76]. It is measured from the inner wall to the inner wall. Any obstruction along this path will lead to biliary ductal dilation, and ultrasound performs well at detecting CBD dilation (76–84% sensitivity, 98% specificity) (Fig. 10.36) [54]. With advancing age, the normal CBD can increase in diameter, though most remain less than 7–8 mm [77, 78]. Patients who are post-cholecystectomy often have CBD dilation up to 10 mm [79].

As it is not common to directly visualize a stone within the CBD, choledocholithiasis is usually inferred from a dilated CBD even if the stone is not visualized. However, it is important to consider other important causes of CBD dilation, including intrinsic obstruction (e.g., cholangiocarcinoma) and extrinsic compression (e.g., pancreatic tumor, lymphadenopathy). Mirizzi syndrome occurs when an impacted stone lies within the cystic duct and extrinsically compresses the adjacent common hepatic duct. If the CBD is not specifically seen but the portal vein and common hepatic artery are seen, it is likely not dilated. Alternatively, prior studies have shown that, among patients with normal liver function tests and no evidence of cholelithiasis, the incidence of a solitary stone obstructing the CBD is exceedingly uncommon (<1%) [80, 81].

Pancreas

Normal Anatomy

Pancreatic parenchyma is generally homogenous or marginally lobulated in texture and slightly more hyperechoic than the liver parenchyma (Fig. 10.37). The echogenicity of the pancreas can be variable but tends to become more echogenic with age [82]. The most prominent landmark in the transverse view of the pancreas is the superior mesenteric vein at the confluence with the splenic vein. These vessels run directly posterior to the neck and body of the pancreas and continue adjacent to the pancreatic tail. Graded compression can improve visualization by reducing overlying air in the stomach. Additional strategies for optimizing pancreatic imaging include controlling respirations through held inspiration or exhalation, Valsalva maneuver, or drinking water to create an acoustic window through the stomach [83].

Acute Pancreatitis

The most common ultrasound finding in mild acute pancreatitis is enlargement of the pancreas. Generally, when the pancreas is measured in the anterior-posterior dimension, the pancreatic head is less than 3 cm, the body less than 2.5 cm, and the tail less than 2.0 cm; however, the normal range can vary widely [84]. Enlargement from acute pancreatitis may occur diffusely or focally. Another common finding is decreased echogenicity from the edema, resulting in either diffusely or in focally scattered hypoechoic areas. Secondary ultrasound findings are more subtle, including ill-defined margins of the pancreas and small fluid collections near the pancreas (Fig. 10.38) [85]. In one study of 48 patients with pancreatitis, decreased pancreatic echogenicity compared with the liver was noted in 21 patients (44%), heterogeneous echogenic pattern was detected in 27 patients (56%), focal intrapancreatic regions of abnormal echogenicity were seen in 11 patients (23%), focal masses were seen in 8 patients (17%), hypoechoic peripancreatic areas of inflammation were seen in 29 patients (60%), and acute peripancreatic fluid collections were seen in 10 patients (21%) [86].

Pancreatic Calculi

Pancreatic calculi can form within the duct in the setting of chronic pancreatitis. These calculi can obstruct primary and secondary ducts, as well as make the tissue appear dense and difficult to visualize (Fig. 10.39) [86]. The main pancreatic duct joins the CBD before entering the duodenum via the

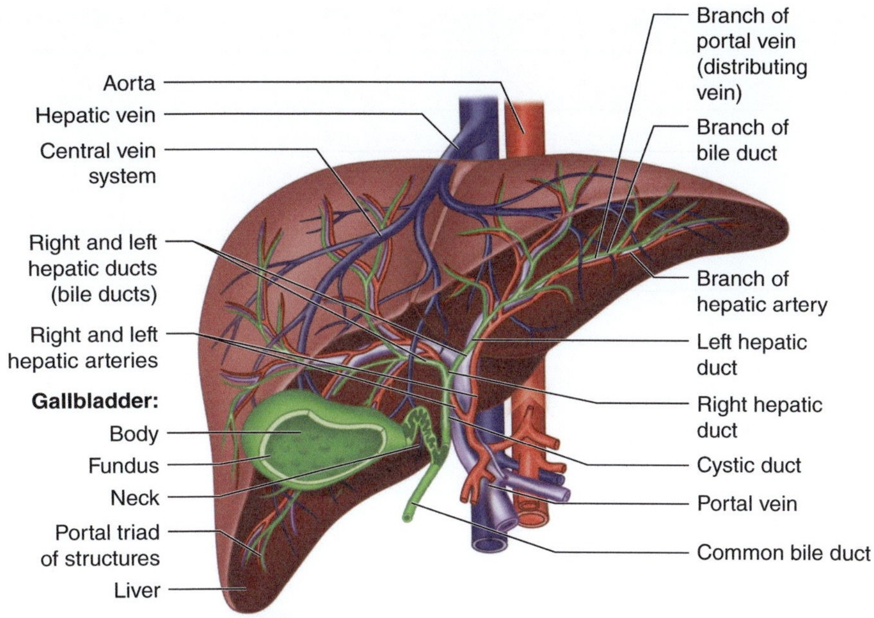

Fig. 10.35 Biliary duct anatomy

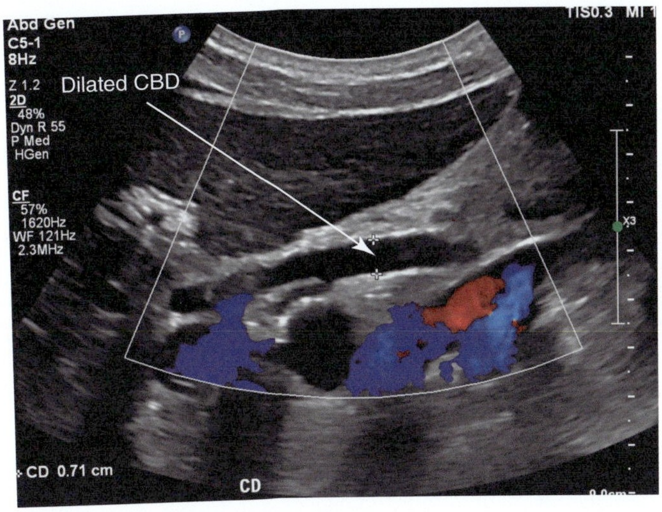

Fig. 10.36 Common bile duct dilation

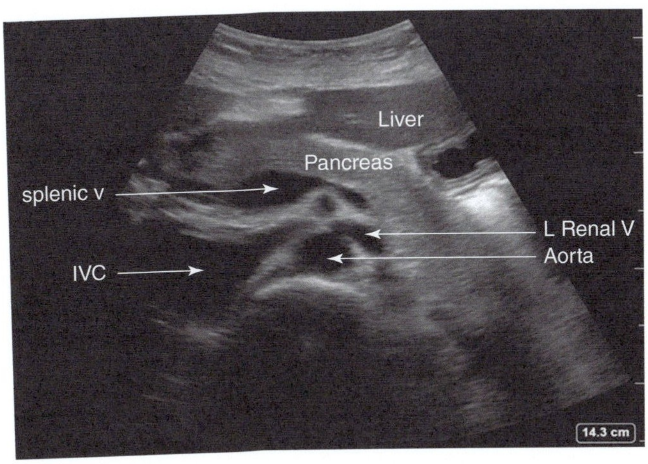

Fig. 10.37 Normal pancreas

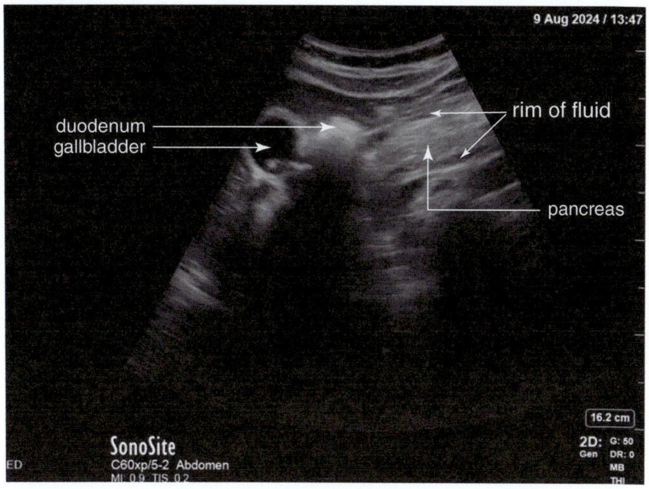

Fig. 10.38 Enlarged heterogeneous pancreas with rim of peripancreatic fluid consistent with acute pancreatitis. (*Image courtesy of Benjamin C Smith 3rd, MD*)

Ampulla of Vater. The normal diameter of this duct should be less than 2.5 mm (Fig. 10.40) [86]. Dilation can occur from intraductal causes such as an obstructing gallstone or extraductal causes such as malignancy [86].

Pancreatic Pseudocysts

Pseudocysts are a known complication of acute and chronic pancreatitis, accounting for 75–90% of all cystic lesions seen in the pancreas [87, 88]. These typically are not diagnosed until four weeks after the onset of symptoms due to the time it takes for the fluid to become fully encapsulated. Pseudocysts develop in 5–16% of patients with acute pancreatitis and increase to 20–40% of patients with chronic pancreatitis [85, 88]. Pseudocysts can be difficult to distinguish

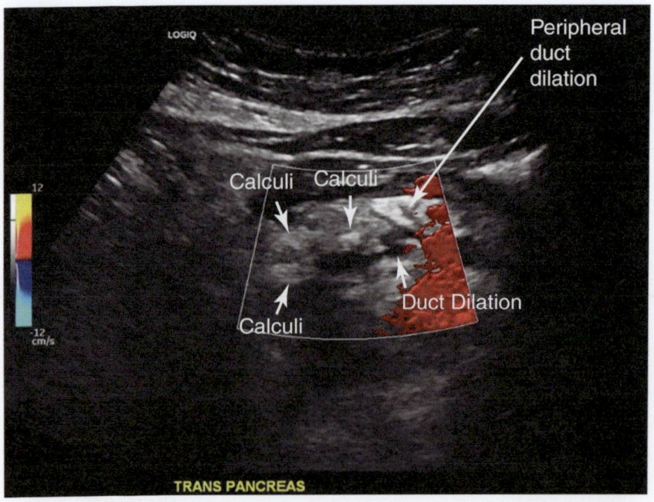

Fig. 10.39 Pancreatic calculi

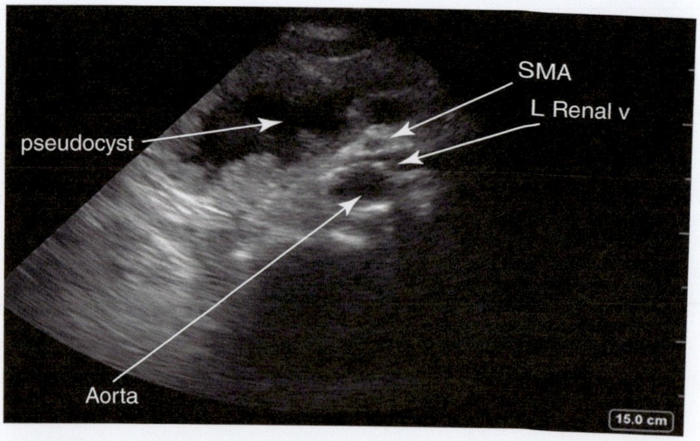

Fig. 10.41 Pancreatic pseudocyst

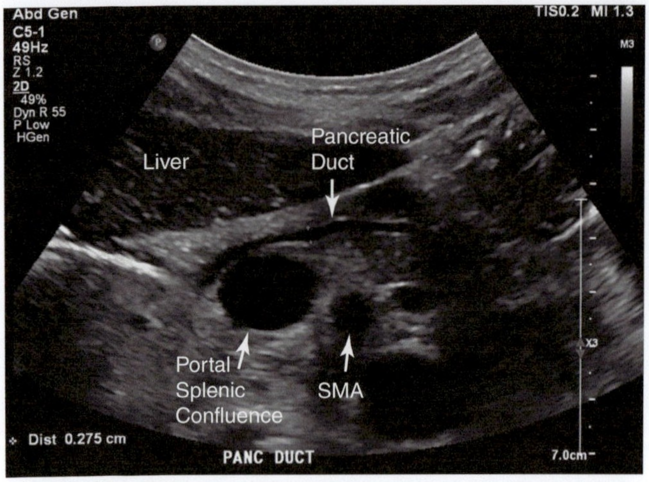

Fig. 10.40 Pancreatic duct dilation

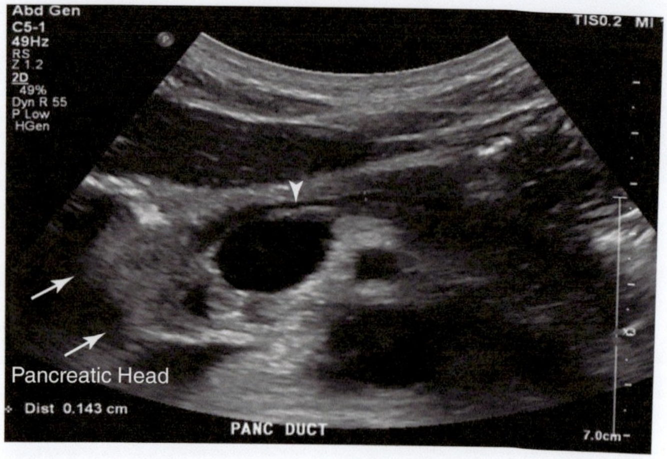

Fig. 10.42 Pancreatic head mass causing pancreatic ductal dilation (arrow)

from pancreatic neoplasms; therefore, clinical correlation is essential. A history of pancreatitis and temporal proximity to an episode of pancreatitis support pseudocyst over neoplasm. Pseudocysts are encapsulated, internally anechoic with posterior acoustic enhancement, and have no blood flow with color Doppler (Fig. 10.41). Pseudocysts that appear after episodes of necrotizing pancreatitis can be more complex and heterogeneous with thick septations, referred to as walled-off necrosis [85, 88]. In these cases, contrast-enhanced computed tomography can be helpful due to the potential for adverse outcomes [89].

Pancreatic Masses

There are multiple types of masses that can be seen in the pancreas. Pancreatic masses generally appear hypoechoic compared to adjacent pancreatic tissue [89]. Pancreatic head masses can create a "double duct sign," where the common bile duct on the periampullary side of the pancreatic head and the pancreatic duct in the body are both dilated due to obstruction of both ducts (Fig. 10.42). The presence of this sign should warrant further investigation with contrast-enhanced CT to rule out extrinsic compression of the pancreas, especially if a mass is not apparent, as masses are often difficult to identify [90]. It is important to note that the double duct sign can also occur from gallbladder or pancreas calculi obstruction [90].

Pancreatic ductal adenocarcinoma (PDA) is the most common solid malignant neoplasm in the pancreas, with 60–70% developing in the pancreatic head [90]. PDA is hypoechoic in appearance with ill-defined margins as the tumor infiltrates into surrounding tissue. PDA often involves the pancreatic duct, which results in the dilation of the duct beyond the tumor. Aggressive PDAs can mimic cystic lesions due to the anechoic center that develops with necrosis of lesion tissue. Calcifications can help distinguish chronic pancreatitis from PDA. In chronic pancreatitis, the calcifications tend to be multiple and situated around the duct, whereas in PDA, calcifications are rare and have no association with ductal dilation [91].

The second most common solid pancreatic tumors are neuroendocrine tumors. Neuroendocrine tumors, such as insulinomas, appear as benign nodules that are well-defined, small, hypervascular, and hypoechoic (Fig. 10.43). They typically are less than 1.5 cm in diameter at diagnosis but can grow to over 3 cm. Larger tumors are at higher risk of malignancy [90, 92].

Cystic lesions comprise 10–15% of all pancreatic tumors [85, 93]. The most common is a benign serous cystadenoma, occurring in about 20% of pancreatic cystic neoplasms. These are usually asymptomatic, found incidentally, and occur in older women [85, 94]. They consist of several small cysts clustered together that do not communicate with the pancreatic duct (Fig. 10.44) [85, 94].

Mucinous cystadenomas and cystadenocarcinomas are largely indistinguishable from each other and comprise 10% of all cystic lesions [85, 94]. They typically involve the body or tail of the pancreas, and 95% occur in women between the 4th and 6th decade [87]. Secondary signs such as invasion into adjacent organs or vasculature and eggshell calcifications (fine calcifications at the periphery of a mass) are highly suggestive of mucinous cystadenocarcinoma when present [85, 87, 94].

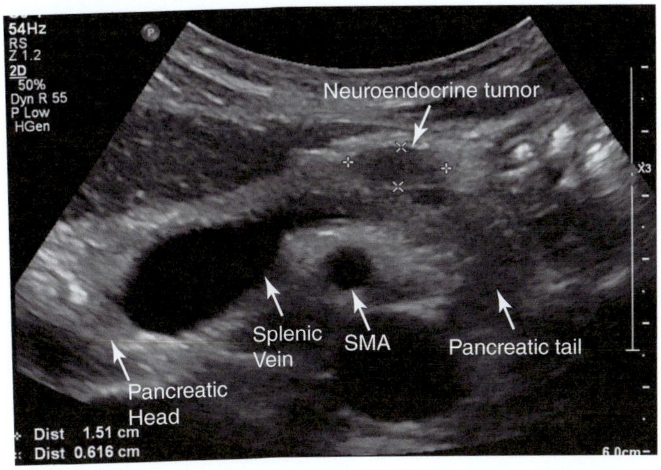

Fig. 10.43 Neuroendocrine tumor

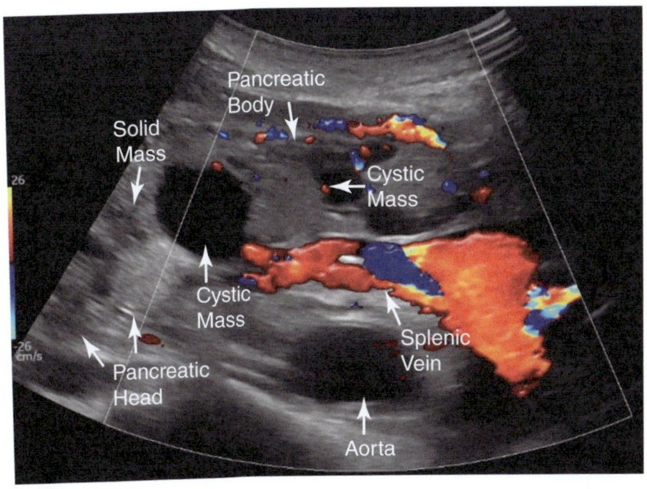

Fig. 10.44 Pancreatic serous cystadenoma

Intraductal papillary mucinous tumors represent 20% of all cystic pancreatic lesions and typically affect elderly men [87, 94]. This tumor causes hyperproduction of mucous cells, which can lead to dilation of the main pancreatic duct and its branches. Sonographic findings include communication of the lesion with the pancreatic duct and pancreatic duct dilation. Invasion into the main pancreatic duct is associated with a higher risk of malignancy [87, 94].

Spleen

Normal Anatomy

The spleen is located in the left upper quadrant of the abdomen. Because it is located underneath the diaphragm and posterior to the stomach, the spleen can be more challenging to visualize. Ultrasound can evaluate splenic echotexture, size, and presence of masses. The spleen has a homogenous echotexture and is isoechoic or slightly hyperechoic when compared to the liver. The spleen should appear hyperechoic when compared with the cortex of the left kidney. The homogenous echotexture makes splenic pathology more prominent and easy to identify. Placing the patient in the right lateral decubitus position can help with visualization and allow the probe to slide more posteriorly. Sustained deep inspiration or expiration can aid in visualizing the spleen in both the long and short axes.

Splenomegaly

Splenic size can vary significantly among individuals and is dependent on several factors, including sex, height, and age. For this reason, cutoffs for determining normal spleen size can be unreliable [95, 96]. Therefore, when measuring the spleen, these factors and clinical history need to be taken into account. The upper limit of normal for splenic length is 13 cm in the craniocaudal measurement or 6 mm in the transverse orientation. When evaluating for splenomegaly, the measurement should be taken in both the long and short axes at the level of the splenic hilum. If the spleen is too large to image in one view, the full length can be captured and measured in two views with one image superior to the hilum and the second view inferior to the hilum.

Splenomegaly refers to enlargement of the spleen (Fig. 10.45). There are multiple etiologies for splenomegaly and in the majority of these, splenomegaly is a diagnostic indicator for other diseases [97]. Splenomegaly can result from systemic processes such as congestive or inflammatory diseases. Other causes can be hematologic, infectious, or

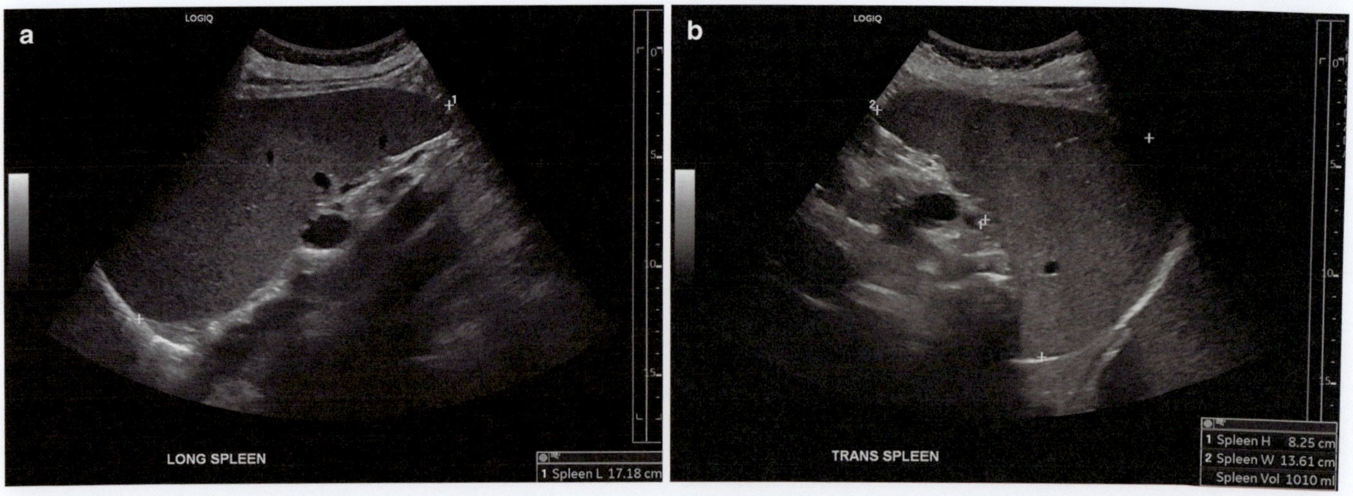

Fig. 10.45 (**a**) Splenomegaly viewed in a long axis. (**b**) Splenomegaly views in a short axis

infiltrative in nature. In cases of severe splenomegaly (>18 cm), the physician should consider the possibility of spontaneous rupture, a rare but life-threatening complication [97].

Splenic Cysts

Splenic cysts are often asymptomatic and present as incidental findings on ultrasound. They can arise from a variety of etiologies and can present as singular or multiple cystic lesions. Simple cysts present as thin-walled, anechoic ovoid lesions and should demonstrate posterior acoustic enhancement (Fig. 10.46). Simple cysts can be divided into two categories: true cysts and pseudocysts. True cysts, also known as primary cysts, are either non-parasitic or parasitic. Parasitic splenic cysts are most commonly caused by an *Echinococcus granulosus* infection that can result in hydatid disease [99].The majority of non-parasitic cysts are congenital in origin and are more likely to be seen in the upper pole of the spleen [99, 100]. When simple cysts are found incidentally in asymptomatic patients, they do not need to be followed up with further evaluation [98]. After traumatic injury, the spleen can form pseudocysts or secondary cysts, which tend to be simple in nature. Even when there is a thick outer wall calcification, these are rarely concerning [98].

Whenever a cyst is seen in the spleen, splenic abscess or pseudoaneurysm should be considered. Color Doppler can quickly resolve the question of pseudoaneurysm (absence of Doppler signal should rule this out), and in the absence of fever, pain, or vomiting, abscess is highly unlikely. When cystic lesions develop thick-walled septations with solid components, they are considered cystic masses and are usually due to infectious processes or neoplasms.

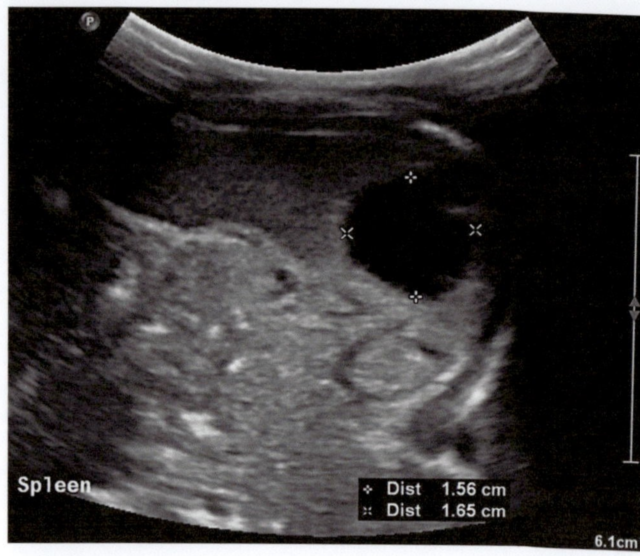

Fig. 10.46 Splenic cyst

Splenic Calcifications

Microlithiasis of the spleen is noted when multiple small calcifications are present. This creates a “starry sky” pattern with ultrasound, which presents as multiple hyperechoic foci within the spleen (Fig. 10.47). These calcifications can be caused by infectious agents, with the most common being histoplasmosis, tuberculosis, brucellosis, candidiasis, or pneumocystis. In tuberculosis infections, calcifications tend to be larger in size and fewer in number but may still present

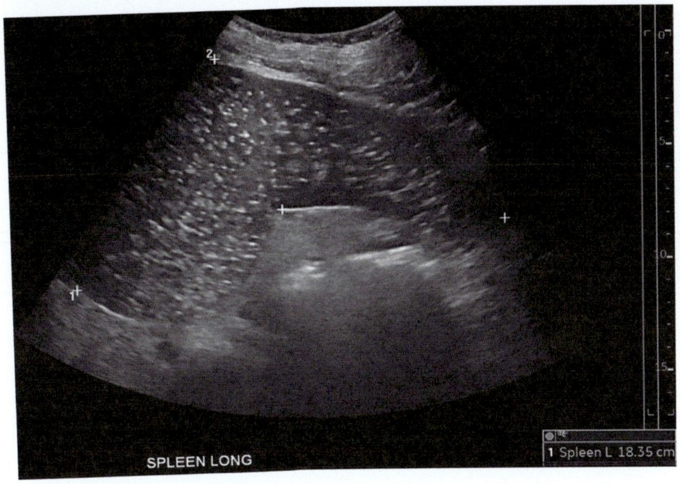

Fig. 10.47 Microlithiasis of the spleen

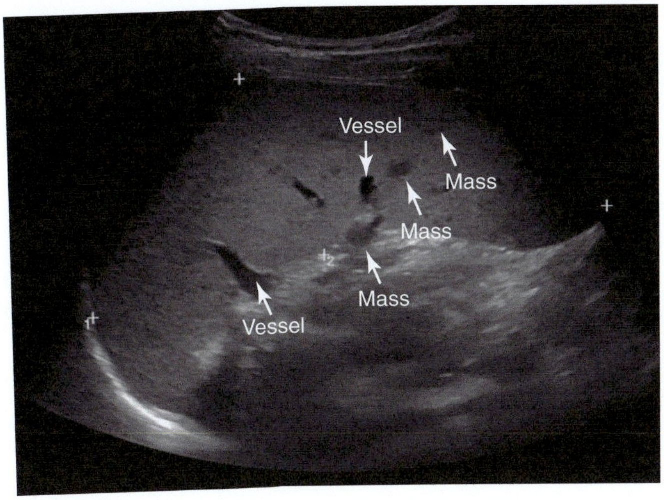

Fig. 10.48 Splenic masses

diffusely throughout the spleen [101]. Other causes of calcifications beyond infectious processes include sickle cell disease and trauma with splenic infarction. Splenic calcifications can be seen with hemangiomas as well. However, these are often incidental findings among asymptomatic patients, and no follow-up is necessary [98, 101].

Splenic Masses

Splenic masses can have cystic components or be completely solid (Fig. 10.48). Benign masses in the spleen are common, with hemangioma as the most common, occurring in 0.1–14% of the population [102]. Hemangiomas and hamartomas are both benign vascular tumors that are well-defined. The main sonographic difference is that hemangiomas appear hyperechoic and hamartomas appear slightly hypoechoic on ultrasound [103]. Both lesions may contain cystic components as well. Other benign lesions, such as sclerosing angiomatoid nodular transformation and inflammatory pseudotumors, occur much less frequently.

Primary malignancies are rare in the spleen, but the most common is primary lymphoma in patients with Hodgkin's disease, followed by angiosarcoma, which appears complex, heterogeneous, and highly vascular [98, 103, 104]. The sonographic appearance can vary from multiple small masses to larger and bulky masses. All nodules typically appear anechoic to hypoechoic but may occasionally display an echogenic target sign with a hypoechoic ring [103].

Much like primary tumors, metastases to the spleen are also uncommon and tend to only appear in advanced stages of disease. These lesions often appear solid and hypoechoic compared to surrounding tissues but can present in a number of ways, including hyperechoic, cystic, or heterogeneous. Melanoma will metastasize to the spleen in many cases, though metastases to the spleen can come from any malignant source in the body [103].

Splenic Infarction

Splenic infarction occurs when a thrombus occludes the splenic artery in the spleen. Due to the high volume of blood entering the spleen, it is susceptible to embolism from any location (though most originate from the heart). Autoimmune disorders such as rheumatoid arthritis and systemic lupus erythematosus can lead to splenic infarction. Sickle cell disease can also have areas of infarction that can lead to "auto-splenectomy" if enough of the splenic tissue is damaged that it ceases functioning [105].

Infarcts occur at the outer margins of the spleen and appear either as hypoechoic, wedge-shaped lesions or as multiple cystic structures within a hypoechoic area in early stages (Fig. 10.49). In some cases, infarcted areas may appear irregularly shaped with ill-defined borders. As the infarct progresses over time, fibrosis may develop, giving the infarct an overall hyperechoic appearance without cystic structures [105].

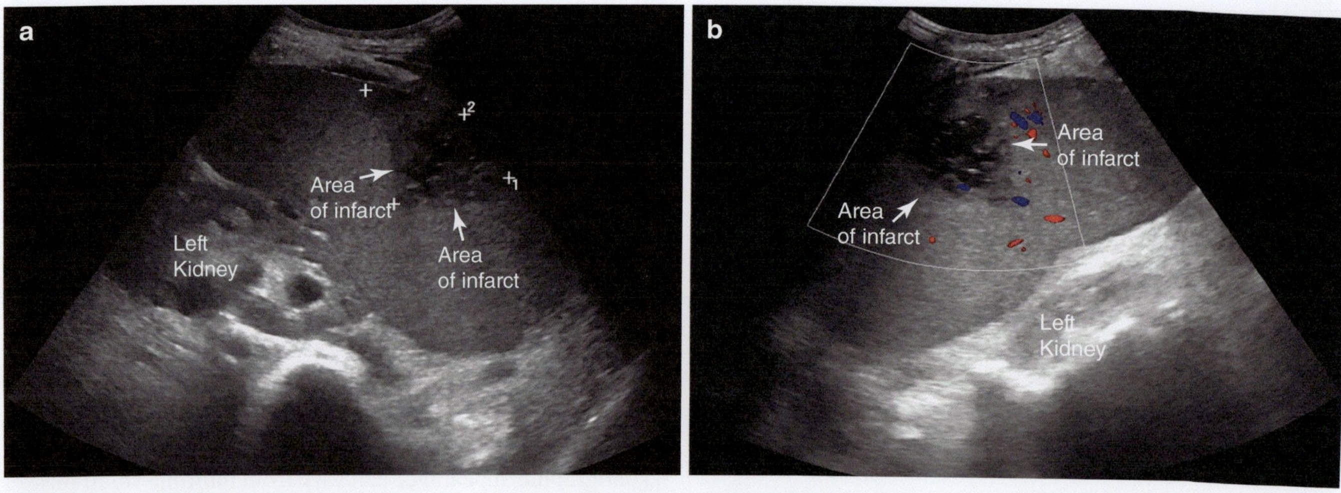

Fig. 10.49 (**a**) Short-axis view of a splenic infarct viewed in B-mode. (**b**) Long-axis view of a splenic infarct with color Doppler

Key Ultrasound Findings

Pathology	Key ultrasound findings
Steatosis	Hyperechoic liver parenchyma similar to cirrhosis.
Cirrhosis	Hyperechoic liver parenchyma; ascites.
Acute Hepatitis	Hepatomegaly, decreased echogenicity of the liver parenchyma with increased echogenicity of portal venous structures ("starry night").
Intrahepatic Ductal Dilation	Hyperechoic tubular channels within the liver parenchyma. No signal with color Doppler assessment.
Liver cyst	Round anechoic mass with smooth edges, epithelial lining; posterior acoustic enhancement.
Hemangioma	Hyperechoic, round mass.
Hepatocellular carcinoma	Single, heterogenous mass.
Metastatic disease to the Liver	Multiple, heterogenous, scattered masses; cannonball lesions.
Portal Hypertension	Splenomegaly, ascites, and visualization of portosystemic venous collaterals.
Portal Vein Thrombosis	Echogenic thrombus seen in the portal vein; portal vein diameter >13 mm; decreased Doppler signal.
Portal Venous Gas	Reverberation artifact in the peripheral vasculature of the liver.
Hepatic Vein Obstruction (Budd-Chiari Syndrome)	Hepatic vein occlusion; intrahepatic collaterals; reversal of portal venous flow; disruption of IVC flow; presence of liver mass.
Pneumobilia	Reverberation artifact in the central regions of the liver, intrahepatic ducts.
Intrahepatic Infections	Cystic lesions containing simple or complex fluid, lack an epithelial lining, irregular in shape.
Gallbladder sludge	Gravity-dependent echogenic fluid in the gallbladder.

Pathology	Key ultrasound findings
Cholelithiasis	Mobile echogenic stones within the gallbladder lumen.
Acute Cholecystitis	Gallstones, sonographic Murphy's sign, gallbladder wall thickening (>3 mm), pericholecystic fluid.
Acalculous Cholecystitis	Findings consistent with cholecystitis in the absence of gallstones.
Porcelain Gallbladder	Complete or partial highly echogenic wall with dense posterior shadowing.
Gallbladder polyp	Non-shadowing mass (can be multiple).
Gallbladder carcinoma	Increased risk with non-shadowing mass greater than 10 mm; pedunculated, solitary, adjacent wall thickening; patient older than 50 years.
Adenomyomatosis	Gallbladder wall thickening (>3 mm) with focal posterior reverberation artifacts.
Biliary Ductal Dilation	Common bile duct diameter >6 mm.
Acute Pancreatitis	Diffuse or focal enlargement of pancreas; fluid around pancreas.
Pancreatic Calculi	Dilated pancreatic duct beyond stone; echogenic stone with posterior shadowing; double duct sign.
Pancreatic Masses	Solid masses seen most commonly in pancreatic head; Cystic lesions more common in body or tail of pancreas; Double duct sign; Invasion of adjacent organs or vasculature highly suggestive of malignancy.
Pancreatic Pseudocyst	Encapsulated cyst with anechoic areas and posterior acoustic enhancement; located in or adjacent to pancreas; often complex with septations.
Splenomegaly	>13 cm in long axis, >6 cm in short axis.
Splenic Cysts	Primary cysts are thin-walled and contain cellular epithelial lining; secondary or pseudocysts are thick-walled with calcified outer rim; cystic masses have multiple thick septations with solid components.

Pathology	Key ultrasound findings
Splenic Masses	Well-defined solid mass with variable echogenicity; can be homogeneous or heterogeneous; may or may not be cystic components; solid malignant tumors tend to be highly vascular.
Splenic calcification	"Starry night" appearance; multiple hyperechoic foci; can appear as larger hypoechoic lesions as well.
Splenic Infarction	Hypoechoic area on periphery of spleen; typically wedge-shaped in appearance; irregular borders with multiple cystic appearing areas; hyperechoic areas of fibrosis may develop over time.

IVC, inferior vena cava

Pearls and Pitfalls

- Steatosis and cirrhosis both appear diffusely hyperechoic, so further investigation with hepatic vein Doppler analysis or contrast-enhanced ultrasound should be used to differentiate when clinically appropriate.
- Focal nodular hyperplasia and adenoma can have similar appearances and should be evaluated with further imaging.
- Pneumobilia is usually iatrogenic. Portal venous gas is rare, more in the periphery compared to pneumobilia, and typically associated with high mortality conditions such as sepsis, ischemia, or necrotizing disease.
- Findings that suggest cholecystitis when coupled with gallstones or sludge: sonographic Murphy's sign, gallbladder wall thickening, and pericholecystic fluid.
- Gallbladder wall thickening can occur outside of cholecystitis in fluid overload, ascites, and postprandial settings (a contracted gallbladder may appear to have a thickened wall but is not pathologic).
- Be sure to evaluate the entire gallbladder in multiple planes with careful evaluation to avoid missing a stone impacted in the neck.
- Focal enlargement of the pancreatic head due to acute pancreatitis can mimic a pancreatic mass.
- Pseudocysts can be difficult to distinguish from pancreatic mass; clinical correlation is imperative due to adverse outcomes if mistaken.
- Pseudocysts develop four weeks after onset of symptoms of acute pancreatitis.
- Walled-off necrosis of the pancreas should be followed by contrast-enhanced computed tomography.
- Invasion of cystic lesions into surrounding organs or vasculature is highly suspicious for malignancy.
- Spleen dimensions depend on patient size and gender; tall or large patients may have a normal spleen over 13 cm.
- Always use color Doppler to evaluate splenic cysts to rule out pseudoaneurysm.
- Many splenic ultrasound findings are asymptomatic and incidental.

Disclosures/Conflicts of Interest Christine M Schutzer: Consultant, Vave Health Inc.

References

1. Cozzi D, Agostini S, Bertelli E, Galluzzo M, Papa E, Scevola G, Trinci M, Miele V. Contrast-Enhanced Ultrasound (CEUS) in non-traumatic abdominal emergencies. Ultrasound Int Open. 2020;6(3):E76–86. https://doi.org/10.1055/a-1347-5875.
2. Liu GJ, Lu MD. Diagnosis of liver cirrhosis with contrast-enhanced ultrasound. World J Radiol. 2010;2(1):32–6. https://doi.org/10.4329/wjr.v2.i1.32.
3. Kratzer W, Fritz V, Mason RA, Haenle MM, Kaechele V, Roemerstein Study Group. Factors affecting liver size: a sonographic survey of 2080 subjects. J Ultrasound Med. 2003;22(11):1155–61.
4. Idilman IS, Ozdeniz I, Karcaaltincaba M. Hepatic steatosis: etiology, patterns, and quantification. Semin Ultrasound CT MR. 2016;37(6):501–10.
5. Ferraioli G, Berzigotti A, Barr RG, et al. Quantification of liver fat content with ultrasound: a WFUMB position paper. Ultrasound Med Biol. 2021;47(10):2803–20.
6. Dasarathy S, Dasarathy J, Khiyami A, Joseph R, Lopez R, McCullough AJ. Validity of real time ultrasound in the diagnosis of hepatic steatosis: a prospective study. J Hepatol. 2009;51(6):1061–7. https://doi.org/10.1016/j.jhep.2009.09.001. Epub 2009 Sep 20. PMID: 19846234; PMCID: PMC6136148.
7. Hernaez R, Lazo M, Bonekamp S, Kamel I, Brancati FL, Guallar E, Clark JM. Diagnostic accuracy and reliability of ultrasonography for the detection of fatty liver: a meta-analysis. Hepatology. 2011;54(3):1082–90. https://doi.org/10.1002/hep.24452. PMID: 21618575; PMCID: PMC4197002.
8. Anthony PP, Ishak KG, Nayak NC, Poulsen HE, Scheuer PJ, Sobin LH. The morphology of cirrhosis. Recommendations on definition, nomenclature, and classification by a working group sponsored by the World Health Organization. J Clin Pathol. 1978;31(5):395–414.
9. Aubé C, Bazeries P, Lebigot J, Cartier V, Boursier J. Liver fibrosis, cirrhosis, and cirrhosis-related nodules: imaging diagnosis and surveillance. Diagn Interv Imaging. 2017;98(6):455–68. https://doi.org/10.1016/j.diii.2017.03.003.

10. Theise ND. Macroregenerative (dysplastic) nodules and hepatocarcinogenesis: theoretical and clinical considerations. Semin Liver Dis. 1995;15(4):360–71. https://doi.org/10.1055/s-2007-1007287.
11. Tanaka S, Kitamra T, Fujita M, Kasugai H, Inoue A, Ishiguro S. Small hepatocellular carcinoma: differentiation from adenomatous hyperplastic nodule with color Doppler flow imaging. Radiology. 1992;182(1):161–5. https://doi.org/10.1148/radiology.182.1.1309217.
12. Colli A, Cocciolo M, Riva C, et al. Abnormalities of Doppler waveform of the hepatic veins in patients with chronic liver disease: correlation with histologic findings. AJR Am J Roentgenol. 1994;162(4):833–7.
13. Barr RG, Ferraioli G, Palmeri ML, Goodman ZD, Garcia-Tsao G, Rubin J, Garra B, Myers RP, Wilson SR, Rubens D, Levine D. Elastography assessment of liver fibrosis: Society of Radiologists in ultrasound consensus conference statement. Radiology. 2015;276(3):845–61. https://doi.org/10.1148/radiol.2015150619.
14. Albrecht T, Blomley MJ, Cosgrove DO, Taylor-Robinson SD, Jayaram V, Eckersley R, Urbank A, Butler-Barnes J, Patel N. Non-invasive diagnosis of hepatic cirrhosis by transit-time analysis of an ultrasound contrast agent. Lancet. 1999;353(9164):1579–83. https://doi.org/10.1016/S0140-6736(98)06373-9.
15. Kaneko T, Teshigawara O, Sugimoto H, Hirota M, Inoue S, Takeda S, Nakao A. Signal intensity of the liver parenchyma in microbubble contrast agent in the late liver phase reflects advanced fibrosis of the liver. Liver Int. 2005;25(2):288–93. https://doi.org/10.1111/j.1478-3231.2005.01025.x.
16. Zwiebel WJ. Sonographic diagnosis of diffuse liver disease. Semin Ultrasound CT MR. 1995;16(1):8–15. https://doi.org/10.1016/0887-2171(95)90011-x.
17. Pitchaimuthu M, Duxbury M. Cystic lesions of the liver-a review. Curr Probl Surg. 2017;54(10):514–42. https://doi.org/10.1067/j.cpsurg.2017.09.001.
18. Tsuruya K, Nishizaki Y, Tatemichi M, Mishima Y, Shimma Y, Arase Y, Hirose S, Shiraishi K, Kagawa T. The prevalence and natural history of hepatic cysts examined by ultrasound: a health checkup population retrospective cohort study. Sci Rep. 2022;12(1):12797. https://doi.org/10.1038/s41598-022-16875-z.
19. Rawla P, Sunkara T, Muralidharan P, Raj JP. An updated review of cystic hepatic lesions. Clin Exp Hepatol. 2019;5(1):22–9. https://doi.org/10.5114/ceh.2019.83153.
20. Moorthy K, Mihssin N, Houghton PW. The management of simple hepatic cysts: sclerotherapy or laparoscopic fenestration. Ann R Coll Surg Engl. 2001;83(6):409–14.
21. Leon M, Chavez L, Surani S. Hepatic hemangioma: what internists need to know. World J Gastroenterol. 2020;26(1):11–20. https://doi.org/10.3748/wjg.v26.i1.11.
22. Ross D, Pina J, Mirza M, Galvan A, Ponce L. Letter: regression of focal nodular hyperplasia after discontinuation of oral contraceptives. Ann Intern Med. 1976;85(2):203–4. https://doi.org/10.7326/0003-4819-85-2-203.
23. Chang CY, Hernandez-Prera JC, Roayaie S, Schwartz M, Thung SN. Changing epidemiology of hepatocellular adenoma in the United States: review of the literature. Int J Hepatol. 2013;2013:604860. https://doi.org/10.1155/2013/604860.
24. Khan AR, Wei X, Xu X. Portal vein tumor thrombosis and hepatocellular carcinoma - the changing tides. J Hepatocell Carcinoma. 2021;8:1089–115. https://doi.org/10.2147/JHC.S318070.
25. Claudon M, Dietrich CF, Choi BI, Cosgrove DO, Kudo M, Nolsøe CP, et al. World Federation for Ultrasound in medicine; European Federation of Societies for ultrasound. Guidelines and good clinical practice recommendations for Contrast Enhanced Ultrasound (CEUS) in the liver - update 2012: a WFUMB-EFSUMB initiative in cooperation with representatives of AFSUMB, AIUM, ASUM, FLAUS and ICUS. Ultrasound Med Biol. 2013;39(2):187–210. https://doi.org/10.1016/j.ultrasmedbio.2012.09.002.
26. Chammas MC, Bordini AL. Contrast-enhanced ultrasonography for the evaluation of malignant focal liver lesions. Ultrasonography. 2022;41(1):4–24. https://doi.org/10.14366/usg.21001.
27. Berzigotti A, Seijo S, Reverter E, Bosch J. Assessing portal hypertension in liver diseases. Expert Rev Gastroenterol Hepatol. 2013;7(2):141–55. https://doi.org/10.1586/egh.12.83.
28. Suk KT. Hepatic venous pressure gradient: clinical use in chronic liver disease. Clin Mol Hepatol. 2014;20(1):6–14. https://doi.org/10.3350/cmh.2014.20.1.6.
29. Maruyama H, Yokosuka O. Ultrasonography for noninvasive assessment of portal hypertension. Gut Liver. 2017;11(4):464–73.
30. Trebicka J, Strassburg CP. Etiology and complications of portal vein thrombosis. Viszeralmedizin. 2014;30(6):375–80. https://doi.org/10.1159/000369987.
31. Minoda AM, Cadete RBF, Teixeira SR, Muglia VF, Elias Junior J, de Melo-Leite AF. The ABCD of portal vein thrombosis: a systematic approach. Radiol Bras. 2020;53(6):424–9.
32. Geleto G, Getnet W, Tewelde T. Mean normal portal vein diameter using sonography among clients coming to Radiology Department of Jimma University Hospital, Southwest Ethiopia. Ethiop J Health Sci. 2016;26(3):237–42.
33. Menu Y, Alison D, Lorphelin JM, Valla D, Belghiti J, Nahum H. Budd-Chiari syndrome: US evaluation. Radiology. 1985;157(3):761–4. https://doi.org/10.1148/radiology.157.3.3903857.
34. Sagoo MG, Aland RC, Gosden E. Morphology and morphometry of the caudate lobe of the liver in two populations. Anat Sci Int. 2018;93(1):48–57. https://doi.org/10.1007/s12565-016-0365-7.
35. Millener P, Grant EG, Rose S, et al. Color Doppler imaging findings in patients with Budd-Chiari syndrome: correlation with venographic findings. AJR Am J Roentgenol. 1993;161(2):307–12.
36. Huang J, Stone MB. Ultrasound identification of traumatic pneumobilia. Am J Emerg Med. 2010;28(2):255.e5–6. https://doi.org/10.1016/j.ajem.2009.05.007.
37. Mohsen AH, Green ST, Read RC, McKendrick MW. Liver abscess in adults: ten years experience in a UK centre. QJM. 2002;95(12):797–802. https://doi.org/10.1093/qjmed/95.12.797.
38. Barosa R, Pinto J, Caldeira A, Pereira E. Modern role of clinical ultrasound in liver abscess and echinococcosis. J Med Ultrason (2001). 2017;44(3):239–45. https://doi.org/10.1007/s10396-016-0765-2.
39. Roediger R, Lisker-Melman M. Pyogenic and Amebic infections of the liver. Gastroenterol Clin N Am. 2020;49(2):361–77. https://doi.org/10.1016/j.gtc.2020.01.013.
40. Fiore M, Cascella M, Bimonte S, et al. Liver fungal infections: an overview of the etiology and epidemiology in patients affected or not affected by oncohematologic malignancies. Infect Drug Resist. 2018;11:177–186. Published 2018 Jan 29. https://doi.org/10.2147/IDR.S152473.
41. Pastakia B, Shawker TH, Thaler M, O'Leary T, Pizzo PA. Hepatosplenic candidiasis: wheels within wheels. Radiology. 1988;166(2):417–21. https://doi.org/10.1148/radiology.166.2.3275982.
42. Del Carpio M, Moguilansky S, Costa M, et al. Diagnosis of human hydatidosis. Predictive value of a rural ultrasonographic survey in an apparently healthy population. Medicina (B Aires). 2000;60(4):466–8.
43. Sayek I, Tirnaksiz MB, Dogan R. Cystic hydatid disease: current trends in diagnosis and management. Surg Today. 2004;34(12):987–96. https://doi.org/10.1007/s00595-004-2830-5.
44. Zuluaga-Gómez M, Orjuela-Correa RA, González-Arroyave D, Naranjo-Hernández D, Ardila CM. Point-of-care ultrasound for the diagnosis of liver abscess in a patient with HIV in the emergency department: a case report. Med Int (Lond). 2023;3(1):5.

45. Malik AA, Bari SU, Rouf KA, Wani KA. Pyogenic liver abscess: changing patterns in approach. World J Gastrointest Surg. 2010;2:395–401.
46. McNeil T, Daniel S, Gordon DL. Management of pyogenic liver abscess: a South Australian experience. ANZ J Surg. 2020;90:2274–8.
47. Kim M, Kang TW, Jang KM, Kim YK, Kim SH, Ha SY, Sinn DH, Gu S. Tumefactive Gallbladder Sludge at US: prevalence and clinical importance. Radiology. 2017;283(2):570–9.
48. Ross M, Brown M, McLaughlin K, Atkinson P, Thompson J, Powelson S, Clark S, Lang E. Emergency physician-performed ultrasound to diagnose cholelithiasis: a systematic review. Acad Emerg Med. 2011;18(3):227–35.
49. Kim HC, Yang DM, Jin W, Ryu JK, Shin HC. Color Doppler twinkling artifacts in various conditions during abdominal and pelvic sonography. J Ultrasound Med. 2010;29(4):621–32. https://doi.org/10.7863/jum.2010.29.4.621.
50. Huerta S, Kakati R, Lanier H. Gas-containing Biliary Calculi: case series and a systematic review. Am Surg. 2023;89(6):2656–64. https://doi.org/10.1177/00031348221121553.
51. Sitaridis K, Domi I, Nathanailidou M, Chatzigiannis G, Boulas KA, Sourtse G, Hatzigeorgiadis A. Air in gallbladder: emphysematous cholecystitis or else? Clin Case Rep. 2023;11(3):e6391. https://doi.org/10.1002/ccr3.6391.
52. Jahantab MB, Salehi V, Mehrabi S, Abedini L, Yavari Barhaghtalab MJ. Cholecystomegaly: a case report and review of the literature. Case Rep Gastrointest Med. 2020;2020:8825167.
53. Gupta P, Marodia Y, Bansal A, Kalra N, Kumar-M P, Sharma V, Dutta U, Sandhu MS. Imaging-based algorithmic approach to gallbladder wall thickening. World J Gastroenterol. 2020;26(40):6163–81.
54. Wilson SJ, Thavanathan R, Cheng W, Stuart J, Kim DJ, Glen P, Duigenan S, Shorr R, Woo MY, Perry JJ. Test characteristics of emergency medicine-performed point-of-care ultrasound for the diagnosis of acute Cholecystitis: a systematic review and meta-analysis. Ann Emerg Med. 2024;83(3):235–46.
55. Villar J, Summers SM, Menchine MD, Fox JC, Wang R. The absence of gallstones on point-of-care ultrasound rules out acute Cholecystitis. J Emerg Med. 2015;49(4):475–80.
56. Nelson M, Ash A, Raio C, et al. Stone-in-neck phenomenon: a new sign of cholecystitis. Crit Ultrasound J. 2011;3:115–7. https://doi.org/10.1007/s13089-011-0071-6.
57. Elwood DR. Cholecystitis. Surg Clin North Am. 2008;88(6):1241–52., viii. https://doi.org/10.1016/j.suc.2008.07.008.
58. Sharma R, Stead TS, Aleksandrovskiy I, Amatea J, Ganti L. Gallbladder Hydrops Cureus. 2021;13(9):e18159.
59. Jain A, Mehta N, Secko M, Schechter J, Papanagnou D, Pandya S, Sinert R. History, physical examination, laboratory testing, and emergency department ultrasonography for the diagnosis of acute Cholecystitis. Acad Emerg Med. 2017;24(3):281–97.
60. Huang SS, Lin KW, Liu KL, Wu YM, Lien WC, Wang HP. Diagnostic performance of ultrasound in acute cholecystitis: a systematic review and meta-analysis. World J Emerg Surg. 2023;18(1):54.
61. Engel JM, Deitch EA, Sikkema W. Gallbladder wall thickness: sonographic accuracy and relation to disease. AJR Am J Roentgenol. 1980;134(5):907–9.
62. Simeone JF, Brink JA, Mueller PR, Compton C, Hahn PF, Saini S, Silverman SG, Tung G, Ferrucci JT. The sonographic diagnosis of acute gangrenous cholecystitis: importance of the Murphy sign. AJR Am J Roentgenol. 1989;152(2):289–90. https://doi.org/10.2214/ajr.152.2.289.
63. Derici H, Kara C, Bozdag AD, Nazli O, Tansug T, Akca E. Diagnosis and treatment of gallbladder perforation. World J Gastroenterol. 2006;12(48):7832–6.
64. Huffman JL, Schenker S. Acute acalculous cholecystitis: a review. Clin Gastroenterol Hepatol. 2010;8(1):15–22.
65. Smith EA, Dillman JR, Elsayes KM, Menias CO, Bude RO. Cross-sectional imaging of acute and chronic gallbladder inflammatory disease. AJR Am J Roentgenol. 2009;192(1):188–96.
66. Yeo DM, Jung SE. Differentiation of acute cholecystitis from chronic cholecystitis: determination of useful multidetector computed tomography findings. Medicine (Baltimore). 2018;97(33):e11851. https://doi.org/10.1097/MD.0000000000011851.
67. Machado NO. Porcelain gallbladder: decoding the malignant truth. Sultan Qaboos Univ Med J. 2016;16(4):e416–21. https://doi.org/10.18295/squmj.2016.16.04.003.
68. Morimoto M, Matsuo T, Mori N. Management of Porcelain Gallbladder, its risk factors, and complications: a review. Diagnostics (Basel). 2021;11(6):1073. https://doi.org/10.3390/diagnostics11061073.
69. Schnelldorfer T. Porcelain gallbladder: a benign process or concern for malignancy? J Gastrointest Surg. 2013;17(6):1161–8. https://doi.org/10.1007/s11605-013-2170-0.
70. Myers RP, Shaffer EA, Beck PL. Gallbladder polyps: epidemiology, natural history and management. Can J Gastroenterol. 2002;16(3):187–94. https://doi.org/10.1155/2002/787598.
71. Corwin MT, Siewert B, Sheiman RG, Kane RA. Incidentally detected gallbladder polyps: is follow-up necessary?--Long-term clinical and US analysis of 346 patients. Radiology. 2011;258(1):277–82.
72. https://www.cancer.org/cancer/types/gallbladder-cancer/about/key-statistics.html. Accessed April 2024.
73. Boscak AR, Al-Hawary M, Ramsburgh SR. Best cases from the AFIP: Adenomyomatosis of the gallbladder. Radiographics. 2006;26(3):941–6.
74. Yu MH, Lee JY, Yoon JH, Baek JH, Han JK, Choi BI. Color Doppler twinkling artifacts from gallbladder adenomyomatosis with 1.8 MHz and 4.0 MHz color Doppler frequencies. Ultrasound Med Biol. 2012;38(7):1188–94.
75. Boscak AR, Al-Hawary M, Ramsburgh SR. Best cases from the AFIP: Adenomyomatosis of the gallbladder. Radiographics. 2006;26(3):941–6. https://doi.org/10.1148/rg.263055180.
76. Worku MG, Enyew EF, Desita ZT, Moges AM. Sonographic measurement of normal common bile duct diameter and associated factors at the University of Gondar comprehensive specialized hospital and selected private imaging center in Gondar town, North West Ethiopia. PLoS One. 2020;15(1):e0227135.
77. Perret RS, Sloop GD, Borne JA. Common bile duct measurements in an elderly population. J Ultrasound Med. 2000;19(11):727–30.; quiz 731. https://doi.org/10.7863/jum.2000.19.11.727.
78. Bachar GN, Cohen M, Belenky A, Atar E, Gideon S. Effect of aging on the adult extrahepatic bile duct: a sonographic study. J Ultrasound Med. 2003;22(9):879-82; quiz 883–5. https://doi.org/10.7863/jum.2003.22.9.879.
79. Park SM, Kim WS, Bae IH, Kim JH, Ryu DH, Jang LC, Choi JW. Common bile duct dilatation after cholecystectomy: a one-year prospective study. J Korean Surg Soc. 2012;83(2):97–101. https://doi.org/10.4174/jkss.2012.83.2.97.
80. Lahham S, Becker BA, Gari A, Bunch S, Alvarado M, Anderson CL, Viquez E, Spann SC, Fox JC. Utility of common bile duct measurement in ED point of care ultrasound: a prospective study. Am J Emerg Med. 2018;36(6):962–6.
81. Becker BA, Chin E, Mervis E, Anderson CL, Oshita MH, Fox JC. Emergency biliary sonography: utility of common bile duct measurement in the diagnosis of cholecystitis and choledocholithiasis. J Emerg Med. 2014;46(1):54–60.
82. Glaser J, Stienecker K. Pancreas and aging: a study using ultrasonography. Gerontology. 2000;46(2):93–6. https://doi.org/10.1159/000022141.

83. Abu-Yousef MM, El-Zein Y. Improved US visualization of the pancreatic tail with simethicone, water, and patient rotation. Radiology. 2000;217(3):780–5.
84. Kreel L, Haertel M, Katz D. Computed tomography of the normal pancreas. J Comput Assist Tomogr. 1977;1(3):290–9. https://doi.org/10.1097/00004728-197707000-00002.
85. Finstad TA, Tchelepi H, Ralls PW. Sonography of acute pancreatitis: prevalence of findings and pictorial essay. Ultrasound Q. 2005;21(2):95–104; quiz 150, 153-4.
86. Kim SW, Kim SH, Lee DH, Lee SM, Kim YS, Jang JY, Han JK. Isolated main pancreatic duct dilatation: CT differentiation between benign and malignant causes. AJR Am J Roentgenol. 2017;209(5):1046–55.
87. Hammond N, et al. Imaging of cystic diseases of the pancreas. Radiol Clin North Am. 2002;40(6):1243–62.
88. Draganov P, Habashi S. Pancreatic Pseudocyst. World J Gastroenterol. 2009;15(1):38–47.
89. Hocke M, Dietrich CF. New technology-combined use of 3D contrast enhanced endoscopic ultrasound techniques. Ultraschall Med. 2011;32(3):317–8.
90. Scialpi M, Reginelli A, D'Andrea A, Gravante S, Falcone G, Baccari P, Manganaro L, Palumbo B, Cappabianca S. Pancreatic tumors imaging: an update. Int J Surg. 2016;28(Suppl 1):S142–55.
91. Sarantis P, Koustas E, Papadimitropoulou A, Papavassiliou AG, Karamouzis MV. Pancreatic ductal adenocarcinoma: treatment hurdles, tumor microenvironment and immunotherapy. World J Gastrointest Oncol. 2020;12(2):173–81. https://doi.org/10.4251/wjgo.v12.i2.173.
92. Shah S, Mortele KJ. Uncommon solid pancreatic neoplasms: ultrasound, computed tomography and magnetic resonance imaging features. Semin Ultrasound CT MR. 2007;28(5):357–70. https://doi.org/10.1053/j.sult.2007.08.002.
93. Al-Haddad M, Schmidt MC, Sandrasegaran K, Dewitt J. Diagnosis and treatment of cystic pancreatic tumors. Clin Gastroenterol Hepatol. 2011;9(8):635–48. https://doi.org/10.1016/j.cgh.2011.03.005. Epub 2011 Mar 11
94. Elsayes KM, Narra VR, Abou El Abbass HA, Aly TS, Radwan SM, Chen ZM. Pancreatic tumors: diagnostic patterns by 3D gradient-echo post contrast magnetic resonance imaging with pathologic correlation. Curr Probl Diagn Radiol. 2006;35(4):125–39. https://doi.org/10.1067/j.cpradiol.2006.02.002.
95. Hosey RG, et al. Ultrasound assessment of spleen size in collegiate athletes. Br J Sports Med. 2006;40:251–4. https://doi.org/10.1136/bjsm.2005.022376.
96. Morozov S, Izranov V. Methods of ultrasound Spleen Morphometry. J Ultrasound Med. 2022;41:2123–33.
97. Pozo AL, Godfrey EM, Bowles KM. Splenomegaly: investigation, diagnosis and management. Blood Rev. 2009;23:105–11.
98. Trenker C, et al. WFUMB position paper – incidental findings, how to manage: spleen. Ultrasound Med Biol. 2021;47(8):2017–32.
99. Adas G, et al. Diagnostic problems with parasitic and non-parasitic splenic cysts. BMC Surg. 2009;9:9. https://doi.org/10.1186/1471-2482-9-9.
100. Golmohammadzadeh H, Maddah G, Shams Hojjati Y, Abdollahi A, Shabahang H. Splenic cysts: analysis of 16 cases. Caspian. J Intern Med. 2016 Summer;7(3):217–21.
101. Fyfe AJ, Gallipoli P. Multiple splenic calcifications. Br J Haematol. 2009;144(6):808.
102. Weerakkody Y, Ranchod A, Yap J, et al. Splenic Hemangioma. Reference Article, Radiopaedia.org. https://doi.org/10.53347/rID-17918
103. Srivastava A, Beland M. Ultrasound of the liver and spleen. Ultrasound Clin. 2014;9(4):545–65. https://doi.org/10.1016/j.cult.2014.o6.001.
104. Juin Hsien BL, Shelat VG. Spleen Angiosarcoma: a world review. Expert Rev Gastroenterol Hepatol. 2021;15(10):1115–41. https://doi.org/10.1080/17474124.2021.
105. Schattner A, Adi M, Kitroser E, Klepfish A. Acute splenic infarction at an academic general hospital over 10 years: presentation, etiology, and outcome. Medicine (Baltimore). 2015;94(36):e1363.
106. Tamarozzi F. Ultrasound diagnosis of cystic echinococcosis: updates and implications for clinical management. J Helminthol. 2024;98:e34. https://doi.org/10.1017/S0022149X2400021X

Gastrointestinal Ultrasound

11

Margaret Lin-Martore and Keith Boniface

Background

Point-of-care ultrasound (POCUS) has been increasingly used to diagnose gastrointestinal pathologies. While other types of imaging such as computed tomography (CT) and magnetic resonance imaging (MRI) are often used for bowel-related concerns, these modalities have limitations such as ionizing radiation or limited availability. Ultrasound has been used to assess the bowel for a multitude of conditions, but historically has been primarily in the domain of radiology. However, radiology-performed ultrasound is not universally available and may increase patient length of stay. POCUS allows assessment of the bowel in real time by the clinician at bedside. Several organizations have recommended ultrasound as first-line testing for multiple gastrointestinal conditions in an effort to reduce potential harm and improve diagnosis and treatment [1, 2].

There are some technical challenges specific to gastrointestinal ultrasound, including bowel gas limiting visualization, inadequate fasting state, and patient tolerance of the study. However, numerous studies have shown that POCUS can be used to diagnose a variety of bowel pathologies accurately and efficiently [3–10]. In this chapter, we will describe various POCUS modalities for assessing the gastrointestinal tract, from the esophagus through to the large intestine, as well as extraperitoneal applications.

Supplementary Information The online version contains supplementary material available at https://doi.org/10.1007/978-3-031-85308-1_11.

M. Lin-Martore (✉)
Departments of Emergency Medicine and Pediatrics, University of California, San Francisco, San Francisco, CA, USA
e-mail: margaret.lin-martore@ucsf.edu

K. Boniface
Department of Emergency Medicine, George Washington University, Washington, DC, USA
e-mail: kboniface@mfa.gwu.edu

M. Gottlieb, N. Panebianco (eds.), *Advanced Point-of-Care Ultrasound*, https://doi.org/10.1007/978-3-031-85308-1_11

Indications and Diagnoses by Anatomical Region

Anatomical region	Diagnosis	Indication
Esophagus	Zenker's diverticulum	Neck swelling Dysphagia
	Esophageal foreign body and food impaction	Dysphagia Odynophagia Esophageal obstruction
Stomach	Hiatal hernia	Abdominal pain Gastroesophageal reflux Dyspepsia
	Gastric volume	Evaluation of stomach volume and contents prior to procedural sedation
	Hypertrophic pyloric stenosis	Infants with nonbilious, projectile vomiting
Bowel	Small bowel obstruction	Abdominal pain Distension Vomiting Obstipation
	Malrotation and volvulus	Typically neonates with bilious emesis
	Appendicitis	Children and adults with: Right lower quadrant pain Fever Nausea
	Mesenteric adenitis	Children and young adults with: Right lower quadrant pain Fever Nausea
	Intussusception	Young children with: Colicky abdominal pain, lethargy, vomiting, or bloody stools Occasionally, adults with abdominal pain and vomiting
	Large bowel obstruction	Abdominal pain Abdominal distension Vomiting Obstipation
	Diverticulitis	Adult patients with: Abdominal pain especially in left lower quadrant Fever Nausea/vomiting Constipation and/or diarrhea
	Pneumatosis intestinalis	Neonates with suspected necrotizing enterocolitis Adults (typically 5th to 8th decade) presenting with abdominal pain
	Inflammatory bowel disease	Adults and children with: Abdominal pain Diarrhea Lower gastrointestinal bleeding Suspected inflammatory bowel disease
Extra-intestinal and other Miscellaneous Applications	Hernia	Abdominal pain and swelling, especially in the inguinal or umbilical region or at areas of prior surgery
	Pneumoperitoneum	Abdominal pain and acute abdomen suspected of hollow viscus perforation from: Peptic ulcer disease Endoscopy Surgical dehiscence
	Mesenteric ischemia	Abdominal pain in patients with: Vascular disease or atrial fibrillation Pain out of proportion to the physical exam findings

Core Views

View	Image	Approach
Esophagus	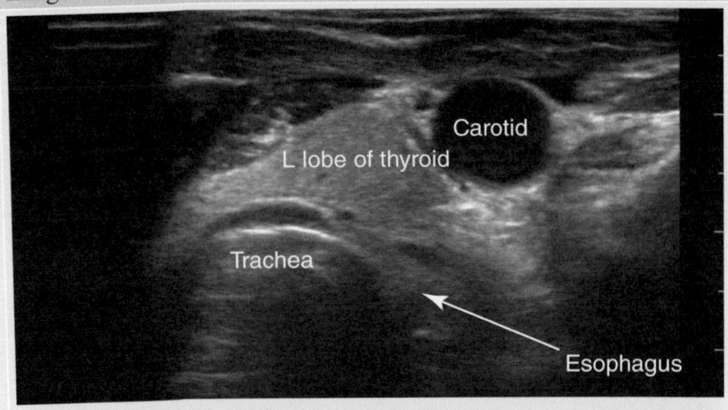 Transverse view of esophagus 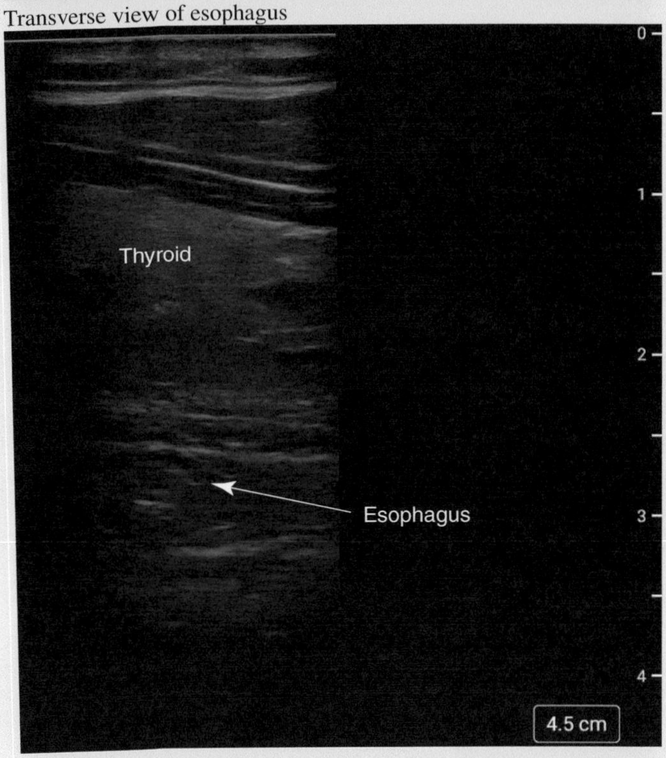 Long axis view of esophagus	Place the probe on the anterior neck and visualize the esophagus in the longitudinal and transverse planes. The esophagus is typically located to the left of and posterior to the trachea. Can improve visualization by having the patient swallow.
Stomach	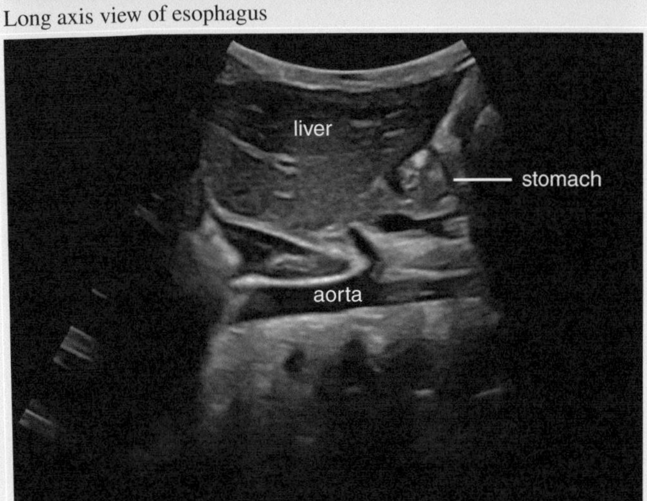 Stomach antrum labeled in green. *Image courtesy of Maytal Firnberg, MD*	Place the probe in the epigastric region in the sagittal plane with the patient in the right lateral decubitus position. Sweep the probe to the right until the gastric antrum is identified posterior to the left lobe of the liver.

View	Image	Approach
Pylorus	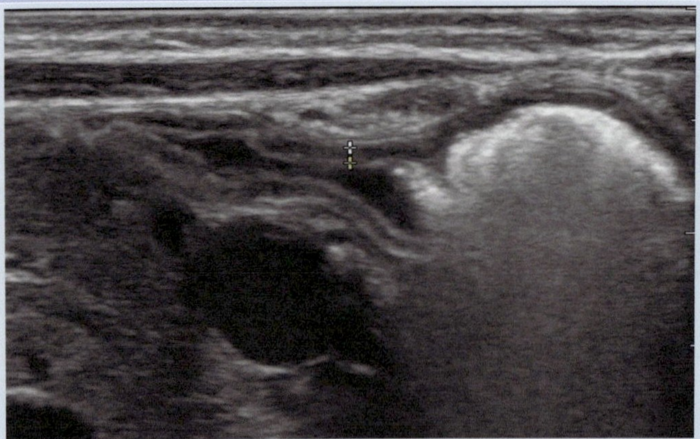 Normal Pylorus. *Image courtesy of Matthew Moake, MD, PhD.*	Place the probe in the transverse orientation in the epigastrium and slide to the right until the gastric wall is visualized. Rotate the probe to view the pylorus in the long axis.
Small Bowel	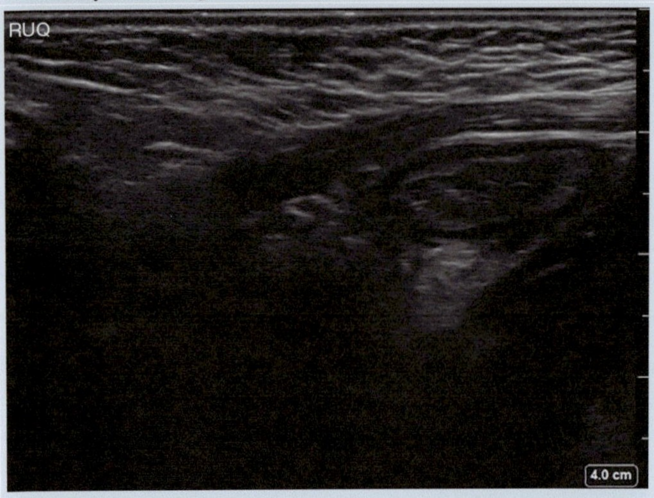 Normal small bowel	All four quadrants of the abdomen must be examined in multiple planes to evaluate the small bowel for pathologies such as: small bowel obstruction and intussusception. For the lawnmower technique, place the probe in the right lower quadrant and sweep up to the right upper quadrant. Then, slide laterally and sweep inferiorly. This approach is repeated until the entire abdomen is interrogated. The bowel may be assessed for distension and peristalsis pattern, wall thickness, luminal diameter, air in the wall, free air or fluid, a target sign (seen in intussusception), and other signs of pathology. Graded compression may assist in displacing bowel gas. Color Doppler can be used to assess for flow within the bowel when ischemia is suspected.
Appendix	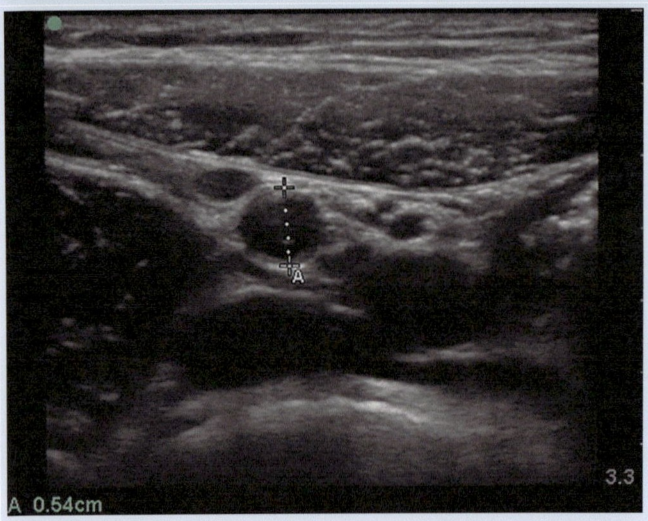 Normal appendix	There are three techniques for identifying the appendix: 1. Place the probe at the point of maximum tenderness and evaluate the region in several planes. 2. Place the probe in a transverse orientation in the right lower quadrant below McBurney's point and sweep the probe cephalad. to caudad, moving laterally (similar to a localized version of the lawnmower technique). 3. Identify the cecum and then locate the appendix which arises from the cecum. The appendix typically is found within the triangle formed by the iliopsoas muscle, rectus muscles, and iliac vessels. Graded compression may assist in displacing bowel gas.

View	Image	Approach
Large Bowel	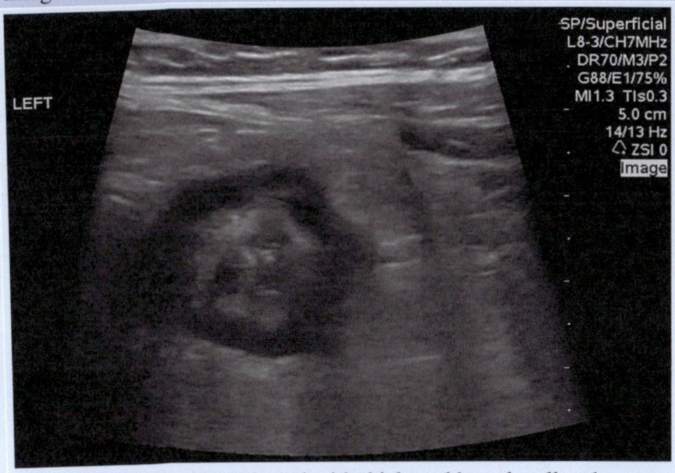 Transverse view of large bowel with thickened bowel wall and surrounding stranding	Sweep through the large bowel systematically using graded compression, following its course around the periphery of the abdomen and extending to trace the sigmoid colon. Evaluate the colon in several planes, including the short and long axes relative to the bowel. Pay particular attention to the point of maximum tenderness.

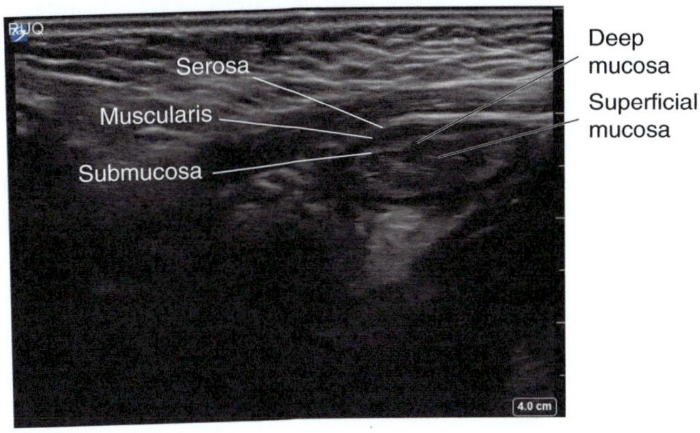

Fig. 11.1 Layers of the bowel

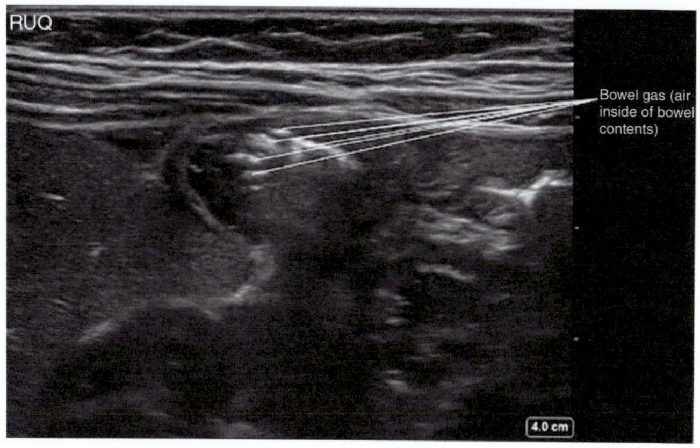

Fig. 11.2 Bowel gas inside of bowel contents

General Approach

The wall of the gastrointestinal tract has five distinct layers (Fig. 11.1), each alternating in a hyper- and hypo-echoic appearance on ultrasound. This pattern is referred to as the "gut signature." The layers from internal to external are: superficial mucosa, deep mucosa, submucosa, muscularis propria, and serosa. Often, not all the layers are visualized.

While individual scanning protocols vary based upon the organ and pathology, one important technique for viewing the gastrointestinal tract (particularly bowel) is to apply graded compression. Graded compression mitigates the effect of air in the bowel obscuring ultrasound images deep to this (Fig. 11.2, Video 11.1). To do this, the operator slowly and gently presses on the abdomen with the ultrasound probe over the area of interest. Then, pressure is steadily increased while waiting for normal bowel (typically air-filled) to move out of the way with peristalsis, thereby allowing affected bowel (typically dilated, fluid-filled, or inflamed) to come into view. This slow and gentle approach is effective for bowel visualization and also minimizes patient discomfort.

Clinical Applications

Zenker's Diverticulum

A pharyngoesophageal diverticulum, also known as Zenker's diverticulum, typically occurs at the level of the cricopharyngeus muscle and can cause dysphagia, neck swelling, and regurgitation of food [11]. It can be seen as an outpouching of the esophagus with a well-defined hypoechoic border filled with mixed densities of food and air. It typically extends to the left of the trachea, deep to the left lobe of thyroid gland where it can be mistaken for a thyroid nodule. Dynamic scanning while the patient swallows water or com-

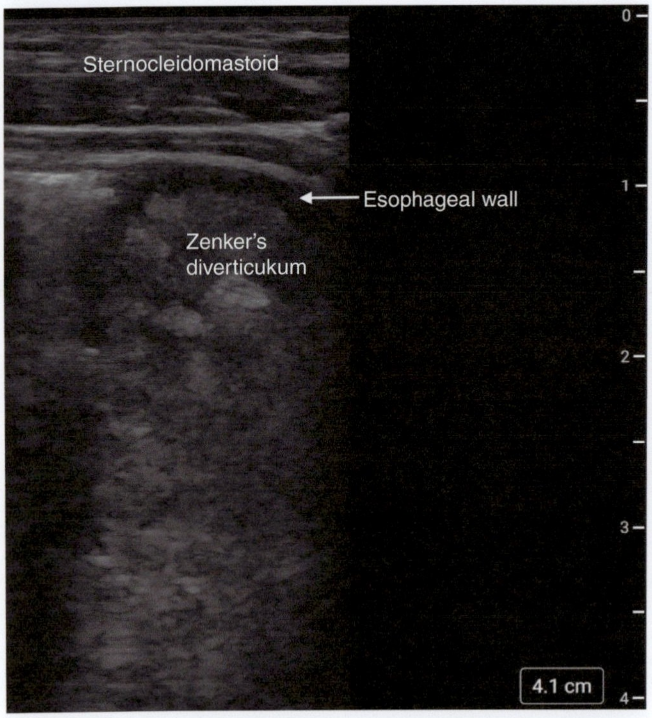

Fig. 11.3 Zenker's diverticulum. This food-containing outpouching of the mucosal and submucosal layers of the esophagus is seen in the left side of the neck

pression sonography may reveal changes in echogenicity of the lesion [12, 13] (Fig. 11.3, Video 11.2).

Esophageal Foreign Bodies and Food Bolus Impaction

Esophageal foreign bodies and food bolus impactions present with dysphagia, odynophagia, and inability to swallow secretions. Ultrasound of the esophagus can reveal a dilated esophagus containing contents of mixed echogenicity, without a change in the diameter with swallowing efforts. One study reported the diameter of the esophagus in healthy controls was 9.3 mm compared with 17.5 mm in those with esophageal foreign body impaction [14]. Some foreign bodies may also be directly visualized. Metallic foreign bodies (e.g., coins, button batteries) may be seen as linear hyperechoic structures with posterior reverberation artifacts, while food boluses may be seen as hyper- to hypo-echoic structures with variable degrees of fluid and air [15–17].

Hiatal Hernia

More distally, the esophagus can be visualized just lateral and anterior to the proximal abdominal aorta in either the transverse or sagittal plane, using the left lobe of the liver as

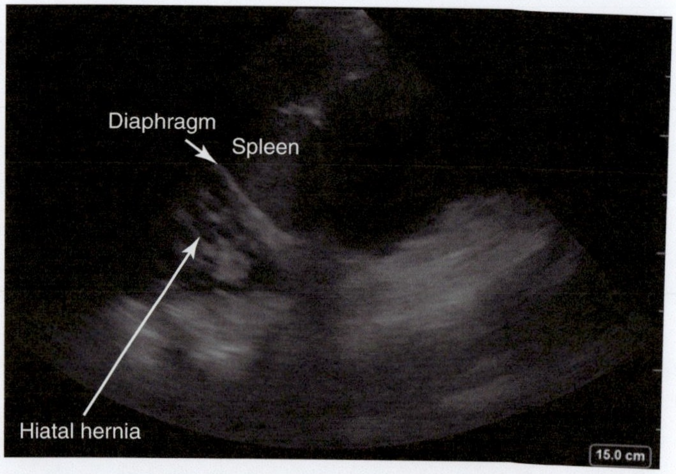

Fig. 11.4 Hiatal hernia visualized from the left upper quadrant view of FAST examination

an acoustic window. Hiatal hernias can be seen proximal to the diaphragmatic hiatus with an increased esophageal diameter. The esophageal diameter should be measured from outer wall to outer wall while visualized in the long axis just anterior to the aorta. One study reported a sensitivity of 86% and specificity of 96% for hiatal hernia, using an esophageal diameter threshold of 18 mm [18]. Hiatal hernias can also be visualized behind the heart on cardiac ultrasound as well as in the left upper quadrant view of the FAST examination above the diaphragm (Fig. 11.4).

Gastric Volume

Fasting times prior to sedation for emergent procedures and the association between fasting duration and risk of aspiration are unclear [19]. Sonography can be used to assess the volume as well as consistency (e.g., liquid, solid, air) of gastric contents in real time. This information can then help guide decisions on timing of procedural sedation and aspiration risk [20–23]. Additional research is still needed to determine its best use and relationship to clinical outcomes [20, 24]. Visually, the stomach has a similar "gut signature" with alternating hypo- and hyper-echoic layers as described above; however, the muscularis layer is thicker in comparison to the bowel, which can assist with identification. The mucosal surface of the stomach also has distinctive rugal folds which can be visualized by ultrasound.

Begin with a qualitative visual assessment of the stomach to determine if it is empty, has liquid (anechoic) contents, or has solid (echogenic) contents. Place the patient in the right lateral decubitus position as this uses gravity to assist with gastric content flow into the gastric antrum. A curvilinear or linear probe can be used depending on the patient's body habitus. The probe is placed in the epigastric region in a sag-

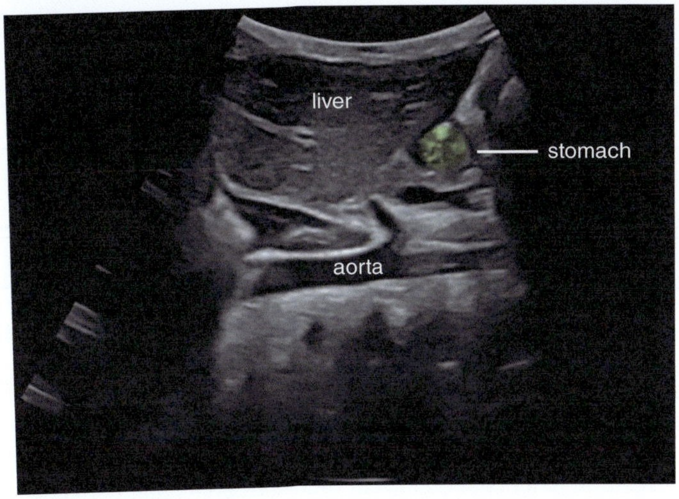

Fig. 11.5 Gastric antrum

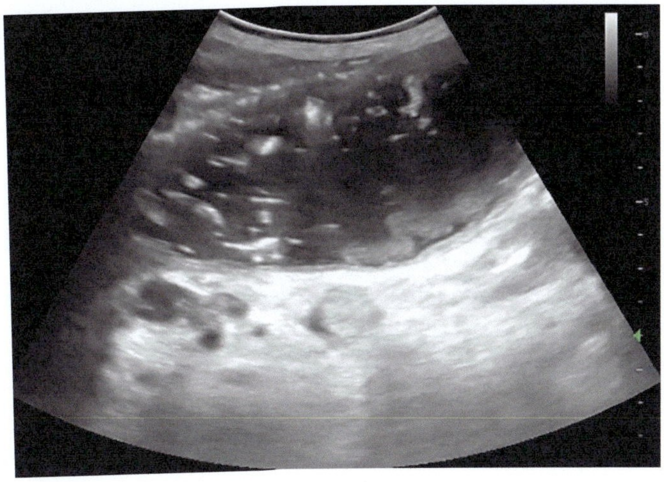

Fig. 11.6 Distended stomach with echogenic stomach contents

ittal plane and swept to the right until the gastric antrum is identified posterior to the left lobe of the liver (Fig. 11.5). The gastric antrum typically has less gas and, therefore, is easier to visualize than the gastric body. When empty, the gastric antrum appears as a small round structure with clear wall layers and no peristalsis. When not empty, it appears distended with peristalsis. Contents typically include gas (hyperechoic, nondependent), fluid (anechoic) and solid (varying degrees of echogenicity) components that are gravity dependent and may form a meniscus (Fig. 11.6, Video 11.3). The inferior vena cava and aorta can be visualized posterior to the antrum.

An empty stomach would be considered low risk, whereas thick/solid contents would be considered high risk. For patients with liquid stomach contents, the next step is to measure the gastric antrum cross-sectional area (CSA) according to the formula: [(anterior–posterior antrum diameter × cephalo-caudal antrum diameter × π)/4].

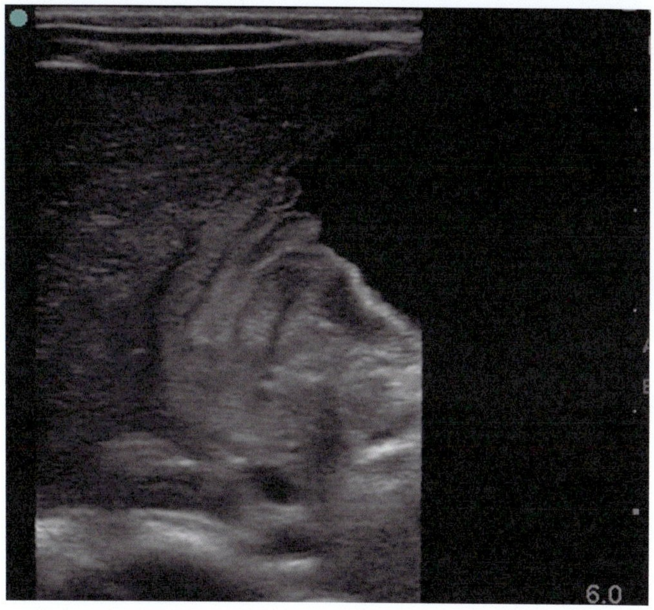

Fig. 11.7 Hypertrophic pyloric stenosis

One formula for nonpregnant adults is [Volume (mL) = 27 + 14.6 × CSA − 1.28 × age in years], with a cutoff of 1.5 mL/kg for low risk for aspiration [25]. For pediatric patients [Volume = −7.8 + (3.5 × CSA) + (0.127) × age (months)] can be used, with volume cutoff of 1.25 mL/kg for liquid contents being low risk for aspiration [26].

Hypertrophic Pyloric Stenosis

Hypertrophic pyloric stenosis (HPS) is a common cause of obstruction in infants 2–8 weeks of age but can occur up to 6 months, where the gastric pylorus hypertrophy does not allow gastric contents to exit the stomach. Infants often present with projectile, nonbilious emesis. POCUS performed by emergency physicians is 98% sensitive and 94% specific for HPS [3]. There is also evidence that POCUS decreases the length of stay for emergency department (ED) patients with suspected HPS [27].

A high-frequency (5–10 MHz) wide footprint linear probe is typically utilized. The patient is held either in a supine or right lateral decubitus position by a parent or guardian. The right lateral decubitus position is preferred to displace bowel gas and to allow fluid to enter the antrum. In the setting of an over-distended stomach, which can make visualization of the pylorus difficult, turning the patient to a left lateral decubitus position can improve visualization.

Start with the probe in a transverse orientation (indicator directed to the patient's right) in the epigastric region. Then, slide to the patient's right until the gastric wall comes into view. Rotate the probe as needed to view the pylorus in the long axis (Fig. 11.7). In the absence of pathology, stomach

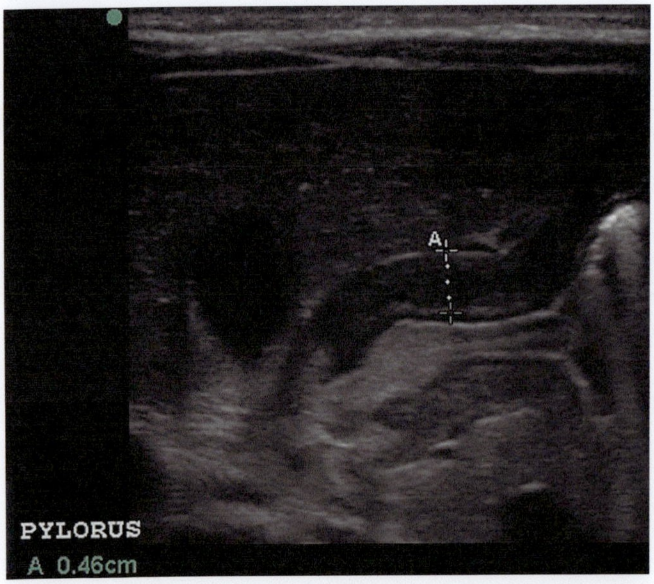

Fig. 11.8 Hypertrophic pyloric stenosis with a pyloric muscle width measuring >3 mm

contents can be visualized passing through the pylorus, especially if the patient is feeding during the examination (Video 11.4).

In HPS, the stomach contents do not typically pass, as they are blocked by the hypertrophic pyloric muscle. Pyloric thickness of a single muscle wall >3 mm in diameter or pyloric transverse diameter >14 mm suggests HPS [28]. There is debate over cutoffs for pylorus channel lengths, with thresholds ranging from >10 mm to ≥20 mm [29]. Given the variability in thresholds and greater diagnostic accuracy using pyloric muscle thickness, we recommend using muscle thickness over channel length [28] (Figs. 11.8 and 11.9; Videos 11.5 and 11.6). Studies have shown that there is variation in where calipers are placed for measurements, which can lead to poor interrater reliability [30]. One common practice is to measure the hypoechoic muscularis externa layer for the pyloric muscle thickness from the first part of the duodenum to the gastric antrum for the channel length [28].

Other findings suggestive of HPS include extension of the thickened pylorus in longitudinal view resembling the appearance of the uterine cervix on ultrasound (Fig. 11.7), and a "target" or "donut" sign where the hypoechoic muscle surrounded by the hyperechoic mucosa appears like a target or donut in the transverse axis (Fig. 11.9b) [31–33].

Small Bowel Obstruction

Small bowel obstruction (SBO) can occur from adhesions, hernias, masses, and inflammation. Ultrasound was first used to demonstrate SBO in 1979 [34]. Since then, multiple prospective studies have assessed the role of POCUS for SBO [35–38]. A systematic review and meta-analysis reported 92% sensitivity and 97% specificity for the diagnosis of SBO using POCUS, which is similar to CT and MRI [4]. In this study, the operator must know the sonographic difference between small and large bowel. The small bowel has plicae circulares, whereas the large bowel has haustra. The primary criterion for SBO is a dilated small bowel, with a diameter ≥2.5 cm (Fig. 11.10). Other criteria can include a zone of transition to a distal collapsed lumen or abnormal peristalsis (consisting of alternating, decreased, or absent peristalsis) (Video 11.7). There are no clearly defined ultrasound criteria for ileus, but dilated loops of bowel ≥2.5 cm with no clear transition zone and diminished peristalsis should raise suspicion for ileus.

The findings of free intraperitoneal fluid between bowel loops or bowel wall thickness (>4 mm) have been correlated with the need for surgery in radiology studies [39, 40]. POCUS studies have not had similar findings with regard to need for surgery but have found correlations between interluminal fluid, bowel wall edema, and the presence of SBO [37, 38]. Absence of Doppler signal in the bowel wall should raise concern for ischemia and complicated closed-loop obstruction.

The curvilinear probe is typically used for SBO diagnosis, whereas a high-frequency (5–10 MHz) linear probe is used for bowel wall assessment. Small bowel loops are recognized by their characteristic plicae circulares, as opposed to large bowel which have haustra and are typically filled with stool and gas. Systematic scanning in multiple imaging planes in all four quadrants of the abdomen should be performed, using sweeping movements and graded compression until dilated loops come into view, which are then measured from outer wall to outer wall at the widest diameter, making sure that measurements are taken perpendicular to the lumen of the bowel. In the setting of bowel gas obscuring views, roll the patient into a lateral decubitus position or approach the small bowel from the lateral abdomen. Color Doppler can be applied using a linear probe to assess perfusion of the bowel wall.

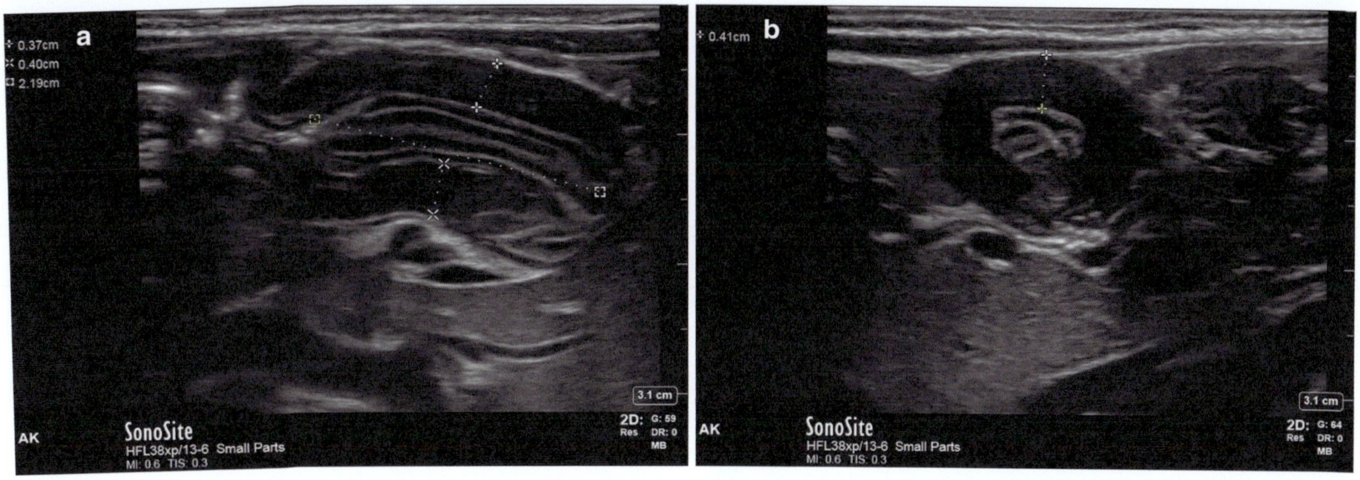

Fig. 11.9 Hypertrophic pyloric stenosis with thickened pyloric muscle width >3 mm and channel length >20 mm seen in (**a**) long-axis and (**b**) short-axis. (*Images courtesy of Matthew Moake, MD, PhD*)

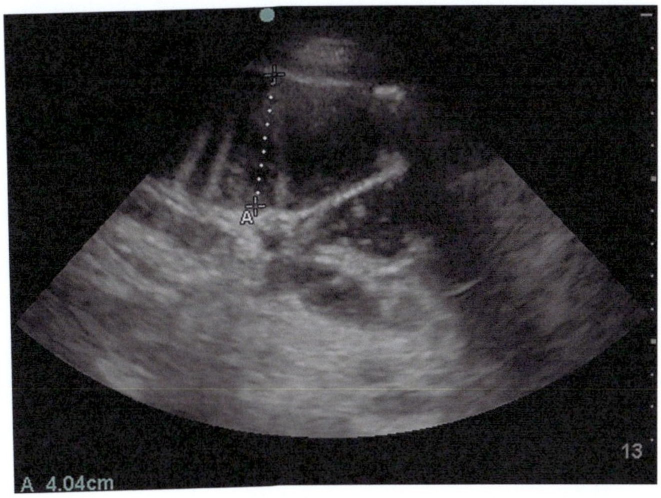

Fig. 11.10 Small bowel obstruction with dilated loops measuring 4.0 cm in diameter

Malrotation and Volvulus

Malrotation is a congenital condition that predisposes to midgut volvulus. Volvulus is a surgical emergency, where the bowel can twist on itself and become ischemic. While malrotation with volvulus is most commonly diagnosed within the first month of life, it can present at any age [41]. Neonates who present with bilious emesis are considered to have malrotation until proven otherwise. Studies evaluating ultrasound for malrotation and volvulus have had high diagnostic accuracy and some have advocated for ultrasound as a primary screening tool [5, 42, 43]. While radiology-performed ultrasound is most commonly used, POCUS has also been shown to accurately identify malrotation and volvulus [44, 45].

To evaluate for malrotation and volvulus, the patient should be in the supine position. A high-frequency linear probe is often used for evaluation, though a curvilinear probe may also be used. Place the probe transversely over the right hypochondrium with the indicator directed to the patient's right. The stomach and small bowel may be prominent if there is obstruction. The vertebral body should be identified posterior to the stomach, near the bottom of the screen. The probe is then swept toward the patient's midline and the aorta, inferior vena cava, celiac artery, superior mesenteric artery (SMA), and superior mesenteric vein (SMV) are identified anterior to the vertebral body.

Sonographic findings of malrotation include inversion of the SMA and SMV and an abnormal position of the duodenum [46]. Normally, the SMV is to the anatomic right of the SMA and both vessels run parallel with each other (Fig. 11.11a). The third part of the duodenum should be retroperitoneal between the SMA and aorta. In malrotation, this normal orientation is disrupted and the SMV can be seen to the anatomic left of the SMA, while the duodenum is intraperitoneal and may be seen anterior to the mesenteric vessels. The whirlpool sign refers to a swirling appearance of the SMA, SMV, and mesentery suggestive of volvulus (Fig. 11.11b, Video 11.8). Color Doppler can be applied to better visualize the whirlpool sign and assess the blood flow (Fig. 11.11c, Video 11.9). The relationship between SMA and SMV can be difficult to discern due to compression, described as the SMA cutoff sign, or interruption of the SMA at the level of the whirlpool [43]. The stomach may also be dilated proximal to the volvulus (Fig. 11.12).

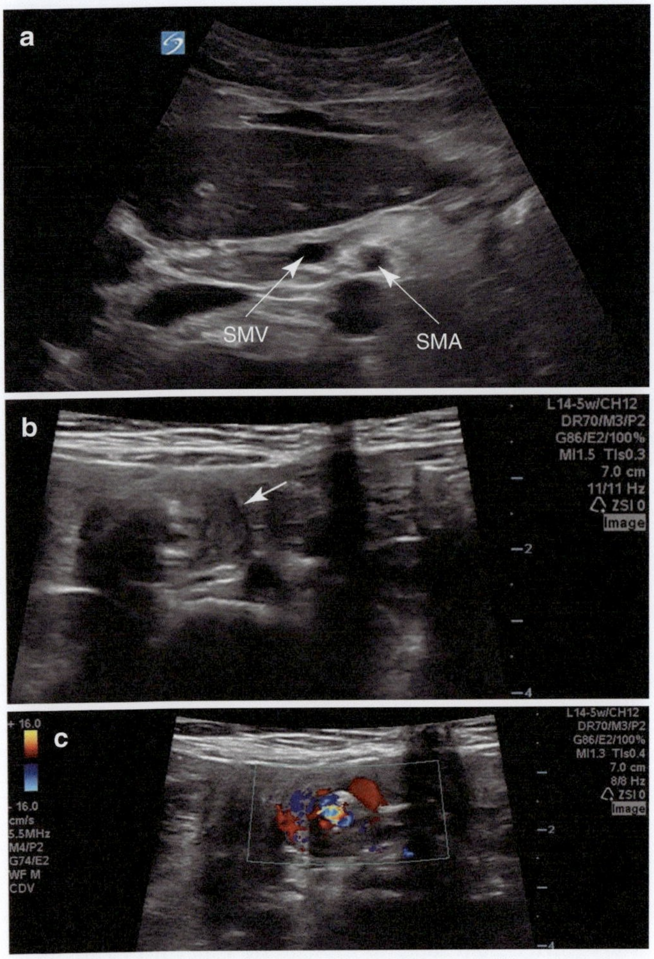

Fig. 11.11 (**a**) Normal relationship of SMA and SMV with the probe in the transverse orientation. (**b**) Whirlpool sign (arrow) in a patient with malrotation and volvulus on B-mode ultrasound. (**c**) Whirlpool sign in a patient with malrotation and volvulus with color Doppler (*Images (b) and (c) are Images courtesy of Charisse Kwan, MD*)

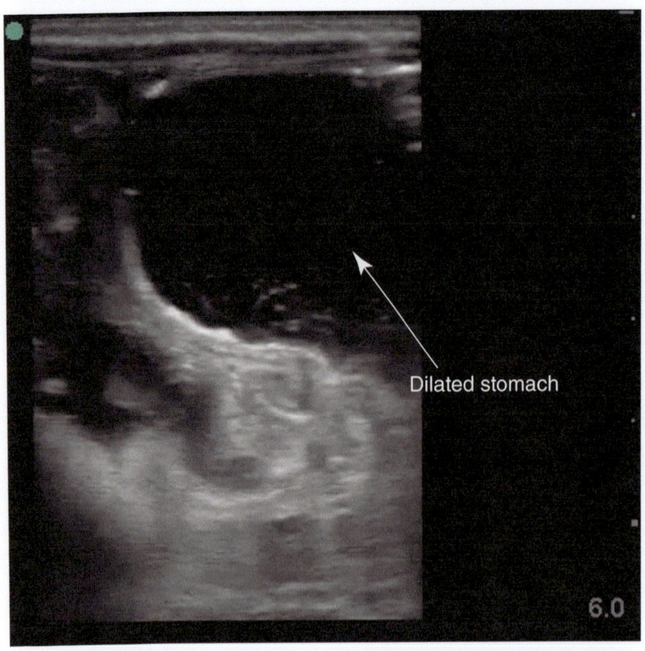

Fig. 11.12 Dilated stomach in patient with malrotation with volvulus

Appendicitis

Appendicitis is a common surgical emergency encountered in the emergency department (ED) [47]. POCUS is 91% sensitive and 97% specific for appendicitis [6]. POCUS also reduces CT utilization and decreases ED length of stay [48, 49]. Unfortunately, non-diagnostic imaging may occur in approximately half of cases; thus, POCUS is best used as a "rule-in" than "rule-out" study [50]. A non-inflamed appendix can be very challenging to identify, and patient factors, location of the appendix, and operator comfort can influence visualization [51–53]. A nonvisualized appendix examination can pose a diagnostic dilemma particularly when alternative diagnoses are being considered [6, 54]; however, absence of secondary signs of inflammation coupled with a reassuring exam and laboratory values can appropriately decrease suspicion for appendicitis [50].

Probe selection is based on patient size and habitus, with linear, high-frequency probes often used in children and adults with a body mass index <25 mg/kg^2, whereas a curvilinear, low-frequency probe is more commonly used in larger patients. One of the most common techniques is to start at the point of maximal tenderness. Have the patient point with one finger over the area of maximal discomfort, and apply graded compression over that area assessing for a tubular, noncompressible structure. This area should be interrogated in multiple planes. Another method is to place the probe in a transverse orientation (indicator to patient's right) in the right lower quadrant below McBurney's point. The probe should be inferior enough that no bowel should be seen initially. Slide the probe cephalad and the first loop that comes into view should be the cecum. The appendix arises from the cecum and typically is found within the triangle formed by the iliopsoas muscle, rectus muscle, and iliac vessels. Another approach, referred to as the lawnmower technique, involves starting at the umbilicus in the transverse view, moving laterally to the ascending colon, sweeping down to the cecum, moving medially, and then moving up and down the border of the cecum. The probe is then placed in the sagittal orientation laterally and swept through the area with the cecum in view [54]. Graded compression is often needed to view the appendix, regardless of the approach.

A normal appendix can be identified as a tubular, aperistaltic, blind-ending structure with a diameter ≤6 mm, deriving from the cecum (Fig. 11.13). Appendicitis is diagnosed when there is a noncompressible appendix >6 mm in diameter (Fig. 11.14, Videos 11.10–11.12), with secondary findings of inflammation such as hyperemia (Fig. 11.15), free fluid (Fig. 11.16), or surrounding hyperechoic fat [55–57]. Visualization of an appendicolith can be seen in approximately 30% of appendicitis cases [58]. Ruptured appendicitis may appear as a complex right lower quadrant mass with localized free fluid, extraluminal air, and hyperechoic fat (Fig. 11.17).

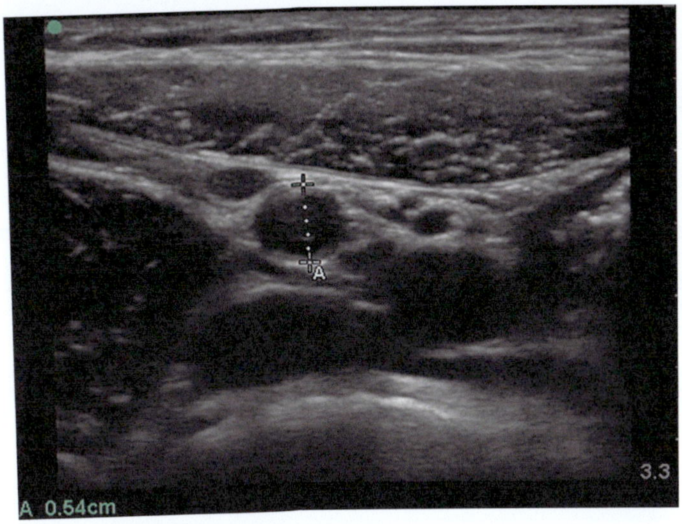

Fig. 11.13 Normal appendix

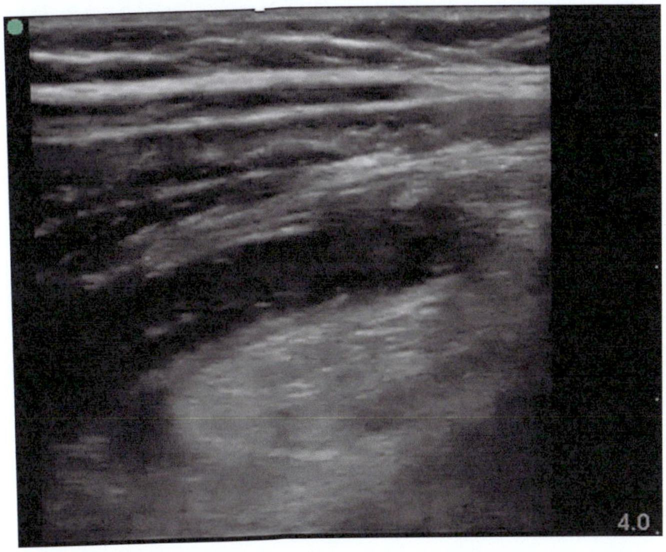

Fig. 11.14 Appendicitis surrounded by hyperechoic fat

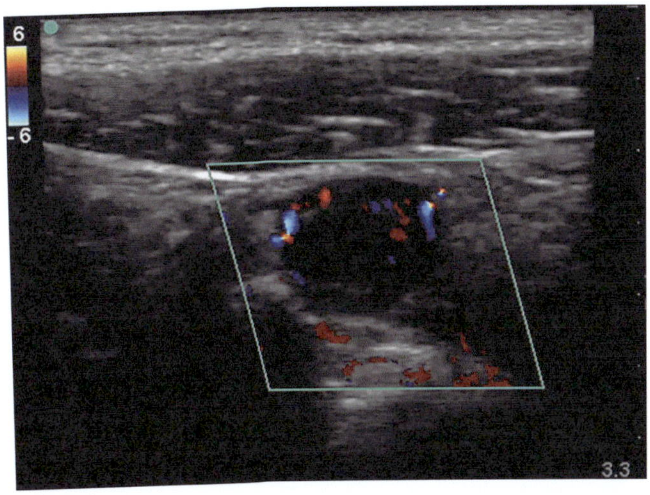

Fig. 11.15 Appendicitis with hyperemia

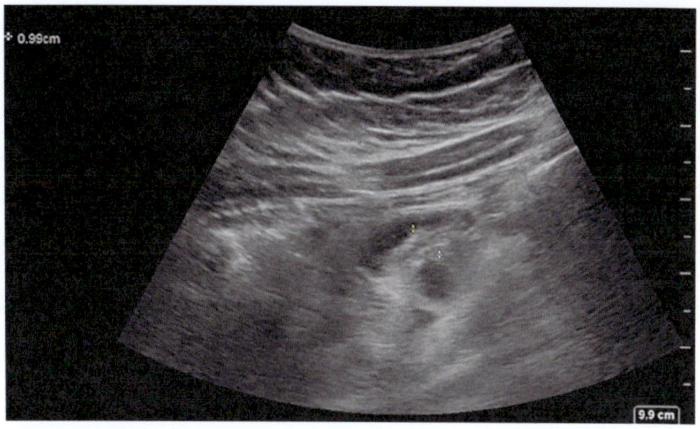

Fig. 11.16 Ruptured appendicitis. Tubular structure measuring approximately 1 cm, surrounded by free fluid

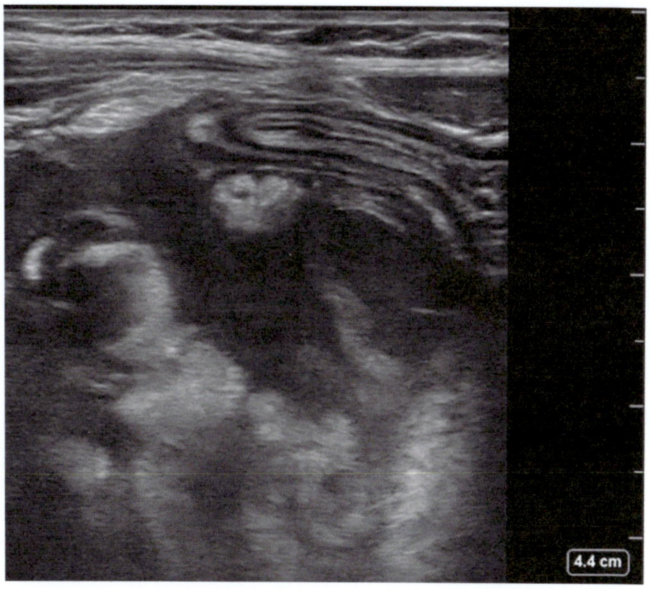

Fig. 11.17 Complex right lower quadrant mass in a patient with ruptured appendicitis. (*Image courtesy of Ashkon Shaahinfar, MD*)

Mesenteric Adenitis

Primary mesenteric lymphadenitis (also known as mesenteric adenitis) is characterized by tender enlarged intra-abdominal lymph nodes in the absence of an identifiable cause such as inflammatory bowel disease or appendicitis. Mesenteric adenitis is most common in the pediatric population and shares many symptoms and signs with acute appendicitis, but is self-limited and benign. Mesenteric lymphadenopathy can also be found in cases of appendicitis, so it is important to identify a normal appendix before reaching this diagnosis [55].

Similar to the appendix examination, use a linear or curvilinear probe based on body habitus. Scan through the right lower quadrant as described in the appendicitis section, including localizing and compressing the appendix. Mesenteric adenitis is typically found in the right lower quadrant anterior to the right psoas muscle or in the small bowel mesentery. Multiple criteria for mesenteric adenitis have been published, including identification of three or more lymph nodes >4–10 mm in short axis [59, 60], >10 mm in long axis [61], or multiple enlarged lymph nodes >10–15 mm [62] in the setting of a normal appendix. Color Doppler over the lymph nodes should demonstrate hypervascular flow.

Intussusception

Ileocolic intussusception typically occurs in children under 3 years when the ileum (intussusceptum) telescopes into the colon (intussuscipiens), leading to bowel obstruction [63]. While other types of intussusception can occur, ileocolic is important to quickly diagnose, as it requires an emergent reduction to prevent ischemia and bowel necrosis [64]. POCUS is accurate for ileocolic intussusception with a recent systematic review and meta-analysis reporting a sensitivity of 95.1% and specificity of 98.1% [7]. POCUS also reduces ED length-of-stay and time to management for this condition [65].

To perform this exam, evaluate the large bowel in an upside-down "U" manner, starting at the right lower quadrant using a high-frequency linear probe. Important anatomical landmarks are the rectus abdominis muscle, peritoneal line, iliopsoas, iliac vessels, and the bladder. Begin with the probe in a transverse orientation (indicator directed to the patient's right) in the right lower quadrant, just superior to the inguinal ligament. Sweeping superiorly, the first part of bowel encountered should be the cecum. The ascending colon is then traced from the right lower quadrant to the right upper quadrant. The probe is then rotated to the sagittal position to trace the transverse colon across to the left upper quadrant. The probe is then rotated back to transverse and the descending colon is traced down to the left lower quadrant. Ileocolic intussusception includes the ileum and is typically seen on the right upper quadrant of the abdomen.

Ileocolic intussusception can appear as a >2.5 cm "target" sign in the short axis [66] (Fig. 11.18, Video 11.13) or a "sandwich" sign in the long axis (Fig. 11.19). Graded compression optimizes visualization. Ileocolic intussusceptions often contain a large central core (containing fat and lymph nodes) that is larger in size when compared to the wall (core-to-wall ratio >1) (Fig. 11.20). In addition to visualizing the intussusception in short axis, it can be helpful to measure the length of the intussusception in the long axis and note which abdominal quadrant it is located, as well as evaluate for signs of ischemia (e.g., presence of free fluid, absence of color Doppler signal). This information can help indicate the likelihood of success of reduction and complications [67].

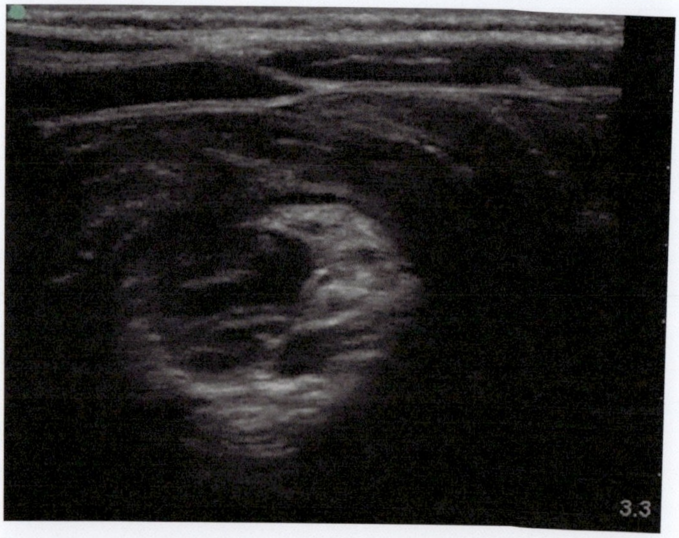

Fig. 11.18 Short axis view of ileocolic intussusception with target sign. Note the size of the intussusception is larger than 2.5 cm in diameter, suggesting ileocolic intussusception

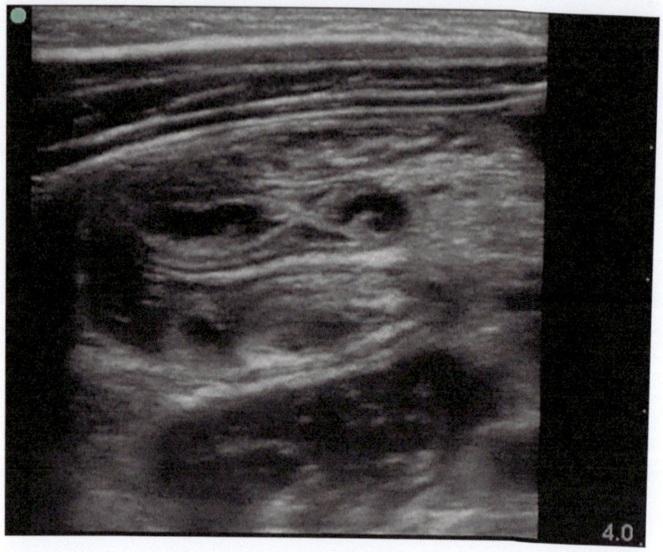

Fig. 11.19 Longitudinal view of ileocolic intussusception with sandwich sign

Small bowel-small bowel intussusception also appears as a target or sandwich lesion but tends to be smaller (<2.5 cm in diameter) (Fig. 11.21, Video 11.14) and can be located anywhere in the abdomen (as opposed to the right side for ileocolic intussusception) [66]. These cases typically resolve on their own (sometimes under ultrasound visualization) and do not require a procedural intervention. Their core-to-wall ratio is usually <1. Evaluating these findings with ultrasound should always be done in the context of the patient's clinical status and presentation.

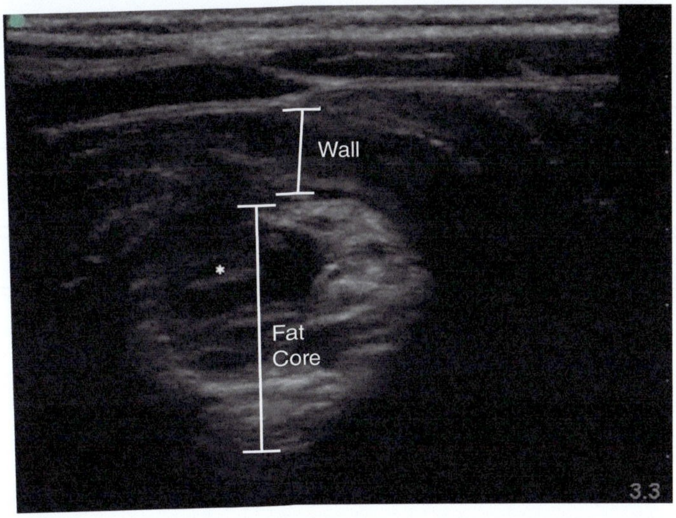

Fig. 11.20 Ileocolic intussusception with Core:Wall ratio >1. Note also the lymph node in the fat core (*)

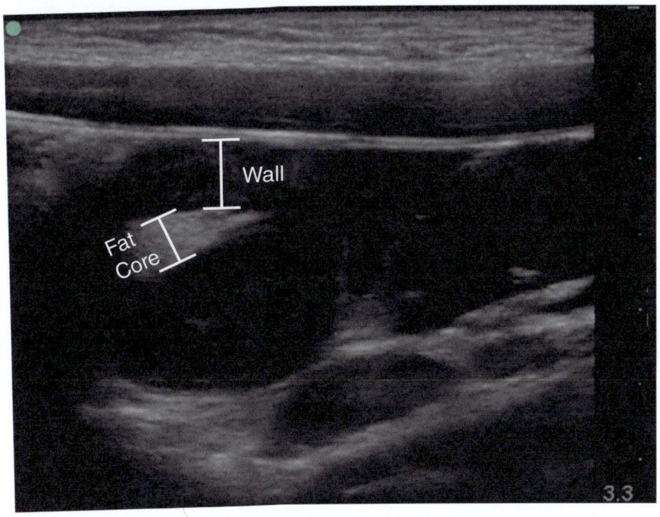

Fig. 11.21 Small bowel-small bowel intussusception which is <2 cm in diameter with Core:Wall ratio <1

Large Bowel Obstruction

The use of ultrasound for the identification of large bowel obstruction (LBO) has been less studied than other portions of the bowel. Clinical guidelines from the European Federation of Societies for Ultrasound in Medicine and Biology suggest that ultrasound criteria for LBO are challenging due to abundant gas in the obstructed colon but state an abrupt transition from dilated (>4.5 cm) colon to a non-dilated segment is suggestive of the diagnosis [2].

Using a curvilinear probe and graded compression, a "picture frame" technique can be used to scan the ascending, transverse, and descending colon around the perimeter of the abdomen, similar to that used for intussusception. In addition, patients with LBO and an incompetent ileocecal valve may demonstrate dilated loops of distal small intestine.

Diverticulitis

Diverticulosis refers to small outpouchings through the muscular wall of the large bowel and affects over 50% of Americans older than 60 years of age [68]. Diverticulitis involves inflammation of these diverticula, and is a common cause of abdominal pain. In North America, diverticulitis typically affects the sigmoid colon, causing left lower quadrant pain, while in Asia, the majority of diverticulitis affects the cecum and ascending colon, causing right-sided pain [69].

The use of ultrasound for suspected diverticulitis was first described in 1985 [70], and since then emergency medicine studies have reported sensitivities of 92–95% and specificities of 76–97% [71–73].

To perform this, use a low-frequency curvilinear probe and scan in a transverse orientation over the point of maximal tenderness. Apply graded compression to displace overlying bowel gas, and sweep down the descending colon (or ascending colon if suspecting right-sided diverticulitis). A full bladder may optimize visualization of the lower sigmoid colon. The sonographic hallmark of diverticulitis is the visualization of a hypoechoic thickened colonic wall with air-containing diverticula, focal tenderness over the area, and adjacent inflamed fat. Bowel wall thickening has been defined as either >4 or >5 mm in studies evaluating ultrasound for diverticulitis [72, 74] (Fig. 11.22, Video 11.15).

Complicated diverticulitis (e.g., abscess, perforation, fistula, stenosis) is more challenging to identify, with sensitivities as low as 50–55% [71, 73]. Abscesses resulting from perforation have a hypoechoic rounded walled-off appearance; however, gas within the abscess may make it difficult to distinguish from surrounding inflamed bowel. Perforation resulting in pneumoperitoneum can be detected, as described later in this chapter.

Pneumatosis Intestinalis

Pneumatosis intestinalis is the presence of gas in the extraluminal space, typically involving the wall of the gastrointestinal tract (Fig. 11.23). It is most often seen in the setting of necrotizing enterocolitis in infants [75], but can be seen in adults with bowel ischemia, trauma, or infection. It can also be an asymptomatic finding in adults with chronic obstructive pulmonary disease or those taking certain medications or immunosuppressive therapy. Aside from case reports,

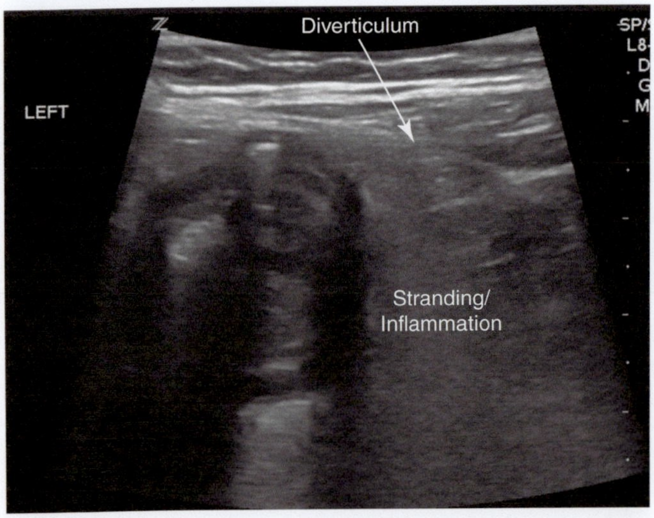

Fig. 11.22 Short-axis view of sigmoid colon with anterior air-filled diverticulum and surrounding hyperechoic stranding and inflammation

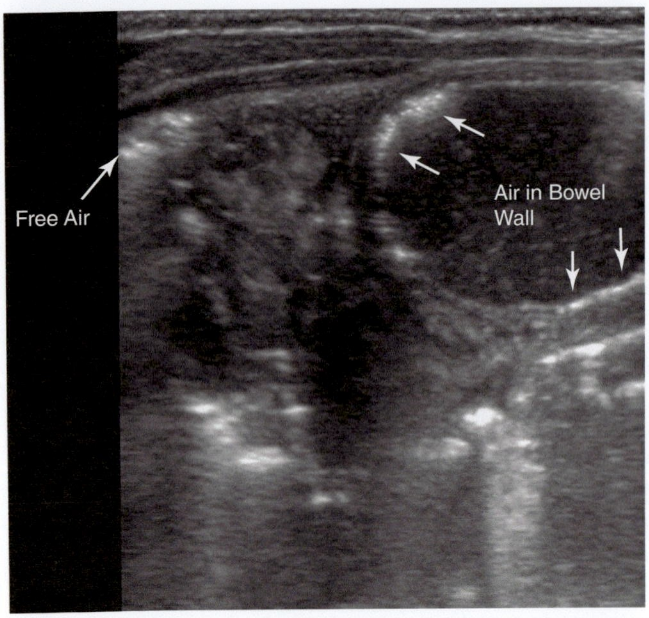

Fig. 11.23 Pneumatosis intestinalis with air in bowel wall. This patient also has pneumoperitoneum. (*Image Courtesy of Jim Tsung, MD*)

there are limited data on the use and accuracy of POCUS for pneumatosis intestinalis [76, 77].

The bowel can then be interrogated using a "lawnmower" technique, as described earlier. Pneumatosis intestinalis will appear as an echogenic foci within the bowel wall. Two common mimics of this include intraluminal air and pneumoperitoneum. Intraluminal air will move with peristalsis, pneumoperitoneum will displace with graded compression. In contrast, pneumatosis intestinalis will not move or displace.

Hernia

Hernias involve a defect in the abdominal wall through which abdominal contents may protrude. While this can occur anywhere throughout the abdomen, they are most commonly seen in the inguinal canal, femoral canal, umbilicus, and incisional sites. Hernias may incarcerate (defined as unable to be reduced) or strangulate (defined as incarceration that impairs blood flow leading to bowel wall ischemia), and can lead to bowel obstruction. Valsalva maneuvers may make hernias more pronounced, facilitating diagnosis clinically and sonographically. The use of ultrasound to identify abdominal hernias was first reported in 1975 [78]. POCUS is limited primarily to case reports [79–81], but a meta-analysis of radiology ultrasound for the diagnosis of hernias demonstrated sensitivity of 97% and specificity of 85% for inguinal hernias [9].

Scanning for hernias is best accomplished with the linear, high-frequency probe with the depth set so that the peritoneal line is at the middle of the screen. A curvilinear probe is used when the depth exceeds the limits of the linear probe. For incisional, umbilical, and other ventral abdominal hernias, start at the point of maximal tenderness or at the area of swelling. Scan in multiple planes to identify the peritoneal line. Then, identify the fascial defect in the abdominal wall with herniating fat or bowel loops. Applying gentle but firm pressure with the probe over the defect can accomplish focused reduction under direct visualization.

An indirect inguinal hernia in males involves bowel and fat passing through the internal inguinal ring, the inguinal canal, and the external inguinal ring into the scrotum (Fig. 11.24). In females, the ovary and fallopian tube tend to herniate instead of bowel and follow the same path toward the labia majora instead of the scrotum. The key landmark to identify an inguinal hernia is the inferior epigastric artery, which originates at the external iliac artery and courses superomedially along the posterior aspect of the rectus sheath. Trace the inferior epigastric artery caudally to the level of its juncture with the external iliac artery at the inguinal ligament. Normally, the inferior epigastric artery is anterior to the bowel and the peritoneum. In indirect hernias, bowel or fat can be seen sliding anteriorly to the inferior epigastric artery with Valsalva (Fig. 11.25) [82]. An additional technique includes applying color or power Doppler to the herniated bowel wall to assess blood flow. The absence of flow raises the concern for strangulation.

Pneumoperitoneum

Hollow viscus perforation with resulting pneumoperitoneum is a surgical emergency. Ultrasound to identify pneumoperitoneum was first described in 1982 and performed with 91%

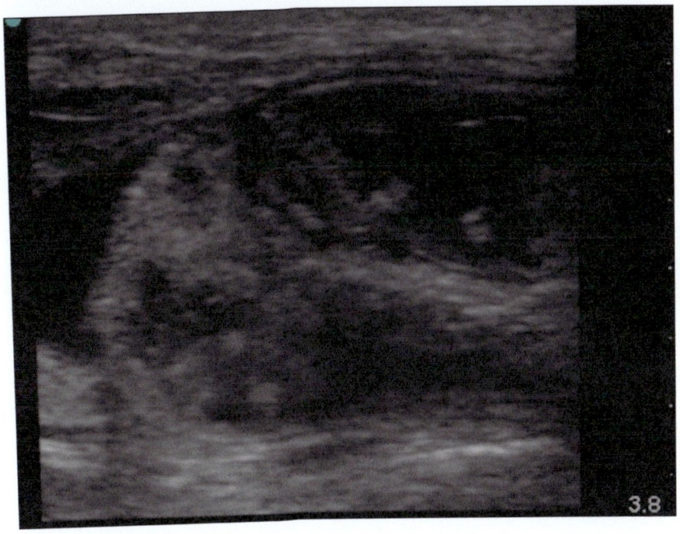

Fig. 11.24 Herniated loop of small bowel with a small amount of extraluminal fluid in inguinal canal. The probe is aligned with the left inguinal ligament

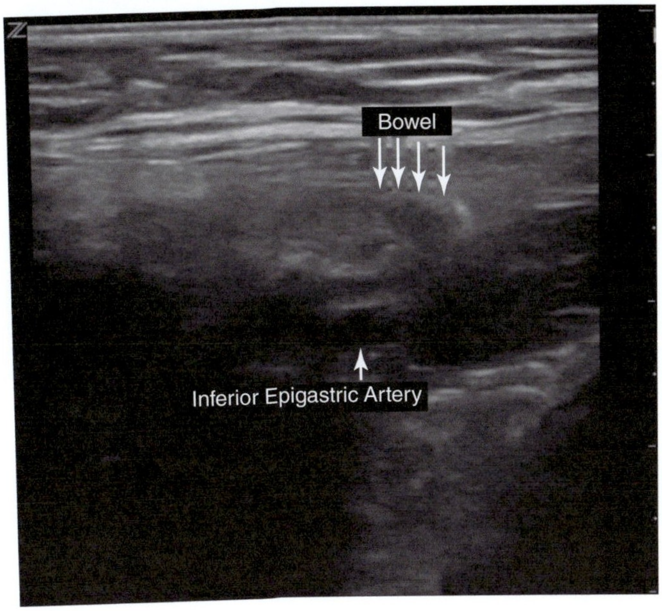

Fig. 11.25 Inguinal hernia (bowel) passing anteriorly to inferior epigastric artery. The probe is at the level of the right inguinal ligament over the femoral artery and vein (obscured by bowel shadow)

sensitivity and 96% specificity in radiology studies [83]. Emergency physicians have been able to identify pneumoperitoneum by detecting the enhanced peritoneal stripe sign or reverberation artifact with 96% sensitivity and 82% specificity [84].

Begin by placing the patient supine in the reverse Trendelenburg position so that any extraluminal gas moves anterior to the liver. Place a linear, high-frequency probe in a sagittal position over the right upper quadrant. Adjust the

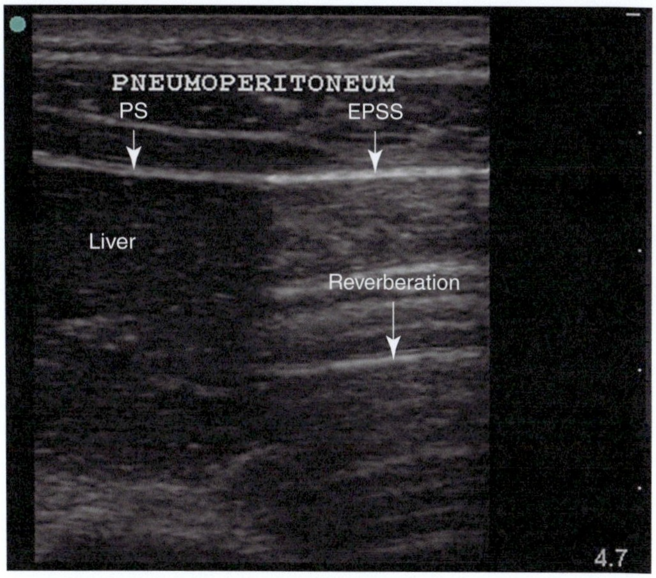

Fig. 11.26 Free intraperitoneal air collecting between the liver and the anterior abdominal wall of the right upper quadrant which demonstrates an increased echogenicity contiguous with the peritoneal stripe (PS) known as the enhanced peritoneal stripe sign (EPSS). Reverberation artifacts are seen deep to the EPSS

depth so that the peritoneal line is across the center of the screen. If this is not possible with a linear probe, change to the curvilinear probe. The liver can also be imaged through the right mid-axillary line with the patient in a left lateral decubitus position (while remaining in reverse Trendelenburg) [85]. Air is anti-dependent, hugging the anterior peritoneal line in a supine patient and shifts depending on the patient's position.

Pneumoperitoneum appears as a hyperechoic dot or line that is seemingly contiguous with the peritoneal line, known as enhancement of the peritoneal stripe sign (EPSS) [86]. Air also creates a posterior reverberation artifact, similar to A-lines seen on lung ultrasound (Fig. 11.26, Video 11.16) This is easiest to identify in the right upper quadrant, where the fluid-rich, hypoechoic liver provides a backdrop to highlight the abnormal appearance of air. Use caution when scanning outside of the right upper quadrant, as normal intraluminal bowel gas can easily be confused with pneumoperitoneum on ultrasound. Identifying the peritoneal line can help distinguish between free intraperitoneal and contained intraluminal air, as bowel gas is "offset" from the peritoneal stripe by the thickness of the bowel wall (Fig. 11.27). The scissors maneuver consists of applying pressure over a single area of pneumoperitoneum so that the liver comes into contact with the peritoneal line, thereby displacing the pneumoperitoneum. When performed, this appears as a real-time absence (with compression) and return (with relaxation) of the EPSS and associated reverberation artifact (Video 11.17) [87].

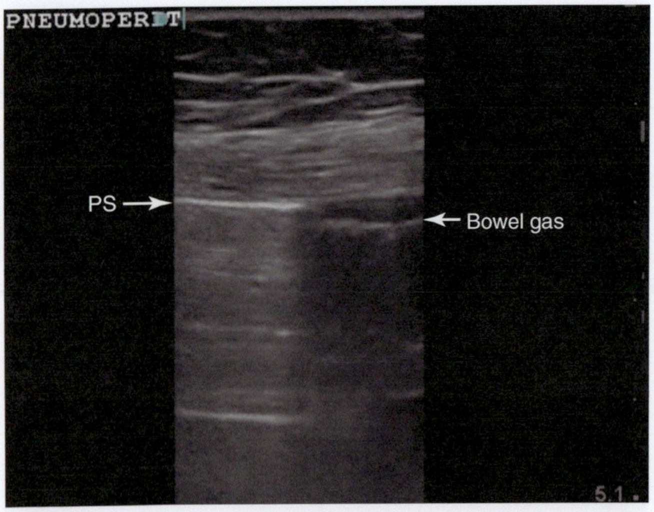

Fig. 11.27 This image illustrates the difference between the enhancement of the peritoneal stripe (PS) and adjacent intraluminal bowel gas, offset from the peritoneal stripe by the bowel wall thickness

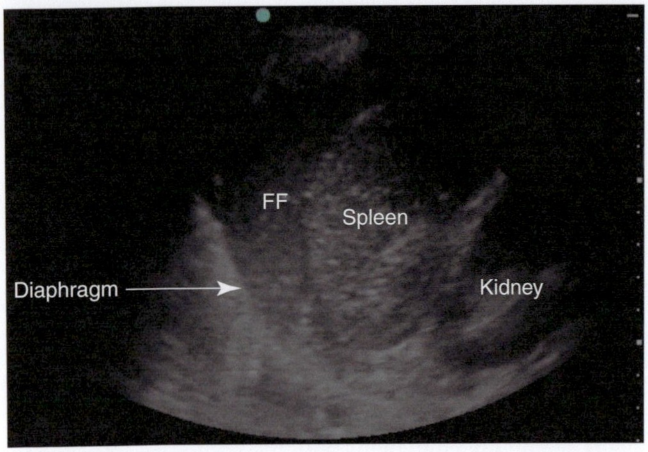

Fig. 11.28 Echogenic free fluid (FF) is found between the diaphragm (D) and spleen in the left upper quadrant view of the FAST exam

Free fluid can also be seen with hollow viscus perforation [88]. This fluid is more echogenic and heterogeneous than simple ascites given intestinal fluid contains partially digested food and has been referred to as "dirty fluid" (Fig. 11.28, Video 11.18) [89].

Mesenteric Ischemia

Acute ischemia of the mesentery is caused by embolism in 40–50% of cases, thrombosis in 20–30% of cases, and dissection in less than 5% of cases [90]. Chronic mesenteric ischemia is caused by progressive atherosclerosis in over 90% of cases [90]. Ultrasound of the mesenteric vasculature can identify proximal stenoses and occlusions using Doppler over the celiac artery and SMA. Ultrasound of the mesenteric vasculature can be limited by overlying bowel gas, and good interpretability has been shown in only 66–68% of cases [91]. Significant stenosis (>70%) is indicated by elevated peak systolic velocities in the celiac artery and SMA (with cutoffs in the literature ranging from 200–320 cm/s and 205–400 cm/sec, respectively) [92]. End-diastolic velocity can also be used to identify narrowing of the abdominal vasculature, with an end-diastolic velocity of >45 cm/sec indicating at least 50% stenosis of the SMA [93, 94].

A low-frequency curvilinear probe is placed in a sagittal orientation over the proximal and mid-aorta to view the celiac artery and SMA take-off anteriorly, respectively. Fasting facilitates visualization, but is not always feasible in the acute care setting. Chronic stenoses of the celiac and SMA are typically identified within 2–3 cm of their origin [95]. Once an adequate B-mode image of the aorta and anterior branches are obtained, color Doppler can be used to see if there is narrowing or complete absence of blood flow. Spectral Doppler with a small sample gate is placed in the branch vessel and advanced slowly every few millimeters. Breath-holding may facilitate tracing of the vessels.

Inflammatory Bowel Disease

Patients with inflammatory bowel disease (IBD), such as Crohn's disease and ulcerative colitis may present with flares of their disease and are at risk for abscess formation and other complications. In Crohn's disease, all bowel regions may be affected, but disease can primarily be seen at the ileocecal region, while in ulcerative colitis, the left colon is often primarily affected [96]. Ultrasound can provide diagnostic information and risk assessment in place of other imaging modalities that expose these patients to radiation. Intestinal POCUS has been suggested as a method of evaluating for and monitoring of IBD especially among gastroenterologists [97]. POCUS by emergency physicians has also been proposed as a tool to evaluate for IBD and associated complications, such as intra-abdominal abscesses [96, 98, 99]. One recent systematic review and meta-analysis found bowel ultrasound was 89% sensitive and 86% specific for assessing IBD disease activity [100].

Intestinal ultrasound for IBD requires assessment of both the large and small bowel. One described method to assess the large bowel is with a low-frequency curvilinear probe using the upside-down U technique previously described. Here, in IBD assessment, the probe typically starts in the left lower quadrant, first evaluating the rectum and distal sigmoid colon and then sweeps up to the left upper quadrant, evaluating the transverse colon, then to the right upper and lower quadrants and the corresponding ascending colon and cecum. The ileocecal valve and terminal ileum are typically located near the iliac vessels and psoas muscle.

The small intestine can then be assessed using the previously described "lawn-mower" technique. While a low-frequency curvilinear probe allows for a more global assessment, switching to a higher-frequency probe when possible can be used to better interrogate an area of interest. Typically, the small bowel has increased peristalsis compared to large bowel, while the large bowel is relatively stationary [97, 101]. Furthermore, the small bowel mucosa has plicae circulares, which begin in the second part of the duodenum, become more prominent in the jejunum, and disappear in the distal ileum.

In adults, bowel wall thickness >3 mm from the mucosa–lumen interface (hyperechoic layer) to serosa–muscle interface (hyperechoic layer) in any segment is concerning for active disease. In children, a bowel wall thickness of 1.9 mm is typically considered the upper limit of normal [10, 101].

Color Doppler can be applied to assess for hyperemia (Figs. 11.29 and 11.30; Videos 11.19 and 11.20), which indicates active inflammation. Bowel wall stratification can be disrupted or lost in active IBD, so evaluating for a classic multilayered gut signature is helpful, while the absence of a typical gut signature would support an IBD) diagnosis. Strictures (wall thickening resulting in a narrow lumen), fistulas (hypoechoic tract within the bowel wall), ulcers (depressions in the mucosa), and perianal abscesses may also be seen (Fig. 11.31, Video 11.21) [102, 103]. An intraabdominal abscess appears as a rounded, hypoechoic lesion with surrounding hyperemia, hyperechoic fat, and free fluid. Of note, sonographic mimics of IBD include non-IBD colitis (e.g., ischemic or bacterial), diverticulitis, and carcinoma.

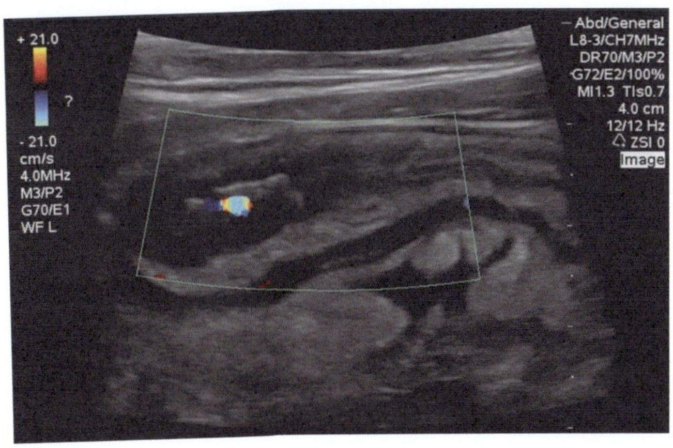

Fig. 11.29 Inflamed bowel with bowel wall thickening in Crohn's disease

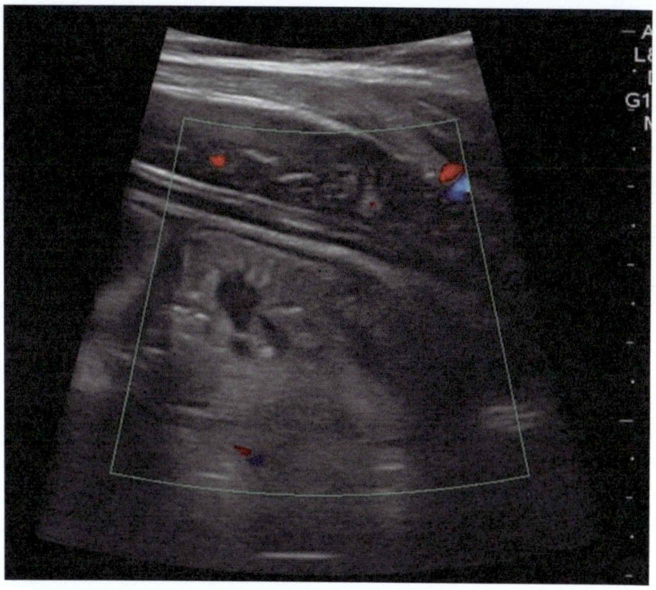

Fig. 11.30 Bowel wall thickening and inflammation in a patient with ulcerative colitis

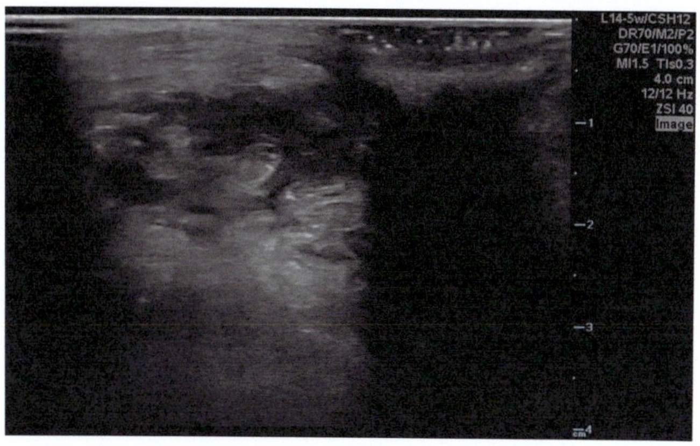

Fig. 11.31 Perianal abscess in a patient with inflammatory bowel disease. (*Image courtesy of Charisse Kwan, MD*)

Key Ultrasound Findings

Diagnosis	Key ultrasound findings
Zenker's diverticulum	Outpouching of the esophagus found posterior to the left lobe of the thyroid gland containing mixed echogenicities of air and food particles. Dynamic scanning of the area of concern with patient swallowing and probe compression can reveal changes in echogenicity to help distinguish this from a thyroid nodule.
Esophageal foreign body or food impaction	Dilation of the esophagus containing echodensities of food and liquid within. Scanning while the patient swallows does not cause the contents to move or the esophagus to change diameter.

(continued)

Diagnosis	Key ultrasound findings
Hiatal hernia	Sagittal view through left lobe of liver to identify esophageal hiatus in the diaphragm, anterior to and slightly to the left of the aorta. Increased diameter of diaphragmatic hiatus >18 mm. Gastric contents visualized in the left hemithorax behind the heart.
Gastric volume	Visualization of the gastric antrum and measurement of its cross-sectional area. Adult volume formula (mL) $= 27 + 14.6 \times \text{RLD-CSA} - 1.28 \times \text{age}$ in years, with a cutoff of 1.5 mL/kg for low risk for aspiration. Pediatric volume formula (mL) $= -7.8 + (3.5 \times \text{RLD-CSA}) + 0.127 \times \text{age}$ (months), with volume cutoff of 1.25 mL/kg for liquid contents being low risk for aspiration. Visualization of the stomach and the state of its contents (e.g., solid, liquid, air).
Hypertrophic Pyloric Stenosis	Visualization of hypertrophied pylorus with width >3 mm. Lack of passage of stomach contents through pylorus.
Small bowel obstruction	Dilation of small bowel loops >2.5 cm. To-and-fro peristalsis of the bowel contents. Decreased or absent color flow in the bowel wall and inter-luminal fluid raises concern for high-grade obstruction.
Malrotation and Volvulus	Abnormal position of SMV to SMA. Visualization of SMA cut off sign. Whirlpool sign—clockwise rotation of SMV around the SMA. Abnormal position of third portion of the duodenum.
Appendicitis	Tubular, aperistaltic, noncompressible blind-ending structure arising from the cecum, measuring >6 mm in diameter. Secondary findings include: visualization of an appendicolith, free fluid, increased blood flow, or hyperechoic fat stranding. To identify appendix utilize multiple different techniques including identifying the point of maximal tenderness, starting inferior to McBurney's Point in the right lower quadrant and identifying anatomical landmarks while sweeping cephalad, and graded compression.
Mesenteric adenitis	Enlarged lymph nodes >8–10 mm in short axis with increased flow on color Doppler, found anterior to the psoas muscle in the right lower quadrant or in the small bowel mesentery. Identify a normal appendix before making a diagnosis of mesenteric adenitis.
Intussusception	Visualization of target sign or sandwich sign. In the short axis, the target sign diameter is typically >2.5 cm for ileocolic intussusception, and on the right side of the abdomen and may have fat and lymph nodes in its core with a core:wall >1. Secondary signs of ischemia include free fluid and poor flow in color Doppler.
Large bowel obstruction	Abrupt transition from dilated (>4.5 cm) colon to a nondilated segment.
Diverticulitis	Visualization of the hyperechoic outpouching of the diverticula through the thickened (>4 mm) colonic wall. Hyperechoic inflammation/stranding surrounding the diverticula. A fluid collection adjacent to an inflamed diverticulum, with or without contained gas, may represent an abscess.
Pneumatosis Intestinalis	Echogenic foci in the bowel wall. Confirm location of air is in the bowel wall and not inside the bowel contents or outside the bowel in the peritoneum.
Hernia	Visualization of bowel protruding through fascial defect or adjacent to umbilicus (in ventral hernia) or through inguinal canal superficial to the inferior epigastric artery (in indirect hernia). Begin scanning with the patient in the supine position, then have the patient Valsalva to identify sliding of hernia contents.
Pneumoperitoneum	Visualization of free intraperitoneal air as enhancement of the peritoneal stripe between the liver and anterior abdominal wall. Air, when appreciated, is mobile with patient position and probe pressure. In cases of hollow viscus rupture, FAST exam may reveal echogenic fluid consistent with intestinal contents.
Mesenteric ischemia	Doppler of the longitudinal axis of the celiac trunk and the SMA. Peak systolic velocities of >200 cm/sec in the celiac or SMA, or peak diastolic velocities of >45 cm/sec should raise concern for chronic mesenteric ischemia and should be followed by computed tomography angiography.
Inflammatory bowel disease	Evaluation of extraintestinal manifestations of IBD such as abscess, stricture, and fistula. Evaluation of bowel wall thickening (>3 mm) and other signs of inflammation.

RLD right lateral decubitus, *CSA* cross-sectional area, *SMV* superior mesenteric vein, *SMA* superior mesenteric artery

Pearls and Pitfalls

- Graded compression, or steady probe pressure to the abdomen, can be helpful to visualize structures obscured by intestinal air.
- Patient positioning may improve visualization of structures. Right lateral decubitus is ideal for HPS and gastric antrum evaluation. Left lateral decubitus is helpful for HPS evaluation with an over-distended stomach. Reverse Trendelenburg shifts free intraperitoneal air cephalad.
- The point of maximal tenderness is often a high-yield site to begin a gastrointestinal ultrasound examination.
- Use protocolized techniques to best visualize bowel (e.g., upside-down U for colon, lawnmower technique for small bowel).
- Utilize dynamic scanning techniques. Have the patient swallow or compress the area to assess for Zenker's diverticulum or esophageal foreign body. Have the patient Valsalva while looking for hernia. Use the scissors technique when assessing for pneumoperitoneum.

References

1. Ultrasound guidelines: emergency, point-of-care, and clinical ultrasound guidelines in medicine. American College of Emergency Physicians. Revised 2023. https://www.acep.org/siteassets/new-pdfs/policy-statements/ultrasound-guidelines%2D%2Demergency-point-of-care-and-clinical-ultrasound-guidelines-in-medicine.pdf. Accessed 5 Feb 2024.
2. Hollerweger A, Maconi G, Ripolles T, Nylund K, Higginson A, Serra C, Dietrich C, Dirks K, Gilja O. Gastrointestinal ultrasound (GIUS) in intestinal emergencies—an EFSUMB position paper. Ultraschall Med - Eur J Ultrasound. 2020;41(06):646–57. https://doi.org/10.1055/a-1147-1295.
3. Hom J, Lam SHF, Delaney KM, Koos JA, Kunkov S. Vomiting, pyloric mass, and point-of-care ultrasound: diagnostic test accuracy for hypertrophic pyloric stenosis-a meta-analysis. J Emerg Med. 2023;65(5):e427–31. https://doi.org/10.1016/j.jemermed.2023.06.001.
4. Gottlieb M, Peksa GD, Pandurangadu AV, Nakitende D, Takhar S, Seethala RR. Utilization of ultrasound for the evaluation of small bowel obstruction: a systematic review and meta-analysis. Am J Emerg Med. 2017; https://doi.org/10.1016/j.ajem.2017.07.085.
5. Nguyen HN, Kulkarni M, Jose J, Sisson A, Brandt ML, Sammer MBK, Pammi M. Ultrasound for the diagnosis of malrotation and volvulus in children and adolescents: a systematic review and meta-analysis. Arch Dis Child. 2021;106(12):1171–8. https://doi.org/10.1136/archdischild-2020-321082.
6. Fields JM, Davis J, Alsup C, Bates A, Au A, Adhikari S, Farrell I. Accuracy of point-of-care ultrasonography for diagnosing acute appendicitis: a systematic review and meta-analysis. Acad Emerg Med. 2017;24(9):1124–36. https://doi.org/10.1111/acem.13212.
7. Lin-Martore M, Firnberg MT, Kohn MA, Kornblith AE, Gottlieb M. Diagnostic accuracy of point-of-care ultrasonography for intussusception in children: a systematic review and meta-analysis. Am J Emerg Med. 2022;58:255–64. https://doi.org/10.1016/j.ajem.2022.06.025.
8. Tsou P-Y, Wang Y-H, Ma Y-K, Deanehan JK, Gillon J, Chou EH, Hsu T-C, Huang Y-C, Lin J, Lee C-C. Accuracy of point-of-care ultrasound and radiology-performed ultrasound for intussusception: a systematic review and meta-analysis. Am J Emerg Med. 2019;37(9):1760–9. https://doi.org/10.1016/j.ajem.2019.06.006.
9. Robinson A, Light D, Nice C. Meta-analysis of sonography in the diagnosis of inguinal hernias. J Ultrasound Med. 2013;32(2):339–46.
10. Dong J, Wang H, Zhao J, Zhu W, Zhang L, Gong J, Li Y, Gu L, Li J. Ultrasound as a diagnostic tool in detecting active Crohn's disease: a meta-analysis of prospective studies. Eur Radiol. 2014;24(1):26–33. https://doi.org/10.1007/s00330-013-2973-0.
11. Law R, Katzka DA, Baron TH. Zenker's diverticulum. Clin Gastroenterol Hepatol. 2014;12(11):1773–82. https://doi.org/10.1016/j.cgh.2013.09.016.
12. Huang HJ, Chen R, Sheng JG, Cao KK, Zhao JQ. Characteristic analysis of Zenker's diverticulum incidentally detected on multimodal neck ultrasound. J Méd Ultrason. 2020;47(2):279–85. https://doi.org/10.1007/s10396-019-00992-w.
13. Wang Y, Song Y. Sonographic characteristics of pharyngoesophageal diverticula: report of 14 cases and review of the literature. J Clin Ultrasound. 2016;44(6):333–8. https://doi.org/10.1002/jcu.22321.
14. Singleton J, Schafer JM, Hinson JS, Kane EM, Wright S, Hoffmann B. Bedside sonography for the diagnosis of esophageal food impaction. Am J Emerg Med. 2017;35(5):720–4. https://doi.org/10.1016/j.ajem.2017.01.008.
15. Ahn JH, Sohn Y. Application of point-of-care ultrasound for different types of esophageal foreign bodies: three case reports. Medicine. 2020;99(4):e18893. https://doi.org/10.1097/md.0000000000018893.
16. Kawai Y, Ogawa O, Hirose Y. Point-of-care ultrasound for an Esophageal foreign body. J Emerg Med. 2022;63(2):e53–6. https://doi.org/10.1016/j.jemermed.2022.04.035.
17. Buonsenso D, Chiaretti A, Curatola A, Morello R, Giacalone M, Parri N. Pediatrician performed point-of-care ultrasound for the detection of ingested foreign bodies: case series and review of the literature. J Ultrasound. 2021;24(1):107–14. https://doi.org/10.1007/s40477-020-00452-z.
18. Barone M, Lernia PD, Carbonara M, Ladisa R, Donno A, Amoruso A, Leo AD, Francavilla A. Sliding gastric hiatal hernia diagnosis by transabdominal ultrasonography: an easy, reliable and non-invasive procedure. Scand J Gastroenterol. 2006;41(7):851–5. https://doi.org/10.1080/00365520500453408.
19. Godwin SA, Burton JH, Gerardo CJ, Hatten BW, Mace SE, Silvers SM, Fesmire FM. Clinical policy: procedural sedation and analgesia in the emergency department. Ann Emerg Med. 2014;63(2):247–258.e18. https://doi.org/10.1016/j.annemergmed.2013.10.015.
20. Perlas A, Arzola C, de Putte PV. Point-of-care gastric ultrasound and aspiration risk assessment: a narrative review. Can J Anesth J Can d'anesthésie. 2018;65(4):437–48. https://doi.org/10.1007/s12630-017-1031-9.
21. Leviter J, Steele DW, Constantine E, Linakis JG, Amanullah S. "Full stomach" despite the wait: point-of-care gastric ultrasound at the time of procedural sedation in the pediatric emergency department. Acad Emerg Med. 2019;26(7):752–60. https://doi.org/10.1111/acem.13651.
22. Miller AF, Levy JA, Krauss BS, Gravel CA, Vieira RL, Neuman MI, Monuteaux MC, Rempell RG. Does point-of-care gastric ultrasound correlate with reported fasting time? Pediatr Emerg Care. 2021;37(12):e1265–9. https://doi.org/10.1097/pec.0000000000001997.

23. Moake MM, Presley BC, Hill JG, Wolf BJ, Kane ID, Busch CE, Jackson BF. Point-of-care ultrasound to assess gastric content in pediatric emergency department procedural sedation patients. Pediatr Emerg Care. 2022;38(1):e178–86. https://doi.org/10.1097/pec.0000000000002198.
24. Valla FV, Tume LN, Chaparro CJ, Arnold P, Alrayashi W, Morice C, Nabialek T, Rouchaud A, Cercueil E, Bouvet L. Gastric point-of-care ultrasound in acutely and critically ill children (POCUS-ped): a scoping review. Front Pediatr. 2022;10:921863. https://doi.org/10.3389/fped.2022.921863.
25. Perlas A, Mitsakakis N, Liu L, Cino M, Haldipur N, Davis L, Cubillos J, Chan V. Validation of a mathematical model for ultrasound assessment of gastric volume by gastroscopic examination. Anesthesia Analg. 2013;116(2):357–63. https://doi.org/10.1213/ane.0b013e318274fc19.
26. Spencer AO, Walker AM, Yeung AK, Lardner DR, Yee K, Mulvey JM, Perlas A. Ultrasound assessment of gastric volume in the fasted pediatric patient undergoing upper gastrointestinal endoscopy: development of a predictive model using endoscopically suctioned volumes. Pediatr Anesth. 2015;25(3):301–8. https://doi.org/10.1111/pan.12581.
27. Park JS, Byun Y-H, Choi SJ, Lee JS, Ryu J-M, Lee J-Y. Feasibility of point-of-care ultrasound for diagnosing hypertrophic pyloric stenosis in the emergency department. Pediatr Emerg Care. 2021;37(11):550–4. https://doi.org/10.1097/pec.0000000000002532.
28. van den Bunder FA, Derikx JP, Kiblawi R, van Rijn RR, Dingemann J. Diagnostic accuracy of palpation and ultrasonography for diagnosing infantile hypertrophic pyloric stenosis: a systematic review and meta-analysis. Br J Radiol. 2022;95(1139):20211251. https://doi.org/10.1259/bjr.20211251.
29. Piotto L, Gent R, Taranath A, Bibbo G, Goh DW. Ultrasound diagnosis of hypertrophic pyloric stenosis—time to change the criteria. Australas J Ultrasound Med. 2022;25(3):116–26. https://doi.org/10.1002/ajum.12305.
30. Calle-Toro JS, Kaplan SL, Andronikou S. Are we performing ultrasound measurements of the wall thickness in hypertrophic pyloric stenosis studies the same way? Pediatr Surg Int. 2020;36(3):399–405. https://doi.org/10.1007/s00383-019-04601-2.
31. Haller JO, Cohen HL. Hypertrophic pyloric stenosis: diagnosis using US. Radiology. 1986;161(2):335–9. https://doi.org/10.1148/radiology.161.2.3532185.
32. Indiran V, Selvaraj V. The cervix sign and other sonographic signs of hypertrophic pyloric stenosis. Abdom Radiol. 2016;41(10):2085–6. https://doi.org/10.1007/s00261-016-0809-5.
33. Dias SC, Swinson S, Torrão H, Gonçalves L, Kurochka S, Vaz CP, Mendes V. Hypertrophic pyloric stenosis: tips and tricks for ultrasound diagnosis. Insights Imaging. 2012;3(3):247–50. https://doi.org/10.1007/s13244-012-0168-x.
34. Pon MS, Scudamore C, Harrison RC, Cooperberg PL. Ultrasound demonstration of radiographically obscure small bowel obstruction. AJR Am J Roentgenol. 1979;133(1):145–6.
35. Unlüer EE, Yavaşi O, Eroğlu O, Yilmaz C, Akarca FK. Ultrasonography by emergency medicine and radiology residents for the diagnosis of small bowel obstruction. Eur J Emerg Med. 2010;17(5):260–4. https://doi.org/10.1097/mej.0b013e328336c736.
36. Jang TB, Schindler D, Kaji AH. Bedside ultrasonography for the detection of small bowel obstruction in the emergency department. Emerg Med J. 2011;28(8):676–8. https://doi.org/10.1136/emj.2010.095729.
37. Becker BA, Lahham S, Gonzales MA, Nomura JT, Bui MK, Truong TA, Stahlman BA, Fox JC, Kehrl T. A prospective, multicenter evaluation of point-of-care ultrasound for small-bowel obstruction in the emergency department. Acad Emerg Med. 2019;26(8):921–30. https://doi.org/10.1111/acem.13713.
38. Boniface KS, King JB, LeSaux MA, Haciski SC, Shokoohi H. Diagnostic accuracy and time-saving effects of point-of-care ultrasonography in patients with small bowel obstruction: a prospective study. Ann Emerg Med. 2020;75(2):246–56. https://doi.org/10.1016/j.annemergmed.2019.05.031.
39. Grassi R, Romano S, D'Amario F, Rossi AG, Romano L, Pinto F, Mizio RD. The relevance of free fluid between intestinal loops detected by sonography in the clinical assessment of small bowel obstruction in adults. Eur J Radiol. 2004;50(1):5–14. https://doi.org/10.1016/j.ejrad.2003.11.009.
40. Silva AC, Pimenta M, Guimaraes LS. Small bowel obstruction: what to look for. Radiographics. 2009;29(2):423–39. https://doi.org/10.1148/rg.292085514.
41. Nagdeve NG, Qureshi AM, Bhingare PD, Shinde SK. Malrotation beyond infancy. J Pediatr Surg. 2012;47(11):2026–32. https://doi.org/10.1016/j.jpedsurg.2012.06.013.
42. Zhang W, Sun H, Luo F. The efficiency of sonography in diagnosing volvulus in neonates with suspected intestinal malrotation. Medicine. 2017;96(42):e8287. https://doi.org/10.1097/md.0000000000008287.
43. Wong K, Tassel DV, Lee J, Buchmann R, Riemann M, Egan C, Youssfi M. Making the diagnosis of midgut volvulus: limited abdominal ultrasound has changed our clinical practice. J Pediatr Surg. 2020;55(12):2614–7. https://doi.org/10.1016/j.jpedsurg.2020.04.012.
44. Sivitz AB, Lyons R. Mid-gut volvulus identified by pediatric emergency ultrasonography. J Emerg Med. 2013;45(5):e173–4. https://doi.org/10.1016/j.jemermed.2013.05.048.
45. Garcia AM, Asad I, Tessaro MO, Sivitz A, Osborn K, Shaahinfar A, Leung SK, Rowe E, Riera A. A multi-institutional case series with review of point-of-care ultrasound to diagnose Malrotation and Midgut volvulus in the pediatric emergency department. Pediatr Emerg Care. 2019;35(6):443–7. https://doi.org/10.1097/pec.0000000000001737.
46. Zhou L, Li S, Wang W, Shan Q, Pan F, Liu J, Xie X. Usefulness of sonography in evaluating children suspected of Malrotation. J Ultrasound Med. 2015;34(10):1825–32. https://doi.org/10.7863/ultra.14.10017.
47. Addis DG, Shaffer N, Fowler BS, Tauxe RV. The epidemiology of appendicitis and appendectomy in the United States. Am J Epidemiol. 1990;132(5):910–25. https://doi.org/10.1093/oxfordjournals.aje.a115734.
48. Doniger SJ, Kornblith A. Point-of-care ultrasound integrated into a staged diagnostic algorithm for pediatric appendicitis. Pediatr Emerg Care. 2018;34(2):109–15. https://doi.org/10.1097/pec.0000000000000773.
49. Elikashvili I, Tay ET, Tsung JW. The effect of point-of-care ultrasonography on emergency department length of stay and computed tomography utilization in children with suspected appendicitis. Acad Emerg Med. 2014;21(2):163–70. https://doi.org/10.1111/acem.12319.
50. Cohen B, Bowling J, Midulla P, Shlasko E, Lester N, Rosenberg H, Lipskar A. The non-diagnostic ultrasound in appendicitis: is a non-visualized appendix the same as a negative study? J Pediatr Surg. 2015;50(6):923–7. https://doi.org/10.1016/j.jpedsurg.2015.03.012.
51. Abo A, Shannon M, Taylor G, Bachur R. The influence of body mass index on the accuracy of ultrasound and computed tomography in diagnosing appendicitis in children. Pediatr Emerg Care. 2011;27(8):731–6. https://doi.org/10.1097/pec.0b013e318226c8b0.
52. Binkovitz LA, Unsdorfer KML, Thapa P, Kolbe AB, Hull NC, Zingula SN, Thomas KB, Homme JL. Pediatric appendiceal ultrasound: accuracy, determinacy and clinical outcomes.

Pediatr Radiol. 2015;45(13):1934–44. https://doi.org/10.1007/s00247-015-3432-7.
53. Bachur RG, Dayan PS, Bajaj L, Macias CG, Mittal MK, Stevenson MD, Dudley NC, Sinclair K, Bennett J, Monuteaux MC, Kharbanda AB, Pediatrics PEMCRC of the AA of. The effect of abdominal pain duration on the accuracy of diagnostic imaging for pediatric appendicitis. Ann Emerg Med. 2012;60(5):582–590.e3. https://doi.org/10.1016/j.annemergmed.2012.05.034.
54. Sivitz AB, Cohen SG, Tejani C. Evaluation of acute appendicitis by pediatric emergency physician sonography. Ann Emerg Med. 2014;64(4):358–364.e4. https://doi.org/10.1016/j.annemergmed.2014.03.028.
55. Sivit CJ. Diagnosis of acute appendicitis in children: spectrum of sonographic findings. Am J Roentgenol. 1993;161(1):147–52. https://doi.org/10.2214/ajr.161.1.8517294.
56. Vasavada P. Ultrasound evaluation of acute abdominal emergencies in infants and children. Radiol Clin North Am. 2004;42(2):445–56. https://doi.org/10.1016/j.rcl.2004.01.003.
57. Estey A, Poonai N, Lim R. Appendix Not Seen. Pediatr Emerg Care. 2013;29(4):435–9. https://doi.org/10.1097/pec.0b013e318289e8d5.
58. Ramdass MJ, Sing QY, Milne D, Mooteeram J, Barrow S. Association between the appendix and the fecalith in adults. Can J Surg. 2015;58(1):10–4. https://doi.org/10.1503/cjs.002014.
59. Simanovsky N, Hiller N. Importance of sonographic detection of enlarged abdominal lymph nodes in children. J Ultrasound Med. 2007;26(5):581–4. https://doi.org/10.7863/jum.2007.26.5.581.
60. Karmazyn B, Werner EA, Rejaie B, Applegate KE. Mesenteric lymph nodes in children: what is normal? Pediatr Radiol. 2005;35(8):774–7. https://doi.org/10.1007/s00247-005-1462-2.
61. Sung T, Callahan MJ, Taylor GA. Clinical and imaging mimickers of acute appendicitis in the pediatric population. Am J Roentgenol. 2006;186(1):67–74. https://doi.org/10.2214/ajr.04.1380.
62. Sanchez TR, Corwin MT, Davoodian A, Stein-Wexler R. Sonography of abdominal pain in children. J Ultrasound Med. 2016;35(3):627–35. https://doi.org/10.7863/ultra.15.04047.
63. Waseem M, Rosenberg HK. Intussusception. Pediatr Emerg Care. 2008;24(11):793–800. https://doi.org/10.1097/pec.0b013e31818c2a3e.
64. Marsicovetere P, Ivatury S, White B, Holubar S. Intestinal intussusception: etiology, diagnosis, and treatment. Clin Colon Rectal Surg. 2017;30(01):030–9. https://doi.org/10.1055/s-0036-1593429.
65. Kim JH, Lee J-Y, Kwon JH, Cho H-R, Lee JS, Ryu J-M. Point-of-care ultrasound could streamline the emergency department workflow of clinically nonspecific intussusception. Pediatr Emerg Care Publish Ahead of Print. 2017;(2):1. https://doi.org/10.1097/pec.0000000000001283.
66. Subramaniam S, Chen AE, Khwaja A, Rempell R. Point-of-care ultrasound for differentiating ileocolic from small bowel-small bowel intussusception. J Emerg Med. 2022;62(1):72–82. https://doi.org/10.1016/j.jemermed.2021.07.002.
67. Gondek AS, Riaza L, Cuadras D, Castellarnau XT, Krauel L. Ileocolic intussusception: predicting the probability of success of ultrasound guided saline enema from clinical and sonographic data. J Pediatr Surg. 2018;53(4):599–604. https://doi.org/10.1016/j.jpedsurg.2017.10.050.
68. Strate LL, Morris AM. Epidemiology, pathophysiology, and treatment of diverticulitis. Gastroenterology. 2019;156(5):1282–1298.e1. https://doi.org/10.1053/j.gastro.2018.12.033.
69. Chiu T-C, Chou Y-H, Tiu C-M, Chiou H-J, Wang H-K, Lai Y-C, Chiou Y-Y. Right-sided colonic diverticulitis: clinical features, sonographic appearances, and management. J Méd Ultrasound. 2017;25(1):33–9. https://doi.org/10.1016/j.jmu.2016.10.007.
70. Parulekar SG. Sonography of colonic diverticulitis. J Ultrasound Med. 1985;4(12):659–66. https://doi.org/10.7863/jum.1985.4.12.659.
71. Nazerian P, Gigli C, Donnarumma E, de Curtis E, Bribani A, Lanzi S, Rovida S, Magazzini S, Grifoni S, Perani C. Diagnostic accuracy of point-of-care ultrasound integrated into clinical examination for acute diverticulitis: a prospective multicenter study. Ultraschall Med - Eur J Ultrasound. 2020;42(06):614–22. https://doi.org/10.1055/a-1161-0780.
72. Cohen A, Li T, Stankard B, Nelson M. A prospective evaluation of point-of-care ultrasonographic diagnosis of diverticulitis in the emergency department. Ann Emerg Med. 2020;76(6):757–66. https://doi.org/10.1016/j.annemergmed.2020.05.017.
73. Shokoohi H, Selame LA, Loesche MA, Almulhim A, Saud AAA, Goldsmith A, Eke O, Springer C, Arru CD, Gullikson J, McKaig B, Liteplo AS, Huang C. Accuracy of "TICS" ultrasound protocol in detecting simple and complicated diverticulitis: a prospective cohort study. Acad Emerg Med. 2022; https://doi.org/10.1111/acem.14628.
74. Dirks K, Calabrese E, Dietrich C, Gilja O, Hausken T, Higginson A, Hollerweger A, Maconi G, Maaser C, Nuernberg D, Nylund K, Pallotta N, Ripolles T, Romanini L, Saftoiu A, Serra C, Wüstner M, Sporea I. EFSUMB position paper: recommendations for gastrointestinal ultrasound (GIUS) in acute appendicitis and diverticulitis. Ultraschall Med - Eur J Ultrasound. 2019;40(02):163–75. https://doi.org/10.1055/a-0824-6952.
75. Pear BL. Pneumatosis intestinalis: a review. Radiology. 1998;207(1):13–9. https://doi.org/10.1148/radiology.207.1.9530294.
76. James V, Warier A, Lee KP, Ong GY-K. Point-of-care ultrasound identification of pneumatosis intestinalis in pediatric abdominal pain: a case report. Crit Ultrasound J. 2017;9(1):2. https://doi.org/10.1186/s13089-017-0057-0.
77. Tan SW, James V, Warier A, Ong GY. Point-of-care ultrasound identification of pneumatosis intestinalis associated with Henoch-Schönlein purpura gastrointestinal involvement: a case report. World J Emerg Med. 2021;12(1):76. https://doi.org/10.5847/wjem.j.1920-8642.2021.01.013.
78. Spangen L. Ultrasound as a diagnostic aid in ventral abdominal hernia. J Clin Ultrasound. 1975;3(3):211–3. https://doi.org/10.1002/jcu.1870030311.
79. Jalbout NA, Liteplo A, Shokoohi H. Point-of care ultrasound in stratifying clinically evolving inguinal and femoral hernias. J Emerg Med. 2022;63(2):257–64. https://doi.org/10.1016/j.jemermed.2022.04.034.
80. Jacomino K, Frasure SE, Boniface KS, Shokoohi H. Point-of-care ultrasound in the diagnosis of an incarcerated inguinal hernia. Cureus. 2021;13(7):e16281. https://doi.org/10.7759/cureus.16281.
81. Siadecki SD, Frasure SE, Saul T, Lewiss RE. Diagnosis and reduction of a hernia by bedside ultrasound: a case report. J Emerg Med. 2014;47(2):169–71. https://doi.org/10.1016/j.jemermed.2013.09.026.
82. Stavros AT, Rapp C. Dynamic ultrasound of hernias of the groin and anterior abdominal wall. Ultrasound Q. 2010;26(3):135–69. https://doi.org/10.1097/ruq.0b013e3181f0b23f.
83. Jiang L, Wu J, Feng X. The value of ultrasound in diagnosis of pneumoperitoneum in emergent or critical conditions: a meta-analysis. Hong Kong J Emerg Med. 2019;26(2):111–7. https://doi.org/10.1177/1024907918805668.
84. Nazerian P, Tozzetti C, Vanni S, Bartolucci M, Gualtieri S, Trausi F, Vittorini M, Catini E, Cibinel GA, Grifoni S. Accuracy of abdominal ultrasound for the diagnosis of pneumoperitoneum in patients with acute abdominal pain: a pilot study. Crit Ultrasound J. 2015;7(1):15. https://doi.org/10.1186/s13089-015-0032-6.
85. Grechenig W, Peicha G, Clement H-G, Grechenig M. Detection of pneumoperitoneum by ultrasound examination: an experimental and clinical study. Inj. 1999;30(3):173–8. https://doi.org/10.1016/s0020-1383(98)00248-4.

86. Muradali D, Wilson S, Burns PN, Shapiro H, Hope-Simpson D. A specific sign of pneumoperitoneum on sonography: enhancement of the peritoneal stripe. Am J Roentgenol. 1999;173(5):1257–62. https://doi.org/10.2214/ajr.173.5.10541100.
87. Karahan OI, Kurt A, Yikilmaz A, Kahriman G. New method for the detection of intraperitoneal free air by sonography: scissors maneuver. J Clin Ultrasound. 2004;32(8):381–5. https://doi.org/10.1002/jcu.20055.
88. Chen S, Wang H, Chen W, Lin F, Hsu C, Chang K, Chen W. Selective use of ultrasonography for the detection of Pneumoperitoneum. Acad Emerg Med. 2002;9(6):643–5. https://doi.org/10.1197/aemj.9.6.643.
89. Shokoohi H, Boniface KS, Abell BM, Pourmand A, Salimian M. Ultrasound and perforated viscus; dirty fluid, dirty shadows, and peritoneal enhancement. Emerg (Tehran, Iran). 2016;4(2):101–5.
90. Campion EW, Clair DG, Beach JM. Mesenteric Ischemia. N Engl J Med. 2016;374(10):959–68. https://doi.org/10.1056/nejmra1503884.
91. van Petersen AS, Meerwaldt R, Kolkman JJ, Huisman AB, van der Palen J, van Bockel JH, Zeebregts CJ, Geelkerken RH. The influence of respiration on criteria for transabdominal duplex examination of the splanchnic arteries in patients with suspected chronic splanchnic ischemia. J Vasc Surg. 2013;57(6):1603–1611.e10. https://doi.org/10.1016/j.jvs.2012.11.120.
92. Terlouw LG, Moelker A, Abrahamsen J, Acosta S, Bakker OJ, Baumgartner I, Boyer L, Corcos O, Dijk LJ, Duran M, Geelkerken RH, Illuminati G, Jackson RW, Kärkkäinen JM, Kolkman JJ, Lönn L, Mazzei MA, Nuzzo A, Pecoraro F, Raupach J, Verhagen HJ, Zech CJ, Noord D, Bruno MJ. European guidelines on chronic mesenteric ischaemia – joint United European Gastroenterology, European Association for Gastroenterology, Endoscopy and Nutrition, European Society of Gastrointestinal and Abdominal Radiology, Netherlands Association of Hepatogastroenterologists, Hellenic Society of Gastroenterology, Cardiovascular and Interventional Radiological Society of Europe, and Dutch Mesenteric Ischemia Study group clinical guidelines on the diagnosis and treatment of patients with chronic mesenteric ischaemia. UEG J. 2020;8(4):371–95. https://doi.org/10.1177/2050640620916681.
93. Zwolak RM, Fillinger MF, Walsh DB, LaBombard FA, Musson A, Darling CE, Cronenwett JL. Mesenteric and celiac duplex scanning: a validation study. J Vasc Surg. 1998;27(6):1078–88. https://doi.org/10.1016/s0741-5214(98)60010-0.
94. Bowersox JC, Zwolak RM, Walsh DB, Schneider JR, Musson A, LaBombard FE, Cronenwett JL. Duplex ultrasonography in the diagnosis of celiac and mesenteric artery occlusive disease. J Vasc Surg. 1991;14(6):780–8. https://doi.org/10.1067/mva.1991.33215.
95. Oderich GS. Current concepts in the management of chronic mesenteric ischemia. Curr Treat Options Cardiovasc Med. 2010;12(2):117–30. https://doi.org/10.1007/s11936-010-0061-1.
96. Granat N, Gabrieli S, Alpert EA. Point-of-care ultrasound to diagnose colitis in the emergency department: a case series and review of the literature. J Emerg Med. 2020;58(1):77–84. https://doi.org/10.1016/j.jemermed.2019.08.035.
97. Dolinger MT, Kayal M. Intestinal ultrasound as a non-invasive tool to monitor inflammatory bowel disease activity and guide clinical decision making. World J Gastroenterol. 2023;29(15):2272–82. https://doi.org/10.3748/wjg.v29.i15.2272.
98. Esterson A, Alpert EA, Gabrieli S, Granat N. Sonographic assessment of inflammatory bowel disease in the emergency department: a case series and review of the literature. J Clin Ultrasound. 2021;49(3):277–81. https://doi.org/10.1002/jcu.22946.
99. Rivera K, Cabrera G, Kalivoda EJ. Point-of-care ultrasound diagnosis of a Crohn's disease-related Intraabdominal abscess in the emergency department. Cureus. 2021;13(4):e14290. https://doi.org/10.7759/cureus.14290.
100. Malik S, Venugopalan S, Tenorio BG, Khan SR, Loganathan P, Navaneethan U, Mohan BP. Diagnostic accuracy of bowel ultrasonography in patients with inflammatory bowel disease: a systematic review and meta-analysis. Ann Gastroenterol. 2024;37(1):54–63. https://doi.org/10.20524/aog.2024.0842.
101. Dolinger MT, Kellar A. Point-of-care intestinal ultrasound in pediatric inflammatory bowel disease. Curr Gastroenterol Rep. 2023;25(11):355–61. https://doi.org/10.1007/s11894-023-00892-7.
102. Lin W-C, Chang C-W, Chen M-J, Wang H-Y. Intestinal ultrasound in inflammatory bowel disease: a novel and increasingly important tool. J Méd Ultrasound. 2023;31(2):86–91. https://doi.org/10.4103/jmu.jmu_84_22.
103. Allocca M, Furfaro F, Fiorino G, Peyrin-Biroulet L, Danese S. Point-of-care ultrasound in inflammatory bowel disease. J Crohns Colitis. 2020;15(1):143–51. https://doi.org/10.1093/ecco-jcc/jjaa151.

Obstetric Ultrasound

12

Alexis Salerno, Samantha A. King, and Eileen Y. Wang

Background

With the rise in chronic conditions and the increasing age of first-time mothers, a growing number of individuals are entering pregnancy with complex healthcare needs. An average of 1-in-3 pregnancies are referred to non-obstetricians and approximately one-third of women will present for an emergency department (ED) visit during their pregnancy [1]. Though these numbers may vary significantly depending on factors such as access to prenatal care and geographical location, most clinicians will inevitably encounter the responsibility of caring for a pregnant patient [2]. The use of obstetric point-of-care ultrasound (POCUS) has been shown to decrease length of stay and lower overall costs associated with ED visits [3].

In early pregnancy, the most critical question that clinicians attempt to answer is if there is an intrauterine pregnancy (IUP) [4]. Ectopic pregnancies are a leading cause of morbidity and mortality worldwide [5]. They account for approximately 2% of all pregnancies, though can be as high as 6–16% in symptomatic ED patients [6]. Since the late 1990s, POCUS has been essential in the evaluation of pregnant patients. An IUP demonstrated on obstetric POCUS, in the absence of assisted reproductive therapy, is 99.3% sensitive with nearly a 100% negative predictive value for ruling out an ectopic pregnancy [7]. In cases where an IUP is not visualized, there should be increased suspicion of an ectopic pregnancy. In otherwise stable patients, a lack of IUP may result in further imaging, serial examinations, or close follow-up. However, in cases with hemodynamic instability or evidence of rupture on ultrasound, POCUS can expedite consultation and operative management [8].

Over time, obstetric POCUS has expanded to encompass a more comprehensive obstetrical evaluation, extending beyond mere assessment for an IUP. In the first trimester, POCUS can estimate gestational age, identify failed pregnancies, and detect multiple and molar pregnancies. During the second and third trimester, bedside clinicians can use POCUS to determine fetal position, placental location, cervical length, amniotic fluid levels, and signs of fetal distress. Finally, postpartum obstetric POCUS can assess for retained products of conception (RPOC) and endometritis.

Indications

Indications
- Positive pregnancy test
- Abdominal pain during pregnancy
- Vaginal bleeding during pregnancy
- Evaluate fetal status
- Postpartum abdominal pain or vaginal bleeding

Diagnoses
- Intrauterine pregnancy
- Gestational age
- Fetal heart rate
- Ectopic pregnancy
- Multiple gestations
- Gestational trophoblastic disease
- Subchorionic hemorrhage
- Pregnancy failure
- Ovarian hyperstimulation syndrome
- Placental location and complications
- Fetal presentation
- Amniotic fluid status
- Cervical length
- Retained products of conception

Supplementary Information The online version contains supplementary material available at https://doi.org/10.1007/978-3-031-85308-1_12.

A. Salerno (✉)
Department of Emergency Medicine, University of Maryland School of Medicine, Baltimore, MD, USA
e-mail: Alexis.Salerno@som.umaryland.edu

S. A. King
Department of Emergency Medicine, University of Texas Medical Branch, Galveston, TX, USA
e-mail: saaking@utmb.edu

E. Y. Wang
Department of Obstetrics and Gynecology, University of Pennsylvania, Philadelphia, PA, USA
e-mail: Eileen.Wang@pennmedicine.upenn.edu

M. Gottlieb, N. Panebianco (eds.), *Advanced Point-of-Care Ultrasound*, https://doi.org/10.1007/978-3-031-85308-1_12

Core Views

View	Image	Approach
Transabdominal	Uterus Long-Axis 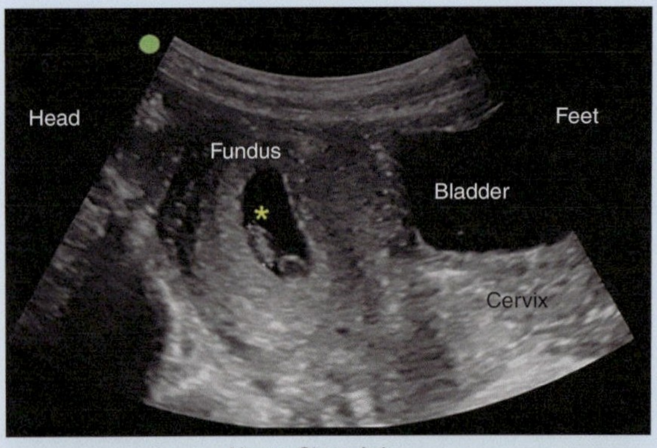 Uterus Short-Axis 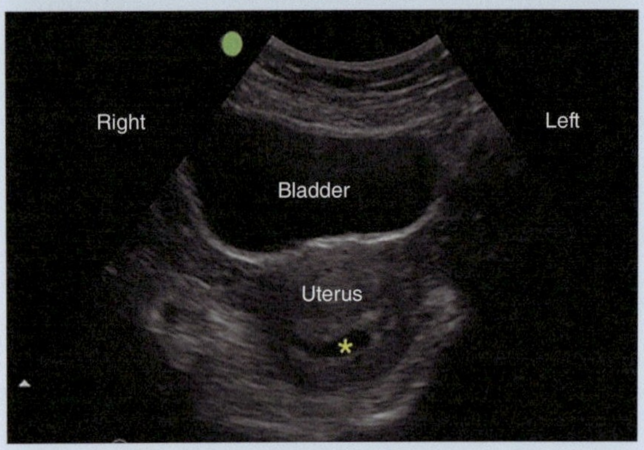 Core View 1 (Asterisk: Gestational Sac) Core Video 12.1. Transabdominal Curvilinear	Place a curvilinear probe superior to the pubic symphysis with the indicator toward the patient's head, to obtain a long-axis view of the uterus. Fan the probe right and left to confirm the full extent and location of the uterus by connecting the vaginal stripe to the cervix and the uterus. Next, rotate the probe counterclockwise towards the patient's right side, to obtain a short-axis view. Fan inferiorly and superiorly to visualize the bladder and the uterus from cervix to fundus. The ovaries will sit lateral to the uterus and medial to the iliac vessels. To better image each individual adnexa, apply graded compression and slide or fan the probe laterally.
Transvaginal	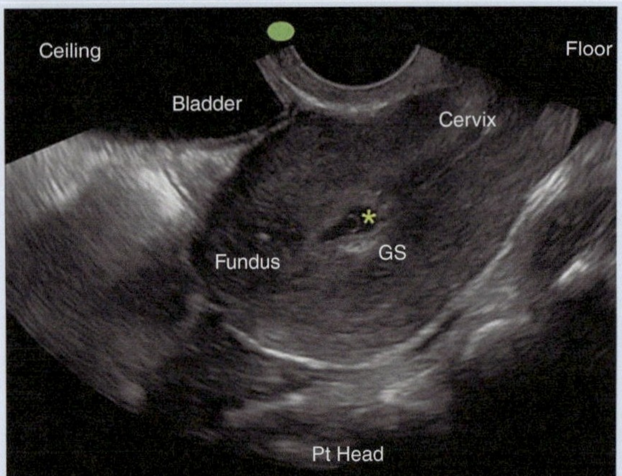 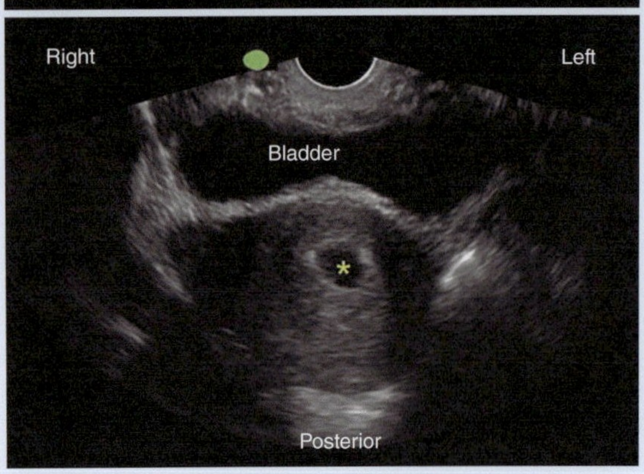 Core View 2 (Asterisk: Gestational Sac) Core Video 12.2. Transvaginal ultrasound	Insert a covered endocavitary probe into the vagina with the probe indicator pointing anteriorly (toward the ceiling in a supine patient) until it rests in the anterior fornix to obtain a sagittal view of the uterus in the long axis. Fan the probe right and left to fully interrogate the uterus and surrounding structures. Next, rotate the probe indicator counterclockwise 90° toward the patient's right side to assess the uterus in a short axis. Interrogate the uterus by fanning anteriorly and posteriorly. At the level of the cornual flares, rock the probe to the patient's right to locate their right ovary. Once identified, rotate the probe indicator 90 degrees clockwise to evaluate the adnexa in the sagittal plane. Repeat with the contralateral side.

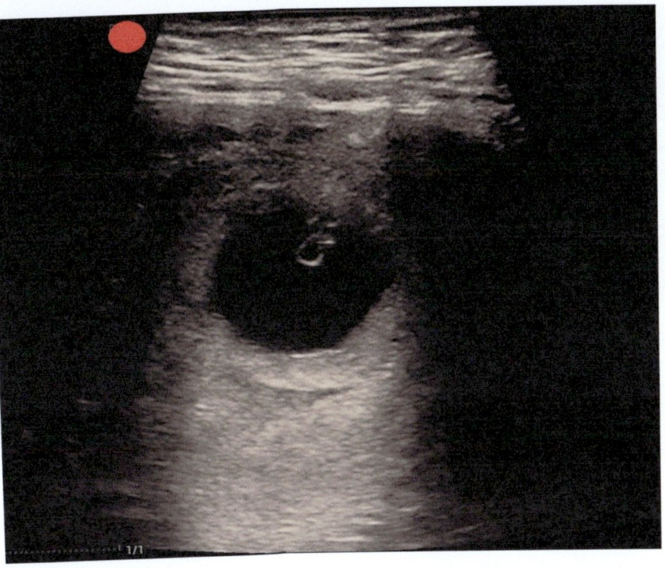

Fig. 12.1 Intrauterine pregnancy evaluated with a linear probe

To begin the POCUS obstetric examination, the ultrasound machine should be set to the obstetric examination preset. This decreases the ultrasound's thermal index to the American Institute of Ultrasound in Medicine recommended threshold of <0.7, helping to prevent biological effects on the fetus [9]. The transabdominal approach should be attempted first in all patients, optimally with a full bladder. Standard views include longitudinal and transverse sweeps through the entire uterus, evaluation of the bilateral adnexa, estimation of gestational age, and fetal heart rate measurement (when present). Although the transabdominal examination is traditionally performed using a curvilinear probe, studies have shown that in patients with a low body mass index, the diagnostic accuracy and sensitivity improve when using a high-frequency linear probe using an obstetrics or small parts examination preset (Fig. 12.1, Video 12.1) [10, 11].

If no definitive IUP is visualized transabdominally, the patient should empty their bladder in preparation for a transvaginal examination. Studies have shown that among patients with an indeterminate transabdominal ultrasound, a viable IUP can be identified transvaginally approximately 50% of the time [3]. Patients should be informed that if the transvaginal ultrasound is nondiagnostic for IUP a comprehensive radiology exam may be recommended, allowing the patient to decide their comfort with potentially having a rapid diagnosis versus the potential for two invasive exams. Importantly, endocavitary probes require a high level of disinfection, and therefore clinicians should follow institutional guidelines for cleaning and disinfection after the examination [12].

Clinical Applications

Intrauterine Pregnancy Criteria

The primary goal of POCUS in early pregnancy is to determine if the patient has an IUP [13]. In early pregnancy, some classic sonographic signs such as the "double decidual sac sign" (a round fluid collection bounded by two concentric hyperechoic rings within the uterus) or the "intradecidual sign" (a small fluid sac on one side of the thickened decidual line) may not be visualized [14]. At approximately 5 weeks, the most frequent finding is a gestational sac (a fluid-filled circular sac within the central portion of the uterus) [13]. However, a gestational sac alone does not confirm an IUP. To confirm an IUP, there must also be a yolk sac (a small circular hyperechoic structure within the gestational sac; Fig. 12.2; Video 12.2). The yolk sac appears at approximately 5 ½ weeks gestation and by 6 weeks a fetal pole with a heartbeat can be visualized (Table 12.1) [13].

The fetal heart rate (FHR) can be calculated using M-mode or pulsed-wave Doppler; however, M-mode is preferred because of the theoretical risk of mechanical and thermal damage of Doppler to fetal tissue [15]. To assess FHR, place the M-mode line through the flickering fetal heartbeat. A repeated pattern of movements on the M-mode tracing (appearing similar to a sine wave) located at the same depth as it appears on the B-mode image represents the systolic and diastolic movements of the fetal heart (Fig. 12.3). Using the calculation function on the ultrasound machine, place one of two calipers at the beginning of one heartbeat and the other at the beginning of the next heartbeat. The machine will calculate the FHR based on that distance. Often, the ultrasound machine settings calculate the FHR using the distance between two fetal heartbeats to reduce the effect of beat-to-beat variability. However, the number of fetal heartbeats used for this calculation can also be manually adjusted. The normal FHR range varies based on gestational age (Table 12.2) [16–19].

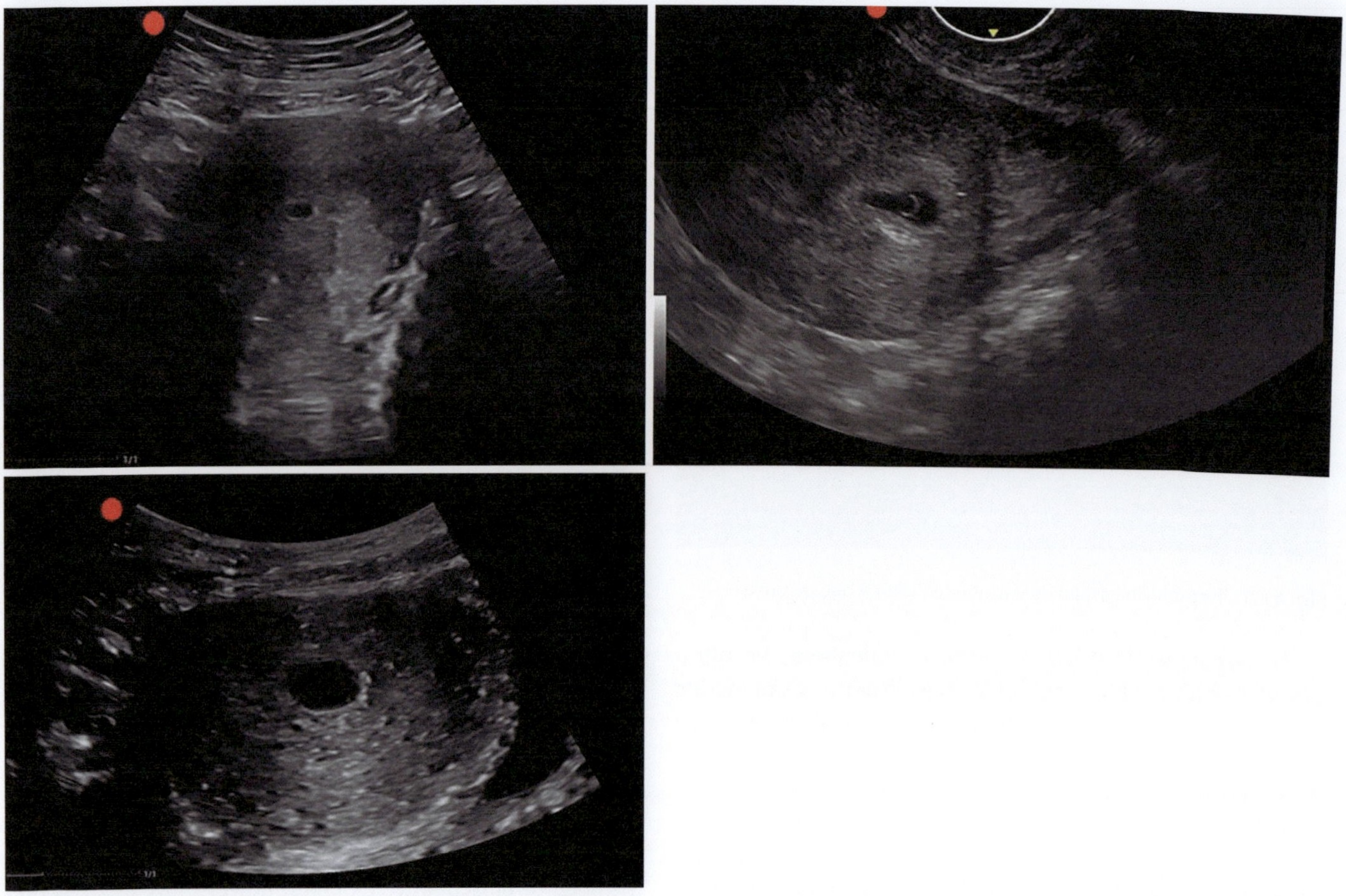

Fig. 12.2 Early intrauterine pregnancy. This figure shows examples of early pregnancy findings. On the left, the two images have small gestational sacs without yolk sacs. These are not confirmed intrauterine pregnancies. The image on the right shows a transvaginal ultrasound with a gestational sac and a yolk sac, confirming an intrauterine pregnancy

Table 12.1 Estimated gestational age and transvaginal ultrasound findings [13]

Estimated gestational age	Ultrasound findings
4.5–5 weeks	Gestational sac
5.5 weeks	Gestational sac with yolk sac
6 weeks	Fetal pole with heartbeat

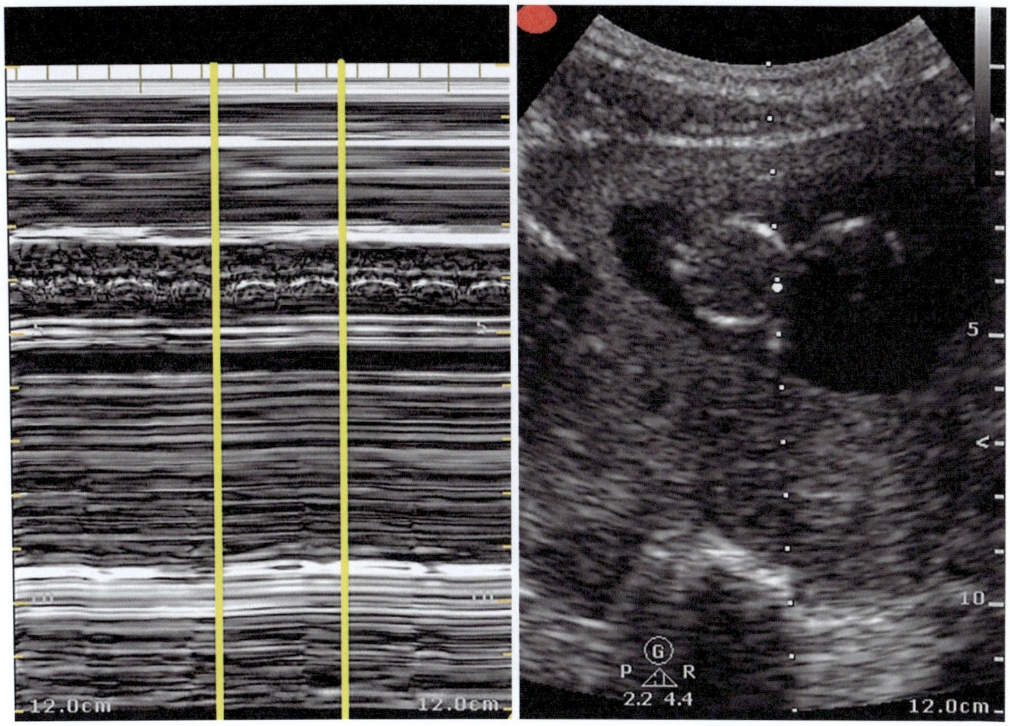

Fig. 12.3 Fetal heart rate measurement. This image shows the M-mode tracing for a fetal heart rate. Based on the ultrasound calculator settings, the distance between two heartbeats was measured to estimate a fetal heart rate

Table 12.2 Normal values for fetal heart rate [16–19]

Gestational age	Range of fetal heart rate
5–6 weeks	90–135 beats/min
6–7 weeks	120–155 beats/min
8–12 weeks	140–180 beats/min
13–27 weeks	135–155 beats/min
>27 weeks	120–160 beats/min

First Trimester Pregnancy

Gestational Age Estimation

The date of the last menstrual period often serves as the initial gestational age estimation. However, ultrasound measurements can supersede this estimate in the setting of significant discrepancy [20]. First trimester ultrasound dating is considered the most accurate [20].

Prior to detecting a fetal pole, an estimation of gestational age can be derived from the mean gestational sac diameter (MSD) (Fig. 12.4). This process involves identifying the gestational sac in its largest diameter. Utilizing calipers, in conjunction with software packages on the ultrasound machine, measure the height and width of the gestational sac. The ultrasound probe is then rotated 90° and the gestational sac's length is measured. The ultrasound software package will use these three measurements to calculate an estimated MSD. While MSD can offer an estimate before the fetal pole is detectable, these measurements should not be used for determinative dating or to rule in an IUP [20]. A gestational sac without definitive evidence of an IUP is a pregnancy of unknown location until proven otherwise.

The most accurate ultrasonographic measurement of gestational age before the 14th week of gestation is the crown-rump length (CRL) [21, 22]. To perform this measurement, identify the fetal pole and align it in a longitudinal plane with the fetal spine in neutral position. Utilizing the calculation function, place calipers at the crown (head) and the rump (bottom) of the fetal pole excluding the yolk sac and any fetal extremities (Fig. 12.5). The ultrasound software package will use this measurement to estimate gestational age. After the first trimester, the accuracy of the CRL measurement diminishes as the fetus begins to flex and extend the spine, leading to a preference for other anatomical measurements (e.g., head circumference, biparietal diameter, femur length) to estimate gestational age in the second and third trimesters [20].

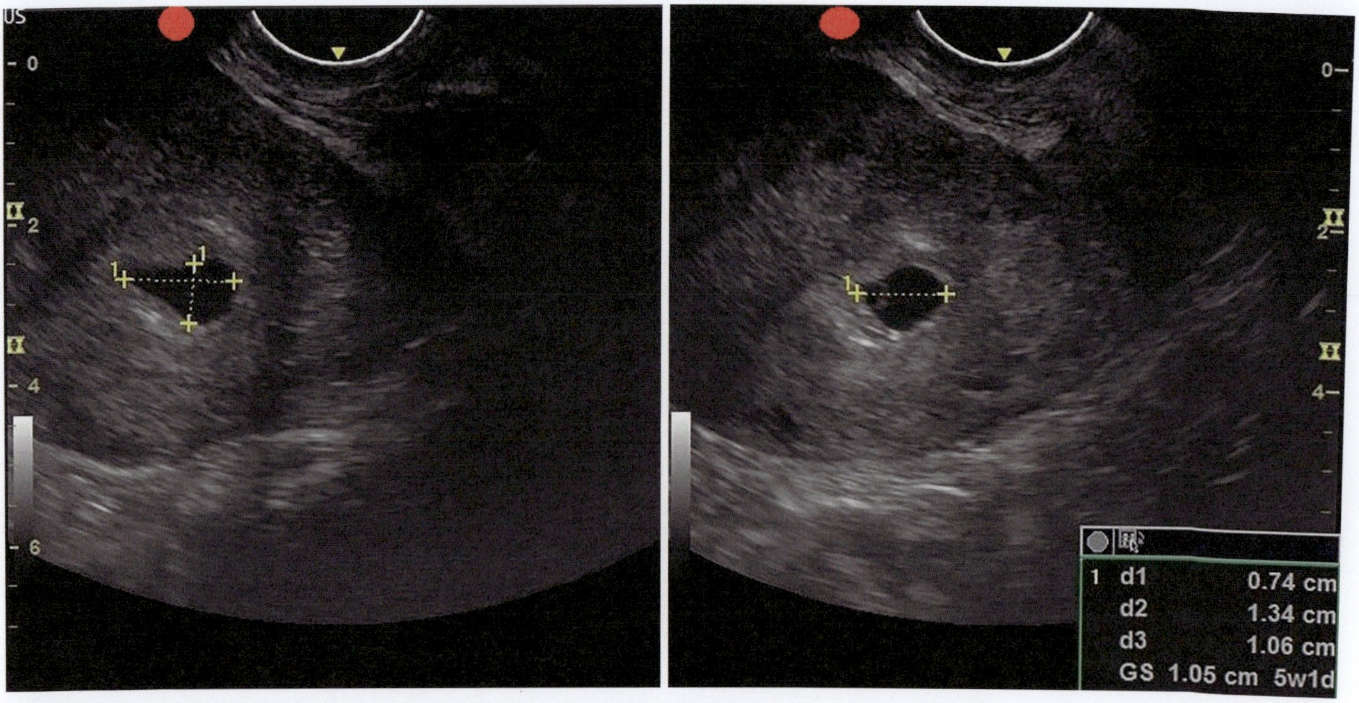

Fig. 12.4 Mean sac diameter. This image shows an example of early pregnancy gestational age estimation using mean sac diameter on a transvaginal ultrasound examination

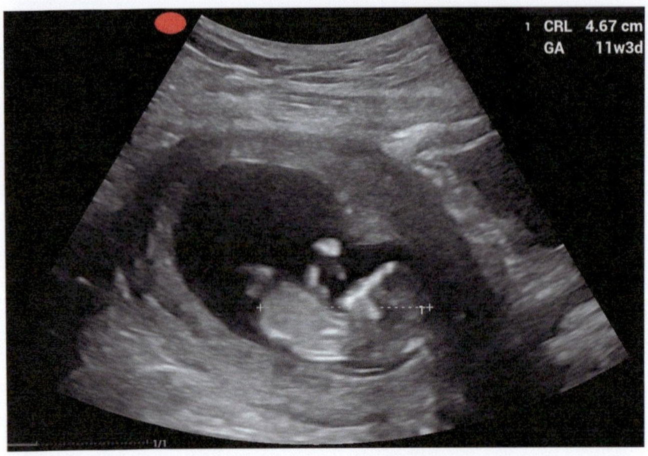

Fig. 12.5 Crown-rump length. This image shows an example of 1st trimester pregnancy gestational age estimation using crown-rump length on a transabdominal ultrasound examination

Multiple Gestations

Multiple gestations can be divided into three main categories according to the number of chorionic and amniotic sacs: dichorionic–diamniotic, monochorionic–diamniotic, and monochorionic–monoamniotic [23]. The amniotic sac is the innermost layer adjacent to the amniotic fluid, appearing as a thin wall on ultrasound. The chorion is the outermost fetal layer and has a much thicker appearance. Similar to gestational age estimation, determination of the chorionicity and amnionicity is most accurate in the first trimester [23].

Chorionicity is ascertained by identification of two or more thick-walled gestational sacs or the identification of multiple placentae later in the first trimester [24]. Early in the first trimester, a triangular-shaped extension of the chorion between the pregnancies ("lambda sign" or "twin peak sign") is associated with dichorionic twins (Fig. 12.6; Video 12.3) [25]. In comparison, the absence of a lambda sign and more perpendicular appearance of a thin separating membrane support a monochorionic–diamniotic pregnancy.

Amniotic sacs can be identified as thin-walled sacs within the chorionic sacs. Monoamniotic twins occur when there is no membrane separating the fetuses. Evaluation of the number of amniotic sacs may need to be repeated on multiple scans due to potential misidentification [24].

Pregnancy of Unknown Location

Early in pregnancy, individuals without an identifiable pregnancy (either intrauterine or ectopic location) on ultrasound are referred to as a pregnancy of unknown location (PUL). Previous studies have evaluated a "discriminatory zone," the beta-human chorionic gonadotropin (hCG) level at which one would expect to visualize a double decidual sign (not yolk sac) on ultrasound (1500 mIU/mL for transvaginal, 5000 mIU/mL for transabdominal). However, more recent

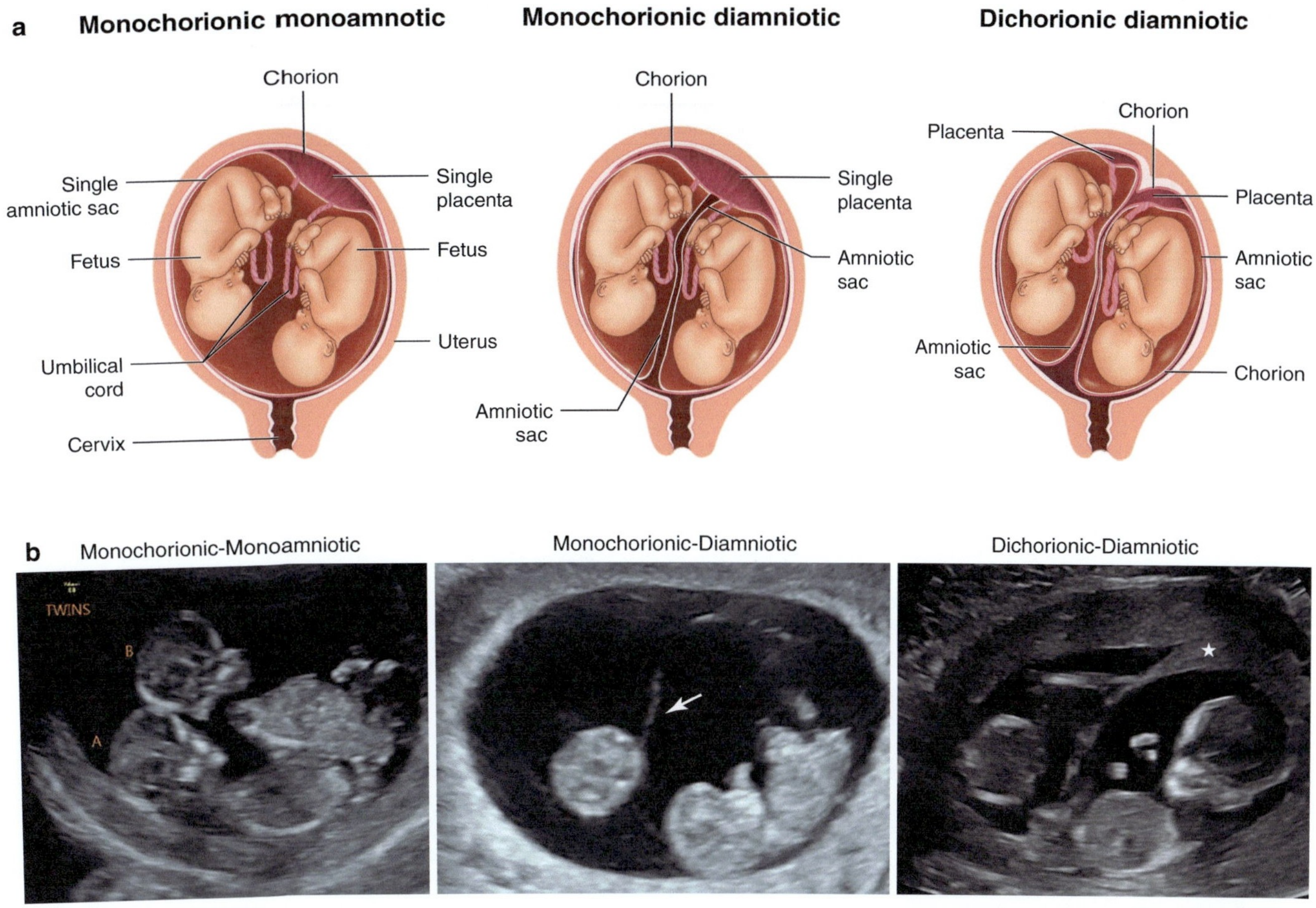

Fig. 12.6 Multiple gestation evaluation (**a**) Illustration of chorionicity and amniotic sac. (**b**) Multiple gestations on ultrasound. The arrow points to the thin amniotic membrane between the fetuses. The asterisk points to the thick chorionic sac between the fetuses

literature indicates that both IUPs and ectopic pregnancies can have values that fall outside the discriminatory zone [26]. Therefore, utilizing the hCG level may provide false reassurance or assume pathology in a normal early pregnancy, though remains useful for trending laboratory values in the setting of a PUL [13, 26–28].

In the setting of a PUL, an ectopic pregnancy should be strongly considered. Hemodynamically stable patients with PUL and no intraperitoneal free fluid should be referred for repeat hCG level testing within 48 hours (with or without repeat imaging) in addition to close follow-up with an obstetrician to determine early pregnancy, nonviable pregnancy, or ectopic pregnancy [29]. At discharge, patients should be given strict return precautions, specifically for pain and vaginal bleeding.

Ectopic Pregnancy

An ectopic pregnancy is any pregnancy that develops in a location other than within the endometrial cavity, most commonly occurring within the fallopian tubes (95%), and rarely within the ovary (<3%), interstitium (2–4%), cesarean scar (<1%), cervix (<1%) and abdomen (<1%) [30]. (Fig. 12.7).

Sonographic findings of a tubal ectopic pregnancy on ultrasound most commonly include an empty uterus with a heterogeneous adnexal mass (Fig. 12.8; Videos 12.4 and 12.5) [31]. Placing color Doppler over the mass may reveal surrounding hyperemia, referred to as a "ring of fire." Identifying a gestational sac with a yolk sac or heartbeat within the adnexal mass confirms an ectopic pregnancy. Ectopic pregnancies of advanced gestational age may be misinterpreted as intrauterine because the placenta and surrounding color flow may look uterine. Careful attention must be paid to confirm the landmarks of the uterus, in two planes, connecting the vaginal stripe to the cervix, and the cervix to the uterus before making any decisions on the location of the pregnancy.

Intra-ovarian ectopic pregnancies are rare and sonographically appear similar to tubal ectopic pregnancies. It may be difficult to distinguish an adnexal ectopic pregnancy from an ovarian corpus luteum. In early pregnancy, even before an

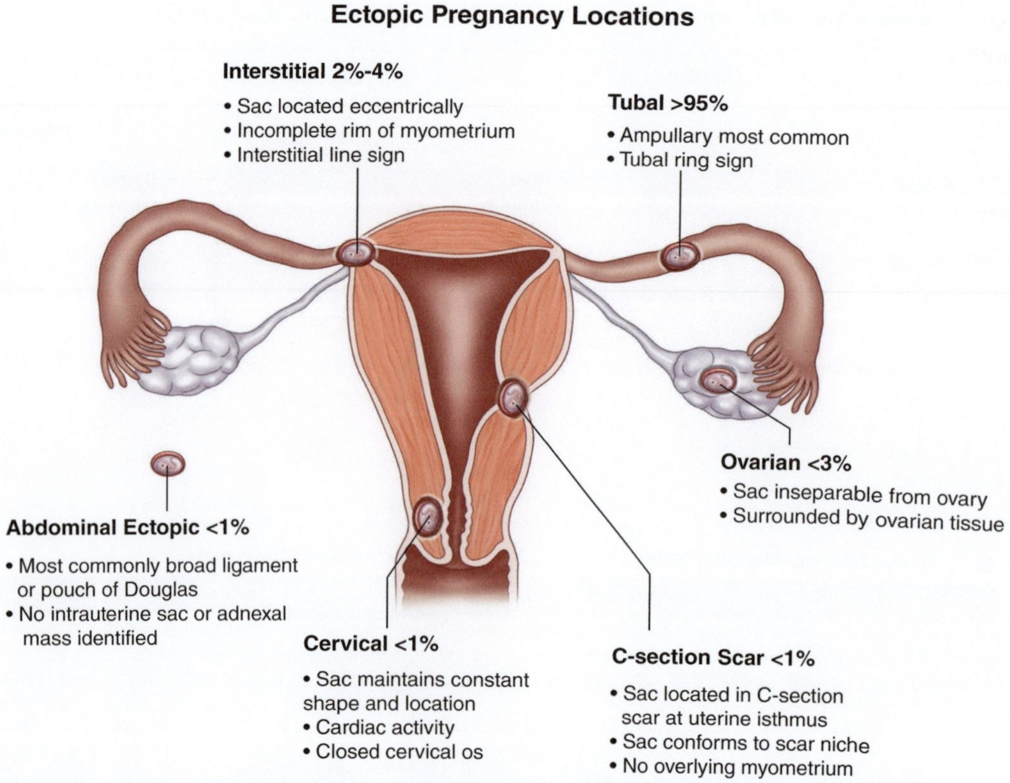

Fig. 12.7 Locations of ectopic pregnancy

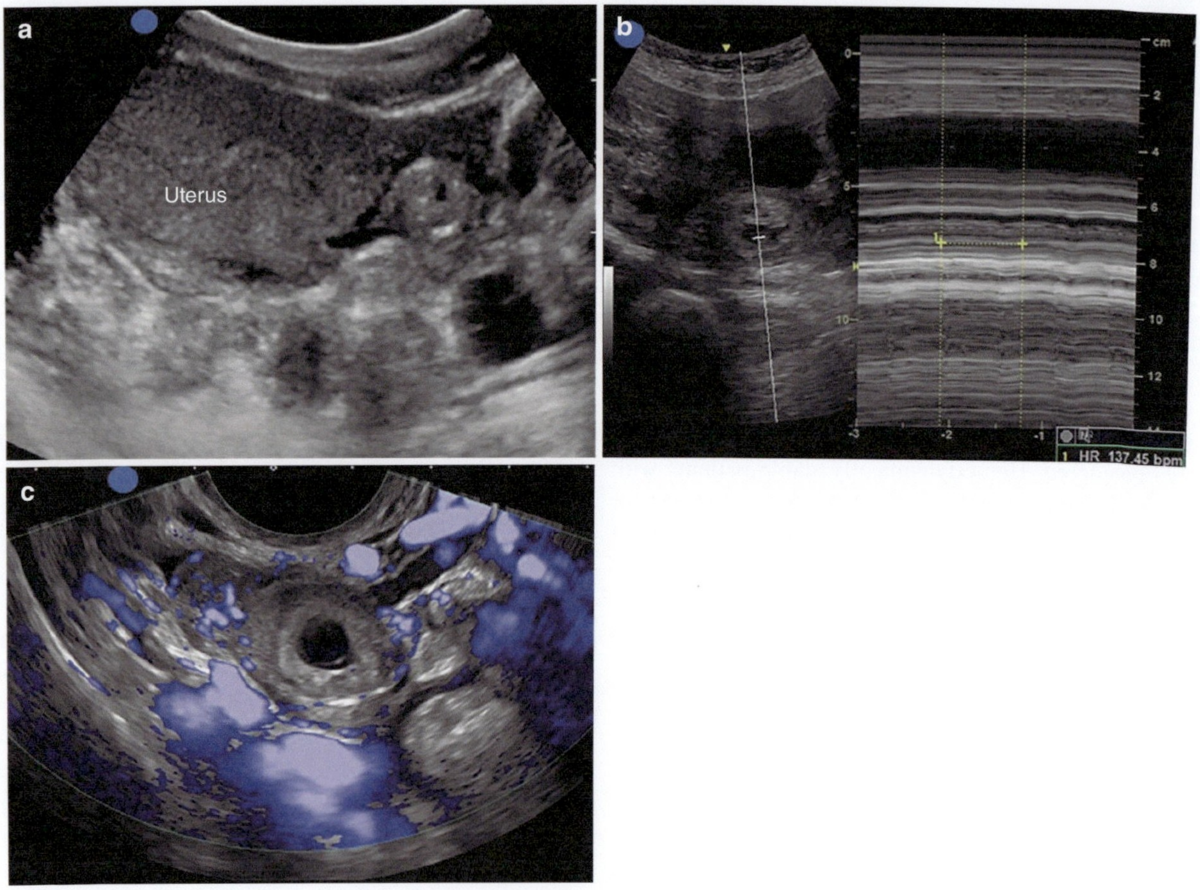

Fig. 12.8 Findings of a tubal ectopic pregnancy. (**a**) Adnexal mass concerning for an ectopic pregnancy. (**b**) Fetal pole and heart tracing outside of the uterus. (**c**) Adnexal mass with a yolk sac and "ring of fire" with color Doppler

IUP is visualized, the corpus luteum acts as an endocrine organ secreting progesterone until placentation occurs (Fig. 12.9; Video 12.6) [32]. A corpus luteum is anechoic, thick walled, and highly vascular. Therefore, it can also have a "ring of fire" appearance on color Doppler (Video 12.7) [32]. One way to distinguish an intra-ovarian mass from a tubal ectopic is to apply manual pressure over the adnexa transabdominally while viewing the ovary with transvaginal ultrasound. A mass that moves with the ovary is intraovarian whereas a mass that slides against or independent of the ovary is tubal.

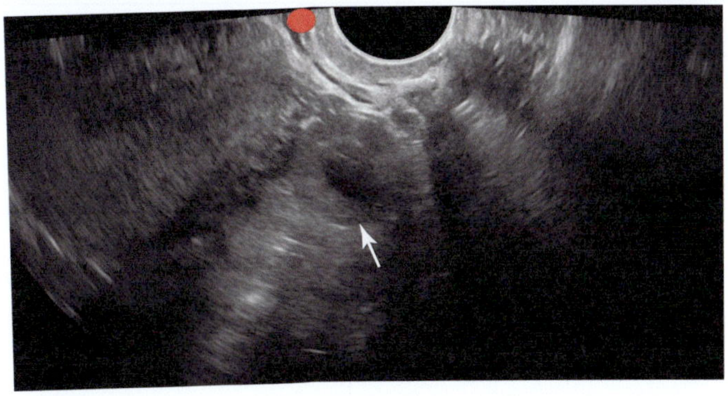

Fig. 12.9 Corpus luteum. This image shows a corpus luteum in the left ovary. Arrow points to a corpus luteum

Ectopic pregnancies outside of the fallopian tubes may present with a variety of findings depending on the location (Fig. 12.10) [33]. Interstitial and cornual ectopic pregnancies will appear on ultrasound as an asymmetrically located gestational sac with less than 8 mm of endomyometrium surrounding it on any side [34]. The endometrial mantle thickness is measured at the thinnest uterine rim from the gestational sac to the outer edge of the myometrium (Fig. 12.11; Video 12.8) [34]. Other ultrasound findings include free fluid in the abdomen and the "interstitial line sign," which refers to an echogenic line that can be seen extending from the endometrial cavity to the uterine cornu abutting the gestational sac (Fig. 12.12) [35, 36].

A Cesarean scar pregnancy develops at the lower uterine segment along scar tissue from a prior Cesarean section. On

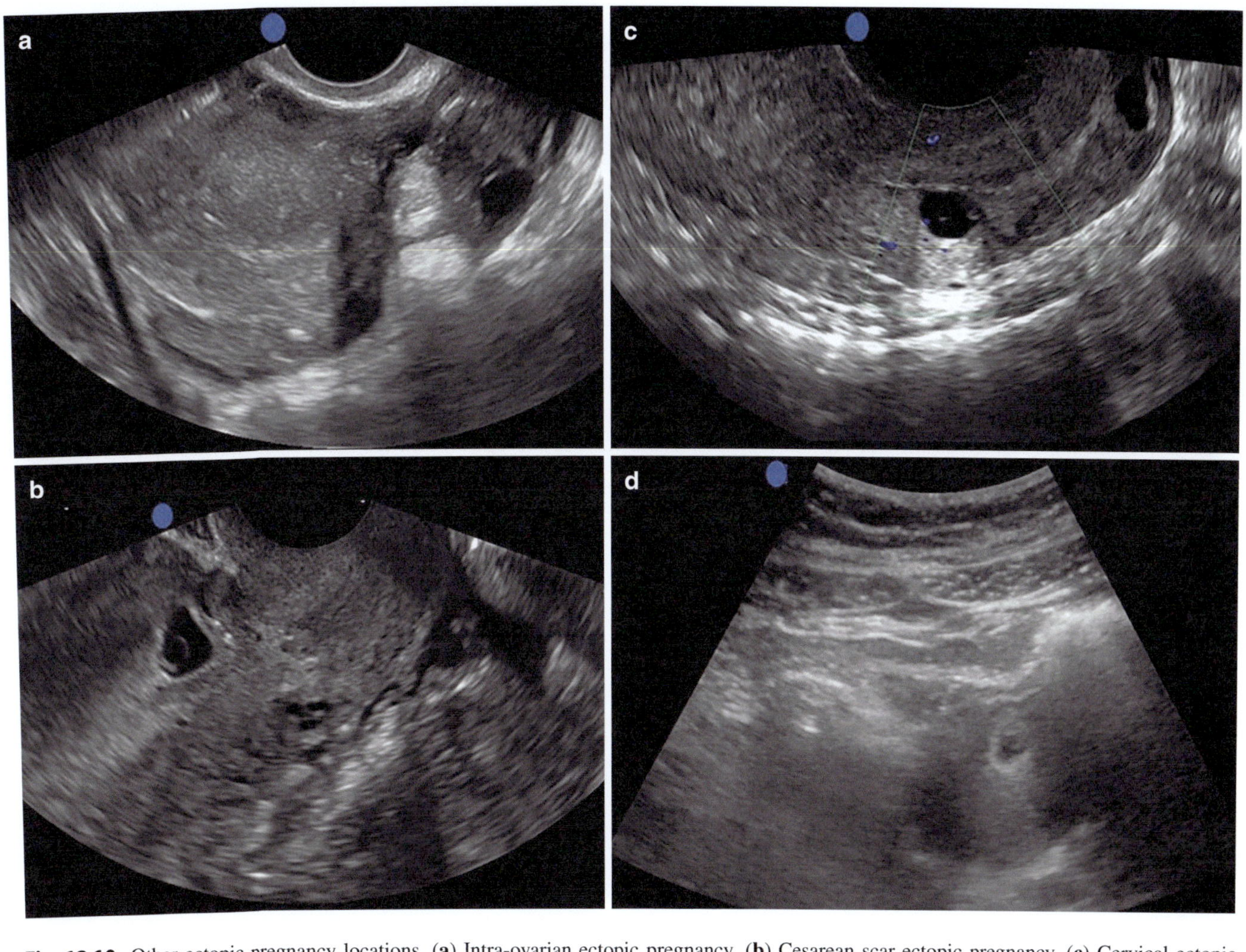

Fig. 12.10 Other ectopic pregnancy locations. (**a**) Intra-ovarian ectopic pregnancy. (**b**) Cesarean scar ectopic pregnancy. (**c**) Cervical ectopic pregnancy. (**d**) Interstitial pregnancy

ultrasound, the gestational sac can appear attached to the scar with myometrial thinning, enhanced blood flow on color Doppler, and a closed internal os (Video 12.9) [31, 37].

A cervical pregnancy will also be located within the lower uterine segment. As the embryo grows, the uterus becomes hourglass shaped with a normal uterine body size and an enlarged cervix [31, 37]. Nabothian cysts, benign fluid-filled structures in the cervix, can mimic cervical ectopic pregnancy. A cervical pregnancy should additionally be distinguished from an active miscarriage. An active miscarriage can be detected by an irregular gestational sac shape and no trophoblastic blood flow, but often patients will need close follow-up.

When an ectopic pregnancy is suspected, it is important to look for evidence of rupture resulting in free fluid in the peritoneal space. This may also be helpful when the ectopic pregnancy is not well-visualized. While a small amount of physiological pelvic fluid (<4 mm stripe in the pelvis) can be normal in young females, moderate-to-large amounts of free fluid in the pelvis or any free fluid in Morison's pouch should be considered a ruptured ectopic pregnancy until proven otherwise [38]. Identification of free fluid in Morison's pouch carries a 99.5% positive predictive value for operative intervention (Video 12.10) [39]. Clotted blood in the pelvis secondary to a slow rupture may be heterogeneously gray instead of the typical black appearance of free intraperitoneal blood.

Finally, a heterotopic pregnancy, defined as a concurrent intrauterine and extrauterine pregnancy, should be considered in any patient who has received reproductive assistance or is under the care of a reproductive endocrinologist (Fig. 12.13) [40]. In this setting, the risk of a heterotopic pregnancy can be up to 1-in-100 to 1-in-500 pregnancies, whereas the risk from natural conception is 1-in-10,000 to 1-in-30,000 pregnancies [40]. Patients with heterotopic pregnancies may present similarly to those with ectopic pregnancy, and the sensitivity of transvaginal ultrasound diagnosis in the first six weeks is only 50–60% [40]. Therefore, any symptomatic patient at risk for a heterotopic pregnancy necessitates an evaluation for an ectopic pregnancy even when an IUP is present.

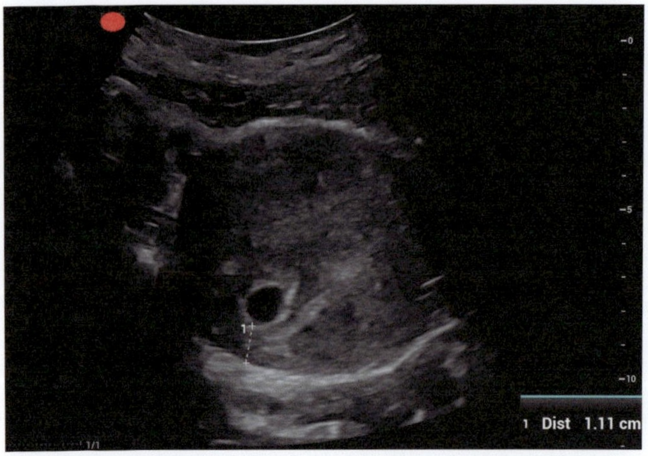

Fig. 12.11 Endometrial mantle thickness measurement. This image shows an example of an eccentrically located pregnancy with the endometrial mantle thickness measured > 8 mm (normal)

First Trimester Complications

Subchorionic Hemorrhage

Subchorionic hemorrhage is a common complication in the first trimester, reported in over 18% of pregnant women [41]. It refers to a crescent-shaped, hypoechoic fluid collection representing blood between the chorionic membrane and the uterine wall (Fig. 12.14; Video 12.11). While there is mixed evidence regarding whether or not a subchorionic hemorrhage poses an increased risk for pregnancy loss, the literature suggests a higher risk of pregnancy loss with increasing size of hemorrhage. One study reported that pregnancy loss rates increased from 7.7% when the subchorionic hemorrhage was small (less than one-third of the chorionic sac circumference) to 18.9% when the subchorionic hemorrhage was large (greater than two-thirds of the circumference) [42].

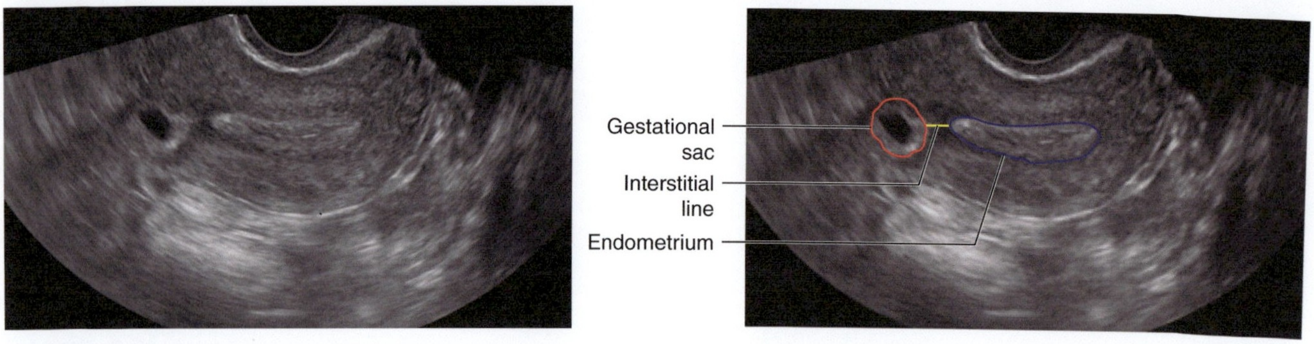

Fig. 12.12 Interstitial line sign

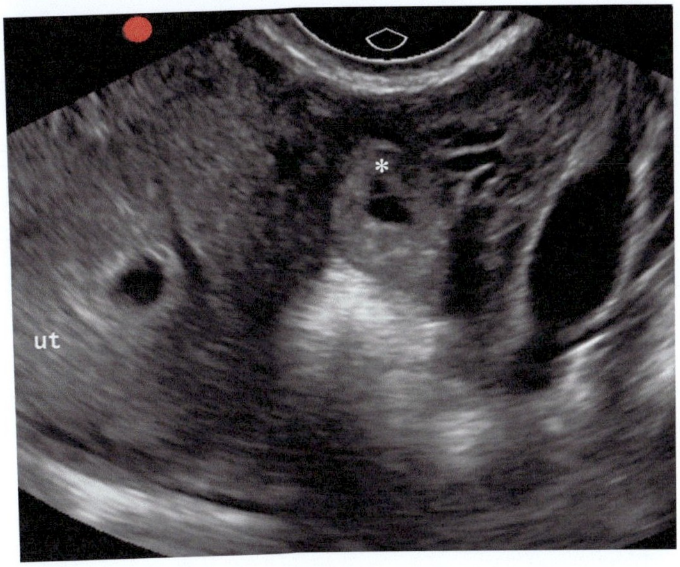

Fig. 12.13 Heterotopic pregnancy. This image demonstrates the simultaneous presence of an intrauterine and an extrauterine pregnancy. The asterisk points to the tubal ectopic pregnancy

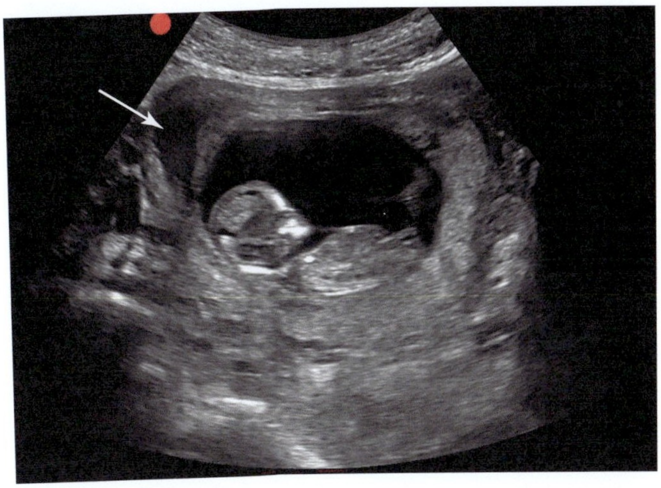

Fig. 12.14 Subchorionic hemorrhage. This image shows an intrauterine pregnancy with an arrow pointing to a subchorionic hemorrhage

Failed Pregnancy

The diagnosis of a failed pregnancy may be made on ultrasound according to various criteria, though the Doubilet Criteria are among the most commonly utilized (Table 12.3) [13]. After an ultrasound concerning for pregnancy failure, a follow-up ultrasound should be completed in 7 to 10 days (Fig. 12.15) [13].

An ultrasound with a loss of fetal heartbeat after previously identified fetal heartbeat on ultrasound should be concerning for an incomplete miscarriage. Patients should be given strict discharge instructions and follow-up. A low-lying gestational sac or clotted blood within the endometrium or vaginal canal may also indicate an incomplete miscarriage. Clotted blood within the endometrium following a miscarriage may also signify RPOC present two or more weeks after a spontaneous or treated abortion [43]. In a complete miscarriage, the ultrasound examination should reveal an empty uterus after having previously identified an IUP.

Ovarian Hyperstimulation Syndrome

Patients receiving *in vitro* fertilization are at risk for ectopic pregnancy, multiple gestations, heterotopic pregnancy, and ovarian hyperstimulation syndrome (OHSS). Patients with OHSS may present with symptoms spanning from abdominal distension, nausea, and vomiting, to life-threatening conditions marked by the third spacing of fluid, leading to massive ascites and pleural effusions [44, 45]. On ultrasound, OHSS is characterized by bilateral enlarged ovaries with multiple enlarged follicles, ascites, and pleural effusions (Fig. 12.16; Video 12.12) [44, 45]. OHSS is graded on the ovarian size and associated symptoms and complications, often using the 2009 updated Golan criteria [46]. Mild OHSS (grade 1 or 2) is associated with ovaries <5 cm in diameter) and lab abnormalities [46]. Moderate OHSS (grade 3 or 4) is associated with ovaries 5 to 12 cm in diameter with abdominal symptoms. Severe OHSS (grade 5 or 6) is associated with ovaries >12 cm in diameter with ascites or pleural effusion [46].

Table 12.3 Guidelines for diagnosis of failed pregnancy on transvaginal ultrasound [13]

Findings diagnostic of failed pregnancy	Findings concerning for but NOT diagnostic of failed pregnancy
• Mean sac diameter ≥25 mm without fetal pole • CRL ≥7 mm without heartbeat • Absence of an embryo WITH a heartbeat ≥2 weeks after a prior ultrasound with a GS without YS • Absence of an embryo WITH a heartbeat ≥11 days after a prior ultrasound with a GS and YS	• Mean sac diameter 16–24 mm without a fetal pole • CRL <7 mm without heartbeat • Absence of an embryo WITH a heartbeat 7–13 days after a prior ultrasound with a GS without YS • Absence of an embryo WITH a heartbeat 7–10 days after a prior ultrasound with a GS and YS • Absence of an embryo ≥6 weeks since LMP • Enlarged YS (≥7 mm) • Empty amnion (amnion seen next to YS without fetal pole) • Small GS relative to fetal pole size (<5 mm difference between mean sac diameter and fetal pole length)

Adapted from Doubilet et al. [13]
CRL crown-rump length, *GS* gestational sac, *YS* yolk sac, *LMP* last menstrual period

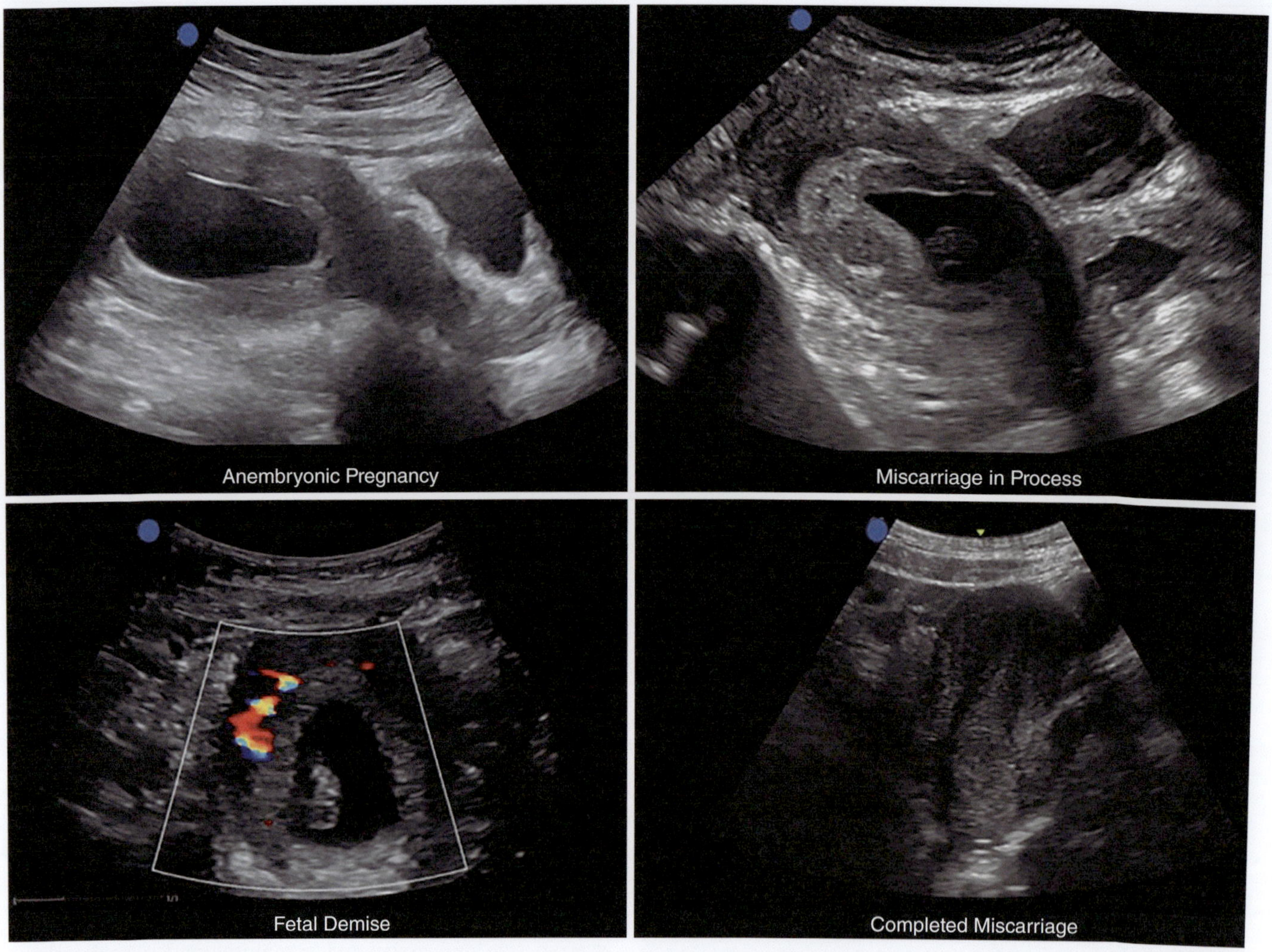

Fig. 12.15 Pregnancy failure

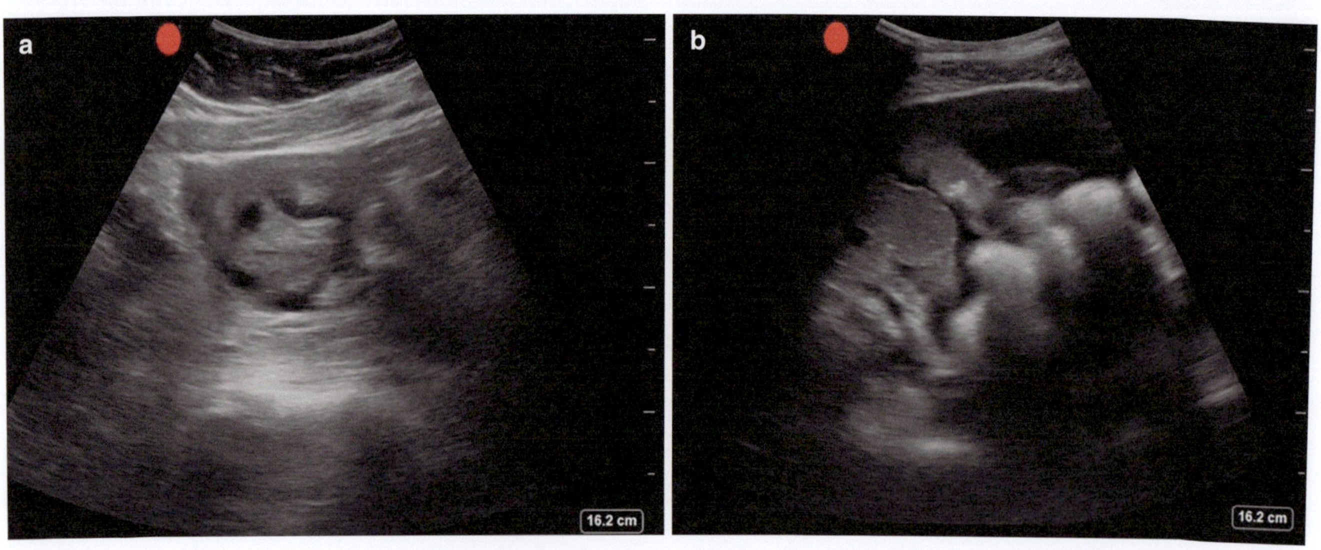

Fig. 12.16 Ovarian hyperstimulation syndrome. (**a**) Ovary with multiple enlarged follicles. (**b**) Ascites from third spacing of fluid

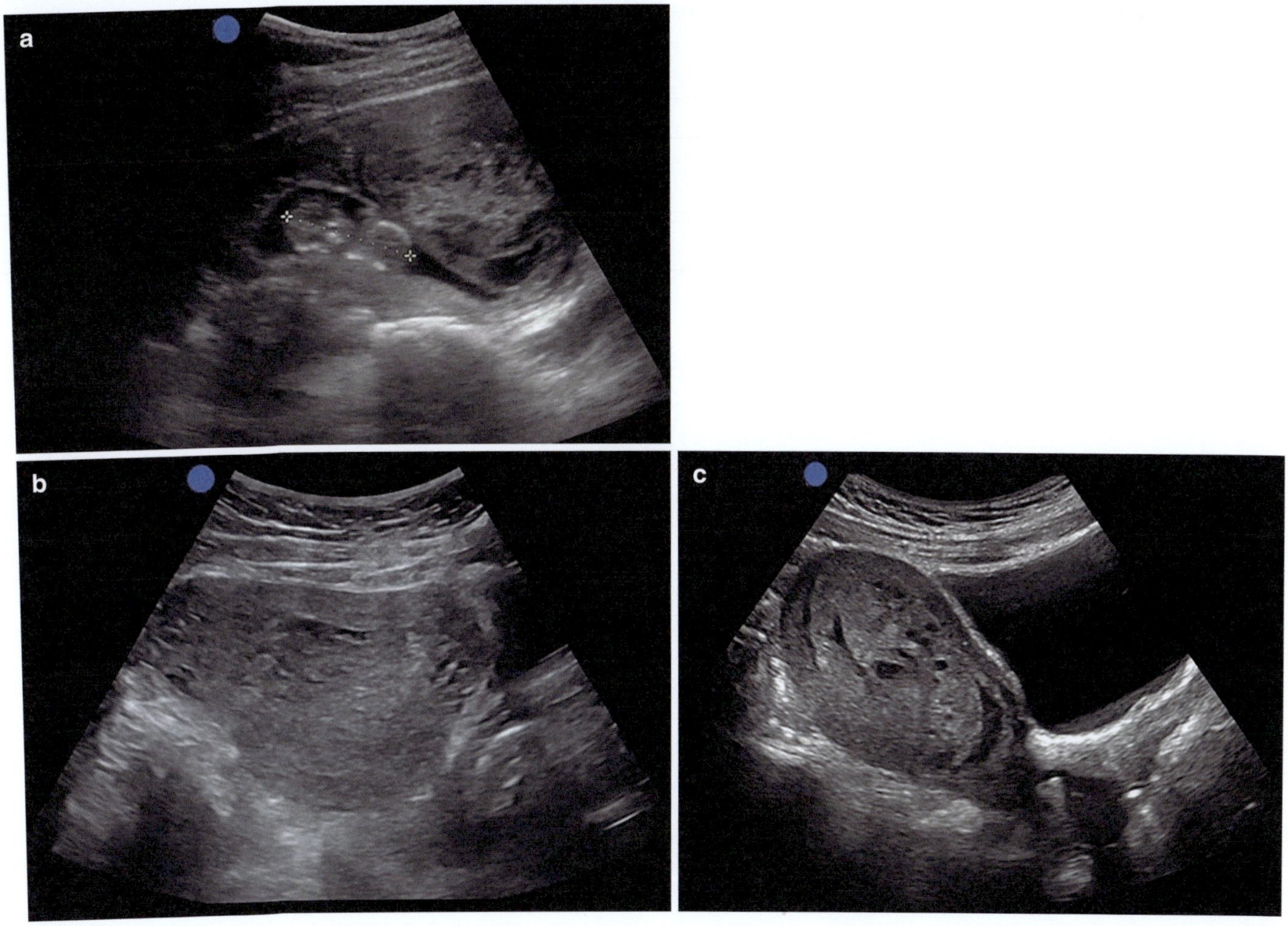

Fig. 12.17 Gestational trophoblastic disease. (**a**) A partial molar pregnancy with the "Swiss Cheese" appearance of the placenta and a fetus. (**b**) Complete molar pregnancy. (**c**) Complete molar pregnancy with a cystic uterine mass

Gestational Trophoblastic Disease

Gestational trophoblastic disease is a spectrum of diseases originating from the placenta [47]. The most common is a hydatidiform mole, which occurs in approximately 1-in-1200 pregnancies [47]. There are two distinct forms of hydatidiform moles: complete and partial. The classic clinical symptoms include vaginal bleeding, hyperemesis, an enlarged uterus, and disproportionately elevated hCG levels for the gestational age. However, due to earlier ultrasound imaging, many patients will present asymptomatically [48].

Ultrasound characteristics of a complete mole typically include an enlarged uterus filled with an echogenic mass. This echogenic mass may contain several hypoechoic and anechoic structures of varying sizes, giving rise to a characteristic "snowstorm" or a "cluster of grapes" appearance (Fig. 12.17; Video 12.13) [48].

In contrast, the ultrasound characteristics of a partial mole may be more subtle. In a partial mole, the placenta is enlarged compared to the uterine cavity, and it may contain internal cystic changes resulting in a "Swiss cheese pattern" [48]. Additionally, a fetus may be present.

Second and Third Trimesters

Gestational Age Assessment

The standard fetal parameters typically measured to assess the gestational age during the second and third trimester include biparietal diameter (BPD), head circumference (HC), abdominal circumference (AC), and femur length (FL) [49].

BPD is obtained at the level of the thalami and cavum septi pellucidi without the presence of cerebellar hemispheres in the image, measuring from the outer edge of the proximal skull to the inner edge of the distal skull

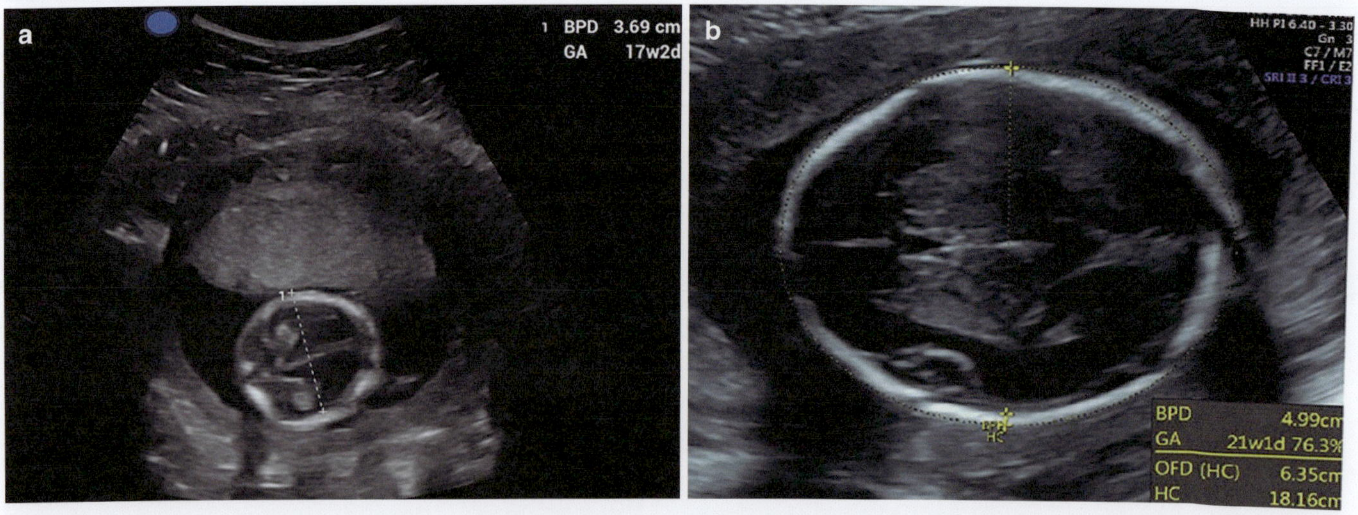

Fig. 12.18 Gestational age using cranial measurements (**a**) Biparietal diameter. (**b**) Head circumference

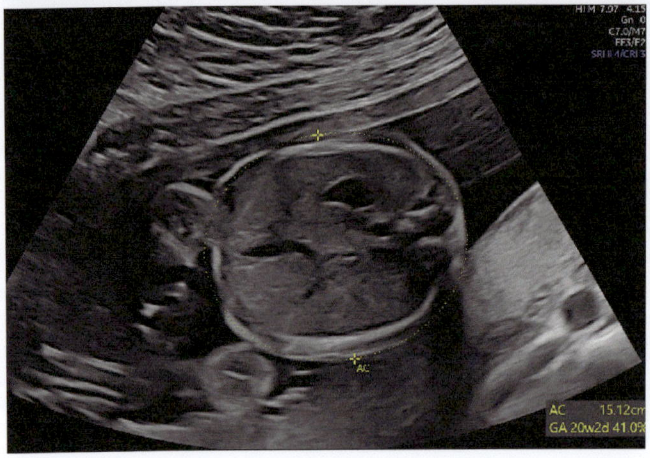

Fig. 12.19 Abdominal circumference

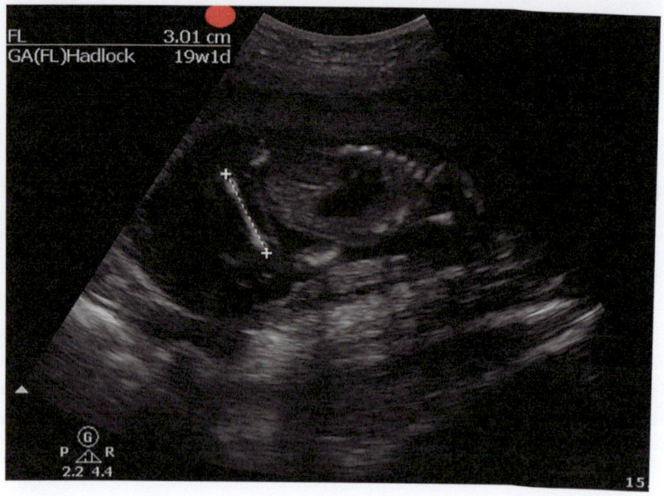

Fig. 12.20 Femur length

(Fig. 12.18a) [50]. HC is obtained at the same level as the BPD, drawing a circle around the outer edge of the skull (Fig. 12.18b) [49]. AC is obtained at the level of the junction of the umbilical vein, portal sinus, and fetal stomach, drawing a circle around the outer edge of the abdominal cavity (Fig. 12.19) [49]. It is important to stay parallel to fetal ribs to avoid oblique over measurement. FL is measured as a single linear measurement of the femoral diaphysis (Fig. 12.20) [49]. When measuring the FL, it is important to exclude cartilage; measuring only the hyperechoic shaft and not the hypoechoic ends.

Dating in the second and third trimester is less accurate than dating in the first trimester [49]. Without prior dating confirmation, the average gestational age of the fetus should be derived from the average gestational age associated with each fetal measurement [49]. When rapid information is needed (e.g., impending delivery or the need to go to the operating room), the easiest measurement to obtain may be the femur length as a single linear measurement.

While AC is a poor parameter for dating, it is a reliable reflection of growth, such that a fetus in a diabetic pregnancy may have a larger liver and more subcutaneous fat resulting in a larger AC, while a growth-restricted fetus will have a HC appropriate for gestational age but may have an AC that lags by 2–3 weeks in size [51]. If there are fetal growth abnormalities such as fetal growth restriction, suggested by a smaller AC than anticipated according to HC dating, an estimated fetal weight (EFW) calculation can be performed using the obstetrics examination preset and the fetal measurements [51].

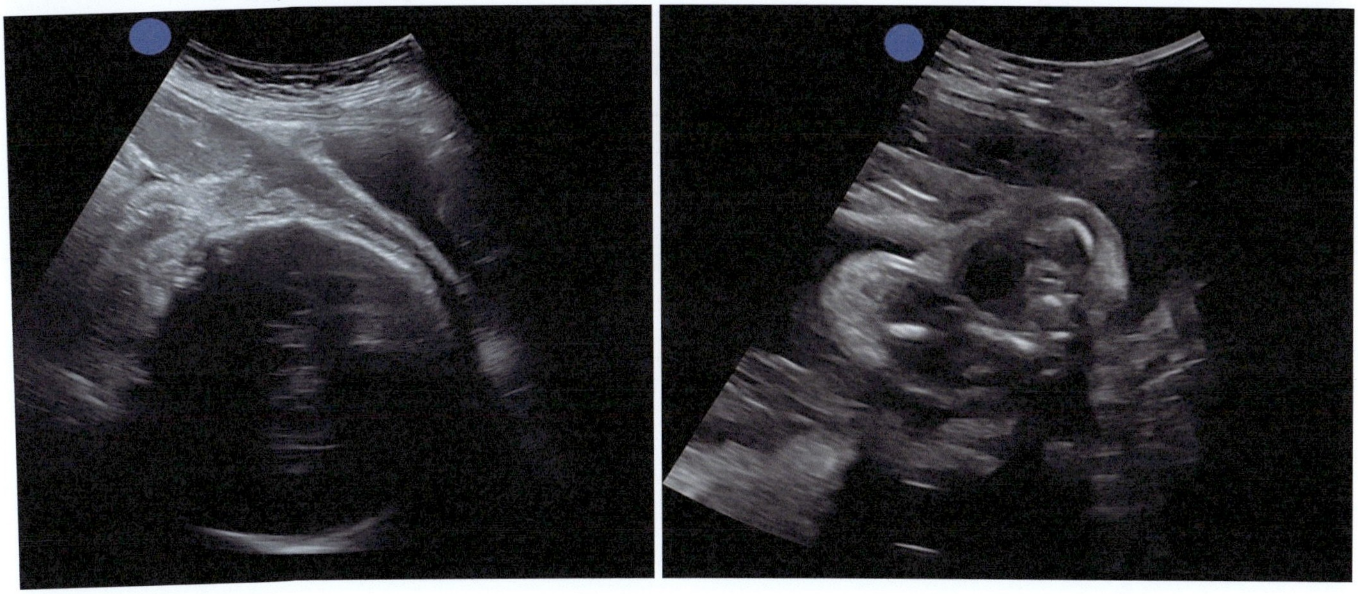

Fig. 12.21 Fetal presentation. This image shows an example of a fetus in cephalic position (left) and breech position (right)

Fetal Presentation

Fetal presentation is the position of the leading part of the fetus or anatomical structure closest to the cervix. To evaluate the fetal presentation, the curvilinear probe is placed in a sagittal orientation superior to the pubic symphysis [52]. The fetal part that overlies the cervix determines the presentation (Fig. 12.21).

The three fetal presentations are cephalic, breech, and transverse [53]. In a cephalic presentation, the fetus is vertically oriented with the fetal head seen over the cervix. In a breech presentation, the fetal feet or rump are seen over the cervix. In a transverse presentation, the fetus will lie with its spine horizontal to the maternal spine with the fetal abdomen seen over the cervix. Breech and transverse fetuses carry a high risk of cord prolapse and typically require Cesarean delivery [54]. Therefore, knowing the fetal position is critical for delivery planning.

Multiple Gestations

With multiple gestations such as twins, the following components should be identified in the second and third trimester: position of each fetus, FHR for each fetus, number and location of placentae, twin membrane to determine chorionicity (as described above) and deepest vertical pocket for each fetus (see below) [55]. Ideally, the twin membrane is identified and the respective pocket of fluid for each twin is measured on either side of the membrane. Twin A is typically defined as the fetus closest to the cervix.

Second and Third Trimester Complications

Placental Complications

In the setting of vaginal bleeding in the second or third trimester, it is important to assess placenta location. To obtain a good view of the placenta and cervical canal, the patient's bladder should be full in order to provide an enhanced acoustic window. The placenta appears as a slightly hyperechoic, homogenous mass adherent to the uterine wall [56]. The location of the placenta can be anterior, posterior, fundal, or lateral in relation to the uterine myometrium (Fig. 12.22; Video 12.14). The placenta may also have accessory lobes, and therefore it is important to fully interrogate the entire uterine cavity when assessing the placenta.

In placenta previa, there is evidence of placental tissue over the cervix (Fig. 12.23). A complete previa occurs when the placenta directly covers the internal os. A low-lying placenta or marginal placenta previa is when the placental edge is <2 cm from the internal os [57]. Over time, the placenta moves superiorly with the stretching of the lower uterine segment; therefore, a placenta overlying the cervix in the first or early second trimester may not be present by the third trimester ultrasound. If a pregnancy approaches 37 weeks with a known placenta previa, a Cesarean delivery is recommended as labor can precipitate vaginal bleeding [58].

In placenta accreta, there is a morbidly adherent placenta that grows into the uterine wall and remains attached after birth. On ultrasound, this can appear as irregularly shaped placental lacunae and increased vascularity at the uterine–placental interface (Figure 12.24). The risk of placenta

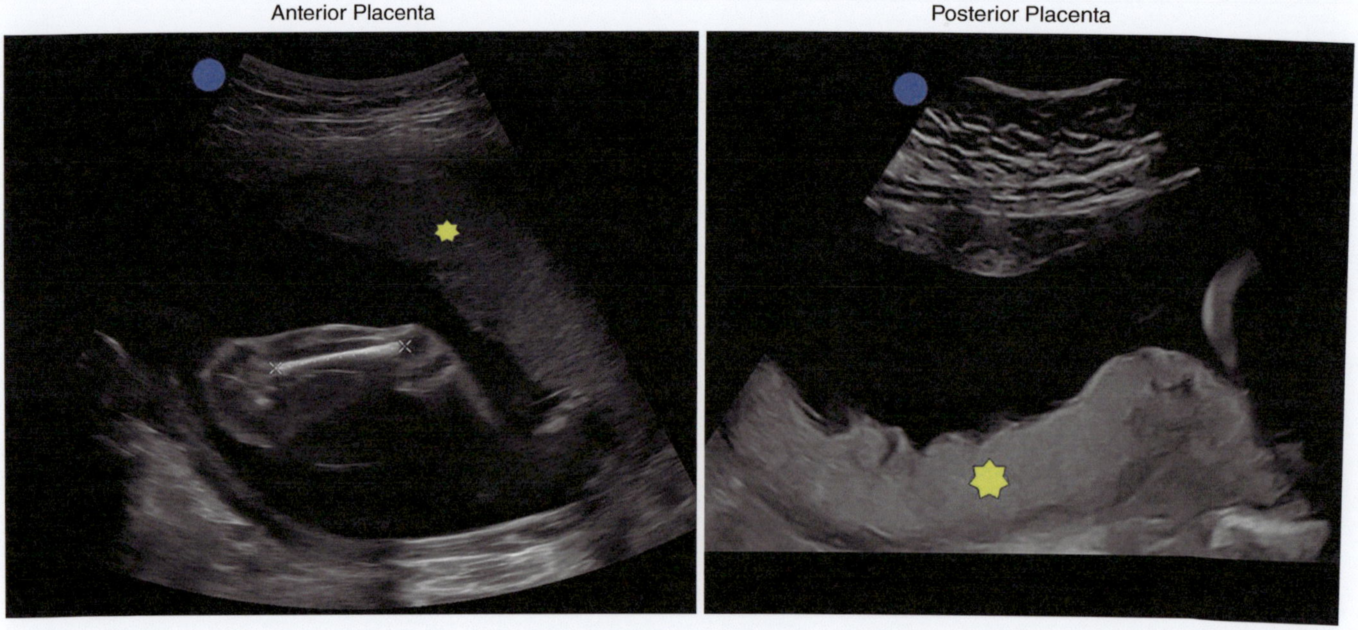

Fig. 12.22 Placental location. This image shows an example of an anterior (left) and a posterior (right) placenta location. Star indicates the placenta

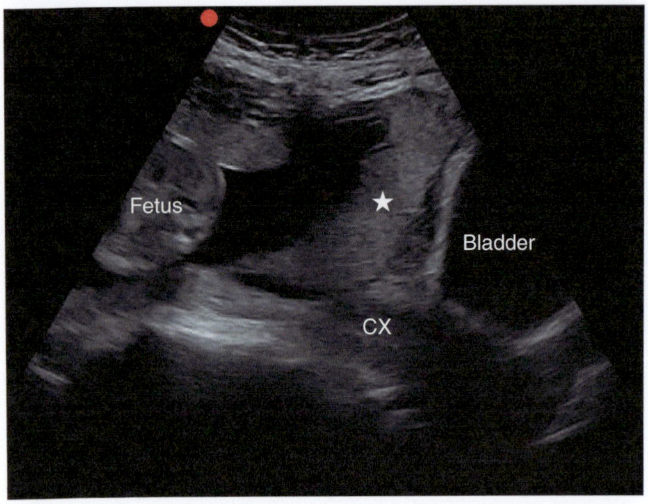

Fig. 12.23 Placenta previa. This image shows a placenta in close proximity to the internal os. *CX* cervix

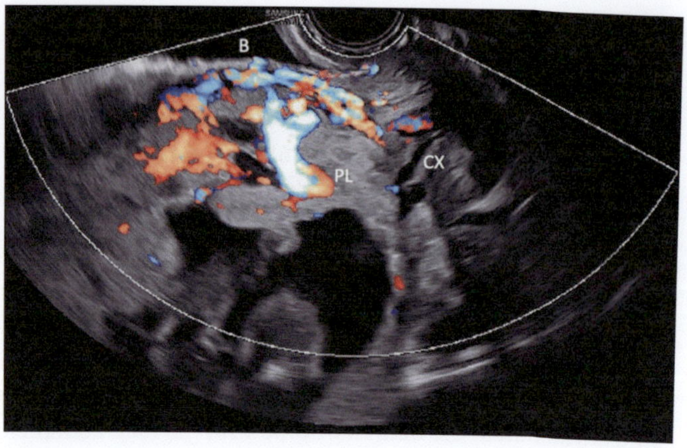

Fig. 12.24 Placenta Accreta. This image shows an example of placenta accreta. *CX* cervix, *PL* placenta, *B* bladder

accreta is increased in patients with a history of Cesarean section and previa during the index pregnancy [59].

In vasa previa, there is evidence of the fetal vessels overlying the cervix. To evaluate for this, a transvaginal ultrasound examination is necessary to evaluate the lower uterine segment above the cervix. Confirmation of a fetal vessel can be obtained by color Doppler and documenting the FHR with pulsed-wave Doppler [60]. While there is no standard prescribed pulse repetition frequency used for this, a frequency lower than 1.3 kHz can lead to artifacts from fetal movement. Additionally, a funic cord presentation (i.e., the presence of the umbilical cord between the cervix and fetal presenting part) can lead to a false positive finding of vasa previa. As with placenta previa, an internal digital examination should not be performed in patients with vasa previa, as disruption of these vessels could lead to fetal bleeding and even exsanguination [61].

In placental abruption, there is a premature placental separation. This may be difficult to visualize on ultrasound (sen-

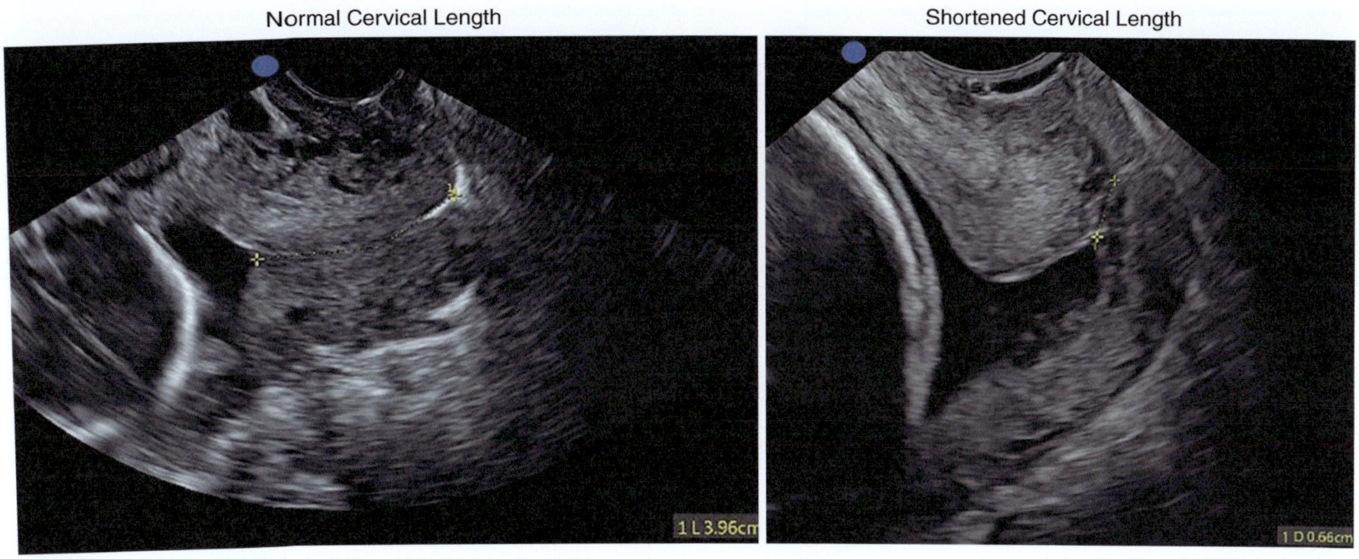

Fig. 12.25 Cervical length. This image shows an example of a normal cervical length (left) as compared to a shortened cervical length (right)

sitivity of 57%) and should be considered in any patient with painful vaginal bleeding without an obvious cause [62, 63]. Findings of placental abruption include pre-placenta hematoma, movement of the placenta when pressure is applied ("jello sign"), increased placental thickness, and intra-amniotic hematoma [63]. One key finding is a retroplacental hematoma volume larger than 50 mL, which signifies a significant placental abruption and higher risk of poor fetal outcome [64]. However, on ultrasound this may sometimes only appear as a thickened placenta [63].

Cervical Length

Cervical lengths are typically monitored in patients at risk of preterm birth to determine if further treatment is indicated. The cervix is viewed using an endocavitary probe when the bladder is empty. The sonographer identifies and measures the closed aspect of the cervical canal from the internal os to the external os (Fig. 12.25) [65]. Excessive pressure on the cervix should be avoided as it can falsely elongate the cervix.

While transvaginal cervical length measurements help to reduce unnecessary resources, the evidence for their role alone in the management of threatened preterm labor is unclear [66–68]. Prior to 23 weeks gestation, a transvaginal cervical length <25 mm may be associated with a higher risk of preterm birth [69]. If the cervix is short and the patient is asymptomatic, she may be evaluated for vaginal progesterone or cerclage prior to 23 weeks depending on prior obstetrical history. While a digital examination provides extensive information on cervical consistency, position, effacement, and dilation after 24 weeks [70], the sonographic cervical length may have a role when a digital examination is contraindicated.

Amniotic Fluid Status

Amniotic fluid is a marker of fetal well-being. During the second half of pregnancy, it is predominantly composed of fetal urine and reflects adequate fetal renal perfusion by the placenta [71]. Amniotic fluid can be assessed at any gestational age by the single deepest vertical pocket (DVP) without any fetal parts or umbilical cord in the measurement. The DVP normally ranges from 2 cm to 8 cm with a pocket width of 1 cm [72]. After 24 weeks gestational age, an amniotic fluid index (AFI) can be obtained by using the patient's umbilicus as the center of a crux, such that there is a right and left lower quadrant below the umbilicus and a right and left upper quadrant above it (Fig. 12.26). The sum of the DVP from each of the four quadrants is used to assess fluid status.

A DVP <2 cm or an AFI <5 cm is suspicious for oligohydramnios, and typically results from loss of fluid (e.g., premature rupture of membranes (PROM), preterm premature rupture of membranes (PPROM)) or poor production of fluid (e.g., placental insufficiency, renal agenesis, posterior urethral valves) [71]. Polyhydramnios is defined as a DVP >8 cm or an AFI >25 cm and is usually idiopathic but can also occur with diabetes with poor glucose control or fetal structural anomalies such as esophageal atresia [73].

Uterine Rupture

Uterine rupture is a rare event that carries high morbidity and mortality for both the fetus and the mother. Women with prior uterine scarring are at an increased risk for rupture, with most of the events occurring during labor [74]. On ultrasound, fetal membranes may be seen through the uterine defect (or in the abdomen with full rupture), and free intra-abdominal fluid may also be present [74].

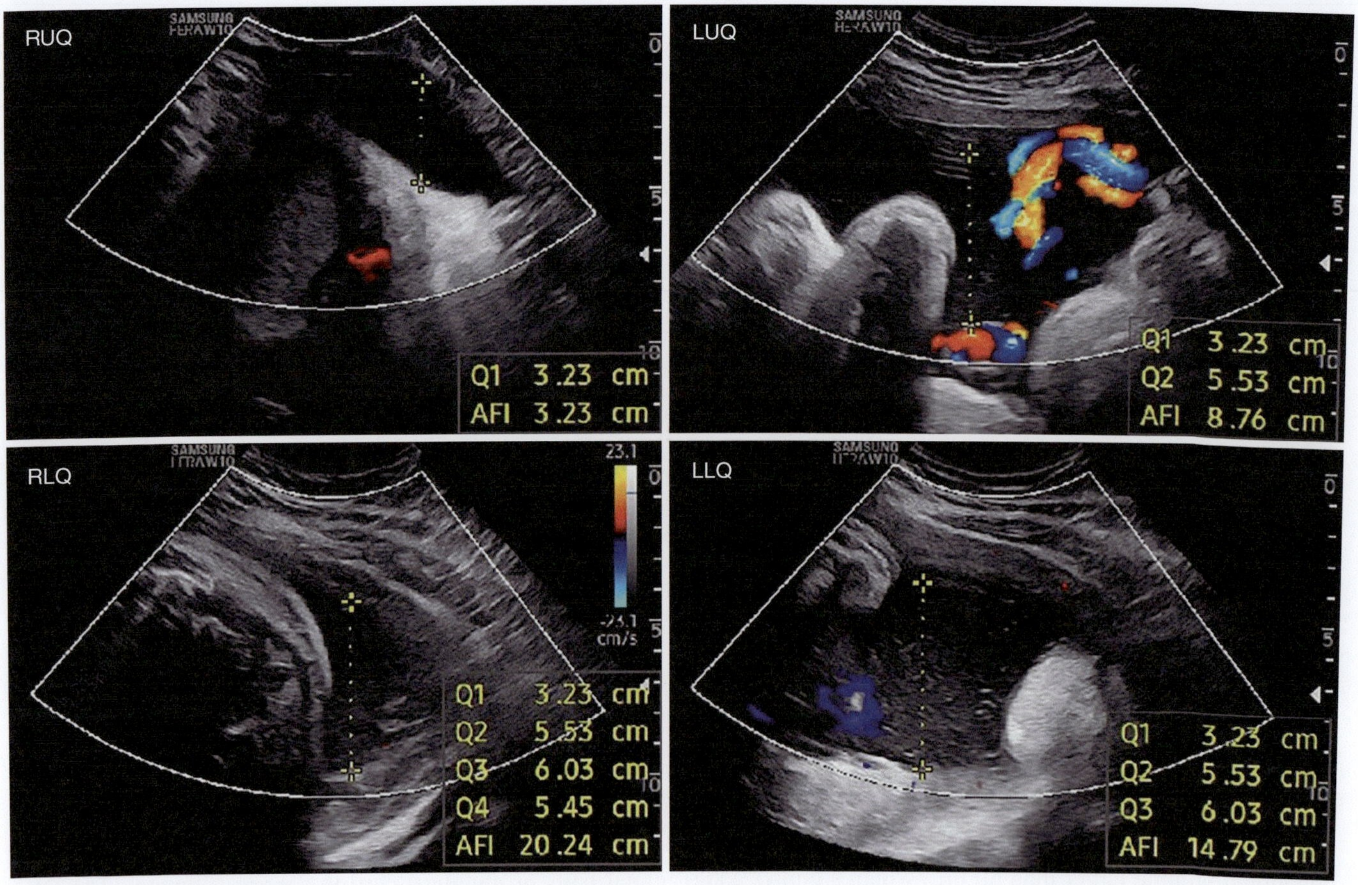

Fig. 12.26 Amniotic fluid index. This image shows the 4 quadrant measurements of an amniotic fluid index. *LUQ* left upper quadrant, *RUQ* right upper quadrant, *LLQ* left lower quadrant, *RLQ* right lower quadrant

Fetal Heart Rate Abnormalities

Beyond 24 weeks gestation, it is critical to confirm the FHR is within normal range (Table 12.2). Transient fetal tachycardia can result from fetal activity or maternal tachycardia. Sustained fetal tachycardia can result from maternal fever or fetal arrhythmias that can produce an FHR >200 beats per minute. Sustained rates this high can lead to high-output cardiac failure and fetal hydrops (interstitial fluid build-up in at least 2 fetal organ systems, including fetal pleural effusions, pericardial effusions, and ascites) [75].

Fetal bradycardias can be transient, spontaneous, self-limiting, or associated with fetal decelerations. Sustained fetal bradycardia (less than 100 beats per minute for 10 minutes or more) is concerning for maternal hypotension, umbilical cord compression, uterine hyperstimulation, or rapid descent of the fetal head into the pelvis [75]. Less common causes of fetal bradycardia include placental abruption, placental infarction, uterine rupture, or maternal hypoxia, and rarely fetal arrhythmias. For this reason, it is important to involve an obstetrician early in case emergent Cesarean delivery is needed.

Preterm Birth

If there is concern for imminent preterm birth, the FHR, fetal presentation, amniotic fluid status, location of the placenta, and estimated gestational age (if time allows) should be determined. Once a previa has been excluded, the cervix should be directly assessed to determine if delivery is impending. The evaluation of fetal presentation will help to determine Cesarean delivery (transverse presentation) versus vaginal delivery (breech, cephalic).

Fetal Demise

In the setting of fetal demise, where no fetal cardiac activity is observed, it is important to determine the following information: gestational age, fetal presentation, and AFI. The gestational age will determine whether a dilation and evacuation procedure or vaginal delivery is the best next step. Fetal demise before 24 weeks is best managed by dilation and evacuation [76]. The Spalding sign (overlapping of the fetal skull bones due to fetal brain collapse) or skin edema may be noted in fetal demise which has been present for over a week [77].

Retained Products of Conception

Abnormal postpartum bleeding or concern for uterine infection after delivery merits assessment of the intrauterine cavity for RPOC. To evaluate for RPOC, assess the uterus in both a long and short axis and apply color Doppler with the pulse repetition frequency set between 2 to 9 cm/s over the area of concern (Fig. 12.27) [78]. In the early postpartum period, the endometrium is thickened, heterogenous, and gradually decreases in size over time. By one month postpartum, the upper limit of normal for endometrial thickness has been reported as 1.2 cm [79]. An echogenic heterogeneous mass within the endometrium that is >1.5 cm, with surrounding color Doppler signal and a pulsed-wave Doppler with a resistive index <0.45 is supportive of RPOC [78]. After a miscarriage, visualization of a gestational sac or fetal parts within this region is strongly supportive of RPOC. Endometrial fluid alone or a thickened endometrium can be present without RPOC. Color Doppler signals in the uterine myometrium, particularly greater than 20 cm/s, could suggest an acquired enhanced myometrial vascularity (EMV) [80]. In EMV, there are notable color signals of tortuous vessels within the myometrium adjacent to the endometrial cavity, which reflect a vascular malformation arising from the myometrial venous plexus or uterine artery branches. EMVs are associated with heavy postpartum bleeding and require alternative management such as uterine artery embolization [80].

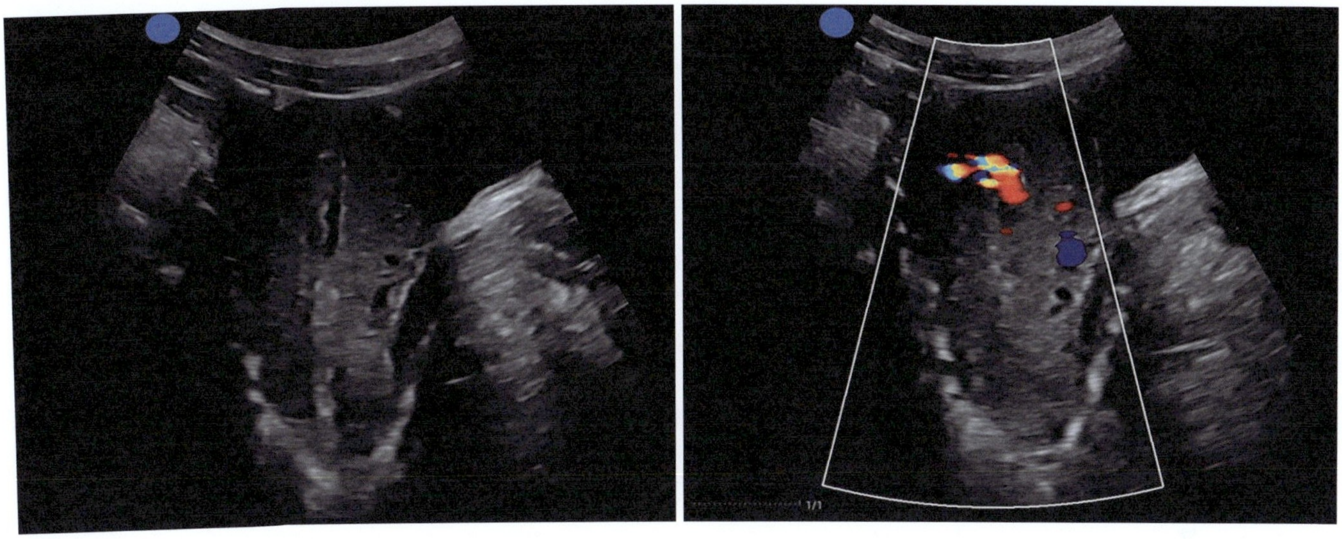

Fig. 12.27 Retained products of conception. Notice the thickened endometrium on the left and increase in color Doppler over the endometrium on the right

Key Ultrasound Findings

Gestational age measurements	
Mean sac diameter	Measured by taking mean diameter of length, width, and height of GS. Utilized for estimation of gestational age when no FP is present.
Crown-rump length	Measure length from the head to the rump of the FP excluding YS and limbs. Utilized for estimation of gestational age in the first trimester.
Abdominal circumference	Circumference of the fetal abdomen at the level of the umbilical vein, portal sinus, and fetal stomach. Utilized for estimation of gestational age in second/third trimester.
Biparietal diameter	Diameter of the fetal skull at the level of the thalami and cavum septi pellucidi without cerebellum. Measured from the outer table to the inner table of the skull. Utilized for estimation of gestational age in second/third trimester.
Head circumference	Measure circumference of head utilizing ellipse tool at same level as biparietal diameter. Utilized for estimation of gestational age in second/third trimester.
Femur length	Measurement of length of the long axis of the femur excluding cartilage. Estimation of gestational age in second/third trimester.
Ectopic pregnancies by location	
Tubal	Appears within adnexa as: Complex mass with or without peripheral hyperemia (ring of fire). GS with YS or FP in adnexa.
Ovarian	Similar in appearance to tubal but found within ovary. Need to distinguish from corpus luteum.
Interstitial	Appears as IUP with a myometrial thickness < 8 mm. Eccentric within the uterus. Interstitial line sign.
Cesarean scar	Low-lying pregnancy at site of prior Cesarean section with myometrial thinning.
Cervical	Low-lying pregnancy with myometrial thinning and surrounding blood flow. Distinguish from miscarriage, which will have irregular shape sac.
Heterotopic	Twin pregnancy with IUP plus ectopic pregnancy. High index of suspicion, especially in patients with history of IVF.
First trimester pregnancy complications	
Subchorionic hemorrhage	Crescent-shaped hypoechoic collection of fluid surrounding IUP. Possible increased risk of miscarriage.
Failed pregnancy	GS >25 mm without YS or FP. FP >7 mm without heartbeat. Absence of an embryo WITH a heartbeat ≥2 weeks after a scan with a GS without YS. Absence of an embryo WITH a heartbeat ≥11 days after a scan with a GS and YS.
Ovarian hyperstimulation syndrome	Typically, in patients undergoing fertility treatments. Bilateral enlarged ovaries with multiple follicles and abdominal symptoms, can develop massive ascites and pleural effusions in severe cases.
Gestational trophoblastic disease	Associated with significantly higher beta-human chorionic gonadotropin than expected for pregnancy duration. "Snowstorm" appearance in uterus.
Second and third trimester assessments	
Placental location	Slightly hyperechoic, homogenous mass adherent to the GS. Anterior, posterior, fundal or lateral position.
Fetal presentation	Determined by fetal part closest to the cervix. Presentations include cephalic, breech, and transverse.
Amniotic fluid status	DVP is the depth measured in an area without fetal parts or umbilical cord. AFI is the sum of the DVP in 4 abdominal quadrants.
Cervical length	Measured transvaginal from internal os to external os. <25 mm associated with preterm birth.
Second and third trimester complications	
Oligohydramnios	DVP <2 cm or AFI <5 cm.
Polyhydramnios	DVP >8 cm or AFI >24 cm.
Placenta previa	Complete previa—placental coverage over the cervical os. Marginal previa—placenta <2 cm away from the cervical os.
Placenta accreta	Placenta adherence to the myometrium.
Vasa previa	Fetal vessels overlying the cervical os.
Fetal heart rate	FHR >200 bpm can lead to fetal high-output cardiac failure. FHR <100 bpm for more than 10 minutes is concerning for fetal distress.
Fetal demise	No FHR present. Obtain gestational age, fetal presentation, and AFI.
Preterm labor	Obtain FHR, fetal presentation, placental location, and AFI.
RPOC	Heterogeneous mass in the endometrium >1.5 cm thick with surrounding color Doppler flow.

GS gestational sac, *YS* yolk sac, *IUP* intrauterine pregnancy, *IVF* in vitro fertilization, *DVP* deepest vertical pocket, *AFI* amniotic fluid index, *FHR* fetal heart rate, *BPD* biparietal diameter

Pearls and Pitfalls

- A transvaginal ultrasound should be performed with an empty bladder, while a transabdominal ultrasound is best performed with a full bladder.
- Minimum criteria for an intrauterine pregnancy are an intrauterine gestational sac containing a yolk sac or fetal pole.
- Intrauterine pregnancy should be surrounded by at least 8 mm of myometrium.
- Gestational dating is more accurate the earlier it is performed; crown-rump length is best in the first trimester, while biparietal diameter and femur length are best in the second and third trimesters.
- Suspect heterotopic pregnancy even after identifying an intrauterine pregnancy in patients receiving fertility treatments.
- In patients with vaginal bleeding after the second trimester, evaluate the placental position to look for signs of placenta previa.
- In patients with impending delivery, evaluate fetal presentation.
- On ultrasound, patients with RPOC have a heterogeneously enlarged endometrium.

References

1. Geissler KH, Pearlman J, Attanasio LB. Physician referrals during prenatal care. Matern Child Health J. 2021;25(12):1820–8. https://doi.org/10.1007/s10995-021-03236-x.
2. Matenchuk BA, Rosychuk RJ, Rowe BH, et al. Emergency department visits during pregnancy. Ann Emerg Med. 2023;81(2):197–208. https://doi.org/10.1016/j.annemergmed.2022.06.021.
3. Panebianco NL, Shofer F, Fields JM, et al. The utility of transvaginal ultrasound in the ED evaluation of complications of first trimester pregnancy. Am J Emerg Med. 2015;33(6):743–8. https://doi.org/10.1016/j.ajem.2015.02.023.
4. Ultrasound guidelines: emergency, point-of-care, and clinical ultrasound guidelines in medicine. Ann Emerg Med. 2023;82(3):e115–55. https://doi.org/10.1016/j.annemergmed.2023.06.005.
5. Mann LM, Kreisel K, Llata E, et al. Trends in ectopic pregnancy diagnoses in United States emergency departments, 2006–2013. Matern Child Health J. 2020;24(2):213–21. https://doi.org/10.1007/s10995-019-02842-0.
6. Murray H, Baakdah H, Bardell T, et al. Diagnosis and treatment of ectopic pregnancy. CMAJ. 2005;173(8):905–12. https://doi.org/10.1503/cmaj.050222.
7. Stein JC, Wang R, Adler N, et al. Emergency physician ultrasonography for evaluating patients at risk for ectopic pregnancy: a meta-analysis. Ann Emerg Med. 2010;56(6):674–83. https://doi.org/10.1016/j.annemergmed.2010.06.563.
8. Burgher SW, Tandy TK, Dawdy MR. Transvaginal ultrasonography by emergency physicians decreases patient time in the emergency department. Acad Emerg Med. 1998;5(8):802–7. https://doi.org/10.1111/j.1553-2712.1998.tb02507.x.
9. Prudent use and safety of diagnostic ultrasound in pregnancy. www.aium.org. Accessed 27 March 2024. https://www.google.com/url?q=https://www.aium.org/resources/official-statements/view/prudent-use-and-safety-of-diagnostic-ultrasound-in-pregnancy&sa=D&source=docs&ust=1711567547296282&usg=AOvVaw3mizVeFk5E9jr-drRNQ4VX.
10. Çelik A, Yazıcı MM, Oktay M. The impact of high-frequency linear transducer on the accuracy of pelvic ultrasound in early pregnancy pelvic pain and bleeding. Am J Emerg Med. 2022;61:105–10. https://doi.org/10.1016/j.ajem.2022.08.045.
11. Tabbut M, Harper D, Gramer D, et al. High-frequency linear transducer improves detection of an intrauterine pregnancy in first-trimester ultrasonography. Am J Emerg Med. 2016;34(2):288–91. https://doi.org/10.1016/j.ajem.2015.11.001.
12. Guideline for Ultrasound Transducer Cleaning and Disinfection. Ann Emerg Med. 2018;72(4):e45–7. https://doi.org/10.1016/j.annemergmed.2018.07.035.
13. Doubilet PM, Benson CB, Bourne T, et al. Diagnostic criteria for nonviable pregnancy early in the first trimester. N Engl J Med. 2013;369(15):1443–51. https://doi.org/10.1056/NEJMra1302417.
14. Phillips CH, Benson CB, Durfee SM, et al. "Pseudogestational Sac" and other 1980s-era concepts in early first-trimester ultrasound: are they still relevant today? J Ultrasound Med. 2020;39(8):1547–51. https://doi.org/10.1002/jum.15243.
15. Aiken CE, Lees CC. Long-term effects of in utero Doppler ultrasound scanning – a developmental programming perspective. Med Hypotheses. 2012;78(4):539–41. https://doi.org/10.1016/j.mehy.2012.01.030.
16. Ogenyi P, Chiegwu HU, England A, et al. Appraisal of trimester-specific fetal heart rate and its role in gestational age prediction. Radiography (Lond). 2022;28(4):926–32. https://doi.org/10.1016/j.radi.2022.06.015.
17. Smrcek JM, Berg C, Geipel A, et al. Early fetal echocardiography: heart biometry and visualization of cardiac structures between 10 and 15 weeks' gestation. J Ultrasound Med. 2006;25(2):173–82. https://doi.org/10.7863/jum.2006.25.2.173.
18. Ouyang Y, Qin J, Lin G, et al. Reference intervals of gestational sac, yolk sac, embryonic length, embryonic heart rate at 6-10 weeks after in vitro fertilization-embryo transfer. BMC Pregnancy Childbirth. 2020;20(1):533. https://doi.org/10.1186/s12884-020-03186-2.
19. Doubilet PM, Benson CB, Chow JS. Outcome of pregnancies with rapid embryonic heart rates in the early first trimester. AJR Am J Roentgenol. 2000;175(1):67–9. https://doi.org/10.2214/ajr.175.1.1750067.
20. Committee Opinion No 700: methods for estimating the due date. Obstet Gynecol. 2017;129(5):e150–4. https://doi.org/10.1097/AOG.0000000000002046.
21. Bailey C, Carnell J, Vahidnia F, et al. Accuracy of emergency physicians using ultrasound measurement of crown-rump length to estimate gestational age in pregnant females. Am J Emerg Med. 2012;30(8):1627–9. https://doi.org/10.1016/j.ajem.2011.12.002.
22. Saul T, Lewiss RE, Rivera MDR. Accuracy of emergency physician performed bedside ultrasound in determining gestational age in first trimester pregnancy. Crit Ultrasound J. 2012;4(1):22. https://doi.org/10.1186/2036-7902-4-22.
23. Monteagudo A, Roman AS. Ultrasound in multiple gestations: twins and other multifetal pregnancies. Clin Perinatol. 2005;32(2):329–54. https://doi.org/10.1016/j.clp.2005.02.006.
24. Jha P, Morgan TA, Kennedy A. US evaluation of twin pregnancies: importance of chorionicity and amnionicity. Radiographics. 2019;39(7):2146–66. https://doi.org/10.1148/rg.2019190042.
25. Maruotti GM, Saccone G, Morlando M, et al. First-trimester ultrasound determination of chorionicity in twin gestations using the lambda sign: a systematic review and meta-analysis. Eur J Obstet

Gynecol Reprod Biol. 2016;202:66–70. https://doi.org/10.1016/j.ejogrb.2016.04.023.
26. Wang R, Reynolds TA, West HH, et al. Use of a β-hCG discriminatory zone with bedside pelvic ultrasonography. Ann Emerg Med. 2011;58(1):12–20. https://doi.org/10.1016/j.annemergmed.2010.12.023.
27. Robertson JJ, Long B, Koyfman A. Emergency medicine myths: ectopic pregnancy evaluation, risk factors, and presentation. J Emerg Med. 2017;53(6):819–28. https://doi.org/10.1016/j.jemermed.2017.08.074.
28. Condous G, Kirk E, Lu C, et al. Diagnostic accuracy of varying discriminatory zones for the prediction of ectopic pregnancy in women with a pregnancy of unknown location. Ultrasound Obstet Gynecol. 2005;26(7):770–5. https://doi.org/10.1002/uog.2636.
29. Pereira PP, Cabar FR, Gomez ÚT, Francisco RPV. Pregnancy of unknown location. Clinics (Sao Paulo). 2019;74:e1111. https://doi.org/10.6061/clinics/2019/e1111.
30. Chukus A, Tirada N, Restrepo R, et al. Uncommon implantation sites of ectopic pregnancy: thinking beyond the complex Adnexal mass. Radiographics. 2015;35(3):946–59. https://doi.org/10.1148/rg.2015140202.
31. Lee R, Dupuis C, Chen B, et al. Diagnosing ectopic pregnancy in the emergency setting. Ultrasonography. 2018;37(1):78–87. https://doi.org/10.14366/usg.17044.
32. Bonde AA, Korngold EK, Foster BR, et al. Radiological appearances of corpus luteum cysts and their imaging mimics. Abdom Radiol. 2016;41(11):2270–82. https://doi.org/10.1007/s00261-016-0780-1.
33. Scibetta EW, Han CS. Ultrasound in early pregnancy: viability, unknown locations, and ectopic pregnancies. Obstet Gynecol Clin N Am. 2019;46(4):783–95. https://doi.org/10.1016/j.ogc.2019.07.013.
34. Lewiss RE, Shaukat NM, Saul T. The endomyometrial thickness measurement for abnormal implantation evaluation by pelvic sonography. J Ultrasound Med. 2014;33(7):1143–6. https://doi.org/10.7863/ultra.33.7.1143.
35. Schraft E, Gottlieb M. Near fatal interstitial pregnancy. Am J Emerg Med. 2022;57:235.e5–8. https://doi.org/10.1016/j.ajem.2022.04.007.
36. Malinowski A, Bates SK. Semantics and pitfalls in the diagnosis of cornual/interstitial pregnancy. Fertil Steril. 2006;86(6):1764.e11–4. https://doi.org/10.1016/j.fertnstert.2006.03.073.
37. Feng H, Zheng Y, Ke Y. Ultrasound vs. histologic findings in 40 patients with special types of ectopic pregnancy. Am J Transl Res. 2021;13(7):7829–38.
38. Hussain ZJ, Figueroa R, Budorick NE. How much free fluid can a pregnant patient have? Assessment of pelvic free fluid in pregnant patients without antecedent trauma. J Trauma. 2011;70(6):1420–3. https://doi.org/10.1097/TA.0b013e3181edc4fe.
39. Moore C, Todd WM, O'Brien E, et al. Free fluid in Morison's Pouch on bedside ultrasound predicts need for operative intervention in suspected ectopic pregnancy. Acad Emerg Med. 2007;14(8):755–8. https://doi.org/10.1197/j.aem.2007.04.010.
40. Hassani KM, El Bouazzaoui A, Khatouf M, et al. Heterotopic pregnancy: a diagnosis we should suspect more often. J Emerg Trauma Shock. 2010;3(3):304. https://doi.org/10.4103/0974-2700.66563.
41. Naert MN, Khadraoui H, Muniz Rodriguez A, et al. Association between first-trimester subchorionic hematomas and pregnancy loss in singleton pregnancies. Obstet Gynecol. 2019;134(2):276–81. https://doi.org/10.1097/AOG.0000000000003360.
42. Bennett GL, Bromley B, Lieberman E, et al. Subchorionic hemorrhage in first-trimester pregnancies: prediction of pregnancy outcome with sonography. Radiology. 1996;200(3):803–6. https://doi.org/10.1148/radiology.200.3.8756935.
43. Hamel CC, van Wessel S, Carnegy A, et al. Diagnostic criteria for retained products of conception-a scoping review. Acta Obstet Gynecol Scand. 2021;100(12):2135–43. https://doi.org/10.1111/aogs.14229.
44. Frasure SE, Rempell JS, Noble VE, et al. Emergency ultrasound diagnosis of ovarian Hyperstimulation syndrome: case report. J Emerg Med. 2012;43(2):e129–32. https://doi.org/10.1016/j.jemermed.2011.06.148.
45. Bellapu S, Guttman J. Use of point-of-care ultrasound for the diagnosis of ovarian hyperstimulation syndrome. J Emerg Med. 2017;52(4):e101–4. https://doi.org/10.1016/j.jemermed.2016.11.026.
46. Golan A, Weissman A. A modern classification of OHSS. Reprod Biomed Online. 2009;19(1):28–32. https://doi.org/10.1016/S1472-6483(10)60042-9.
47. Soper JT. Gestational trophoblastic disease: current evaluation and management. Obstet Gynecol. 2021;137(2):355–70. https://doi.org/10.1097/AOG.0000000000004240.
48. Lukinovic N, Malovrh EP, Takac I, et al. Advances in diagnostics and management of gestational trophoblastic disease. Radiol Oncol. 2022;56(4):430–9. https://doi.org/10.2478/raon-2022-0038.
49. AIUM–ACR–ACOG–SMFM–SRU practice parameter for the performance of standard diagnostic obstetric ultrasound examinations. J Ultrasound Med. 2018;37(11):E13–24. https://doi.org/10.1002/jum.14831.
50. Salerno A, Flanagan K, Ghaffarian K, et al. Quantitative and qualitative analysis of emergency physician performed Biparietal diameter estimate for gestational age. J Emerg Med. 2022;62(3):342–7. https://doi.org/10.1016/j.jemermed.2021.09.001.
51. Martins JG, Biggio JR, Abuhamad A. Society for Maternal-Fetal Medicine Consult Series #52: diagnosis and management of fetal growth restriction. Am J Obstet Gynecol. 2020;223(4):B2–B17. https://doi.org/10.1016/j.ajog.2020.05.010.
52. Ramphul M, Ooi P, Burke G, et al. Instrumental delivery and ultrasound : a multicentre randomized controlled trial of ultrasound assessment of the fetal head position versus standard care as an approach to prevent morbidity at instrumental delivery. BJOG. 2014;121(8):1029–38. https://doi.org/10.1111/1471-0528.12810.
53. Pilliod RA, Caughey AB. Fetal Malpresentation and malposition: diagnosis and management. Obstet Gynecol Clin N Am. 2017;44(4):631–43. https://doi.org/10.1016/j.ogc.2017.08.003.
54. Dilbaz B, Ozturkoglu E, Dilbaz S, et al. Risk factors and perinatal outcomes associated with umbilical cord prolapse. Arch Gynecol Obstet. 2006;274(2):104–7. https://doi.org/10.1007/s00404-006-0142-2.
55. Multifetal gestations: twin, triplet, and higher-order multifetal pregnancies: ACOG practice bulletin, number 231. Obstet Gynecol. 2021;137(6):e145–62. https://doi.org/10.1097/AOG.0000000000004397.
56. Schiffer V, van Haren A, De Cubber L, et al. Ultrasound evaluation of the placenta in healthy and placental syndrome pregnancies: a systematic review. Eur J Obstet Gynecol Reprod Biol. 2021;262:45–56. https://doi.org/10.1016/j.ejogrb.2021.04.042.
57. Jansen CHJR, Kleinrouweler CE, Kastelein AW, et al. Follow-up ultrasound in second-trimester low-positioned anterior and posterior placentae: prospective cohort study. Ultrasound Obstet Gynecol. 2020;56(5):725–31. https://doi.org/10.1002/uog.21903.
58. Lee SU, Jo JH, Lee H, et al. A Multicenter, retrospective comparison study of pregnancy outcomes according to placental location in placenta Previa. J Clin Med. 2024;13(3) https://doi.org/10.3390/jcm13030675.
59. Silver RM, Landon MB, Rouse DJ, et al. Maternal morbidity associated with multiple repeat Cesarean deliveries. Obstet Gynecol. 2006;107(6):1226–32. https://doi.org/10.1097/01.AOG.0000219750.79480.84.
60. Ranzini AC, Oyelese Y. How to screen for vasa previa. Ultrasound Obstet Gynecol. 2021;57(5):720–5. https://doi.org/10.1002/uog.23520.

61. Oyelese Y, Javinani A, Shamshirsaz AA. Vasa Previa. Obstet Gynecol. 2023;142(3):503–18. https://doi.org/10.1097/AOG.0000000000005287.
62. Glantz C, Purnell L. Clinical utility of sonography in the diagnosis and treatment of placental abruption. J Ultrasound Med. 2002;21(8):837–40. https://doi.org/10.7863/jum.2002.21.8.837.
63. Shinde GR, Vaswani BP, Patange RP, et al. Diagnostic performance of ultrasonography for detection of abruption and its clinical correlation and maternal and foetal outcome. J Clin Diagn Res. 2016;10(8):QC04–7. https://doi.org/10.7860/JCDR/2016/19247.8288.
64. Fadl SA, Linnau KF, Dighe MK. Placental abruption and hemorrhage-review of imaging appearance. Emerg Radiol. 2019;26(1):87–97. https://doi.org/10.1007/s10140-018-1638-3.
65. Iams JD, Grobman WA, Lozitska A, et al. Adherence to criteria for transvaginal ultrasound imaging and measurement of cervical length. Am J Obstet Gynecol. 2013;209(4):365.e1–5. https://doi.org/10.1016/j.ajog.2013.07.032.
66. Melamed N, Hiersch L, Domniz N, et al. Predictive value of cervical length in women with threatened preterm labor. Obstet Gynecol. 2013;122(6):1279–87. https://doi.org/10.1097/AOG.0000000000000022.
67. Sanin-Blair J, Palacio M, Delgado J, et al. Impact of ultrasound cervical length assessment on duration of hospital stay in the clinical management of threatened preterm labor. Ultrasound Obstet Gynecol. 2004;24(7):756–60. https://doi.org/10.1002/uog.1766.
68. Ness A, Visintine J, Ricci E, et al. Does knowledge of cervical length and fetal fibronectin affect management of women with threatened preterm labor? A randomized trial. Am J Obstet Gynecol. 2007;197(4):426.e1–7. https://doi.org/10.1016/j.ajog.2007.07.017.
69. Crane JMG, Hutchens D. Transvaginal sonographic measurement of cervical length to predict preterm birth in asymptomatic women at increased risk: a systematic review. Ultrasound Obstet Gynecol. 2008;31(5):579–87. https://doi.org/10.1002/uog.5323.
70. Belics Z, Papp Z. Ultrasonographic assessment of the cervix for prediction of spontaneous preterm birth in singleton pregnancies. Donald School J Ultrasound Obstet Gynecol. 2021;15(1):49–63. https://doi.org/10.5005/jp-journals-10009-1683.
71. Magann EF, Sandlin AT, Ounpraseuth ST. Amniotic fluid and the clinical relevance of the sonographically estimated amniotic fluid volume: oligohydramnios. J Ultrasound Med. 2011;30(11):1573–85. https://doi.org/10.7863/jum.2011.30.11.1573.
72. Magann EF, Sanderson M, Martin JN, et al. The amniotic fluid index, single deepest pocket, and two-diameter pocket in normal human pregnancy. Am J Obstet Gynecol. 2000;182(6):1581–8. https://doi.org/10.1067/mob.2000.107325.
73. Sandlin AT, Chauhan SP, Magann EF. Clinical relevance of sonographically estimated amniotic fluid volume: polyhydramnios. J Ultrasound Med. 2013;32(5):851–63. https://doi.org/10.7863/ultra.32.5.851.
74. Heemskerk SG, Ten Eikelder MLG, Janssen CAH. Uterine rupture in pregnancy after an intervention complicated by uterine perforation: case report and systematic review of literature. Sex Reprod Healthc. 2019;19:9–14. https://doi.org/10.1016/j.srhc.2018.11.001.
75. Donofrio MT, Moon-Grady AJ, Hornberger LK, et al. Diagnosis and treatment of fetal cardiac disease: a scientific statement from the American Heart Association. Circulation. 2014;129(21):2183–242. https://doi.org/10.1161/01.cir.0000437597.44550.5d.
76. Maslovich MM, Burke LM. Intrauterine Fetal Demise. In: StatPearls [Internet]. Treasure Island: StatPearls Publishing; 2024. https://www.ncbi.nlm.nih.gov/books/NBK557533/.
77. Matsunaga F, Tirumani SH. Spalding sign. Abdoml Radiol. 2021;46(3):1278–9. https://doi.org/10.1007/s00261-020-02769-z.
78. Sundararajan S, Roy S, Polanski LT. The accuracy of ultrasound scan in diagnosing retained products of conception: a systematic review and meta-analysis. Am J Obstet Gynecol Epub ahead of print. 2023:S0002-9378(23)02057-4. https://doi.org/10.1016/j.ajog.2023.11.1243.
79. Ucci MA, Di Mascio D, Bellussi F, et al. Ultrasound evaluation of the uterus in the uncomplicated postpartum period: a systematic review. Am J Obstet Gynecol MFM. 2021;3(3):100318. https://doi.org/10.1016/j.ajogmf.2021.100318.
80. Timor-Tritsch IE, Haynes MC, Monteagudo A, et al. Ultrasound diagnosis and management of acquired uterine enhanced myometrial vascularity/arteriovenous malformations. Am J Obstet Gynecol. 2016;214(6):731.e1–731.e10. https://doi.org/10.1016/j.ajog.2015.12.024.

Gynecological Ultrasound

13

Maya Y. Lin, Meghan Herbst, and Monica R. Saxena

Background

Pelvic pain from a gynecologic source is common; one-in-seven women will experience acute or chronic pelvic pain in their lifetime [1]. Among reproductive-age women with acute lower abdominal pain, over 10% may be gynecologic in origin [2]. Accurate and timely diagnosis is crucial given gynecological emergencies can be life-threatening and result in permanent loss of fertility [3, 4].

Pelvic pain can be diagnostically difficult to differentiate, given the broad differential that spans genitourinary, gastrointestinal, and gynecological etiologies. Despite a thorough examination and laboratory evaluation, imaging is often required to make an accurate diagnosis. While computed tomography (CT) is commonly performed among adults with abdominal pain, ultrasound is the recommended first-line imaging modality for pelvic pain due to its excellent test characteristics, availability, and lack of radiation [5–7].

One of the earliest ultrasound applications was in 1956 by Professor Ian Donald, using ultrasonic metal flaw detectors to attempt viewing a uterine fibroid [8]. Since that time, ultrasound imaging has become more accessible, portable, affordable, and easier to use. Advancing technology has allowed for higher-resolution imaging, both transabdominally and transvaginally. Ultrasound is the gold standard for diagnosing ovarian cysts and uterine fibroids, and sensitive for ovarian torsion and secondary findings of pathology such as free fluid in the pelvis [9, 10]. Knowledge of pelvic ultrasound applications allows for early and accurate diagnosis, expediting appropriate management.

Indications

Indications
- Abdominal pain
- Pelvic pain
- Vaginal bleeding
- Vaginal discharge
- Miscarriage
- Infertility

Diagnoses
- Müllerian duct anomalies
- Hematocolpos
- Nabothian cysts
- Fibroid
- Adenomyosis
- Endometrial polyps
- Endometriosis
- Intrauterine device malpositioning
- Pelvic congestion syndrome
- Simple cyst
- Hemorrhagic cyst
- Ovarian cyst rupture
- Polycystic ovarian syndrome
- Cystadenoma
- Cystadenocarcinoma
- Ovarian torsion
- Hydrosalpinx
- Pelvic inflammatory disease
- Endometritis

Supplementary Information The online version contains supplementary material available at https://doi.org/10.1007/978-3-031-85308-1_13.

M. Y. Lin (✉)
Department of Emergency Medicine, NYU Langone Health, New York, NY, USA
e-mail: maya.lin@nyulangone.org

M. Herbst
Department of Emergency Medicine, University of Connecticut School of Medicine, Farmington, CT, USA
e-mail: meherbst@uchc.edu

M. R. Saxena
Department of Emergency Medicine, Stanford University, Palo Alto, CA, USA
e-mail: saxenam@stanford.edu

M. Gottlieb, N. Panebianco (eds.), *Advanced Point-of-Care Ultrasound*, https://doi.org/10.1007/978-3-031-85308-1_13

Core Views

<table>
<tr><th>View</th><th>Images</th><th>Approach</th></tr>
<tr><td>Transabdominal Uterus Long Axis</td><td>

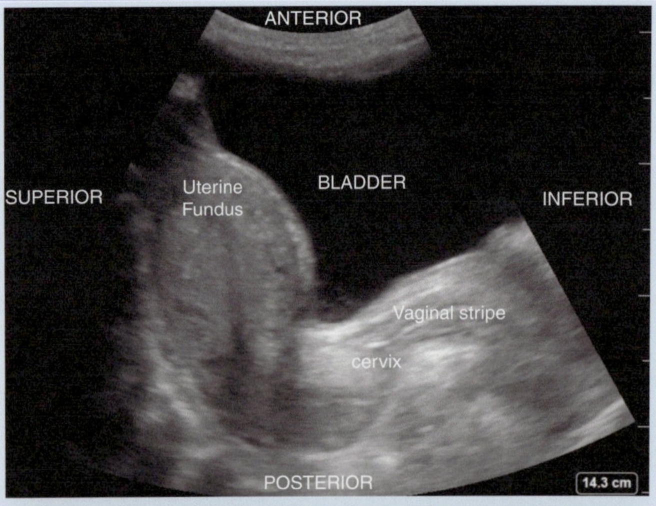

Core View 1. Transabdominal Uterus Long Axis

</td><td>With the patient in a supine position, place a curvilinear probe just above the pubic symphysis in the sagittal plane with the indicator directed cephalad. The bladder (anterior/inferior to the uterus) and vaginal stripe (posterior to the bladder and inferior to the cervix) can be seen in this view and act as sonographic landmarks for the uterus. Fan through the entirety of the uterus in both directions (right and left).</td></tr>
<tr><td>Transabdominal Uterus Short Axis</td><td>

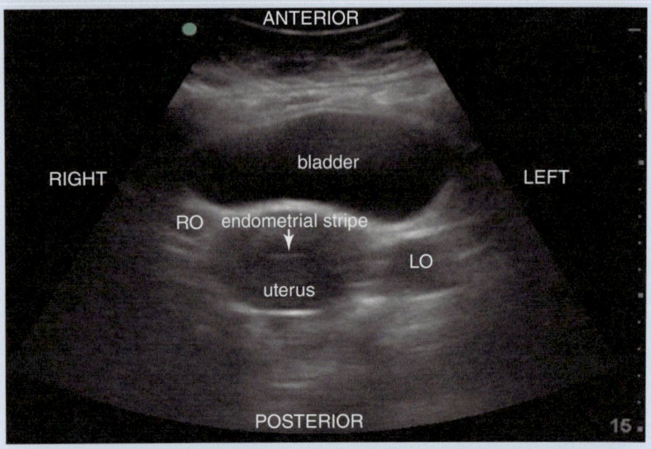

Core View 2. Transabdominal Uterus Short Axis

</td><td>Rotate the probe counterclockwise 90 degrees (indicator pointed to the patient's right side) to view the uterus in the short axis. In this view, the uterus appears “lemon” shaped with the fundus in the center and the cornua appearing as tapered horns on either side. Fan through the entirety of the uterus in both directions (superior and inferior).</td></tr>
<tr><td>Transabdominal Ovary</td><td>

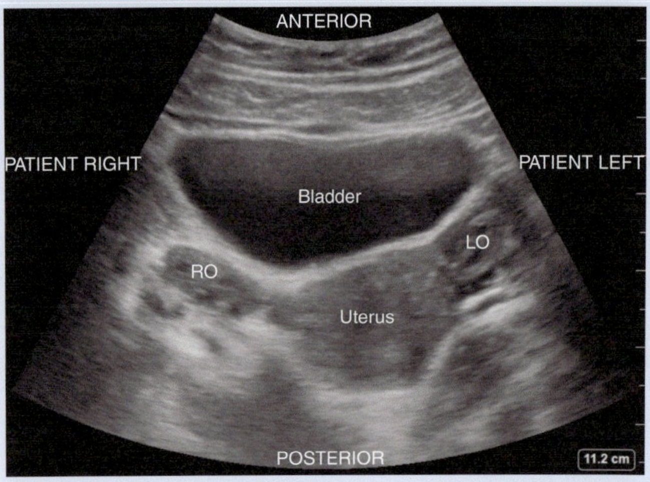

Core View 3. Transabdominal Ovary

</td><td>Follow the cornua and ovarian ligament laterally. The ovaries are usually just lateral to the cornua and anteromedial to the iliac vessels. They appear slightly hypoechoic relative to the uterus and surrounding bowel. Apply graded compression to displace overlying bowel gas, and once identified, fan through the ovary in two orthogonal planes.</td></tr>
</table>

View	Images	Approach
Transvaginal Uterus Long Axis	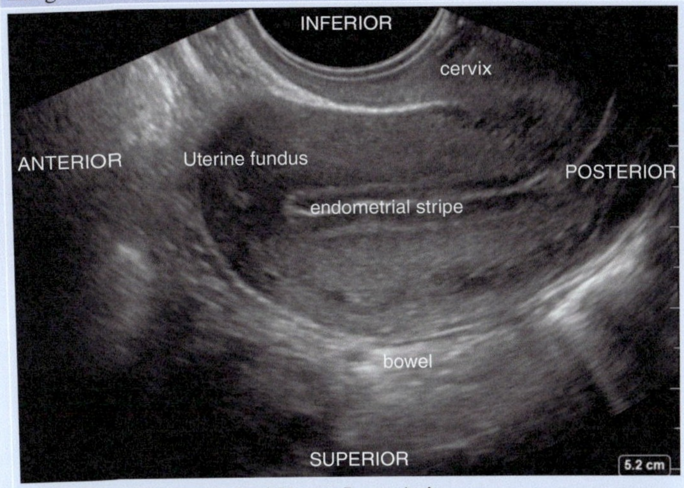 Core View 4. Transvaginal Uterus Long Axis	With the patient in a lithotomy position and an empty bladder, insert a covered endocavitary probe with the indicator directed anteriorly (toward the ceiling) and advance slowly until it is almost past the decompressed bladder. The probe should naturally slip into the anterior fornix. Fan through the entirety of the uterus in both directions (right and left). Attempt to keep the patient covered with a blanket following insertion of the probe. The operator should keep their thumb over the indicator side of the probe so as not to lose track of which way it is directed during the examination.
Transvaginal Uterus Short Axis	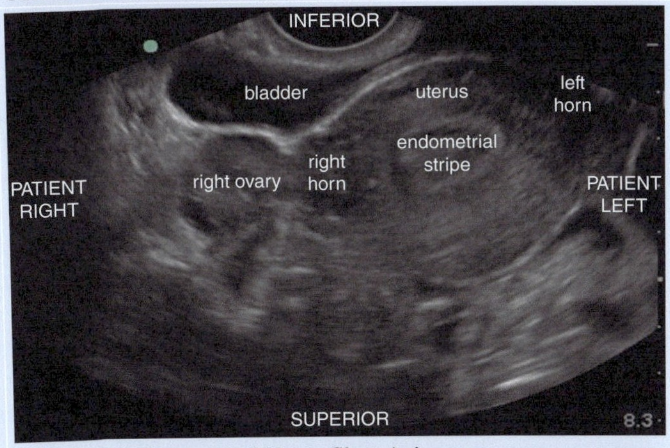 Core View 5. Transvaginal Uterus Short Axis	Rotate the probe 90 degrees counterclockwise to obtain a coronal view (short axis of the uterus), with the indicator pointed towards the patient's right side, and fan anteriorly and posteriorly through the uterus.
Transvaginal Ovary	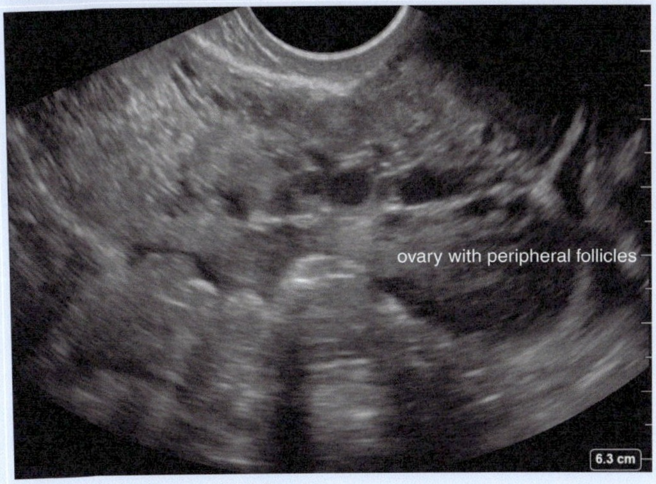 Core View 6. Transvaginal Ovary	Slide the probe horizontally to the patient's right side and fan anteriorly and posteriorly through the area between the cornua and iliac vessels. Similar to the transabdominal approach, the ovary often appears hypoechoic relative to the surrounding hyperechoic bowel gas (displaced by applying gentle pressure over any hypoechoic region until the ovarian shape and details such as follicles come into view). Once identified, fan through the ovary completely in two orthogonal planes. Then, keeping the probe indicator to the patient's right, and at the same level, slide past the uterus to the left side and repeat.

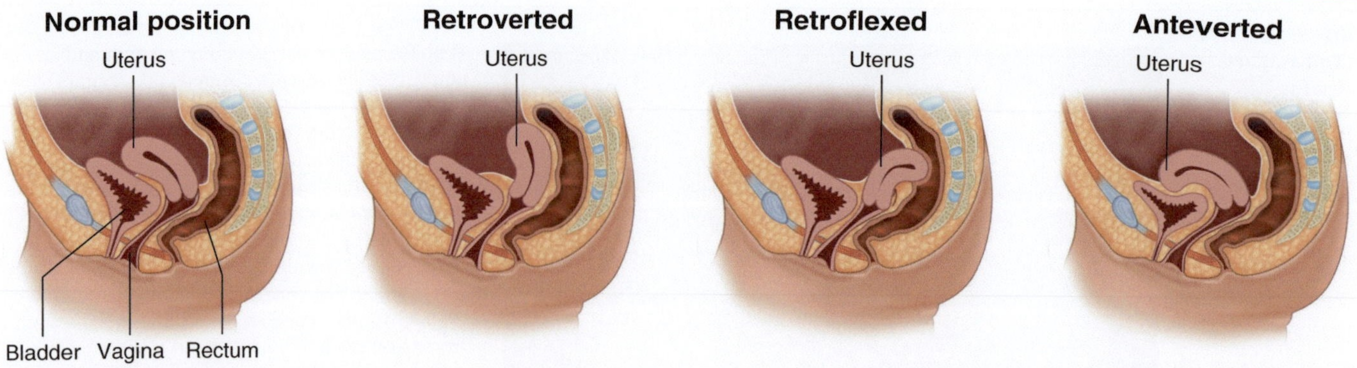

Fig. 13.1 Uterine version and flexion

Normal Anatomy

The uterus is a pear-shaped organ made up of the cervix (most inferior), body (middle), and fundus (most superior, widest portion that includes the uterine horns or cornua, which connect to the fallopian tubes). The mean length of the uterus ranges from 3 cm at birth to 7.5 cm at age 40 years and back to 3 cm at age 90 years [11]. The uterus has a decreasing length-to-width ratio associated with gravidity, ranging from 1.8 in nulliparous women to 1.4 in multiparous women [11]. From deep to superficial, its three tissue layers are the endometrium, myometrium, and serosa. The endometrium, or inner lining, appears hyperechoic relative to the myometrium. The myometrium, or muscular middle layer, contains a network of arcuate vessels arising from the uterine arteries and veins. The serosa is the smooth outer layer that secretes a lubricating fluid to help it slide easily against other structures in the pelvis. The round ligament, uterosacral ligament, and cardinal ligament suspend the uterus in the pelvis. The broad ligament covers the uterus and fallopian tubes.

The fallopian tubes are generally not visible on ultrasound under normal circumstances. The ovaries are oval in shape, with an outer cortex and inner medulla. Their dimensions during reproductive age are approximately 1.5 cm by 1.5 cm by 3 cm, with a mean volume of 0.7 mL at 2 years, peaking at 7.7 mL at 20 years, and then down to 2.8 mL at menopause [12]. Follicles appear as anechoic, thin-walled, well-circumscribed cystic structures in the outer cortex. Typically, follicles are between 2 and 10 mm in size, but can approach up to 30 mm in diameter (dominant follicle) near the time of ovulation [13]. It is normal to see a trace amount (less than 4 mm) of physiologic free fluid in the posterior cul-de-sac [14].

Uterus Position

Uterine version is the angle made by the axis of the cervix and the axis of the vagina and is typically dictated by the direction of the external cervical os. In anteversion, the external os points posteriorly toward the rectum, with the body of the uterus directed anteriorly (Fig. 13.1). In retroversion, the external os points superiorly toward the bladder, with the body of the uterus directed superior or posterior. Retroversion occurs in up to 20% of patients but can transiently occur in the setting of a full bladder [15, 16]. A retroverted uterus may be associated with uterine prolapse due to the closer alignment of the cervix with the vagina [17]. In an axial position, the external os points toward the introitus.

Uterine flexion is the angle made by the axis of the cervix and the axis of the uterine body. With anteflexion, the cervix-to-body angle faces anteriorly. The most common uterine lie is an anteverted slightly anteflexed position, present in approximately 80% of women [18]. Retroflexion is a uterus-to-cervix angle >180 degrees. Retroflexion >210 degrees has been associated with higher-intensity menstrual pain [19]. An anteverted and retroflexed uterine position is common among women who have had a prior Cesarean delivery [20].

Endometrial and Ovarian Cycle

The endometrial cycle has three phases: the proliferative (follicular) phase, the secretory (luteal) phase, and menstruation. During the proliferative phase (days 1–14), estrogen causes vascular and endometrial tissues to undergo extensive proliferation causing thickening of the endometrium. Simultaneously, follicle-stimulating hormone causes the ovarian follicles to grow as large as 2.9 cm, the largest of which is referred to as the dominant follicle. A luteinizing hormone surge leads to rupture of the largest (dominant) follicle and release of an egg (ovulation) around day 14, followed by corpus luteal development. If incomplete follicle rupture occurs, a cyst can develop. During the subsequent luteal phase (days 14–28), progesterone production by the corpus luteum occurs, as well as the endometrial secretory phase where increases in vascularity and mucosal secretions can be visualized as a thickened endometrium [21]. If fertilization does not occur, the corpus luteum involutes and progesterone will drop causing the endometrium to shed in menses.

Premenopausal women can have endometrial thickening up to 8 mm in the proliferative phase and up to 16 mm in the secretory phase [22]. Among postmenopausal women, abnormal endometrial thickening should raise concern for endometrial cancer and prompt follow-up evaluation. The threshold for abnormal endometrial thickening in the postmenopausal woman is greater than 5 mm in the setting of vaginal bleeding and greater than 8–11 mm without vaginal bleeding [22].

Clinical Applications

Müllerian Duct Anomalies

Müllerian duct anomalies are a variety of congenital abnormalities that occur when the pair of Müllerian ducts which form the uterus, cervix, upper vagina, and fallopian tube, do not develop correctly. They are easiest to appreciate when viewing in a short-axis plane through the uterus. Müllerian duct anomalies may be present in up to 7% of the general population and as high as 25% in women with a history of both infertility and miscarriage [23]. Renal anomalies may be associated with uterine anomalies given the close embryonic relationship of the reproductive and urinary systems [24]. The five main types of Müllerian duct anomalies are: septate, bicornuate, unicornuate, didelphys, and arcuate (Fig. 13.2).

Septate Uterus

A septate uterus is the most common Müllerian duct anomaly with a prevalence of up to 35% [25]. It is characterized by normal outer fundal contour (no cleft) with fusion of fundal myometrium creating a septum. A complete septum extends to the external os, whereas a partial septum (subseptate uterus) does not. There is internal fundal indentation of >15 mm and an indentation angle of <90° (Fig. 13.3, Video 13.1) [26]. B-mode ultrasound will demonstrate two distinct endometrial cavities separated by a septum.

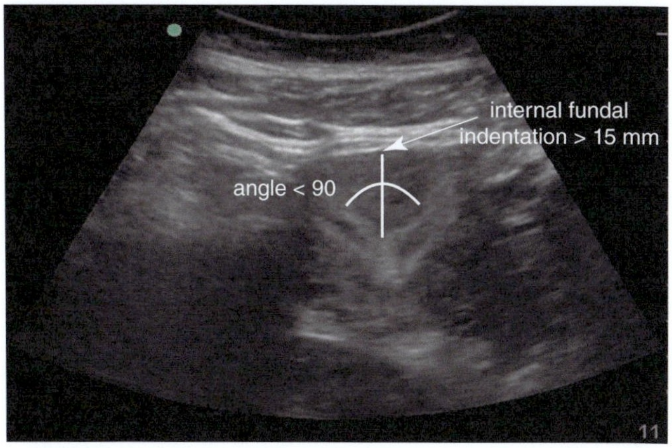

Fig. 13.3 Septate uterus with fundal myometrial fusion and a concave internal fundal indentation >15 mm.

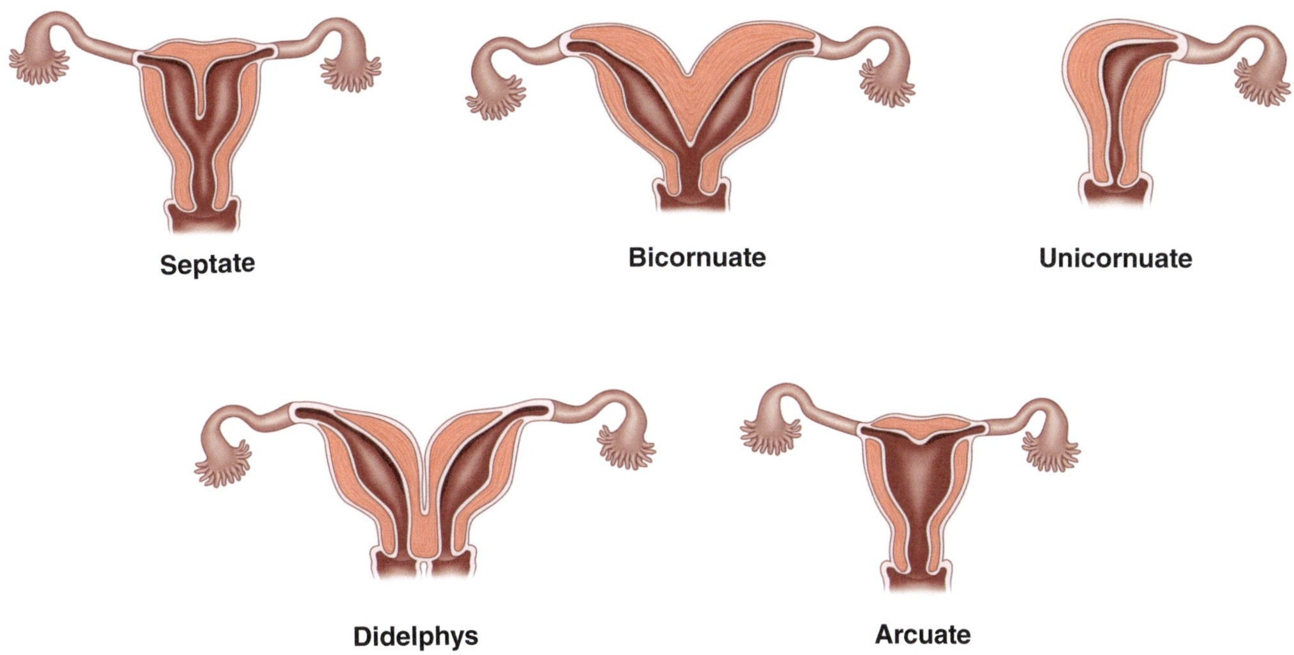

Fig. 13.2 Müllerian duct anomalies

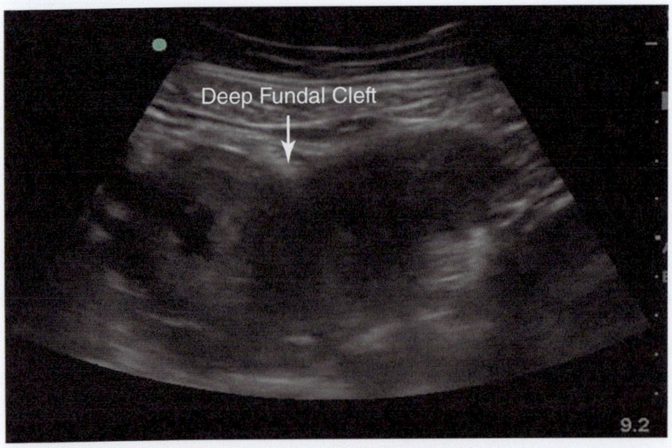

Fig. 13.4 Bicornuate uterus with deep fundal cleft.

Bicornuate Uterus

A bicornuate uterus has a distinct deep fundal cleft >10 mm with two horns that communicate with a single cervical os (Fig. 13.4). The angle of the horns is usually >105° in a bicornuate uterus (compared with an angle of <90° in a septate uterus). On ultrasound, the endometrium converges caudally. The differentiation of the septate uterus (no fundal cleft, complete or near-complete endometrial septum, angle <90°) from bicornuate (fundal cleft >10 mm, converging endometrium, angle >105°) was thought to be important due to a higher risk of pregnancy complications and lower fetal survival among patients with a septate uterus [25]. However, more recent literature suggests rates of preterm delivery, placental abruption, and Cesarean delivery are similar across all congenital anomalies [27].

Didelphys Uterus

A didelphys uterus, which accounts for about 8% of Müllerian duct anomalies [25], has a fundal cleft >10 mm with duplicate uterine horns, duplicate cervices, a longitudinal vaginal septum, and duplicate endometrial cavities with no communication between them. On ultrasound, there are two uterine horns with distinct endometria and two cervices noted. Patients with a didelphys uterus are often asymptomatic but may have dyspareunia, dysmenorrhea, or even hematocolpos in the setting of a thick obstructing vaginal septum [28, 29].

Unicornuate Uterus

A unicornuate uterus accounts for 2–13% of Müllerian duct anomalies [30]. It occurs when there is abnormal development of one of the Müllerian ducts, resulting in only half a uterus and one functional fallopian tube. Ultrasound shows a small rounded asymmetric ellipsoid-shaped uterus with only one horn. It can cause infertility in 15–30% of patients, and among patients who become pregnant, miscarriage and early preterm birth are common with only 30% reaching full term [31].

Arcuate Uterus

An arcuate uterus is characterized by a normal outer fundal contour, no division of the uterine horns, a mild concave internal fundal indentation of <10 mm, and an indentation angle of >90° [26]. This differs from a septate uterus which has an indentation >15 mm and an indentation angle of <90° [26]. Ultrasound may only demonstrate subtle fundal echogenic endometrial thickening on the short-axis view. It may be considered a normal variant and is least associated with reproductive issues [32–34].

Hematocolpos

Hematocolpos typically results from an imperforate hymen and is the most common obstructive anomaly of the female reproductive tract, occurring in 1 per 1000 to 10,000 women [35]. The diagnosis is usually delayed until puberty when this distal vaginal obstruction leads to trapped menstruation in the vaginal canal (hematocolpos) and the uterus (hematometra). Common symptoms include delayed menarche, cyclic lower abdominal pain, and urinary retention, usually presenting between 13 and 15 years of age [36, 37].

Ultrasound is highly accurate for the diagnosis of hematocolpos [38]. Transabdominal ultrasound will show a distended uterus with intraluminal fluid of variable echogenicity occupying the vaginal stripe (Fig. 13.5, Video 13.2) [39]. In the setting of hematometra, clotted blood within the endometrium will appear echogenic and mobile when the patient changes position. To diagnose an imperforate hymen, a transrectal ultrasound can be an alternative to the transvaginal approach [40].

Nabothian Cysts

Nabothian cysts (also called retention cysts or epithelial cysts) are benign mucinous endocervical gland cysts that are formed when squamous epithelium overgrows and causes obstruction at their necks [41]. They are common with a prevalence of 12%, and are typically found in women of reproductive age [42]. Nabothian cysts are best appreciated using transvaginal ultrasound. They will appear close to the probe when placed just inferior to the cervix. They appear as well-circumscribed, unilocular, anechoic cysts located in the endocervical canal and range from a few millimeters to 4 cm in diameter (Fig. 13.6) [43]. If Doppler is used, they will not reveal flow. Occasionally, they can be complex and multiple, and may lead to enlargement of the cervix [42].

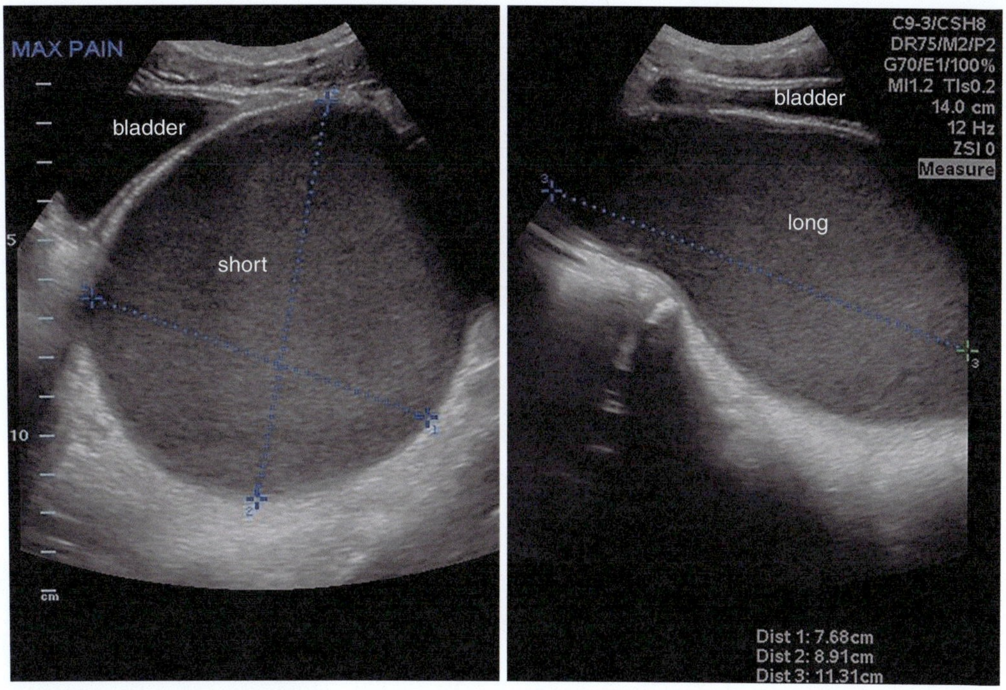

Fig. 13.5 Hematocolpos with trapped menstruation in the vaginal canal.

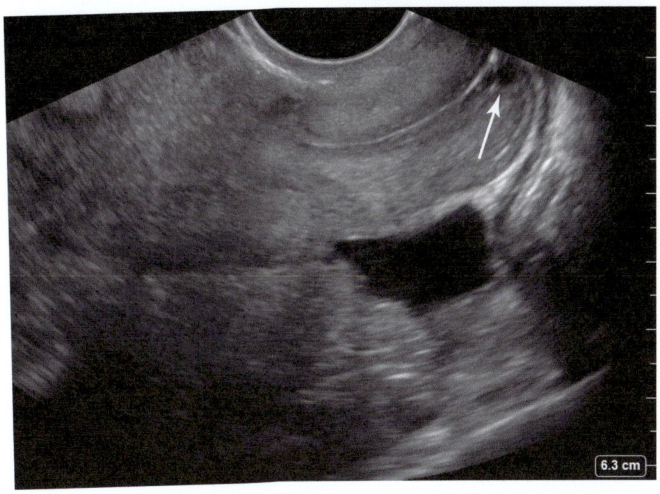

Fig. 13.6 Transvaginal long axis view of the uterus with cervical nabothian cyst

Fibroid (Uterine Leiomyoma)

The most common benign uterine tumor is the uterine leiomyoma, commonly known as a fibroid [44]. These are smooth muscle cell and connective tissue tumors that affect 20–30% of women between 30 and 50 years of age [45]. Growth is associated with higher levels of estrogen, luteinizing hormone, follicle stimulating hormone, and body fat [46, 47].

Fibroids can be asymptomatic or symptomatic and are often incidentally found on ultrasound. Approximately 30% of women experience symptoms from fibroids in the form of pain or vaginal bleeding [48]. Acute pain can result from degeneration (5.1%), rupture (<1%), or torsion (<0.25%) [49, 50]. Large fibroids tend to degenerate when greater than 5–8 cm [51], due to a lack of blood supply and ischemia. Fibroids are classified by their location as submucosal, intramural, and subserosal. Submucosal fibroids close to the endometrium can decrease the success of implantation [52].

Transabdominal ultrasound is 90% sensitive and 85% specific for diagnosing fibroids [53]. This approach (compared to transvaginal ultrasound) allows visualization of the entire uterus, which will generally appear enlarged and lobulated when occupied by fibroids. Fibroids have variable sonographic appearances, including well-defined, homogenous, heterogeneous, or hypoechoic masses (Fig. 13.7a, Video 13.3). Hyperechoic calcifications can sometimes create shadowing. Saline-infusion sonohysterography, a procedure where saline is transcervically instilled into the uterine cavity during the ultrasound, increases the sensitivity for submucosal fibroid detection (sensitivity 94%, specificity 81%) [53, 54].

Color Doppler imaging will demonstrate increased peripheral vascular flow due to the presence of vessels between the subserosal fibroid and the uterus [55]. This finding is called the "bridging vessel sign" and is used to differentiate fibroids from extrauterine tumors [56, 57]. Pulsed-wave Doppler will show high velocity, low resistive index (<0.7), and low pulsatility index (<1.2), which can differentiate a fibroid from adenomyosis [58]. The pulsatility index is a parameter of vascular resistance, defined as the difference between peak systolic and end-diastolic flow velocity, divided by the average flow velocity.

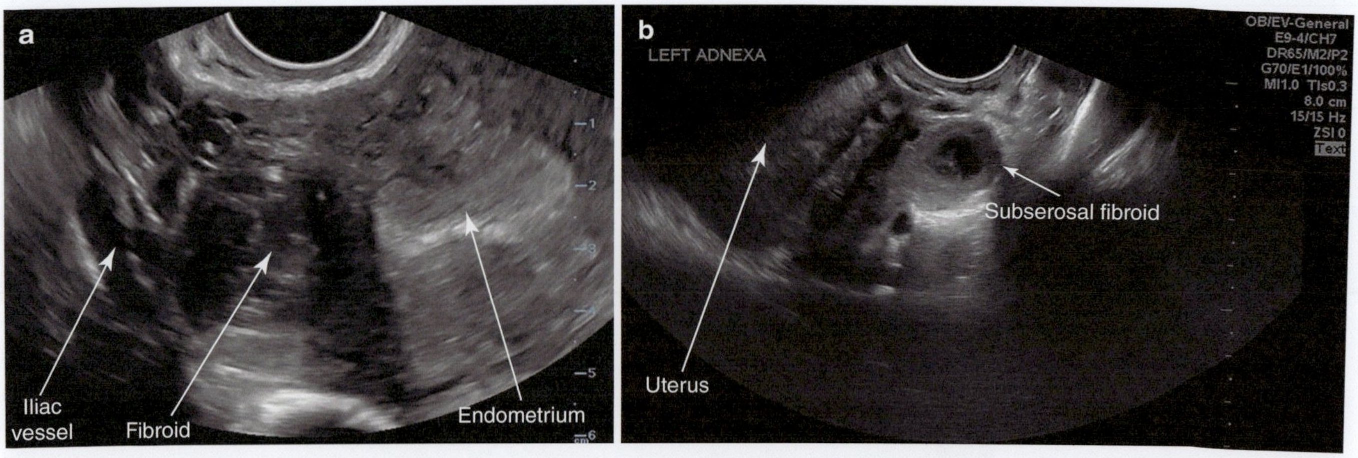

Fig. 13.7 (**a**) Typical appearance of a fibroid. (**b**) Subserosal pedunculated fibroid with central anechoic cystic area which may represent necrosis

A degenerated fibroid will appear as a large, heterogenous, well-circumscribed myometrial mass with anechoic cystic areas that may represent necrosis or infarction (Fig. 13.7, Video 13.3) [59, 60]. Infarcted regions should lack vascularity on Doppler [61]. Torsion can occur in pedunculated fibroids and appears as a hypoechoic avascular mass separate from the ovary that has a pointed peduncle [62].

Adenomyosis

Adenomyosis is a proliferation of endometrial glands and stroma within the myometrium that affects 10–40% of women of reproductive age, especially over the age of 40 years [63, 64]. It causes nonspecific pelvic pain and vaginal bleeding and may be difficult to differentiate from other causes, such as fibroids, endometriosis, and dysfunctional uterine bleeding. Importantly, missed diagnosis can lead to implantation failure and infertility [65].

Transvaginal ultrasound is 82.5% sensitive and 84.6% specific for the diagnosis of adenomyosis, which is comparable to magnetic resonance imaging [66]. A common sonographic finding for adenomyosis is heterogeneous-appearing myometrium with subendometrial echogenic striae ("rainforest sign" or "Venetian blind sign") that appear as finger-like lines due to ectopic endometrium with posterior shadowing (Fig. 13.8). Additional findings include anterior–posterior wall asymmetry of the uterus, loss of endometrial–myometrial interface, and intramural lacunae (e.g., myometrial cysts, engorged cystic glands) <5 mm in size [67]. A heterogeneous uterine appearance carries high sensitivity (80.8%), whereas a globular (rounded) uterus carries high specificity (86.4%) for the diagnosis [68, 69]. Color

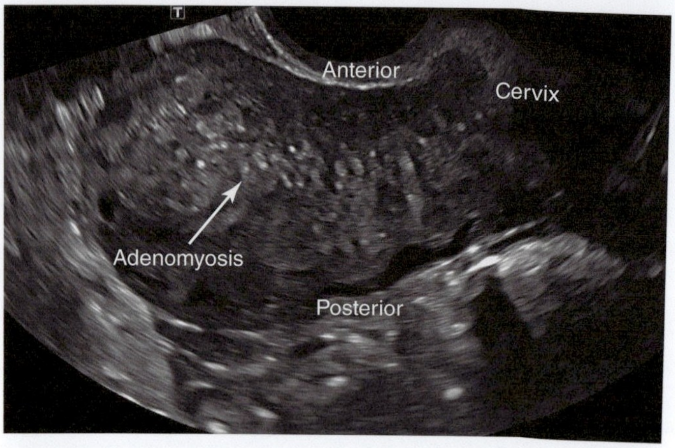

Fig. 13.8 Adenomyosis with a heterogeneous myometrium, anterior–posterior uterine wall asymmetry, and loss of endometrial–myometrial interface

Doppler can be added to differentiate adenomyosis (diffuse scattering of intramural vessels) from fibroids (peripheral vascularization) [70].

An adenomyoma is a concentrated area of adenomyosis that can form an endometrial polyp. Unlike adenomyosis which needs to be treated with a hysterectomy, an adenomyoma may be resected [71–73].

Endometrial Polyps

Endometrial polyps are hyperplastic localized growths in the endometrial stroma. They are most common among women at or near menopause but seen among reproductive-aged and postmenopausal women, usually in the fifth decade of life [74]. Their prevalence is largely unknown because many cases are asymptomatic [75]. When symptomatic, they may present with abnormal uterine bleeding [76], and have been associated with infertility [77].

Using transvaginal ultrasound, polyps appear as hyperechoic, well-defined lesions with smooth borders and a vascular stalk. Polyps are best seen on day 10 of a woman's menstrual cycle when the endometrium is thinnest [78]. They project from the endometrial lining and range from a few millimeters to a few centimeters, with the potential to grow to fill the uterine cavity [79]. Endometrial polyps are either pedunculated or sessile and can be single or multiple. Within the polyp, cystic glands may be visible. Doppler may reveal a characteristic single feeding vessel, differentiating benign polyps from malignant lesions and hyperplasia which otherwise can look similar on B-mode [80, 81]. Malignancy on Doppler has a multivessel appearance (i.e., multiple vessels within the endometrium and in the myometrial–endometrial interface), whereas hyperplasia has a scattered vessel appearance appearing as dispersed flow without a visible origin at the myometrial–endometrial junction [82].

Endometriosis

Endometriosis is an inflammatory condition where endometrial tissue grows outside the uterus, residing most commonly in the pelvic peritoneum and ovary [83]. It affects about 10% of women of reproductive age, leading to symptoms of dysmenorrhea, dyspareunia, chronic pelvic pain, and infertility [84].

Transvaginal ultrasound is the first-line method given its capability for real-time assessment, availability, and cost. The International Deep Endometriosis Analysis (IDEA) group developed a systematic sonographic approach to improve the detection of endometriosis with pelvic ultrasound (Box 13.1) [85]. The recommended steps must all be completed but do not have to be done in order.

Endometriomas are unilocular cystic lesions found in later stages of endometriosis, commonly referred to as chocolate cysts due to the dark endometrial fluid they contain [86]. They are often bilateral. Endometriomas are treated with cystectomy if symptomatic or observed if asymptomatic [87].

On transvaginal ultrasound, endometriomas are homogenous with low-level echoes giving it a ground-glass appearance indicative of chronic repetitive hemorrhages within the cyst [88, 89]. In a minority of endometriomas (<15%), there may be hyperechoic foci (referred to as calcific stippling), fluid-fluid levels, hyperechoic mural irregularity, or general heterogeneity [90, 91]. Application of color Doppler at a low-velocity scale of 5–10 cm/s with low filter settings should demonstrate the absence of vascularity, essential for diagnosis (whereas the presence of vascularity suggests malignancy such as an endometrioid tumor) [92]. Transvaginal ultrasound is 93% sensitive and 96% specific at detecting endometriomas [93]. "Kissing ovaries," when the ovaries are entirely or partly joined together and stabilized behind the uterus in the Pouch of Douglas, suggest pelvic adhesions which increase the risk for bowel and fallopian tube endometriosis (Fig. 13.9) [94].

While small superficial peritoneal endometriosis may be undetectable on ultrasound, "soft markers" such as reduced ovarian mobility and loculated peritoneal fluid with point tenderness may suggest its presence [95].

The "sliding sign" refers to whether the anterior rectum glides freely across the posterior aspect of the cervix, posterior vaginal wall (for an anteverted uterus) or uterine fundus (for a retroverted uterus). The examiner can assess for a sliding sign by balloting the uterus between the abdominal wall and the probe. A positive sliding sign is associated with endometriotic nodule infiltration of the rectal or sigmoid wall as well as obliteration of the pouch of Douglas.

Finally, to look for deep infiltrating endometriosis (DIE) nodules, place the endocavitary probe in the anterior and posterior fornix to assess the anterior and posterior compartments. The nodules appear hypoechoic, linear, or round in

Box 13.1: International Deep Endometriosis Analysis Group Sonographic approach to Improve Detection of Endometriosis with Pelvic Ultrasound [85]

Step 1	Sonographic evaluation of uterus and adnexa for adenomyosis and endometriomas
Step 2	Transvaginal soft markers such as tenderness or fixed ovaries
Step 3	Dynamic imaging of Pouch of Douglas "sliding sign"
Step 4	Assess for Deep Infiltrating Endometriosis (DIE) nodules in anterior and posterior compartments

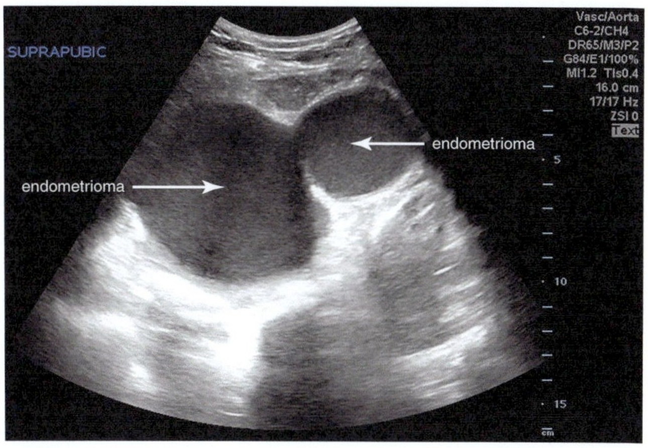

Fig. 13.9 Endometriomas appear homogenous with low-level echoes giving them a ground-glass appearance indicative of chronic repetitive internal hemorrhage

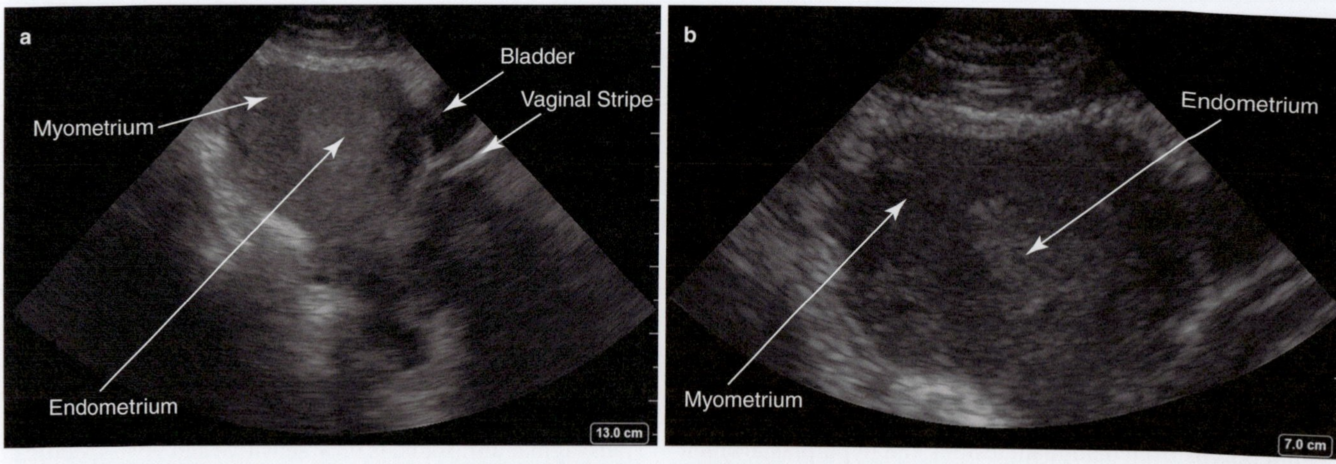

Fig. 13.10 Endometrial cancer viewed in a sagittal plane (**a**) and transverse plane (**b**) with thick endometrial diameter, increased echogenicity, and an ill-defined endometrial-myometrial junction. (*Image courtesy of Jailyn Avila, MD*)

shape with variable borders (smooth or irregular), and demonstrate minimal to no internal flow when using color Doppler [96]. The nodules must extend at least 5 mm into the nearby peritoneum with organ invasion or retroperitoneal involvement to be considered DIE.

Uterine Malignancies

Uterine cancer is the most common cancer of the female genital tract [97]. In postmenopausal women, vaginal bleeding is the most common symptom of uterine cancer [98]. Transvaginal ultrasound is appropriate for the initial evaluation of this subgroup of patients for cancer [99]. A long-axis view of the uterus is used to measure the area with the thickest anterior–posterior diameter. A diameter of ≤4 mm has a high negative predictive value for endometrial cancer [100]. Moreover, when compared to normal uterine tissue, tumors have higher endometrial vascularization, are less likely to have a regular endometrial–myometrial junction, and more likely to have increased echogenicity (Fig. 13.10) [101]. To assess endometrial vascularization, a color score was created by the International Endometrial Tumor Analysis group, where the higher the score, the higher the vascularization, and the more suggestive of a tumor. A score of 1 indicates no color Doppler flow detected, a score of 2 indicates minimal color is detected, a score of 3 indicates moderate color, and a score of 4 indicates abundant color [102].

Intrauterine Devices

An intrauterine device (IUD) is the most commonly used long-acting reversible form of contraception worldwide, used by 10% of women in the United States [103].

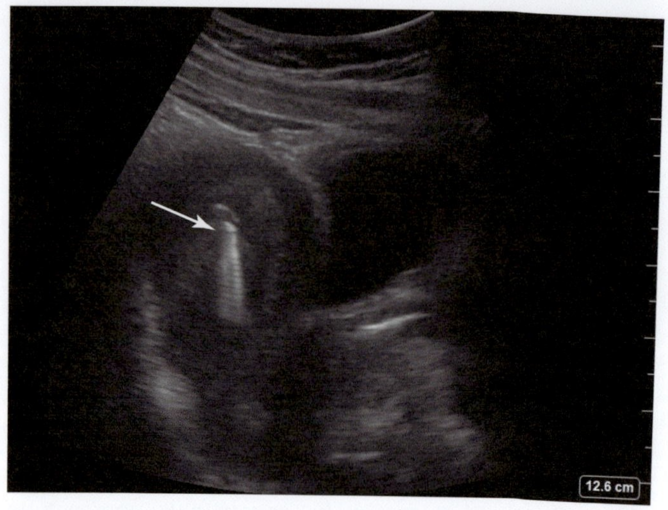

Fig. 13.11 Appropriately positioned intrauterine device in the endometrium, long-axis uterine view.

Complications resulting from malposition may occur in 1 out of 10 women and typically result in vaginal bleeding, discomfort, and decreased efficacy [104–106].

On ultrasound, a long view of the uterus will demonstrate the straight IUD stem as a linear echogenic structure with posterior reverberation artifact in the endometrial cavity, ending 3 mm from the fundal endometrium (Fig. 13.11, Video 13.4). The IUD arms extend laterally to form a T shape. Copper-containing IUDs are more echogenic throughout with a stronger posterior reverberation artifact; in contrast, levonorgestrel-releasing IUDs have a silicone membrane over the stem, leading to central posterior acoustic shadowing with the proximal and distal portions being more echogenic [107, 108].

When evaluating for malposition, the IUD should not extend beyond the endometrium or into the cervix, and the long stem of the IUD should not be transverse or rotated

[109]. Expulsion, when the IUD passes through the external cervical os, typically occurs in the first year after placement, especially when the IUD was placed immediately after vaginal delivery [110]. Displacement, when the IUD is rotated or located in the lower segment of the uterus, should be suspected if the distance between the IUD and the uterine fundus is greater than 3 mm [111]. Sometimes, a low-lying IUD can migrate into the correct position over a period of months [112]. Embedment, when the IUD penetrates the myometrium but does not extend into the serosa, typically occurs at the time of initial placement and is associated with an increased risk of displacement. Embedment of the long IUD stem is easily detectable with 2-dimensional ultrasound, but the use of three-dimensional ultrasound increases sensitivity for detection of embedment of the short arms [113]. Finally, perforation, when the IUD penetrates both the myometrium and serosa, can result in the IUD migrating out of the uterus and into the peritoneum. This complication is rare, occurring only in 1–2 per 1000 insertions [105, 114]. If the IUD is not visible within the uterus and this is suspected, an abdominal radiograph may be needed, as radiographs can identify an extra-peritoneal IUD better than ultrasound [115].

Physiologic Structures: Follicles and the Corpus Luteum

A follicle is a simple cyst ≤3 cm in diameter found in the premenopausal women [13]. It is the fundamental unit of the ovary and contains the oocyte. Most ovaries in women of reproductive age will have 4–24 follicles per ovary; less than 4 follicles per ovary is predictive of menopause in the next 7 years, whereas greater than 24 per ovary suggests a high risk of hyperandrogenic anovulation [116]. Typically, follicles are 4–10 mm in diameter, and they grow approximately 1–2 mm per day, with dominant follicles measuring 20–30 mm just prior to ovulation [13, 117].

A corpus luteum (CL) is a thick-walled cystic structure ≤3 cm present from the time of ovulation and degenerates 10–12 days later if a pregnancy does not occur. On B-mode imaging, CL may appear cystic with crenulated (i.e., irregular or wavy) inner margins and internal echoes (Fig. 13.12). Less commonly, CL may look like a hypoechoic region within the ovary. When applying color Doppler, CL demonstrates intense peripheral color Doppler flow (ring of fire), but no internal Doppler flow [118]. While often referred to as a cyst, and technically a cystic structure, CL is not considered a cyst given: (a) it lacks an epithelial lining, (b) it is a physiologically functional structure that forms from the remnants of the follicle after ovulation, and (c) it acts as a temporary endocrine structure to produce progesterone within the ovary.

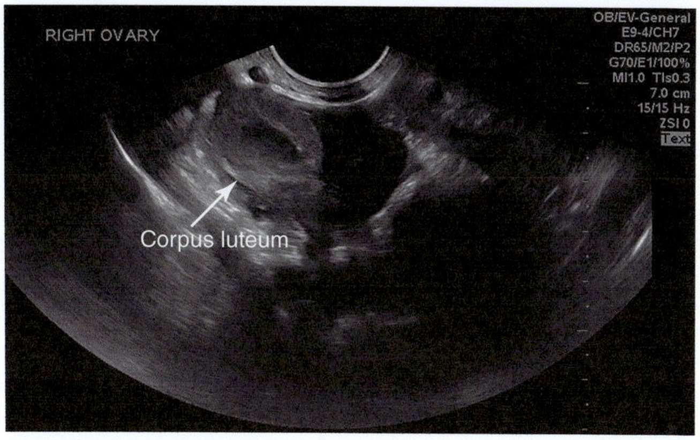

Fig. 13.12 Corpus luteum

Pelvic Congestion Syndrome

Pelvic congestion syndrome (PCS), due to retrograde pelvic venous flow and incompetent uterine and ovarian veins, accounts for approximately one-third of chronic pelvic pain in women [119]. Risk factors include pregnancy, prior pelvic surgery, an enlarged uterus or uterine mass, prolonged standing, heavy lifting, and possibly high levels of estrogen and genetic factors [120]. Pregnancy distends the veins by up to 60%, making the valves incompetent, resulting in venous hypertension and retrograde flow. Weight gain and positional changes of the uterus during pregnancy can also compress and kink the ovarian veins leading to reflux [121]. Nutcracker syndrome, where the left renal vein is compressed by the superior mesenteric artery and aorta, and May–Thurner syndrome, where the left iliac vein is compressed between the right common iliac artery and the lumbar spine, have been thought to lead to ovarian vein dilation and reflux, resulting in PCS; however, studies have shown no association of these syndromes with symptoms [122, 123]. Up to 50% of patients with PCS have polycystic ovarian syndrome but the role of estrogen on PCS is unclear [119]. Genetic factors may additionally predispose to varicosity formation [124].

Ultrasound is the first-line imaging modality when screening for PCS. Findings suggestive of PCS include: (1) tortuous pelvic veins with a diameter >4 mm and slow (<3 cm/s) or retrograde blood flow, and (2) dilated myometrial arcuate veins communicating with the pelvic varicosities [125]. Start with the transabdominal approach to assess for compressive masses such as fibroids or ovarian masses. A transabdominal view also allows visualization of the ovarian veins superior to the pelvis. Attempt viewing the left ovarian vein near its junction with the left renal vein. Place the probe over the upper abdomen in a transverse plane to identify the left renal vein anterior to the abdominal aorta. The left ovarian vein joins the left renal vein just laterally (Fig. 13.13). Rotate

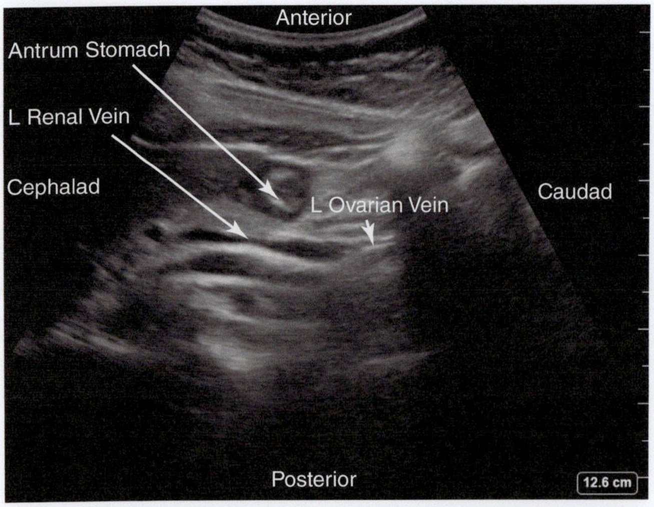

Fig. 13.13 Left ovarian vein viewed on transabdominal ultrasound. (*Image courtesy of Meghan Herbst, MD*)

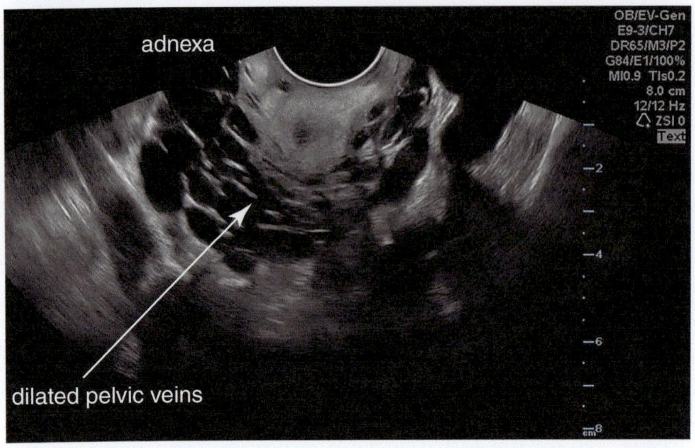

Fig. 13.14 Pelvic congestion syndrome demonstrating dilated arcuate veins and pelvic varicosities

clockwise 90 degrees to align the probe with the left ovarian vein. In this sagittal plane, use pulsed-wave Doppler to assess for retrograde flow. In one study, a left ovarian vein diameter >6 mm carried an 83.3% positive predictive value for PCS, and all patients with PCS had retrograde flow [126].

Transvaginal ultrasound is preferable for evaluation of the pelvic vein diameter and flow, given the higher frequency of the endocavitary probe and proximity of the footprint to the vessel, yielding improved resolution (although this can be attempted using transabdominal ultrasound). In a transverse plane, assess the region between the uterine cornua and ovary for dilated pelvic veins (Fig. 13.14). Have the patient Valsalva to exacerbate pelvic congestion and to help identify the pelvic veins. Color Doppler may help; the vessels should dilate and have an increased color Doppler signal with Valsalva. Once the vessels are identified, measure the vein diameter and apply color Doppler followed by pulsed-wave Doppler to assess the venous velocity [85].

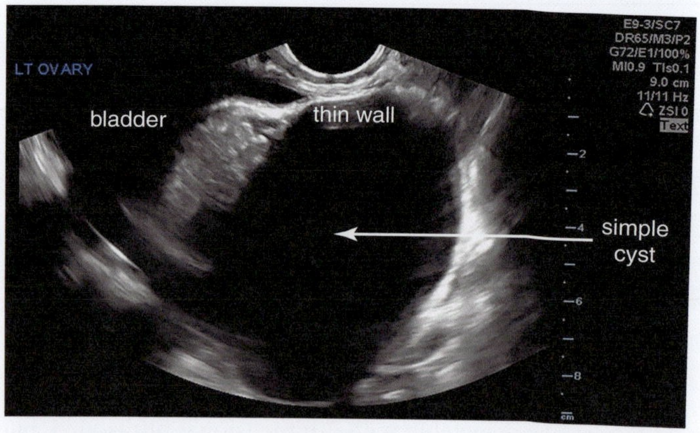

Fig. 13.15 Simple cyst with thin-wall and round or oval shape

Ovarian Cysts and Masses

Ultrasound in the hands of experienced users is both sensitive (77–86%) and specific (94–100%) for adnexal masses [85]. These can be categorized into unilocular or multilocular cysts and those with or without solid components. Unilocular refers to single compartments that may or may not have incomplete septa, wall abnormalities, internal echoes, or solid components (defined as ≥3 mm). Multilocular cysts have more than one compartment. Solid lesions have at least 80% solid components when assessed in two orthogonal planes and lack characteristics of a cyst [127]. A unilocular cyst with solid components has a positive predictive value of 37.1% for malignancy [128]. In contrast, an irregular solid lesion has a positive predictive value for malignancy of 93% [128].

Simple Cysts

Simple cysts are thin-walled, unilocular, round or oval-shaped anechoic fluid collections (Fig. 13.15) [127]. They will demonstrate posterior acoustic enhancement due to their simple fluid content and lack internal color Doppler flow [129]. Simple cysts are often observed and not treated surgically. A "complex cyst," in contrast to a simple cyst, will have thicker walls and may contain septations or solid areas [130]. Importantly, the term "complex cyst" should generally be avoided in favor of the specific diagnosis when available [128].

Hemorrhagic Cyst

A hemorrhagic cyst results from a partial rupture of a mature Graafian follicle. The internal hemorrhage typically gives the cyst a reticular, "spider web" appearance, though intracystic clots can appear as solid components (Fig. 13.16) [131]. Color Doppler can be applied and should not demonstrate blood flow over the internal contents (the peripheral stroma will still have flow). Conversely, flow is often present within

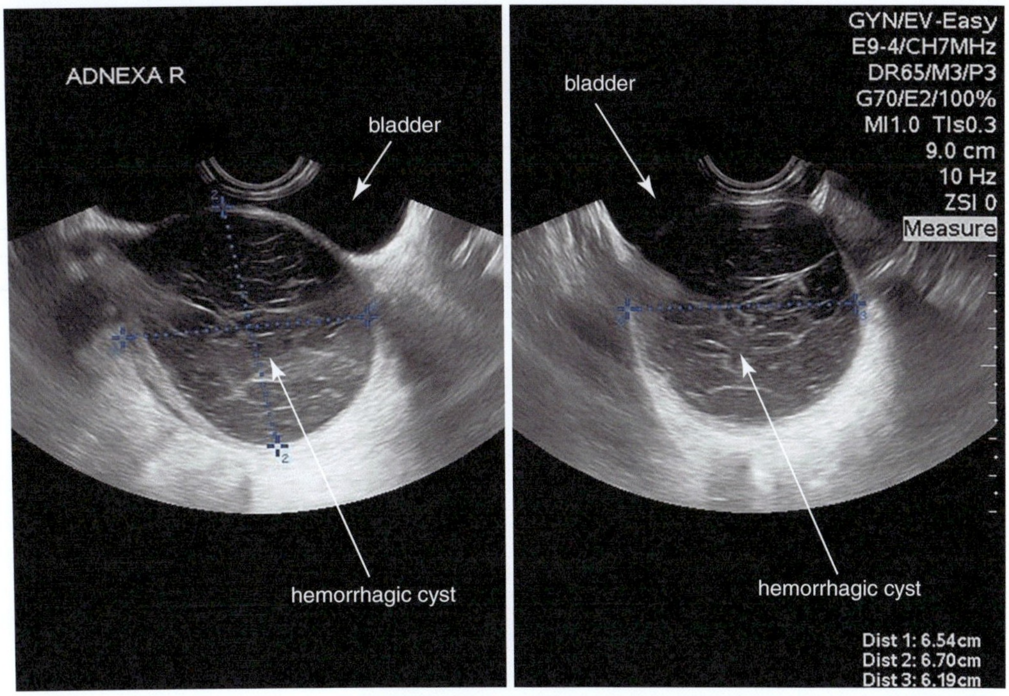

Fig. 13.16 Hemorrhagic cyst with reticular "spider web" internal echoes

cystic tumors that may have a similar appearance. Tapping a hemorrhagic cyst with the endocavitary probe may lead to a jelly-like "wobbling" movement [118]. In most cases, hemorrhagic cysts resolve on their own within 6–12 weeks [13, 132]. They are generally managed with analgesia and a follow-up ultrasound in 6–12 weeks [13, 133].

Cyst Rupture

Ovarian follicular or hemorrhagic cyst rupture is one of the most common causes of acute abdominal pain in young women, typically presenting with an acute onset of severe pain, followed by progressively less pain over subsequent hours [134]. In some cases, severe bleeding can occur, leading to hemorrhagic shock.

Begin by performing a transabdominal ultrasound and assess for free fluid in the pouch of Douglas (Fig. 13.17). This is the easiest and most sensitive finding for cyst rupture [135, 136]. In addition to the pouch of Douglas, fluid may collect around the ovary closest to the ruptured cyst, or extend to the right upper quadrant (Morison's pouch) when bleeding is significant [137, 138]. If the fluid is blood, it may become more echogenic and heterogeneous over time with clot formation either floating or layering within the free fluid. Caution should be taken as clotted blood can often be missed and mistaken for bowel. An associated cyst may or may not be seen on ultrasound [139]. If the transabdominal view is limited, have a low threshold to switch to a transvaginal approach, which can enhance visualization of the ovary and surrounding structures due to the higher resolution and greater proximity.

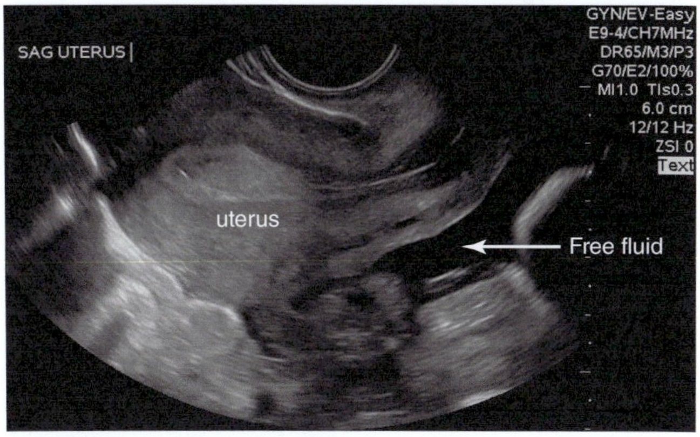

Fig. 13.17 Pelvic free fluid in the pouch of Douglas seen in a transvaginal long-axis view of a patient with a ruptured cyst.

Cystic Teratoma (Dermoid Cyst)

A mature cystic teratoma (also known as a dermoid cyst), is a benign germ cell tumor. Cystic teratomas make up 15–25% of all ovarian neoplasms [140]. Teratomas tend to affect women of reproductive age, are slow-growing, and are bilateral in 8–15% of cases [140, 141].

Ultrasound is moderately sensitive (57.9%) and highly specific (99.7%) for dermoid cysts given their characteristic features [142, 143]. Dermoid cysts are unilocular cysts with echogenic internal content (often appearing as a "white ball" within the lesion) that shadows extensively (Fig. 13.18). When the hyperechoic component takes up a smaller part of the lesion, it is called a Rokitansky nodule (also known as a dermoid plug). When the hyperechoic component of the dermoid cyst takes up the majority of the lesion, distal attenuation results in a "tip of the iceberg" effect (Fig. 13.19). The mixed echoes within the cyst represent fat, bone, fluid, and hair or teeth [144, 145]. Bright echoes with posterior acoustic shadowing typically reflect hair or teeth in the cyst. Dermoid cysts tend to be asymptomatic and are often discovered incidentally. However, a common complication of these cysts is ovarian torsion, occurring in approximately 16% of cases [146].

Polycystic Ovarian Syndrome

Polycystic ovarian syndrome (PCOS) is the most common female endocrine disorder, affecting about 10–13% of women of reproductive age [147]. Manifestations of PCOS include menstrual dysfunction, hirsutism, acne, metabolic alterations, infertility, and ultrasound features of polycystic ovaries [148].

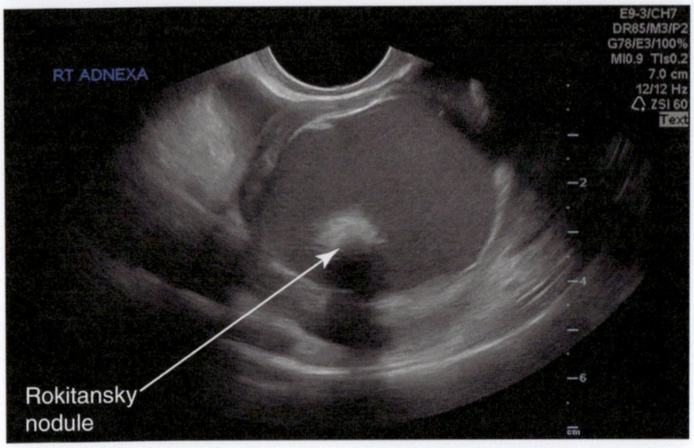

Fig. 13.18 Cystic teratoma with a Rokitansky nodule (dermoid plug)

Transvaginal ultrasound is preferable to transabdominal ultrasound in identifying PCOS given the enhanced resolution images resulting from the higher frequency endocavitary probe, as well as the close proximity of the footprint to the ovary, resulting in less obstruction by intestinal gas or subcutaneous tissues. In an ovulating woman, the best time to assess for PCOS is in the early follicular phase (days 3–5). If there is evidence of a dominant follicle or CL, the ultrasound should be repeated in the next menstrual cycle as it will dissolve and a new one will appear in the next cycle [149]. Inherent in the diagnosis, ovaries tend to be larger and easier to find than the general population. View both ovaries in two orthogonal planes, noting their number of follicles, and measuring each in three dimensions. While many ultrasound devices have a software package that will auto-calculate ovarian volume, a volume can be manually calculated using the ellipsoid formula: $D1 \times D2 \times D3 \times 0.52$.

The 2003 Rotterdam criteria, supported in the 2018 International Evidence-Based Guideline for the Assessment and Management of PCOS, defined PCOS as an ovary with an increased ovarian volume ($\geq$10 mL) and having $\geq$20 follicles in at least one ovary, or $\geq$10 follicles in at least one section of the ovary [147, 150]. The follicles are typically located peripherally, resembling a "string of pearls" (Fig. 13.20, Video 13.5) [151]. If PCOS is suspected, the patient should be referred to an endocrinologist as treatment of PCOS is aimed at preventing and treating the metabolic

Fig. 13.19 Dermoid cysts with "tip of the iceberg" effect

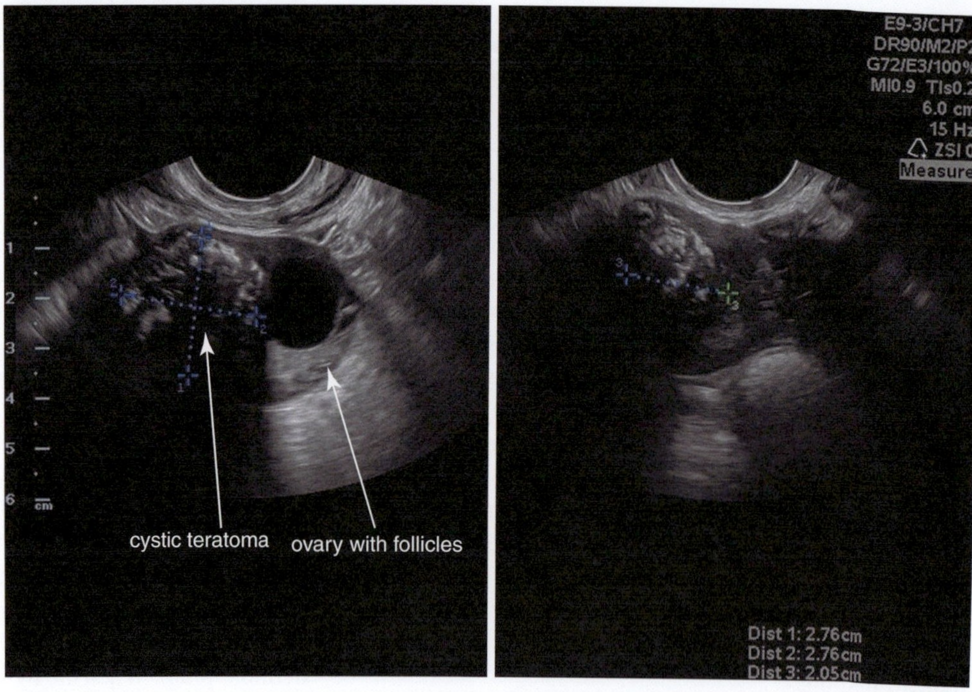

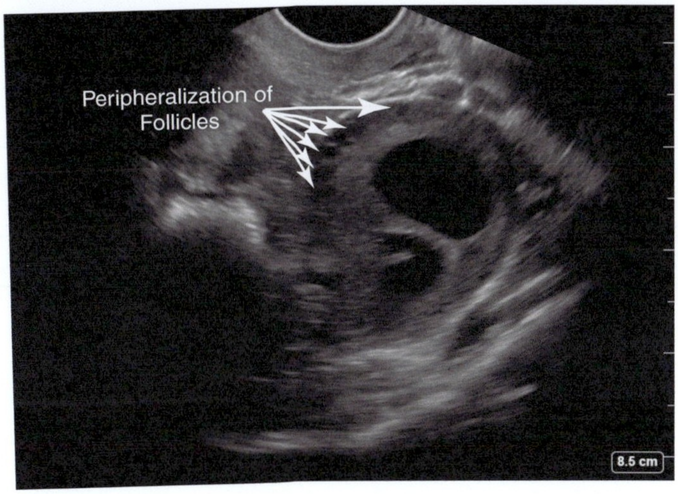

Fig. 13.20 Polycystic left ovary with increased volume, more than 10 follicles in a single section, and peripheralization of the follicles

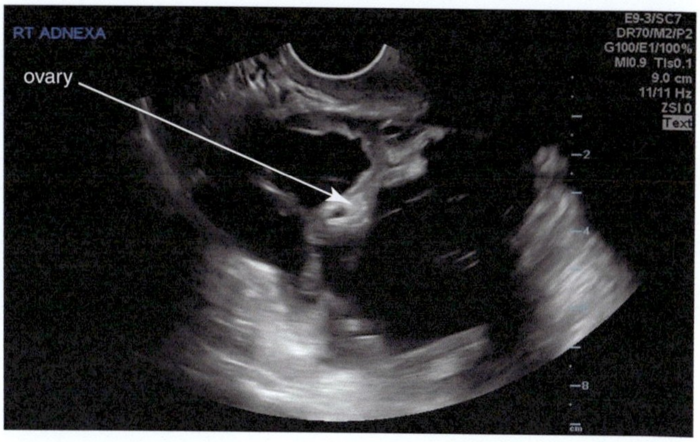

Fig. 13.21 Cystadenocarcinoma with unilocular cysts containing solid components

sequelae of PCOS including diabetes mellitus and cardiovascular disease.

Cystadenoma

Cystadenomas are benign epithelial neoplasms that appear cystic with or without septations and lack vascularity (i.e., there is no internal flow on color Doppler) [152]. Serous cystadenomas are classically smooth, thin-walled, anechoic structures ranging from 5 to 8 cm in diameter [153]. Some serous cystadenomas have fine septations or echogenic areas that look like hemorrhage. Fifteen percent of serous cystadenomas are bilateral [154]. Mucinous cystadenomas are unilateral, thin-walled, and large, ranging from 3 to 30 cm in diameter [155]. Internal thin-walled locules filled with mucin have low-level internal echoes that may vary among tumor locules [156]. Clinical management of cystadenomas is unilateral salpingo-oophorectomy or ovarian cystectomy.

Cystadenocarcinoma

Serous cystadenocarcinomas represent the malignant form of ovarian epithelial tumors, and account for 90% of all ovarian cancers [157]. Given the disease is usually advanced when initially diagnosed, it is associated with high morbidity and mortality [158]. Cystadenocarcinomas consist of unilocular cysts with solid components (Fig. 13.21). Single or multiple papillary projections of the cystic wall represent the solid component. Vascular flow can be detected by placing color Doppler over these projections. Cystadenocarcinomas appear more heterogeneous than cystadenomas and may have associated ascites. Presence of ascites typically indicates tumor extension [159]. Mucinous cystadenocarcinomas appear similar in appearance to serous cystadenocarcinomas, with mixed cystic and solid components. However mucinous cystadenocarcinomas are typically large (>10 cm) and unilateral, whereas serous are typically bilateral with mural thickening [160, 161]. Despite differences in sonographic features and advances in imaging, definitive diagnosis of cystadenomas and cystadenocarcinomas continues to be primarily from histopathology of specimens.

Ovarian Torsion

Ovarian torsion is a gynecological emergency. It occurs when the ovary or fallopian tube has a full or partial twist affecting the ovarian blood supply. Torsion can occur in women of all ages, from infancy through the postmenopausal period, although it is more common in women of reproductive age [162]. Torsion can occur in pregnancy with the highest incidence between the 6th and 14th weeks of gestation [163]. If torsion is suspected clinically, an immediate attempt to diagnose should be made to avoid infarction and preserve ovarian function [164, 165].

Ovarian masses and cysts can act as a fulcrum for torsion and therefore increase risk (Fig. 13.22) [166]. However, because the ovaries are generally mobile and not tightly suspended, torsion can occur without underlying ovarian pathology. Among young adolescent women, torsion without underlying ovarian pathology occurs in close to 50% of cases, leading to delayed diagnosis [167]. More cases of torsion (60%) occur on the right side than the left [168]. This is thought to be due to the higher ovarian venous pressure and longer utero-ovarian ligament on the right, and protection provided by the sigmoid colon on the left.

Ovarian blood supply comes from two sources: the ovarian artery (in the infundibulopelvic ligament) and the uterine artery (in the utero-ovarian ligament). The arteries make an anastomosis (arcade) and enter the uterine capsule. The venous system runs with the arterial system. Initial pain from torsion is from lymphatic and venous stasis. This is followed

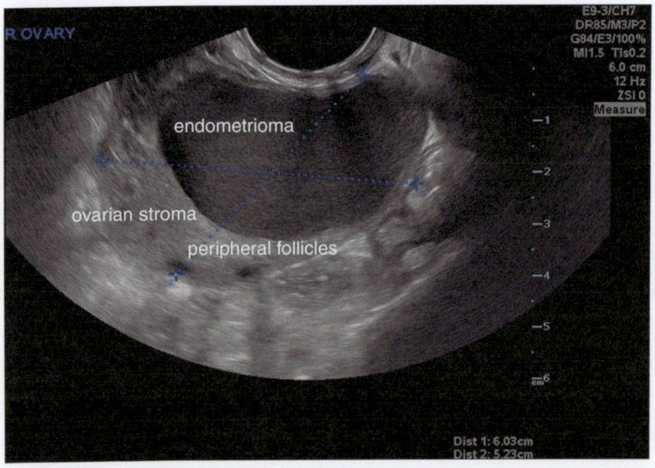

Fig. 13.22 Ovarian torsion with an associated ovarian mass (endometrioma)

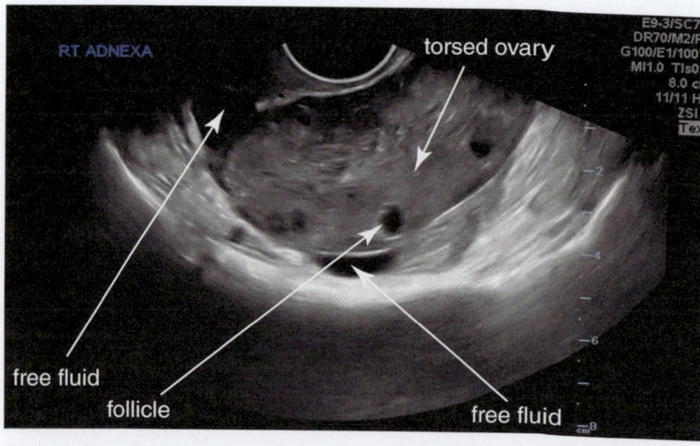

Fig. 13.23 Ovarian torsion with B-mode findings of enlarged size, an edematous ovarian stroma, peripheralization of the follicles, and surrounding free fluid

by edema of the ovarian parenchyma, arterial obstruction, and eventually infarction of the ovary. The ovary can become gangrenous and necrotic with rupture or infection.

Transvaginal ultrasound with Doppler is the imaging of choice. When evaluating the ovaries, start with the unaffected side followed by the painful side. The adnexa should be scanned in B-mode in two planes, followed by a closer examination of the ovary in two planes. The size of the ovary should be measured in three planes.

The most common sonographic finding associated with ovarian torsion is enlarged size >4 cm [169]. Ovarian enlargement is about 80–85% sensitive and 19–65% specific for torsion [170, 171]. Additional findings associated with torsion include ovarian edema, an ovarian cyst or mass, free fluid around the ovary, sites of bleeding within the ovary, free fluid in the pouch of Douglas, distended fallopian tube, abnormal blood flow, and migration to a position more midline and superior to the uterus [171–173]. Presence of any one of these findings carries a sensitivity of close to 90% [171].

The B-mode findings may include an edematous ovarian stroma, peripheralization of the follicles ("string of pearls" sign), free fluid in the peritoneal space, or thickening of the wall of the cystic mass (Fig. 13.23) [167]. Direct visualization of the twisted pedicle in surgery is needed for a definitive diagnosis of torsion [174]. On ultrasound, this will appear as a "target sign" in cross-section with alternating hyperechoic and hypoechoic concentric circles. If color Doppler is added, a "whirlpool" sign may be seen, representing the twisting of the vessels embedded in the thickened pedicle in cross-section with a characteristic spiraling appearance [175]. A whirlpool sign is highly suggestive of torsion [176].

Color Doppler is often incorporated to identify vessels in the setting of torsion assessment [177]. If unable to obtain a color Doppler signal, switching to power Doppler increases the sensitivity for flow. Once vessels are identified with color or power Doppler, apply spectral Doppler to differentiate venous from arterial flow and calculate a resistive index (RI). Place the Doppler gate over the area of interest adjusting the wall filter, gate size, baseline, and scale as needed. If the vessels are hard to identify, lower the filter to increase flow sensitivity. Ovarian vasculature has low resistance and low velocity (10–30 cm/s) requiring the scale to often be lower than other vessels.

An arterial waveform appears triphasic (whereas a venous waveform should appear flat). The RI is calculated by subtracting the end-diastolic velocity from the peak systolic velocity and dividing by the peak systolic velocity. There are normal differences in RI between the dominant and nondominant ovary at baseline and, contrary to some teaching pedagogy, RI should not be used as part of the assessment for torsion [178, 179].

Early stages of torsion may only show loss of venous flow but preserved arterial flow, eventually progressing to loss of both venous and arterial flow (Figs. 13.24 and 13.25). Abnormal or absent venous flow is 100% sensitive and 97% specific for ovarian torsion [180]. Importantly, demonstrating both venous and arterial flow cannot exclude torsion as the ovary has a dual blood supply, and torsion can be intermittent. If there is clinical suspicion of ovarian torsion based on history and physical examination, gynecology should be consulted emergently for time sensitive intra-operative exploration.

Hydrosalpinx

When the fallopian tube is obstructed at either the fimbrial or cornual end, it can fill with fluid and distend, known as hydrosalpinx. This can occur as a result of scarring from pel-

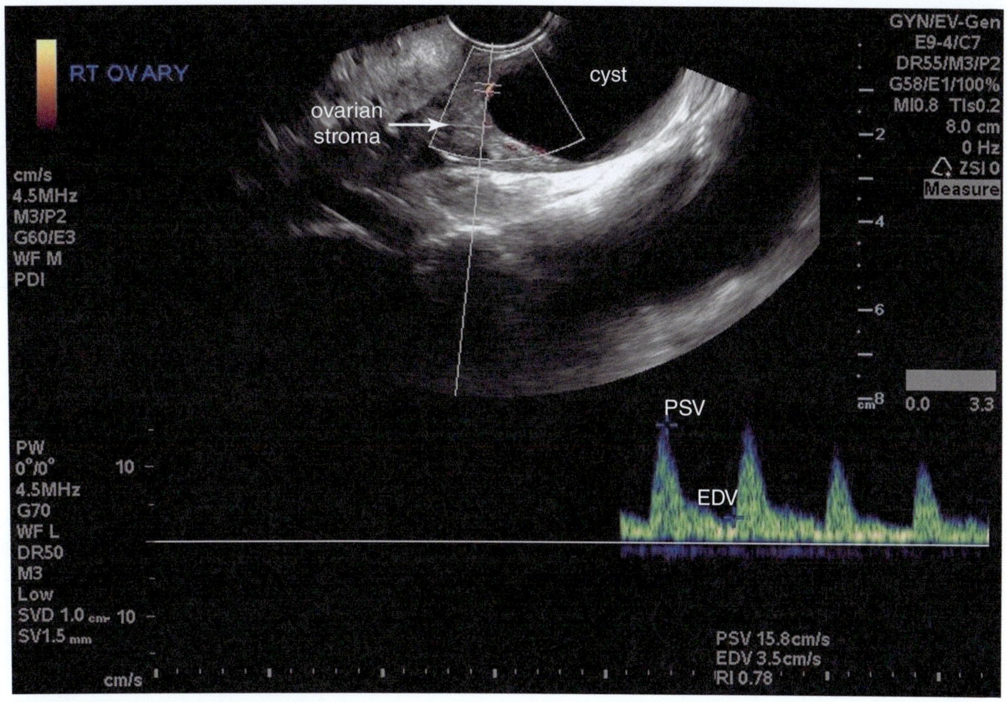

Fig. 13.24 Ovarian torsion with preserved arterial flow on Doppler

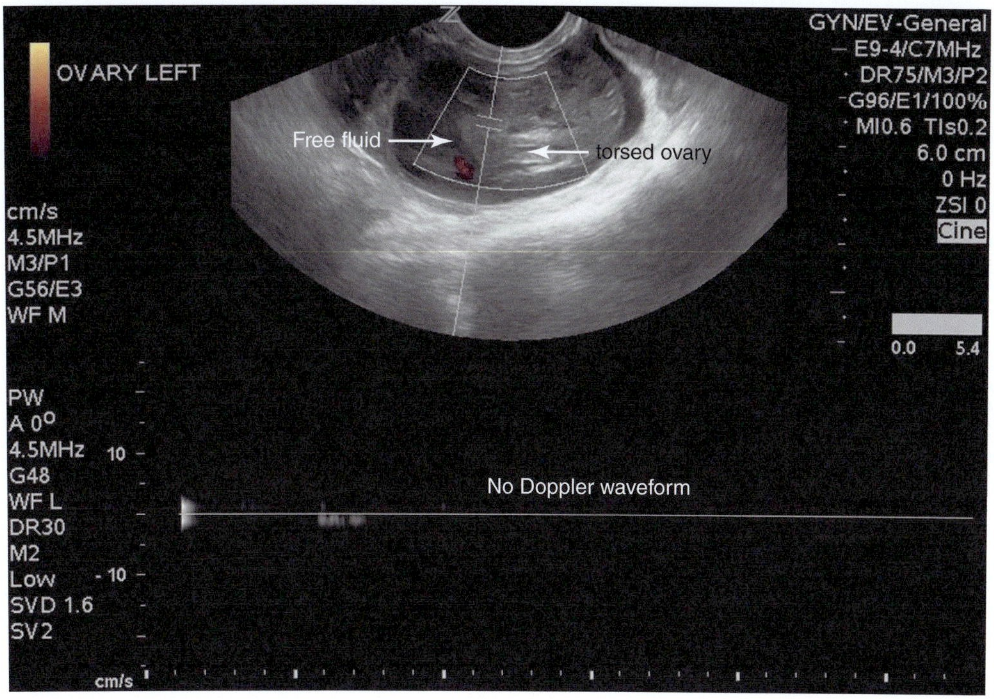

Fig. 13.25 Ovarian torsion demonstrating absence of venous and arterial flow on Doppler

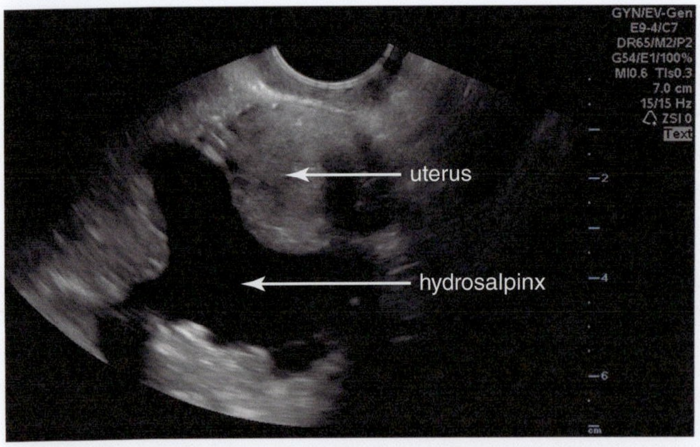

Fig. 13.26 Hydrosalpinx viewed with transvaginal ultrasound

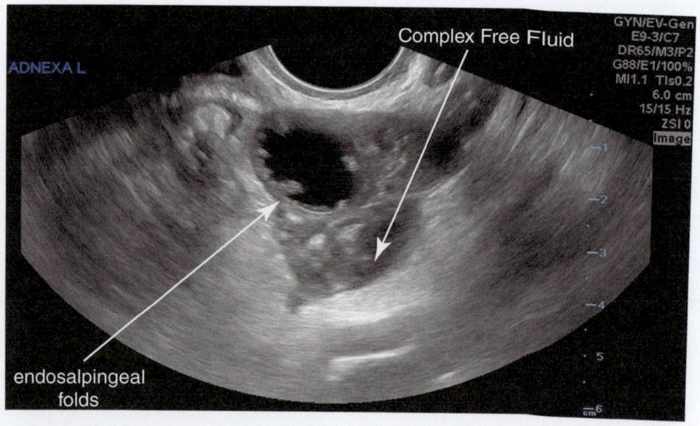

Fig. 13.27 "Cogwheel sign" in a hydrosalpinx

vic surgery and hysterectomy, but symptomatic cases most frequently result from pelvic inflammatory disease [181–183]. Most hydrosalpinges are asymptomatic and commonly seen in postmenopausal women. It is important to diagnose hydrosalpinx when present, as infertility is related to tubal disease in 35% of patients [183, 184].

The normal fallopian tube is rarely appreciated on ultrasound; however, when it is filled with fluid, it is readily appreciated between the ovary and uterine cornua. Hydrosalpinx appears as an elongated cystic mass containing hypo- or anechoic fluid, with intermittent triangular hyperechoic wall protrusions into the lumen (incomplete septa) due to the kinking of the dilated tube (Fig. 13.26) [185, 186]. Hydrosalpinx can easily be confused for ovarian cysts because the tortuous fallopian tube is often visualized in cross-section. However, the longitudinal endosalpingeal folds of the fallopian tube are thick and incomplete, differentiating a hydrosalpinx from an ovarian cyst [185]. When viewing the fallopian tube in short axis, the infolding projections can also look like 2–3 mm hyperechoic nodules, referred to as the "cogwheel sign" given its similarity in appearance to a cogwheel (Fig. 13.27) [187]. Treatment of a symptomatic hydrosalpinx may include salpingectomy or salpingostomy [188]. If asymptomatic hydrosalpinx is diagnosed, a follow-up ultrasound is helpful, as it typically shows no sonographic change in appearance.

Pelvic Inflammatory Disease

Pelvic inflammatory disease (PID) is a spectrum of diseases affecting the female reproductive tract, including the endometrium, fallopian tubes, ovaries, and peritoneal cavity. It encompasses endometritis, salpingitis, pyosalpinx, oophoritis, tubo-ovarian abscess, and pelvic abscess. Patients with PID may have cervical motion tenderness during the insertion of the endocavitary probe at contact with the cervix. In

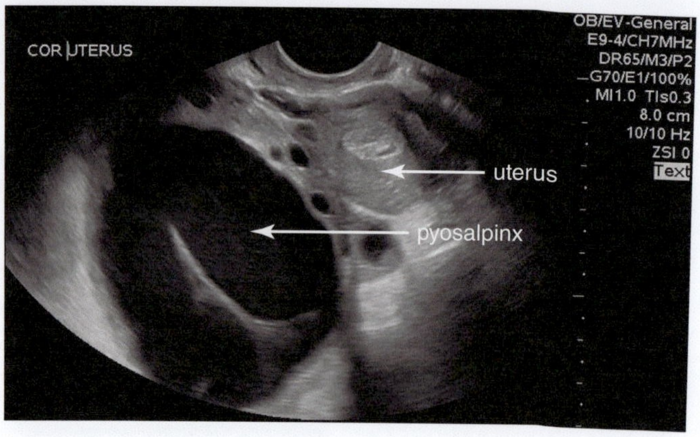

Fig. 13.28 Pyosalpinx demonstrating a thick-walled fallopian tube

early PID, the "indefinite" uterus sign occurs when the margins of the uterus posteriorly are obscured by inflammation and echogenic fluid in the posterior cul de sac.

As PID advances, pyosalpinx occurs where fluid and debris fill the fallopian tube and the wall thickens to >5 mm (Fig. 13.28) [189]. Color Doppler will also show increased flow in the tubal walls.

A tubo-ovarian abscess is a late sequela of PID where the fallopian tube and ovary can no longer be identified as separate structures and become a multilocular cystic mass. There may be septations, solid and cystic components, and surrounding hyperechoic fat enhancement. A ruptured tubo-ovarian abscess can result in the formation of an intra-abdominal abscess.

In Fitz-Hugh–Curtis syndrome, infection spreads up the right paracolic gutter through the peritoneum to the right upper quadrant, which appears as a thickened or three layer hepatic capsule on ultrasonography [190]. The three layers represent the inflamed diaphragm or peritoneum (hyperechoic outermost layer), small ascites (hypoechoic middle layer), and an inflamed hepatic capsule (hyperechoic innermost layer).

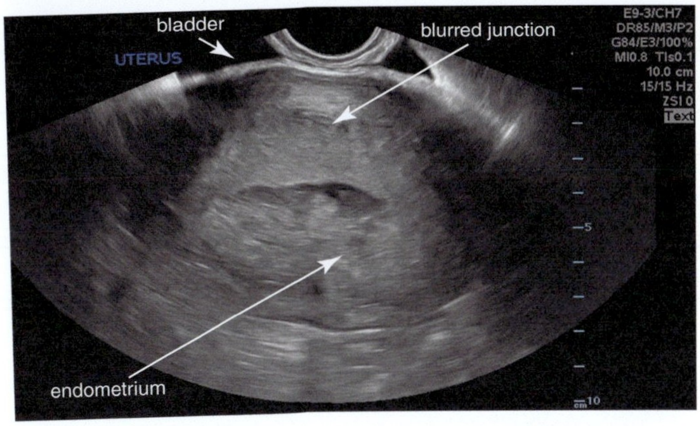

Fig. 13.29 Endometritis characterized by a heterogeneous endometrium with a blurred endometrial junction

Endometritis

Endometritis is inflammation of the endometrium that can occur following up to 2–3% of all vaginal deliveries and 15–20% of Cesarean sections [191, 192]. It can be part of the spectrum of PID and is hard to distinguish sonographically, so it is important to consider in the clinical context [193, 194].

Transabdominal ultrasound can be used initially, followed by transvaginal ultrasound for higher resolution images which allow for a detailed assessment of the endometrium. Sonographic findings include uterine enlargement, a heterogeneous endometrium with a blurred endometrial junction, a subserosal hypoechoic rim (referred to as "hypoechoic rim sign"), echogenic foci with posterior reverberation artifacts from gas-forming bacteria, and increased vascularity on Doppler (Fig. 13.29) [195]. Uterine enlargement and echogenic gas in the postpartum female may not be reliable given these findings may be related to a recent delivery [196]. However, endometrial junctional indistinctness with a hypoechoic rim sign on ultrasound among patients suspected of having endometritis is 80.5% sensitive and 91.7% specific [195].

Key Ultrasound Findings

Hematocolpos	Intraluminal fluid of variable echogenicity occupies the vaginal stripe, and may also appreciate distended uterus with echogenic blood contents
Nabothian Cysts	Simple anechoic cysts in the cervical wall with no color Doppler flow
Fibroid (Leiomyoma)	Heterogeneous appearance within enlarged uterus sometimes with hyperechoic calcifications and shadowing; peripheral vascularity ("bridging vein sign")
Adenomyosis	Ectopic endometrium creates "finger-like" lines in the myometrium ("rainforest" or "Venetian blind" sign)
Endometrial Polyps	Hyperechoic, well-defined lesions with smooth borders and a vascular stalk
Endometriosis	Endometriomas (cysts with isoechoic homogenous echotexture), tender fixed ovaries on transvaginal ultrasound, pouch of Douglas "sliding sign," Deep Infiltrating Endometriosis nodules in anterior and posterior compartments
Intrauterine Device (IUD)	Echogenic linear foreign body with posterior reverberation artifact; appropriate position is in the endometrium, 3 cm from the fundus
Follicle	Simple cyst <3 cm in premenopausal woman
Corpus Luteum	Thick-walled cystic structure ≤3 cm at ovulation, cystic with crenulated inner margins and internal echoes
Pelvic Congestion Syndrome	Pelvic vein diameter >4 mm and slow blood velocity (<3 cm/s)
Simple Cyst	Thin-walled anechoic cyst without septations >2.5 cm with posterior acoustic enhancement.
Hemorrhagic Cyst	May show posterior acoustic enhancement, as well as reticular echoes and intracystic clots
Cystic Teratoma (Dermoid)	Heterogenous mass containing fluid, a large echogenic "ball" with acoustic shadowing, and calcifications
Polycystic Ovarian Syndrome	Increased ovarian volume (≥10 mL) and ≥20 follicles in at least one ovary, or ≥10 follicles in at least one section of the ovary; "string of pearls" appearance of follicles
Cystadenoma	Cystic or anechoic mass with or without septations and no flow on color Doppler
Cystadenocarcinoma	Mixed cystic and solid components with vascularity on Doppler
Ovarian Torsion	Enlarged, edematous ovary with peripheralization of follicles, "whirlpool sign," "string of pearls" appearance of follicles
Hydrosalpinx, Pyosalpinx	Tubular, anechoic adnexal structure with incomplete folds, referred to as "cogwheel sign"
Tubo-ovarian abscess	Multilocular complex cystic adnexal mass
Endometritis	Heterogeneous endometrium with a blurred endometrial junction, "hypoechoic rim sign," echogenic foci with posterior reverberation artifacts and increased vascularity on Doppler

Pearls and Pitfalls

- Transabdominal ultrasound should be attempted first, followed by transvaginal ultrasound when higher resolution images are needed.
- Fan through the entirety of the uterus to avoid missing a uterine abnormality.
- Graded compression is often needed to visualize the ovaries.
- Fibroids (leiomyomas) are common and can have a variable appearance within a large lobulated uterus.
- Free fluid in the peritoneal space is highly sensitive for ovarian cyst rupture, a common cause of acute pelvic pain in young nonpregnant women.
- Blood clots in free fluid can be mistaken for floating bowel.
- Hydrosalpinx and pyosalpinx, when scanned in cross-section, can be mistaken for ovarian cysts or follicles. Scanning in multiple planes and gentle external pressure can help distinguish the separate parts of the fallopian tube.
- Consider adenomyosis and pelvic congestion syndrome as causes of chronic pelvic pain.
- Ovarian torsion is a gynecological emergency and ovarian enlargement with peripheralization of follicles with or without adnexal cyst may be the only sonopathology appreciable.
- Presence of venous and arterial flow does not exclude torsion as the ovary has dual blood supply.
- Pelvic inflammatory disease may exhibit cervical tenderness with insertion of the endocavitary probe with a pyosalpinx or a tubo-ovarian abscess.

References

1. Wilk A, Falk A, DeSilva N. Selected disorders of the female reproductive system. In: Paulman P, Taylor R, Paulman A, Nasir L, editors. Family medicine. New York: Springer; 2020. https://doi.org/10.1007/978-1-4939-0779-3_155-1.
2. Hatipoglu S, Hatipoglu F, Abdullayev R. Acute right lower abdominal pain in women of reproductive age: clinical clues. World J Gastroenterol. 2014;20(14):4043–9. https://doi.org/10.3748/wjg.v20.i14.4043. PMID: 24744594; PMCID: PMC3983461.
3. Cervellin G, Mora R, Ticinesi A, Meschi T, Comelli I, Catena F, Lippi G. Epidemiology and outcomes of acute abdominal pain in a large urban Emergency Department: retrospective analysis of 5,340 cases. Ann Transl Med. 2016;4(19):362. https://doi.org/10.21037/atm.2016.09.10. PMID: 27826565; PMCID: PMC5075866.
4. Fauconnier A, Provot J, Le Creff I, Boulkedid R, Vendittelli F, Doret-Dion M, Sroussi J, Giraudet G, Jacobs R, Bourret A, Bauville E, Carvalho S, Tourette C, Koskas M, Akladios C, Nisolle M, Lejeune C, Huchon C, Alberti C, Dumont A, Bouvier-Colle MH. A framework proposal for quality and safety measurement in gynecologic emergency care. Obstet Gynecol. 2020;136(5):912–21. https://doi.org/10.1097/AOG.0000000000004132. PMID: 33030878; PMCID: PMC7575026.
5. Zafar N, Kupesic PS. Role of ultrasound in the evaluation of acute pelvic pain in nonpregnant reproductive age patients. Reprod Age Patients Donald Sch J Ultrasound Obs Gynecol. 2012;6:207–17. https://doi.org/10.5005/jp-journals-10009-1244.
6. Basta Nikolic M, Spasic A, Hadnadjev Simonji D, Stojanović S, Nikolic O, Nikolic D. Imaging of acute pelvic pain. Br J Radiol. 2021;94(1127):20210281. https://doi.org/10.1259/bjr.20210281. Epub 2021 Sep 7. PMID: 34491817; PMCID: PMC8553212.
7. Bhosale PR, Javitt MC, Atri M, Harris RD, Kang SK, Meyer BJ, Pandharipande PV, Reinhold C, Salazar GM, Shipp TD, Simpson L, Sussman BL, Uyeda J, Wall DJ, Zelop CM, Glanc P. ACR appropriateness criteria® acute pelvic pain in the reproductive age group. Ultrasound Q. 2016;32(2):108–15. https://doi.org/10.1097/RUQ.0000000000000200. PMID: 26588104.
8. Merz E, Evans DH, Dong Y, Jenssen C, Dietrich CF. History of ultrasound in obstetrics and gynaecology from 1971 to 2021 on occasion of the 50 years anniversary of EFSUMB. Med Ultrason. 2023;25(2):175–88. https://doi.org/10.11152/mu-3845. Epub 2022 Aug 22. PMID: 36047427.
9. Estelle Valérie A, Idrissa G, Alihonou S, Anhum K, Simon D. Place of Doppler ultrasound in the characterization of ovarian cysts: about 35 cases. Open J Radiol. 2018;8:167–74. https://doi.org/10.4236/ojrad.2018.83019.
10. Khan AT, Shehmar M, Gupta JK. Uterine fibroids: current perspectives. Int J Women's Health. 2014;6:95–114. https://doi.org/10.2147/IJWH.S51083. PMID: 24511243; PMCID: PMC3914832.
11. Verguts J, Ameye L, Bourne T, Timmerman D. Normative data for uterine size according to age and gravidity and possible role of the classical golden ratio. Ultrasound Obstet Gynecol. 2013;42(6):713–7. https://doi.org/10.1002/uog.12538. PMID: 23754297.
12. Kelsey TW, Dodwell SK, Wilkinson AG, Greve T, Andersen CY, et al. Ovarian volume throughout life: a validated normative model. PLoS One. 2013;8(9):e71465. https://doi.org/10.1371/journal.pone.0071465.
13. Levine D, Patel MD, Suh-Burgmann EJ, Andreotti RF, Benacerraf BR, Benson CB, Brewster WR, Coleman BG, Doubilet PM, Goldstein SR, Hamper UM, Hecht JL, Horrow MM, Hur HC, Marnach ML, Pavlik E, Platt LD, Puscheck E, Smith-Bindman R, Brown DL. Simple adnexal cysts: SRU consensus conference update on follow-up and reporting. Radiology. 2019;293(2):359–71. https://doi.org/10.1148/radiol.2019191354. Epub 2019 Sep 24. PMID: 31549945.
14. Hussain ZJ, Figueroa R, Budorick NE. How much free fluid can a pregnant patient have? Assessment of pelvic free fluid in pregnant patients without antecedent trauma. J Trauma. 2011;70(6):1420–3. https://doi.org/10.1097/TA.0b013e3181edc4fe. PMID: 21817979.
15. Edis-Myers J. Uterine retroversion: a commentary on the indications for the operative correction of retroversion of the uterus, unaccompanied by prolapse- illustrated by six cases. Ind Med Gaz. 1940;75(6):339–44. PMID: 29013983; PMCID: PMC5208011.
16. Haylen BT, McNally G, Birrell W, Logan V, Verity L, Schulz S. Is the retroverted uterus more common in urogynaecology than general gynaecology. Int Urogynecol J Pelvic Floor Dysfunct. 2005;16(Suppl 2):S42.
17. Appelbaum AH, Tirandaz M, Ricci G, Levi D'AR. Alignment of the cervix with the vagina in uterine retroversion: a possible risk factor in uterine prolapse. Diagnostics. 2022;12(6):1428. https://doi.org/10.3390/diagnostics12061428.
18. Muneyyirci-Delale O, Popilevsky F, Zayat N, Vasa R. Lateral, anterior, and posterior displacement of the uterus and its effect on Dysmenorrhea. Womens Health Gyn. 2023;10:1–13.

19. Cagnacci A, Grandi G, Cannoletta M, Xholli A, Piacenti I, Volpe A. Intensity of menstrual pain and estimated angle of uterine flexion. Acta Obstet Gynecol Scand. 2014;93:58–63. https://doi.org/10.1111/aogs.12266.
20. Sanders RC, Parsons AK. Anteverted retroflexed uterus: a common consequence of cesarean delivery. AJR Am J Roentgenol. 2014;203(1):W117–24. https://doi.org/10.2214/AJR.12.10403. PMID: 24951223.
21. Monard M, Marsh C, Schumacher K, Nothnick W. Secretory phase of menstruation and implantation. Front Womens Health. 2018;3 https://doi.org/10.15761/FWH.1000156.
22. Park YR, Lee SW, Kim Y, Bae IY, Kim HK, Choe J, Kim YM. Endometrial thickness cut-off value by transvaginal ultrasonography for screening of endometrial pathology in premenopausal and postmenopausal women. Obstet Gynecol Sci. 2019;62(6):445–53. https://doi.org/10.5468/ogs.2019.62.6.445. Epub 2019 Oct 7. PMID: 31777741; PMCID: PMC6856473.
23. Sugi MD, Penna R, Jha P, Pōder L, Behr SC, Courtier J, Mok-Lin E, Rabban JT, Choi HH. Müllerian duct anomalies: role in fertility and pregnancy. Radiographics. 2021;41(6):1857–75. https://doi.org/10.1148/rg.2021210022. PMID: 34597219.
24. Rackow BW, Arici A. Reproductive performance of women with Müllerian anomalies. Curr Opin Obstet Gynecol. 2007;19:229–37.
25. Grimbizis GF, Camus M, Tarlatzis BC, Bontis JN, Devroey P. Clinical implications of uterine malformations and hysteroscopic treatment results. Hum Reprod Update. 2001;7(2):161–74. https://doi.org/10.1093/humupd/7.2.161.
26. Ludwin A, Martins WP, Nastri CO, Ludwin I, Coelho Neto MA, Leitão VM, Acién M, Alcazar JL, Benacerraf B, Condous G, De Wilde RL, Emanuel MH, Gibbons W, Guerriero S, Hurd WW, Levine D, Lindheim S, Pellicer A, Petraglia F, Saridogan E. Congenital Uterine Malformation by Experts (CUME): better criteria for distinguishing between normal/arcuate and septate uterus? Ultrasound Obstet Gynecol. 2018;51(1):101–9. https://doi.org/10.1002/uog.18923. Erratum in: Ultrasound Obstet Gynecol. 2018;51(2):282. doi: 10.1002/uog.19005. PMID: 29024135
27. Naeh A, Sigal E, Barda S, Hallak M, Gabbay-Benziv R. The association between congenital uterine anomalies and perinatal outcomes - does type of defect matters? J Matern Fetal Neonatal Med. 2022;35(25):7406–11. https://doi.org/10.1080/14767058.2021.1949446. Epub 2021 Jul 8. PMID: 34238096.
28. Heinonen PK. Uterus didelphys: a report of 26 cases. Eur J Obstet Gynecol Reprod Biol. 1984;17(5):345–50.
29. Heinonen PK. Clinical implications of the didelphic uterus: long-term follow-up of 49 cases. Eur J Obstet Gynecol Reprod Biol. 2000;91(2):183–90. https://doi.org/10.1016/S0301-2115(99)00259-6.
30. Heinonen PK. Unicornuate uterus and rudimentary horn. Fertil Steril. 1997;68(2):224–30.
31. Rackow BW, Arici A. Reproductive performance of women with müllerian anomalies. Curr Opin Obstet Gynecol. 2007;19(3):229–37.
32. Isikoglu M. Arcuate uterus: does it really cause pregnancy loss? J Obstet Gynaecol India. 2016;66(1):6–9. https://doi.org/10.1007/s13224-016-0847-5. Epub 2016 Feb 2. PMID: 26924900; PMCID: PMC4755938.
33. Surrey ES, Katz-Jaffe M, Surrey RL, Small AS, Gustofson RL, Schoolcraft WB. Arcuate uterus: is there an impact on in vitro fertilization outcomes after euploid embryo transfer? Fertil Steril. 2018;109(4):638–43. https://doi.org/10.1016/j.fertnstert.2017.12.001. Epub 2018 Mar 30. PMID: 29609956.
34. Donnez J. Arcuate uterus: a legitimate pathological entity? Fertil Steril. 2018;109(4):610. https://doi.org/10.1016/j.fertnstert.2018.01.044. PMID: 29653709.
35. Nasser B, Jerdev M, Nasse H, Nasse W. Hematocolpos-incidence and symptoms in children: a case report. Pediatr Ther. 2022;12:404.
36. Sakalkale R, Samarakkody U. Familial occurrence of imperfurate hymen. J Pediatric Gynecol. 2005;18:427–9.
37. Rabani SM. A rare non urologic cause for urinary retention report of 2 cases. Nephro Urol Mon. 2013;5:766.
38. Lohchab P, Phatak SV, Rajimwale G, Thakur H. Hematocolpos-Ultrasonographic and clinical correlation. J Med Res. 2017;3(6):258–60.
39. Fischer JW, et al. Emergency point of care ultrasound diagnosis of hematocolpometra and imperforate hymen in the pediatric emergency department. Pediatr Emerg Care. 2014;30(2):128–30.
40. Kushnir O, Garde K, Blankstein J. Rectal sonography for diagnosing hematocolpometra. A case report. J Reprod Med. 1997;42(8):519–20.
41. Harou K, Elfarji A, Bassir A, Boukhanni L, Asmouki H, Soummani A. Multiple Nabothian cysts: a cause of cervical obstruction. Open Access Lib J. 2019;6:1–5. https://doi.org/10.4236/oalib.1105212.
42. Fogel SR, Slasky BS. Sonography of Nabothian cysts. Am J Roentgenol. 1982;138:5, 927–30.
43. Okamoto Y, Tanaka YO, Nishida M, Tsunoda H, Yoshikawa H, Itai Y, et al. MR imaging of the uterine cervix: imaging-pathologic correlation. Radiographics. 2003;23:425–45.
44. Stewart EA, Laughlin-Tommaso SK, Catherino WH, Lalitkumar S, Gupta D, Vollenhoven B. Uterine fibroids. Nat Rev Dis Primers. 2016;2:16043.
45. Stewart EA, Cookson C, Gandolfo R, et al. Epidemiology of uterine fibroids: a systematic review. BJOG. 2017;124:1501–12. https://doi.org/10.1111/1471-0528.14640.
46. Commandeur AE, Styer AK, Teixeira JM. Epidemiological and genetic clues for molecular mechanisms involved in uterine leiomyoma development and growth. Hum Reprod Update. 2015;21:593–615. https://doi.org/10.1093/humupd/dmv030.
47. Sato F, Nishi M, Kudo R, et al. Body fat distribution and uterine leiomyomas. J Epidemiol. 1998;8:176–80. https://doi.org/10.2188/jea.8.176.
48. Giuliani E, As-Sanie S, Marsh EE. Epidemiology and management of uterine fibroids. Int J Gynaecol Obstet. 2020;149(1):3–9. https://doi.org/10.1002/ijgo.13102. Epub 2020 Feb 17. PMID: 31960950.
49. Han SC, Kim MD, Jung DC, Lee M, Lee MS, Park SI, Won JY, Lee DY, Lee KH. Degeneration of leiomyoma in patients referred for uterine fibroid embolization: incidence, imaging features and clinical characteristics. Yonsei Med J. 2013;54:215–9.
50. Le D, Dey CB, Byun K. Imaging findings of a torsed pedunculated uterine leiomyoma: a case report. Radiol Case Rep. 2019;15:144–9.
51. Lee HJ, Norwitz ER, Shaw J. Contemporary management of fibroids in pregnancy. Rev Obstet Gynecol. 2010;3:20–7.
52. Carranza-Mamane B, Havelock J, Hemmings R. Reproductive endocrinology and infertility committee. The management of uterine fibroids in women with otherwise unexplained infertility. J Obstet Gynaecol Can. 2015;37:277–85.
53. Levens ED, Wesley R, Premkumar A, Blocker W, Nieman LK. Magnetic resonance imaging and transvaginal ultrasound for determining fibroid burden: implications for research and clinical care. Am J Obstet Gynecol. 2009;200:537.
54. Bittencourt CA, dos Santos Simões R, Bernardo WM, Fuchs LFP, Soares Júnior JM, Pastore AR, Baracat EC. Accuracy of saline contrast sonohysterography in detection of endometrial polyps and submucosal leiomyomas in women of reproductive age with abnormal uterine bleeding: systematic review and

meta-analysis. Ultrasound Obstet Gynecol. 2017;50:32–9. https://doi.org/10.1002/uog.17352.
55. Idowu BM, Ibitoye BO. Doppler sonography of perifibroid and intrafibroid arteries of uterine leiomyomas. Obstet Gynecol Sci. 2018;61:395–403.
56. Kim SH, Sim JS, Seong CK. Interface vessels on color/power Doppler US and MRI: a clue to differentiate subserosal uterine myomas from extrauterine tumors. J Comput Assist Tomogr. 2001;25:36–42.
57. Madan R. The bridging vascular sign. Radiology. 2006;238:371–2.
58. Sharma K, Bora MK, Venkatesh BP, et al. Role of 3D ultrasound and Doppler in differentiating clinically suspected cases of Leiomyoma and Adenomyosis of uterus. J Clin Diagn Res. 2015;9:QC08–12.
59. Kubik-Huch RA, Weston M, Nougaret S, Leonhardt H, Thomassin-Naggara I, Horta M, Cunha TM, Maciel C, Rockall A, Forstner R. European Society of Urogenital Radiology (ESUR) guidelines: MR imaging of Leiomyomas. Eur Radiol. 2018;28:3125–37.
60. Wilde S, Scott-Barrett S. Radiological appearances of uterine fibroids. Indian J Radiol Imaging. 2009;19(3):222–31. https://doi.org/10.4103/0971-3026.54887. PMID: 19881092; PMCID: PMC2766886.
61. Roy C, Bierry G, El Ghali S, Buy X, Rossini A. Acute torsion of uterine leiomyoma: CT features. Abdom Imaging. 2005;30:120–3.
62. Tavernaraki E, Athanasiou S, Ampatzis P. Spontaneous uterine Leiomyoma torsion: a challenging differential diagnosis for radiologists. Eur J Case Rep Intern Med. 2020;7:001586.
63. Filip G, Balzano A, Cagnacci A. Histological evaluation of the prevalence of adenomyosis, myomas and of their concomitance. Minerva Ginecol. 2019;71:177–81. https://doi.org/10.23736/S0026-4784.18.04291-0.
64. Vercellini P, Viganò P, Somigliana E, Daguati R, Abbiati A, Fedele L. Adenomyosis: Epidemiological factors. Best Pract Res Clin Obstet Gynaecol. 2006;20:465–77. https://doi.org/10.1016/j.bpobgyn.2006.01.017.
65. Campo S, Campo V, Benagiano G. Adenomyosis and infertility. Reprod Biomed Online. 2012;24(1):35–46.
66. Meredith SM, Sanchez-Ramos L, Kaunitz AM. Diagnostic accuracy of transvaginal sonography for the diagnosis of adenomyosis: systematic review and metaanalysis. Am J Obstet Gynecol. 2009;201(1):107.e1–6.
67. Haj Hamoud B, Kasoha M, Sillem M, Solomayer EF, Sima RM, Ples L, Schwab R, Olmes GL. Sonographic features of adenomyosis correlated with clinical symptoms and intraoperative findings: a case-control study. Arch Gynecol Obstet. 2023;307(6):1883–9. https://doi.org/10.1007/s00404-022-06852-2. Epub 2023 Mar 11. PMID: 36899194; PMCID: PMC10147740.
68. Kepkep K, Tuncay YA, Göynümer G, Tutal E. Transvaginal sonography in the diagnosis of adenomyosis: which findings are most accurate? Ultrasound Obstet Gynecol. 2007;30:341–5. https://doi.org/10.1002/uog.3985.
69. Andres MP, Borrelli GM, Ribeiro J, et al. Transvaginal ultrasound for the diagnosis of adenomyosis: systematic review and meta-analysis. J Minim Invasive Gynecol. 2018;25:257–64.
70. Arya S, Plavsic SK. Sonographic features of adenomyosis. Donald School J Ultrasound Obstet Gynecol. 2017;11(1):76–81.
71. Brosens JJ, De Souza NM, Barker FG, et al. Endovaginal ultrasonography in the diagnosis of adenomyosis uteri: identifying the predictive characteristics. Br J Obstet Gynaecol. 1995;102:471–4.
72. Fedele L, Bianchi S, Dorta M, et al. Transvaginal ultrasonography in the diagnosis of diffuse adenomyosis. Fertil Steril. 1992;58:94–7.
73. Reinhold C, McCarthy S, Bret PM, et al. Diffuse adenomyosis: comparison of endovaginal US and MR imaging with histopathologic correlation. Radiology. 1996;19:147–60.
74. Sadro CT. Imaging the endometrium: a pictorial essay. Can Assoc Radiol J. 2016;67(3):254–62. https://doi.org/10.1016/j.carj.2015.09.012.
75. Dreisler E, Stampe Sorensen S, Ibsen PH, et al. Prevalence of endometrial polyps and abnormal uterine bleeding in a Danish population aged 20–74 years. Ultrasound Obstet Gynecol. 2009;33(1):102–8.
76. Tjarks M, Van Voorhis BJ. Treatment of endometrial polyps. Obstet Gynecol. 2000;96(6):886–9.
77. Alansari LM, Wardle P. Endometrial polyps and subfertility. Hum Fertil. 2012;15(3):129–33.
78. LaTorre R, De Felice C, De Angelis C, et al. Transvaginal sonographic evaluation of endometrial polyps: a comparison with two dimensional and three dimensional contrast sonography. Clin Exp Obstet Gynecol. 1999;26(3–4):171–3.
79. Reslová T, Tosner J, Resl M, et al. Endometrial polyps. A clinical study of 245 cases. Arch Gynecol Obstet. 1999;262(3–4):133–9.
80. Goldstein SR, Monteagudo A, Popiolek D, et al. Evaluation of endometrial polyps. Am J Obstet Gynecol. 2002;186(4):669–74.
81. Lieng M, Qvigstad E.G.F.D, Lstre O. Flow differences between endometrial polyps and cancer: a prospective study using intravenous contrast-enhanced transvaginal color flow Doppler and three-dimensional Doppler ultrasound. Ultrasound Obstet Gynecol. 2008;32(7):935–40.
82. Alcázar JL, Castillo G, Mínguez JÁ, Galán MJ. Endometrial blood flow mapping using transvaginal power Doppler sonography in women with postmenopausal bleeding and thickened endometrium. Ultrasound Obstet Gynecol. 2003;21:583–8. https://doi.org/10.1002/uog.143.
83. Johnson NP, Hummelshoj L. Consensus on current management of endometriosis. Hum Reprod. 2013;28(6):1552–68.
84. Vigano P, Parazzini F, Somigliana E, Vercellini P. Endometriosis: epidemiology and aetiological factors. Best Pract Res Clin Obstet Gynaecol. 2004;18:177–200.
85. Guerriero S, Condous G, van den Bosch T, Valentin L, Leone FP, Van Schoubroeck D, Exacoustos C, Installé AJ, Martins WP, Abrao MS, Hudelist G, Bazot M, Alcazar JL, Gonçalves MO, Pascual MA, Ajossa S, Savelli L, Dunham R, Reid S, Menakaya U, Bourne T, Ferrero S, Leon M, Bignardi T, Holland T, Jurkovic D, Benacerraf B, Osuga Y, Somigliana E, Timmerman D. Systematic approach to sonographic evaluation of the pelvis in women with suspected endometriosis, including terms, definitions and measurements: a consensus opinion from the International Deep Endometriosis Analysis (IDEA) group. Ultrasound Obstet Gynecol. 2016;48(3):318–32. https://doi.org/10.1002/uog.15955. Epub 2016 Jun 28. PMID: 27349699.
86. Jain S, Dalton ME. Chocolate cysts from ovarian follicles. Fertil Steril. 1999;72(5):852–6. https://doi.org/10.1016/s0015-0282(99)00367-2. PMID: 10560989.
87. Rehmer JM, Flyckt RL, Goodman LR, Falcone T. Management of Endometriomas. Obstet Gynecol Surv. 2019;74(4):232–40. https://doi.org/10.1097/OGX.0000000000000660. PMID: 31344251.
88. Patel MD, Feldstein VA, Chen DC, Lipson SD, Filly RA. Endometriomas: diagnostic performance of US. Radiology. 1999;210:739–45.
89. de Oliveira JGA, Bonfada V, Zanella JFP, Coser J. Transvaginal ultrasound in deep endometriosis: pictorial essay. Radiol Bras. 2019;52(5):337–41. https://doi.org/10.1590/0100-3984.2018.0019. PMID: 31656353; PMCID: PMC6808616.
90. Asch E, Levine D. Variations in appearance of endometriomas. J Ultrasound Med. 2007;26:993–1002.
91. Van Holsbeke C, Van Calster B, Guerriero S, Savelli L, Paladini D, Lissoni AA, et al. Endometriomas: their ultrasound characteristics. Ultrasound Obstet Gynecol. 2010;35:730–40.

92. Chaudhry S, Glanc P, Salem S. Detection and differential diagnosis of suspected malignant transformation of an endometrioma during pregnancy. BMJ Case Rep. 2013;2013:bcr2012007744. https://doi.org/10.1136/bcr-2012-007744. PMID: 23917357; PMCID: PMC3762441.
93. Nisenblat V, Bossuyt PM, Farquhar C, Johnson N, Hull ML. Imaging modalities for the non-invasive diagnosis of endometriosis. Cochrane Database Syst Rev. 2016;2(2):CD009591. https://doi.org/10.1002/14651858.CD009591.pub2. PMID: 26919512; PMCID: PMC7100540.
94. Ghezzi F, Raio L, Cromi A, Duwe DG, Beretta P, Buttarelli M, Mueller MD. "Kissing ovaries": a sonographic sign of moderate to severe endometriosis. Fertil Steril. 2005;83(1):143–7. https://doi.org/10.1016/j.fertnstert.2004.05.094. PMID: 15652900.
95. Okaro E, Condous G, Khalid A, Timmerman D, Ameye L, Huffel SV, et al. The use of ultrasound-based 'soft markers' for the prediction of pelvic pathology in women with chronic pelvic pain: can we reduce the need for laparoscopy? BJOG. 2006;113:251e6.
96. Collins BG, Ankola A, Gola S, McGillen KL. Transvaginal US of endometriosis: looking beyond the Endometrioma with a dedicated protocol. Radiographics. 2019;39(5):1549–68. https://doi.org/10.1148/rg.2019190045. PMID: 31498746.
97. Ferlay J, Soerjomataram I, Dikshit R, Eser S, Mathers C, Rebelo M, Parkin DM, Forman D, Bray F. Cancer incidence and mortality worldwide: sources, methods and major patterns in GLOBOCAN. Int J Cancer. 2012;136:E359–86.
98. ACOG Committee Opinion No. 734: the role of transvaginal ultrasonography in evaluating the endometrium of women with postmenopausal bleeding. Obstet Gynecol. 2018;131(5):e124–9. https://doi.org/10.1097/AOG.0000000000002631. PMID: 29683909.
99. Goldstein RB, Bree RL, Benson CB, Benacerraf BR, Bloss JD, Carlos R, Fleischer AC, Goldstein SR, Hunt RB, Kurman RJ, Kurtz AB, Laing FC, Parsons AK, Smith-Bindman R, Walker J. Evaluation of the woman with postmenopausal bleeding: Society of Radiologists in ultrasound-sponsored consensus conference statement. J Ultrasound Med. 2001;20:1025–36. https://doi.org/10.7863/jum.2001.20.10.1025.
100. The role of transvaginal ultrasonography in evaluating the Endometrium of women with postmenopausal bleeding. www.acog.org. https://www.acog.org/clinical/clinical-guidance/committee-opinion/articles/2018/05/the-role-of-transvaginal-ultrasonography-in-evaluating-the-endometrium-of-women-with-postmenopausal-bleeding.
101. Epstein E, Fischerova D, Valentin L, Testa AC, Franchi D, Sladkevicius P, Frühauf F, Lindqvist PG, Mascilini F, Fruscio R, Haak LA, Opolskiene G, Pascual MA, Alcazar JL, Chiappa V, Guerriero S, Carlson JW, Van Holsbeke C, Giuseppe Leone FP, De Moor B, Bourne T, van Calster B, Installe A, Timmerman D, Verbakel JY, Van den Bosch T. Ultrasound characteristics of endometrial cancer as defined by International Endometrial Tumor Analysis (IETA) consensus nomenclature: prospective multicenter study. Ultrasound Obstet Gynecol. 2018;51:818–28. https://doi.org/10.1002/uog.18909.
102. Leone FP, Timmerman D, Bourne T, Valentin L, Epstein E, Goldstein SR, Marret H, Parsons AK, Gull B, Istre O, Sepulveda W, Ferrazzi E, Van den Bosch T. Terms, definitions and measurements to describe the sonographic features of the endometrium and intrauterine lesions: a consensus opinion from the International Endometrial Tumor Analysis (IETA) group. Ultrasound Obstet Gynecol. 2010;35(1):103–12. https://doi.org/10.1002/uog.7487. PMID: 20014360.
103. Çintesun FNİ, Çintesun E, Esenkaya Ü, Günenc O. Uterine dimensions and intrauterine device malposition: can ultrasound predict displacement or expulsion before it happens? Arch Gynecol Obstet. 2020;302(5):1181–7. https://doi.org/10.1007/s00404-020-05713-0. Epub 2020 Aug 3. PMID: 32748051.
104. Fadiloglu S, Dilbaz B, Fadiloglu E, Dilbaz S. Relationship between copper IUD complications and ultrasonographic findings. Arch Gynecol Obstet. 2018;297(4):989–96.
105. Braaten KP, Benson CB, Maurer R, Goldberg AB. Malpositioned intrauterine contraceptive devices: risk factors, outcomes, and future pregnancies. Obstet Gynecol. 2011;118(5):1014–20.
106. Committee Opinion No 672. Clinical challenges of long-acting reversible contraceptive methods. Obstet Gynecol. 2016;128(3):e69–77.
107. Moschos E, Twickler DM. Does the type of intrauterine device affect conspicuity on 2D and 3D ultrasound? AJR Am J Roentgenol. 2011;196:1439–43. https://doi.org/10.2214/AJR.10.5483.
108. Boortz HE, Margolis DJ, Ragavendra N, Patel MK, Kadell BM. Migration of intrauterine devices: radiologic findings and implications for patient care. Radiographics. 2012;32:335–52.
109. Kerr NK, Dunham R, Wolstenhulme S, Wilson J. Comparison of two- and three-dimensional transvaginal ultrasound in the visualisation of intrauterine devices. Ultrasound. 2014;22(3):141–7. https://doi.org/10.1177/1742271X14532082. Epub 2014 Apr 23. PMID: 27433211; PMCID: PMC4760533.
110. Letti Muller AL, Lopes Ramos JG, Martins-Costa SH, Palma Dias RS, Valerio EG, Hammes LS, et al. Transvaginal ultrasonographic assessment of the expulsion rate of intrauterine devices inserted in the immediate postpartum period: a pilot study. Contraception. 2005;72:192–5.
111. Petta CA, Faundes D, Pimentel E, Diaz J, Bahamondes L. The use of vaginal ultrasound to identify copper T IUDs at high risk of expulsion. Contraception. 1996;54:287–9.
112. Morales-Rosello J. Spontaneous upward movement of lowly placed T-shaped IUDs. Contraception. 2005;72:430–1.
113. Lee A, Eppel W, Sam C, Kratochwil A, Deutinger J, Bernaschek G. Intrauterine device localization by three-dimensional transvaginal sonography. Ultrasound Obstet Gynecol. 1997;10:289–92.
114. Caliskan E, Ozturk N, Dilbaz BO, Dilbaz S. Analysis of risk factors associated with uterine perforation by intrauterine devices. Eur J Contracept Reprod Health Care. 2003;8:150–5.
115. Rowlands S, Oloto E, Horwell DH. Intrauterine devices and risk of uterine perforation: current perspectives. Open Access J Contracept. 2016;7:19–32. https://doi.org/10.2147/OAJC.S85546. PMID: 29386934; PMCID: PMC5683155.
116. Martins WP, Kollmann M, Raine-Fenning N. Counting ovarian follicles: updated threshold for diagnosis of hyperandrogenic anovulation. Ultrasound Obstet Gynecol. 2014;44:131–4.
117. Baerwald AR, Walker RA, Pierson RA. Growth rates of ovarian follicles during natural menstrual cycles, oral contraception cycles, and ovarian stimulation cycles. Fertil Steril. 2009;91(2):440–9.,ISSN 0015-0282. https://doi.org/10.1016/j.fertnstert.2007.11.054.
118. Valentin L. Pattern recognition of pelvic masses by gray-scale ultrasound imaging: the contribution of Doppler ultrasound. Ultrasound Obstet Gynecol. 1999;14:338–47.
119. Ignacio EA, Dua R, Sarin S, et al. Pelvic congestion syndrome: diagnosis and treatment. Semin Intervent Radiol. 2008;25:361–8.
120. Bałabuszek K, Toborek M, Pietura R. Comprehensive overview of the venous disorder known as pelvic congestion syndrome. Ann Med. 2022;54(1):22–36. https://doi.org/10.1080/07853890.2021.2014556. PMID: 34935563; PMCID: PMC8725876.
121. Perry CP. Current concepts of pelvic congestion and chronic pelvic pain. JSLS. 2001;5(2):105–10. PMID: 11394421; PMCID: PMC3015423.
122. Scultetus AH, Villavicencio JL, Gillespie DL. The nutcracker syndrome: its role in the pelvic venous disorders. J Vasc Surg. 2001;34(5):812–9. https://doi.org/10.1067/mva.2001.118802. PMID: 11700480.

123. Aurshina A, Huber S, Deng Y, et al. Correlation of venous symptoms with iliac vein stenosis on magnetic resonance imaging. Proc J Vasc Surg Venous Lymphat Disord. 2021;9(5):1291–1296.e1.
124. Brice G, Mansour S, Bell R, Collin JR, Child AH, Brady AF, Sarfarazi M, Burnand KG, Jeffery S, Mortimer P, Murday VA. Analysis of the phenotypic abnormalities in lymphoedema-distichiasis syndrome in 74 patients with FOXC2 mutations or linkage to 16q24. J Med Genet. 2002;39(7):478–83. https://doi.org/10.1136/jmg.39.7.478. PMID: 12114478; PMCID: PMC1735188.
125. Patel MD, Young SW, Dahiya N. Ultrasound of pelvic pain in the nonpregnant woman. Radiol Clin North Am. 2019;57(3):601–16.
126. Park SJ, Lim JW, Ko YT, Lee DH, Yoon Y, Oh JH, Lee HK, Huh CY. Diagnosis of pelvic congestion syndrome using transabdominal and transvaginal sonography. AJR Am J Roentgenol. 2004;182(3):683–8. https://doi.org/10.2214/ajr.182.3.1820683. PMID: 14975970.
127. Sokalska A, Timmerman D, Testa AC, et al. Diagnostic accuracy of transvaginal ultrasound examination for assigning a specific diagnosis to adnexal masses. Ultrasound Obstet Gynecol. 2009;34:462–70.
128. Andreotti RF. Ovarian-Adnexal reporting lexicon for ultrasound: a white paper of the ACR Ovarian-Adnexal Reporting and Data System Committee. J Am Coll Radiol. 2018;15:1415–29. Copyright ! 2018 American College of Radiology.
129. Timmerman D, Testa AC, Bourne T, Ameye L, Jurkovic D, Van Holsbeke C, et al. Simple ultrasound-based rules for the diagnosis of ovarian cancer. Ultrasound Obstet Gynecol. 2008;31:681–90.
130. Farghaly SA. Current diagnosis and management of ovarian cysts. Clin Exp Obstet Gynecol. 2014;41(6):609–12. PMID: 25551948.
131. Ishihara K, Nemoto Y. Sonographic appearance of hemorrhagic ovarian cyst with acute abdomen by transvaginal scan. Nihon Ika Daigaku Zasshi. 1997;64(5):411–5. https://doi.org/10.1272/jnms1923.64.411. PMID: 9366144.
132. Abbas AM, Amin MT, Tolba SM, Ali MK. Hemorrhagic ovarian cysts: clinical and sonographic correlation with the management options. Middle East Fertil Soc J. 2016;21(1):41–5. ISSN 1110-5690, https://doi.org/10.1016/j.mefs.2015.08.001
133. Kim JH, Lee SM, Lee JH, Jo YR, Moon MH, Shin J, Kim BJ, Hwang KR, Lee TS, Bai KB, Jeon HW. Successful conservative management of ruptured ovarian cysts with hemoperitoneum in healthy women. PLoS One. 2014;9(3):e91171. https://doi.org/10.1371/journal.pone.0091171. PMID: 24608424; PMCID: PMC3946718.
134. Bottomley C, Bourne T. Diagnosis and Management of Ovarian Cyst Accidents. Best Pract Res Clin Obstet Gynaecol. 2009;23:711–24.
135. Von Kuenssberg JD, Stiller G, Wagner D. Sensitivity in detecting free intraperitoneal fluid with the pelvic views of the FAST exam. Am J Emerg Med. 2003;21(6):476–8. https://doi.org/10.1016/s0735-6757(03)00162-1. PMID: 14574655.
136. Mantecon O, George A, DeGeorge C, McCauley E, Mangal R, Stead TS, Peplinski B, Ganti L. A case of Hemorrhagic ovarian cyst rupture necessitating surgical intervention. Cureus. 2022;14(9):e29350. https://doi.org/10.7759/cureus.29350. PMID: 36284799; PMCID: PMC9583282.
137. Amirbekian S, Hooley RJ. Ultrasound evaluation of pelvic pain. Radiol Clin North Am. 2014;52:1215–35.
138. Feng Y, Tamadon A, Hsueh AJW. Imaging the ovary. Reprod Biomed Online. 2018;36:584–93.
139. Hertzberg B, Kliewer M, Paulson E. Ovarian cyst rupture causing hemoperitoneum: imaging features and the potential for misdiagnosis. Abdom Imaging. 1999;24:304–8. https://doi.org/10.1007/s002619900502.
140. Cong L, Wang S, Yeung SY, Lee JHS, Chung JPW, Chan DYL. Mature cystic Teratoma: an integrated review. Int J Mol Sci. 2023;24(7):6141. https://doi.org/10.3390/ijms24076141. PMID: 37047114; PMCID: PMC10093990.
141. Peterson WF, Prevost EC, Edmunds FT, Hundley JM Jr, Morris FK. Benign cystic teratomas of the ovary; a clinico-statistical study of 1,007 cases with a review of the literature. Am J Obstet Gynecol. 1955;70:368–82.
142. Mais V, Guerriero S, Ajossa S, Angiolucci M, Paoletti AM, Melis GB. Transvaginal ultrasonography in the diagnosis of cystic teratoma. Obstet Gynecol. 1995;85(1):48–52. https://doi.org/10.1016/0029-7844(94)00323-6. PMID: 7800323.
143. Ameye L, Timmerman D, Valentin L, et al. Clinically oriented three-step strategy for assessment of adnexal pathology. Ultrasound Obstet Gynecol. 2012;40:582–91.
144. Jermy K, Luise C, Bourne T. The characterization of common ovarian cysts in premenopausal women. Ultrasound Obstet Gynecol. 2001;17:140–4.
145. Cohen L, Sabbagha R. Echo patterns of benign cystic teratomas by transvaginal ultrasound. Ultrasound Obstet Gynecol. 1993;3:120–3.
146. Peterson WF, Prevost EC, Edmunds FT, Hundley JM Jr, Morris FK. Benign cystic teratomas of the ovary; a clinico-statistical study of 1,007 cases with a review of the literature. Am J Obstet Gynecol. 1955;70:368–82. https://doi.org/10.1594/EURORAD/CASE.7708. https://www.eurorad.org/case/7708. ISSN: 1563-4086
147. Teede HJ, Tay CT, Laven JJE, et al. Recommendations from the 2023 international evidence-based guideline for the assessment and management of polycystic ovary syndrome. J Clin Endocrinol Metab. 2023;108(10):2447–69. https://doi.org/10.1210/clinem/dgad463.
148. Diamanti-Kandarakis E, Panidis D. Unravelling the phenotypic map of polycystic ovary syndrome (PCOS): a prospective study of 634 women with PCOS. Clin Endocrinol. 2007;67(5):735–42. https://doi.org/10.1111/j.1365-2265.2007.02954.x. Epub 2007 Aug 29. PMID: 17760884.
149. Fulghesu AM, Canu E, Porru C, Cappai A. Ultrasound diagnosis of polycystic ovarian syndrome: current guidelines, criticism and possible update. Austin J Obstet Gynecol. 2017;4(2):1074.
150. Christ JP, Cedars MI. Current guidelines for diagnosing PCOS. Diagnostics (Basel). 2023;13(6):1113. https://doi.org/10.3390/diagnostics13061113. PMID: 36980421; PMCID: PMC10047373.
151. Ponnatapura J, Dyer RB, Ou JJ. The ovarian "string-of-pearls" sign. Abdom Radiol. 2019;44:1181–2. https://doi.org/10.1007/s00261-018-1830-7.
152. Suh-Burgmann E, Nakhaei M, Gupta S, Brook A, Hecht J, Hung YY, Levine D. Ovarian cystadenomas: growth rate and reliability of imaging measurements. J Ultrasound Med. 2022;41(9):2157–67. https://doi.org/10.1002/jum.15895. Epub 2021 Nov 30. PMID: 34846072.
153. Sayasneh A, Ekechi C, Ferrara L, Kaijser J, Stalder C, Sur S, Timmerman D, Bourne T. The characteristic ultrasound features of specific types of ovarian pathology (review). Int J Oncol. 2015;46(2):445–58. https://doi.org/10.3892/ijo.2014.2764. Epub 2014 Nov 18. PMID: 25406094; PMCID: PMC4277251.
154. Testa AC, Ferrandina G, Timmerman D, et al. Imaging in gynecological disease (1): ultrasound features of metastases in the ovaries differ depending on the origin of the primary tumor. Ultrasound Obstet Gynecol. 2007;29:505–11.
155. Moro F, Esposito R, Landolfo C, Froyman W, Timmerman D, Bourne T, Scambia G, Valentin L, Testa AC. Ultrasound evaluation of ovarian masses and assessment of the extension of ovarian malignancy. Br J Radiol. 2021;94(1125):20201375. https://doi.org/10.1259/bjr.20201375. Epub 2021 Jun 9. PMID: 34106762; PMCID: PMC9327748.

156. Karlan BY, Bristow RE, Li AJ. Gynecologic oncology: clinical practice & surgical atlas. New York: McGraw-Hill Medical; 2012.
157. Liu H, Wang A, Ma Y. Increased expression of LYNX1 in ovarian serous cystadenocarcinoma predicts poor prognosis. Biomed Res Int. 2020;2020:1392674. https://doi.org/10.1155/2020/1392674.
158. Webb PM, Jordan SJ. Epidemiology of epithelial ovarian cancer. Best Pract Res Clin Obstetrics Gynaecol. 2017;41:3–14. https://doi.org/10.1016/j.bpobgyn.2016.08.006.
159. Luis Alcázar J, Ramón Pérez-Vidal J, Tameish S, Chacón E, Manzour N, Ángel MJ. Ultrasound for assessing tumor spread in ovarian cancer. A systematic review of the literature and meta-analysis. Eur J Obstet Gynecol Reprod Biol. 2024;292:194–200. https://doi.org/10.1016/j.ejogrb.2023.11.017. Epub 2023 Nov 18. PMID: 38042117.
160. Laurent P-E, Thomassin-Piana J, Jalaguier-Coudray A. Mucin-producing tumors of the ovary: MR imaging appearance. Diagn Interv Imaging. 2015;96(11):1125–32, ISSN 2211-5684. https://doi.org/10.1016/j.diii.2014.11.034.
161. Brown J, Frumovitz M. Mucinous tumors of the ovary: current thoughts on diagnosis and management. Curr Oncol Rep. 2014;16(6):389. https://doi.org/10.1007/s11912-014-0389-x. PMID: 24777667; PMCID: PMC4261626
162. Robertson JJ, Long B, Koyfman A. Myths in the evaluation and management of ovarian torsion. J Emerg Med. 2017;52(4):449–56, ISSN 0736-4679. https://doi.org/10.1016/j.jemermed.2016.11.012.
163. Young R, Cork K. Intermittent ovarian torsion in pregnancy. Clin Pract Cases Emerg Med. 2017;1(2):108–10. https://doi.org/10.5811/cpcem.2016.12.32932. PMID: 29849404; PMCID: PMC5965408.
164. Dasgupta R, Renaud E, Goldin AB, Baird R, Cameron DB, Arnold MA, Diefenbach KA, Gosain A, Grabowski J, Guner YS, et al. Ovarian torsion in pediatric and adolescent patients: a systematic review. J Pediatr Surg. 2018;53:1387–91.
165. Tielli A, Scala A, Alison M, Vo Chieu VD, Farkas N, Titomanlio L, Lenglart L. Ovarian torsion: diagnosis, surgery, and fertility preservation in the pediatric population. Eur J Pediatr. 2022;181:1405–11.
166. Budhram G, Elia T, Dan J, et al. A case-control study of sonographic maximum ovarian diameter as a predictor of ovarian torsion in emergency department females with pelvic pain. Acad Emerg Med. 2019;26(2):152–9. https://doi.org/10.1111/acem.13523.
167. Karaca SY, İleri A. Ovarian torsion in adolescents with and without ovarian mass: a cross-sectional study. J Pediatr Adolesc Gynecol. 2021;34(6):857–61. https://doi.org/10.1016/j.jpag.2021.05.007. Epub 2021 May 25. PMID: 34044177.
168. Tabbara F, Hariri M, Hitti E. Ovarian torsion: a retrospective case series at a tertiary care center emergency department. PLoS One. 2024;19(3):e0297690. https://doi.org/10.1371/journal.pone.0297690. PMID: 38446824; PMCID: PMC10917280.
169. Albayram F, Hamper UM. Ovarian and adnexal torsion: spectrum of sonographic findings with pathologic correlation. J Ultrasound Med. 2001;20(10):1083–9.
170. Mashiach R, Melamed N, Gilad N, Ben-Shitrit G, Meizner I. Sonographic diagnosis of ovarian torsion. J Ultrasound Med. 2011;30(9):1205–10. https://doi.org/10.7863/jum.2011.30.9.1205.
171. Ghulmiyyah L, Nassar A, Sassine D, Khoury S, Nassif J, Ramadan H, Najem E, Berjawi G. Accuracy of pelvic ultrasound in diagnosing adnexal torsion. Radiol Res Pract. 2019;2019:1406291. https://doi.org/10.1155/2019/1406291. PMID: 31354994; PMCID: PMC6633867.
172. Hiller N, Appelbaum L, Simanovsky N, Lev-Sagi A, Aharoni D, Sella T. CT features of adnexal torsion. AJR Am J Roentgenol. 2007;189(1):124–9.
173. Lee JH, Park SB, Shin SH, et al. Value of intra-adnexal and extra-adnexal computed tomographic imaging features diagnosing torsion of adnexal tumor. J Comput Assist Tomogr. 2009;33(6):872–6.
174. Huang C, Hong MK, Ding DC. A review of ovary torsion. Ci Ji Yi Xue Za Zhi. 2017;29(3):143–7. https://doi.org/10.4103/tcmj.tcmj_55_17. PMID: 28974907; PMCID: PMC5615993.
175. Vijayaraghavan SB. Sonographic Whirlpool sign in ovarian torsion. J Ultrasound Med. 2004;23:1643–9. https://doi.org/10.7863/jum.2004.23.12.1643.
176. Valsky DV, Cohen SM, Hamani Y, Lipschuetz M, Yagel S, Esh-Broder E. Whirlpool sign in the diagnosis of adnexal torsion with atypical clinical presentation. Ultrasound Obstet Gynecol. 2009;34:239–42. https://doi.org/10.1002/uog.7310.
177. Ben-Ami M, Perlitz Y, Haddad S. The effectiveness of spectral and color Doppler in predicting ovarian torsion. A prospective study. Eur J Obstet Gynecol Reprod Biol. 2002;104(1):64–6. https://doi.org/10.1016/s0301-2115(02)00056-8. PMID: 12128265
178. Scholtes MC, Wladimiroff JW, van Rijen HJ, Hop WC. Uterine and ovarian flow velocity waveforms in the normal menstrual cycle: a transvaginal Doppler study. Fertil Steril. 1989;52(6):981–5.
179. Rosado W, Mt T, Gosink B, Pretonius B. Adnexal torsion: diagnosis by using Doppler sonography. AJR. 1992;159:1251–3.
180. Nizar K, Deutsch M, Filmer S, Weizman B, Beloosesky R, Weiner Z. Doppler studies of the ovarian venous blood flow in the diagnosis of adnexal torsion. J Clin Ultrasound. 2009;37:436–9. https://doi.org/10.1002/jcu.20621.
181. Romosan G, Valentin L. The sensitivity and specificity of transvaginal ultrasound with regard to acute pelvic inflammatory disease: a review of the literature. Arch Gynecol Obstet. 2014;289:705–14. https://doi.org/10.1007/s00404-013-3091-6.
182. Taipale P, Tarjanne H, Ylöstalo P. Transvaginal sonography in suspected pelvic inflammatory disease. Ultrasound Obstet Gynecol. 1995;6:430–4.
183. Delgado-Morell A, Nieto-Tous M, Andrada-Ripollés C, Pascual MÁ, Ajossa S, Guerriero S, Alcázar JL. Transvaginal ultrasound accuracy in the Hydrosalpinx diagnosis: a systematic review and meta-analysis. Diagnostics (Basel). 2023;13(5):948. https://doi.org/10.3390/diagnostics13050948. PMID: 36900092; PMCID: PMC10000875
184. Honoré GM, Holden AE, Schenken RS. Pathophysiology and management of proximal tubal blockage. Fertil Steril. 1999;71:785–95.
185. Timor-Tritsch IE, Lerner JP, Monteagudo A, Murphy KE, Heller DS. Transvaginal sonographic markers of tubal inflammatory disease. Ultrasound Obstet Gynecol. 1998;12:56–66. [CrossRef]
186. Molander P, Sjöberg J, Paavonen J, Cacciatore B. Transvaginal power Doppler findings in laparoscopically proven acute pelvic inflammatory disease. Ultrasound Obstet Gynecol. 2001;17:233–8.
187. Guerriero S, Ajossa S, Gerada M, Virgilio B, Pilloni M, Galvan R, Laparte MC, Alcázar JL, Melis GB. Transvaginal ultrasonography in the diagnosis of extrauterine pelvic diseases. Expert Rev Obstet Gynecol. 2008;3:731–52. https://doi.org/10.1586/17474108.3.6.731.
188. Ng KYB, Cheong Y. Hydrosalpinx - Salpingostomy, salpingectomy or tubal occlusion. Best Pract Res Clin Obstet Gynaecol. 2019;59:41–7. https://doi.org/10.1016/j.bpobgyn.2019.01.011. Epub 2019 Jan 29. PMID: 30824209
189. Thomassin-Naggara I, Darai E, Bazot M. Gynecological pelvic infection: what is the role of imaging? Diagn Interv Imaging. 2012;93(6):491–9.,ISSN 2211-5684. https://doi.org/10.1016/j.diii.2012.04.002.
190. Moon YH, Kim JH, Jeong WJ, Park SY. Ultrasonographic findings in Fitz-Hugh-Curtis syndrome: a thickened or three-layer hepatic capsule. Yeungnam Univ J Med. 2018;35(1):127–9. https://doi.org/10.12701/yujm.2018.35.1.127. Epub 2018 Jun 30. PMID: 31620583; PMCID: PMC6784674

191. Rooholamini SA, Au AH, Hansen GC, Kioumehr F, Dadsetan MR, Chow PP, et al. Imaging of pregnancy related complications. Radiographics. 1993;13:753–70.
192. Lev-Toaff AS, Baka JJ, Toaff ME, Friedmas AC, Radecki PD, Caroline RF. Diagnostic imaging in puerperal febrile morbidity. Obstet Gynaecol. 1991;78:50–5.
193. Dalton E, Castillo E. Post partum infections: a review for the non-OBGYN. Obstet Med. 2014;7(3):98–102. Chaim W, Bashiri A, Bar-David J, Shoham-Vardi I, Mazor M. Prevalence and clinical significance of postpartum endometritis and wound infection. Infect Dis Obstet Gynecol. 2000;8(2):77–82.
194. Gupta A, Desai A, Bhatt S. Imaging of the endometrium: physiologic changes and diseases: women's imaging. Radiographics. 2017;37(7):2206–7.
195. Gillies R, Ashley L, Bergin C. Sonographic findings in acute puerperal endometritis: the hypoechoic rim sign and endo-myometrial junction indistinctness. Austr J Ultrasound Med. 2017;20(3):123–8. https://doi.org/10.1002/ajum.12057. PMID: 34760483; PMCID: PMC8409814
196. Mulic-Lutvica A, Axelsson O. Postpartum ultrasound in women with postpartum endometritis, after cesarean section and after manual evacuation of the placenta. Acta Obstet Gynecol Scand. 2007;86(2):210–7. https://doi.org/10.1080/00016340601124086. PMID: 17364285

Male Genitourinary Ultrasound

14

Vietvuong Vo and E. Liang Liu

Background

The male genitourinary tract is comprised of the scrotum, penis, and their corresponding internal structures. Prior to the advent of testicular ultrasonography, diagnosis of many scrotal pathologies relied on surgical evaluation. Applications for scrotal ultrasonography gained momentum in the 1970s when pioneers described grayscale characteristics of various testicular conditions, marking the beginning of the use of ultrasound as a noninvasive tool for evaluating scrotal pathology [1–4]. As ultrasound technology advanced, so did its capabilities in imaging the male genitourinary tract. The introduction of higher frequency probes and real-time ultrasound imaging in the late 1970s provided more detailed and dynamic views of scrotal contents [5, 6]. Doppler assessments were introduced in subsequent years, allowing for the assessment of blood flow within the testicles [7]. While male genitourinary ultrasound initially focused on scrotal pathologies, its applications have expanded over time, and ultrasound is now an integral part of the sonographic assessment of testicular and penile pathology.

Ultrasound is exceptionally useful for prompt diagnosis of time-sensitive conditions such as testicular torsion and allows for noninvasive evaluation of most testicular complaints. The ability to differentiate between various testicular pathologies, characterize masses, and assess blood flow provides clinicians with crucial information for patient management. Ongoing technological advancements continue to increase the capabilities of testicular ultrasound and contribute to even greater diagnostic precision and expanded POCUS applications in both routine clinical practice and emergent urological assessments.

Indications

Indications
- Testicular pain and swelling
- Scrotal pain and swelling
- Testicular trauma
- Penile trauma
- Penile pain

Diagnoses
- Testicular torsion
- Torsion of appendix testis and appendix epididymis
- Epididymo-orchitis
- Scrotal cellulitis and abscess
- Testicular fracture and rupture
- Testicular hematoma
- Hydrocele
- Hematocele
- Pyocele
- Varicocele
- Extratesticular lesions: epididymal cysts, spermatoceles, adenomatoid tumors, papillary cystadenomas, leiomyomas
- Intratesticular lesions: malignancies, cysts, atrophy and fibrosis, microlithiasis
- Penile fracture and hematoma
- Penile foreign body
- High- and low-flow priapism

V. Vo (✉)
Department of Emergency Medicine, University of Texas Southwestern, Dallas, TX, USA
e-mail: vietvuong.vo@utsouthwestern.edu

E. L. Liu
Department of Emergency Medicine, Emory University, Atlanta, GA, USA
e-mail: elliu@emory.edu

M. Gottlieb, N. Panebianco (eds.), *Advanced Point-of-Care Ultrasound*, https://doi.org/10.1007/978-3-031-85308-1_14

Core Views

<table>
<tr><th>View</th><th>Image</th><th>Approach</th></tr>
<tr><td>Buddy View</td><td>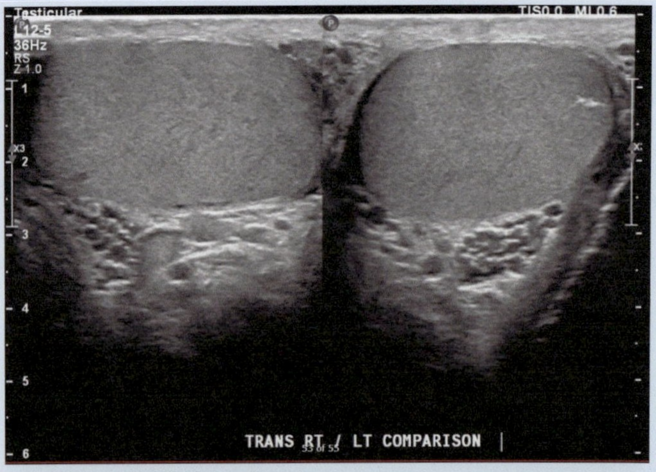

Core View 1. Testicular buddy view</td><td>A linear probe can be used to obtain a side-by-side comparison of bilateral testicles. If the genitalia is edematous or otherwise enlarged, an extended field of view or a curvilinear probe may be used for additional depth. Use the small parts or testes settings on the machine if available.
The probe is placed at the midline and rotated 60 to 75 degrees in the counterclockwise direction to visualize the midpoint of both testicles, as typically, the left testicle lies lower than the right [8].</td></tr>
<tr><td>Testicle</td><td>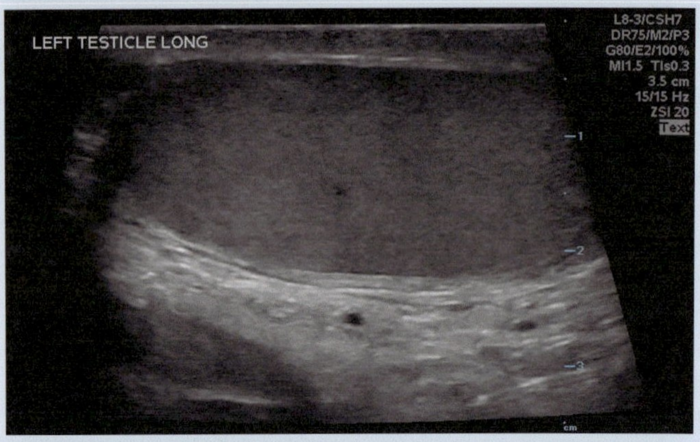

Core View 2. Testicle long-axis
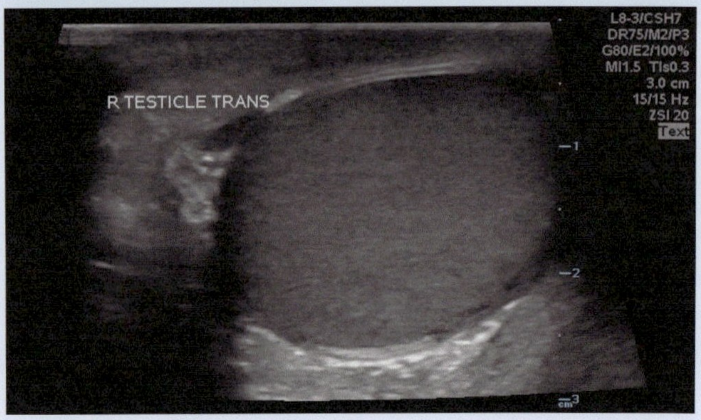

Core View 3. Testicle short-axis</td><td>Evaluate each testicle in two orthogonal planes (long and short axis). Fan or slide from one edge of the testicle to the other. Note any extratesticular structures.</td></tr>
</table>

View	Image	Approach
Epididymis	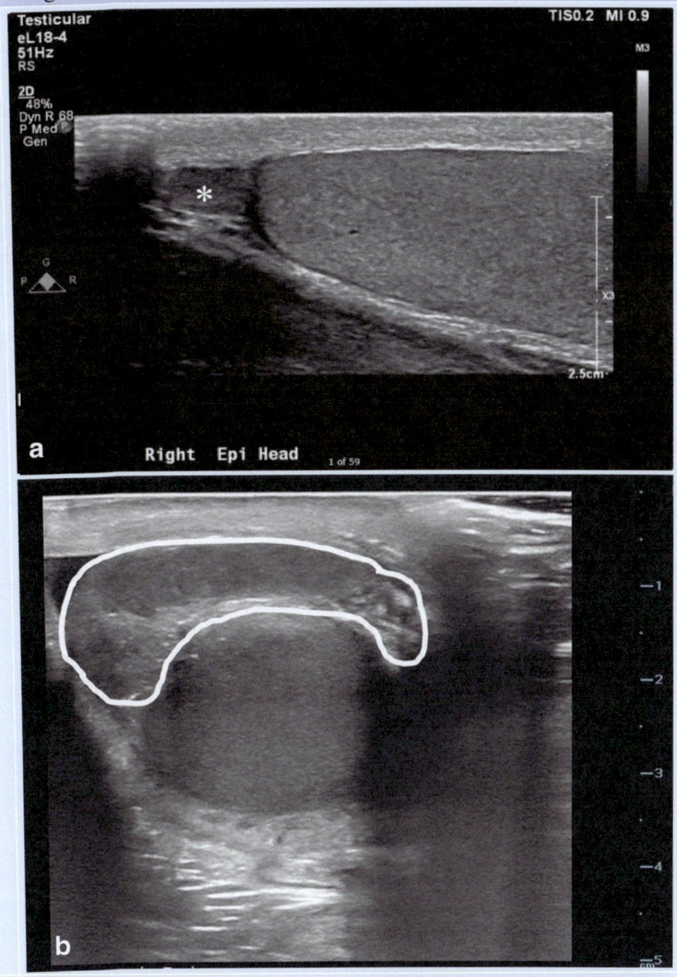	Evaluate the epididymis, which rests at the posterolateral aspect of the testicle. The epididymal head is triangular in shape and isoechoic to the testes. The narrow body and tail are found along the posterior or anterolateral edge and may be indistinguishable from surrounding peritesticular tissue when normal [9]. When normal, the epididymal head (denoted by *) is often all that is seen of the epididymis. In the setting of epididymitis, the body and tail (highlighted in white) found along the posterior or anterolateral edge are more apparent.
	Core View 4. (a) Epididymal head. (b) Body and tail of the epididymis. *Image courtesy of Di Coneybeare, MD, MHPE.*	
Color Doppler	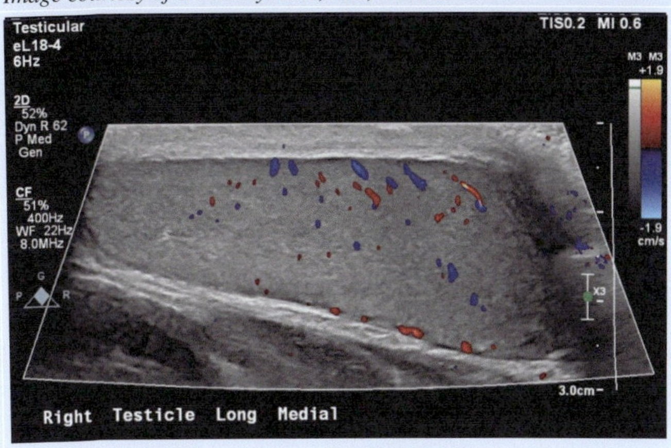	Color Doppler can be used to evaluate perfusion and vascular flow of the testis and aid in detection of hyperemia or ischemia. Evaluate both venous and arterial blood flow using color Doppler. After evaluating testicular perfusion, epididymal blood flow can be evaluated with color Doppler. Given the low flow velocities and volumes of the normal testicles, especially in the pre-pubertal pediatric population, the velocity scale should be set to as low as possible, and wall filters should be removed or set to as low as possible [10]. Color Doppler gain should then be maximized to the point where noise is just noticeable for optimal sensitivity.
	Core View 5. Testicle assessed with color Doppler	

View	Image	Approach
Power Doppler	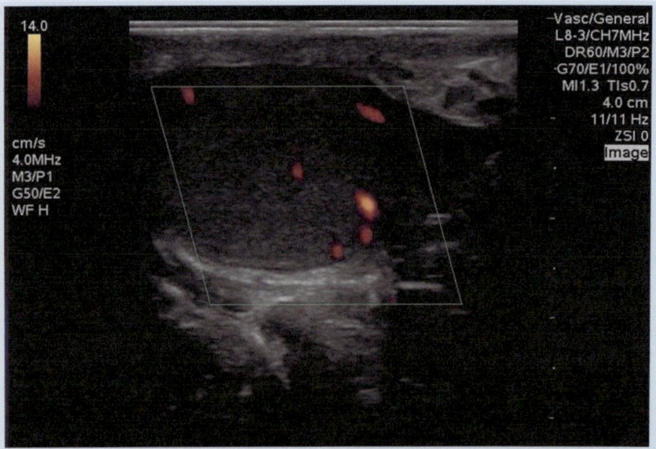 Core View 6. Testicle assessed with power Doppler	Power Doppler can be used to increase sensitivity in detecting vascular signals in low-flow states. The power Doppler box should be superimposed on the B-mode image of the testes. A large box will allow for evaluation of a larger portion of the testicle but will decrease the frame rate and make detection of higher velocities more difficult, so a balance between the two is needed. For the most accurate detection of blood flow, the sensitivity settings should be set as low as possible without introducing artifacts. If machine presets are not already optimized, a low wall filter (100 KHz), low pulse repetition frequency (1–2 Hz), and color gain output settings of 70–90% should be used for testicular scanning [9].
Spectral Doppler	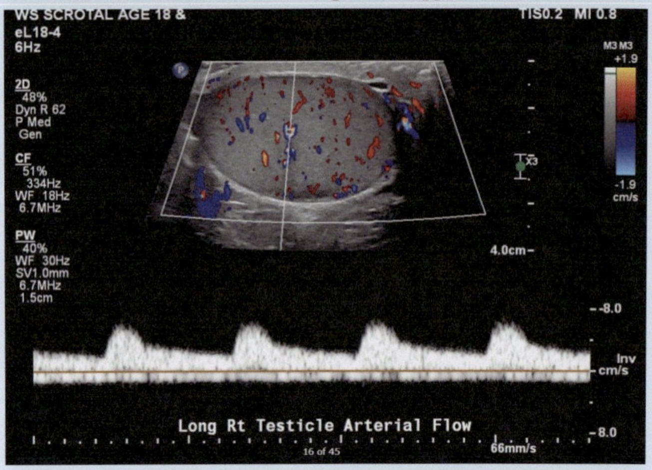 Core View 7. Testicular arterial flow was assessed with spectral Doppler 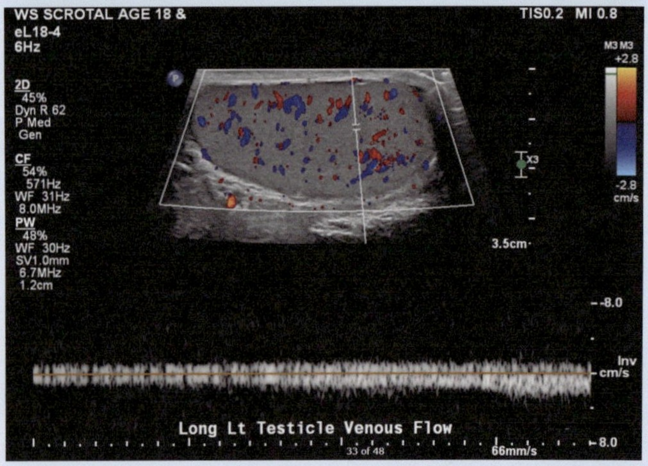 Core View 8. Testicular venous flow was assessed with spectral Doppler	Once a reliable Doppler signal is identified, activate spectral Doppler by placing the Doppler gate over the visualized signal. Set the Doppler gate over both flow toward and away from the probe to evaluate both venous and arterial flow. Set the angle of insonation to less than 60 degrees. Adjust the size of the sampling gate to obtain an optimized waveform and turn up the pulsed-wave Doppler gain until the background shows a small amount of noise without distorting the baseline waveform. Sampling should occur in multiple parts of the testicle and avoid the periphery (the area where arterial anastomoses are located), which can be mistaken as normal parenchymal perfusion. Keep settings the same and switch from the evaluation of the unaffected side to the affected side to compare Doppler signals.

View	Image	Approach
Penis	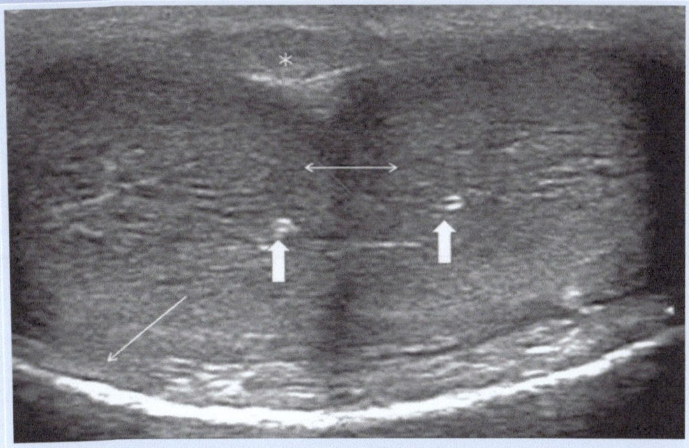 Core View 9. Short-axis view of the penis with the cavernosal arteries (arrows) running through the bilateral corpora cavernosa (double-headed arrow), while the corpus spongiosum (asterisk) is located more superficial. *Images obtained with permission from Fernandes et al.* [90] 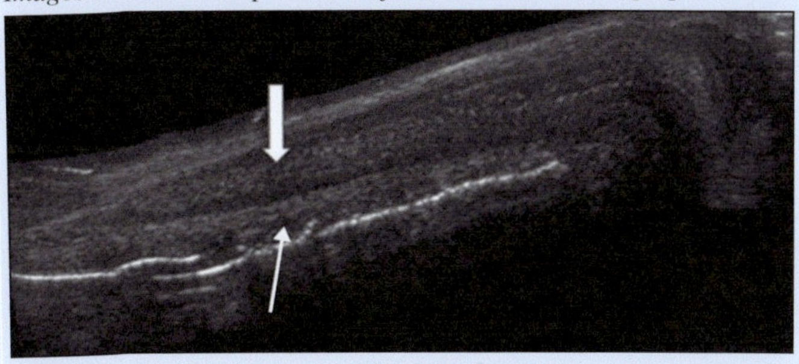 Core View 10. Long-axis view of the penis with the corpus cavernosum (wide arrow) seen in the near field and the corpus spongiosum (thin arrow) seen in the far field. *Images obtained with permission from Fernandes et al.* [90]	Penile ultrasound should be performed via a high-frequency linear probe, and the penis should be evaluated in its entirety in both the long- and short-axis imaging planes. The penis should be in anatomical position, lying superiorly against the anterior abdominal wall. The probe can be placed ventrally or dorsally to evaluate the corporal bodies and urethra. A full evaluation includes placement of the probe in the perineum to visualize the nonexternal portion of the corpora cavernosa [11]. Peak systolic velocity, end-diastolic velocity, and the resistive index of the cavernosal arteries can be evaluated with spectral Doppler at the transition from the proximal third to middle third of the cavernosa. Greater velocities are expected with movement of the probe proximally and on tumescence.

General Approach to Testicular and Penile Ultrasound

In performing a testicular or penile ultrasound examination, the patient should be supine and in a frog-leg position with pillows or blankets supporting each bent knee to help with the relaxation of the legs [9]. The penis is retracted and covered with a towel against the abdomen. A towel roll may be placed under the scrotum to elevate the testicles. In this position, a “buddy” view, longitudinal and transverse view of the testicle, and Doppler evaluation can be obtained. To reduce cremasteric reflex and discomfort to the patient, warmed gel should be used when possible [12].

Ultrasound evaluation of the scrotum is typically performed with a high-frequency (5–12 MHz) linear probe. If the genitalia is edematous or otherwise enlarged, an extended field of view or a curvilinear probe may be used for additional width or depth. Activating the dual screen function can also allow for side-by-side comparison of the testicles. The sonographer should anchor the scanning hand on the patient’s thigh to keep the probe steady and aim the probe marker cephalad or to the patient’s right to follow convention [9]. The asymptomatic side should be evaluated first to optimize B-mode and Doppler settings [13]. Videos in longitudinal and transverse planes should be obtained of the hemiscrotal contents [9]. Focused evaluation of the epididymis should follow in a similar fashion. Perfusion of the testes and epididymides should be evaluated using color, power, and spectral Doppler imaging [9, 13].

Anatomy Overview

The scrotum is a cutaneous pouch that can be divided into halves, each containing testes, epididymis, and components of the spermatic cord (Fig. 14.1). The scrotum is composed of layers, which are a continuation of the abdominal wall. From superficial to deep, the scrotal layers include skin, dartos fascia, external spermatic fascia, cremaster muscle, and internal spermatic fascia. The dartos fascia forms the median raphe, which divides the scrotum into its two halves [8, 9, 14].

Deep to the scrotal wall are the tunica vaginalis and tunica albuginea. The tunica vaginalis is composed of two thin layers (visceral and parietal tunica vaginalis) and surrounds the tunica albuginea. Typically, the layers of the tunica vaginalis produce and resorb a small amount of fluid (1–2 mL) [8], which allows for movement of the testis within the scrotum. This can be seen as a thin anechoic stripe adjacent to the head of the epididymis and should not be mistaken for a hydrocele. The tunica albuginea envelops the testis and is seen as a thin hyperechoic line that surrounds the testis on ultrasound [15]. The testis is found within the tunica albuginea, normally in a vertical lie with a slight anterior tilt, is ovoid in shape, roughly 5 × 3 × 2 cm in size, and should be homogenous and symmetric bilaterally on ultrasound (Fig. 14.2a) [12, 16]. In the postpubertal male, testicular size will decrease with age [8]. The testicle is composed of seminiferous tubules which converge to form the rete testis located at the mediastinum of the testis. This rete testis connects to the epididymis via the efferent ductules. The mediastinum is composed of a fold of the tunica albuginea and can be seen as a hyperechoic linear

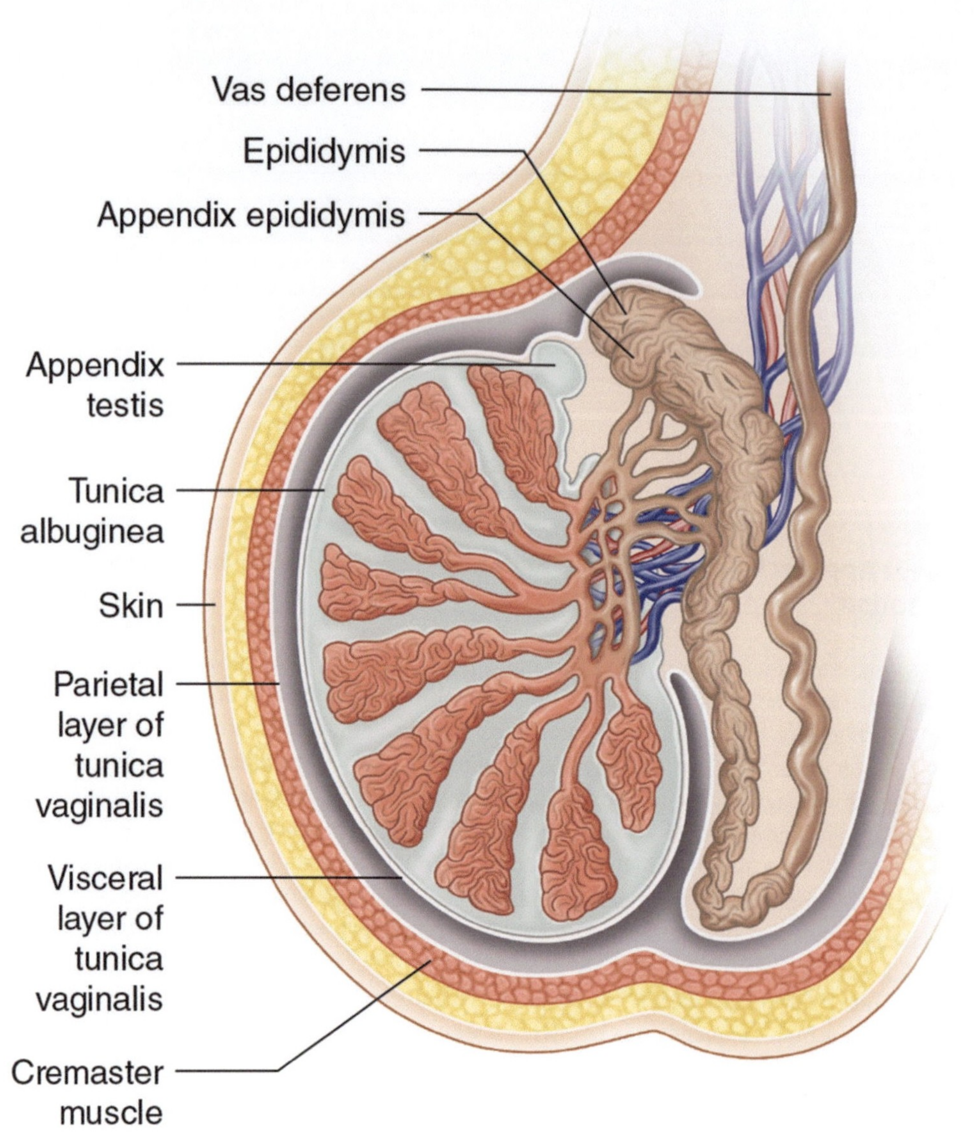

Fig. 14.1 Cross-sectional view of the scrotum depicts the layers of the scrotal sac and its contents including the testes and epididymis

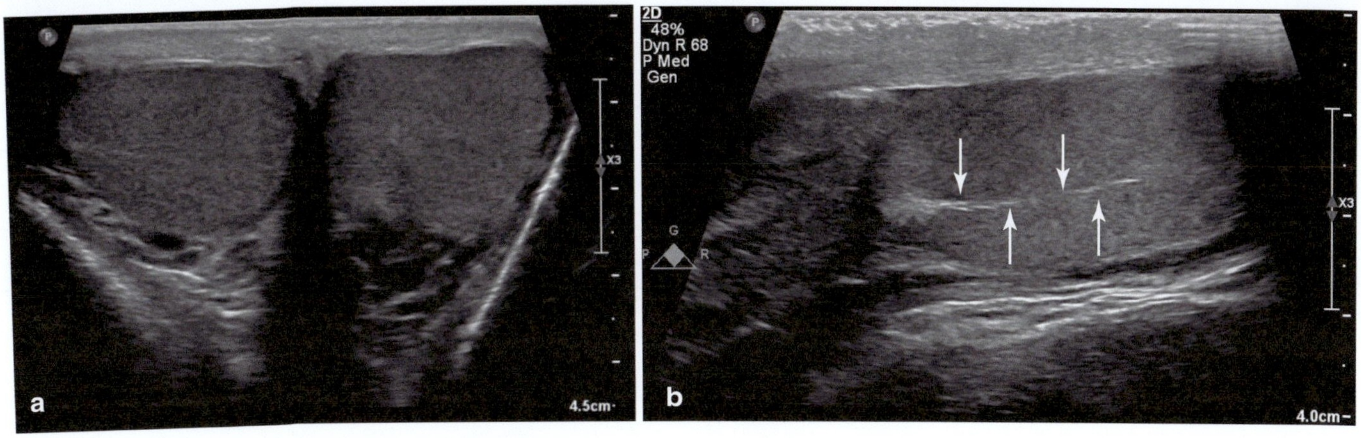

Fig. 14.2 (**a**) Buddy view of both testicles. (**b**) Normal longitudinal view of the right testicle, with the mediastinum testis (white arrows) visualized

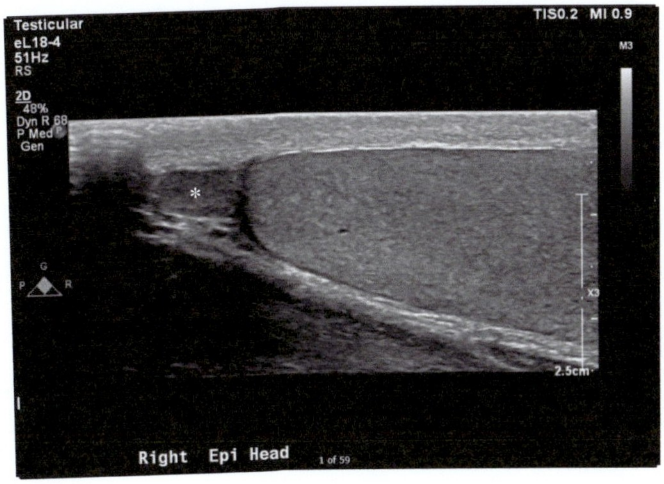

Fig. 14.3 Normal epididymal head denoted with (*)

band along the longitudinal axis (craniocaudal direction) of the testis (Fig. 14.2b) [15].

The epididymis rests at the posterolateral aspect of the testicle and consists of a head, body, and tail (Fig. 14.3). On ultrasound, the epididymal head is triangular in shape, measures 5–12 mm in length, has minimal flow on color Doppler, and has equal or slightly greater echogenicity compared to the testis [8]. The narrow body and tail of the epididymis, each approximately 2–5 mm in diameter, are found along the posterior or anterolateral edge of the testis, hypoechoic to the testis, and indistinguishable from surrounding peritesticular tissue when normal [9]. At the inferior pole of the testis, the epididymal tail connects to the vas deferens and, with its neurovascular bundle, forms the spermatic cord, which traverses through the inguinal canal.

The penis is covered by skin that is continuous with the lower abdominal wall, scrotum, and perineum (Fig. 14.4). From superficial to deep, the fascial layers of the penis are the tunica dartos (superficial) and Buck's fascia (deep), with a loose layer of connective tissue in between. Three cylindrical structures (or corpora) form the penile shaft: the corpus spongiosum ventrally and two corpora cavernosa dorsally. The tunica albuginea surrounds each of the corporal bodies individually [17]. The tunica albuginea and Buck's fascia are typically indistinguishable on ultrasound and noted as a hyperechoic band surrounding the corporal bodies. Penile ultrasound should be performed via a high-frequency linear probe, and the penis should be evaluated in its entirety in both the longitudinal and transverse planes (Fig. 14.5). In a normal ultrasound, the corpora are homogenous, with the corpora cavernosa exhibiting an intermediate to low echogenicity and the corpus spongiosum being slightly hyperechoic [18]. The urethra is contained within the corpus spongiosum and appears as a hypoechoic band or triangular structure within the corpus if distended with fluid [17].

Fig. 14.4 Image demonstrating the anatomy of the penis and associated structures

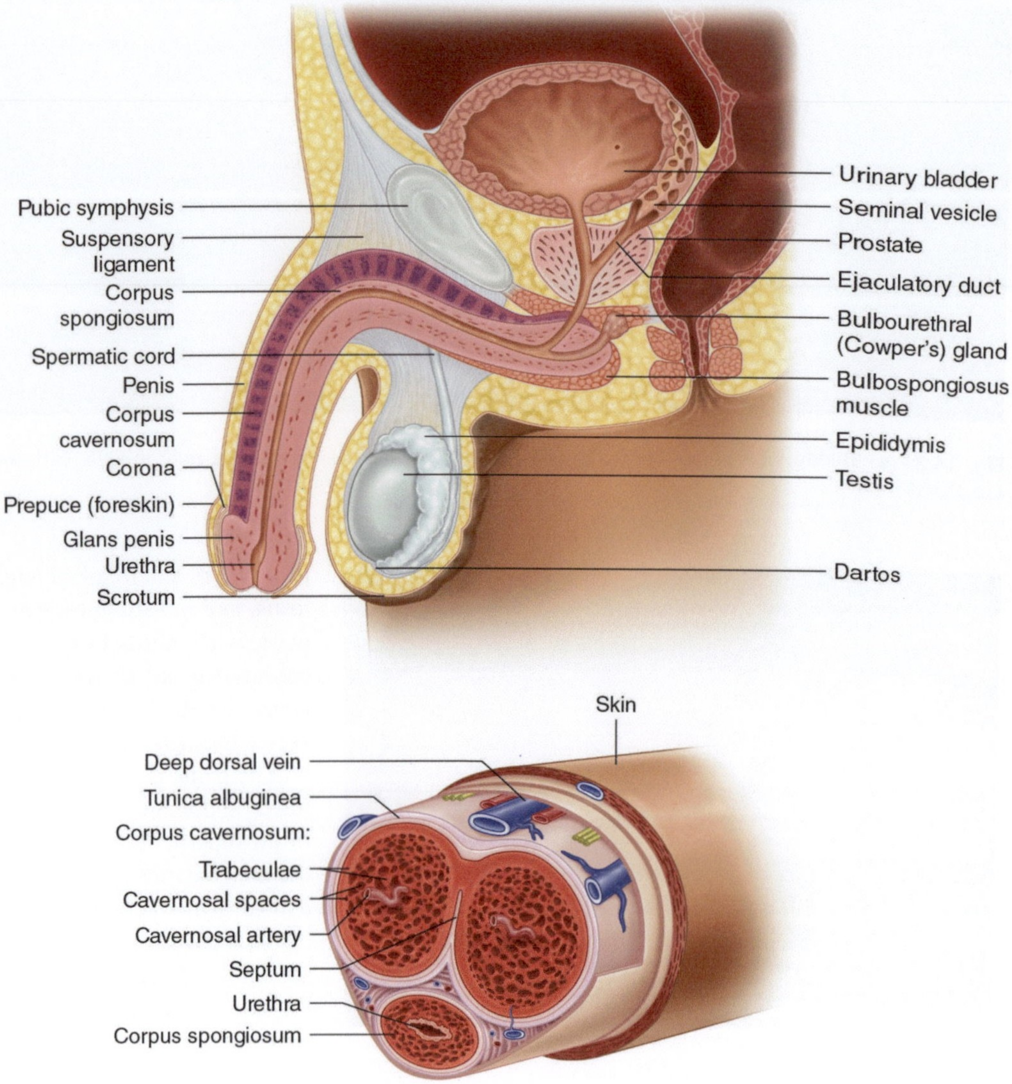

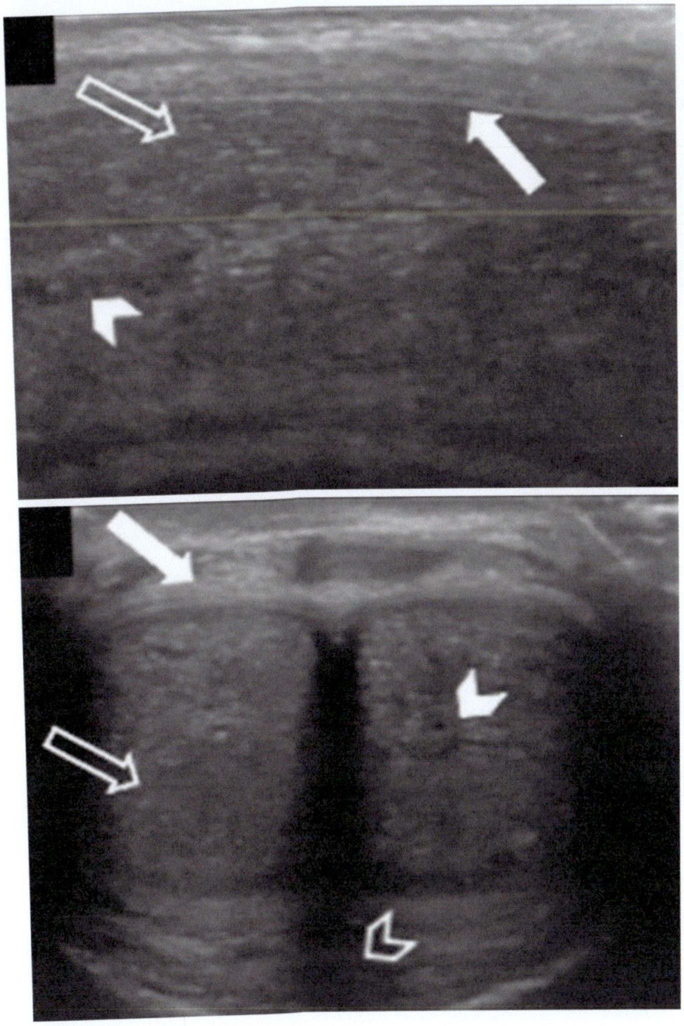

Fig. 14.5 Normal penile sonoanatomy. The longitudinal (upper image) and transverse (lower image) planes of the penis with the following structures labeled: tunica albuginea (solid arrow), corpus cavernosum (open arrow), cavernosal artery (solid arrowhead), and corpus spongiosum (open arrowhead). (*Image obtained with permission from Albasha et al.* [18])

Clinical Applications

Testicular Pathology

Testicular Torsion

Scrotal blood flow is supplied by the testicular, cremasteric, and deferential arteries. The testicular arteries (also known as the internal spermatic arteries) originate from the aorta, just distal to the origin of the renal arteries, and enter the spermatic cord at the internal inguinal ring, where they join the deferential and cremasteric arteries. The testicular arteries primarily supply the testis, while the deferential and cremasteric arteries supply mainly the epididymis and peritesticular tissues. The capsular arteries which are the major arteries of the testis are found in the periphery and give rise to branches that supply the testicular parenchyma traveling toward the mediastinum.

Testicular torsion arises when the spermatic cord undergoes twisting, leading to vascular compromise and subsequent ischemia in the testis. Early detection is crucial to prevent complications such as testicular infarction and infertility [19]. Typically, patients with testicular torsion present with acute unilateral testicular pain, and the affected testis may lie horizontally due to the failure of normal posterior anchoring of the tunica vaginalis [20]. The torsed testicle may become enlarged due to venous congestion.

The sonographic findings of testicular torsion can vary depending on the degree and duration of torsion (Fig. 14.6). The affected testicle may look normal on B-mode imaging early in the disease, though other initial signs can include enlargement of the epididymis with a reactive hydrocele [10]. Continued torsion leads to testicular edema, which may be seen sonographically as testicular enlargement (>5 cm in diameter) and increased heterogeneity with overall decreased echogenicity of the testicular parenchyma [10]. Comparing measured testicular volumes can improve the accuracy of size discrepancy [21]. The presence of a horizontal lie can best be seen as a difference in the orientation of the testes in the buddy view, using the mediastinum as a reference point to confirm positioning [22].

The "whirlpool sign" refers to the twisting of the spermatic cord, resembling a swirling target. One systematic review and meta-analysis found the "whirlpool sign" was 73% sensitive and 99% specific for testicular torsion, though the sensitivity improved to 92% when the neonate population was removed [23]. A redundant spermatic cord, seen as the presence of an excess "bunched up" spermatic cord, can usually be found inferior to the site of torsion [24]. On ultrasound, this may be seen as an ovoid, heterogenous "pseudomass," with the presence of dilated tubular structures representing congested vessels [24].

After infarction, the testicle may increase in echogenicity and become smaller due to atrophy [10]. Heterogeneously hyperechoic areas suggesting hemorrhagic infarction is a late finding and is concerning for a nonviable testicle [25].

Color, power, and spectral Doppler can be used to evaluate perfusion and vascular flow of the testis and aid in the detection of hyperemia or ischemia. Both venous and arterial blood flow should be evaluated using Doppler. Power Doppler is not susceptible to signal aliasing and less dependent on signal angle, which makes it particularly useful in evaluating testicular torsion [26, 27]. It is important to note that while the absence of testicular blood flow confirms a diagnosis of testicular torsion, the presence of flow does not rule out the condition [21]. In the setting of partial torsion, testicular arterial flow may still be present. Hyperemia can also occur in the setting of torsion–detorsion, mimicking

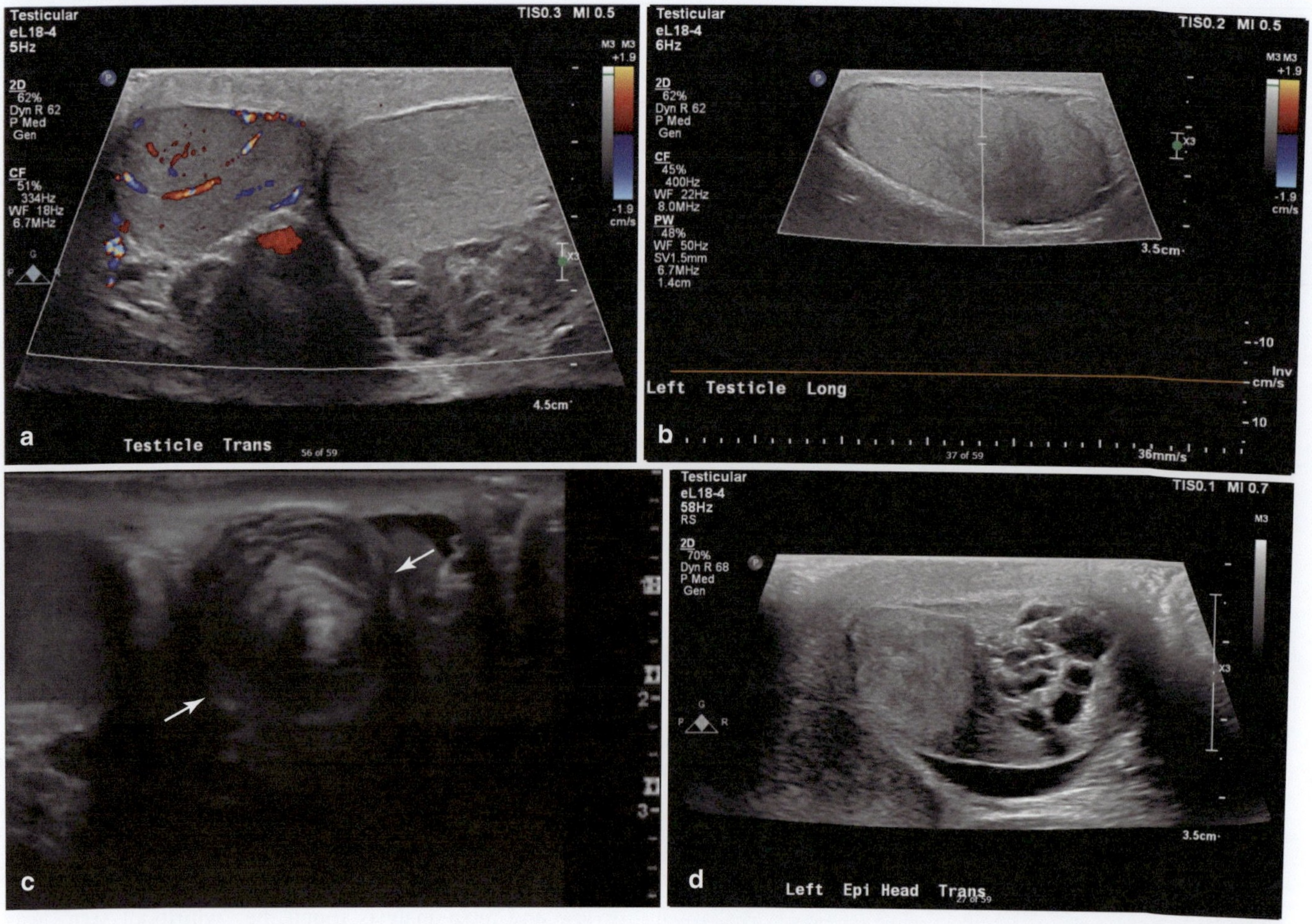

Fig. 14.6 Ultrasound findings of testicular torsion. (**a**) Absence of blood flow in an edematous left testicle (right side of image) compared to the right testicle on buddy view. (**b**) Spectral Doppler showing no flow in the torsed testicle. (**c**) Whirlpool sign (denoted by white arrows). (**d**) Pseudomass (also known as redundant spermatic cord) with a reactive hydrocele

orchitis and making the diagnosis more challenging [28]. On Doppler, the torsed testicle can show reduced blood flow, dampened spectral waveform, and the absence or reversal of diastolic flow (Fig. 14.7) [22]. The amount of perfusion abnormality depends on the duration and degree of torsion with venous flow affected prior to arterial flow [15]. The resultant edema from venous congestion may decrease arterial velocity and diastolic flow, thus increasing the resistive index (RI). The RI is defined as: (peak systolic velocity - end-diastolic velocity)/peak systolic velocity. Most modern ultrasound machines can calculate the RI. Intratesticular arteries have a mean RI of 0.62 (range, 0.48–0.75) [21]. An elevated testicular arterial RI (defined as >0.75) supports the diagnosis of torsion [8]. As torsion progresses, eventually flow is not detected with either color or power Doppler. Together, the findings of an enlarged, edematous, testicle with abnormal Doppler signal (RI > 0.75) should raise the concern for torsion; however, lack of these findings does not exclude the pathology.

Torsion of the Appendix Testis and Appendix Epididymis

Both the epididymis and testis can have appendages located along their upper poles, which may be confused for tumors. The appendix testis is common and seen on ultrasound in 92% of the population [29]. It is found in the upper pole of the testis or in the groove formed between the testis and the head of the epididymis. The appendix testis measures 1–7 mm in length, is isoechoic to the testis, and can range in morphology from ovoid to pedunculated or even cystic (Fig. 14.8) [9]. Visualizing the appendix epididymis is less common (frequency of 23–34%) [29]. The appendix epididymis is found adjacent to the epididymal head, is 3–8 mm in length, and most commonly ovoid in shape [29]. The appendix epididymis is derived from congenital tubular dilatations and is more often cystic-appearing compared to appendix testis (Fig. 14.9). Appendages that are stalk-like or cystic are at increased risk of torsion [30].

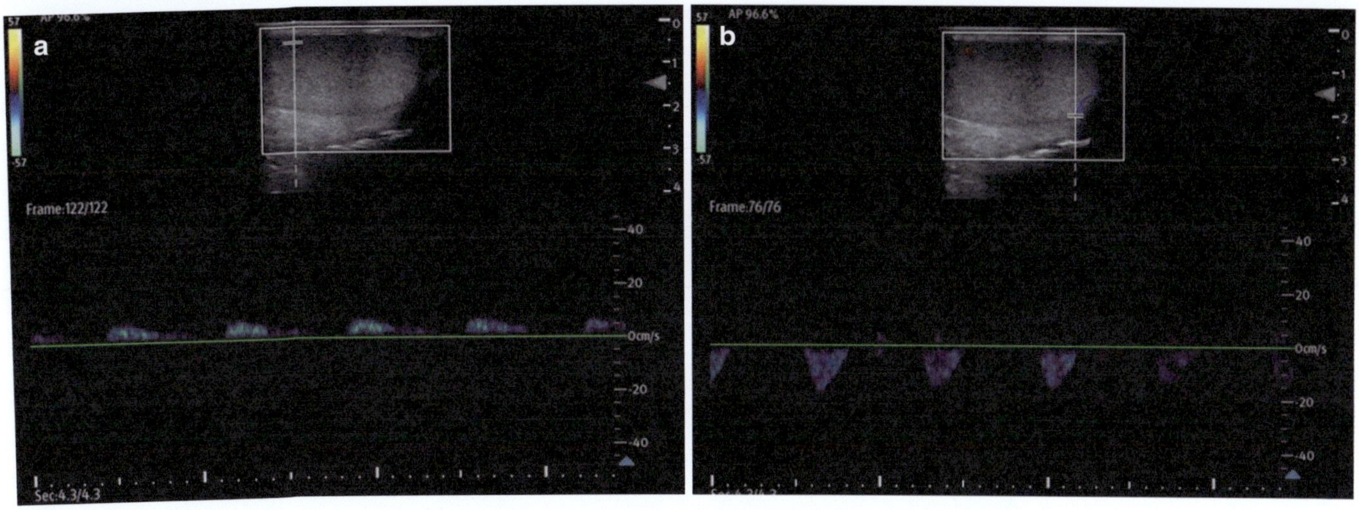

Fig. 14.7 (**a**) Doppler findings of testicular torsion with dampened spectral Doppler waveform. (**b**) Doppler findings of testicular torsion with absence or reversal of diastolic flow

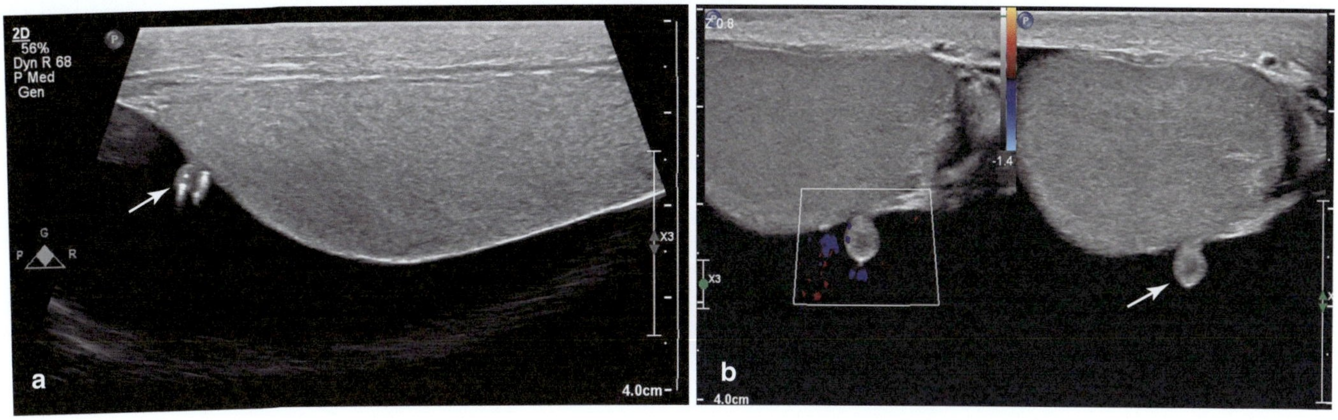

Fig. 14.8 Appendix testis (arrow) seen in the long axis (**a**) and short axis (**b**) in the setting of a hydrocele

Torsion of the testicular appendages is a leading cause of acute scrotal pain in prepubertal children [31, 32]. Trauma and prepubertal enlargement predispose the patient to appendageal torsion [31]. Patients with torsion of the appendix testis or appendix epididymis can present with significant scrotal pain, typically localized to the upper pole of the testis or epididymis, respectively [31]. On examination, a small firm nodule may be palpable at the superior aspect of the testis and may demonstrate the "blue dot" sign, a bluish discoloration secondary to venous congestion noted through the skin [8, 33].

Sonographic findings of torsion of the appendage will demonstrate a normal-appearing testis and epididymis with an enlarged, ovoid, extratesticular hyperechoic mass adjacent to the testis and epididymis with a central hypoechoic area and absent flow (Fig. 14.10) [8, 34, 35]. There can be hyperemia around the appendage noted on color Doppler [10]. Secondary findings include an enlarged epididymal head, reactive hydrocele, and skin thickening [10, 34]. These cases are managed conservatively. Follow-up imaging, while not necessary, can reveal atrophy of the appendix, presence of a scrotolith, or appearance of a scrotal pearl [33].

Over time, these appendages will calcify and become completely separate from the testis or epididymis, resulting in a freely mobile, calcified structure within the scrotum, referred to as a scrotal pearl or scrotal calculus (Fig. 14.11). On ultrasound, these scrotal pearls appear hyperechoic, mobile, and may exhibit acoustic shadows, with or without gravity dependence. The presence of a hydrocele can allow for easier detection and evaluation of appendages and scrotal pearls.

Epididymo-Orchitis

Epididymitis and orchitis are the most common causes of acute scrotal pain, with an estimated annual incidence of

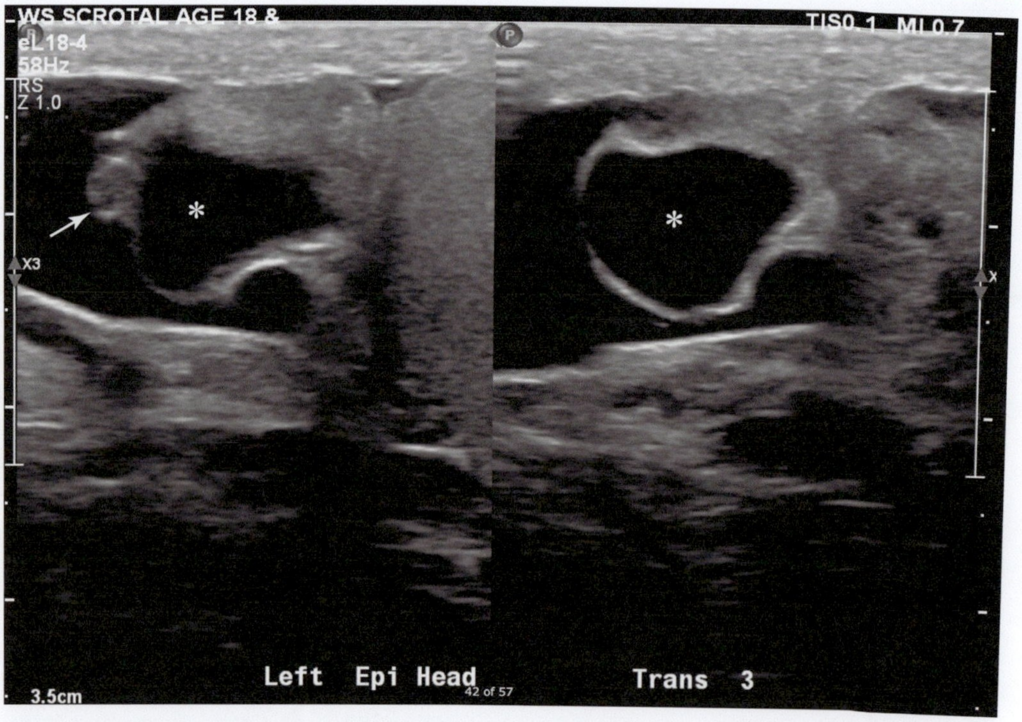

Fig. 14.9 Epididymal cyst (*) with appendix epididymis (arrow) in the setting of a hydrocele

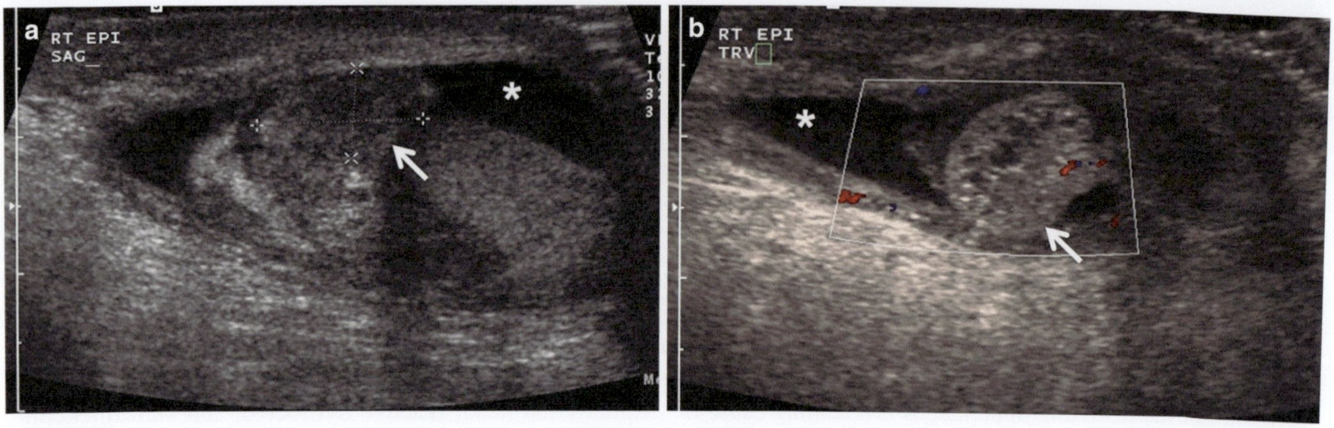

Fig. 14.10 Torsion of the testicular appendage showing a mixed echogenicity lesion anterior to the epididymal head (arrow) with a small hydrocele (*) and minimal internal flow. (*Image obtained with permission from Sweet et al.* [87])

600,000 cases [36]. The clinical presentation of epididymo-orchitis shares similarities with testicular torsion, manifesting as unilateral testicular pain radiating to the lower abdomen, associated with nausea and vomiting. However, those diagnosed with an infectious cause may also exhibit symptoms typical of urinary tract infections (e.g., dysuria, hematuria, urgency, frequency, fevers)—features rarely associated with testicular torsion [37]. Most commonly, the cause is infectious and due to the retrograde ascent of bacteria through the vas deferens [37–39]. Due to the ascending nature of the infection, the epididymal tail is typically the first to be infected, followed by the epididymal body and the head, and eventually the testicular parenchyma [40]. Thus, untreated epididymitis leads to concomitant orchitis in 20–40% of cases [9, 38]. Failure to promptly address acute epididymo-orchitis may result in complications such as sterility, testicular infarction and atrophy, abscess formation, septicemia, and the development of chronic epididymo-orchitis [41, 42]. Isolated orchitis (in the absence of epididymitis) is rare and is usually viral, with mumps being the most notable entity [9, 38].

Epididymitis can exhibit focal or diffuse sonographic involvement of the epididymis, appearing as hypoechoic enlargement and hyperemia (Fig. 14.12). Secondary scrotal wall thickening and reactive hydrocele can be present as well [8–10]. Up to 20% of epididymitis cases may exhibit a nor-

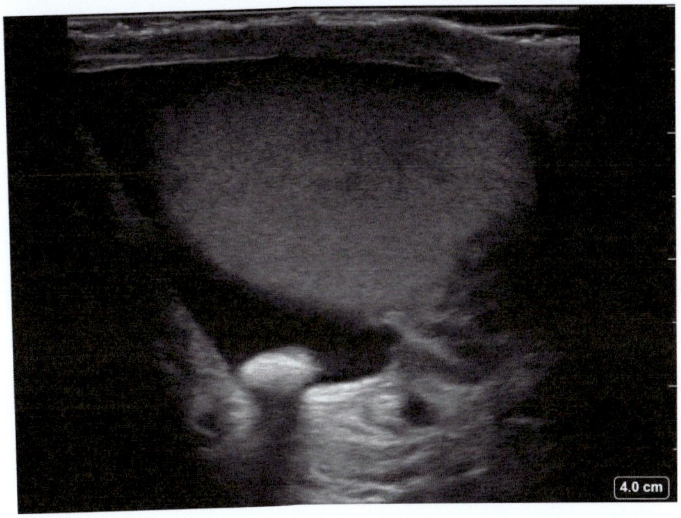

Fig. 14.11 Scrotal pearl. (*Image courtesy of Meghan Herbst, MD*)

mal B-mode appearance, so the utilization of color Doppler is recommended due to improvement in diagnosis when B-mode and color Doppler are combined (87–100% sensitivity, 91–100% specificity) [43, 44]. Normally, minimal blood flow is observed in the epididymis, so the identification of significant vascularity especially when compared to the contralateral epididymis is considered abnormal [9]. Analysis of spectral Doppler of the epididymal artery can also be valuable. The acute inflammatory process seen in epididymitis is characterized by augmentation in vascular flow, with peak systolic velocities exceeding 15 cm/s, which is 84% sensitive and 94% specific for epididymitis [45]. A reduction in vascular resistance is also characteristic of epididymitis, with RI typically falling below 0.5 [9].

An infrequent complication of epididymitis is the formation of an epididymal abscess. An epididymal abscess will exhibit sonographic features akin to other abscesses, including the presence of an avascular anechoic or hypoechoic fluid collection with variable mixed echogenicities representing pus with peripheral hyperemia but no internal vascularity [9]. Internal debris and septations within the layers of the tunica vaginalis suggests a pyocele which can also develop [9].

The inflammatory process of orchitis can lead to edema, appearing as either an enlarged and diffusely hypoechoic testicle or as multiple focal hypoechoic lesions within the testicle [9]. A striated appearance has also been described in orchitis, with multiple hypoechoic bands radiating from the mediastinum testis (Fig. 14.13) [46, 47]. These bands are thought to be bound by the interlobular septa and represent associated fibrosis [47]. The findings of a testicle with heterogeneous echotexture, with involved portions being hypoechoic and hypervascular, are not specific for orchitis and can also be seen in testicular torsion, trauma, and certain testicular tumors making differentiating based solely on B-mode ultrasound images difficult. Moreover, 40% of orchitis may exhibit a normal B-mode appearance, so reliance on B-mode ultrasound alone is often insufficient [8, 44]. Similar to their application in epididymitis, color or power Doppler is recommended to detect significant regional or diffuse hyperemia associated with inflammation [8, 9]. While epididymitis commonly displays focal involvement, orchitis is typically more diffuse. Similar to the assessment of epididymitis, an arterial RI below 0.5 and a peak systolic velocity exceeding 15 cm/s in the testicular arterial supply demonstrate a 97% sensitivity and specificity for orchitis [8, 45]. Comparing the Doppler flow of the affected to the contralateral testicle can also help distinguish orchitis from torsion based on whether the relative hyperemia is on the same or opposite side of the painful testicle. Complications of orchitis, such as testicular necrosis or abscess, may manifest as avascular areas with increased vascularity around the periphery [9]. Venous infarction can also be seen as a reversal of flow during diastole in the setting of acute orchitis [48].

Scrotal Cellulitis and Abscess

Scrotal cellulitis is inflammation of the scrotal wall due to infectious causes. Higher incidences are observed among individuals with diabetes mellitus, obesity, and immunocompromise [49, 50]. This condition can present with scrotal pain and swelling, attributed to edema and hyperemia between Colles' and Buck's fascia [49]. Particularly in immunocompromised patients, the tense swelling associated with scrotal cellulitis can progress to devascularization and potentially advance to necrotizing fasciitis, commonly known as Fournier's gangrene [49]. Unlike the scrotum, the testicles are usually spared, owing to their distinct blood supply. Patients may exhibit symptoms such as scrotal pain, swelling, and systemic signs of infection. Physical examination may reveal erythema, edema, and tenderness of the scrotal skin. Creptius can be noted in patients with Fournier's gangrene. Timely diagnosis and antibiotic therapy are crucial to prevent the escalation of infection, with ultrasound serving as a valuable tool for diagnosis and assessment of testicular involvement.

Normal scrotal wall thickness can vary from 2 to 8 mm depending on the contraction of the muscular layer [8]. Findings of scrotal cellulitis include thickening of the scrotal wall, increased echogenicity, subcutaneous edema, and cobblestoning (Fig. 14.14) [9]. Patients may develop a reactive hydrocele. The presence of thickened and increased echogenicity of the overlying skin combined with hyperemia suggests cellulitis over other noninflammatory causes of edema [51]. In contrast, the presence of edema in soft tissue sites distinctly separate from and in addition to the scrotum would support the diagnosis of noninflammatory causes of edema as a result of low plasma oncotic pressures or venous congestion such as congestive heart failure, vascular insufficiency,

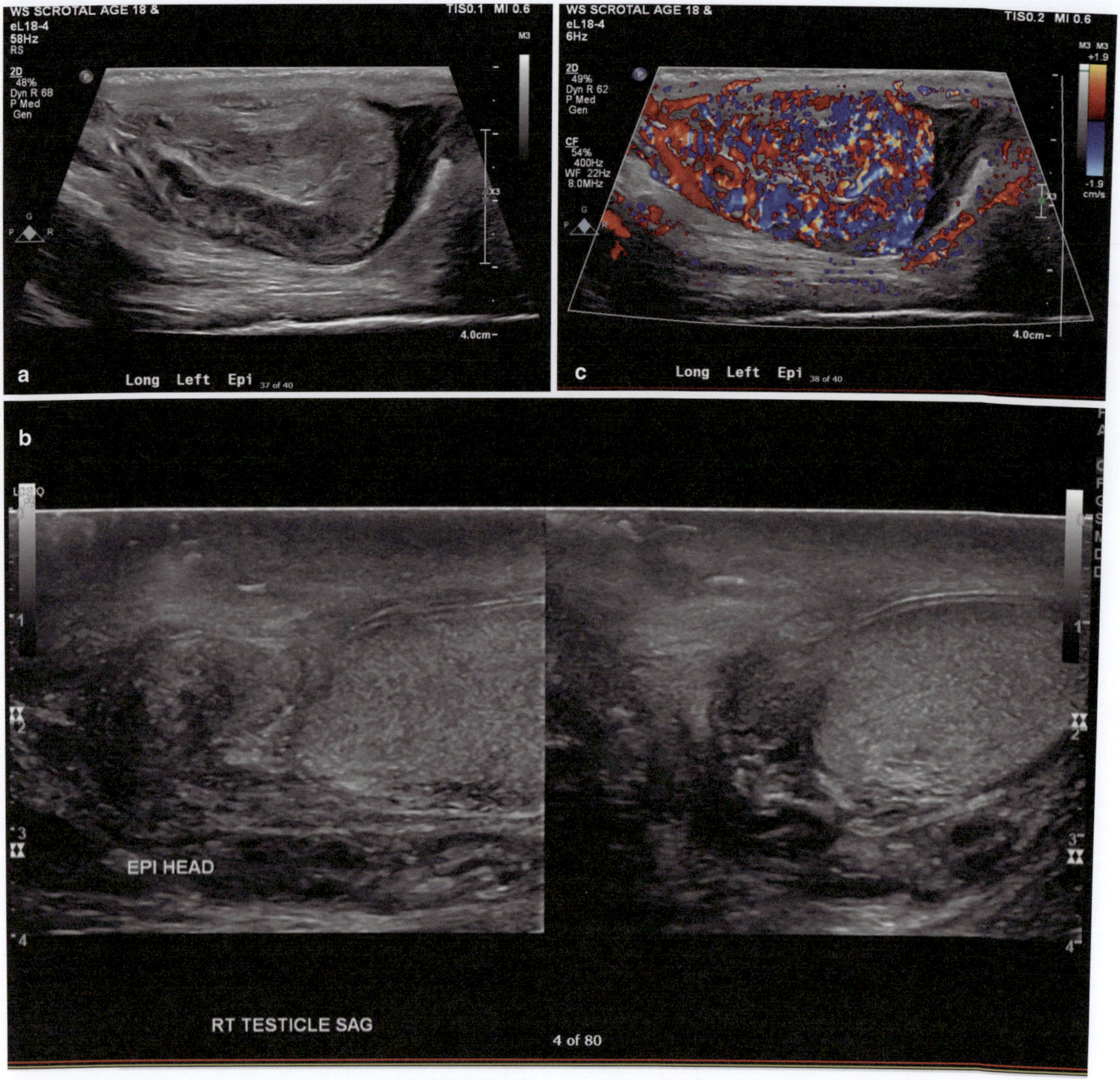

Fig. 14.12 Epididymo-orchitis. (**a**) Heterogeneous appearance of the epididymis in long-axis on B-mode. (**b**) Heterogeneous appearance of the epididymal head in short-axis on B-mode. (**c**) Hyperemia of the epididymis and testicle demonstrated on color Doppler in a patient with epididymo-orchitis

liver failure, and nephrotic syndrome [52]. A phlegmon can manifest as an ill-defined hypoechoic area devoid of flow on color Doppler. As this phlegmon evolves, a fluid collection or abscess can be seen.

Testicular Trauma

Testicular trauma can result in contusion, hematoma, fracture, or rupture of the testis (Fig. 14.15). Approximately 20% of patients seeking medical attention after testicular trauma are found to have testicular rupture [53]. Other pathologic findings that can occur in the setting of testicular trauma include hydroceles, hematoceles, traumatic epididymitis, and traumatic torsion. Scrotal sonography can accurately detect injuries to the testis with 100% sensitivity and 80% specificity for identifying tunica albuginea fractures [54].

Testicular hematomas can vary in appearance with increased echogenicity early in the course, progressing to heterogeneous and hypoechoic fluid collections with septa

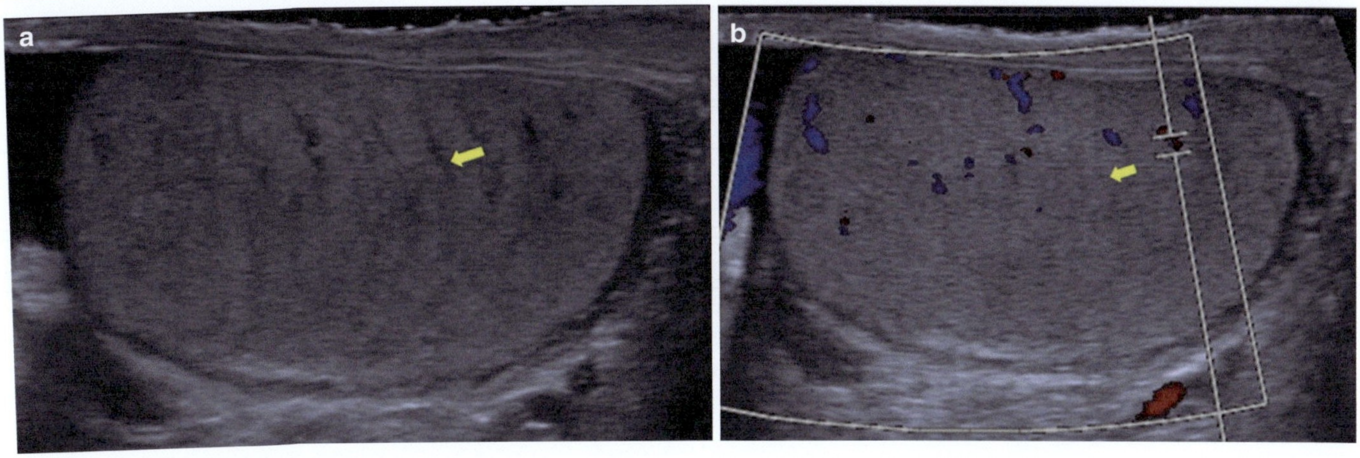

Fig. 14.13 Orchitis. (**a**) Diffuse "striated" appearance, characterized by alternating bands of varying echogenicity (yellow arrow). (**b**) In the same patient, color Doppler image shows that these striations (yellow arrow) are distinct from the normal blood vessels. (*Image obtained with permission from Whitworth and Dyer* [88])

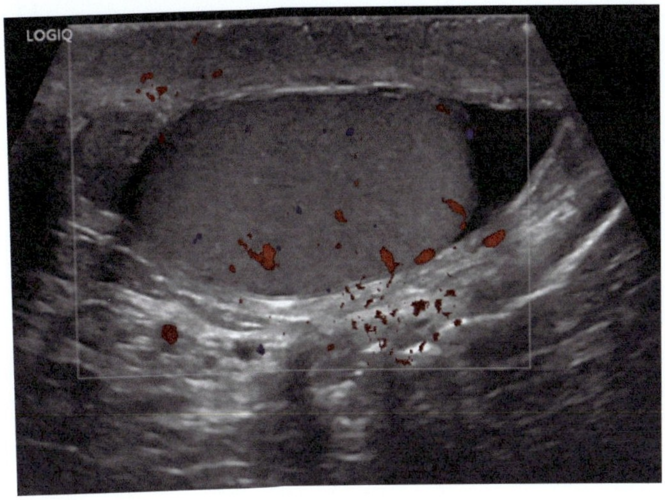

Fig. 14.14 Scrotal cellulitis. (*Image courtesy of Di Coneybeare, MD, MHPE*)

and loculations over time [10]. Testicular hematomas do not exhibit internal or peripheral Doppler flow [33]. Due to the variable echotexture of intratesticular hematomas, they can be difficult to distinguish from parenchymal contusions. Surgical exploration may be needed when there is a high clinical suspicion, as large or expanding intratesticular hematomas are at risk of secondary infection and necrosis [33, 55]. However, no current parameters exist to define what size is considered significant for an intratesticular hematoma [56].

A testicular fracture is a disruption in the usual testicular architecture, visualized as a linear hypoechoic streak extending across the testicular parenchyma. A testicular fracture will have a preserved overall contour maintaining smoothness and typical shape of the testicle as the tunica albuginea is usually intact. There may also be an accompanying hematocele or testicular hematoma. Doppler imaging should be used to assess vascular integrity. The absence of flow is concerning for ischemia [28, 57].

Testicular rupture involves the disruption of the tunica albuginea, resulting in sonographic findings of a heterogeneous-appearing testis with irregular and poorly defined borders, scrotal wall thickening, and an associated hematocele [28, 57]. Both color and power Doppler should be used to aid in detecting disruptions of the normal capsular blood flow of the tunica vasculosa (vascular layer of the testis). Hemorrhage and infarction can appear as heterogeneous intratesticular lesions. Acute hematoceles can make evaluation of the tunica albuginea difficult to appreciate and may necessitate surgical exploration for evaluation of testicular rupture [15]. The direct visualization of a fracture line may be observed in only 17–20% of testicular rupture cases [53, 58]. Because of the limitation of scrotal ultrasound in detecting testicular rupture, emergent surgical exploration may be needed if there is suspicion for testicular rupture as delays in care can increase the risk for infection, necrosis, future infertility, and hormonal dysfunction [33].

Hydrocele, Hematocele, and Pyocele

A hydrocele is an abnormal accumulation of serous fluid between the parietal and visceral layers of the tunica vaginalis and is the most common cause of painless scrotal swelling [9]. Hydroceles can be unilateral or bilateral and typically present in the anterolateral aspect of the scrotum, corresponding to the tunica's attachment to the testicle [9]. The etiology of hydroceles may stem from a persistently patent processus vaginalis communicating with the intra-abdominal cavity, or it may arise due to various factors such as trauma, torsion, malignancy, surgery, radiation, infection, or other inflammatory etiologies [59]. Clinically, hydroceles are painless, fluctuant, soft scrotal masses [59]. Persistent and

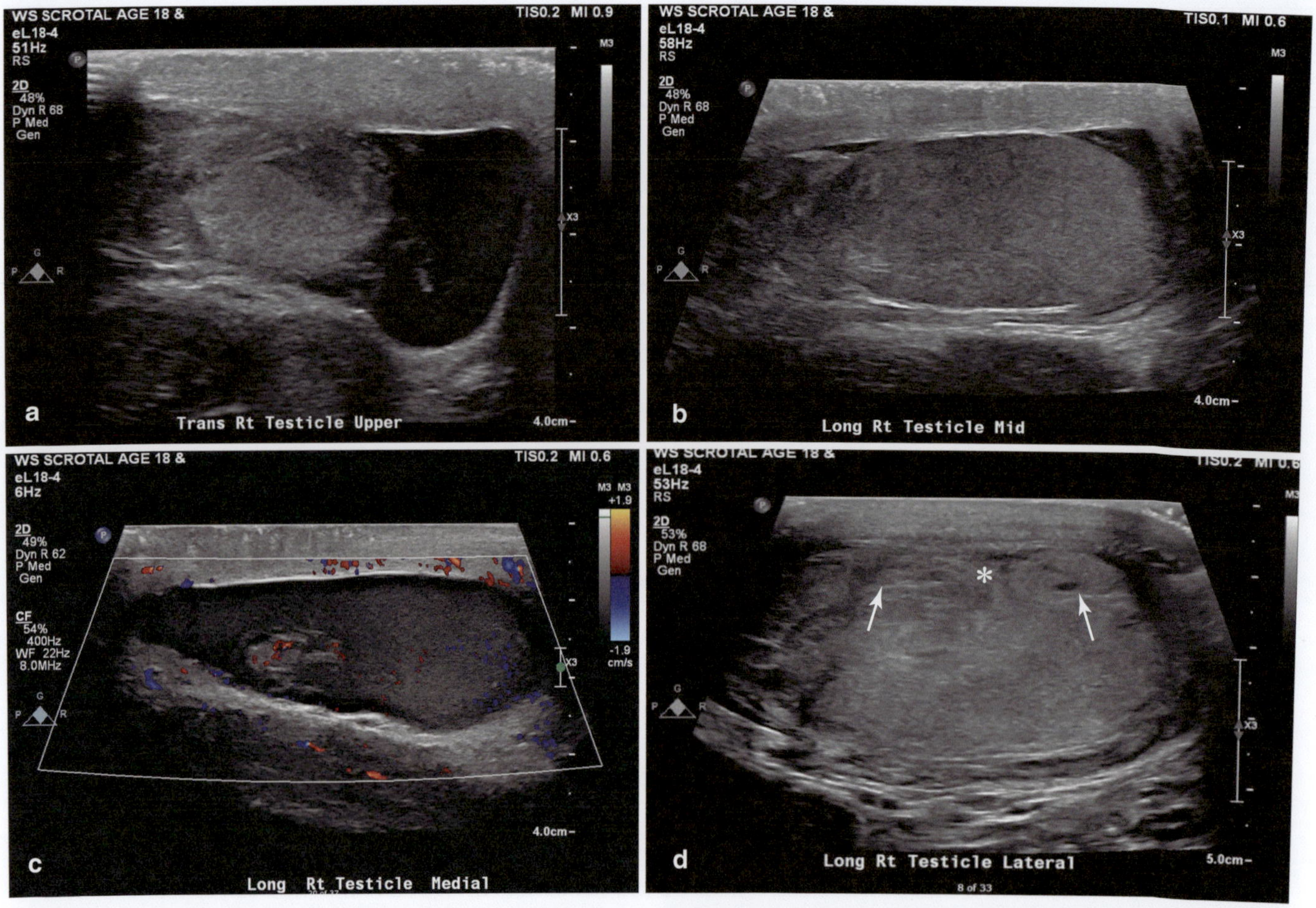

Fig. 14.15 Sonographic findings of testicular rupture and fracture. (**a**) Heterogeneous appearance of the testicle in the transverse plane with associated hydrocele. (**b**) Heterogeneous appearance of the testicle in the sagittal plane. (**c**) Hydrocele with evidence of testicular infarction. (**d**) Hematoma with visible fracture line (arrows) and rupture of tunica albuginea (*)

symptomatic hydroceles may necessitate intervention through hydrocelectomy.

Ultrasound plays a crucial role in diagnosing hydroceles and assessing the underlying causes. On ultrasound, a simple hydrocele appears as an anechoic fluid collection encircling the anterolateral aspect of the testicle and may extend into the inguinal canal (Fig. 14.16). Low-level internal echoes may occasionally be present due to elevated protein content or the deposition of cholesterol crystals [60, 61]. These reactive hydroceles typically present with thin walls [9].

Hematoceles are a result of blood collecting within the visceral and parietal tunica vaginalis and will vary in echotexture depending upon the chronicity of the trauma (Fig. 14.17). Hematoceles can occur due to extratesticular or intratesticular bleeding and can be a consequence of previous trauma, surgery, or malignancy. In the hyperacute stage, hematoceles will appear as an anechoic fluid collection with unclotted blood, though low-level echoes may be appreciated if the gain is increased [62]. As the blood clots, hyperechoic collections will appear within the scrotal sac, and then over time; clot lysis can also occur resulting in either reduction in size and echogenicity of the fluid collection (more common) or the development of a chronic hematocele [62]. Chronic hematoceles are more complex with echogenic debris, septations, or fluid–fluid levels [8, 62].

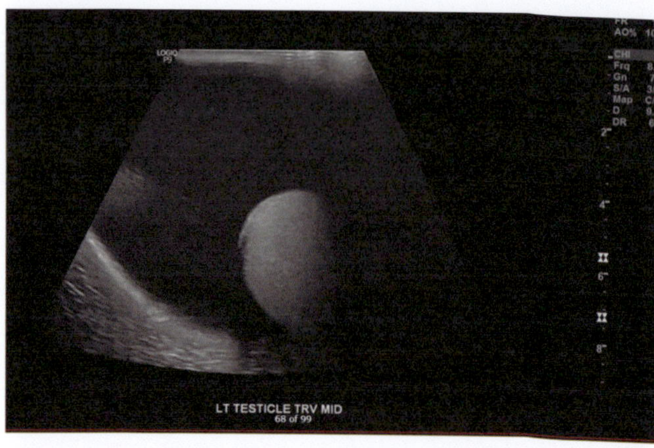

Fig. 14.16 Simple hydrocele

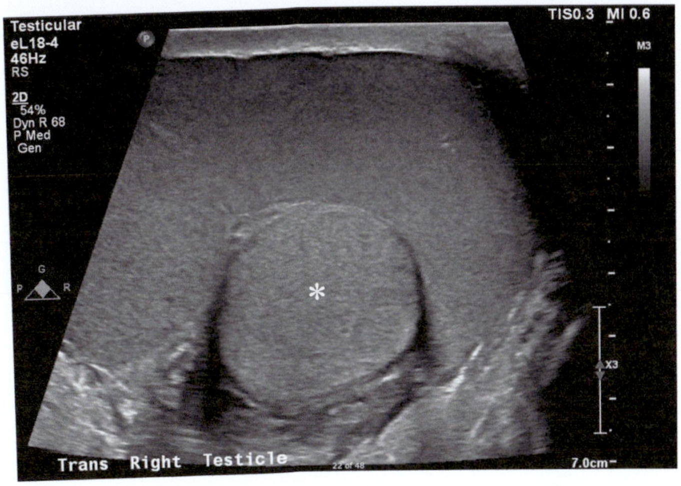

Fig. 14.17 Testicle (*) within a hematocele

Pyoceles are collections of purulent fluid within the tunica vaginalis [62]. Pyoceles can occur after surgery or trauma or from untreated infections like epididymo-orchitis or intratesticular abscess rupture [62]. These processes can create complex cystic structures with internal echoes, irregular septations, or loculations seen on ultrasound (Fig. 14.18) [9]. Distinguishing between blood and fluid can be challenging and relies more on clinical history as hematoceles can have various echotexture depending on its chronicity. Pyoceles can also exhibit peripheral hyperemia [8, 63].

Varicocele

Venous flow drains via the pampiniform plexus, which emerges from the testis through the mediastinum testis and ascends within the spermatic cord. The pampiniform plexus is formed by the internal spermatic veins situated anterior to

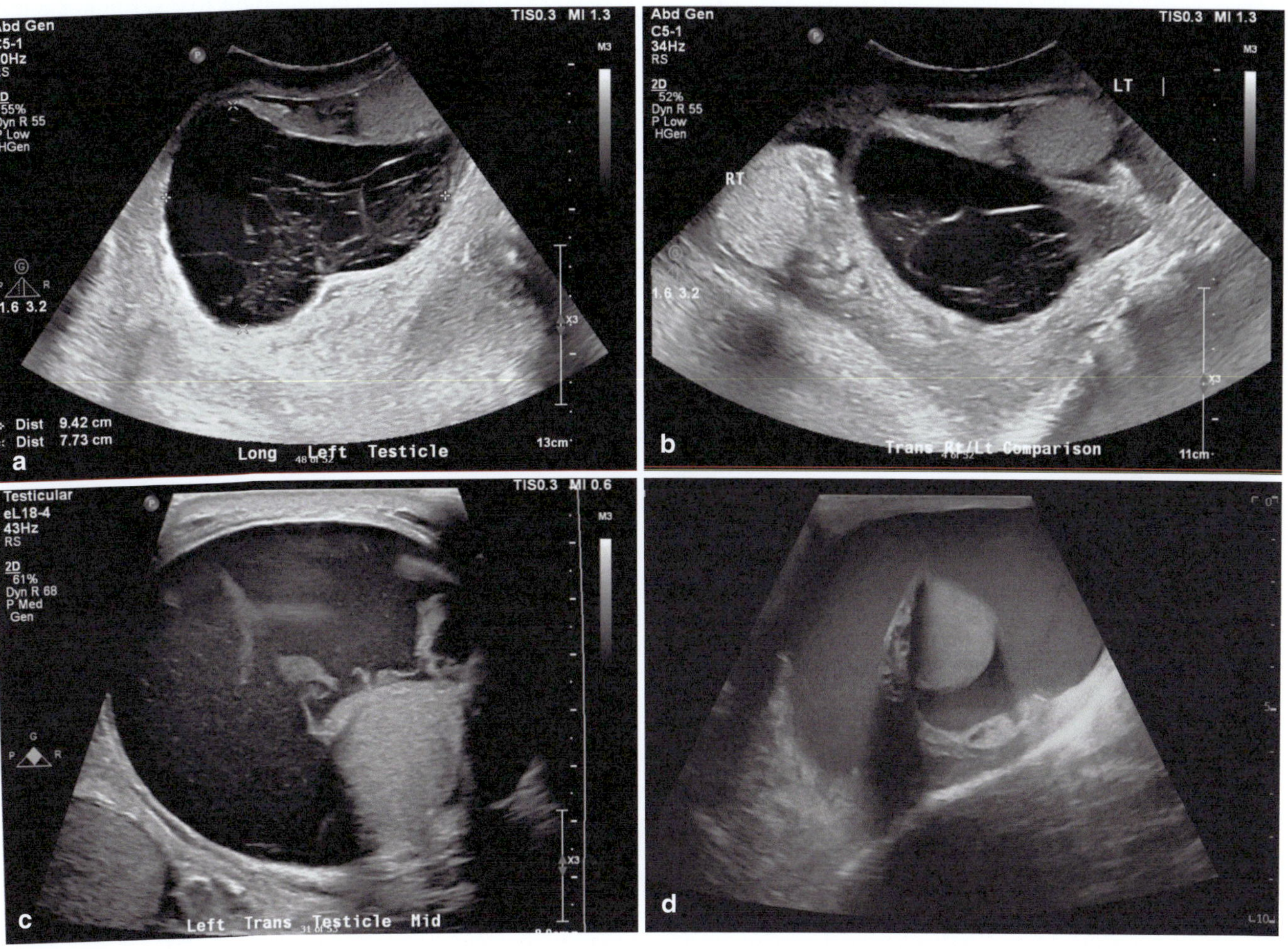

Fig. 14.18 Examples of complex hydroceles with septations, loculations, and internal echoes seen in the long axis

the ductus deferens and enveloping the testicular artery [64]. The normal diameter of pampiniform plexus veins ranges between 0.5 and 1.5 mm [65]. As the pampiniform plexus traverses through the inguinal canal to enter the abdominal cavity, it merges to become the testicular vein. The right testicular vein drains directly into the inferior vena cava, whereas the left testicular vein drains into the left renal vein.

Varicoceles are abnormal dilations of the pampiniform plexus and represent the most prevalent spermatic cord mass [66]. Varicoceles are found in 15% of the general population and are strongly linked to primary and secondary infertility [67, 68]. Patients typically present with a palpable scrotal mass, dull pain, sensation of heaviness, or infertility. On examination, low-grade varicoceles may exhibit a thickened spermatic cord, while high-grade varicoceles may feel like a 'bag of worms' [69]. Infertility is primarily attributed to the elevated temperature caused by engorged veins, impacting spermatogenesis and testicular endocrine function, potentially reversible through embolization or varicocelectomy [70].

Primary varicoceles are often left-sided and attributed to incompetent valves in the internal spermatic vein, leading to retrograde blood flow into the pampiniform plexus. Eighty-five percent of varicoceles are left-sided, while 15% are bilateral [12]. Isolated right-sided varicoceles are rare [12]. The left-sided predominance is due to the length of the left internal spermatic vein and its drainage into the left renal vein at an acute angle, causing increased venous pressure and retrograde flow (Fig. 14.19). Secondary varicoceles result from increased pressure on the spermatic vein due to various causes, including hydronephrosis, cirrhosis, an extrinsic mass, thrombosis of the inferior vena cava, and "nutcracker" phenomenon (i.e., compression of the left renal vein by the superior mesenteric artery and the abdominal aorta) [68, 71]. Varicoceles that are right-sided, noncompressible, or diagnosed in patients over 40 are associated with an increased likelihood of malignancy [67].

Ultrasound can be helpful in diagnosing clinical and subclinical varicoceles [72]. In addition to the typical view of the scrotum, sonographers should obtain a focused evaluation of the pampiniform plexus, which can be found posterior and lateral to the testis. Sonographic assessment involves measuring individual vein diameters, the total diameter of the venous plexus, and using color and spectral Doppler to evaluate for flow reversal with the Valsalva maneuver.

Varicoceles will appear as multiple anechoic or hypoechoic, serpiginous tubular structures with individual diameters exceeding 2.5 mm, best visualized superolateral to the testis (Fig. 14.20) [73, 74]. Additional criteria for the diagnosis of varicoceles include total diameter of the plexus greater than 3 mm and change in flow velocity on Valsalva maneuver of >2 cm/s [74]. Combining these three criteria improves the diagnostic accuracy of varicoceles to a sensitivity of 93% and specificity of 85% when compared to physical exams alone [73, 74].

With varicoceles, color Doppler will show phasic variation and retrograde flow or increased flow and vessel enlargement during Valsalva [73]. These maneuvers are crucial to differentiate varicoceles from other inflammatory conditions, as reflux is not typically seen in other inflammatory conditions. Spectral Doppler of varicoceles should display a venous phase blood flow pattern at rest with intermittent-to-continuous reversal of flow with Valsalva [10]. Intratesticular varicoceles are sometimes associated with extra-testicular varicoceles, though the latter is rare and generally benign [75].

Extratesticular Lesions

Extratesticular lesions are lesions involving the epididymis, spermatic cord, tunica vaginalis, or paratesticular area. The majority (97%) of extratesticular masses are benign, whereas those that are intratesticular are more likely to be malignant (95%) [15]. Therefore, it is important to determine the location of the mass relative to the testicle and whether it is cystic or solid.

Cysts within the epididymis include spermatoceles (most common) and epididymal cysts (less common). Spermatoceles typically are cystic lesions at the head of the epididymis with fluid containing spermatozoa (Fig. 14.21). Spermatoceles are typically anechoic, unilocular, and may have low-level echoes in the lumen representing proteinaceous fluid and spermatozoa [8]. Spermatoceles can be multilocular and tend to be larger than epididymal cysts [8]. While spermatoceles are found only at the head of the epididymis, epididymal cysts can be present anywhere within the epididymis [8]. Epididymal cysts are cystic dilations of the tubules in the epididymis, appearing on ultrasound as well-defined, anechoic structures. However, due to overlapping components, epididymal cysts and spermatoceles cannot be reliably differentiated from each other on imaging alone.

The most common epididymal tumors are adenomatoid tumors, which are benign [8, 15]. They most commonly originate in the tail of the epididymis and are round, well-defined lesions that can be hypoechoic, hyperechoic, or isoechoic compared to adjacent tissue (Fig. 14.22) [8, 15]. Other rarer tumors include papillary cystadenomas and leiomyomas [8]. Papillary cystadenomas are associated with von Hippel–Lindau disease and often are incidental ultrasound findings in patients that cause minimal or no discomfort [8]. The sonographic appearance can range from predominantly cystic lesions with some intramural solid components to completely solid masses and are typically 1.5 to 2 cm in size [8]. Leiomyomas can arise in any smooth muscle in the body. In the scrotum, they can arise from the epididymis, spermatic cord, tunica albuginea, and tunica dartos and may appear as solid, hypoechoic, heterogeneous masses that can have cystic components and calcifications [8, 15].

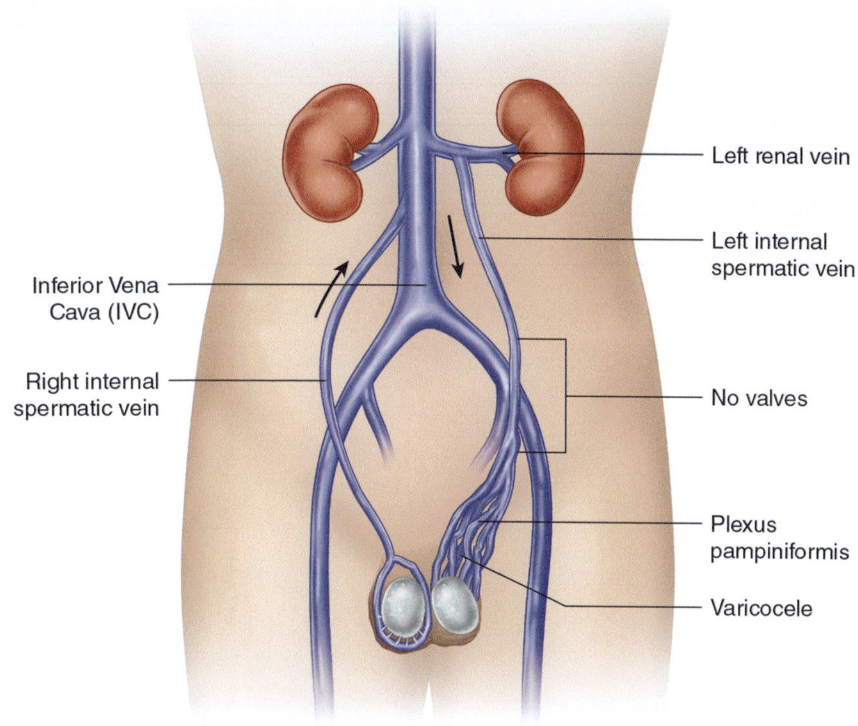

Fig. 14.19 Anatomic depiction of testicular venous flow. Varicoceles are predominantly left-sided due to the length of the left internal spermatic vein and its drainage into the left renal vein at an acute angle, causing increased venous pressure and retrograde flow

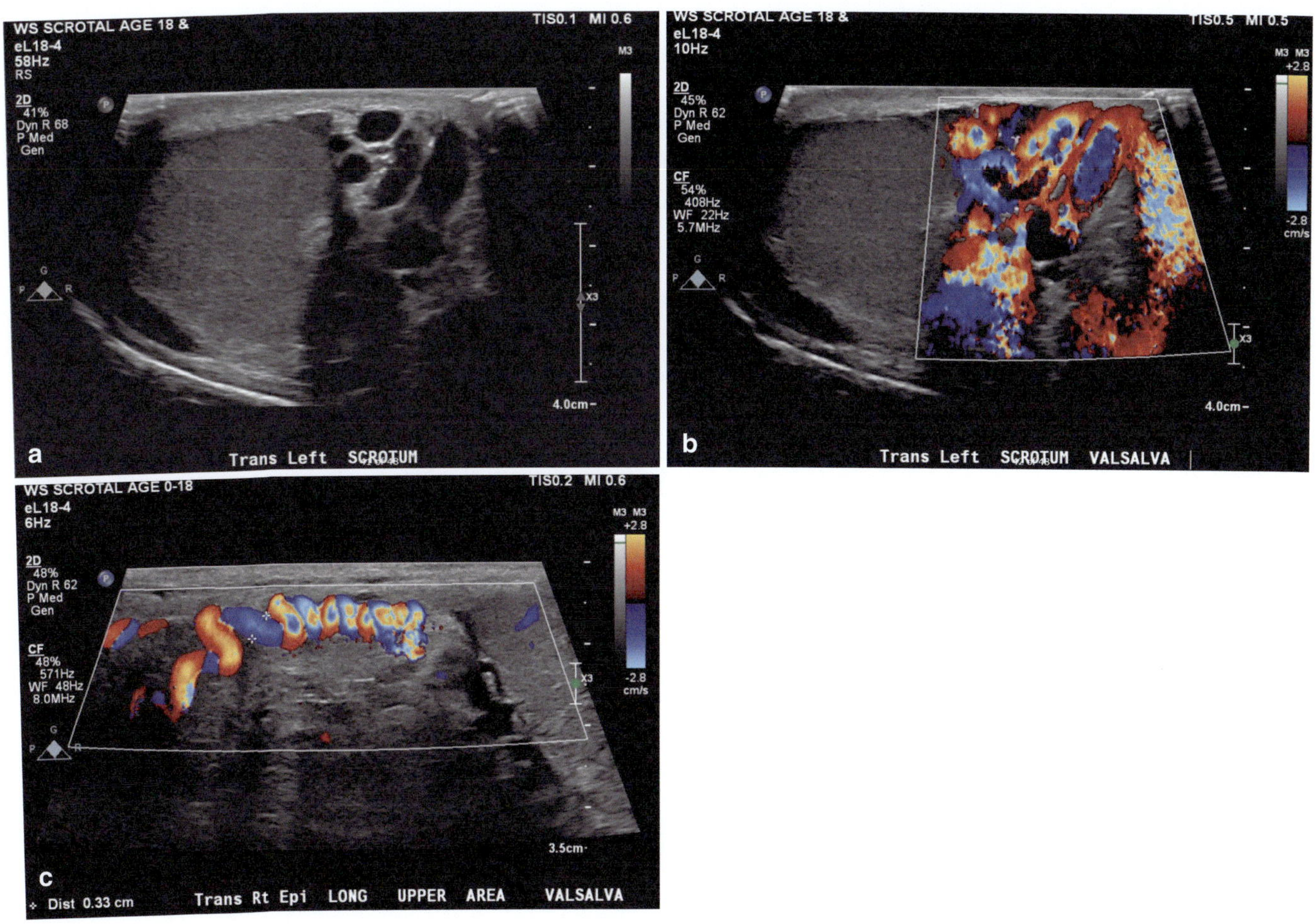

Fig. 14.20 Varicocele. (**a**) B-mode ultrasound demonstrating dilated vessels. (**b**) Color Doppler demonstrating vascular flow in the vessels seen in image (**a**). (**c**) Color Doppler demonstrating the classic tubular appearance of a varicocele

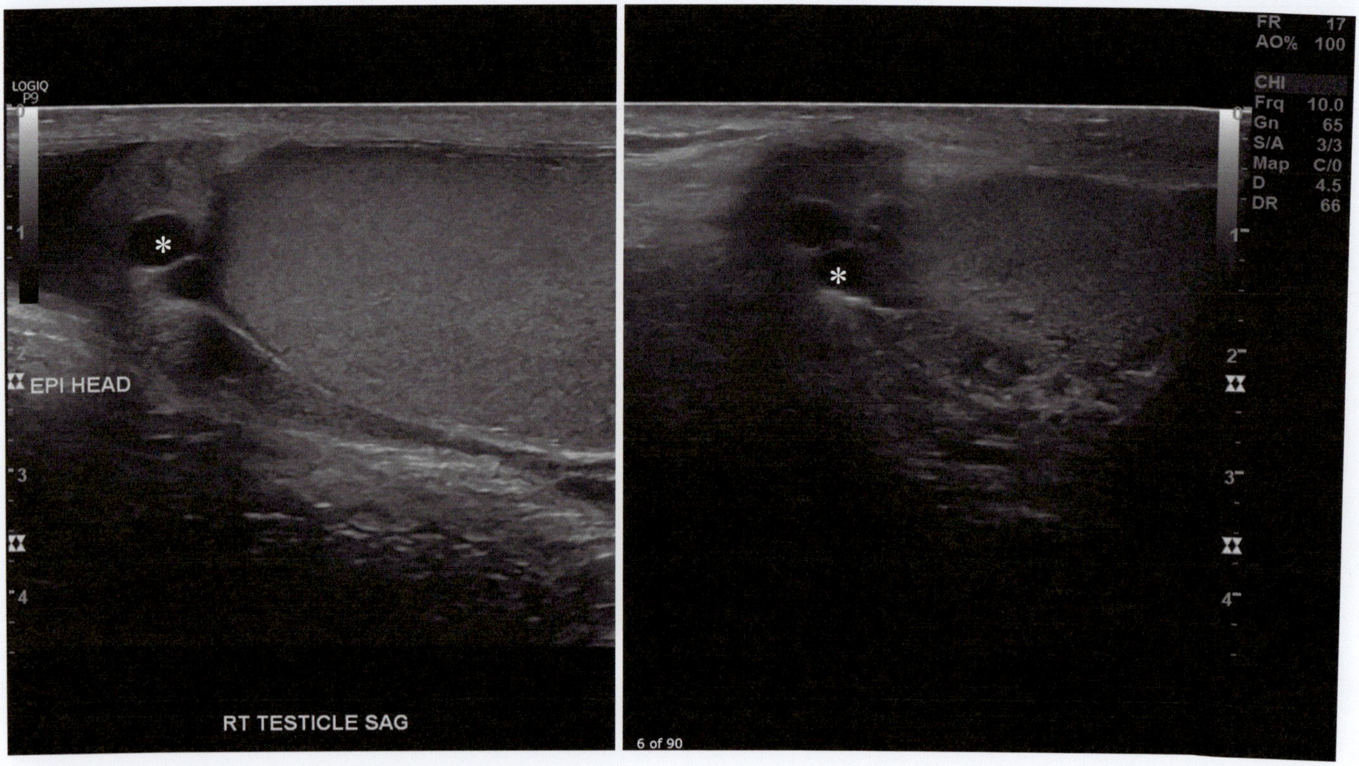

Fig. 14.21 Spermatocele denoted with an (*)

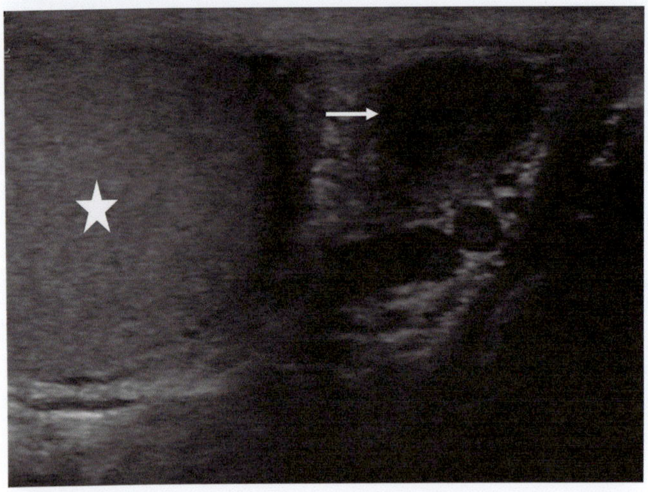

Fig. 14.22 Adenomatoid tumor (arrow) displacing the testicle (star) superiorly. (*Image courtesy of Rafailidis et al.* [89])

Intratesticular Lesions

Simple testicular cysts are well-defined, homogeneous, and anechoic or hypoechoic with posterior acoustic enhancement on ultrasound. The differential for testicular cysts includes tunica albuginea cysts, simple cysts, and tubular ectasia of the rete testis. Tunica albuginea cysts are typically palpable, less than 5 mm in size, and appear simple on ultrasound evaluation [16]. Intratesticular simple cysts are generally not palpable, idiopathic, often post-traumatic or post-inflammatory, range from 2 mm to 2 cm in size, can be single or multiple, and do not generally have a perceptible wall [15].

On ultrasound, the rete testis can appear as numerous spherical or tubular anechoic structures in the region of the mediastinum. Rete testis ectasia, typically found in older men, manifests as a cluster of multiple small cysts and tubules along the testicular mediastinum causing enlargement of the mediastinum [62]. These are bilateral in one-third of cases but can be asymmetric and are often associated with spermatoceles [8]. The condition is most often due to obliteration of the efferent ductules and over half of patients will have a history of spermatic duct obstruction resulting from vasectomy or inguinal hernia repair [15].

The majority of intratesticular solid tumors are malignancies and include germ cell tumors (90–95% of all testicular tumors), sex-cord and stromal tumors, lymphoma, leukemia, and metastatic disease [8, 15]. Testicular cancer is the most common solid tumor malignancy diagnosed in men less than 34 years old, with an incidence of 5.6 cases per 100,000 per year [76]. Ultrasound has a sensitivity of up to 98% and specificity of up to 99.8% in diagnosing malignancy [77]. Testicular hematomas and abscesses, featuring substantial cystic components, warrant careful monitoring. While cystic changes can occur in testicular malignancies, purely cystic cancers are exceptionally rare [8]. Testicular malignancies can be variable in appearance (Fig. 14.23). Common features seen in testicular malignancies include distinct lesions that are frequently lobulated, solid, or complex cystic in nature, display heterogeneously hypoechoic

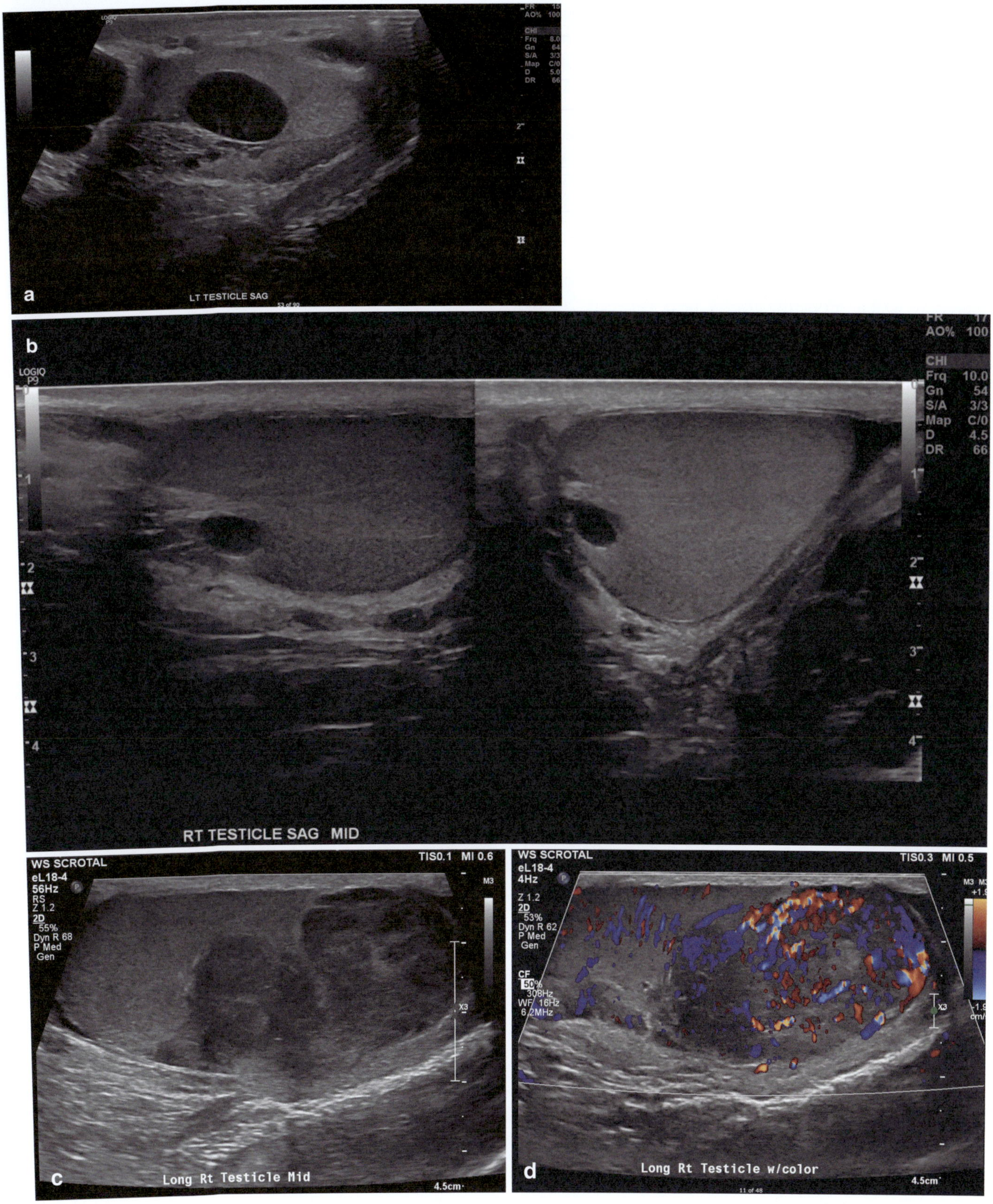

Fig. 14.23 Testicular masses. (**a**) Cystic mass within the testicle. (**b**) Smaller cystic mass exhibiting posterior acoustic enhancement. (**c**) B-mode image of a heterogenous mass found to be a germ cell tumor on pathology. (**d**) Color Doppler image of the heterogeneous mass in image (**c**)

patterns, have irregular or ill-defined margins, have echogenic foci, or possess internal blood flow observed through Doppler ultrasound [8]. The echogenic foci seen in many testicular tumors correspond to local hemorrhage, calcification, or fibrosis but can also represent cartilage or immature bone in teratomas [8]. As heterogeneous echotexture of the testis can also be found in the setting of orchitis or testicular trauma, patients should be followed for complete resolution with serial ultrasounds to rule out tumors and metastasis [8].

Testicular atrophy and fibrosis can be confused for a tumor as they will also appear as hypoechoic regions of the testis. One common cause of this is segmental testicular infarction which primarily affects men between 20 and 40 years of age with underlying hematologic disorders (e.g., vasculitis, sickle cell disease) or in the setting of epididymo-orchitis [15]. The testicle has a triple arterial blood supply from the testicular artery, cremasteric artery, and artery of ductus deferens. When interruption of one of these arteries occurs, an infarct can result. This will commonly appear as a wedge-shaped or triangular morphology with the vertex directed toward the rete testis which is similar in morphology to focal infarcts seen in other organs [78]. In one series, more than 80% of patients with segmental testicular infarction had infarcts located in the upper hemisphere of the testis [78]. While there is some overlap, the presence of a wedge-shaped abnormality with a lack of internal enhancements, often radiating from the mediastinum, helps distinguish segmental testicular infarction from a potential mass [15].

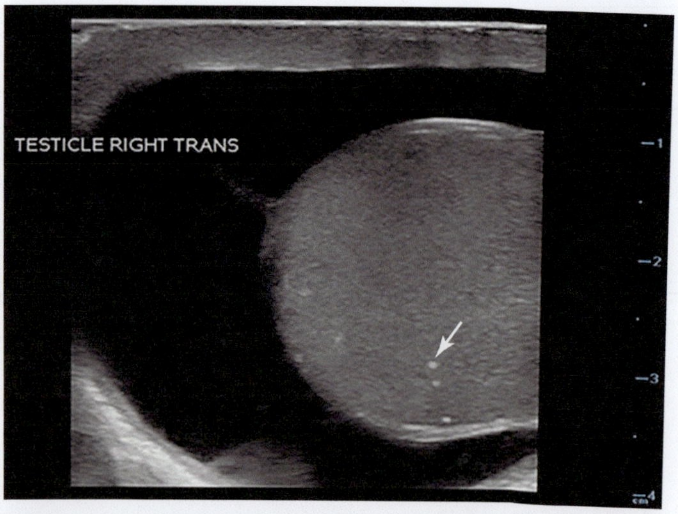

Fig. 14.24 Microlithiasis. Hyperechoic calcifications (arrow) consistent with testicular microlithiasis

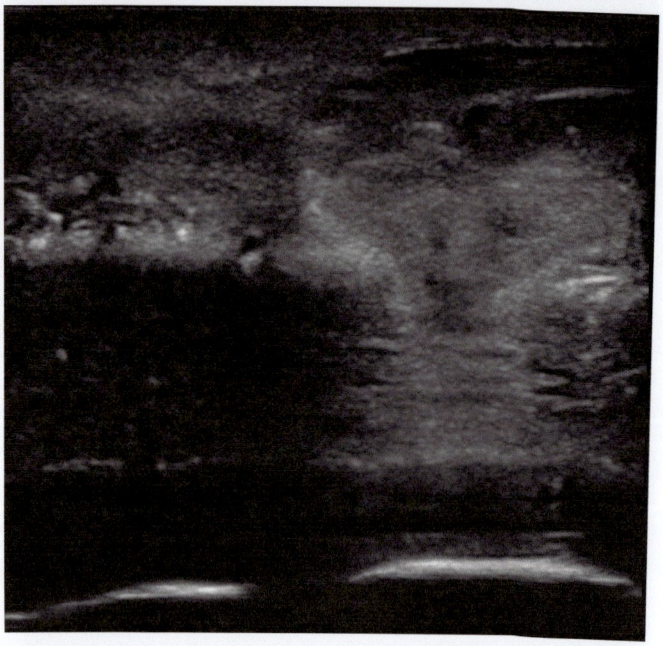

Fig. 14.25 Penile fracture. (*Image courtesy of Michael Gottlieb, MD*)

Microlithiasis

Testicular microlithiasis is defined as intratubular calcifications within the testis due to degeneration of the cells lining the seminiferous tubules [10]. This is an uncommon condition with a reported prevalence of 0.6% of patients undergoing scrotal ultrasound [79]. These are usually incidentally noted on ultrasound and characterized by the intratesticular presence of multiple, randomly distributed, small, hyperechoic foci without acoustic shadowing, each typically measuring 1–3 mm (Fig. 14.24) [80, 81]. Counts may range from a few to over 60 testicular microliths on a single image [81]. Five or more microliths per ultrasound field are considered abnormal and associated with an increased risk of testicular neoplasm, varicoceles, testicular atrophy, Klinefelter syndrome, torsion, cryptorchism, and infertility [8]. Microlithiasis is found in approximately half of all germ cell tumors, though the majority of patients (66%) with microlithiasis do not develop malignancy [10, 15].

Penile Ultrasound

Penile Trauma

Emergency department presentations of acute penile traumas are rare with an incidence of 1 in 175,000 hospital admissions in the United States [82]. Both penetrating and blunt trauma can occur, and ultrasound can help identify hematomas, foreign bodies, and associated vascular injuries.

Penile fractures occur most often due to an external bending force applied to an erect penis which results in rupture of one or both corpora cavernosa due to a tear in the tunica albuginea [18]. The patient can experience a cracking sensation, severe penile pain, swelling, ecchymosis, and detumescence. Between 10 and 20% of cases are associated with urethral injury [28]. The diagnosis is often made clinically, but ultrasound can be used in cases of uncertainty. A disruption in the tunica albuginea along the long axis of the tunica suggests a penile fracture (Fig. 14.25). The presence of a

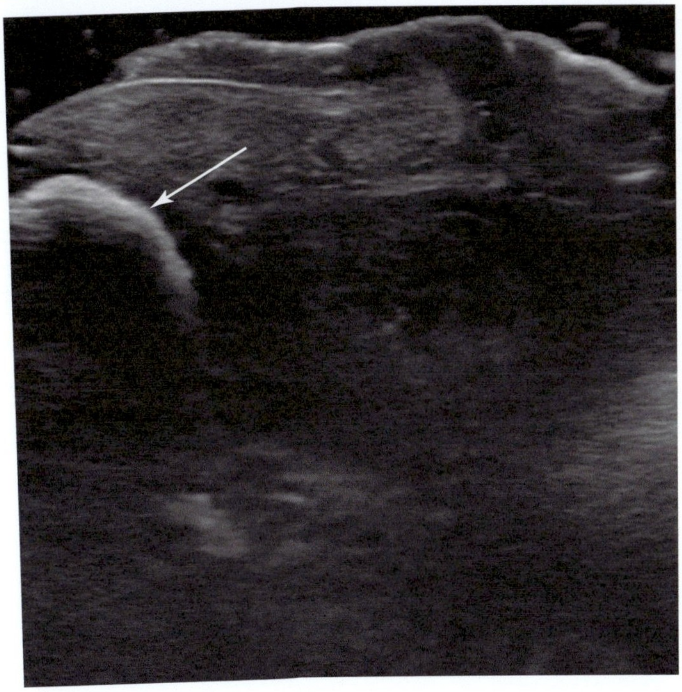

Fig. 14.26 Penile Foreign Body. A retained foreign body (arrow) is visible in the tip of the penis. (*Image courtesy of Michael Gottlieb, MD*)

hematoma deep to the skin or Buck's fascia also supports a diagnosis [33]. Air in the corpora cavernosa would suggest an associated urethral injury [33].

Much like soft tissue evaluations elsewhere in the body, penile foreign bodies may be seen as objects embedded in the penis or within the urethra with various echogenicities depending on the object's composition. The body will naturally mount a granulomatous reaction by either absorbing the material or encapsulating it. If this reaction fails, the foreign body can mount an inflammatory response and erode through tissue causing local damage including rupture of the tunica albuginea or urethra [18]. Ultrasound can be useful to help identify the foreign body, its size, and its relative location (Fig. 14.26).

Priapism

Priapism refers to abnormally prolonged erection (greater than 3 hours) due to vascular pathology rather than sexual arousal [82]. It can be classified as low- or high-flow [17]. High-flow priapism is secondary to arterial trauma resulting in abnormal arterial inflow which causes a nonpainful erection. Low-flow priapism is more common than high-flow and is a medical emergency because impaired venous drainage can result in penile ischemia [18]. The etiology of low-flow priapism is often idiopathic but can be due to hypercoagulable states such as sickle cell disease, trauma, medications, neurologic disorders, infections, and malignancies. Untreated, low-flow priapism can result in infarction, fibrosis, and erectile dysfunction [17].

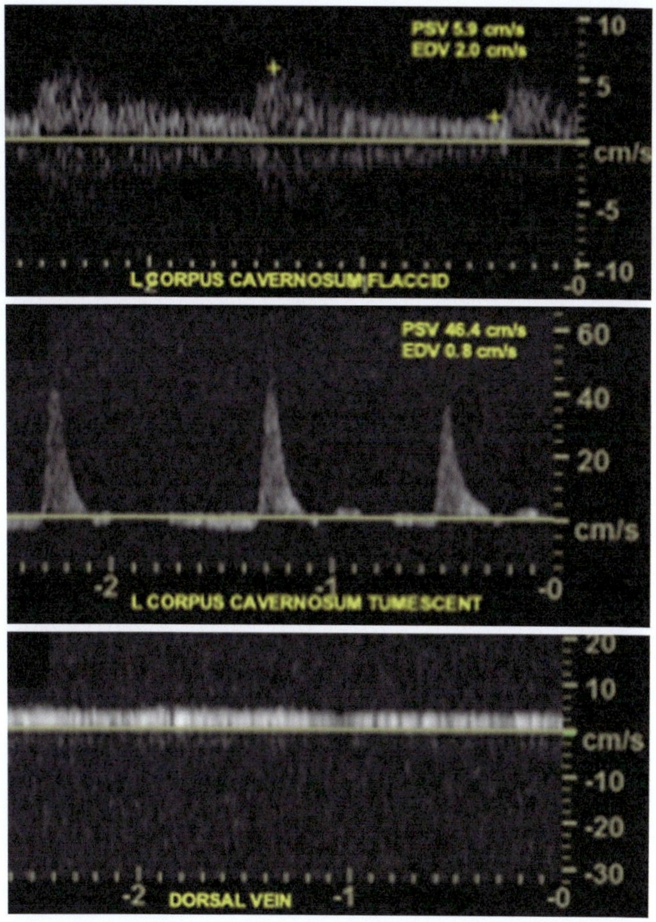

Fig. 14.27 Spectral Doppler demonstrating lower peak systolic and end-diastolic velocities in the flaccid penis (top image). With tumescence, both systolic and diastolic flow increase, and then diastolic flow decreases to zero and undergoes flow reversal (middle image). Spectral Doppler of the dorsal vein should demonstrate a monophasic waveform (bottom image). (*Image obtained with permission from Albasha et al. [18]*)

The diagnosis is often made based on the clinical presentation and evaluation of the aspirated corporeal blood. Ultrasound can be helpful as a less invasive technique. The flaccid penis demonstrates monophasic waveforms with minimal diastolic flow [17]. With tumescence, both systolic and diastolic flow increase [17]. Diastolic flow then decreases to zero and undergoes flow reversal [17]. Normal peak systolic velocity ranges from 5 to 15 cm/s in the flaccid penis and greater than 35 cm/s in the tumescent state [18]. Normal end-diastolic velocity throughout the erection cycle should be below 3–5 cm/s [18]. Spectral Doppler of the dorsal vein should show a monophasic waveform (Fig. 14.27) [18].

Doppler flow can be used to evaluate occult arteriovenous fistulas in the setting of high-flow priapism, which is denoted by an arterial color blush or extravasation of blood from an injured artery (Fig. 14.28). If a fistula is present, ultrasound will show high velocity and turbulent flow within the corpus

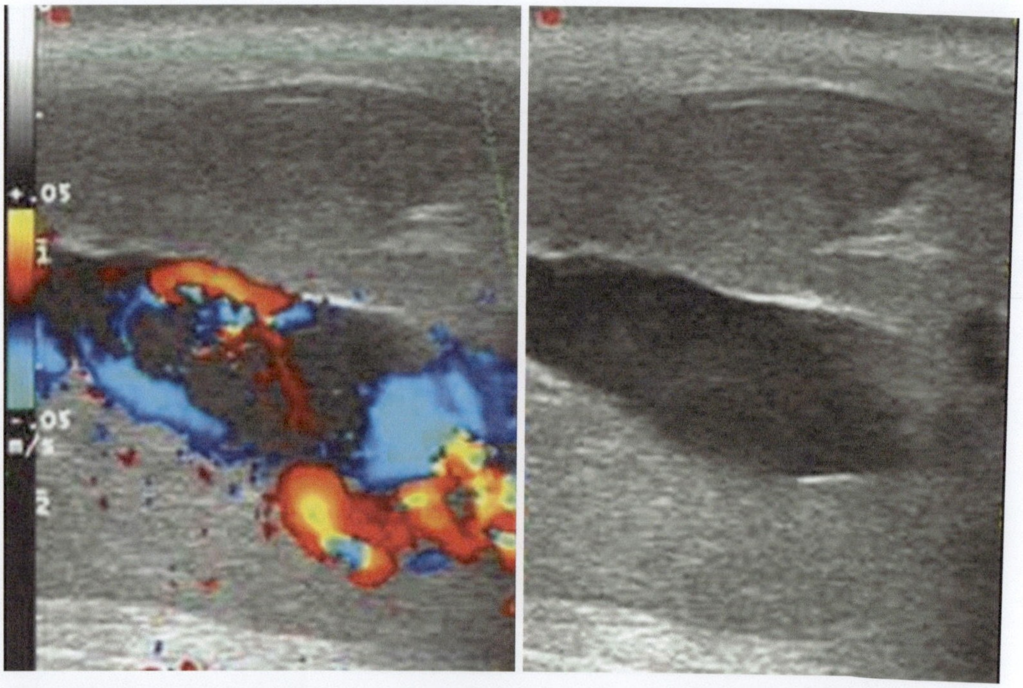

Fig. 14.28 A hematoma with an arteriovenous fistula causing high-flow priapism in the setting of penile trauma. (*Image obtained with permission from Fernandes et al.* [90])

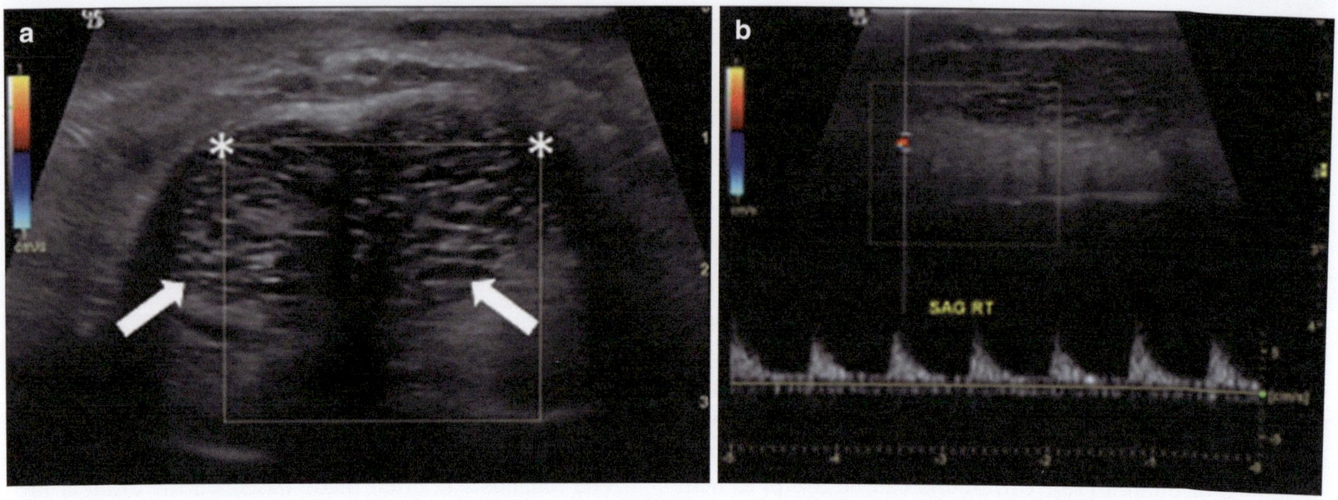

Fig. 14.29 (**a**) Image of low-flow priapism with no Doppler flow in the corpora cavernosa (asterisks) and ischemic changes of increased echotexture and heterogeneity of the cavernosa (solid arrows). (**b**) Where flow is detected in the cavernosa, the velocity will be low rather than the greater than 35 cm/s expected in the corpora cavernosa in the tumescent state. (*Image obtained with permission from Albasha et al.* [18])

cavernosa [82]. In low-flow priapism, there may be low or no Doppler flow in the corpora cavernosa with ischemic changes such as increased echotexture and heterogeneity of the cavernosa (Fig. 14.29). Evidence of high intracavernous resistance can be seen in low systolic peak velocities and the loss of the diastolic component of the cavernous arteries' flow [82]. Flow is often seen in the dorsal penile veins, but thrombosis or low flow of the dorsal penile veins can support a diagnosis of low-flow priapism [18].

Ultrasound-Guided Dorsal Penile Nerve Block

The penis is innervated by the left and right dorsal nerves which are branches of the pudendal nerves. These nerves run lateral to and alongside the paired dorsal arteries, and are found along the base of the penis at the penoscrotal junction. An ultrasound-guided dorsal penile nerve block deposits local anesthetic deep to Buck's fascia where the dorsal nerves of the penis emerge from under the pubic bone (Fig. 14.30). Ultrasound guidance allows for higher block

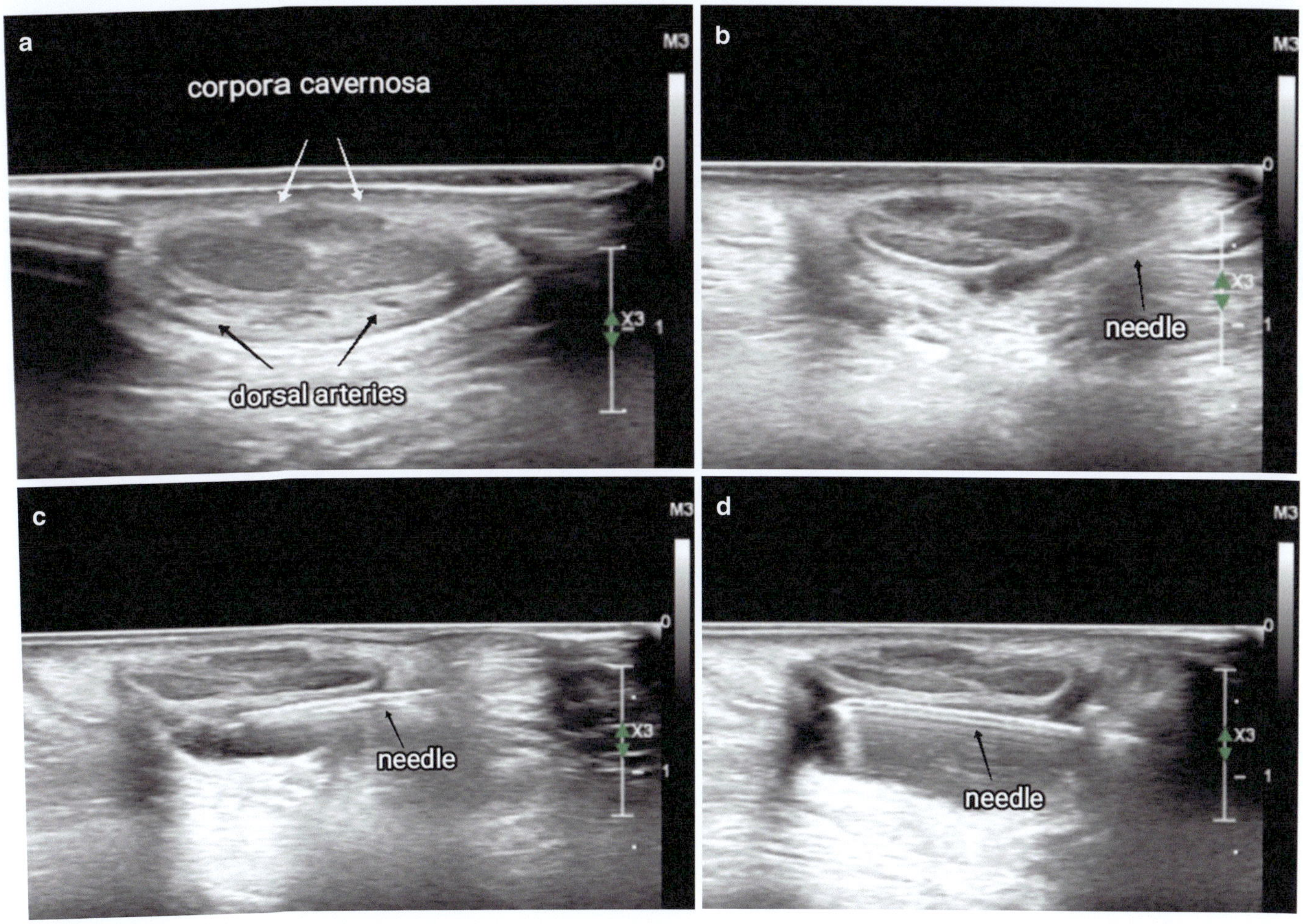

Fig. 14.30 Ultrasound-guided dorsal penile nerve block. (*Image obtained with permission from Dottore et al.* [85])

success rates, shorter block onset times, reduced total volume of local anesthetic used, visualization of the anatomy of the region of interest with confirmation of the distribution of the local anesthetic in real time, and avoidance of structures that may be damaged by the needle [83]. These blocks are ideal for situations in which pain control to the penis is indicated. To perform the block, a high frequency linear probe is placed transversely at the base of the penis. Identify the corpora cavernosa, dorsal arteries and veins, and superficial and deep Buck's fascia. Advance the needle using an in-plane technique through the hyperechoic superficial layer of Buck's fascia lateral to the dorsal artery [84]. After negative aspiration, inject local anesthetic deep into Buck's fascia and visualize the anechoic spread of anesthetic. Retract the needle slightly and hydrodissect to advance the needle toward the contralateral nerve [85]. Once under the fascia and after negative aspiration, inject local anesthetic around the contralateral nerve [86]. The procedure has also been described in an out-of-plane approach [86]. To block the scrotal branches of the pudendal nerve which provides sensory innervation to the ventral midline penile skin to the frenulum, a small ventral bleb is placed at the peno-scrotal junction [86].

Key Ultrasound Findings

Location	Pathology	Ultrasound findings
Scrotum	Scrotal cellulitis	Cobblestoning and scrotal thickness >8 mm.
	Scrotal pearl or scrotal calculus	Hyperechoic with or without acoustic shadows. Mobile, gravity dependent.
	Hydrocele	Anechoic fluid collection encircling the anterolateral aspect of the testicle, may extend into the inguinal canal. Low-level echoes may be present. No internal flow.
	Pyocele	Complex cystic structures with internal echoes and irregular septations and loculations with peripheral wall hyperemia. May note skin thickening, calcifications.
	Hematocele	Variable echotexture based on chronicity. Hyperechoic collections (early). More organized, hypoechoic fluid with septations or fluid-fluid levels (later). No internal flow.
Testicle	Normal testis	Vertical lie with a slight anterior tilt, homogenous, ovoid, 5 × 3 × 2 cm, symmetric bilaterally. Low resistance pattern (RI 0.48–0.75).
	Mediastinum	Hyperechoic linear band along the longitudinal axis of the testis.
	Appendix testis	Upper pole of testis or between the testis and epididymal head, 1–7 mm, isoechoic to the testis. Morphology varies (ovoid, pedunculated, cystic).
	Torsion of the appendix testis	Hyperechoic mass with a central hypoechoic area adjacent to the testis. Absent internal flow and noted peripheral flow. Reactive hydrocele and skin thickening.
	Testicular torsion	Various echotexture. Normal appearance on B-mode (early). Enlarged testis, decreased echogenicity. Heterogenous (after 24 h). Smaller size and increase echogenicity (infarct). Transverse lie. Doppler: absent flow is pathognomonic. Reduced blood flow, dampened spectral waveform, and the absence or reversal of diastolic flow. Elevated testicular arterial RI > 0.75. Hyperemia in the setting of torsion/detorsion. Whirlpool sign and redundant spermatic cord - ovoid, heterogenous pseudomass with dilated tubular structures. Reactive hydrocele, scrotal skin thickening, hyperemic paratesticular tissue.
	Orchitis	Various appearance. Can have normal B-mode appearance. Enlarged testis. Diffuse or focal hypoechoic lesions. Heterogeneous echotexture with hypervascular affected regions. Scrotal wall thickening and reactive hydrocele. Regional or diffuse hyperemia. High Doppler blood flow (peak systolic velocity >15 cm/s). RI of the testicular artery <0.5.
	Testicular abscess	Focal, complex fluid collection with peripheral but no internal vascularity.
	Infarction or contusion	Focal areas of heterogeneous testicular tissue with peripheral but no internal vascularity. Reversal of diastolic flow.
	Testicular fracture	Linear hypoechoic streak extending across the testicular parenchyma. Overall smooth contour and shape of testis maintained. Accompanying hematocele or testicular hematoma.
	Testicular hematoma	Increased echogenicity (early). Heterogeneous and hypoechoic fluid collections with septa and loculations (later). No internal or peripheral Doppler flow.
	Testicular rupture	Heterogeneous testis with irregular and poorly defined borders. Scrotal wall thickening and presence of hematocele. Discrete fracture line noted (less common).
	Testicular tumors	Variable appearance. Distinct lesions that are frequently lobulated. Solid or complex cystic in nature. Heterogeneously hypoechoic. Irregular or ill-defined margins. Echogenic foci. Internal blood flow.
	Testicular cyst	Well-defined, homogeneous, and anechoic to hypoechoic with posterior acoustic enhancement. Lack of internal vascularity. *Tunica albuginea cysts*: <5 mm, simple. *Intratesticular simple cysts*: 2 mm–2 cm, single or multiple, simple without a perceptible wall. *Rete testis ectasia*: cluster of multiple spherical or tubular anechoic structures in the region of the mediastinum.
	Testicular atrophy and fibrosis	Hypoechoic regions arranged in a linear pattern and wedge shaped, often radiate from the mediastinum. Lack of internal enhancements.
	Testicular microlithiasis	Multiple, randomly distributed, small, hyperechoic foci without acoustic shadowing, each typically measuring 1–3 mm.

(continued)

Location	Pathology	Ultrasound findings
Epididymis	Epididymal head	Posterolateral aspect of the testicle. Triangular, 5–12 mm in length, equal or slightly greater echogenicity compared to testis. Minimal internal flow.
	Epididymal body and tail	Posterior or anterolateral edge of testis. 2–5 mm in diameter each, hypoechoic to the testis. Indistinguishable from surrounding peritesticular tissue.
	Appendix epididymis	Adjacent to epididymal head, 3–8 mm in length, most commonly ovoid, more often cystic.
	Torsion of the appendix epididymis	Hyperechoic mass with central hypoechoic area adjacent to the epididymis with reactive hydrocele and skin thickening. Absent internal flow and noted peripheral flow.
	Epididymitis	Can have normal B-mode appearance or hypoechoic enlargement. Hyperemia. Associated with scrotal wall thickening, reactive hydrocele, orchitis, pyocele, and scrotal abscess.
	Epididymal cysts	Well-defined, anechoic cystic structures, unilocular. Found anywhere within the epididymis.
	Spermatocele	Anechoic, well-defined cystic structures, unilocular or multilocular, can have low-level echoes within lumen. Found at the head of the epididymis.
	Epididymal tumors	Round, well-defined lesions of variable echogenicity. Range from cystic with intramural solid components to solid masses, can have calcifications.
Spermatic cord	Pampiniform plexus	Veins normally 0.5–1.5 mm.
	Varicocele	Posterior and lateral to the testis. Multiple anechoic to hypoechoic, serpiginous tubular structures >2 mm in diameter. Venous phase blood flow pattern at rest with intermittent to continuous reversal of flow with Valsalva. Phasic variation and retrograde flow or increased flow and vessel enlargement during Valsalva.
Penis	Normal	Homogenous corpora. Intermediate to low echogenicity (corpora cavernosa). Slightly hyperechoic (corpus spongiosum). Flaccid: Monophasic waveforms with minimal diastolic flow, normal peak systolic velocity 5–15 cm/s. Tumescent: Systolic and diastolic flow increases initially then diastolic flow decreases to zero and undergoes flow reversal, normal peak systolic velocity >35 cm/s. Dorsal vein—monophasic waveform.
	Penile fracture	Disruption in the tunica albuginea. Presence of a hematoma deep to the skin or Buck's fascia. Presence of air (dirty shadowing) in the corpora cavernosa suggests urethral injury.
	Penile foreign body	Masses with various sizes and echogenicities.
	High-flow priapism	Arterial color blush or extravasation of blood from an injured artery. High velocity and turbulent flow within the corpus cavernosa.
	Low-flow priapism	Low or no Doppler flow in the corpora cavernosa with ischemic changes (increased echotexture and heterogeneity of the cavernosa). Low systolic peak velocities and loss of the diastolic component of the cavernous arteries' flow. May see thrombosis or low flow of the dorsal penile veins.

RI resistive index

Pearls and Pitfalls

- Compare the bilateral testes and obtain views in two orthogonal planes. Make sure to use the "buddy view" when evaluating differences in color flow and echotexture.
- Use color Doppler, power Doppler, and spectral Doppler to evaluate perfusion and vascular flow of the testis and aid in detection of hyperemia or ischemia.
- Employ dynamic imaging and Valsalva technique to differentiate between varicoceles and other inflammatory processes.
- Consider that hyperemia may be present in torsion/detorsion as well as orchitis and that testicular infarct, a mimic of torsion, can occur both in the setting of trauma and infection.
- Look for secondary signs of testicular fracture and rupture as fracture lines are observed in a minority of cases. Surgical exploration may be needed to confirm the diagnosis.
- Incidental testicular tumors may mimic findings for testicular cysts, atrophy, fibrosis, trauma, or infection. Make sure patients with testicular trauma and infection receive repeat imaging to not miss testicular tumors.
- If the clinical picture is clear for emergent pathologies such as testicular torsion, testicular trauma, penile fracture, and priapism, ultrasound should not delay management.

References

1. Miskin M, Bain J. B-mode ultrasonic examination of the testes. J Clin Ultrasound. 1974;2(4):307–11. https://doi.org/10.1002/jcu.1870020412.
2. Gottesman JE, Sample WF, Skinner DG, Ehrlich RM. Diagnostic ultrasound in the evaluation of scrotal masses. J Urol. 1977;118(4):601–3. https://doi.org/10.1016/s0022-5347(17)58117-3.
3. Sample WF, Gottesman JE, Skinner DG, Ehrlich RM. Gray scale ultrasound of the scrotum. Radiology. 1978;127(1):225–8. https://doi.org/10.1148/127.1.225.
4. Shawker TH. B-mode ultrasonic evaluation of scrotal swellings. Radiology. 1976;118(2):417–9. https://doi.org/10.1148/118.2.417.
5. Kossoff G. Technology of real-time ultrasound. Part I. Contrib Gynecol Obstet. 1979;6:2–10.
6. Leopold GR, Woo VL, Scheible FW, Nachtsheim D, Gosink BB. High-resolution ultrasonography of scrotal pathology. Radiology. 1979;131(3):719–22. https://doi.org/10.1148/131.3.719.
7. Saitoh M, Ohe H, Tanaka S, Mishina T, Watanabe H. Ultrasonic diagnosis of intrascrotal contents. Tohoku J Exp Med. 1977;123(4):337–41. https://doi.org/10.1620/tjem.123.337.
8. Dogra VS, Gottlieb RH, Oka M, Rubens DJ. Sonography of the scrotum. Radiology. 2003;227(1):18–36. https://doi.org/10.1148/radiol.2271001744.
9. Adhikari S. Testicular. In: Ma O, Mateer JR, Reardon RF, Byars DV, Knapp BJ, Laudenbach AP, editors. Ma and Mateer's emergency ultrasound. 4th ed. McGraw Hill; 2021.
10. Ragheb D, Higgins JL Jr. Ultrasonography of the scrotum: technique, anatomy, and pathologic entities. J Ultrasound Med. 2002;21(2):171–85. https://doi.org/10.7863/jum.2002.21.2.171.
11. AIUM practice parameter for the performance of penile ultrasound. J Ultrasound Med. 2023;42(9):E45–8. https://doi.org/10.1002/jum.16235.
12. Hertzberg BS, Middleton WD. Ultrasound : the requisites. Philadelphia: Elsevier; 2016.
13. Rebik K, Wagner JM, Middleton W. Scrotal ultrasound. Radiol Clin North Am. 2019;57(3):635–48. https://doi.org/10.1016/j.rcl.2019.01.007.
14. McAchran SE, Dogra V, Resnick MI. Office urologic ultrasound. Urol Clin North Am. 2005;32(3):337–vii. https://doi.org/10.1016/j.ucl.2005.03.005.
15. Aganovic L, Cassidy F. Imaging of the scrotum. Radiol Clin North Am. 2012;50(6):1145–65. https://doi.org/10.1016/j.rcl.2012.08.003.
16. Carkaci S, Ozkan E, Lane D, Yang WT. Scrotal sonography revisited. J Clin Ultrasound. 2010;38(1):21–37. https://doi.org/10.1002/jcu.20642.
17. Shenoy-Bhangle A, Perez-Johnston R, Singh A. Penile imaging. Radiol Clin North Am. 2012;50(6):1167–81. https://doi.org/10.1016/j.rcl.2012.08.009.
18. Albasha H, Wang SS, Revels JW, Beckett K, Flink CC. Imaging review of penile pathologies encountered in the emergency department. Emerg Radiol. 2022;29(1):147–59. https://doi.org/10.1007/s10140-021-01988-1.
19. Sharp VJ, Kieran K, Arlen AM. Testicular torsion: diagnosis, evaluation, and management. Am Fam Physician. 2013;88(12):835–40.
20. Kass EJ, Lundak B. The acute scrotum. Pediatr Clin N Am. 1997;44(5):1251–66. https://doi.org/10.1016/s0031-3955(05)70556-3.
21. Bandarkar AN, Blask AR. Testicular torsion with preserved flow: key sonographic features and value-added approach to diagnosis. Pediatr Radiol. 2018;48(5):735–44. https://doi.org/10.1007/s00247-018-4093-0.
22. Prando D. Torsion of the spermatic cord: the main gray-scale and doppler sonographic signs. Abdom Imaging. 2009;34(5):648–61. https://doi.org/10.1007/s00261-008-9449-8.
23. McDowall J, Adam A, Gerber L, Enyuma COA, Aigbodion SJ, Buchanan S, Laher AE. The ultrasonographic "whirlpool sign" in testicular torsion: valuable tool or waste of valuable time? A systematic review and meta-analysis. Emerg Radiol. 2018;25(3):281–92. https://doi.org/10.1007/s10140-018-1579-x. Epub 2018 Jan 15. PMID: 29335899.
24. Munden MM, Williams JL, Zhang W, Crowe JE, Munden RF, Cisek LJ. Intermittent testicular torsion in the pediatric patient: sonographic indicators of a difficult diagnosis. AJR Am J Roentgenol. 2013;201(4):912–8. https://doi.org/10.2214/AJR.12.9448.
25. Kaye JD, Shapiro EY, Levitt SB, et al. Parenchymal echo texture predicts testicular salvage after torsion: potential impact on the need for emergent exploration. J Urol. 2008;180(4 Suppl):1733–6. https://doi.org/10.1016/j.juro.2008.03.104.
26. Luker GD, Siegel MJ. Scrotal US in pediatric patients: comparison of power and standard color Doppler US. Radiology. 1996;198(2):381–5. https://doi.org/10.1148/radiology.198.2.8596836.
27. Babcock DS, Patriquin H, LaFortune M, Dauzat M. Power doppler sonography: basic principles and clinical applications in children. Pediatr Radiol. 1996;26(2):109–15. https://doi.org/10.1007/BF01372087.
28. Uyeda JW, Gans BS, Sodickson A. Imaging of acute and emergent genitourinary conditions: what the radiologist needs to know. AJR Am J Roentgenol. 2015;204(6):W631–9. https://doi.org/10.2214/AJR.14.14117.
29. Rafailidis V, Apostolou D, Charsoula A, Rafailidis D. Sonography of the scrotum: from appendages to scrotolithiasis. J Ultrasound Med. 2015;34(3):507–18. https://doi.org/10.7863/ultra.34.3.507.
30. Sellars ME, Sidhu PS. Ultrasound appearances of the testicular appendages: pictorial review. Eur Radiol. 2003;13(1):127–35. https://doi.org/10.1007/s00330-002-1387-1.
31. Mushtaq I, Fung M, Glasson MJ. Retrospective review of paediatric patients with acute scrotum. ANZ J Surg. 2003;73(1–2):55–8. https://doi.org/10.1046/j.1445-2197.2003.02612.x.
32. Fujita N, Tambo M, Okegawa T, Higashihara E, Nutahara K. Distinguishing testicular torsion from torsion of the appendix testis by clinical features and signs in patients with acute scrotum. Res Rep Urol. 2017;9:169–174. Published 2017 Aug 28. https://doi.org/10.2147/RRU.S140361.
33. McAdams CR, Del Gaizo AJ. The utility of scrotal ultrasonography in the emergent setting: beyond epididymitis versus torsion. Emerg Radiol. 2018;25(4):341–8. https://doi.org/10.1007/s10140-018-1606-y.
34. Baldisserotto M, de Souza JC, Pertence AP, Dora MD. Color Doppler sonography of normal and torsed testicular appendages in children. AJR Am J Roentgenol. 2005;184(4):1287–92. https://doi.org/10.2214/ajr.184.4.01841287.
35. Lev M, Ramon J, Mor Y, Jacobson JM, Soudack M. Sonographic appearances of torsion of the appendix testis and appendix epididymis in children. J Clin Ultrasound. 2015;43(8):485–9. https://doi.org/10.1002/jcu.22265.
36. National Center for Health Statistics. National Ambulatory Medical Care Survey, 2002. Available at: http://www.cdc.gov/nchs/about/major/ahcd/ahcd1.htm. Accessed 23 Jan 2009.
37. Trojian TH, Lishnak TS, Heiman D. Epididymitis and orchitis: an overview. Am Fam Physician. 2009;79(7):583–7.
38. Avery LL, Scheinfeld MH. Imaging of penile and scrotal emergencies. Radiographics. 2013;33(3):721–40. https://doi.org/10.1148/rg.333125158.

39. Turgut AT, Bhatt S, Dogra VS. Acute painful scrotum. Ultrasound Clin. 2008;3(1):93–107. https://doi.org/10.1016/j.cult.2007.12.004.
40. Berger RE, Alexander ER, Harnisch JP, et al. Etiology, manifestations and therapy of acute epididymitis: prospective study of 50 cases. J Urol. 1979;121(6):750–4. https://doi.org/10.1016/s0022-5347(17)56978-5.
41. Schuppe HC, Pilatz A, Hossain H, et al. Orchitis und Infertilität [Orchitis and male infertility]. Urologe A. 2010;49(5):629–35. https://doi.org/10.1007/s00120-010-2256-1.
42. Ludwig M. Diagnosis and therapy of acute prostatitis, epididymitis and orchitis. Andrologia. 2008;40(2):76–80. https://doi.org/10.1111/j.1439-0272.2007.00823.x.
43. McLaren PSM. A systematic review on the utility of ultrasonography in the diagnosis of testicular torsion in acute scrotum patients. Radiography (Lond). 2021;27(3):943–9. https://doi.org/10.1016/j.radi.2020.12.012.
44. Coley BD. The acute pediatric scrotum. Ultrasound Clin. 2006;1(3):485–96. https://doi.org/10.1016/j.cult.2006.05.002.
45. Brown JM, Hammers LW, Barton JW, et al. Quantitative Doppler assessment of acute scrotal inflammation. Radiology. 1995;197(2):427–31. https://doi.org/10.1148/radiology.197.2.7480687.
46. Cook JL, Dewbury K. The changes seen on high-resolution ultrasound in orchitis. Clin Radiol. 2000;55(1):13–8. https://doi.org/10.1053/crad.1999.0372.
47. Casalino DD, Kim R. Clinical importance of a unilateral striated pattern seen on sonography of the testicle. AJR Am J Roentgenol. 2002;178(4):927–30. https://doi.org/10.2214/ajr.178.4.1780927.
48. Sanders LM, Haber S, Dembner A, Aquino A. Significance of reversal of diastolic flow in the acute scrotum. J Ultrasound Med. 1994;13(2):137–9. https://doi.org/10.7863/jum.1994.13.2.137.
49. Haury B, Rodeheaver G, Stevenson T, Bacchetta C, Edgerton MT, Edlich RF. Streptococcal cellulitis of the scrotum and penis with secondary skin gangrene. Surg Gynecol Obstet. 1975;141(1):35–9.
50. Conzi R, Damasio MB, Bertolotto M, et al. Scrotal imaging group of the european society of urogenital radiology. Sonography of scrotal wall lesions and correlation with other modalities. J Ultrasound Med. 2017;36:2149–63.
51. Hayeri MR, Ziai P, Shehata ML, Teytelboym OM, Huang BK. Soft-tissue infections and their imaging mimics: from cellulitis to necrotizing fasciitis. Radiographics. 2016;36(6):1888–910. https://doi.org/10.1148/rg.2016160068.
52. Mesquita RD, Rosas JL. Adult acute scrotal Edema - when radiologists can help to avoid unnecessary surgical treatment. J Radiol Case Rep. 2017;11(8):24–30. Published 2017 Aug 31. https://doi.org/10.3941/jrcr.v11i8.3165.
53. Lewis CA, Michell MJ. The use of real-time ultrasound in the management of scrotal trauma. Br J Radiol. 1991;64(765):792–5. https://doi.org/10.1259/0007-1285-64-765-792.
54. Sasso F, Gulino G, Di Pinto A, Alcini E. Correlazione tra immagine ultrasonografica e quadro chirurgico nei traumi scrotali [Correlation between ultrasonography imaging and surgical findings in scrotal trauma]. Arch Ital Urol Androl. 1995;67(2):159–62.
55. Lynch TH, Martínez-Piñeiro L, Plas E, et al. EAU guidelines on urological trauma. Eur Urol. 2005;47(1):1–15. https://doi.org/10.1016/j.eururo.2004.07.028.
56. Bowen DK, Gonzalez CM. Intratesticular hematoma after blunt scrotal trauma: a case series and algorithm-based approach to management. Cent Eur J Urol. 2014;67(4):427–9. https://doi.org/10.5173/ceju.2014.04.art24.
57. Siegel MJ. The acute scrotum. Radiol Clin North Am. 1997;35(4):959–76.
58. Jeffrey RB, Laing FC, Hricak H, McAninch JW. Sonography of testicular trauma. AJR Am J Roentgenol. 1983;141(5):993–5. https://doi.org/10.2214/ajr.141.5.993.
59. Keihani S, Hojjat A, Kajbafzadeh AM. Abdominoscrotal hydrocele: role of physical exam and Transillumination in diagnosis. J Pediatr. 2015;167(6):1448–e1. https://doi.org/10.1016/j.jpeds.2015.08.047.
60. Collings C, Cronan JJ, Grusmark J. Diffuse echoes within a simple hydrocele: an imaging caveat. J Ultrasound Med. 1994;13(6):439–42. https://doi.org/10.7863/jum.1994.13.6.439.
61. Gooding GA, Leonhardt WC, Marshall G, Seltzer MA, Presti JC Jr. Cholesterol crystals in hydroceles: sonographic detection and possible significance. AJR Am J Roentgenol. 1997;169(2):527–9. https://doi.org/10.2214/ajr.169.2.9242769.
62. Patil V, Shetty SM, Das S. Common and uncommon presentation of fluid within the scrotal spaces. Ultrasound Int Open. 2015;1(2):E34–40. https://doi.org/10.1055/s-0035-1555919.
63. Akin EA, Khati NJ, Hill MC. Ultrasound of the scrotum. Ultrasound Q. 2004;20(4):181–200. https://doi.org/10.1097/00013644-200412000-00004.
64. Benson CB, Doubilet PM, Richie JP. Sonography of the male genital tract. AJR Am J Roentgenol. 1989;153(4):705–13. https://doi.org/10.2214/ajr.153.4.705.
65. Metin A, Bulut O, Temizkan M. Relationship between the left spermatic vein diameter measured by ultrasound and palpated varicocele and Doppler ultrasound findings. Int Urol Nephrol. 1991;23(1):65–8. https://doi.org/10.1007/BF02549730.
66. Woodward PJ, Schwab CM, Sesterhenn IA. From the archives of the AFIP: extratesticular scrotal masses: radiologic-pathologic correlation. Radiographics. 2003;23(1):215–40. https://doi.org/10.1148/rg.231025133.
67. Alsaikhan B, Alrabeeah K, Delouya G, Zini A. Epidemiology of varicocele. Asian J Androl. 2016;18(2):179–81. https://doi.org/10.4103/1008-682X.172640.
68. de Los RT, Locke J, Afshar K. Varicoceles in the pediatric population: diagnosis, treatment, and outcomes. Can Urol Assoc J. 2017;11(1-2Suppl1):S34–9. https://doi.org/10.5489/cuaj.4340.
69. Lomboy JR, Coward RM. The Varicocele: clinical presentation, evaluation, and surgical management. Semin Intervent Radiol. 2016;33(3):163–9. https://doi.org/10.1055/s-0036-1586143.
70. Goldstein M, Eid JF. Elevation of intratesticular and scrotal skin surface temperature in men with varicocele. J Urol. 1989;142(3):743–5. https://doi.org/10.1016/s0022-5347(17)38874-2.
71. Reddy DK, Shekar PA. Nutcracker syndrome-A rare but important cause of Varicocele in adolescent boys. Urology. 2020;141:143–6. https://doi.org/10.1016/j.urology.2020.04.008.
72. Trum JW, Gubler FM, Laan R, van der Veen F. The value of palpation, varicoscreen contact thermography and colour Doppler ultrasound in the diagnosis of varicocele. Hum Reprod. 1996;11(6):1232–5. https://doi.org/10.1093/oxfordjournals.humrep.a019362.
73. Lee J, Binsaleh S, Lo K, Jarvi K. Varicoceles: the diagnostic dilemma. J Androl. 2008;29(2):143–6. https://doi.org/10.2164/jandrol.107.003467.
74. Chiou RK, Anderson JC, Wobig RK, et al. Color Doppler ultrasound criteria to diagnose varicoceles: correlation of a new scoring system with physical examination. Urology. 1997;50(6):953–6. https://doi.org/10.1016/S0090-4295(97)00452-4.
75. Das KM, Prasad K, Szmigielski W, Noorani N. Intratesticular varicocele: evaluation using conventional and Doppler sonography. AJR Am J Roentgenol. 1999;173(4):1079–83. https://doi.org/10.2214/ajr.173.4.10511183.
76. Baird DC, Meyers GJ, Hu JS. Testicular cancer: diagnosis and treatment. Am Fam Physician. 2018;97(4):261–8.
77. Coursey Moreno C, Small WC, Camacho JC, et al. Testicular tumors: what radiologists need to know--differential diagnosis, staging, and management. Radiographics. 2015;35(2):400–15. https://doi.org/10.1148/rg.352140097.

78. Fernández-Pérez GC, Tardáguila FM, Velasco M, et al. Radiologic findings of segmental testicular infarction. AJR Am J Roentgenol. 2005;184(5):1587–93. https://doi.org/10.2214/ajr.184.5.01841587.
79. Cast JE, Nelson WM, Early AS, et al. Testicular microlithiasis: prevalence and tumor risk in a population referred for scrotal sonography. AJR Am J Roentgenol. 2000;175(6):1703–6. https://doi.org/10.2214/ajr.175.6.1751703.
80. Janzen DL, Mathieson JR, Marsh JI, et al. Testicular microlithiasis: sonographic and clinical features. AJR Am J Roentgenol. 1992;158(5):1057–60. https://doi.org/10.2214/ajr.158.5.1566667.
81. Bennett HF, Middleton WD, Bullock AD, Teefey SA. Testicular microlithiasis: US follow-up. Radiology. 2001;218(2):359–63. https://doi.org/10.1148/radiology.218.2.r01fe25359.
82. Cozzi D, Verrone GB, Agostini S, et al. Acute penile trauma: imaging features in the emergency setting. Radiol Med. 2019;124(12):1270–80. https://doi.org/10.1007/s11547-019-01065-1.
83. Yildirim SA, Ozcan H, Turkoz A. Ultrasound-guided penile block for circumcision instead of anatomical landmark method in newborn babies. Ain-Shams J Anesthesiol. 2021;13:39. https://doi.org/10.1186/s42077-021-00158-2.
84. Suleman MI, Akbar Ali AN, Kanarek V, Li M, Patel A. Ultrasound guided in-plane penile nerve block for circumcision: a new, modified technique suggests lower anesthetic volume and narcotic use. Middle East J Anaesthesiol. 2016;23:647–53.
85. Dottore B, Meroi F, Tomasino S, et al. Pediatric ultrasound-guided dorsal penile nerve block and sedation in spontaneous breathing: a prospective observational study. Front Med (Lausanne). 2023;10:1268594. Published 2023 Dec 4. https://doi.org/10.3389/fmed.2023.1268594.
86. Sandeman DJ, Dilley AV. Ultrasound guided dorsal penile nerve block in children. Anaesth Intensive Care. 2007;35:266–9. https://doi.org/10.1177/0310057X0703500217.
87. Sweet DE, Feldman MK, Remer EM. Imaging of the acute scrotum: keys to a rapid diagnosis of acute scrotal disorders. Abdom Radiol (NY). 2020;45(7):2063–81. https://doi.org/10.1007/s00261-019-02333-4.
88. Whitworth PW 3rd, Dyer RB. The "striated" testis. Abdom Radiol (NY). 2019;44(8):2943–4. https://doi.org/10.1007/s00261-019-02046-8.
89. Rafailidis V, Huang DY, Sidhu PS. Paratesticular lesions: aetiology and appearances on ultrasound. Andrology. 2021;9(5):1383–94. https://doi.org/10.1111/andr.13021.
90. Fernandes MAV, de Souza LRMF, Cartafina LP. Ultrasound evaluation of the penis. Radiol Bras. 2018;51(4):257–61. https://doi.org/10.1590/0100-3984.2016.0152.

15 Ocular Ultrasound

Daniel J. Kim, Gillian Sheppard, and Rajiv Thavanathan

Background

Eye-related complaints are a common reason for patients to seek emergency care, comprising 1.5% of presentations to the emergency department (ED), of which one-third are secondary to trauma [1]. In the ED, the ocular examination can be challenging as ambient lighting, facial trauma, and poor patient tolerance can impact the accuracy of direct ophthalmoscopy, especially in the hands of non-ophthalmologists [2]. For these reasons, agreement between emergency physician and ophthalmologist diagnosis may align in only two-thirds of cases [3]. As such, clinicians developed an interest in point-of-care ultrasound (POCUS) of the eye. The first report of diagnostic ocular ultrasound was published in 1956 using A-mode scanning, and improvements rapidly occurred with the development of ocular B-mode scanning in the late 1950s and high-frequency ultrasound probes in the 1960s [4]. With technological improvements and the increasing portability of ultrasound machines in the 1980s and 1990s, emergency medicine has embraced POCUS, extending the use of its diagnostic applications to the eye in 2000 [5]. Since then, the evidence base for ocular POCUS has grown dramatically, supporting its use to accurately diagnose both traumatic ocular pathology and posterior chamber abnormalities [6, 7]. This is relevant both to clinicians practicing in a busy ED who need to make accurate diagnoses and triage appropriate ophthalmology referrals, as well as to clinicians practicing in clinic settings, the hospital, or resource-limited environments where there may be limited access to ophthalmology or advanced imaging like computed tomography (CT) [8].

Supplementary Information The online version contains supplementary material available at https://doi.org/10.1007/978-3-031-85308-1_15.

D. J. Kim (✉)
Department of Emergency Medicine, University of British Columbia, Vancouver, BC, Canada

G. Sheppard
Discipline of Emergency Medicine, Memorial University of Newfoundland, St. John's, NL, Canada
e-mail: gsheppard@mun.ca

R. Thavanathan
Department of Emergency Medicine, University of Ottawa, Ottawa, ON, Canada
e-mail: rthavanathan@toh.ca

Indications

Indications
- Vision impairment/loss
- Eye pain
- Trauma
- Concern for increased intracranial pressure

Diagnoses
- Retinal detachment
- Posterior vitreous detachment
- Vitreous hemorrhage
- Asteroid hyalosis
- Choroidal detachment
- Lens dislocation
- Intraocular foreign body
- Dilated optic nerve sheath
- Optic disc elevation
- Central retinal artery occlusion
- Pupillary assessment
- Retrobulbar hematoma
- Globe rupture
- Periorbital cellulitis
- Orbital cellulitis
- Endophthalmitis
- Posterior scleritis
- Ocular mass

Core Views

Patients can be placed in a semi-seated or supine position for the ultrasound examination [9]. Gel can be applied either directly onto the closed eyelid or onto a translucent adhesive dressing (e.g., Tegaderm™) that can be applied over the eyelid prior to the application of gel [10]. Use of an adhesive

M. Gottlieb, N. Panebianco (eds.), *Advanced Point-of-Care Ultrasound*, https://doi.org/10.1007/978-3-031-85308-1_15

dressing has been shown to reduce image quality without any significant improvement to patient discomfort during the scan, suggesting it may not be necessary [11]. Sterile gel should be used if applied directly to the closed eye [12, 13]. It is important to use a large amount of gel to ensure adequate contact between the ultrasound probe and the eye and to minimize any air artifact [10].

A high-frequency linear probe (7.5–15 MHz) is used for ocular ultrasound [14, 15]. The absorption of ultrasound energy generates heat in the adjacent tissue, and the thermal index (TI) indicates the potential for heating during diagnostic ultrasound. Additionally, mechanical tissue damage can occur from the interactions of ultrasound waves with tiny gas bubbles in tissue, and the mechanical index (MI) indicates the potential for sonographically adverse nonthermal bioeffects. In keeping with the as low as reasonably achievable (ALARA) principle, the TI should be ≤1 and the MI should be ≤0.3 when performing ocular imaging [15–17]. Many modern ultrasound machines allow the user to select an "ophthalmic" or "small parts" setting, and this should be used if available [15, 16]. If these settings are not available or cannot be manually adjusted, the patient should be informed that the scan is an off-label use, and appropriate consent should be obtained prior to sonographic examination of the eye; reassuringly, there has never been evidence of diagnostic ultrasound leading to injury in humans [16]. There is a theoretical risk of both thermal and non-thermal related deleterious effects on eye tissue that may be exacerbated with Doppler compared to B-mode imaging. As such, Doppler examination of the eye should be as short as possible [15–17].

The depth should be set so the optic nerve can be visualized, and the gain should be set to achieve a hypoechoic posterior chamber. If the gain is too low, subtle pathology may be missed, while if the gain is too high, artifacts may appear in the posterior chamber and be mistaken for pathology [13]. Higher gain settings have been shown to improve sensitivity for posterior chamber pathology but at the expense of lower specificity [18].

There are two common ways for the operator to position themselves while doing the scan. The most common approach involves the sonographer standing or sitting facing the patient and bracing their hand holding the probe on the bridge of the patient's nose or cheek to minimize pressure transmitted from the probe to the eye (Fig. 15.1) [13]. Alternatively, using the posterior technique, the sonographer stands facing the patient's feet and uses the patient's forehead to brace the hand holding the probe [9]. Regardless of technique, it is important to minimize the amount of pressure applied to the probe as this force will be transmitted directly to the eye. Excess pressure on the eye will be uncomfortable for the patient and may exacerbate conditions such as globe rupture [13, 19, 20].

The ultrasound examination should be performed in both the transverse view, sweeping cephalad to caudad, as well as the sagittal view, sweeping left and right [21]. When assessing for retinal pathology, first obtain views with the patient

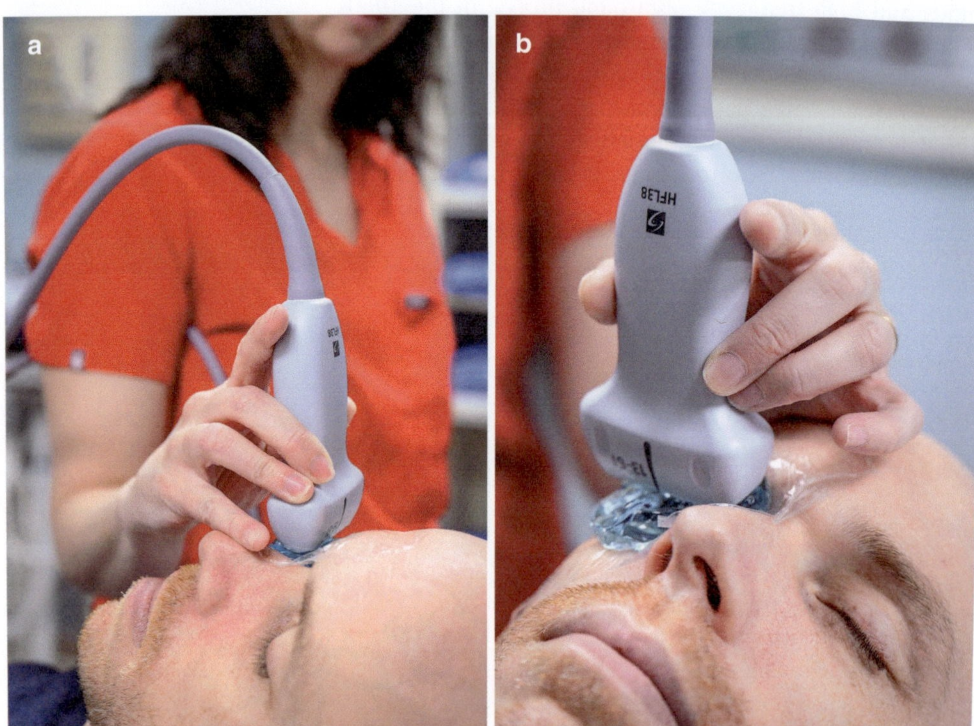

Fig. 15.1 Demonstration of the standard scanning technique and the posterior scanning technique. (**a**) With the standard scanning technique, the sonographer is positioned facing the patient and braces their hand holding the probe on the patient's cheek or maxilla to minimize pressure transmitted from the probe to the eye. (**b**) The posterior technique positions the sonographer behind the patient's head, facing the patient's feet with their hand holding the probe braced on the patient's forehead. Although this image depicts the use of an adhesive dressing, it is not needed, as it degrades image quality without improving patient discomfort during the scan. (*Image courtesy of Ritche Perez*)

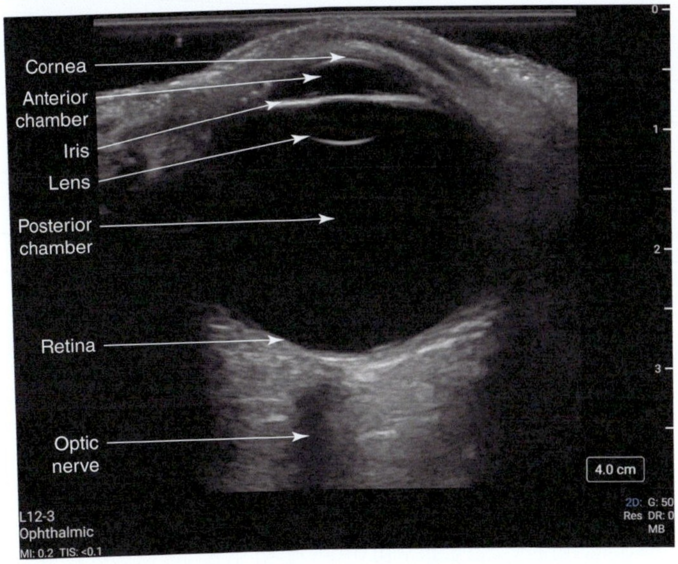

Fig. 15.2 Sonographic appearance of a normal eye. The smaller anterior chamber is bound by the thin cornea and the lens in the near field, and the larger spherical posterior chamber in the far field. (A) cornea. (B) anterior chamber. (C) iris. (D) lens. (E) posterior chamber. (F) retina. (G) optic nerve

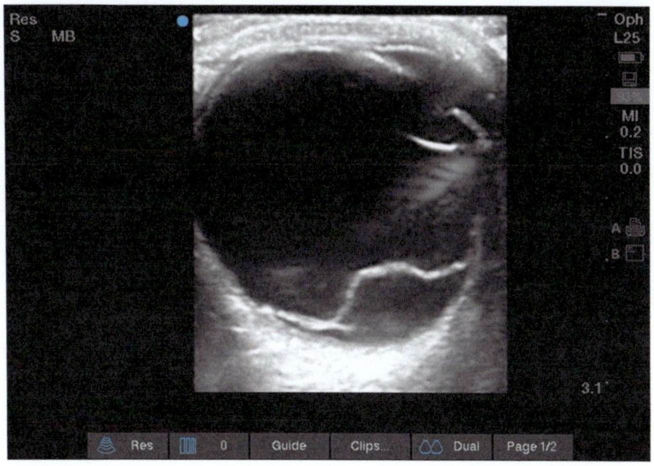

Fig. 15.3 Ultrasound image of retinal detachment with the hyperechoic, thick linear membrane lying anterior to and separated from the choroid. (*Image courtesy of David Smith, MBChB*)

looking forward; then, have the patient look in the extremes of view to examine the sides of the globe that may initially be missed due to edge artifact. Dynamic scanning should also be performed, with the patient moving their eye left and right in the transverse plane, and up and down in the sagittal plane while the probe remains stationary. Dynamic scanning allows for the assessment of echoes in the posterior chamber and can help differentiate retinal detachment from vitreous detachment [22].

Sonographically, the normal eye is composed of two anechoic areas: the smaller anterior chamber bound by the thin cornea and the lens in the near field, and the larger spherical posterior chamber in the far field (Fig. 15.2). The optic nerve has a hypoechoic linear appearance where it lies just posterior to the globe [13, 20].

Clinical Applications

Retinal Detachment

Retinal detachment is the separation of the neurosensory retina from the choroid [23]. It is estimated to occur at an incidence of 6.3 to 17.9 per 100,000 population [24], with a higher incidence in patients referred from the ED to ophthalmology [25]. Retinal detachment is an ophthalmologic emergency and can be challenging to diagnose as history is insufficient for the diagnosis, and physical examination of the posterior chamber with direct ophthalmoscopy outside the ophthalmology setting is difficult [26]. POCUS provides clinicians with a tool that doesn't require pupillary dilation to assess posterior chamber pathology. A systematic review and meta-analysis included 9 studies with 1189 eyes and demonstrated that POCUS had a sensitivity of 94% and specificity of 94% for retinal detachment [7].

Sonographically, a retinal detachment appears as a hyperechoic, linear membrane lying in an anterior or oblique position and separated from the choroid (Fig. 15.3). The retina is typically tethered to the optic nerve. It should be readily visualized on a standard ophthalmic ultrasound setting which generally defaults to a low to mid-range gain setting [18]. On dynamic assessment, the detached retina will have restricted, taut mobility with minimal movement (Video 15.1) [27]. Once a retinal detachment is diagnosed, determine if the retina is attached to the macular region of the choroid, which is located just lateral to the optic nerve [28]. If the retina is attached to the macula, it is referred to as a macula-on detachment, and the patient requires acute ophthalmologic intervention to prevent the detachment from moving centrally and causing irreversible vision loss. If the retina is not attached to the macula, it is a macula-off detachment, and outcomes with vision are not significantly improved with urgent repair [29]. If there is any ambiguity as to macular involvement, emergent ophthalmology consultation should be obtained.

The entire posterior chamber should be interrogated slowly and in both horizontal and vertical planes to avoid missing a small retinal detachment or tear [27, 28]. It is important to note that in patients presenting with acute onset of floaters or flashing lights, up to 14% may have a retinal tear which puts the patient at high risk for progression to a retinal detachment [26]. Unfortunately, POCUS is only 48% sensitive for diagnosing retinal tear [30], so patients with new floaters or flashing lights and a POCUS examination that does not demonstrate a retinal detachment need timely ophthalmologic assessment.

Posterior Vitreous Detachment

Posterior vitreous detachment is the separation of the posterior vitreous from the retina due to vitreous degeneration, most commonly associated with aging [31]. If symptomatic, patients will often report painless, acute onset floaters or flashing lights [26]. Unlike retinal detachment, posterior vitreous detachment has a sonographic appearance of a thin, smooth curved membrane with low to medium echogenicity, without tethering to the optic nerve. It can often be subtle and even imperceptible at low gain and usually requires increasing the gain to adequately visualize this finding [18]. Most vitreous detachments occur posteriorly, so the thin membrane is typically positioned horizontally, just superficial to the retina (Fig. 15.4). With ocular movement, the vitreous is highly mobile, and a posterior vitreous detachment will demonstrate undulating mobility with significant swaying after movement (Video 15.2) [27]. POCUS is less accurate for making the diagnosis of posterior vitreous detachment. A systematic review and meta-analysis that included 4 studies with 388 eyes found POCUS to be only 67% sensitive but 89% specific for posterior vitreous detachment [7]. Fortunately, posterior vitreous detachment is a benign condition in the absence of an associated retinal tear. However, these patients will still need ophthalmology follow-up, as some patients may have an associated retinal tear [26], and up to 3% of patients with uncomplicated posterior vitreous detachment will develop a new retinal tear within 6 weeks [33].

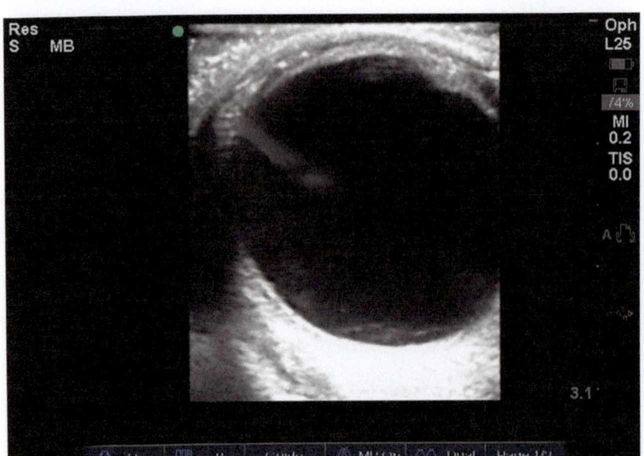

Fig. 15.4 Ultrasound image of posterior vitreous detachment with the thin membrane positioned horizontally just above the retina. (*Image credit: Stringer et al.* [32])

Vitreous Hemorrhage

Vitreous hemorrhage is the presence of extravasated blood in the vitreous cavity. It most commonly occurs due to bleeding from abnormal blood vessels such as neovascularization in diabetic retinopathy, posterior vitreous detachment with or without retinal detachment, and ocular trauma [34].

On ultrasound, the appearance of vitreous hemorrhage will depend on the acuity of the bleeding. New vitreous hemorrhage will have the appearance of diffuse low-level echoes suspended within the vitreous, suggestive of particles in a snow globe. With time, vitreous hemorrhage will develop multiple heterogeneous echogenic layers in the posterior chamber of the eye (Fig. 15.5) [20, 27]. With dynamic sonography, this material will appear to "tumble," drawing comparisons to clothes in a washing machine (Video 15.3) [27]. Similar to posterior vitreous detachment, the gain will often need to be increased to better visualize vitreous hemorrhage. On some high-quality machines, the normal vitreous matrix may also be visible at higher gains and can be mistaken for pathology [18]. Based on a systematic review and meta-analysis including 5 studies and 739 eyes, POCUS has a sensitivity of 90% and specificity of 92% for diagnosing vitreous hemorrhage [7].

Asteroid Hyalosis

Asteroid hyalosis is an idiopathic condition in which multiple yellow-white particles or asteroid bodies composed of calcium and complex phospholipids develop within the otherwise homogeneous and proteinaceous vitreous [35]. It is named due to the asteroid bodies resembling a starry night

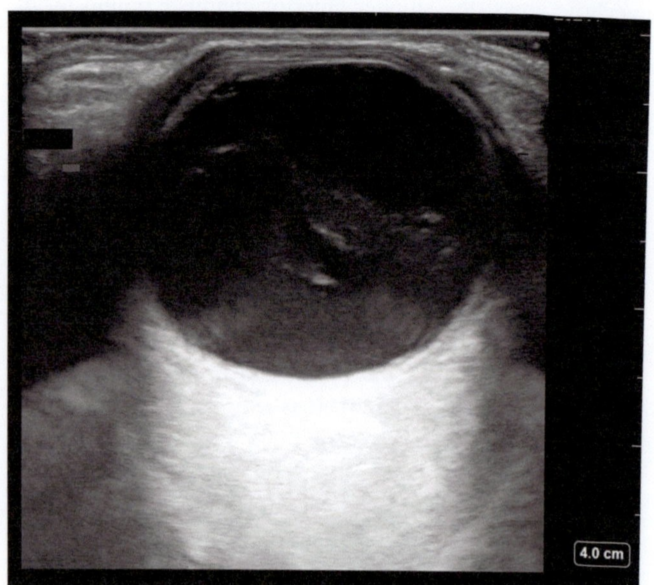

Fig. 15.5 Ultrasound image of vitreous hemorrhage, represented by multiple heterogeneous echoes suspended within the posterior chamber

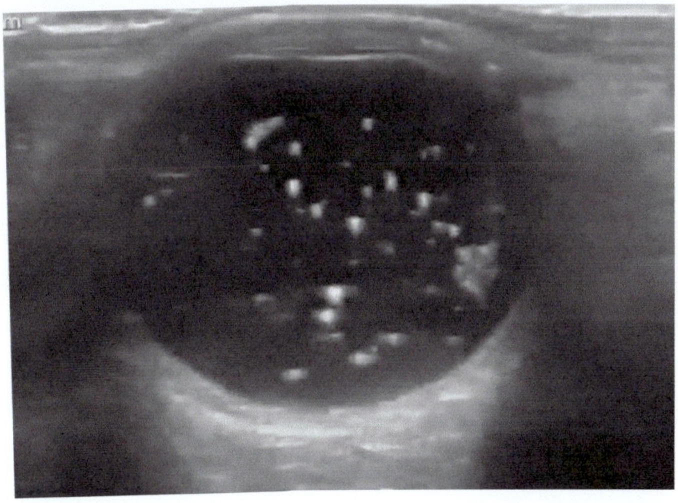

Fig. 15.6 Sonographic findings of asteroid hyalosis include mobile hyperechoic opacities in the posterior chamber that appear like discrete mobile points without posterior acoustic shadowing. These opacities have a striking amount of after-movement on dynamic scanning. (*Image credit: Gros and Mccafferty* [38])

sky on ophthalmoscopy [36]. The prevalence of asteroid hyalosis has been reported to be 0.86%, and it is commonly associated with advanced age, male sex, and hypertension [35, 37]. It is usually asymptomatic, but ophthalmoscopy will demonstrate multiple yellow-white, iridescent opacifications in the vitreous that are mobile with eye movement and do not settle inferiorly with rest [35]. The ultrasound findings of asteroid hyalosis include mobile hyperechoic opacities in the posterior chamber that appear like discrete mobile points without posterior acoustic shadowing (Fig. 15.6) [39]. The striking after-movements of asteroid hyalosis with dynamic scanning are similar to that observed with vitreous hemorrhage, though the latter forms more heterogeneous echogenic layers as opposed to discrete points. As the eye ceases rotation, the echogenic material from both asteroid hyalosis and vitreous hemorrhage swirl in a characteristic pattern that has been described as a "washing machine" sign [32, 39].

Choroidal Detachment

Choroidal detachment occurs when fluid or blood accumulates in the potential space between the choroid and the sclera and is a rare cause of painless or painful vision loss. The choroid is a vascular layer between the retina and the sclera that provides oxygen and nutrients to the retina [40]. Unlike the retina, the choroid attaches anteriorly near the ciliary bodies and posteriorly near the exit foramina of the veins, anterior to the optic disc. As a result, choroidal detachment appears as a thick hyperechoic convex protrusion into the vitreous that does not extend to the optic disc, analogous to the seams of a baseball (Fig. 15.7). On dynamic scanning, choroid detachment generally appears fixed, unlike the

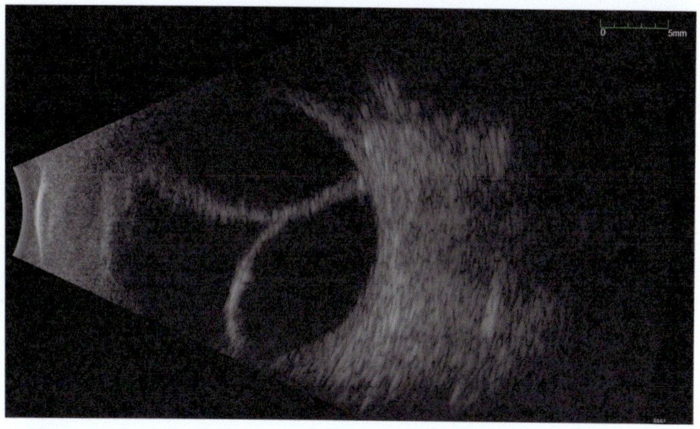

Fig. 15.7 Ultrasound image of choroidal detachment with thick hyperechoic convex protrusions into the vitreous that do not extend to the optic disc. (*Image courtesy of Adriane Santa Croce*)

mobility that retinal detachment demonstrates [41]. The seams may appear to "kiss" one another if they touch in the middle of the vitreous. Ultrasound can also distinguish between serous or hemorrhagic choroidal detachment. In serous detachment, fluid is less echo-dense than the fluid in hemorrhagic detachment. Both types require urgent ophthalmology referral for definitive management [40].

Lens Dislocation

Ectopia lentis is a dislocation or malposition of the lens due to disruption of the zonular fibers that normally hold the lens in place [42]. The most common cause is trauma; in the absence of trauma, there should be prompt consideration of other systemic disorders (e.g., connective tissue disorders) and other primary ocular disorders [43]. Most commonly, the lens dislocates into the posterior chamber; anterior chamber dislocation is rare as the iris limits ectopic movement of the lens [44]. There are multiple potential complications of lens dislocation including secondary glaucoma, retinal detachment, cataract, and vision loss [43].

Ultrasound will demonstrate the hyperechoic oval- or circular-shaped lens displaced from its usual position in the hyaloid fossa into the posterior or anterior chamber of the eye (Fig. 15.8). The lens may demonstrate an anechoic center and move freely in the posterior chamber if the patient is asked to move the affected eye [44]. Given that lens dislocation is most commonly traumatic, it is prudent to minimize pressure if there is any suspicion of globe rupture. A systematic review and meta-analysis that included 2 studies with 400 eyes and 31 cases of lens dislocation found that POCUS had a sensitivity of 97% and specificity of 99% [7].

The direction of lens dislocation dictates management. Generally, anterior dislocations require surgical management with lens removal to avoid complications, such as acute angle closure glaucoma. Posterior dislocations can be managed con-

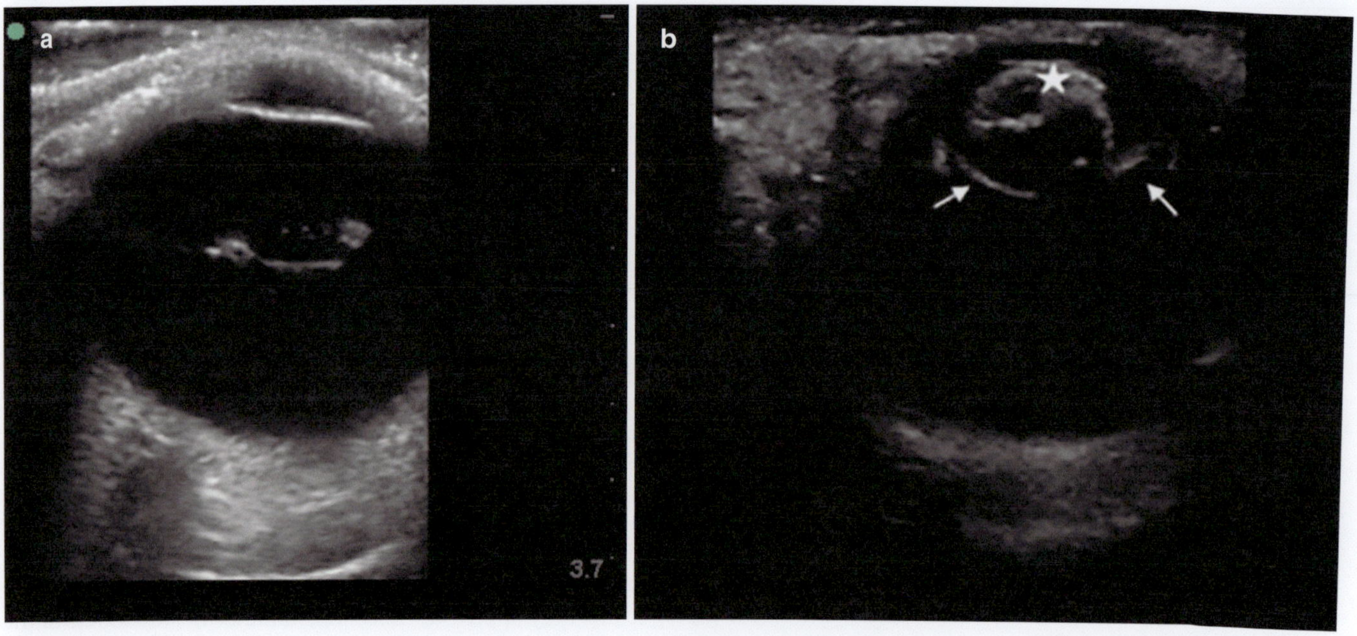

Fig. 15.8 Ultrasound image of lens dislocation with a hyperechoic oval-shaped lens is displaced into the (**a**) posterior chamber or (**b**) anterior chamber of the eye. (*Image* (**a**) *courtesy of Justin Ahn, MD. Image credit* (**b**): *Shirke et al.* [45])

servatively with a trial of corrective contact lenses and careful monitoring, although surgical removal may be considered if complications such as glaucoma or uveitis develop [46].

Intraocular Foreign Body

Intraocular foreign bodies (IOFBs) account for 16–41% of open globe injuries and require urgent diagnosis as they can frequently cause vision loss [47]. Vision loss may be caused by direct laceration or hemorrhage from the IOFB at the time of injury, or from subsequent development of endophthalmitis or retinal damage. Clinical examination alone may be insufficient to identify IOFB, especially if there is concomitant corneal damage or ocular media clouding (e.g., hyphema or vitreous hemorrhage) [47]. As such, other imaging modalities may be necessary to confirm and localize the IOFB. Noncontrast CT of the orbits with thin cuts (1.0–1.5 mm) is often used for primary diagnosis, with a sensitivity of 95% [48]. However, POCUS can offer another option for diagnosis in resource-limited settings. One systematic review and meta-analysis reporting POCUS for IOFB had a sensitivity of 100% and specificity of 99% based on 2 studies with 400 eyes and 17 cases of IOFB [7].

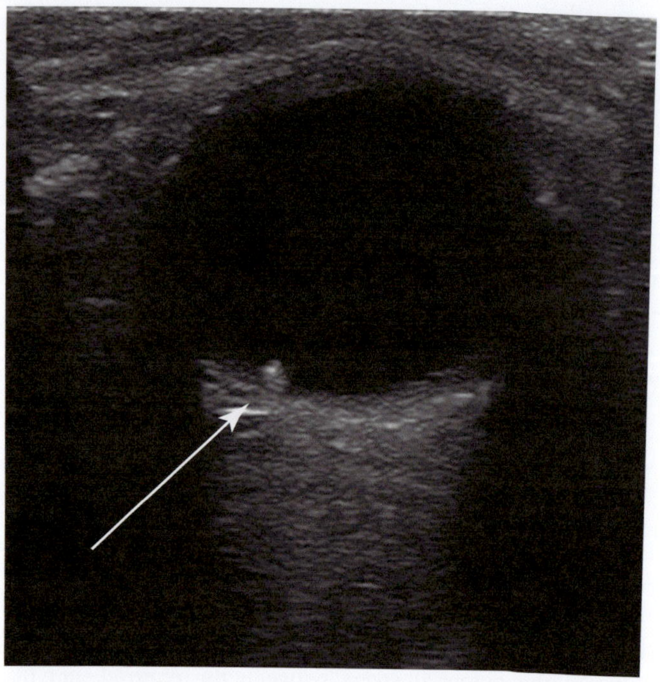

Fig. 15.9 Ultrasound image of an intraocular foreign body (arrow), appearing as an echogenic object in the bottom left quadrant of the posterior chamber. (*Image courtesy of Michael Woo, MD*)

On ultrasound, IOFB will typically appear as highly reflective echogenic objects and may be accompanied by comet-tail artifacts (Fig. 15.9) [13]. If scanning with color Doppler, IOFBs may have a twinkling artifact seen as a colorful reverberation posterior to the foreign body [49]. Against the anechoic background of the posterior vitreous, IOFBs composed of metal and glass produce reverberations as compared to plastic particles which may appear as discrete objects without reverberations [50].

Sonographic assessment for IOFB is operator-dependent, with one study of emergency medicine residents showing increasing accuracy by year of training [51]. IOFBs located in areas subject to acoustic shadowing from adjacent structures (e.g., directly behind the crystalline lens or embedded in the retina) may elude detection with ultrasound [52]. Dynamic sonography may be beneficial here to shift the position or angle to enhance the visibility of the IOFB. It is also imperative when assessing for IOFB that clinicians use copious amounts of gel and avoid placing any undue pressure on the eye, as this could lead to extrusion of intraocular contents in the setting of globe rupture [19–21].

Most patients with IOFB will require surgical removal of the IOFB to restore ocular anatomy and to treat or prevent associated complications. The exact timing of operative intervention depends on several factors such as the composition of the IOFB and the availability of appropriate equipment and personnel [47].

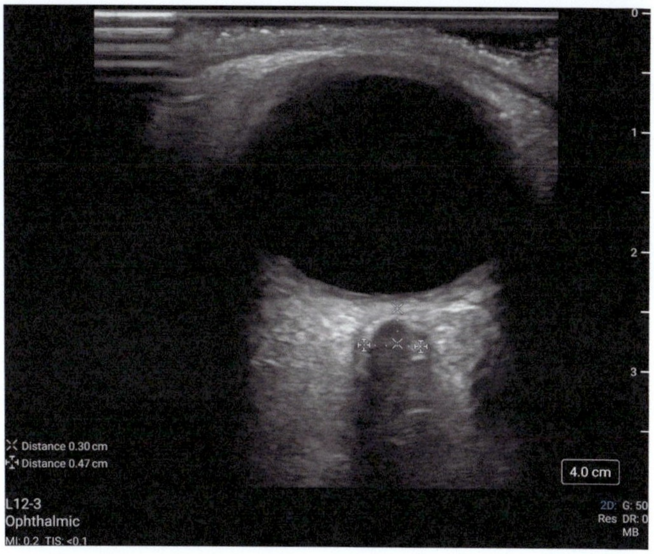

Fig. 15.10 Normal sonographic measurement of the optic nerve sheath diameter 3 mm behind the globe, with the measurement taken orthogonal to the optic nerve long axis and from the outer edges of the hyperechoic striped bands

Ocular Nerve Sheath Diameter

The optic nerve is surrounded by a sheath that is an extension of the dura mater containing cerebrospinal fluid [53]. Increases in volume or pressure within the cranium will raise intracranial pressure (ICP); because the optic nerve sheath is distensible, it will distend and increase in size [54, 55]. Accurate measurement of raised ICP in critically ill patients has traditionally required invasive neuromonitoring techniques. Ultrasound of the optic nerve sheath diameter (ONSD) has been proposed as an adjunctive monitoring tool [56]. Additional studies have suggested there may be utility in ONSD assessment for diagnosing pathology including idiopathic intracranial hypertension [57], optic neuritis [58], acute mountain sickness [59], and ventriculoperitoneal shunt dysfunction [60], but the current literature base is small, of heterogeneous quality, and demonstrates mixed diagnostic accuracy for these conditions.

The intraocular portion of the optic nerve is visible with traditional fundoscopy, while the intraorbital segment of the optic nerve is best visualized with ultrasound or other diagnostic imaging [53]. The optic nerve is identifiable on ultrasound as a homogeneous hypoechoic linear structure extending beyond the posterior segment of the eye (Fig. 15.10). The optic nerve sheath is a hyperechoic band circumferentially surrounding the optic nerve [13]. The ultrasound probe often needs to be angled approximately 10–15° medially and inferiorly to ensure the optic nerve is parallel to the length of the probe. Alternatively, the patient can be instructed to adjust their gaze to optimize the image [61]. Once an adequate view is obtained in the transverse orientation, the operator should freeze the image and measure the ONSD 3 mm posterior to the globe, taking care to measure orthogonal to the long axis of the optic nerve from the outer edges of the hyperechoic striped bands. This 3 mm distance behind the globe was chosen because ultrasound contrast is the greatest and the optic nerve sheath is most distensible at this point [54, 62, 63]. Because the optic nerve is not perfectly round and artifact may be generated by an oblique incidence of ultrasound waves on the border of the optic nerve, measurement in different planes will yield slightly different results [64]. However, there is no clear evidence that averaging multiple measurements improves the accuracy of ONSD estimation. As such, repeating these measurements in the sagittal plane and averaging the results can be considered, but is not required [65]. Application of color Doppler to correctly discern the course of the optic nerve, given the central retinal artery and vein run in the middle of the nerve, increases accurate identification of ONSD margins with good intra-rater reliability (Fig. 15.11) [61, 66].

The mean size of the ONSD in healthy patients is 4.1 mm [67]. In the literature, optimal ONSD cut-off values in adults for raised ICP range from 4.1 mm to 7.2 mm, with this wide range likely resulting from variation in operator technique and experience, patient positioning, and quality of ultrasound technology employed between studies [68]. A commonly accepted upper limit of normal value is 5 mm [69]. A systematic review and meta-analysis compared cut-off values in the 25th–75th percentile range (4.9–5.5 mm) with cut-off values in the 75th–90th percentile range (5.6–6.3 mm), and found similar sensitivity (95% versus 92%) but improved specificity for the higher cut-off group (78% versus 93%). Given this finding, the optimal cut-off value for abnormal ONSD is likely between 5.6 and 6.3 mm (Fig. 15.12) [68]. In the pediatric population, ONSD is affected by age and may be affected by the patency of the anterior fontanelle [70]. It will increase with age, most rapidly in the first year of life.

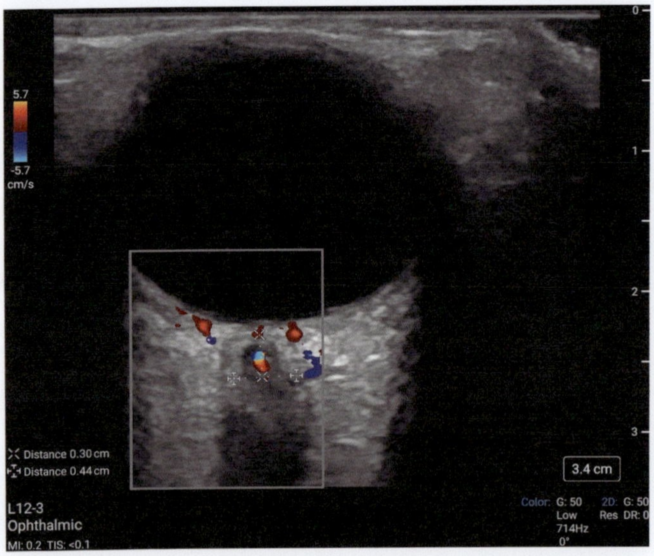

Fig. 15.11 Use of color Doppler to visualize the central retinal artery and vein running in the middle of the nerve to more accurately discern the course of the optic nerve as well as the optic nerve sheath margins

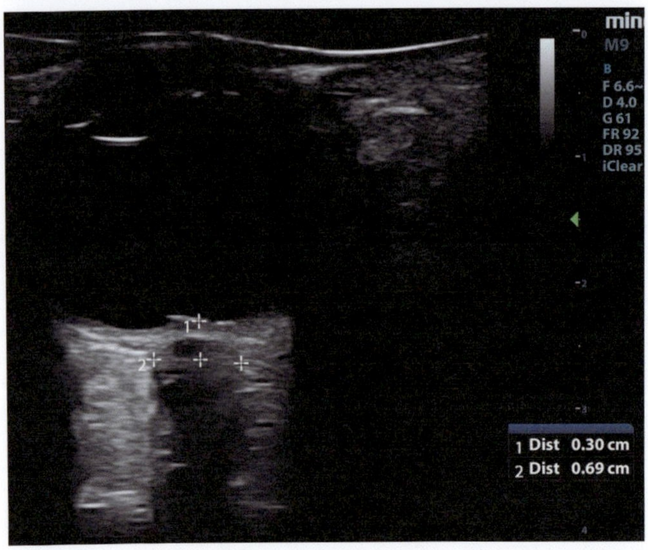

Fig. 15.12 Abnormally dilated optic nerve sheath diameter of 6.9 mm. (*Image courtesy of Jeffrey Kramer, MD*)

Generally cited cut-off values for ONSD are 4.0 mm in infants ≤1 year of age, 4.5 mm in children 1–15 years of age, and 5 mm in children >15 years of age [71].

Optic Disc Elevation

When there is persistently elevated ICP, a congested papilla develops, leading to optic disc elevation (ODE). While slight bulging of the optic nerve into the globe is normal, ODE refers to a pathologically pronounced degree of elevation

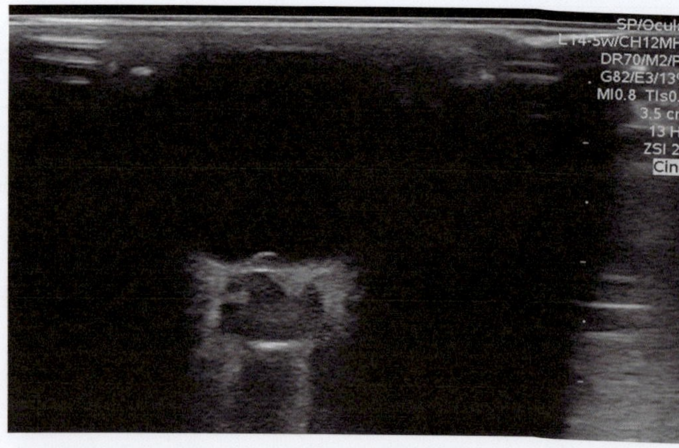

Fig. 15.13 Ultrasound image of optic disc elevation with a contoured hyperechoic prominence into the vitreous originating from the location of the optic nerve. The optic nerve sheath diameter is also abnormally dilated. (*Image courtesy of Michael Gottlieb, MD*)

[72]. It is important to recognize that patients with an acute insult to the brain (e.g., traumatic brain injury, hemorrhagic stroke) may not have ODE immediately. It can take hours to days for papilledema to develop, so assessing for ODE may not be accurate in these acute settings [73].

Sonographically, ODE will appear as a contoured hyperechoic prominence into the vitreous originating from the location of the optic nerve (Fig. 15.13) [74]. ODE should be measured from the anterior-most peak of the optic disc to its intersection with the arc of the posterior surface of the globe [73]. ODE in patients with papilledema can range between 0.6 mm and 1.2 mm with a sensitivity of 70–90% and specificity of 69–100% [74]. Using 0.6 mm as the cut-off increases the sensitivity by 9–20%, at the expense of reducing the specificity by 0–24% [74]. There is no clear consensus on cut-off values for ODE, so clinicians should exercise caution when interpreting these measurements in clinical practice [74].

Other conditions can mimic papilledema on ultrasound, referred to as pseudopapilledema. Pseudopapilledema can be caused by inflammatory diseases, infection, infiltrative conditions, microvascular infarction, and optic disc drusen [73, 75]. Optic disc drusen is the deposit of hyaline-containing bodies within the optic nerve head that can become calcified and swollen. On ultrasound, the optic disc drusen appears as an ovoid hyperechoic entity at the margin of the optic nerve and the retina, which may also have posterior shadowing if calcified (Fig. 15.14) [77]. However, buried optic disc drusen may have a sonographic appearance mimicking ODE without a hyperechoic mass; this may be seen in up to 70% of patients with optic disc drusen [74]. Combining ONSD and ODE assessment may help the clinician distinguish true papilledema from ODE secondary to buried optic disc drusen, as ODE seen in the setting of elevated ICP should be accompanied by increased ONSD measurements [74].

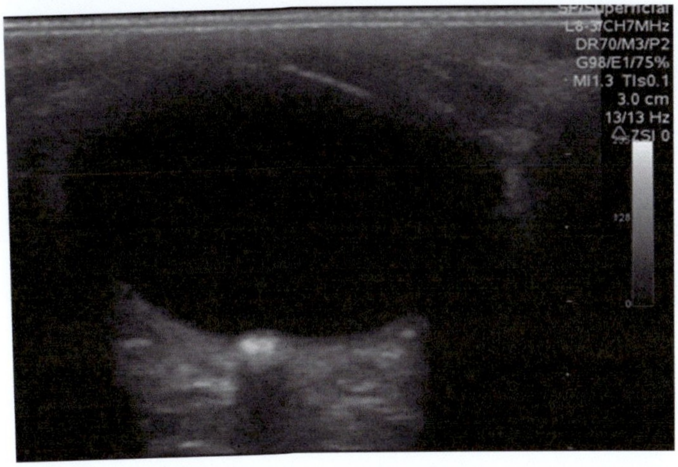

Fig. 15.14 Ultrasound image of optic disc drusen, the ovoid hyperechoic entity at the margin of the optic nerve and the retina; in this case, there is posterior shadowing due to calcification. The normal appearance of the optic nerve sheath diameter supports that this finding is not a case of true papilledema. (*Image credit: Rifenburg and Williams* [76])

Central Retinal Artery Occlusion

Central retinal artery occlusion (CRAO) is an ophthalmologic emergency that presents with sudden, painless vision loss and should be considered an acute stroke of the eye. The monocular vision loss can be profound and enduring, with resultant long-term visual acuity of 20/400 or worse in up to 80% of patients [78].

POCUS can play a role in the evaluation and risk stratification of CRAO, and it may be more accurate than dilated fundoscopic examination alone [79]. In a small study of 29 patients with confirmed CRAO without visible emboli on ophthalmologist fundoscopic examination, 31% had retrobulbar plaques visible on orbital color Doppler imaging [80]. The retrobulbar spot sign (RBSS) (initially termed "Hollenhorst plaque") consists of a bright white echogenic spot visualized in the central retinal artery reflecting so-called "white thrombi" of cholesterol and fibrin deposits of thromboembolic disease (Fig. 15.15) [79, 81]. The RBSS should be differentiated from optic disc drusen, deposits of hyaline-containing bodies within the optic nerve that can become calcified. Although drusen may be sonographically hyperechoic (similar to RBSS), they should generally be located more superficially at the margin of the optic nerve and the retina [82].

There are no high-quality studies evaluating the accuracy of the RBSS, although several small studies have found the RBSS for thromboembolic CRAO to be 31–83% sensitive and 100% specific [80, 83, 84]. RBSS appears to be a poor prognostic factor and is associated with secondary retinal ischemia [84]. For patients presenting outside the window for acute stroke treatment, presence of a RBSS may point away from an arteritic cause of CRAO (such as giant cell arteritis) and may help avoid the complications associated with high-dose corticosteroids. However, this approach has yet to be prospectively validated [79].

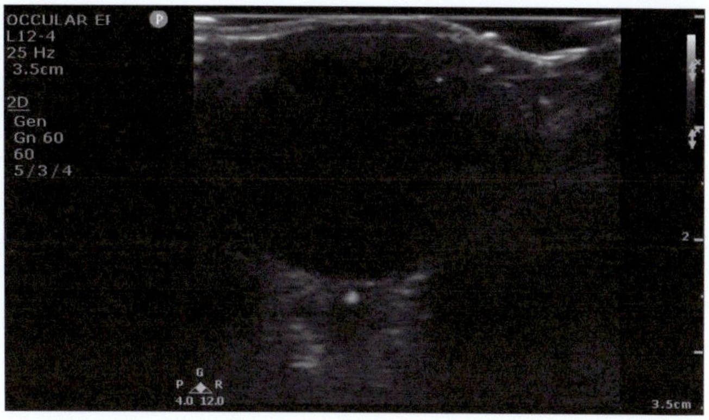

Fig. 15.15 Ultrasound image of the retrobulbar spot sign, consisting of a bright white echogenic spot visible in the central retinal artery representing the cholesterol and fibrin deposits of thromboembolic disease. (*Image courtesy of Wilson Lam, MD*)

POCUS evaluation with color Doppler may also be useful for the diagnosis of CRAO. In a normal eye, color Doppler should demonstrate the paired central retinal artery and vein running parallel to the optic nerve, with bidirectional spectral Doppler flow (Fig. 15.16) [21]. In CRAO, there may be minimal or absent blood flow in the central retinal artery [13]. Similarly, dampened waveforms on spectral Doppler of the affected artery may also be consistent with flow-limiting occlusion [81]. Doppler examination of the eye should be as brief as possible to avoid potential deleterious thermal and nonthermal effects [15–17].

Pupillary Assessment

Pupillary assessment using POCUS is simple and convenient, particularly in patients who have barriers to direct visualization such as in the setting of severe soft tissue swelling of the eyelids [85]. Ultrasound can be used to elicit both the direct and consensual pupillary light reflex (PLR) [86]. Monitoring the PLR is important in critically ill patients with traumatic brain injury or other intracranial pathology that may lead to rapid neurologic deterioration [87].

The linear probe should be placed on the eyelid in the transverse orientation, and the beam should be directed at 45 degrees in a superior or inferior orientation [85]. The ultrasound probe should be fanned until it is directed through the lens and into the iris. Having the patient adjust their gaze upward or downward may improve the image quality. The goal is to generate a coronal view of the round anechoic pupil surrounded by the round hyperechoic iris (Fig. 15.17). Shining a light on the same pupil elicits the direct PLR, while shining a light on the opposite pupil elicits a consensual PLR (Video 15.4) [86]. The PLR can also be docu-

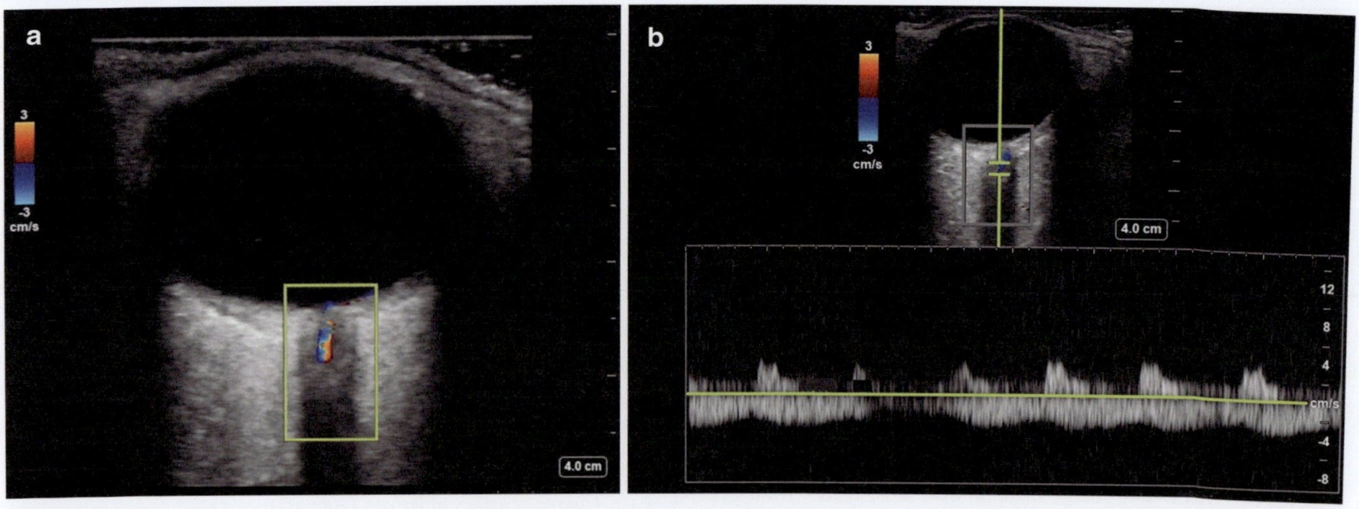

Fig. 15.16 (**a**) Normal color Doppler of the paired central retinal artery and vein running in the middle of the optic nerve. (**b**) Normal bidirectional flow pattern on spectral Doppler

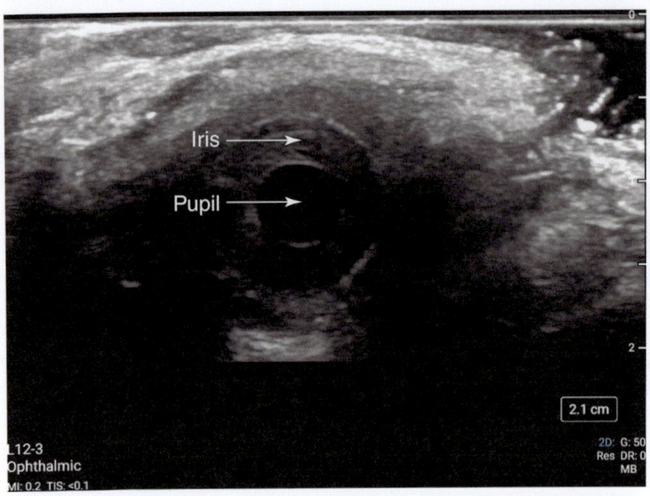

Fig. 15.17 Ultrasound image of a coronal view of the round anechoic pupil surrounded by the round hyperechoic iris. (A) iris. (B) pupil

mented using M-mode if the M-mode line is placed through the largest diameter of the pupil and iris (Fig. 15.18) [85]. This can be a useful means to compare the PLR bilaterally.

A study of 100 healthy subjects found that pupillary diameter constricts 1.8 ± 0.4 mm with an ipsilateral light stimulus, and constricts 2.0 ± 0.4 mm with a contralateral light stimulus [86]. The time it takes for the pupil to constrict sonographically with an ipsilateral or contralateral light stimulus is <1 second [86]. In another study of 200 subjects, there was substantial agreement between clinical assessment and ultrasound assessment of the pupillary reflex, with a kappa of 0.74 [88].

Retrobulbar Hematoma

Traumatic retrobulbar hematoma is a rare, vision-threatening emergency resulting from ocular trauma and occurring in 0.3% of orbital wall fractures [89]. Without prompt intervention, a permanent reduction in visual acuity can develop in as little as 90 minutes [90]. Diagnosis may be challenging as the typical clinical features and the presence of increased intraocular pressure make it difficult to assess, particularly given the significant associated eyelid swelling. Ultrasound allows for dynamic evaluation of the posterior chamber and retrobulbar structures when other conditions such as lid edema may render an examination difficult if not impossible [6, 13].

Reports describing the sonographic diagnosis of retrobulbar hematoma have been published as early as 1971 [91]. Retrobulbar hematoma may appear as a relatively hypoechoic area posterior to the globe [5]. The term "guitar pick sign" has been coined to describe the conical deformation of the posterior globe due to the mass effect from the retrobulbar hematoma (Fig. 15.19). The deformation of the posterior globe is not specific to a retrobulbar hematoma, and other causes such as globe rupture or posterior staphyloma (i.e., bulging of the posterior sclera) should be considered in the differential diagnosis [92].

The diagnostic test characteristics of POCUS for retrobulbar hematoma are uncertain. A prospective cohort study of 351 eyes with suspected traumatic eye injury being evaluated with both POCUS and orbital CT imaging found that POCUS was 96% sensitive and 100% specific for retrobulbar hematoma. However, this was based on a total of only 23 cases of retrobulbar hematoma [6]. Although CT or magnetic resonance imaging (MRI) may subsequently be necessary to assess the extent of ocular injuries, detect other associated injuries, and assist in planning operative management, POCUS may have a role in rapid identification to expedite lateral canthotomy and inferior cantholysis to decompress the orbit [93]. POCUS may also be beneficial for assessing response to treatment. In the original report of the "guitar pick sign," the patient had normalization of the shape of the poste-

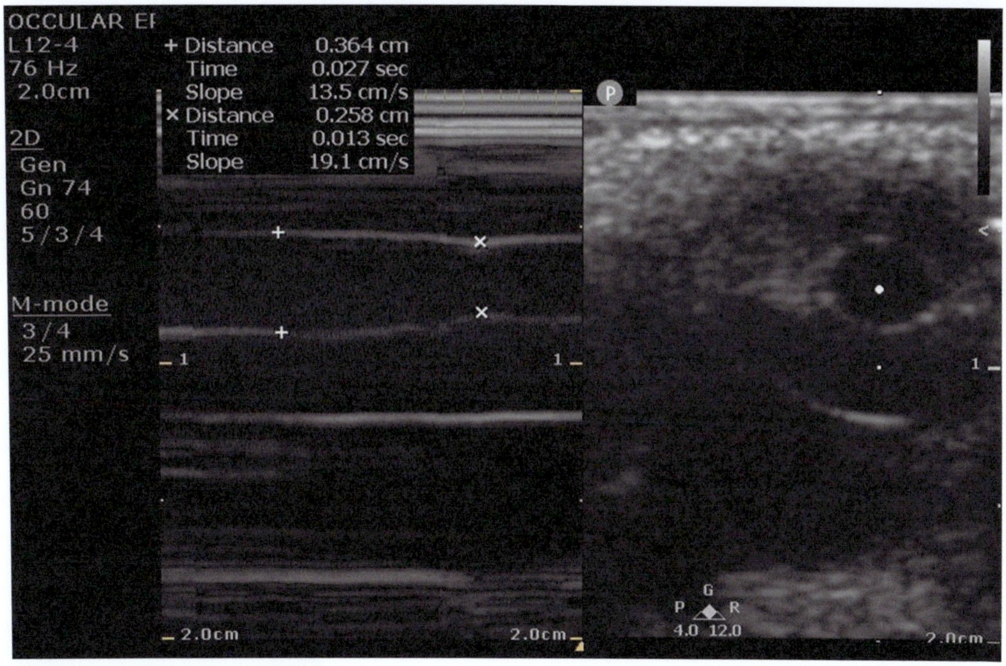

Fig. 15.18 Pupillary light reflex in M-mode where the M-mode line is placed through the largest diameter of the pupil and iris

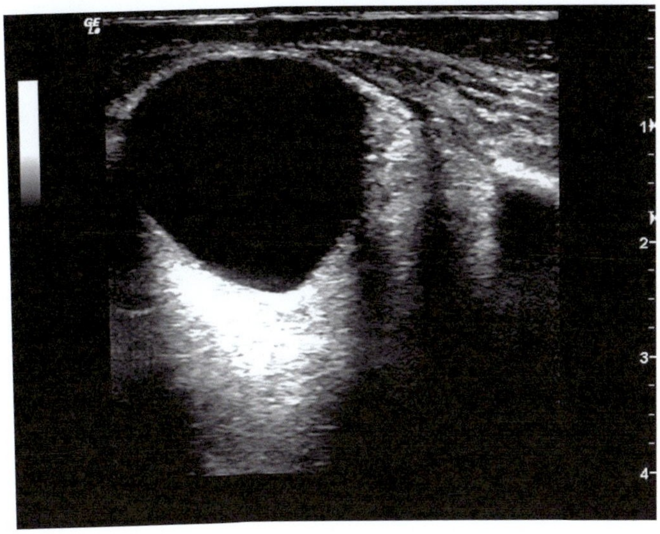

Fig. 15.19 Ultrasound image of the "guitar pick sign," the conical deformation of the posterior ocular globe due to mass effect from a retrobulbar hematoma. (*Image credit: Theoret et al.* [92])

rior globe on repeat sonographic assessment after the performance of a lateral canthotomy and inferior cantholysis [92].

Globe Rupture

Globe rupture is one of the more severe sequelae of ocular trauma and can occur as a result of either blunt or penetrating eye trauma [94]. Open globe injury refers to the complete penetration of all the layers of the eye wall [95]. Patients present with eye pain, redness, and vision loss. Although the ocular examination may suggest the diagnosis (e.g., shallow anterior chamber, peaked or irregular pupil, positive Seidel sign), physical assessment of the eye is often limited due to the associated periorbital swelling after trauma [94]. In this setting, the eye can be further assessed with imaging. CT has been shown to have a sensitivity of only 75–76% and a specificity of 85–94% [96, 97]. As such, a negative CT is insufficiently sensitive to rule out globe rupture.

Ultrasound assessment of suspected globe rupture is controversial, as there is a theoretical risk of extrusion of intraocular contents with pressure from the ultrasound probe. Case reports and studies of POCUS used to diagnose globe rupture in the setting of trauma have not reported this complication or any other adverse effects from the ultrasound examination [5, 6, 98–100]. Although this does not prove safety, it is reassuring when combined with evidence that a probe placed gently on a closed lid with a large amount of gel does not increase the intraocular pressure beyond that of normal diurnal variation [19]. In cases of clinically obvious globe rupture, the risk of worsening the ocular injury outweighs the benefit of performing ocular POCUS. However, in uncertain cases or when physical examination of the eye is limited or impossible due to periorbital swelling, POCUS of the eye is a reasonable strategy as the benefits of establishing the diagnosis of globe rupture in a timely manner outweigh the risks. A copious amount of sterile gel should be used, and the hand should be braced on the bony bridge of the nose or on the forehead to prevent direct pressure on the eye [9, 21].

Sonographic findings of globe rupture include decrease in globe volume, loss of normal spherical globe shape, heterogenous mixture of hemorrhage and vitreous in the posterior chamber, scleral buckling, anterior chamber collapse, and presence of

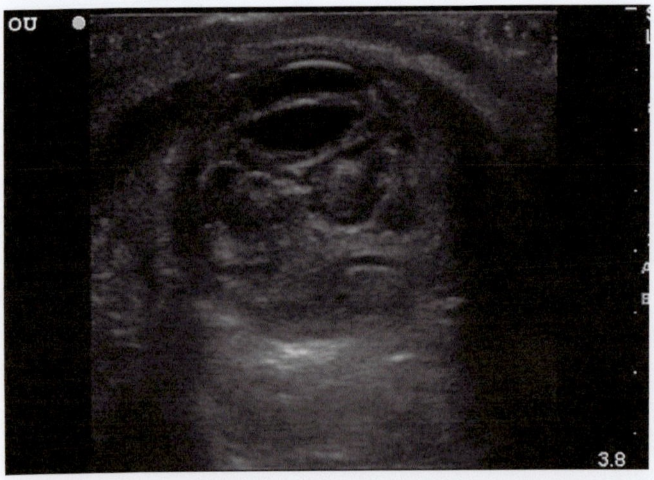

Fig. 15.20 Ultrasound image of globe rupture, represented by decrease in globe volume, loss of normal spherical globe shape, and a heterogenous mixture of hemorrhage and vitreous in the posterior chamber. (*Image credit: Wu et al.* [100])

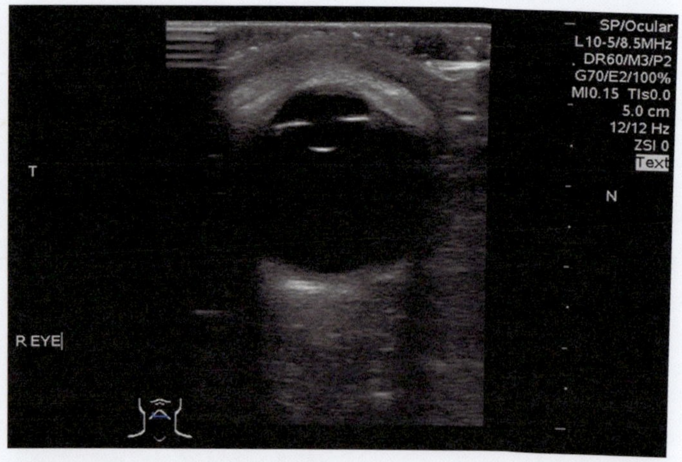

Fig. 15.21 Ultrasound image of periorbital cellulitis, suggested by the hyperechoic thickening of the soft tissues of the eyelid. (*Image courtesy of Elaine Situ-LaCasse, MD*)

an IOFB as a cause of the rupture (Fig. 15.20) [14, 21]. A systematic review and meta-analysis reported POCUS had a sensitivity of 100% and specificity of 99% [7]; however, this was based on only two studies that enrolled 400 eyes, of which there were only 8 cases of globe rupture [6, 98]. Because of the small numbers, the confidence in these diagnostic test characteristics is low [7]. However, in the hands of an experienced POCUS user, it may have better diagnostic accuracy than CT.

Orbital and Periorbital Cellulitis

Orbital and periorbital cellulitis are inflammatory processes involving the soft tissue overlying the orbit and are usually due to infection caused by hematogenous seeding, direct inoculation, or contiguous spread from a sinus infection [101]. The spectrum of disease can range from periorbital (also known as preseptal) cellulitis affecting structures superficial to the orbital septum (e.g., eyelid and periorbital skin and soft tissue) to orbital (also known as postseptal) cellulitis. Orbital cellulitis is a medical emergency that, if left untreated, can potentially lead to permanent vision loss, intracranial abscess, meningitis, or cavernous sinus thrombosis [102].

Ultrasound findings of periorbital cellulitis are analogous to other sites of skin and soft tissue infection (discussed in Chap. 18), including hyperechoic infiltration of the soft tissues of the eyelid accompanied by hyperemia seen on color Doppler, or hypoechoic inflammatory changes of edema (Fig. 15.21). In orbital cellulitis, there can be hyperechoic swelling of the periorbital fat associated with thickening and loss of definition of the extraocular muscles due to inflammatory edema (Fig. 15.22) [101]. In some cases, an anechoic mass extending from the orbital wall may be visible, which can represent a subperiosteal or retrobulbar abscess [103].

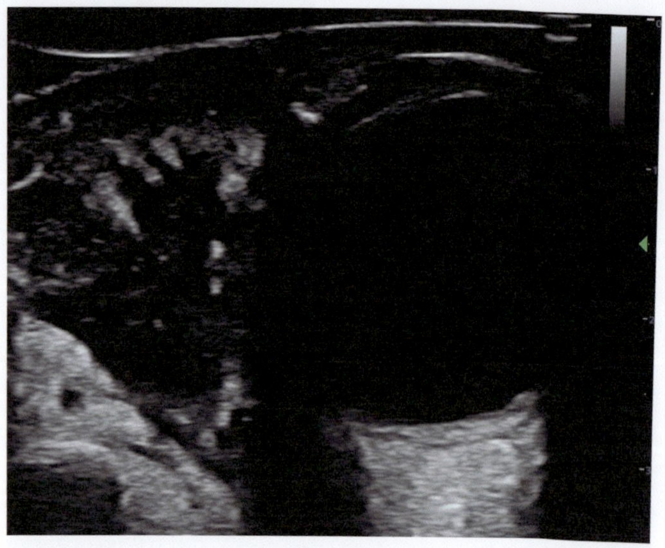

Fig. 15.22 Ultrasound image of an orbital abscess, consisting of an anechoic mass extending from the lateral and posterior orbital walls. This may be seen in cases of orbital cellulitis. (*Image courtesy of Kyle Flattery, MD*)

Some sonographers have described a modification to the usual POCUS technique, involving angling of the probe towards the nasal or temporal periorbital tissues to better visualize the periorbital fat [104].

Endophthalmitis

Endophthalmitis is a vision-threatening condition associated with severe inflammation of intraocular tissue usually due to infection within the vitreous cavity [105]. The most common etiologies are either postoperative or iatrogenic, but it can also be associated with penetrating trauma or open globe injury, particularly if there is a retained IOFB [95]. This rare but devastating disease may quickly lead to irreversible blindness if not promptly diagnosed and treated [106]. Unfortunately, establishing the diagnosis clinically is difficult as physical examination of the posterior chamber can be challenging, results of aqueous and vitreous culture are unlikely to be available during the initial assessment, and laboratory results including inflammatory markers can be falsely reassuring if negative [106]. To this end, sonographic evaluation of the globe may be helpful as an adjunct to the history, physical examination, and laboratory testing [13].

Ultrasound may demonstrate direct signs of intraocular inflammation, such as vitreous or chorioretinal exudates appearing as increased echogenic debris in the normally anechoic vitreous. In more advanced cases, this may progress to chorioretinal thickening (Fig. 15.23) [106]. These features are highly suggestive of infectious endophthalmitis, although definitive diagnosis requires fluid culture. Importantly, the absence of these findings is insufficient to exclude the diagnosis [105]. No studies have assessed the diagnostic test characteristics of these findings for endophthalmitis in a population of patients presenting with undifferentiated eye complaints. There may be some correlation between the specific causative microorganism and the corresponding ultrasound findings: streptococcal species are more likely to be associated with severe vitreous opacities, whereas gram-negative species and aseptic inflammation are more likely to be associated with minimal vitreous opacities [107]. CT or MRI may still be necessary to assess the extent of disease, complications, alternate diagnoses, and the presence of an IOFB [106].

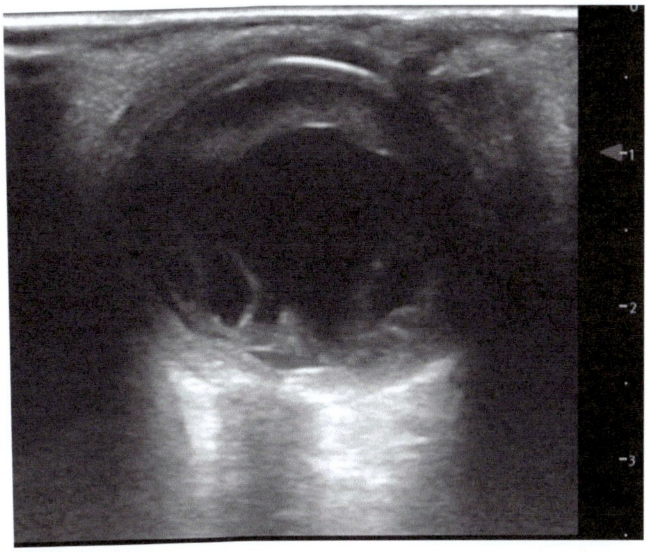

Fig. 15.23 Ultrasound image of endophthalmitis with vitreous exudates appearing as increased echogenic debris in the normally anechoic vitreous as well as chorioretinal thickening. (*Image courtesy of Jailyn Avila, MD*)

Posterior Scleritis

Posterior scleritis is an inflammatory process affecting the sclera or adjacent vasculature posterior to the junction between the choroid and the ciliary body. It is the least common type of scleritis, accounting for 2–12% of cases of scleritis in the literature [108]. Patients can present with a variety of symptoms including eye pain, periocular pain, or vision loss, but milder cases can be associated with atypical symptoms. Delayed diagnosis or treatment can lead to inflammation of the optic disc and sclera, macular edema, and vision loss [108]. On ultrasound, posterior scleritis most commonly manifests as thickening of the posterior wall of the globe >2 mm [109]. A difference of ≥20% in posterior wall thickness between the symptomatic eye and the asymptomatic eye is also suggestive of the diagnosis [108]. Posterior scleritis may also present with fluid in Tenon's space, the potential space between the outer surface of the sclera and the Tenon's sheath which covers the globe from the limbus to the optic nerve; this finding is known as the "T-sign" (Fig. 15.24) [109].

Ocular Masses

Ultrasound can be used to detect intraocular and extraocular masses. Approximately two-thirds of orbital lesions are benign and one-third are malignant, though both can cause significant morbidity [110]. Intraocular pathologies may include melanoma, ocular metastasis, hemangioblastoma, and retinoblastoma. Extraocular masses may include optic nerve glioma, optic nerve sheath meningioma, lymphoma, cavernous hemangioma, schwannoma, or idiopathic orbital inflammatory syndrome [111]. Recognizing an ocular mass with POCUS can expedite care for patients affected by these conditions [112].

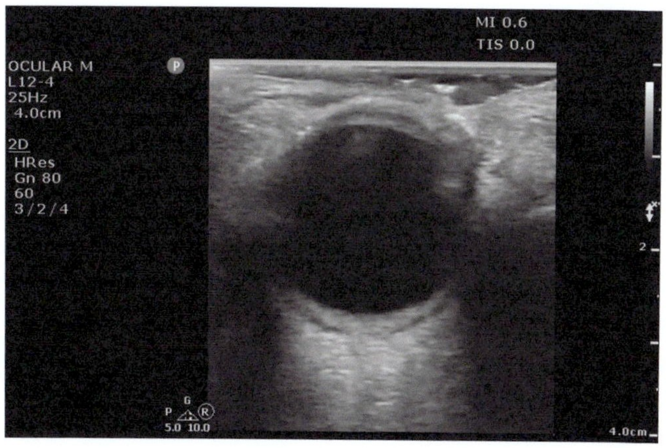

Fig. 15.24 Ultrasound image of posterior scleritis, with thickening of the posterior wall of the globe and fluid in Tenon's space, the area between the outer surface of the sclera and the Tenon's sheath covering the globe from the limbus to the optic nerve. (*Image credit: Tabbut et al.* [109])

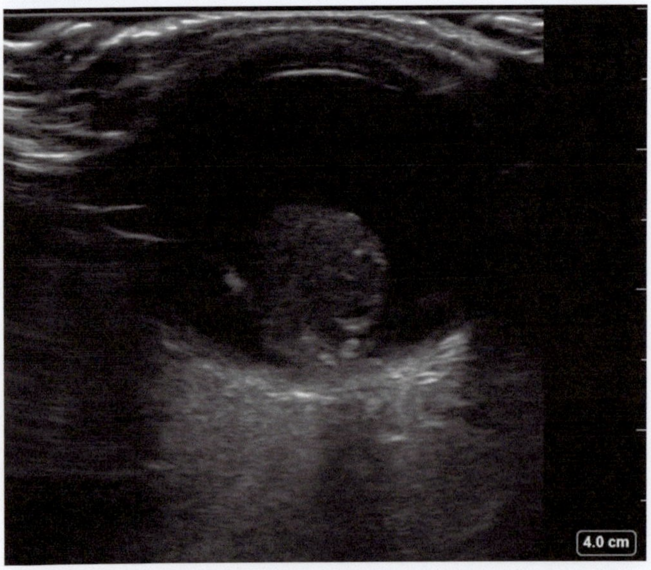

Fig. 15.25 Ultrasound image of intraocular mass with an echogenic mushroom-shaped appearance. (*Image courtesy of Meghan Herbst, MD*)

Melanoma appears as an echogenic mass that can have a dome-shaped or mushroom-like appearance (Fig. 15.25) [113]. It may be associated with retinal detachment, subretinal fluid, scleral erosion, or extraocular extension [114]. Choroidal metastasis has a well-circumscribed echogenic lenticular appearance, arising from the choroid [115]. Retinoblastoma is the most common ocular malignancy in children [116]. Sonographically, retinoblastoma appears as a heterogeneous echogenic soft tissue mass [117], often has calcifications [113], and can invade the optic nerve [114]. Optic nerve lesions, like optic nerve glioma and optic nerve sheath meningioma, are well-circumscribed hypoechoic intraconal lesions [115]. They may also cause enlarged optic nerve shadowing [113].

Ultrasound is effective in demonstrating and localizing orbital masses. However, ocular ultrasound is only 54% accurate in determining the exact nature of the mass [118]. No studies have assessed the diagnostic test characteristics of POCUS specifically for identifying ocular masses. Identification of an ocular mass on ultrasound generally requires further investigation with multimodal imaging including CT and MRI, as well as prompt ophthalmology referral [111].

Key Ultrasound Findings

Ocular condition	Key ultrasound findings
Retinal Detachment	Hyperechoic, thick linear membrane lying anterior to and separated from the choroid, typically tethered to the optic nerve. On dynamic scanning, this membrane will have restricted, taught mobility with minimal after-movement.
Posterior Vitreous Detachment	Thin, smooth, curved membrane with low-to-medium echogenicity, without tethering to the optic nerve. On dynamic scanning, this membrane will have undulating mobility with significant swaying after movement.
Vitreous Hemorrhage	Either low-level echoes suspended within the vitreous or multiple heterogeneous echogenic layers in the posterior chamber. On dynamic scanning, this material appears to "tumble."
Asteroid Hyalosis	Mobile hyperechoic opacities in the posterior chamber that appear like discrete mobile points without posterior acoustic shadowing and have significant after-movements on dynamic scanning that do not settle inferiorly with rest.
Choroidal Detachment	Thick hyperechoic convex protrusion into the vitreous that does not extend to the optic disc and does not have mobility on dynamic scanning.
Lens Dislocation	Hyperechoic, oval- or circular-shaped lens displaced from its usual position in the hyaloid fossa into the posterior or anterior chamber of the eye.
Ocular Foreign Body	Highly reflective echogenic objects within the eye which may be accompanied by comet-tail or reverberation artifacts.
Ocular Nerve Sheath Diameter	Homogeneous hypoechoic linear structure extending beyond the posterior segment of the eye whose diameter should be measured orthogonally to the long axis of the optic nerve 3 mm behind the globe (normal ≤5 mm).
Optic Disc Elevation	Contoured hyperechoic prominence into the vitreous originating from the location of the optic nerve that should be measured from its anterior-most peak to its intersection with the arc of the posterior surface of the globe (normal <0.6–1.2 mm).
Central Retinal Artery Occlusion	Suggested by the retrobulbar spot sign, a bright white echogenic spot in the central retinal artery, as well as decreased or absent flow in the central retinal artery on Doppler.
Pupillary Assessment	Coronal view of the round anechoic pupil surrounded by the round hyperechoic iris. The pupil should normally constrict with both a direct and consensual pupillary light reflex.

(continued)

Ocular condition	Key ultrasound findings
Retrobulbar Hematoma	Relatively hypoechoic area posterior to the globe. May demonstrate the "guitar pick sign," a conical deformation of the posterior ocular globe due to mass effect from the retrobulbar hematoma.
Globe Rupture	Decrease in globe volume, loss of normal spherical globe shape, heterogenous mixture of hemorrhage and vitreous in the posterior chamber, scleral buckling.
Periorbital Cellulitis	Hyperechoic infiltration of the soft tissues of the eyelid with hyperemia on color Doppler.
Orbital Cellulitis	Hyperechoic swelling of periorbital fat with thickening and loss of definition of the extraocular muscles due to inflammatory edema.
Endophthalmitis	Increased echogenic debris in the normally anechoic vitreous. Chorioretinal thickening may be present in advanced disease.
Posterior Scleritis	Thickening of the posterior wall of the globe >2 mm or ≥20% compared to the asymptomatic eye. Fluid may be present in Tenon's space, the potential space between the outer surface of the sclera and the Tenon's sheath which covers the globe from the limbus to the optic nerve.
Ocular Mass	*Intraocular*: Intraocular echogenic mass, may be hyperechoic or hypoechoic depending on the exact pathology. *Extraocular*: Well-circumscribed hypoechoic intraconal lesion with enlarged optic nerve shadowing.

Pearls and Pitfalls

- A high-frequency linear probe (7.5–15 MHz) using the ophthalmic preset with lowered acoustic power should be used for imaging the eye.
- Use of an adhesive dressing is not needed, as it degrades image quality without improving patient discomfort during the scan.
- A large amount of sterile gel should be used.
- The sonographer should brace the hand holding the probe on the bony prominences of the patient's face (i.e., bridge of nose, cheek, forehead) to minimize pressure transmitted from the probe to the eye.
- The eye should be scanned at both low and high gain settings: low gain may miss subtle pathology, while overly high gain may result in an artifact being over-called as pathology.
- Have the patient look straight ahead as well as in their extremes of view to evaluate for subtle wall findings that could be obscured by edge artifact.
- Dynamic scanning assesses the pattern of movement of echoes in the posterior chamber and can help differentiate retinal detachment from vitreous detachment.

References

1. Vaziri K, Schwartz SG, Flynn HW, Kishor KS, Moshfeghi AA. Eye-related emergency department visits in the United States, 2010. Ophthalmology. 2016;123(4):917–9. https://doi.org/10.1016/j.ophtha.2015.10.032.
2. Bruce BB, Thulasi P, Fraser CL, et al. Diagnostic accuracy and use of nonmydriatic ocular fundus photography by emergency physicians: phase II of the FOTO-ED study. Ann Emerg Med. 2013;62(1):28–33.e1. https://doi.org/10.1016/j.annemergmed.2013.01.010.
3. Oliver C, Tadrous C, Docherty G, Warner S. Retrospective analysis of ophthalmology consults to a tertiary academic teaching centre. Can J Ophthalmol. 2019;54(4):484–8. https://doi.org/10.1016/j.jcjo.2018.08.010.
4. Lizzi FL, Coleman DJ. History of ophthalmic ultrasound. J Ultrasound Med. 2004;23(10):1255–66. https://doi.org/10.7863/jum.2004.23.10.1255.
5. Blaivas M. Bedside emergency department ultrasonography in the evaluation of ocular pathology. Acad Emerg Med. 2000;7(8):947–50. https://doi.org/10.1111/j.1553-2712.2000.tb02080.x.
6. Ojaghihaghighi S, Lombardi KM, Davis S, Vahdati SS, Sorkhabi R, Pourmand A. Diagnosis of traumatic eye injuries with point-of-care ocular ultrasonography in the emergency department. Ann Emerg Med. 2019;74(3):365–71. https://doi.org/10.1016/j.annemergmed.2019.02.001.
7. Propst SL, Kirschner JM, Strachan CC, et al. Ocular point-of-care ultrasonography to diagnose posterior chamber abnormalities: a systematic review and meta-analysis. JAMA Netw Open. 2020;3(2):e1921460. https://doi.org/10.1001/jamanetworkopen.2019.21460.
8. Scholtz LC, Rosenberg J, Robbins MS, et al. Ultrasonography in neurology: a comprehensive analysis and review. J Neuroimaging. 2023;33(4):511–20. https://doi.org/10.1111/jon.13124.
9. Khattab E, Hoffmann B, Schafer J, et al. Examiner position in ocular point-of-care ultrasound: a proposed technique. J Emerg Med. 2019;56(6):684–6. https://doi.org/10.1016/j.jemermed.2019.03.027.
10. Roth KR, Gafni-Pappas G. Unique method of ocular ultrasound using transparent dressings. J Emerg Med. 2011;40(6):658–60. https://doi.org/10.1016/j.jemermed.2009.10.020.
11. Marks A, Patel D, Chottiner M, Kayarian F, Peksa GD, Gottlieb M. Covered or uncovered: a randomized control trial of Tegaderm versus no Tegaderm for ocular ultrasound. Am J Emerg Med. 2022;61:87–9. https://doi.org/10.1016/j.ajem.2022.08.044.
12. AIUM Official Statement. Guidelines for cleaning and preparing external- and internal-use ultrasound transducers and equipment between patients as well as safe handling and use of ultrasound coupling gel. J Ultrasound Med. 2023;42(7):E13–22. https://doi.org/10.1002/jum.16167.
13. Kilker BA, Holst JM, Hoffmann B. Bedside ocular ultrasound in the emergency department. Eur J Emerg Med. 2014;21(4):246–53. https://doi.org/10.1097/MEJ.0000000000000070.
14. Skidmore C, Saurey T, Ferre RM, Rodriguez-Brizuela R, Spaulding J, Lundgreen MN. A narrative review of common uses of ophthalmic ultrasound in emergency medicine. J Emerg Med. 2021;60(1):80–9. https://doi.org/10.1016/j.jemermed.2020.08.003.
15. Abramowicz JS, Adhikari S, Dickman E, et al. Ocular ultrasound: review of bioeffects and safety, including Fetal and point of care perspective: review of bioeffects and safety, including Fetal and point-of-care perspective. J Ultrasound Med. 2022;41(7):1609–22. https://doi.org/10.1002/jum.15864.

16. Miller DL, Abo A, Abramowicz JS, et al. Diagnostic ultrasound safety review for point-of-care ultrasound practitioners. J Ultrasound Med. 2020;39(6):1069–84. https://doi.org/10.1002/jum.15202.
17. Safety Group of the British Medical Ultrasound Society. Guidelines for the safe use of diagnostic ultrasound equipment. Ultrasound. 2010;18(2):52–9. https://doi.org/10.1258/ult.2010.100003.
18. Chang M, Finney N, Baker J, et al. Optimal image gain intensity of point-of-care ultrasound when screening for ocular abnormalities in the emergency department. West J Emerg Med. 2023;24(3):622–8. https://doi.org/10.5811/westjem.59714.
19. Berg C, Doniger SJ, Zaia B, Williams SR. Change in intraocular pressure during point-of-care ultrasound. West J Emerg Med. 2015;16(2):263–8. https://doi.org/10.5811/westjem.2015.1.24150.
20. Roque PJ, Hatch N, Barr L, Wu TS. Bedside ocular ultrasound. Crit Care Clin. 2014;30(2):227–41., v. https://doi.org/10.1016/j.ccc.2013.10.007.
21. Tandon A, Khullar T, Bhatt S. Sonography in acute ocular pathology: a kaleidoscopic view. Emerg Radiol. 2019;26(2):241–8. https://doi.org/10.1007/s10140-018-1655-2.
22. Lorente-Ramos RM, Armán JA, Muñoz-Hernández A, Gómez JMG, de la Torre SB. US of the eye made easy: a comprehensive how-to review with ophthalmoscopic correlation. Radiographics. 2012;32(5):E175–200. https://doi.org/10.1148/rg.325115105.
23. Kang HK, Luff AJ. Management of retinal detachment: a guide for non-ophthalmologists. BMJ. 2008;336(7655):1235–40. https://doi.org/10.1136/bmj.39581.525532.47.
24. Mitry D, Charteris DG, Fleck BW, Campbell H, Singh J. The epidemiology of rhegmatogenous retinal detachment: geographical variation and clinical associations. Br J Ophthalmol. 2010;94(6):678–84. https://doi.org/10.1136/bjo.2009.157727.
25. Docherty G, Hwang J, Yang M, et al. Prospective analysis of emergency ophthalmic referrals in a Canadian tertiary teaching hospital. Can J Ophthalmol. 2018;53(5):497–502. https://doi.org/10.1016/j.jcjo.2018.01.008.
26. Hollands H, Johnson D, Brox AC, Almeida D, Simel DL, Sharma S. Acute-onset floaters and flashes: is this patient at risk for retinal detachment? JAMA. 2009;302(20):2243–9. https://doi.org/10.1001/jama.2009.1714.
27. Gandhi K, Shyy W, Knight S, Teismann N. Point-of-care ultrasound for the evaluation of non-traumatic visual disturbances in the emergency department: the VIGMO protocol. Am J Emerg Med. 2019;37(8):1547–53. https://doi.org/10.1016/j.ajem.2019.04.049.
28. Lahham S, Ali Q, Palileo BM, Lee C, Fox JC. Role of point of care ultrasound in the diagnosis of retinal detachment in the emergency department. OAEM. 2019;11:265–70. https://doi.org/10.2147/OAEM.S219333.
29. Ross WH, Stockl FA. Visual recovery after retinal detachment. Curr Opin Ophthalmol. 2000;11(3):191–4. https://doi.org/10.1097/00055735-200006000-00007.
30. Woo MY, Hecht N, Hurley B, Stitt D, Thiruganasambandamoorthy V. Test characteristics of point-of-care ultrasonography for the diagnosis of acute posterior ocular pathology. Can J Ophthalmol. 2016;51(5):336–41. https://doi.org/10.1016/j.jcjo.2016.03.020.
31. Margo CE, Harman LE. Posterior vitreous detachment. How to approach sudden-onset floaters and flashing lights. Postgrad Med. 2005;117(3):37–42. https://doi.org/10.3810/pgm.2005.03.1599.
32. Stringer CEA, Ahn JS, Kim DJ. Asteroid Hyalosis: a mimic of vitreous Hemorrhage on point of care ultrasound. CJEM. 2017;19(4):317–20. https://doi.org/10.1017/cem.2016.358.
33. Dayan MR, Jayamanne DG, Andrews RM, Griffiths PG. Flashes and floaters as predictors of vitreoretinal pathology: is follow-up necessary for posterior vitreous detachment? Eye (Lond). 1996;10(Pt 4):456–8. https://doi.org/10.1038/eye.1996.100.
34. Spraul CW, Grossniklaus HE. Vitreous Hemorrhage. Surv Ophthalmol. 1997;42(1):3–39. https://doi.org/10.1016/s0039-6257(97)84041-6.
35. Duong R, Abou-Samra A, Bogaard JD, Shildkrot Y. Asteroid Hyalosis: an update on prevalence, risk factors, emerging clinical impact and management strategies. Clin Ophthalmol. 2023;17:1739–54. https://doi.org/10.2147/OPTH.S389111.
36. Yazar Z, Hanioglu S, Karakoç G, Gürsel E. Asteroid hyalosis. Eur J Ophthalmol. 2001;11(1):57–61. https://doi.org/10.1177/112067210101100111.
37. Fawzi AA, Vo B, Kriwanek R, et al. Asteroid hyalosis in an autopsy population: the University of California at Los Angeles (UCLA) experience. Arch Ophthalmol. 2005;123(4):486–90. https://doi.org/10.1001/archopht.123.4.486.
38. Gros EC, Mccafferty LR. Asteroid hyalosis: a mimicker of vitreous hemorrhage on point of care ultrasound: a case report. POCUS J. 2023;8(2):113–5. https://doi.org/10.24908/pocus.v8i2.16391.
39. Kachewar SG, Kulkarni DS. An imaging review of intra-ocular calcifications. J Clin Diagn Res. 2014;8(1):203–5. https://doi.org/10.7860/JCDR/2014/4475.3904.
40. Diep MQ, Madigan MC. Choroidal detachments: what do optometrists need to know? Clin Exp Optom. 2019;102(2):116–25. https://doi.org/10.1111/cxo.12807.
41. Jarrett B, Secko M. Choroid detachment, a rare cause of vision loss diagnosed by point-of-care ultrasound. J Emerg Med. 2017;52(4):527–9. https://doi.org/10.1016/j.jemermed.2016.07.115.
42. Bord SP, Linden J. Trauma to the globe and orbit. Emerg Med Clin North Am. 2008;26(1):97–123, vi-vii. https://doi.org/10.1016/j.emc.2007.11.006.
43. Lee S, Hayward A, Bellamkonda VR. Traumatic lens dislocation. Int J Emerg Med. 2015;8:16. https://doi.org/10.1186/s12245-015-0064-5.
44. Pyle M, Gallerani C, Weston C, Frasure SE, Pourmand A. Point of care ultrasound and ocular injuries: a case of lens dislocation and a comprehensive review of the literature. J Clin Ultrasound. 2021;49(3):282–5. https://doi.org/10.1002/jcu.22904.
45. Shirke T, Wilcox K, Luong T. Traumatic anterior dislocation of ocular cataract lens. Clin Pract Cases Emerg Med. 2021;5(4):485–7. https://doi.org/10.5811/cpcem.2021.7.52725.
46. Salehi-Had H, Turalba A. Management of traumatic crystalline lens subluxation and dislocation. Int Ophthalmol Clin. 2010;50(1):167–79. https://doi.org/10.1097/IIO.0b013e3181c567de.
47. Jung HC, Lee SY, Yoon CK, Park UC, Heo JW, Lee EK. Intraocular foreign body: diagnostic protocols and treatment strategies in ocular trauma patients. J Clin Med. 2021;10(9):1861. https://doi.org/10.3390/jcm10091861.
48. Patel SN, Langer PD, Zarbin MA, Bhagat N. Diagnostic value of clinical examination and radiographic imaging in identification of intraocular foreign bodies in open globe injury. Eur J Ophthalmol. 2012;22(2):259–68. https://doi.org/10.5301/EJO.2011.8347.
49. Ustymowicz A, Krejza J, Mariak Z. Twinkling artifact in color Doppler imaging of the orbit. J Ultrasound Med. 2002;21(5):559–63. https://doi.org/10.7863/jum.2002.21.5.559.
50. Nouby-Mahmoud G, Silverman RH, Coleman DJ. Using high-frequency ultrasound to characterize intraocular foreign bodies. Ophthalmic Surg. 1993;24(2):94–9.
51. Pfeiffer P, Marco CA. 348: Ultrasonographic detection of intraocular foreign bodies. Ann Emerg Med. 2008;52(4, Supplement):S148. https://doi.org/10.1016/j.annemergmed.2008.06.374.
52. Bryden FM, Pyott AA, Bailey M, McGhee CN. Real time ultrasound in the assessment of intraocular foreign bodies. Eye (Lond). 1990;4(Pt 5):727–31. https://doi.org/10.1038/eye.1990.103.
53. Lau T, Ahn JS, Manji R, Kim DJ. A narrative review of point of care ultrasound assessment of the optic nerve in emergency

medicine. Life (Basel). 2023;13(2):531. https://doi.org/10.3390/life13020531.
54. Hansen HC, Helmke K. The subarachnoid space surrounding the optic nerves. An ultrasound study of the optic nerve sheath. Surg Radiol Anat. 1996;18(4):323–8. https://doi.org/10.1007/BF01627611.
55. Liu D, Kahn M. Measurement and relationship of subarachnoid pressure of the optic nerve to intracranial pressures in fresh cadavers. Am J Ophthalmol. 1993;116(5):548–56. https://doi.org/10.1016/s0002-9394(14)73195-2.
56. Aletreby W, Alharthy A, Brindley PG, et al. Optic nerve sheath diameter ultrasound for raised intracranial pressure: a literature review and meta-analysis of its diagnostic accuracy. J Ultrasound Med. 2022;41(3):585–95. https://doi.org/10.1002/jum.15732.
57. del Saz-Saucedo P, Redondo-González O, Mateu-Mateu Á, Huertas-Arroyo R, García-Ruiz R, Botia-Paniagua E. Sonographic assessment of the optic nerve sheath diameter in the diagnosis of idiopathic intracranial hypertension. J Neurol Sci. 2016;361:122–7. https://doi.org/10.1016/j.jns.2015.12.032.
58. Lochner P, Cantello R, Brigo F, et al. Transorbital sonography in acute optic neuritis: a case-control study. AJNR Am J Neuroradiol. 2014;35(12):2371–5. https://doi.org/10.3174/ajnr.A4051.
59. Fagenholz PJ, Gutman JA, Murray AF, Noble VE, Camargo CA, Harris NS. Optic nerve sheath diameter correlates with the presence and severity of acute mountain sickness: evidence for increased intracranial pressure. J Appl Physiol (1985). 2009;106(4):1207–11. https://doi.org/10.1152/japplphysiol.01188.2007.
60. Lin SD, Kahne KR, El Sherif A, et al. The use of ultrasound-measured optic nerve sheath diameter to predict ventriculoperitoneal shunt failure in children. Pediatr Emerg Care. 2019;35(4):268–72. https://doi.org/10.1097/PEC.0000000000001034.
61. Aspide R, Bertolini G, Albini Riccioli L, Mazzatenta D, Palandri G, Biasucci DG. A proposal for a new protocol for sonographic assessment of the optic nerve sheath diameter: the CLOSED protocol. Neurocrit Care. 2020;32(1):327–32. https://doi.org/10.1007/s12028-019-00853-x.
62. Newman WD, Hollman AS, Dutton GN, Carachi R. Measurement of optic nerve sheath diameter by ultrasound: a means of detecting acute raised intracranial pressure in hydrocephalus. Br J Ophthalmol. 2002;86(10):1109–13. https://doi.org/10.1136/bjo.86.10.1109.
63. Helmke K, Hansen HC. Fundamentals of transorbital sonographic evaluation of optic nerve sheath expansion under intracranial hypertension. I. Experimental study. Pediatr Radiol. 1996;26(10):701–5. https://doi.org/10.1007/BF01383383.
64. Blehar DJ, Gaspari RJ, Montoya A, Calderon R. Correlation of visual axis and coronal axis measurements of the optic nerve sheath diameter. J Ultrasound Med. 2008;27(3):407–11. https://doi.org/10.7863/jum.2008.27.3.407.
65. Hirzallah MI, Lochner P, Hafeez MU, et al. Quality assessment of optic nerve sheath diameter ultrasonography: scoping literature review and Delphi protocol. J Neuroimaging. 2022;32(5):808–24. https://doi.org/10.1111/jon.13018.
66. Aspide R, Bertolini G, Belotti LMB, et al. The CLOSED protocol to assess optic nerve sheath diameter using color-Doppler: a comparison study in a cohort of idiopathic normal pressure hydrocephalus patients. Ultrasound J. 2022;14(1):43. https://doi.org/10.1186/s13089-022-00291-5.
67. Kim DH, Jun JS, Kim R. Ultrasonographic measurement of the optic nerve sheath diameter and its association with eyeball transverse diameter in 585 healthy volunteers. Sci Rep. 2017;7(1):15906. https://doi.org/10.1038/s41598-017-16173-z.
68. Berhanu D, Ferreira JC, Abegão Pinto L, Aguiar de Sousa D, Lucas Neto L, Tavares FJ. The role of optic nerve sheath ultrasonography in increased intracranial pressure: a systematic review and meta analysis. J Neurol Sci. 2023;454:120853. https://doi.org/10.1016/j.jns.2023.120853.
69. Koziarz A, Sne N, Kegel F, et al. Bedside optic nerve ultrasonography for diagnosing increased intracranial pressure: a systematic review and meta-analysis. Ann Intern Med. 2019;171(12):896–905. https://doi.org/10.7326/M19-0812.
70. Padayachy LC, Padayachy V, Galal U, Pollock T, Fieggen AG. The relationship between transorbital ultrasound measurement of the optic nerve sheath diameter (ONSD) and invasively measured ICP in children. : part II: age-related ONSD cut-off values and patency of the anterior Fontanelle. Childs Nerv Syst. 2016;32(10):1779–85. https://doi.org/10.1007/s00381-016-3068-4.
71. Lin JJ, Chen AE, Lin EE, Hsia SH, Chiang MC, Lin KL. Point-of-care ultrasound of optic nerve sheath diameter to detect intracranial pressure in neurocritically ill children - a narrative review. Biom J. 2020;43(3):231–9. https://doi.org/10.1016/j.bj.2020.04.006.
72. Lochner P, Czosnyka M, Naldi A, et al. Optic nerve sheath diameter: present and future perspectives for neurologists and critical care physicians. Neurol Sci. 2019;40(12):2447–57. https://doi.org/10.1007/s10072-019-04015-x.
73. Teismann N, Lenaghan P, Nolan R, Stein J, Green A. Point-of-care ocular ultrasound to detect optic disc swelling. Acad Emerg Med. 2013;20(9):920–5. https://doi.org/10.1111/acem.12206.
74. Ghanem G, Haase D, Brzezinski A, Ogawa R, Asachi P, Chiem A. Ultrasound detected increase in optic disk height to identify elevated intracranial pressure: a systematic review. Ultrasound J. 2023;15(1):26. https://doi.org/10.1186/s13089-023-00324-7.
75. Cheong I, Bermeo M, Tamagnone FM. Transorbital ultrasonography used to detect papilledema, in a patient with intracranial hypertension. J Diagn Med Sonogr. 2023;39(3):289–92. https://doi.org/10.1177/87564793231153866.
76. Rifenburg RP, Williams JJ. Optic nerve head drusen: a case of false-positive papilledema discovered by ocular ultrasound in the emergency department. Crit Ultrasound J. 2010;2(2):75–6. https://doi.org/10.1007/s13089-010-0036-1.
77. Braun A, Doniger SJ. Point-of-care ultrasonography for the identification of 2 children with optic disc drusen mimicking papilledema. Pediatr Emerg Care. 2014;30(7):505–7. https://doi.org/10.1097/PEC.0000000000000172.
78. Varma DD, Cugati S, Lee AW, Chen CS. A review of central retinal artery occlusion: clinical presentation and management. Eye (Lond). 2013;27(6):688–97. https://doi.org/10.1038/eye.2013.25.
79. Smith AT, Wilbert CD, Ferre RM. Using the Retrobulbar spot sign to assist in diagnosis and management of central retinal artery occlusions. J Ultrasound Med. 2020;39(1):197–202. https://doi.org/10.1002/jum.15073.
80. Foroozan R, Savino PJ, Sergott RC. Embolic central retinal artery occlusion detected by orbital color Doppler imaging. Ophthalmology. 2002;109(4):744–47; discussion 747-748. https://doi.org/10.1016/s0161-6420(01)01011-9.
81. Cozzi N, Stevens K, Pillay Y, et al. Diagnosis of central retinal artery occlusion in the emergency department using POCUS: a case series. POCUS J. 2021;6(2):73–5. https://doi.org/10.24908/pocus.v6i2.14974.
82. Gise R, Gaier ED, Heidary G. Diagnosis and imaging of optic nerve head Drusen. Semin Ophthalmol. 2019;34(4):256–63. https://doi.org/10.1080/08820538.2019.1620804.
83. Ertl M, Altmann M, Torka E, et al. The retrobulbar "spot sign" as a discriminator between vasculitic and thrombo-embolic affections of the retinal blood supply. Ultraschall Med. 2012;33(7):E263–7. https://doi.org/10.1055/s-0032-1312925.
84. Nedelmann M, Graef M, Weinand F, et al. Retrobulbar spot sign predicts thrombolytic treatment effects and etiology in central retinal artery occlusion. Stroke. 2015;46(8):2322–4. https://doi.org/10.1161/STROKEAHA.115.009839.

85. Sargsyan AE, Hamilton DR, Melton SL, Amponsah D, Marshall NE, Dulchavsky SA. Ultrasonic evaluation of pupillary light reflex. Crit Ultrasound J. 2009;1(2):53. https://doi.org/10.1007/s13089-009-0012-9.
86. Schmidt FA, Ruprecht K, Connolly F, et al. B-mode ultrasound assessment of pupillary function: feasibility, reliability and normal values. PLoS One. 2017;12(12):e0189016. https://doi.org/10.1371/journal.pone.0189016.
87. Yic CD, Prada G, Paz SI, et al. Comparison of ultrasonographic versus infrared pupillary assessment. Ultrasound J. 2020;12(1):38. https://doi.org/10.1186/s13089-020-00188-1.
88. Modi P, Bhoi S, Aggarwal P, et al. Feasibility of USG-guided objective initial assessment of pupillary size and pupillary reflexes versus clinical examination in patients with altered mental status: a cross-sectional study. J Ultrasound Med. 2024;43(2):335–46. https://doi.org/10.1002/jum.16366.
89. Rosdeutscher JD, Stadelmann WK. Diagnosis and treatment of retrobulbar hematoma resulting from blunt periorbital trauma. Ann Plast Surg. 1998;41(6):618–22. https://doi.org/10.1097/00000637-199812000-00006.
90. Hislop WS, Dutton GN, Douglas PS. Treatment of retrobulbar haemorrhage in accident and emergency departments. Br J Oral Maxillofac Surg. 1996;34(4):289–92. https://doi.org/10.1016/s0266-4356(96)90004-2.
91. Till P. Ultrasonic diagnosis of retrobulbar hematomas. Klin Monatsbl Augenheilkd. 1971;158(5):723–7.
92. Theoret J, Sanz GE, Matero D, et al. The "guitar pick" sign: a novel sign of retrobulbar hemorrhage. CJEM. 2011;13(3):162–4. https://doi.org/10.2310/10.2310/8000.2011.110279.
93. Murali S, Davis C, McCrea MJ, Plewa MC. Orbital compartment syndrome: pearls and pitfalls for the emergency physician. J Am Coll Emerg Phys Open. 2021;2(2):e12372. https://doi.org/10.1002/emp2.12372.
94. Romaniuk VM. Ocular trauma and other catastrophes. Emerg Med Clin North Am. 2013;31(2):399–411. https://doi.org/10.1016/j.emc.2013.02.003.
95. Pelletier J, Koyfman A, Long B. High risk and low prevalence diseases: open globe injury. Am J Emerg Med. 2023;64:113–20. https://doi.org/10.1016/j.ajem.2022.11.036.
96. Chou C, Lou YT, Hanna E, et al. Diagnostic performance of isolated orbital CT scan for assessment of globe rupture in acute blunt facial trauma. Injury. 2016;47(5):1035–41. https://doi.org/10.1016/j.injury.2016.01.014.
97. Yuan WH, Hsu HC, Cheng HC, et al. CT of globe rupture: analysis and frequency of findings. AJR Am J Roentgenol. 2014;202(5):1100–7. https://doi.org/10.2214/AJR.13.11010.
98. Blaivas M, Theodoro D, Sierzenski PR. A study of bedside ocular ultrasonography in the emergency department. Acad Emerg Med. 2002;9(8):791–9. https://doi.org/10.1111/j.1553-2712.2002.tb02166.x.
99. Humniski N, Ahn JS, Manji R, Kim DJ. Globe rupture diagnosed with point-of-care ultrasound. J Emerg Med. 2023;65(5):e453–6. https://doi.org/10.1016/j.jemermed.2023.06.002.
100. Wu TS, Dommer P, Pearson TC. Images in emergency medicine. Woman with right eye pain and swelling. Partial globe rupture. Ann Emerg Med. 2011;57(6):703, 708. https://doi.org/10.1016/j.annemergmed.2010.08.033.
101. Derr C, Shah A. Bedside ultrasound in the diagnosis of orbital cellulitis and orbital abscess. Emerg Radiol. 2012;19(3):265–7. https://doi.org/10.1007/s10140-011-0993-0.
102. Pelletier J, Koyfman A, Long B. High risk and low prevalence diseases: orbital cellulitis. Am J Emerg Med. 2023;68:1–9. https://doi.org/10.1016/j.ajem.2023.02.024.
103. Falticeanu A, Tritschler P, Dumitriu D. Ultrasound in pediatric orbital cellulitis. Med Ultrason. 2020;22(2):253–4. https://doi.org/10.11152/mu-2438.
104. Beam G, Check R, Denne N, Minardi J, End B. Point-of-care ultrasound findings in a case of orbital cellulitis: a case report. J Emerg Med. 2021;61(2):157–60. https://doi.org/10.1016/j.jemermed.2021.03.033.
105. Lemley CA, Han DP. Endophthalmitis: a review of current evaluation and management. Retina. 2007;27(6):662–80. https://doi.org/10.1097/IAE.0b013e3180323f96.
106. Gunalda J, Williams D, Koyfman A, Long B. High risk and low prevalence diseases: Endophthalmitis. Am J Emerg Med. 2023;71:144–9. https://doi.org/10.1016/j.ajem.2023.06.029.
107. Kohanim S, Daniels AB, Huynh N, Eliott D, Chodosh J. Utility of ocular ultrasonography in diagnosing infectious endophthalmitis in patients with media opacities. Semin Ophthalmol. 2012;27(5–6):242–5. https://doi.org/10.3109/08820538.2012.711417.
108. Maleki A, Ruggeri M, Colombo A, et al. B-scan ultrasonography findings in unilateral posterior Scleritis. J Curr Ophthalmol. 2022;34(1):93–9. https://doi.org/10.4103/joco.joco_267_21.
109. Tabbut M, Bates A, Marple G, Gramer D, Tabbut B. Point-of-care ultrasound in the evaluation of the acutely painful red eye. J Emerg Med. 2019;57(5):705–9. https://doi.org/10.1016/j.jemermed.2019.04.034.
110. Shields JA, Shields CL, Scartozzi R. Survey of 1264 patients with orbital tumors and simulating lesions: the 2002 Montgomery lecture, part 1. Ophthalmology. 2004;111(5):997–1008. https://doi.org/10.1016/j.ophtha.2003.01.002.
111. Purohit BS, Vargas MI, Ailianou A, et al. Orbital tumours and tumour-like lesions: exploring the armamentarium of multiparametric imaging. Insights Imaging. 2016;7(1):43–68. https://doi.org/10.1007/s13244-015-0443-8.
112. Loe S, Dinh V. Intra-ocular mass diagnosed with bedside ultrasound. Hong Kong J Emerg Med. 2014;21(1):48–50. https://doi.org/10.1177/102490791402100110.
113. Kendall CJ, Prager TC, Cheng H, Gombos D, Tang RA, Schiffman JS. Diagnostic ophthalmic ultrasound for radiologists. Neuroimaging Clin N Am. 2015;25(3):327–65. https://doi.org/10.1016/j.nic.2015.05.001.
114. Kadakia A, Zhang J, Yao X, Zhou Q, Heiferman MJ. Ultrasound in ocular oncology: technical advances, clinical applications, and limitations. Exp Biol Med (Maywood). 2023;248(5):371–9. https://doi.org/10.1177/15353702231169539.
115. Nagaraju RM, Gurushankar G, Bhimarao KB. Efficacy of high frequency ultrasound in localization and characterization of orbital lesions. J Clin Diagn Res. 2015;9(9):TC01-06. https://doi.org/10.7860/JCDR/2015/13021.6428.
116. Dimaras H, Corson TW. Retinoblastoma, the visible CNS tumor: a review. J Neurosci Res. 2019;97(1):29–44. https://doi.org/10.1002/jnr.24213.
117. Presley BC, Flannigan MJ. Emergency department bedside ultrasound diagnosis of retinoblastoma in a child. Pediatr Emerg Care. 2013;29(10):1128–31. https://doi.org/10.1097/PEC.0b013e3182a64234.
118. Lanni V, Iuliano A, Fossataro F, et al. The role of ultrasonography in differential diagnosis of orbital lesions. J Ultrasound. 2021;24(1):35–40. https://doi.org/10.1007/s40477-020-00443-0.

Central Nervous System Ultrasound

16

Tim Montrief, Ee Tein Tay, and Aarti Sarwal

Background

Over the last decade, there has been rising interest in using point-of-care ultrasound (POCUS) to assess central nervous system (CNS) pathology, with emerging literature supporting its use in the evaluation of a wide range of acute neurological emergencies [1–5]. While neuroimaging modalities like computed tomography (CT) and magnetic resonance imaging (MRI) are often the imaging modality of choice, these are not universally available, particularly in lower-resourced or austere settings. Moreover, some patients may not be sufficiently stable to leave the clinical care area or require rapid reassessment necessitating a bedside modality, such as POCUS. In scenarios like multi-trauma, mass casualties, or global pandemic/pandemic-induced restrictions, clinicians may also need to prioritize resources, utilizing a limited number of CTs available for more emergent indications.

Depending upon the application, POCUS can be definitive or assist in triaging resource-demanding alternative neuroimaging. POCUS may also be helpful in allowing for serial, non-invasive, and radiation-free data. This imaging modality may be particularly beneficial for specific populations, such as pediatric patients, where POCUS can reduce exposure to radiation, and patients on mechanical circulatory support, where transport is challenging and risky.

T. Montrief (✉)
Division of Critical Care Medicine, DeWitt-Daughtry Family Department of Surgery, University of Miami Miller School of Medicine, Miami, FL, USA
e-mail: T.montrief@umiami.edu

E. T. Tay
Ronald O. Perelman Department of Emergency Medicine, New York University Grossman School of Medicine, New York, NY, USA
e-mail: ee.tay@langone.org

A. Sarwal
Department of Neurology, Virginia Commonwealth University, Richmond, VA, USA
e-mail: Aarti.Sarwal@vcuhealth.org

With increasing incorporation of POCUS into acute and critical care settings, CNS applications now extend beyond traditional use in the evaluation of acute ischemic stroke or vasospasm in subarachnoid hemorrhage [6, 7]. POCUS includes B-mode evaluation for intracranial pathology, including intracranial hemorrhage, subdural hemorrhage, hydrocephalus, midline shift, acute ischemic stroke, intracranial hypertension, as well as extracranial pathologies such as skull fractures, extracranial hemorrhage, temporal arteritis, and subgaleal hematomas [2, 4, 7–14]. Given the need to evaluate extracranial carotid vascular pathology in acute cerebrovascular disorders, POCUS has further expanded to include carotid pathologies, including assessment for carotid stenosis, thrombus, dissection, pseudoaneurysm, and steal phenomena [15, 16]. Several organizations have incorporated POCUS into societal guidelines, defining indications, standardized techniques, and various levels of skills/competencies required for clinical applications [14, 17–19].

Indications

Indications
- Headache
- Head trauma
- Altered mental status
- Neurologic complaints concerning stroke
- Serial assessment in high-risk patients to avoid risk of repeated head CT

Diagnosis
- Acute ischemic stroke
- Subarachnoid hemorrhage
- Intracranial hemorrhage (intra and extra-axial hemorrhage)
- Extracranial hemorrhage, cephalohematoma, and subgaleal hematomas
- Skull Fracture
- Intracranial hypertension
- Temporal arteritis
- Hydrocephalus and ventriculoperitoneal shunt functionality
- Carotid arterial disease (stenosis, thrombus, pseudoaneurysm, dissection)
- Ancillary test for death by neurological criteria

M. Gottlieb, N. Panebianco (eds.), *Advanced Point-of-Care Ultrasound*, https://doi.org/10.1007/978-3-031-85308-1_16

Core Views

<table>
<tr><th>View</th><th>Image</th><th>Approach</th></tr>
<tr><td>Transtemporal</td><td></td><td></td></tr>
<tr><td>Mesencephalic</td><td>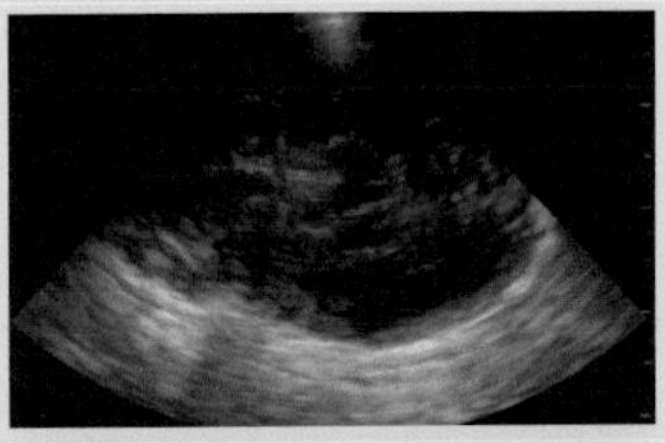</td><td>Use the phased array probe on the temporal window with the indicator to the patient's eyes and depth set to 12–15 cm. Identify the butterfly-shaped midbrain.</td></tr>
<tr><td>Diencephalic</td><td>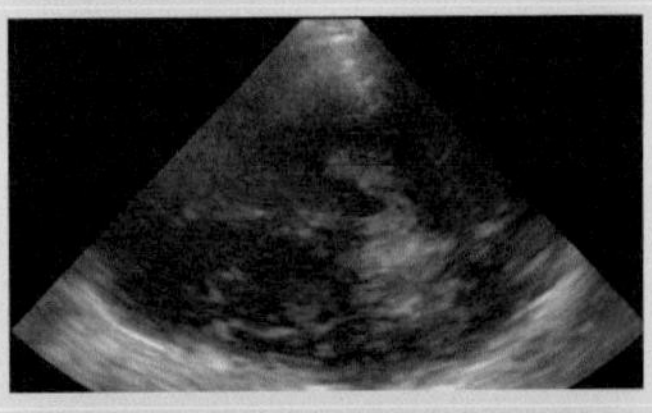</td><td>Using the same technique as above, fan cephalad to identify the third ventricle.</td></tr>
<tr><td>Ventricular</td><td>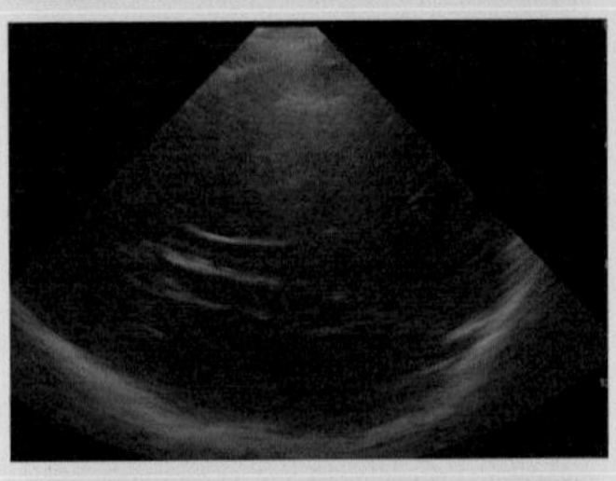</td><td>Using the same technique as above, fan cephalad to identify the frontal horns of the lateral ventricles.</td></tr>
<tr><td>Submandibular</td><td>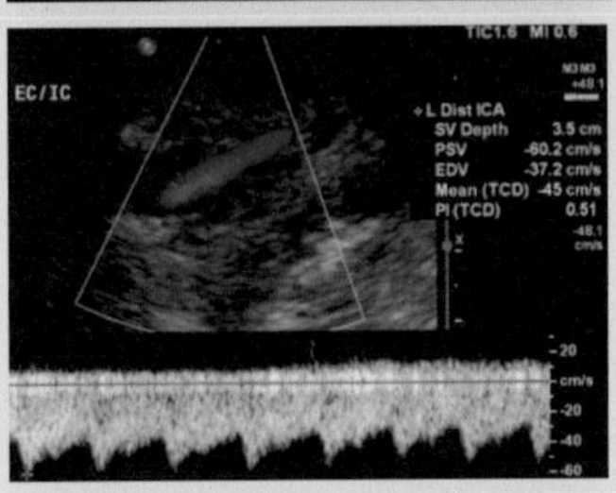</td><td>Place the phased array probe, using the transcranial Doppler preset, laterally under the jaw anterior and medial to the sternocleidomastoid muscle, aiming upwards and slightly medially to evaluate the internal carotid artery. The probe indicator is up toward the head.</td></tr>
<tr><td>Suboccipital</td><td>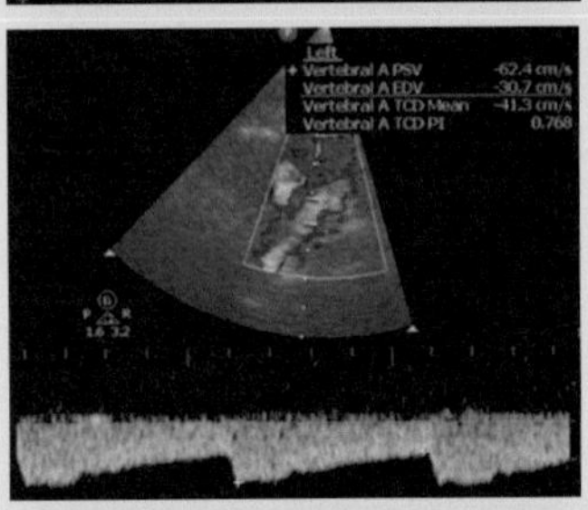</td><td>Place the phased array probe inferior and medial to the mastoid process, indicator facing horizontal, depth set at about 10 cm, with the beam angled toward the bridge of the nose or contralateral eye.</td></tr>
<tr><td>Transorbital</td><td>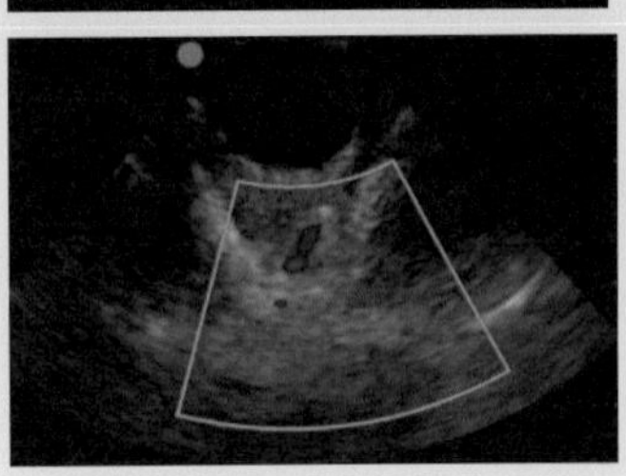</td><td>Place the phased array probe, using the ophthalmic preset, over the closed eyelid with the indicator toward the patient's right and copious amounts of gel. Identify the ophthalmic artery and internal carotid artery.</td></tr>
</table>

Transcranial Ultrasound

POCUS is performed using a low-frequency phased array probe with the transcranial Doppler (TCD) preset. If the TCD preset is unavailable, an abdominal preset can substitute for TCD during B-mode imaging. For vessel imaging using Doppler (when TCD is not available), the abdominal preset can serve as a substitute provided tissue harmonic imaging is turned off [2, 20]. The linear probe may be used for transcranial insonation in the neonatal and younger pediatric populations.

The POCUS examination is typically performed using three classic 'windows' to insonate the brain and intracranial arteries in the circle of Willis: the transtemporal window, the suboccipital window, the submandibular, and the transorbital window [20]. B-mode examination of the brain is typically reserved for the transtemporal window, including the mesencephalic, diencephalic, and ventricular planes in adult and pediatric patients, while the transfontanellar approach is used in neonates. Transcranial color-coded duplex sonography (TCCS) is a subset of TCD that utilizes B-mode color Doppler assistance to visualize the circle of Wills and guide the placement of the sampling gate for pulse Doppler insonation (Fig. 16.1) [11].

Color and pulsed-wave Doppler can be used to insonate the circle of Willis using the transtemporal windows, suboc-

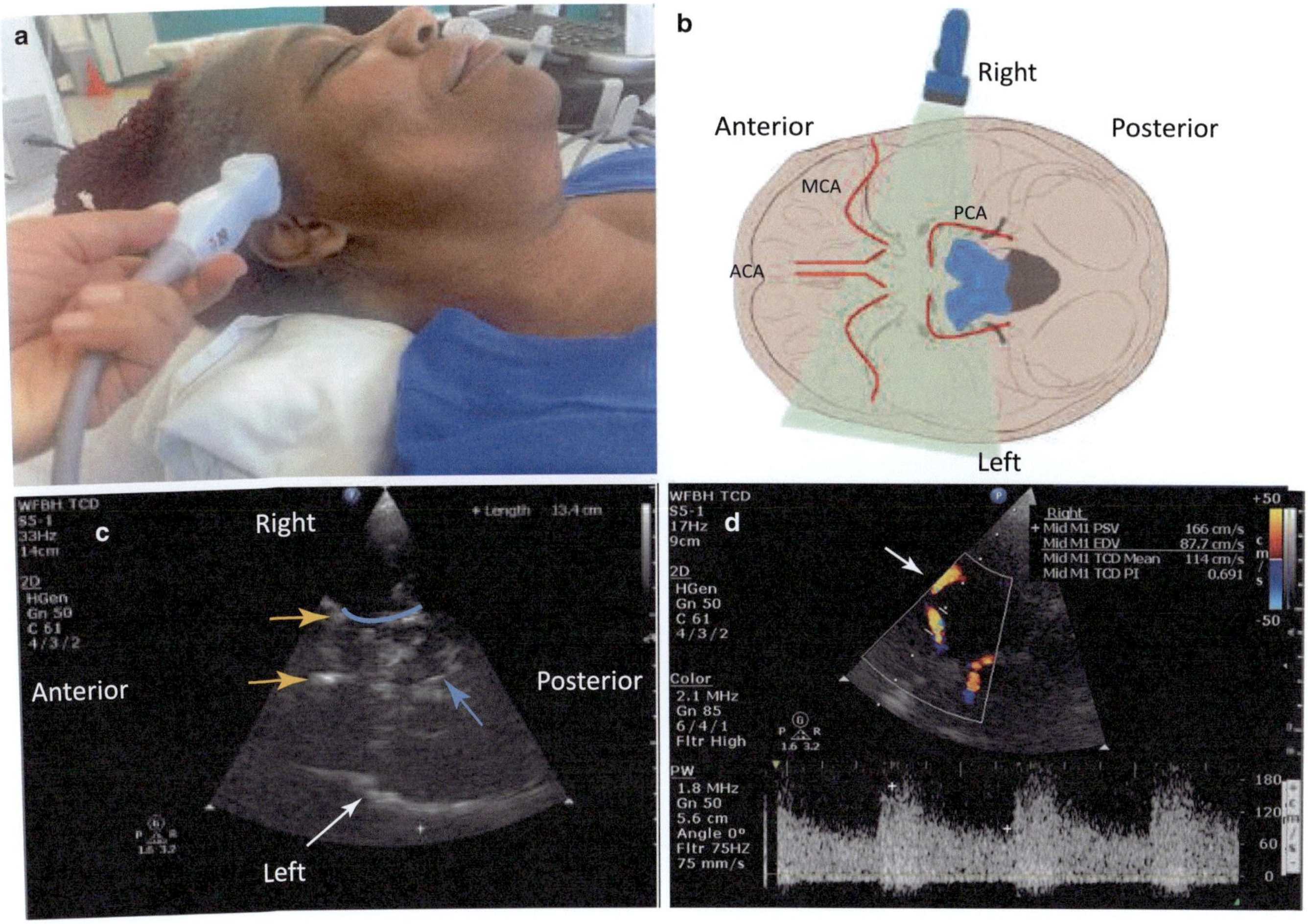

Fig. 16.1 Transcranial ultrasound of the circle of Willis using the transtemporal window. (**a**) Placement of a phased array probe on the right temporal bone with index marker pointed anteriorly toward the right temporal bone with index marker pointed anteriorly toward the eyes. (**b**) Cross-section through the human skull at the level of the basal cistern shows the relative placement of intracranial vessels and the insonation plane of an ultrasound probe placed on the temporal bone. Midbrain is shown as a blue structure posterior to the circle of Willis (marked with red lines). *Skull illustration courtesy Patrick J. Lynch,* http://patricklynch.net *Creative Commons Attribution 2.5 License 2006*. (**c**) B-mode image of the brain at the level of basal cisterns showing the opposite skull (white arrow), butterfly-shaped midbrain in the center (blue arrow), and an ipsilateral bony ridge created by the petrous part of the temporal bone and lesser wing of the sphenoid (blue line). The clinoid processes are visible as two hyperechoic signals anterior to the midbrain (yellow arrows). By convention, the anterior part of the head is aligned on the left of the screen, with the posterior/occipital part aligned on the right of the screen on ultrasound of the brain. (**d**) Pulsed-wave Doppler of the middle cerebral artery showing placement of gate in the middle segment of the vessel (white arrow) at a depth of 5.6 cm to show spectral Doppler waveforms at the bottom of the image. Quantitative analysis of these waveforms shows the mean flow velocity (114 cm/s) and pulsatility index (0.691) on the right upper part of the image

cipital windows, orbital windows, or submandibular windows. In general, TCD refers to spectral pulsed-wave Doppler to insonate the intracranial vasculature to monitor cerebral blood flow velocity (CBF-V) and intracranial vessel pulsatility [2, 4, 11]. In contrast, carotid Doppler assessment is performed in the neck using the linear high-frequency probe in a vascular preset to insonate the extracranial internal carotid artery, external carotid artery, and vertebral arteries.

Transtemporal Window

The temporal bone is thin enough in 80–90% of adults to provide an acoustic window to the brain. However, this may be affected by machine limitations, patient factors, and operator skill [2, 21–23]. For the temporal windows, place the probe on the temporal bone with the probe marker facing the patient's eyes, and fan the probe inferiorly from the lateral canthus downward toward the ear. The ultrasound depth should be increased to allow visualization of the contralateral skull as a hyperechoic convex structure in the far field (usually seen at 12–15 cm depth). Brain parenchyma is ordinarily gray or hypoechoic on ultrasound, while white matter and choroid has a higher attenuation than gray matter. Due to artifacts created by the base of the skull, ipsilateral brain parenchyma can be difficult to visualize. Hence, B-mode assessment focuses on the contralateral parenchyma or midline structures. As the probe is tilted cephalad, several planes are visible: the mesencephalic, diencephalic, and ventricular planes (Fig. 16.2).

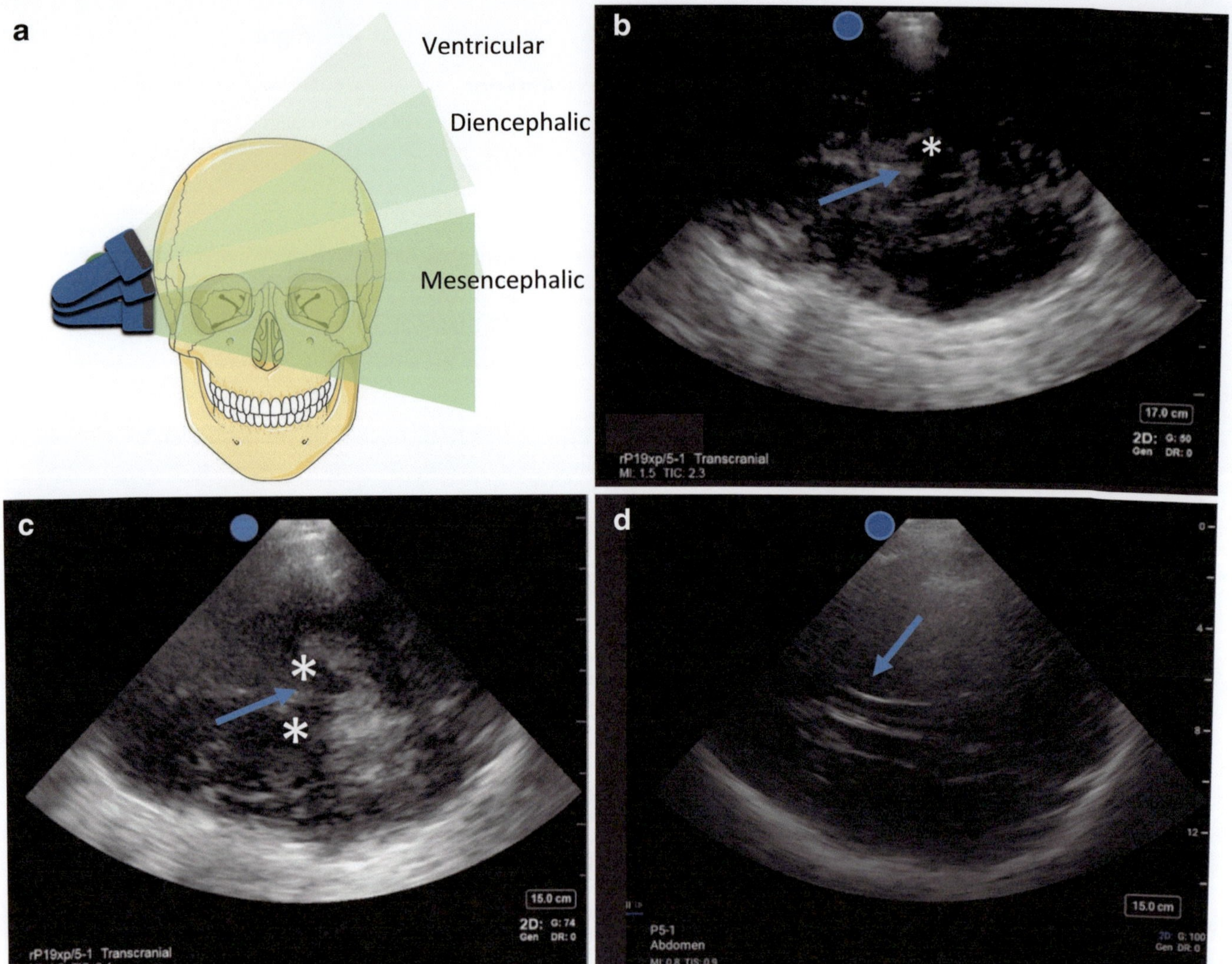

Fig. 16.2 Different planes visualized through the temporal window. (**a**) Schematic of the skull showing the relative direction of the probe to show different planes of insonation for cranial imaging: mesencephalic, diencephalic, and ventricular plane. *Servier Medical Art is licensed under CC BY 4.0*. (**b**). B-mode cranial ultrasound of the mesencephalic plane showing the midbrain (asterisk) with cerebral peduncles and colliculi surrounded by hyperechoic basal cisterns. The cerebral aqueduct (arrow) is visible in the posterior part of the midbrain between the colliculi. (**c**) Cross-section shows the diencephalic plane with the third ventricle (arrow) separating the two thalami (asterisks). (**d**) Cross-section shows the ventricular plane and the outline of the lateral ventricles (arrow) seen as the choroid/ependymal layer lining it

1. *Mesencephalic*: The midbrain appears as a central hypoechoic butterfly-shaped structure with cerebral peduncles and colliculi surrounded by hyperechoic basal cisterns. The cerebral aqueduct and hyperechoic pineal gland can also be seen as a hyperechoic structure posterior to the midbrain.
2. *Diencephalic*: Cephalad movement of probe from the midbrain allows visualization of the pulsating third ventricle, which appears as central parallel hyperechoic lines with hypoechoic thalami on each side.
3. *Ventricular plane*: The most cephalad view includes the frontal horns of the lateral ventricles appearing as hypoechoic structures lined by a hyperechoic choroid plexus. Temporal horns typically appear hyperechoic due to the presence of choroid, with their boundaries marked by the splenium of corpus callosum. The lateral ventricle and septum pellucidum can also be identified in patients with favorable anatomy.

Submandibular Window

The submandibular window for insonation of the extracranial internal carotid artery can be performed with a TCD preset and phased array probe (in contrast to the linear probe, which is classically used to insonate the neck when evaluating for carotid artery stenosis) (Fig. 16.3). This window is obtained by placing the probe laterally under the jaw anterior and medial to the sternocleidomastoid muscle, aiming the probe upwards and slightly medially to evaluate the internal carotid artery.

Suboccipital Window

The suboccipital window is obtained by placing the probe inferior and medial to the mastoid process and directing the probe toward the bridge of the nose or contralateral eye. The probe can also be placed in the posterior neck in the midline and directed towards the middle of the forehead. The index marker is pointed cephalad (Fig. 16.4). Pulsed-wave Doppler can be used to look at the vertebral and basilar arteries through the hypoechoic foramen magnum in this window.

Transorbital Window

A transorbital window is used to insonate the ophthalmic artery and internal carotid artery (Fig. 16.5). The probe is placed gently over the closed eyelid with the marker pointed toward the patient's midline and angled slightly medial and upward to obtain the transorbital window, which visualizes the orbital fossa [2]. Orbital insonation should only be performed using the ocular preset, which reduces the power of the ultrasound beam to lower the mechanical index and thermal index. The index marker on the probe points in the same direction as the index marker on the screen, typically 9 o'clock in the ophthalmic preset.

Doppler Ultrasound

Color Doppler Through the transtemporal window, color Doppler can help insonate the middle cerebral artery (MCA), anterior cerebral arteries (ACA), internal carotid artery (ICA), anterior communicating artery (AComm), posterior communicating artery (PComm), and posterior cerebral arteries (PCA) based on published practice standards for image acquisition (Fig. 16.6) [24, 25]. Ipsilateral to the probe, the MCA is visible as the artery with flow going towards the probe anterior to the midbrain. The ACA can be visualized by pointing the probe more anteriorly and will

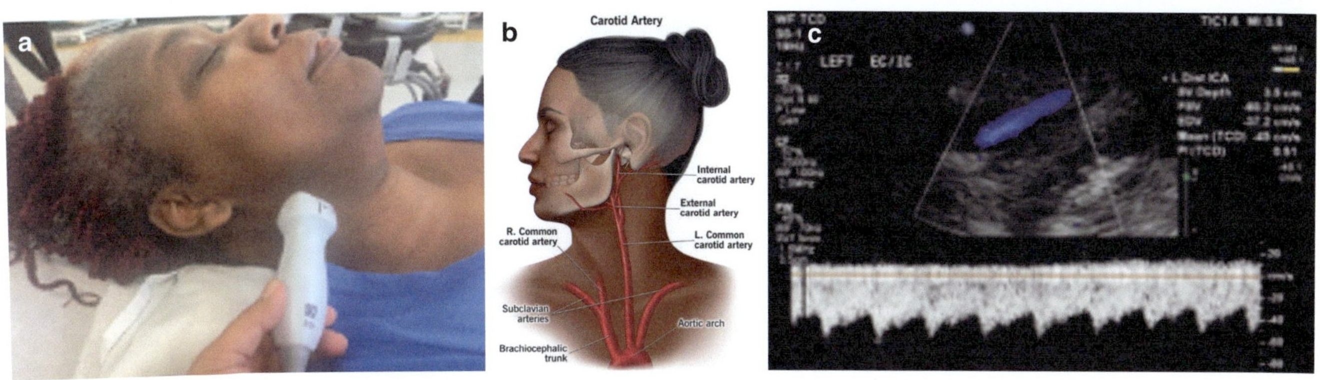

Fig. 16.3 Submandibular window. (**a**) Probe placement for the submandibular window with index marker pointed toward 12 o'clock. This allows visualization of the internal carotid artery in the neck along the long axis. (**b**) Relative position of the internal carotid artery (ICA) and external carotid artery (ECA) in the neck. (**c**) The internal carotid artery is identified by color Doppler signal with flow away from the probe. Pulsed-wave Doppler demonstrates its low resistance waveforms. The internal carotid artery differs from the external carotid artery by its postero-lateral position and low resistance waveforms (compared to the external carotid artery that is anteromedial and has high resistance waveforms)

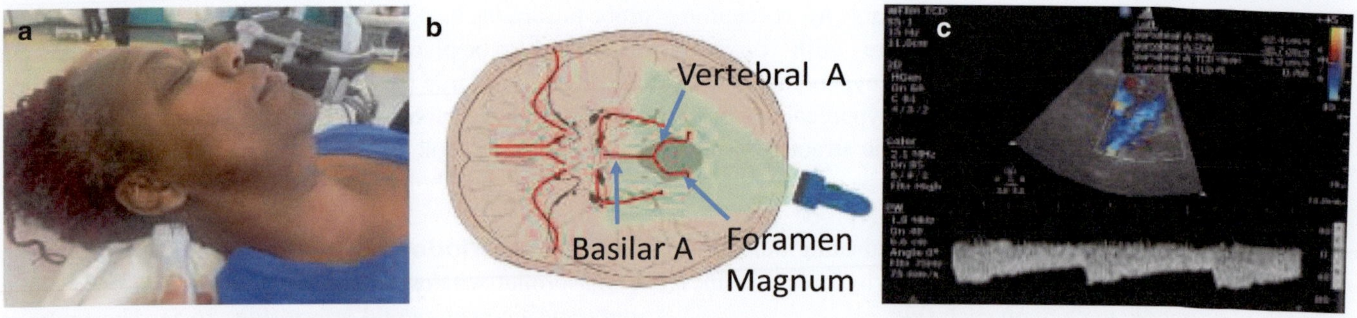

Fig. 16.4 Suboccipital window. (**a**) Placement of the probe in the suboccipital area in a supine patient with index marker pointed cephalad. (**b**) Identification of the round foramen magnum (dark green structure in the base of the skull). *Skull illustration courtesy Patrick J. Lynch,* http://patricklynch.net *Creative Commons Attribution 2.5 License 2006.* (**c**) Color Doppler is used to visualize the Y-shaped vertebrobasilar arteries with flow away from the probe. Pulsed-wave Doppler insonation is then performed by placing the Doppler gate on the segment of interest

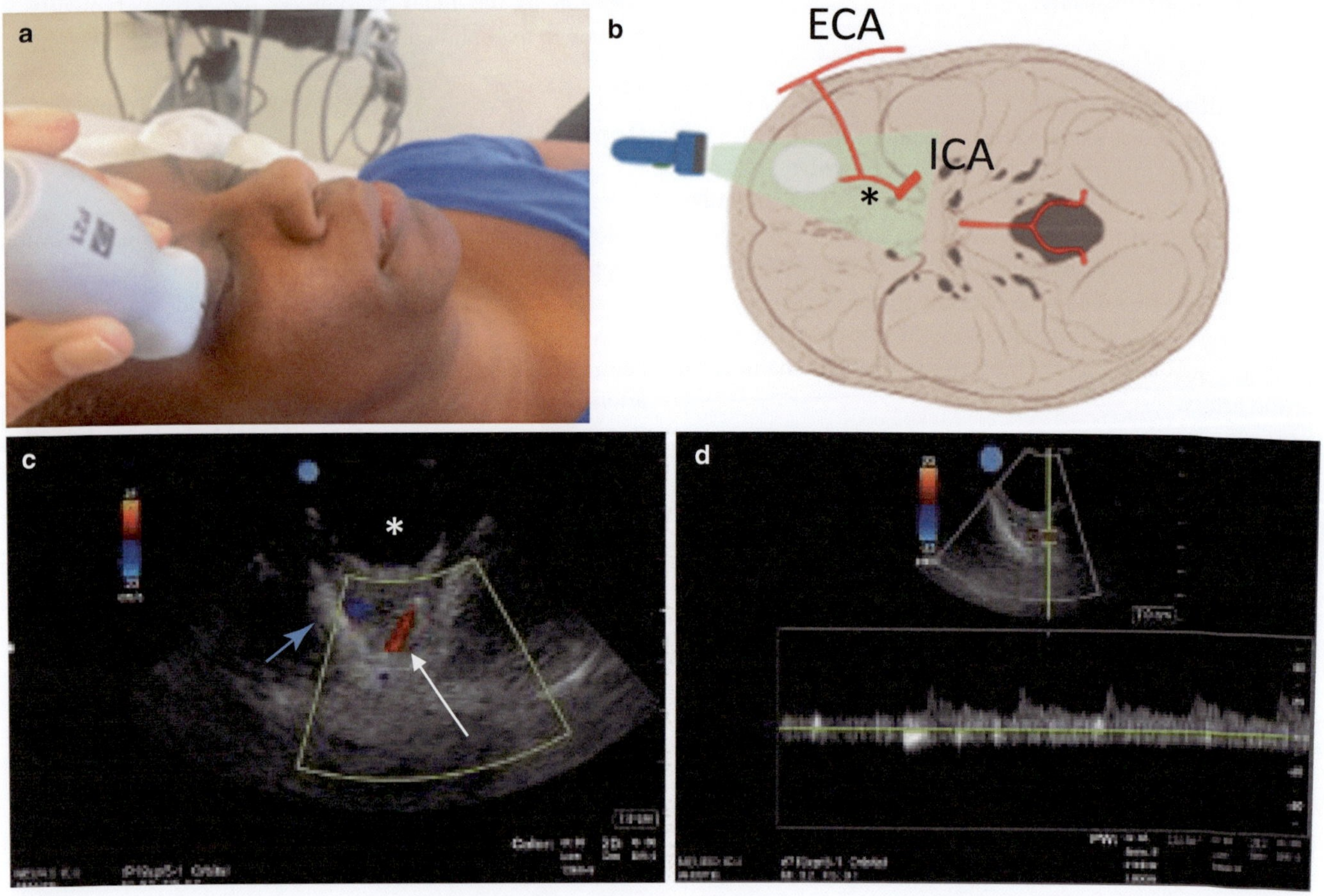

Fig. 16.5 Transorbital window. (**a**) Phased array probe placed on the lateral part of closed eyelid to visualize the orbital fossa with index marker pointed toward the 9 o'clock position. (**b**) Cross-section of the skull showing relative anatomy of the external carotid artery (ECA) connecting to the ophthalmic artery (asterisk) branch from the internal carotid artery (ICA). *Skull illustration courtesy Patrick J. Lynch, http://patricklynch.net Creative Commons Attribution 2.5 License 2006.* (**c**) Using the eye (asterisk) as an acoustic window with color Doppler signal corresponding to the ophthalmic artery (white arrow) within the orbital fossa (blue arrow). Normal ophthalmic artery flow is toward the probe. (**d**) Pulsed-wave Doppler can then be used at depth of 3.5-4.5 cm to interrogate the spectral Doppler waveforms

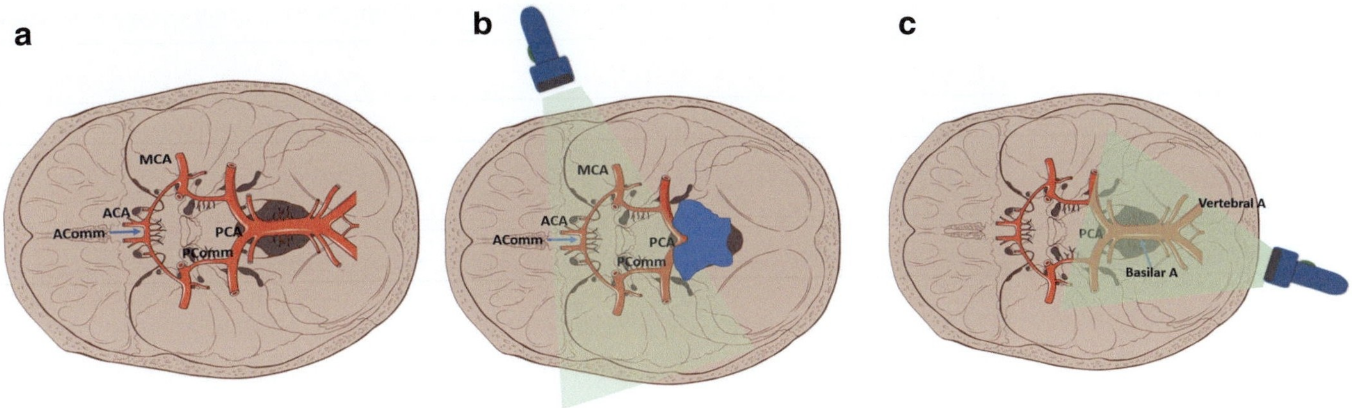

Fig. 16.6 Circle of Willis vessel anatomy. (**a**) Cross-section of the skull showing the vessels that make up the circle of Willis. (**b**) Temporal window insonation to visualize the circle of Willis. The relative position of each vessel in relation to the midbrain and probe is demonstrated. (**c**) Occipital window insonation of the circle of Willis. *ACA* anterior cerebral artery, *AComm* anterior communicating artery, *MCA* middle cerebral artery, *PComm* posterior communicating artery, *PCA* posterior cerebral artery. *Servier Medical Art is licensed under CC BY 4.0*

Table 16.1 Characteristics of selected cerebral vasculature

Window	Artery	Probe angle	Depth (mm) from the probe	Flow direction relative to the probe	Adult MFV (cm/s)
Transtemporal	MCA	Straight/anterior-superior	30–65	Towards	55 ± 12
Transtemporal	ACA	Straight/anterior-superior	60–75	Away	50 ± 11
Transtemporal	PCA-segment 1	Straight/posterior	60–70	Towards	39 ± 10
Transtemporal	PCA- segment 2	Straight/ posterior-superior	60–70	Away	40 ± 10
Suboccipital	BA	Superior	80–120	Away	41 ± 10
Suboccipital	VA	Superior lateral	60–75	Away	38 ± 10
Transorbital	OA	Straight	45–55	Towards	21 ± 5

MCA middle cerebral artery, *MFV* mean flow velocity, *ACA* anterior cerebral artery, *PCA* posterior cerebral artery, *BA* basilar artery, *VA* vertebral artery, *OA* ophthalmic artery

appear as flow going away from the probe. The PCA is identified by its location around the midbrain and can be seen by pointing the probe more posteriorly.

Spectral Doppler The Spectral Doppler waveform provides vital information regarding an arterial segment's flow characteristics. The sample volume gate of the pulsed-wave Doppler is adjusted to 5–10 mm to ensure appropriate capture of the typical diameter of the intracranial arteries (approximately 3–5 mm) [26]. The pulsed-wave Doppler gate is placed over the segment of interest to provide spectral Doppler parameters of mean flow velocity and the pulsatility index. Proper vessel identification relies on a combination of the relative direction of the probe within the acoustic window, the direction of blood flow relative to the probe's orientation [2]. Relative depth of insonated segments of each vessel where the Doppler gate should be placed and the corresponding normal mean flow velocities at that depth on pulsed-wave Doppler are provided in Table 16.1. For example, the proximal MCA can be insonated by placing the Doppler gate at 55-65 mm depth, while the distal MCA can be insonated at 35-40 mm and the middle MCA segment around 40-55 mm depth. A complete TCCS examination includes Doppler measurements of each major vessel in the circle of Willis, requiring all core POCUS views: (1) temporal window for ACA, MCA, ICA, and PCA insonation; (2) suboccipital window for vertebrobasilar insonation; and (3) orbital window for ophthalmic artery insonation [18]. Contrast agent microbubbles may improve vessel identification in cases with inadequate temporal bone windows, but data are limited [27, 28].

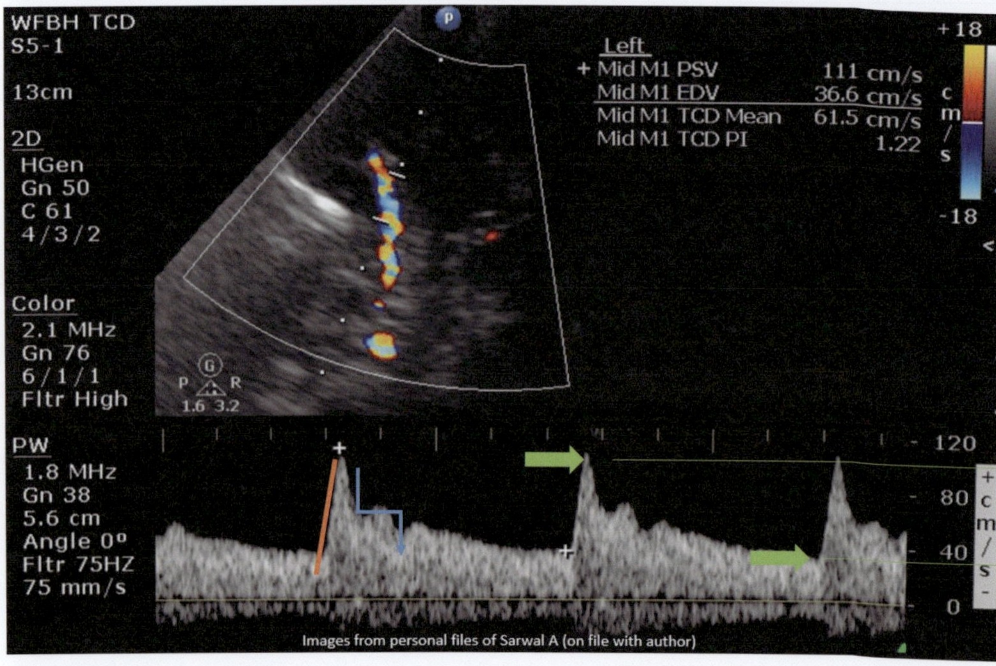

Fig. 16.7. Left middle cerebral artery (M1) spectral Doppler waveform. The Doppler waveform is characterized by a sharp systolic upstroke (orange line) followed by stepwise deceleration (blue line) with positive robust end-diastolic flow velocity that is one-third to one-half of the peak systolic flow velocity (green arrows and lines). Note the depth of the gate and zero presumed angle of insonation. *PSV* peak systolic velocity (cm/s), *EDV* end diastolic velocity (cm/s), *MFV* mean flow velocity (cm/s), *PI* Pulsatility Index

The normal spectral Doppler waveform for intracranial vessels is a low-resistance waveform characterized by a sharp systolic upstroke followed by stepwise deceleration with positive robust end-diastolic flow velocity that is one-third to one-half of the peak systolic flow velocity (Fig. 16.7.). Several parameters can be measured, including peak systolic velocity (PSV), end-diastolic velocity (EDV), and mean flow velocity (MFV). This is typically measured as the time-averaged mean of maximum velocities. Arterial resistance is measured by using the pulsatility index (PI), calculated by dividing the difference between end-diastolic velocity and peak systolic velocity by the mean flow velocity: PI = (PSV – EDV) / MFV [29]. Alternatively, resistance index (RI) may be calculated by using the formula: RI = (PSV – EDV) / PSV. However, PI is more widely used in TCD compared to systemic vascular Doppler and may have a better correlation with ICP. Normal PI is 0.6 to 1.2. A high PI >1.2 represents high resistance to flow in the insonated artery and can be due to increased age, distal atherosclerotic disease, or increased intracranial pressure [26, 30]. Hypercarbia may lower PI, while hypocarbia or vasoconstriction may increase PI higher than normal limits [31].

The angle of insonation is typically adjusted to be 60 degrees or less relative to the direction of flow in vascular ultrasound. The direction variability in different segments of the circle of Willis makes it difficult to acquire signals at that angle. General consensus is to keep the angle 30-45 degrees, when possible. Despite that, measurements of MFV do not account for the angle adjustment and assume zero angle for correction [25]. Most of the literature in TCD comes from non-imaging TCD where vessel segments are not visualized. Hence, angle adjustment, if not feasible with TCD or TCCS, has followed the convention of not adjusting the angle to allow translation of available data.

Carotid Ultrasound

Extracranial carotid artery imaging may be added to the POCUS examination utilizing a high-frequency linear probe with the vascular or carotid ultrasound preset (Fig. 16.8). Carotid examination should be performed in both the short- and long-axis with B-mode for structural abnormalities, while color and duplex Doppler ultrasound investigate blood flow [16]. Carotid POCUS should begin by placing the probe over the sternocleidomastoid muscle in the transverse plane with appropriate identification of the common carotid artery [20]. The sternocleidomastoid muscle provides a better-quality acoustic window for carotid applications. Once the proximal common carotid artery is identified, the probe should be rotated 90 degrees to the cephalad direction to image the distal common carotid artery, carotid bulb, carotid bifurcation, external carotid artery (ECA), and ICA. The arterial walls and lumen should be imaged in B-mode and evaluated for luminal irregularities, including the presence of thrombus, dissection flaps, pseudoaneurysms, or plaque formation. For comparative purposes, the neck's affected and unaffected sides should both be examined.

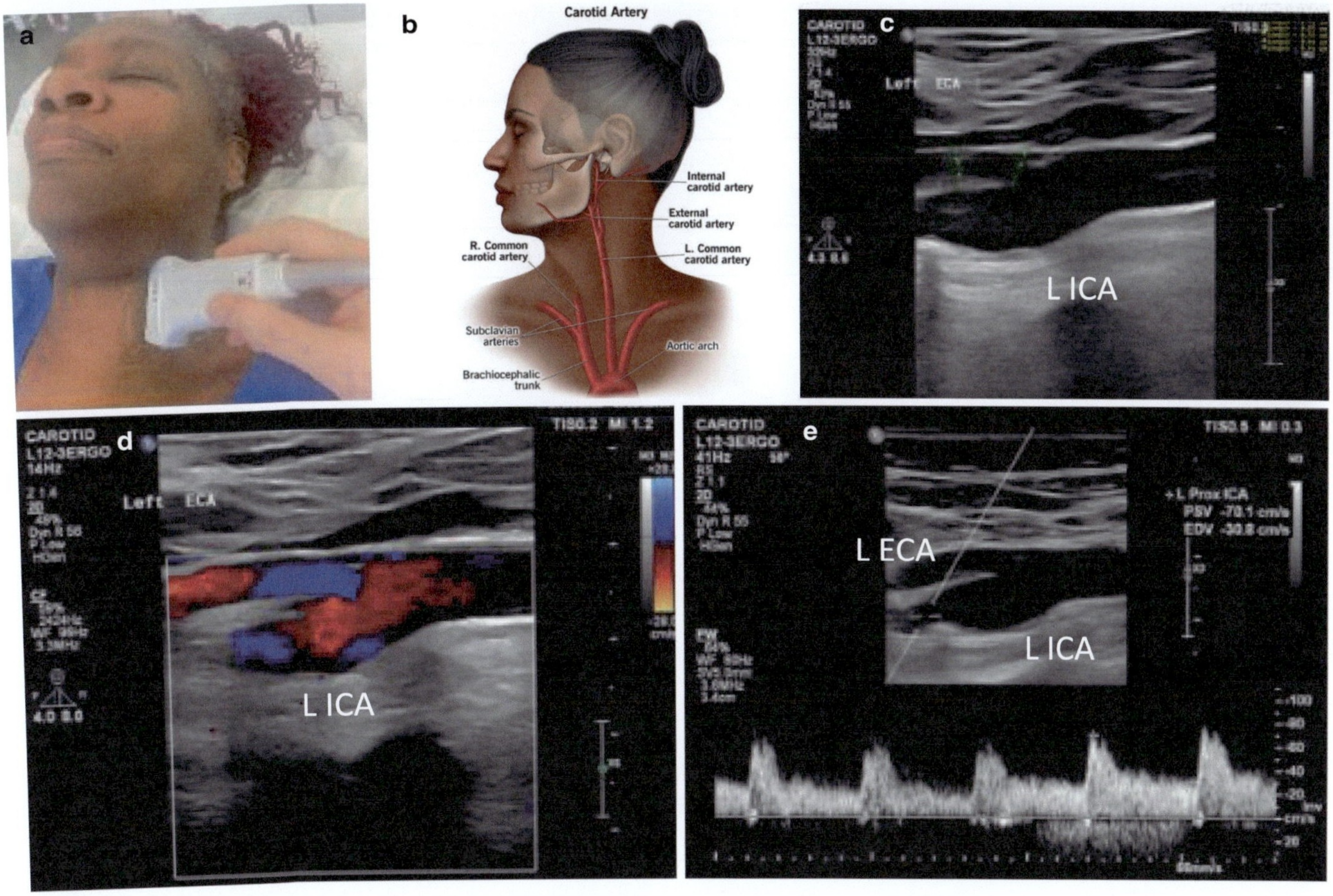

Fig. 16.8 Carotid ultrasound. (**a**) Technique for carotid POCUS. Begin by placing a high-frequency linear probe in the transverse plane at the level of the sternocleidomastoid muscle. Move the probe cephalad and then rotate the probe 90 degrees to image the carotid artery in the longitudinal plane. (**b**) Relative position of the internal carotid artery (ICA) and external carotid artery (ECA) in the neck. (**c**) Normal B-mode image of the long-axis view showing both the ICA and ECA in the same view. Green lines show measurements of plaque and corresponding residual lumen in the ECA. (**d**) Color Doppler images show the turbulence of flow near the flow divider where the common carotid artery divides into ECA and ICA. (**e**) Pulsed-wave Doppler insonation of the proximal ICA at an angle of insonation close to 60 degree with the Doppler gate adjusted to capture most of the blood flow within the lumen excluding the vessel walls. The velocity measured is posted in the right upper corner of the image with a peak systolic velocity of 70.1 cm/s and an end-diastolic velocity of 30.8 cm/s

During carotid artery assessment, it is important to distinguish between the ICA and ECA. The ICA has no branches in the neck and has low resistance waveforms on the pulsed-wave Doppler with an EDV greater than one-fourth of the PSV. In contrast, the ECA has multiple branches in the neck supplying the muscles of the face and neck with high-resistance waveforms on pulsed-wave Doppler that show diastolic flow velocity very low compared to systolic flow velocities. The ECA can also be distinguished by the transmission of temporal artery pulses during a "temporal tap." The temporal tap maneuver consists of tapping over the ipsilateral superficial temporal artery while assessing the carotid bifurcation on Doppler ultrasound, enabling the practitioner to visualize a reflected flow in the ECA. Figure 16.9 demonstrates important distinguishing features between the ICA and ECA.

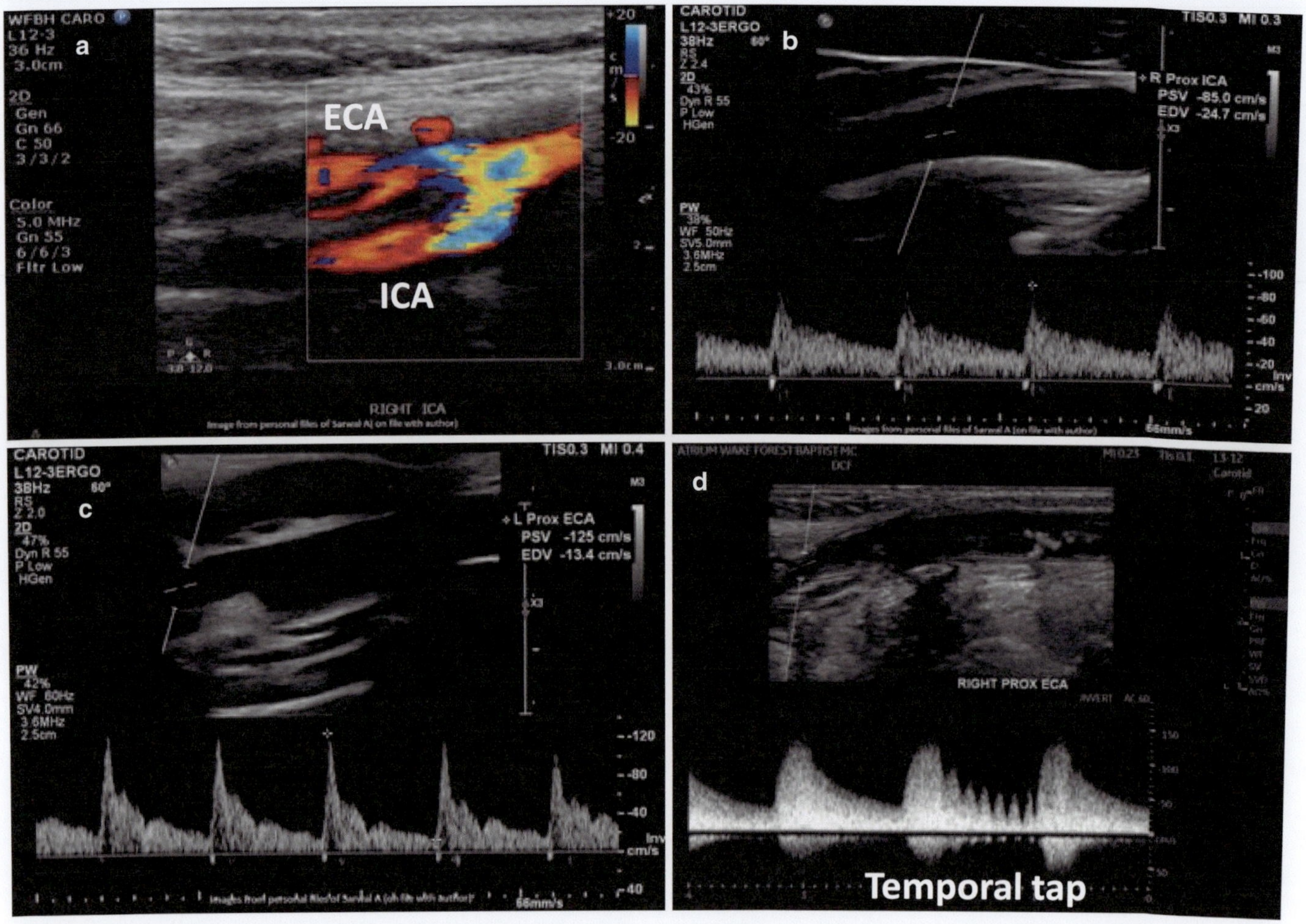

Fig. 16.9 Internal versus external carotid artery sonographic comparison. (**a**) Carotid artery ultrasound examination using color Doppler mode showing the bifurcation of the carotid into internal carotid artery (ICA) and external carotid artery (ECA). (**b**) ICA has no branches in the neck and has low resistance waveforms on the pulsed-wave Doppler with diastolic velocity greater than one-fourth of the peak systolic velocity. (**c**) ECA has multiple branches in the neck supplying the muscles of the face and neck with high resistance waveforms on pulsed-wave Doppler that shows diastolic flow velocity very low compared to systolic flow velocities. (**d**) ECA can also be distinguished by transmission of temporal artery pulses when the temporal artery is tapped in the temple while insonating the ECA in the neck using ultrasound, known as the temporal tap maneuver

Clinical Applications

B-Mode

Intracranial Hemorrhage

While CT remains the gold standard for diagnosing subdural, epidural, and intracerebral hemorrhage, POCUS can be a valuable alternative in resource-limited settings or when CT is unavailable [2, 14, 32]. An exploratory study of 11 patients comparing POCUS to CT or MRI brain for the diagnosis of intracranial hemorrhage found POCUS was 100% sensitive and 50% specific [33]. Similarly, POCUS has been investigated as a monitoring tool for hemorrhagic transformation in patients with acute hemispheric stroke, with a separate study of 11 patients reporting a sensitivity of 91% and specificity of 95% [34]. However, POCUS can have false positives from tumors, chronic white matter disease, calcifications, posterior acoustic enhancement artifacts created by the midbrain, hyperechoic signal artifacts from the basal cisterns, or bony landmarks parallel to the occipital bone, as well as a variety of clinical scenarios, including cerebral edema, evolving subacute ischemic stroke, pneumocephalus, encephalomalacia, arterio-venous malformations, and cistern effacement [25, 29]. Data suggest POCUS is less accurate for intracranial hemorrhage when the hemorrhage is smaller than 1 cm, greater than 5-7 days old, or in poorly insonated areas of the brain (e.g., infratentorial regions) [33–37]. Intraventricular hemorrhage by itself is also difficult to identify due to significant hyper-

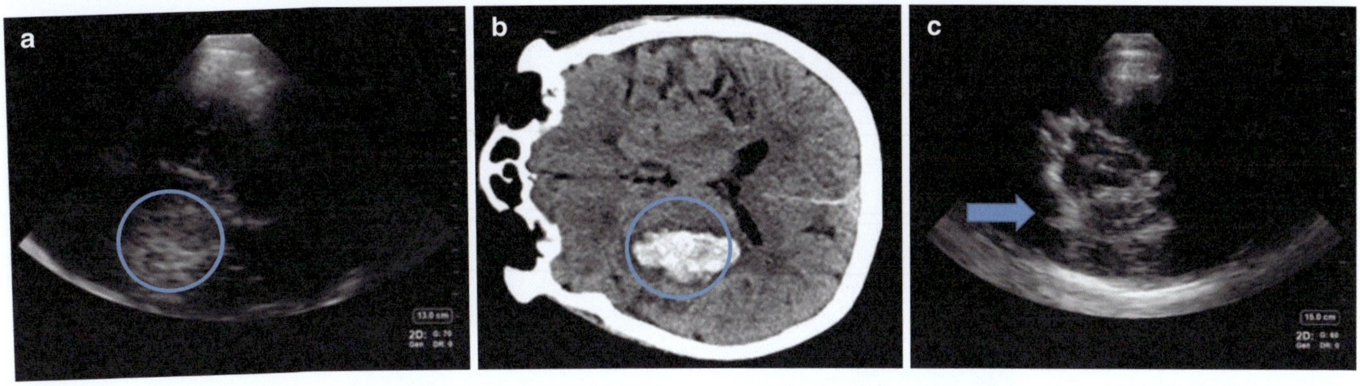

Fig. 16.10 Intraparenchymal hemorrhage. (**a**) Cranial ultrasound image showing a focal area of increased echogenicity (blue circle) reflecting an intracerebral hemorrhage and shadowing from the linear hyperechoic falx cerebri. (**b**) Non-contrast computed tomography of the brain for the same patient in (**a**) showing intracerebral hemorrhage (blue circle). (**c**) Posterior enhancement artifact (arrow) and hyperechoic signals created by choroid in the basal cisterns responsible for a false positive appearance of intracranial hemorrhage

echoic artifacts produced by ependyma and choroid within the ventricles in the transtemporal window.

The size of the intracranial hemorrhage and resultant cerebral edema (assessed via the presence of midline shift) can also be monitored serially over time. The overall diagnostic accuracy of B-mode ultrasound in subdural hemorrhage detection has been low due to the variable densities of most subdural hemorrhages. Of note, the echogenicity of the hematoma is not indicative of chronicity since chronic subdural hematomas can show hyperechoic signals created by the presence of septations. Epidural hemorrhage is typically seen with hyperacute extra-axial bleeds and, when visualized, has a distinct hyperechoic signal of the dura, separating it from the underlying mixed echogenicity brain parenchyma and encasing a hypoechoic area of acute blood.

To visualize an intracranial hemorrhage, the contralateral brain parenchyma is insonated using the transtemporal window described above. Acute intraparenchymal hemorrhage less than one week old appears as a hyperechoic area surrounded by normal brain echogenicity (Fig. 16.10). Suspected hemorrhage should be imaged in multiple planes by rotating the probe to reduce the possibility of false positivity from hyperechoic artifacts [33]. The volume can be measured by obtaining orthogonal images in the axial and coronal planes. One study of 48 patients with acute supratentorial cerebral hemorrhage reported good correlation between POCUS and CT for longitudinal, sagittal, and coronal diameter, as well as hematoma volume ($r = 0.907$; $r = 0.811$, $r = 0.595$, and $r = 0.856$, respectively) [36]. The dural border of the arachnoid space has a highly echogenic structure that defines the dural space's proximal aspect in the brain's contralateral hemisphere. The subdural space lies between this dural border and the hyperechoic skull. Hyperechoic material in this space with obliteration of the fine skull line seen in the contralateral space indicates a subdural hemorrhage (Fig. 16.11).

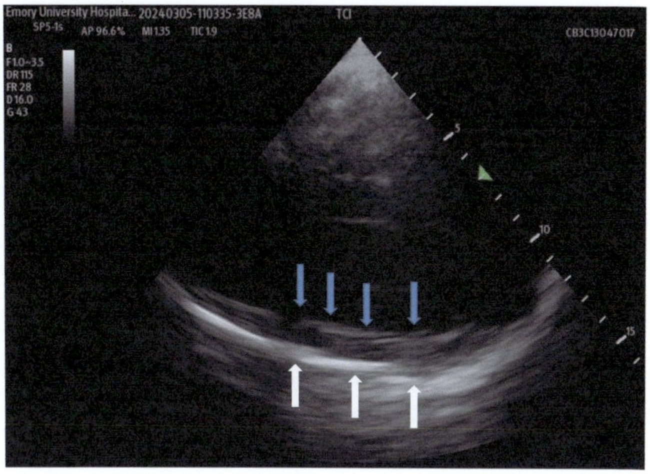

Fig. 16.11 B-mode ultrasound through the right temporal window showing hyperechoic shadowing and left subdural hemorrhage (blue arrows) against the hyperechoic signal of the opposite skull (white arrows). *(Image courtesy of Erika Sigman, MD)*

Midline Shift

Midline shift occurs when mass lesions, bleeding, or acute ischemia lead to cerebral edema and subsequent displacement of brain parenchyma. POCUS may be used to evaluate midline shift in select cases (e.g., limited resource settings, if the patient is too unstable for CT) by identifying displaced anatomic landmarks, although CT remains the gold standard diagnostic modality [2, 4, 7]. It is often difficult to reproduce the same axial section and angle of insonation to image the opposite skull to ensure an accurate measurement. Therefore, serial measurements of midline shift are more helpful than absolute measurements. While any amount of midline shift is considered abnormal, a clinically significant midline shift may be as small as 2 mm [38, 39].

Measurement of midline shift at the midbrain level can be performed through the temporal window in the mesence-

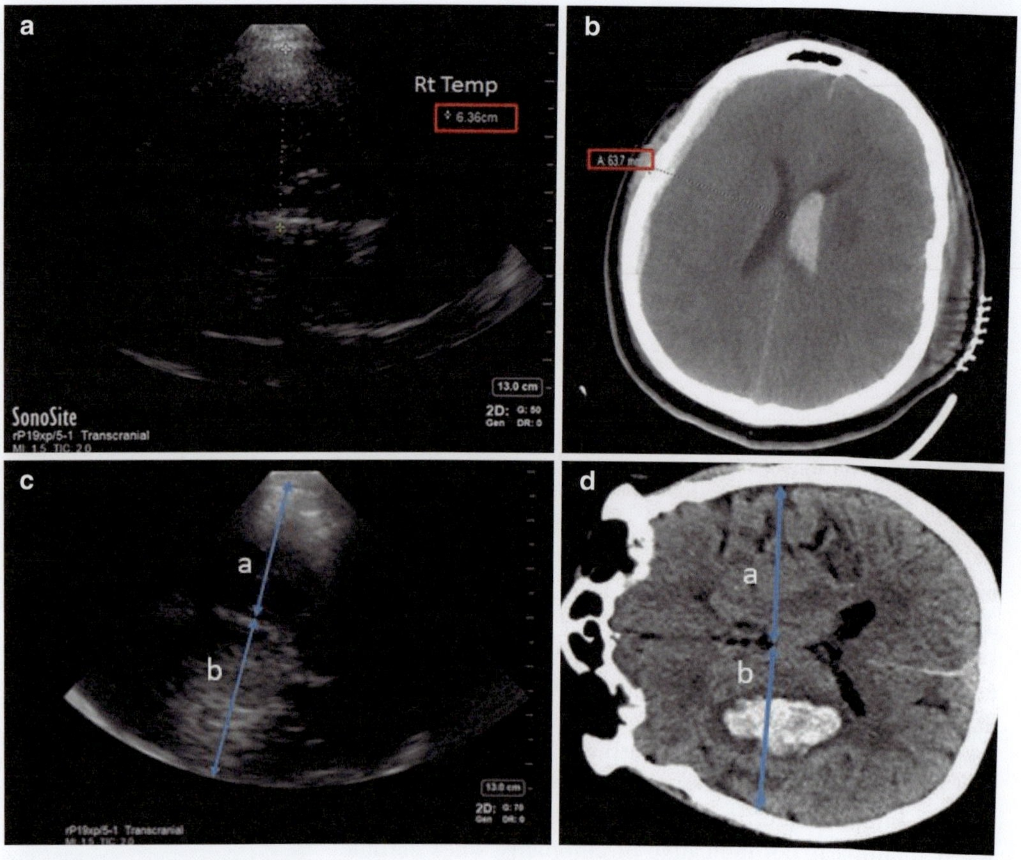

Fig. 16.12 POCUS imaging for midline shift. (**a**) Insonation from right temporal bone to septum pellucidum measuring 6.36 cm. (**b**) CT corresponding to the patient in (**a**) demonstrating a similar distance from the right temporal bone to the septum pellucidum as found on POCUS. (**c**) Cross-sectional image showing use of the temporal window to do ipsilateral and contralateral measurements of the midline structure (third ventricle) to skull distance in a patient with an intraparenchymal hemorrhage in the far field. (**d**) Corresponding CT imaging of the same patient in image (**c**) demonstrating similar measures

phalic, diencephalic, or ventricular plane, depending on the pathology (Fig. 16.12). The septum pellucidum or falx cerebri can be a useful midline marker in frontal lesions, whereas pineal gland or third ventricle displacement may be more appropriate to measure in temporal lesions. Midline shift is best measured as the distance from the ipsilateral temporal bone to the center of the relevant visible midline structure (e.g., third ventricle, septum pellucidum, falx cerebri, or pineal gland) and from that midline structure to the inner margin of the opposite skull. When the inner bone of the ipsilateral skull is not clearly visible, measurements can be performed from the top of the image to the midline structure. Any discrepancies between these two measurements may indicate the presence of midline shift [2]. To increase reliability during serial assessments, insonation should be done using the same temporal window (right or left) to get a cross section showing similar anatomical orientation of visible structures. For example, the most convex portion of the skull can be kept at the bottom part of the screen with midbrain or lateral ventricles visible in the same orientation when reproducing acquisition.

Hydrocephalus

The gold standard imaging modality for hydrocephalus remains CT. B-mode POCUS has been an area of interest due to its repeatability, low radiation exposure, and potential to visualize ventricular size [40, 41]. In one small study, the correlation between POCUS and CT measurements of the third ventricle's width (r = 0.83–0.95), the right (r = 0.86) and left (r = 0.92) frontal horns, and the middle part (r = 0.73) of the lateral ventricles was high, though other studies have shown that adequate visualization of the ventricles remains a concern [41, 42]. The cerebral aqueduct and other anatomic structures may also be mistaken for the third ventricle, leading to false positives.

Hydrocephalus is evaluated using the transtemporal window to visualize the midbrain with the probe tilted upwards approximately 10–15° from the mesencephalic view to obtain a transverse view of the third ventricle. Intracranial ventricles appear as pulsating pairs of hyperechoic lines in B-mode that elongate when rotating the probe. The largest transverse diameter of the third ventricle should be measured with the place of insonation adjusted to obtain an axial section of the midbrain showing symmetrical cerebral peduncles (Fig. 16.13). The angle to the opposite skull should be maintained on serial measurements to increase the accuracy for detecting a change. There is high variability in the normal size of the third ventricles due to the inconsistent plane in which measurements are done and inherent variability in the size of the third ventricle due to age-related cerebral atrophy. Average values vary and can be 1.2–5.1 mm in patients under 60 years of age, and 3.3–9.2 mm in those over 60 years of

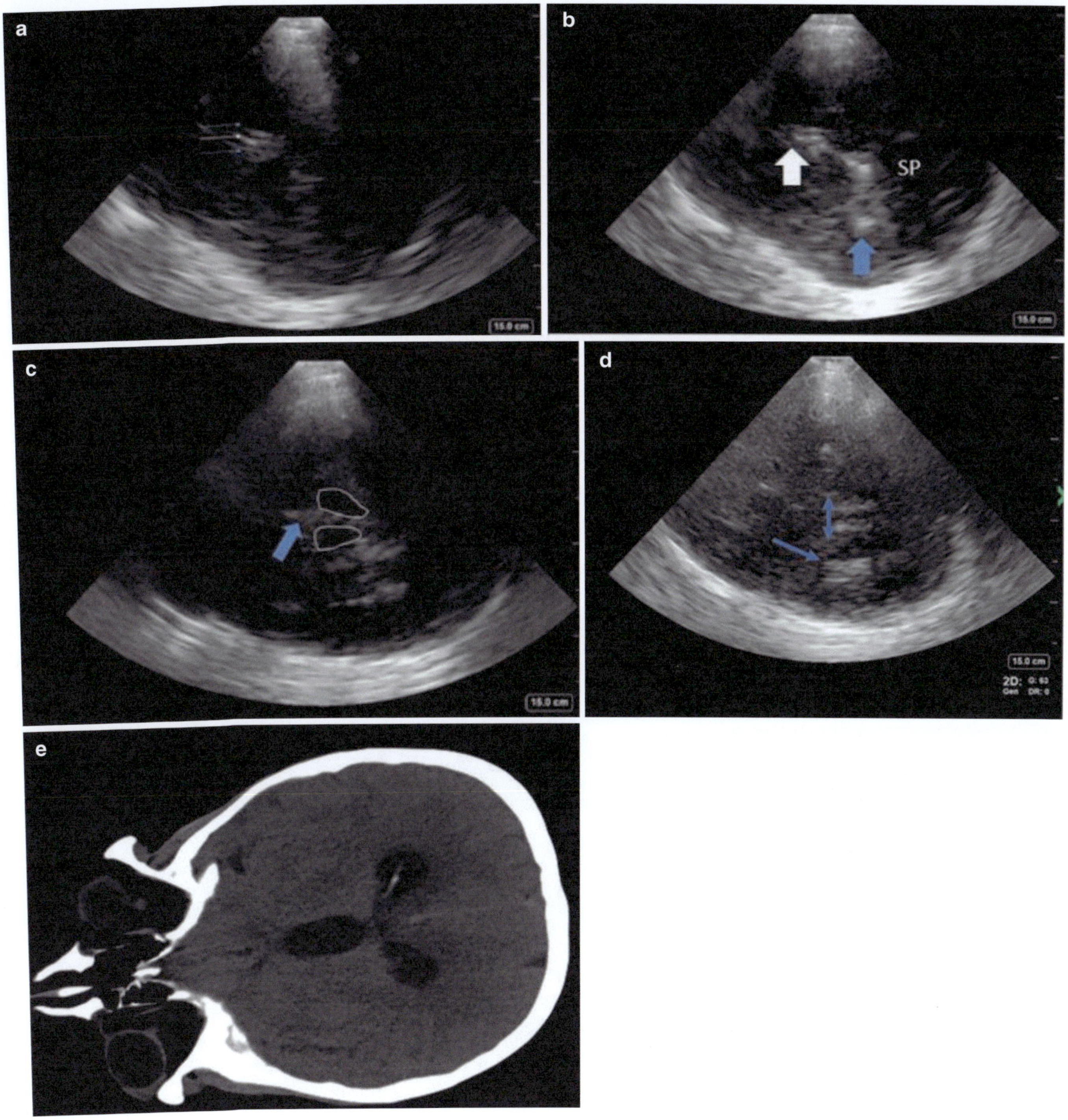

Fig. 16.13 B-mode ultrasound showing different planes in which ventricles can be visualized. (**a**) Cross-section of the brain in the ventricular plane showing the frontal horns of the lateral ventricles (thin blue arrows) separated by the septum pellucidum (white arrow). (**b**) Lateral ventricles are sometimes visible only by the hyperechoic shadows produced by the choroid without obvious visualization of the cerebrospinal fluid-containing hypoechoic ventricular cavity. Arrows represent the frontal (white arrow) and temporal (blue arrow) horns. (**c**) Cross-section in the diencephalic plane demonstrating the thalamus (outlined on each side) with the third ventricle (blue arrow). The cavity of the third ventricle is obscured by the hyperechoic signals from the choroid. (**d**) Third ventricular enlargement (blue arrows) in a patient with acute hydrocephalus on B-mode cranial ultrasound. (**e**) The corresponding cross-sectional imaging on non-contrast computed tomography for the image in (**d**)

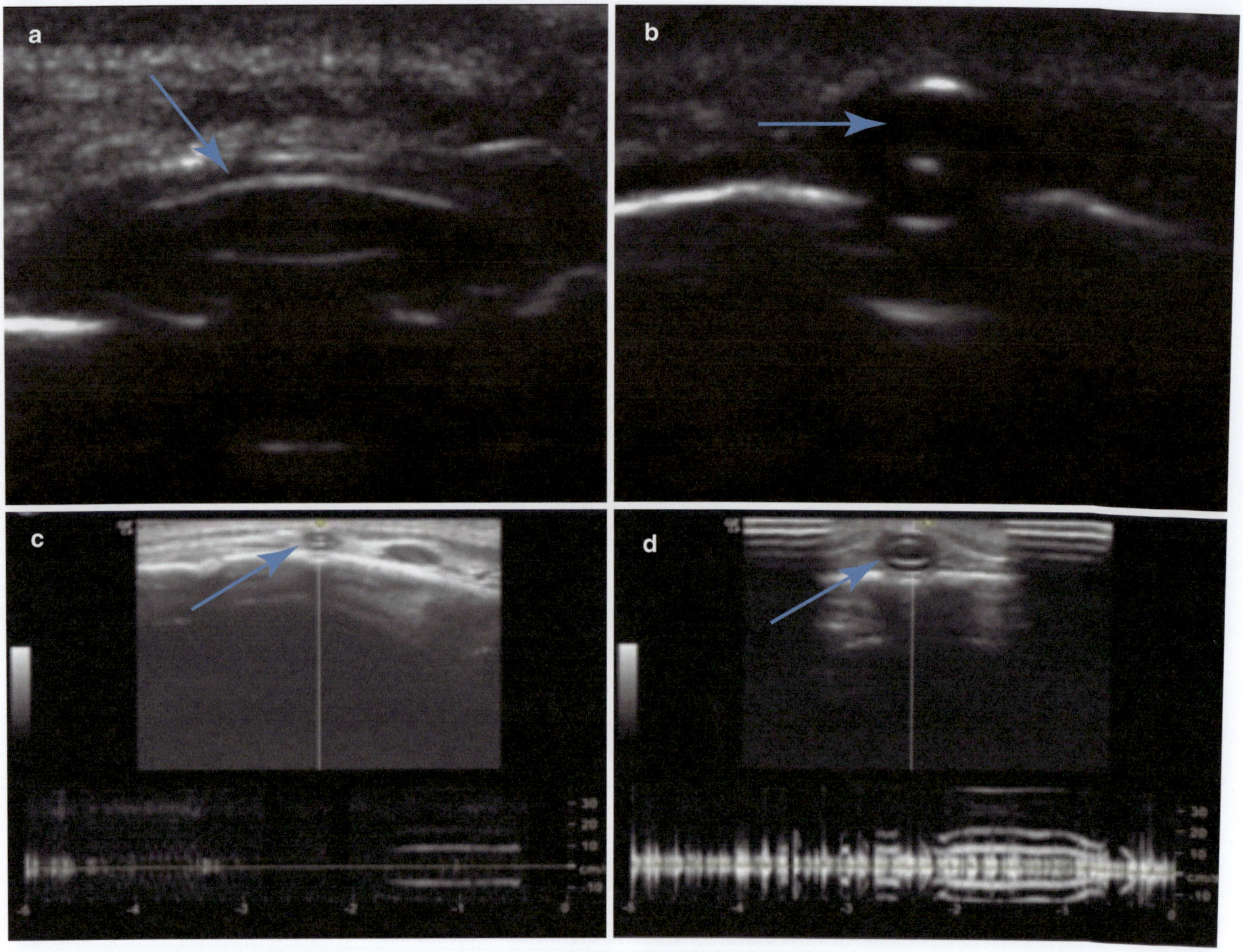

Fig. 16.14 Assessment of ventriculoperitoneal shunt with ultrasound. (**a**) Ultrasound images of the Rickham reservoir (arrow). *Copyright: © 2013 Vega RA Reproduced from Vega et al.* [45]. (**b**) Ultrasound images of the distal catheter tubing (arrow). *Copyright: © 2013 Vega RA Reproduced from Vega et al.* [45]. (**c**) Localization of VP shunt tube (blue arrow) in soft tissue of the scalp. (**d**) Detection of VP shunt flow in M-mode. The flow in the VP shunt is observed distal to the chamber by pressing/releasing the chamber. This presents as fluctuating M-mode signals as CSF flows through the distal section of the VP shunt. In the absence of flow, the M-mode signal shows symmetric signals like a barcode

age [43]. Ventricular measurements should always be obtained and validated with the patient's CT of the head, allowing serial measurements to provide higher accuracy for detecting a change in the ventricular size. Importantly, hydrocephalus evaluation is highly operator-dependent and requires a high level of skill [18].

For patients with known hydrocephalus and a ventriculoperitoneal (VP) shunt, POCUS may be used to assess patency and functionality, although the evidence for this technique is limited [44]. When scalp thickness precludes palpation of the shunt, ultrasound can also facilitate localization of the reservoir to facilitate a VP shunt tap (Fig. 16.14a, b) [45]. After localizing the shunt via palpation or ultrasound, the linear probe is placed distal to the shunt chamber. M-mode or color Doppler can be used to visualize the shunt while the shunt chamber is compressed and released [46]. If the shunt functions properly, the flow will be present in M-mode (Fig. 16.14c, d). Finally, an abdominal ultrasound may reveal free fluid in the peritoneum, indirectly suggesting VP shunt patency.

Post-Hemicraniectomy Assessment

In patients who undergo a hemicraniectomy, underlying neurological deficits may preclude detection of an acute pathology. Hemicraniectomy can be a life-saving decompressive surgery, but can be complicated by intracranial hemorrhage, subdural or epidural hematoma contralateral to the craniectomy defect, and post-traumatic hydrocephalus [47]. Absence

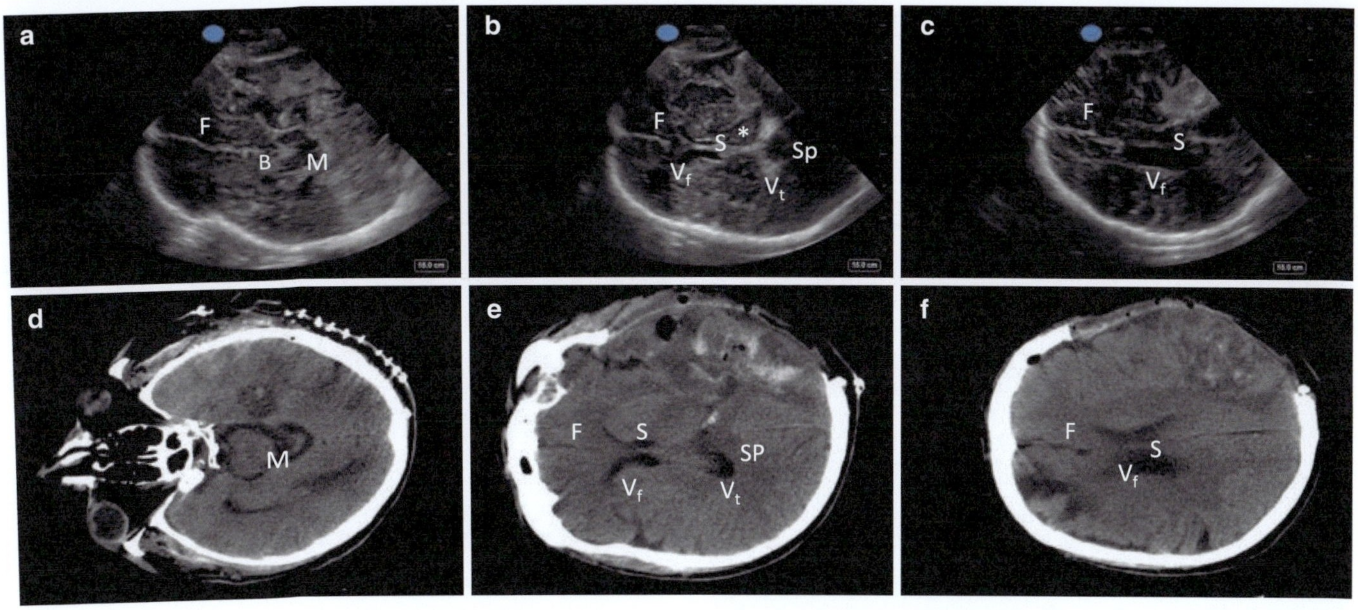

Fig. 16.15 Hemicraniectomy patient with B-mode ultrasound images in the upper panel showing the axial cross section of the brain with a probe placed gently on the craniectomy defect site and corresponding CT brain non-contrast images in the lower panel. (**a**) Mesencephalic plane on ultrasound. F falx cerebri, *B* mammillary bodies, *M* midbrain. (**b**) Diencephalic plane on ultrasound. Thalamic structures are visible as hypoechoic structures on either side of the midline (asterisk). *F* falx cerebri, *S* septum pellucidum, *Sp* splenium of corpus callosum, *Vt* temporal horn of lateral ventricle, *Vf* frontal horn of lateral ventricle. (**c**) Ventricular plane on ultrasound. *F* falx cerebri, *S* septum pellucidum, *Vf* frontal horn of lateral ventricle. (**d**) CT imaging corresponding to Figure (**a**). (**e**) CT imaging corresponding to Figure (**b**). (**f**) CT imaging corresponding to Figure (**c**)

of the skull facilitates ultrasound insonation, which should be performed using the abdominal preset to delineate the anatomical characteristics as well as to reduce the power of ultrasound through reduced mechanical and thermal index. Intracranial structures are more easily discernible in these patients (Fig. 16.15).

Evaluation of Acute Ischemic Stroke

Ultrasound has good test characteristics for detecting large cerebral artery occlusion, with a sensitivity of 81.8% and specificity of 94% [48, 49]. However, Doppler signals can be affected by insufficient acoustic bone windows and operator experience [50]. While CT angiography is the diagnostic modality of choice for large vessel occlusion during acute stroke evaluation, ultrasound can be helpful in patients who have severe contrast allergies or when there are unanticipated delays in obtaining CT angiography. POCUS imaging for acute stroke should include evaluation of all vessels that can be insonated through the temporal and occipital windows, focusing on the vessel suspected to be occluded based on the patient's clinical presentation. Ultrasound can also complement the information obtained from a CT angiography by elaborating the hemodynamic significance of the stenosis. Focal and segmental hemodynamically significant intracranial stenosis can be diagnosed by pulsed-wave Doppler showing a high-resistance waveform proximal to the lesion followed by a post-stenotic waveform, which is characterized by a delayed, slow-rising upstroke with decreased flow velocity (referred to as *parvus et tardus*; Fig. 16.16) [49]. Lesser degrees of stenosis may cause high velocities without any visible change in waveforms [51]. If post-stenotic waveforms are present in all anterior circulation vessels on one side but waveforms on the other side of the brain have normal waveforms, more proximal carotid stenosis (or innominate artery stenosis on the right side) should be suspected. If both the anterior and posterior circulation show post-stenotic waveforms, proximal extracerebral pathology, such as significant aortic stenosis, should be considered [52].

TCCS has been investigated to predict responsiveness and monitor the efficacy of thrombolytics and endovascular thrombectomy [53]. Though TCCS-based prediction of recanalization after thrombolysis in large vessel occlusions has been largely replaced in the thrombectomy era, the role of TCCS post-thrombectomy is still being explored in evaluating early neurological deterioration that occurs in 15–30% of these patients [10, 54–60]. Additionally, hyperperfusion after recanalization post-thrombolysis or post-thrombectomy is an active area of investigation, and TCCS-based flow velocities are being investigated to guide patient-specific blood pressure goals and to reduce the risk of post-reperfusion intracranial hemorrhage [61–64].

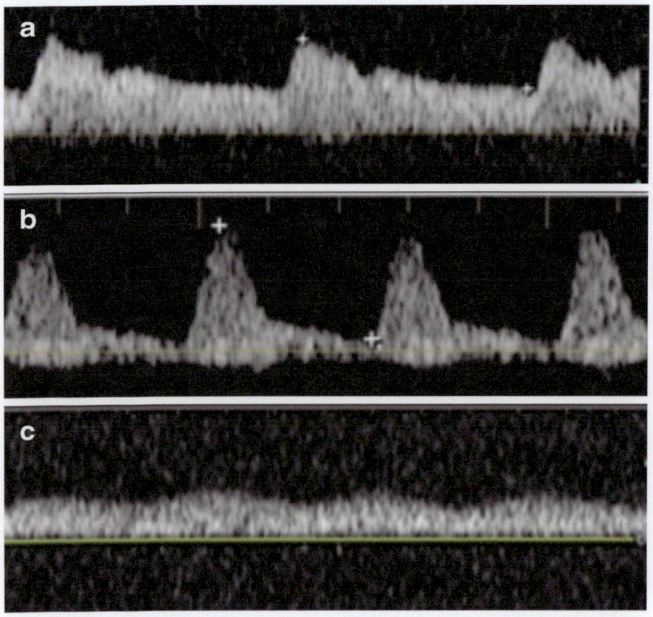

Fig. 16.16 Pulsed-wave Doppler waveforms obtained from insonation of the middle cerebral artery. (**a**) Normal physiological low-resistance waveforms characterized by rapid systolic upstroke, stepwise systolic deceleration, and an end-diastolic velocity one-third to one-half of the peak flow velocity. (**b**) Resistive waveforms showing rapid systolic upstroke as well rapid systolic deceleration with end-diastolic velocity less than one-fourth the peak flow velocity. Resistive waveforms can be caused by focal intramural stenosis or extramural compression of a vessel. (**c**) Post-stenotic waveforms of *parvus et tardus* that can be insonated in segments distal to the area of high-grade stenosis

TCCS can also be used to guide management in stroke patients with radiological-clinical mismatch in consultation with the neuro-interventionalist [65]. TCCS is the only modality that can demonstrate active micro-embolization as an etiology of acute ischemic stroke by the detection of high-intensity transient signals (HITS) (Fig. 16.17) [66]. Circulating microemboli create ultrasound waves that are backscattered from the surface of emboli and manifest as HITS. These are characteristically 3 dB greater than the spectral background with a short duration of less than 300 milliseconds.

Lastly, TCCS-based evaluation of collateralization can be performed via insonation of the ophthalmic artery through the orbital window. Presence of a reversed ophthalmic artery (i.e., blood flow from the ECA branches to the intracranial ICA through the ophthalmic artery, as opposed to expected flow of blood from the ICA to the ophthalmic artery) can be a sign of intracranial stenosis with compensation of blood flow from the opposite hemisphere (Fig. 16.18). The ophthalmic artery is typically the last of the many collaterals that can maintain blood flow through the MCA when the ICA has stenosis or an occlusion proximal to the origin of the ophthalmic artery. The ophthalmic artery pulls blood from the ECA branches to perfuse the MCA via the ICA. Reversal of the ACA can thus be an early sign of collateralization and ipsilateral ICA stenosis or occlusion, if the anterior communicating artery is patent.

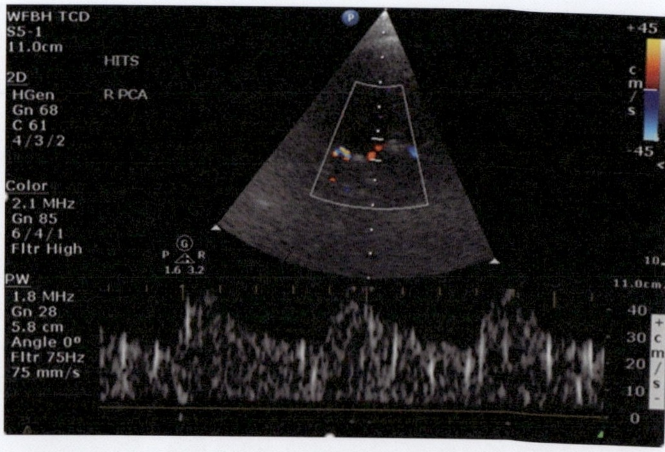

Fig. 16.17 Transcranial Doppler insonation of the posterior cerebral artery through the temporal window. Pulsed-wave Doppler is interpreted by high-intensity transient signals (HITS) which represent active microemboli passing through the insonated vessel at the time of insonation. These can be seen as hyperechoic vertical lines standing out against the backdrop of spectral Doppler waveforms

Intracranial Hypertension

Use of TCCS for intracranial pressure (ICP) estimation can be performed using qualitative waveform analysis or quantitative flow velocities [67]. Increased ICP caused by cerebral edema or hydrocephalus (i.e., perfusion-limiting ICP or oligemic ICP) increases the outflow resistance to cerebral blood flow, which manifests as a high-resistance waveform in the major cerebral arteries. Figure 16.16 shows the transition of waveforms when an intramural compression causes high resistance, where resistive waveforms show low diastolic flow with post-stenotic waveforms downstream. Increased ICP causes a more global increase in outflow resistance by extramural compression and shows changes in waveforms from low resistance to high resistance, as shown in Fig. 16.19, but will generally not result in post-stenotic waveforms [26, 67].

High-resistance patterns may be physiological patterns at baseline seen in patients at older age or with advanced atherosclerosis. Globally, high-resistance patterns can be seen in hyperventilation as well. The high-resistance pattern seen in vessel stenosis caused by vasospasm or thrombus is seen only in affected vessels. Serial acute changes in resistance throughout the circle of Willis are classically more indicative of increased ICP if other factors have been ruled out and baseline TCD waveforms are low resistance. High-resistance patterns reflect increased ICP and should guide the escalation of ICP-lowering therapies, whether these are medical or surgical (depending on the pathophysiology of the acute brain injury).

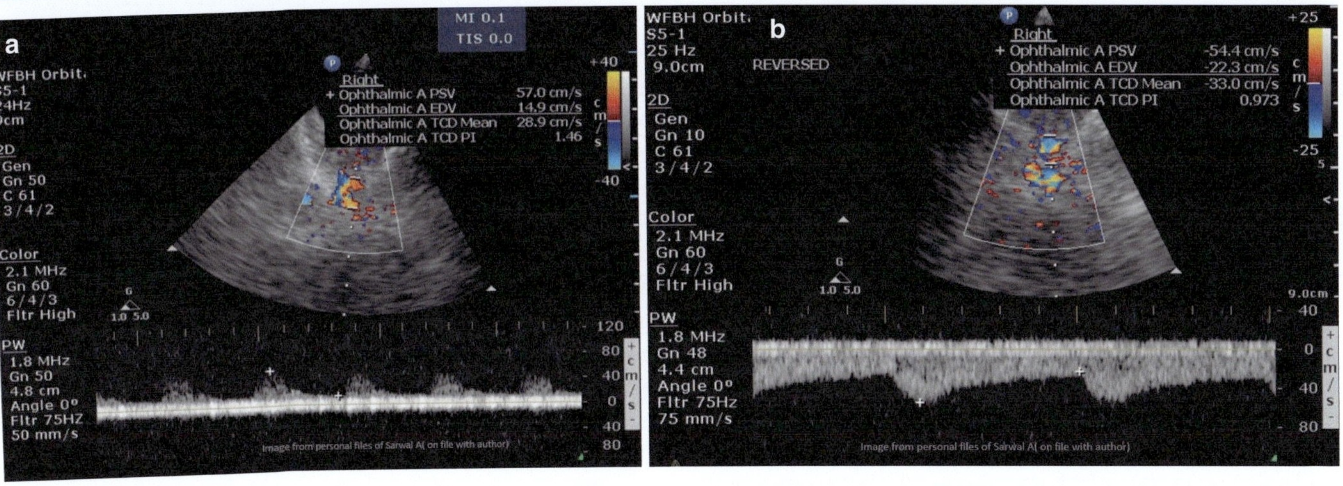

Fig. 16.18 Transcranial Doppler insonation through the orbital window to visualize the flow of the ophthalmic artery. (**a**) The physiological direction of flow of blood in the ophthalmic artery is toward the probe, appearing as a positive Doppler shift. This designates flow from the internal carotid artery to the ophthalmic artery. (**b**) Pathological reversal of flow in the ophthalmic artery occurs when blood flows from the extracranial external carotid artery to the intracranial internal carotid artery (ICA) through the ophthalmic artery due to occlusion or stenosis in ICA proximal to the origin of the ophthalmic artery. This allows the ICA to feed the ipsilateral middle cerebral artery in settings of flow-limiting stenosis or occlusion

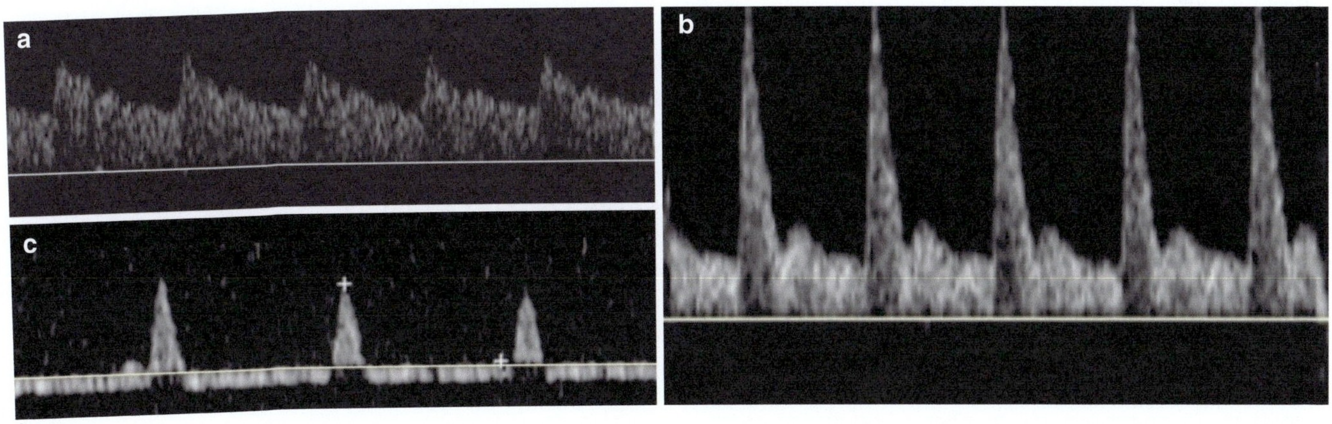

Fig. 16.19 Progression of transcranial Doppler waveforms with increasing intracranial pressure (ICP) after acute brain injury causing decreasing cerebral perfusion pressure in relation to systemic mean arterial pressure (MAP). (**a**) Normal waveforms with sharp systolic upstroke, stepwise systolic deceleration, and robust diastolic flow with end-diastolic velocity one-half to one-third of peak systolic velocity. This suggests ICP are within normal range and much lower than the MAP. (**b**) Increased peak systolic flow with decreasing diastolic flow and eventual blunting of diastolic flow. This suggests ICP is approaching the diastolic pressures and close to the MAP. (**c**) When ICP is significantly higher than diastolic pressure, but below the systemic systolic blood pressure, the heart maintains antegrade flow to brain during the systolic part of the cardiac cycle but cerebral flow is reversed during diastole. This creates an oscillating flow pattern (forward flow in systole and reversed flow in diastole) that denotes no net forward flow or no net cerebral perfusion. Permanence of this flow pattern in a patient with unsalvageable injury denotes impending cerebral circulatory arrest. Further increase in ICP causes flow during only part of systole, appearing as systolic stumps on TCCS waveforms followed by a complete absence of flow and cerebral circulatory arrest

Persistent high-resistance patterns despite ICP-lowering therapies are an ominous sign. Figure 16.19 shows the progression of the waveforms as ICP increases in relation to the patient's systemic blood pressure. Progression of high-resistance waveforms to oscillating patterns with to-and-fro blood flow (i.e., towards the brain during systole and away from the brain during diastole) or systolic stumps (i.e., minimal low velocity blood flow seen only during early systole) suggest impending cerebral circulatory arrest. Persistence of these patterns on serial TCD performed at least 30 minutes apart are the foundational criteria for the use of TCD as an ancillary test to evaluate death by neurological criteria in the appropriate clinical setting.

Giant Cell Arteritis

Giant cell arteritis (GCA), also known as temporal arteritis, is an autoimmune vasculitis affecting medium and large blood vessels, particularly the external carotid artery branches [68]. Temporal artery ultrasound has been an increasingly utilized modality in diagnosing GCA. The most common temporal artery ultrasound protocol utilizes the high-frequency linear probe to scan both superficial temporal arteries (Fig. 16.20) [69]. The probe is placed anterior and superior to the ear, with the indicator towards the patient's eye. The temporal artery is superficial and is typically found at a depth of 4-5 mm. A complete examination includes evaluating the common superficial temporal artery and all three temporal artery branches (superficial, parietal, and frontal) in long- and short-axis views. The exam typically begins with the common superficial branch, sliding superiorly to examine the distal parietal branch, followed by the frontal branch. A normal temporal artery is a thin-walled structure with an anechoic lumen [69]. GCA may present visually with a 'halo sign', defined as reduced luminal size in the presence of circumferential hypoechoic vessel wall thickening [70]. Color Doppler may help differentiate the true lumen from circumferential peri-arterial edema. False positives have been described in a minority of patients [71].

While there are no definitive criteria for temporal artery ultrasound measurements of intimal medial complex thickness in GCA, a normal temporal artery has an intimal medial thickness of 0.2 mm, while an inflamed artery ranges from 0.5 to 0.9 mm [72, 73]. In addition, a normal temporal artery is compressible and will "disappear" when applying pressure with the probe. The 'compression sign' (persistent visualization of the temporal artery during compression) has a specificity of 100% and sensitivity of 75% for the diagnosis of GCA [74]. The current recommended standard is to diagnose vasculitis based on the presence of a 'halo sign', a non-compressible artery ('compression sign'), and a wide intima-media thickness (IMT). In equivocal cases, a thickened IMT of the facial, subclavian, or axillary artery on the same side may support diagnosis of GCA. Recently, an ultrasound score has been proposed to predict the positive likelihood of a positive temporal artery biopsy in a patient with high pre-test probability based on clinical presentation that utilizes IMT in the common superficial temporal artery, frontal temporal artery, parietal temporal artery, temporal, and axillary artery (Table 16.2) [75].

Literature continues to be conflicting on the diagnostic accuracy of temporal artery ultrasound, with multiple systematic reviews over the last two decades showing a sensitivity of 55-77% and a specificity of 81–100% [76–78]. While this is routinely used in rheumatology clinics, there has been recent interest in using this for screening patients in the acute care setting [79]. However, other techniques such as CT, MRI, and temporal artery biopsy remain necessary to confirm the diagnosis or rule out other conditions [68, 79]. Despite this, the use of temporal artery ultrasound for screening has been endorsed by many societies, including the European Alliance of Associations for Rheumatology (EULAR) and the American College of Rheumatology (ACR)/EULAR Classification Criteria. They recommend ultrasound of the temporal and possibly the axillary arteries as the first-line imaging modality in patients with suspected predominantly cranial GCA and that a non-compressible 'halo sign' is the ultrasound finding most suggestive of GCA. Given the challenge of making this diagnosis, multi-modality imaging may enhance diagnostic confidence.

Carotid Artery Pathology

Carotid artery ultrasound is an emerging POCUS application that can be used to evaluate a variety of carotid artery pathology with CNS implications, including thrombus, pseudoaneurysm, dissection flaps, and luminal stenosis, particularly when CT angiography is delayed or not accessible. While diagnostic carotid ultrasound performed by trained sonographers has been the mainstay of carotid stenosis evaluation for

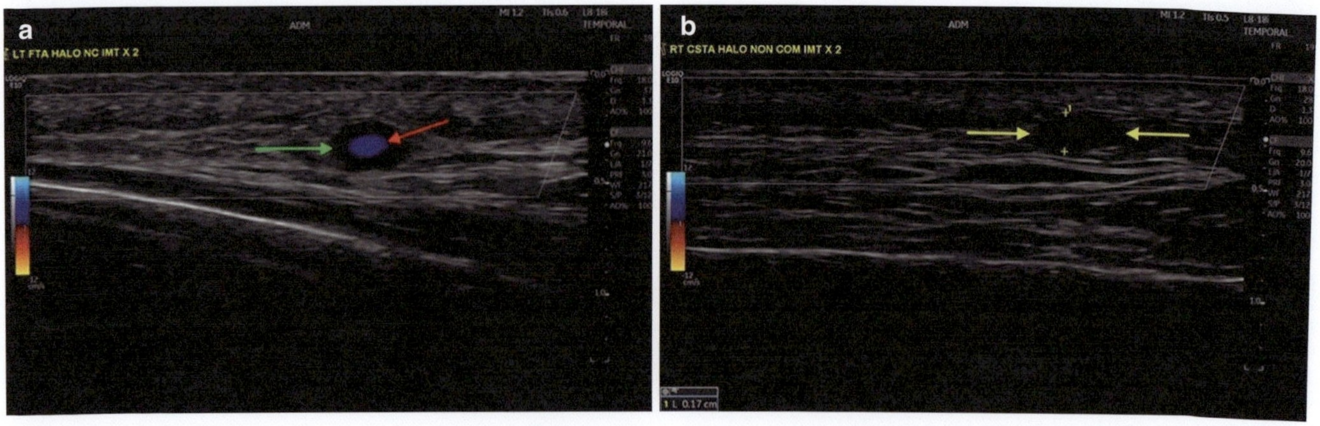

Fig. 16.20 Temporal artery ultrasound. (**a**) Short-axis view of the frontal branch of the superficial temporal artery, demonstrating a "halo sign," as indicated by the anechoic region (green arrow) surrounding the inner Doppler (red arrow) signal. (**b**) "Compression sign" via the short-axis view of the superficial temporal artery. The hypoechoic region between two parallel hyperechoic lines (adventitia) represents an edematous intima-media complex (region between two yellow arrows). *Copyright: © 2022 Kirby, Flood, Mullan, Murphy and Kane* [80]

Table 16.2 Total Halo Score. An ultrasound score incorporating maximal intima-media thickness (IMT) and bilaterality of the superficial temporal artery/axillary artery halos predicting likelihood of a positive temporal artery biopsy

Halo score	Common superficial TA	Frontal TA	Parietal TA	Axillary artery
0	≤0.3	≤0.1	≤0.2	≤0.5
1	0.31–0.4	0.11–0.2	0.21–0.3	0.51–0.6
2	0.41–0.5	0.21–0.3	0.31–0.4	0.61–0.89
3	0.51–0.79	0.31–0.49	0.41–0.59	0.9–1.59
4	≥0.8	≥0.5	≥0.6	≥1.6

Each branch is assigned a score based on the maximal IMT identified in that branch. Scores are added to give a Total Halo Score with a maximum of 48 [75]
TA temporal artery

decades and recommended by several guidelines, use of carotid POCUS in the acute and critical care settings has more limited literature [16, 81]. In one emergency department-based study of 70 patients, carotid POCUS was shown to have a sensitivity of 70% and a specificity of 86% for detecting the presence of >50% carotid stenosis [16].

POCUS applications of carotid ultrasound during an acute neurological crisis include evaluation for the presence of a thrombus, mobile plaque, dissection, or pseudoaneurysm. Evaluation of carotid stenosis and occlusion is typically done using B-mode, color Doppler, and pulsed-wave Doppler. High blood flow velocities allow the carotid arterial plaque or apparent stenosis to be both qualitatively and quantitatively identified.

The bifurcation of the carotid is the typical seat of atherosclerotic disease due to turbulence of flow. While stenosis is a diffuse and circumferential process, an arterial plaque generally presents as an acute area of thickening. Color Doppler is first used to look for the presence of hypoechoic plaques not otherwise visible on B-mode and aliasing that may point towards high velocity and turbulent flow (Fig. 16.21a). A thorough investigation of velocities around the plaque is key to ensuring that the area of highest velocity is not missed. The Society of Radiologists in Ultrasound consensus panel defined six Doppler velocity cut points for classifying internal carotid artery stenosis of 50% and 70% (Table 16.3) [82]. These criteria are based on meta-analyses of clinical trials that show high sensitivity and specificity of velocity-based criteria to categorize the degree of hemodynamically significant stenosis in broad categories of <50% stenosis, 50–69% stenosis, and >70% stenosis that correlate with thresholds for medical and surgical treatment of carotid stenosis [83, 84]. These criteria, initially published in 2003, are undergoing revision by the Intersocietal Accreditation Commission at the time of publication of this chapter [85, 86]. Clinicians should consult their local accredited vascular labs, who validate their ultrasound stenosis criteria against angiography in the local population to address which velocity cutoffs should be used.

Appropriate identification of the ECA is key when evaluating carotid stenosis. In the presence of severe carotid stenosis or occlusion, the ECA may provide a collateral channel to draw blood from the common carotid artery and shunt it to the distal intracranial ICA through a reversed ophthalmic artery or several other collateralization channels between ECA and ICA that cannot be evaluated using ultrasound. This results in the high-resistance ECA waveforms being replaced by low-resistance patterns looking very similar to ICA waveforms. In the presence of collateralization, ECA may appear "internalized," where it takes on the features of the ICA with an end-diastolic velocity much higher than the expected one-third to one-half of the peak systolic velocity. However, it can still be distinguished from ICA by the presence of branches in the neck and the appearance of oscillations in response to temporal tap (Fig. 16.9). In addition, the Intersocietal Accreditation Commission ultrasound labs typically validate carotid stenosis criteria on ultrasound against cerebral angiogram for their local population; hence, clinicians incorporating carotid stenosis assessment in their ultrasound portfolio should consult their institutional or regional vascular or neurodiagnostic laboratory that performs routine carotid ultrasounds [83]. A duplex ultrasound examination, preferably performed in an accredited vascular laboratory, is the initial diagnostic imaging of choice for evaluating the severity of carotid stenosis in both symptomatic and asymptomatic patients who need diagnostic workup for carotid disease [83]. Currently, the United States Preventive Services Task Force recommends against screening for asymptomatic carotid artery stenosis in the general adult population [87].

Carotid dissection flaps will appear as mobile hyperechoic structures within the anechoic tubular structure of the carotid artery and may be further characterized using color Doppler (Fig. 16.21b–d). Typically, dissections occur in the ICA at the base of the skull and are not visible with neck-based, B-mode ultrasound. Linear luminal walls of heterogeneous plaques can be confused with dissections, so a thorough examination in both the short- and long-axis should be performed. Common carotid artery dissections occur at the origin and can be visible on neck ultrasound.

Pseudoaneurysms are communicating channels between the carotid artery and a periarterial collection through which blood flows. Due to the different velocities of blood entering and exiting the pseudoaneurysm, swirling may also be seen on B-mode imaging. Color Doppler will reveal bidirectional, turbulent flow between the arterial lumen and the collection.

In patients presenting with an unknown history, presence of carotid stents on carotid arterial ultrasound can provide evidence of cardiovascular or cerebrovascular risk factors (Fig. 16.21e). A completely occluded carotid artery will show hyperechoic signals filling the entire lumen with no detectable pulsed-wave Doppler signals (Fig. 16.21f).

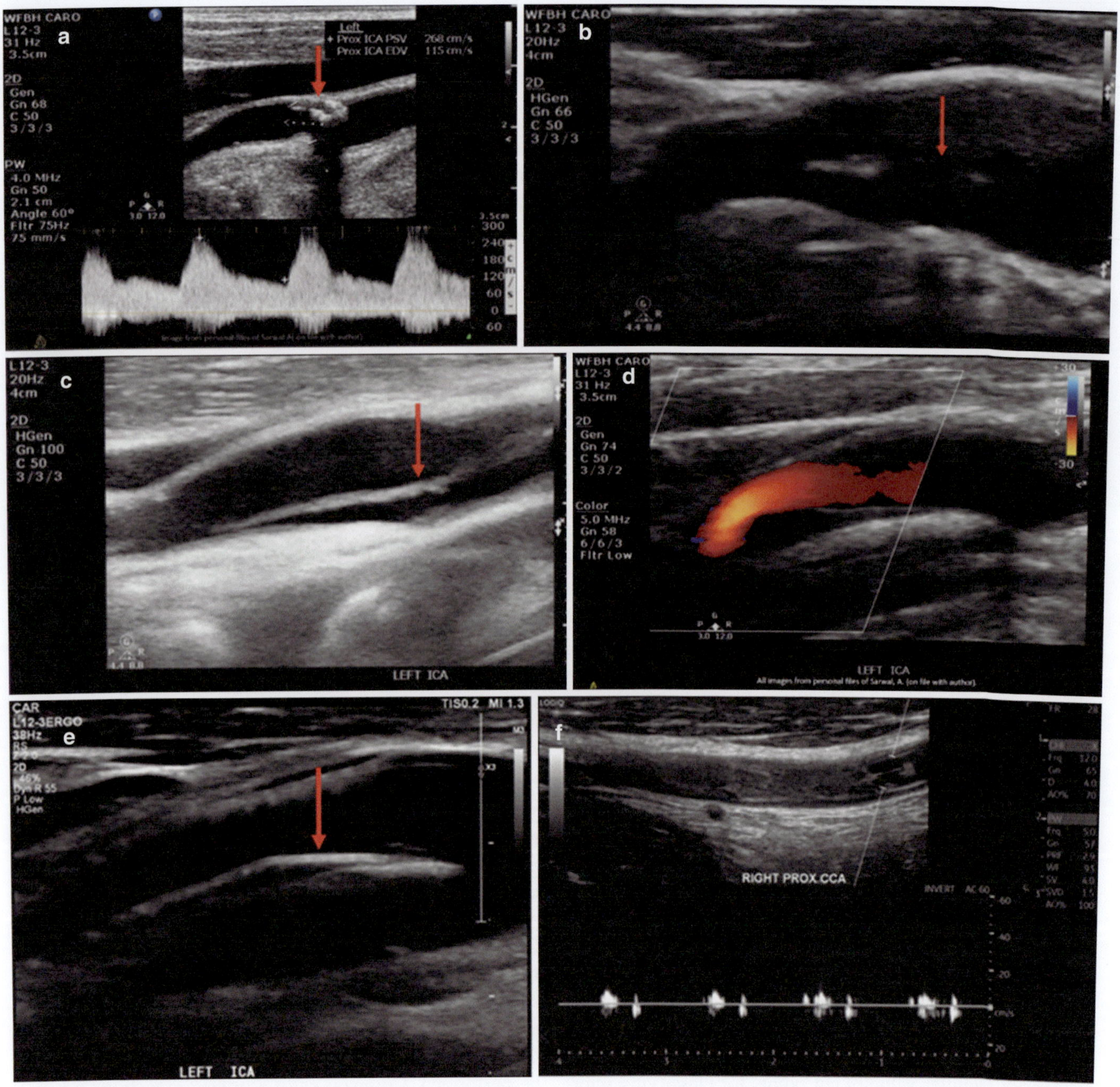

Fig. 16.21 Carotid ultrasound used to visualize various carotid pathologies. (**a**) Hyperechoic calcified carotid plaque (red arrow) at the bifurcation causing acoustic shadows on B-mode and high velocities (peak systolic velocity of 268 cm/s and end-diastolic velocity of 115 cm/s meeting the criteria for 70–99% stenosis). (**b**) Dissection flap in the left internal carotid artery (ICA) with thrombosed false lumen (red arrow). (**c**) Left ICA with an intimal flap concerning for dissection (red arrow). (**d**) Color Doppler of left ICA shows an absence of flow on color Doppler through the false lumen. (**e**) Presence of carotid stent seen as a mechanical artifact lining the carotid artery with distinct margins (Red arrow). (**f**) Complete occlusion of the common carotid artery with hyperechoic plaque filling the lumen and no flow signals insonated on pulsed-wave Doppler

Table 16.3 The Society of Radiologists in Ultrasound consensus panel criteria for diagnosis of internal carotid artery stenosis [82]

Degree of stenosis (%)	ICA PSV (cm/s)	Plaque estimate (%)	ICA/CCA PSV ratio	ICA EDV (cm/s)
Normal	<125	None	<2	<40
< 50	<125	<50	<2	<40
50–69	125–230	≥50	2–4	40–100
≥70 but less than near occlusion	>230	≥50	>4	>100
Near occlusion	High, low, or undetectable	Visible	Variable	Variable
Total occlusion	Undetectable	Visible, no detectable lumen	Not applicable	Not applicable

CCA common carotid artery, *EDV* end-diastolic velocity, *ICA* internal carotid artery, *PSV* peak systolic velocity

Pediatric Applications

Transfontanelle Ultrasound

Transfontanelle ultrasound imaging may be helpful for rapid screening of high-risk pediatric patients with open fontanelles at the bedside for increased intraventricular size or intracranial hemorrhage [88, 89]. POCUS has been shown to have a 60% sensitivity and 94% specificity for detecting intracranial pathologies in early research but has not yet been studied in large, prospective cohorts [7]. Although POCUS imaging can be performed with either a curvilinear, phased array, or linear probe placed over the anterior fontanelle, deeper structures are better visualized using the phased array due to the probe's smaller footprint over an infant's anterior fontanelle (Fig. 16.22). Once the best fontanelle location is determined to visualize the intracranial contents, the probe position should not be moved but tilted anteriorly and posterior and then from side to side.

POCUS can be used to detect hydrocephalus in infants with an increased head circumference or a bulging anterior fontanelle suggestive of increased ICP. Dilatation of the lateral ventricle over 10 mm or the third ventricle on the coronal plane over 1 mm suggests hydrocephalus [88]. Measurements for ventricular dilatation can also be used for patients with increased ventricle size associated with shunt malfunction (Fig. 16.23). Use of transcranial ultrasound to detect intracranial hemorrhage or hydrocephalus continues to be investigational but is an area of active exploration [90].

Skull Fractures

Detection of skull fractures by POCUS may be used in pediatric patients who present with blunt head trauma. Identifying the presence of skull fractures may assist in clinical management decisions for further radiological studies. One meta-analysis of seven studies and 925 patients reported 91% sensitivity and 96% specificity for diagnosing pediatric skull fractures [91].

To evaluate a potential skull fracture, a high-frequency linear probe should be placed over the area of injury, often characterized by a hematoma, abrasion, or soft tissue swelling. Skull fractures are identified as an area of discontinuity of the bony cortex, which is usually in a vertical or oblique line (Fig. 16.24) [9]. For younger children with intact suture lines, it is essential to distinguish fractures from suture lines by identifying the location of sutures and comparing the suture lines to the contralateral side of the skull or following the continuation of the suture lines between the anterior and posterior fontanelles (Figs. 16.25 and 16.26) [9]. Sonographic features of patients with skull fractures may appear similar to those of suture lines. While the presence of soft tissue swelling may assist in indicating the presence of an injury, not all skull fractures have accompanying swelling.

Subgaleal Hematomas and Cephalohematomas

Similar to diagnosing skull fractures, the examination begins with placing a high-frequency linear probe over the area of interest, which is often identified by associated soft tissue swelling. Ultrasound images over scalp hematomas may appear to be hypoechoic or hyperechoic with simultaneous detection on ultrasound. Since scalp hematomas are generally a slow expansion from initial blunt trauma, color Doppler may not detect any flow within the hematomas. Differentiating subgaleal hematomas from cephalohematomas is difficult on POCUS due to the need for identification of suture lines, which may not be discretly visible. Cephalohematomas do not cross suture lines, whereas subgaleal hematomas may cross suture lines (Fig. 16.27) [8].

Subgaleal hematoma is often caused by blunt head trauma and is defined by the presence of blood between the epicranial aponeurosis and the periosteum of the skull (Fig. 16.28). Cephalohematoma may be caused by birth traumas, mainly when forceps are used for delivery, and is defined by blood trapped under the periosteum. POCUS use as an adjunct to traditional diagnostic neuroimaging modalities is limited to case reports in the acute care setting and needs further investigation [8].

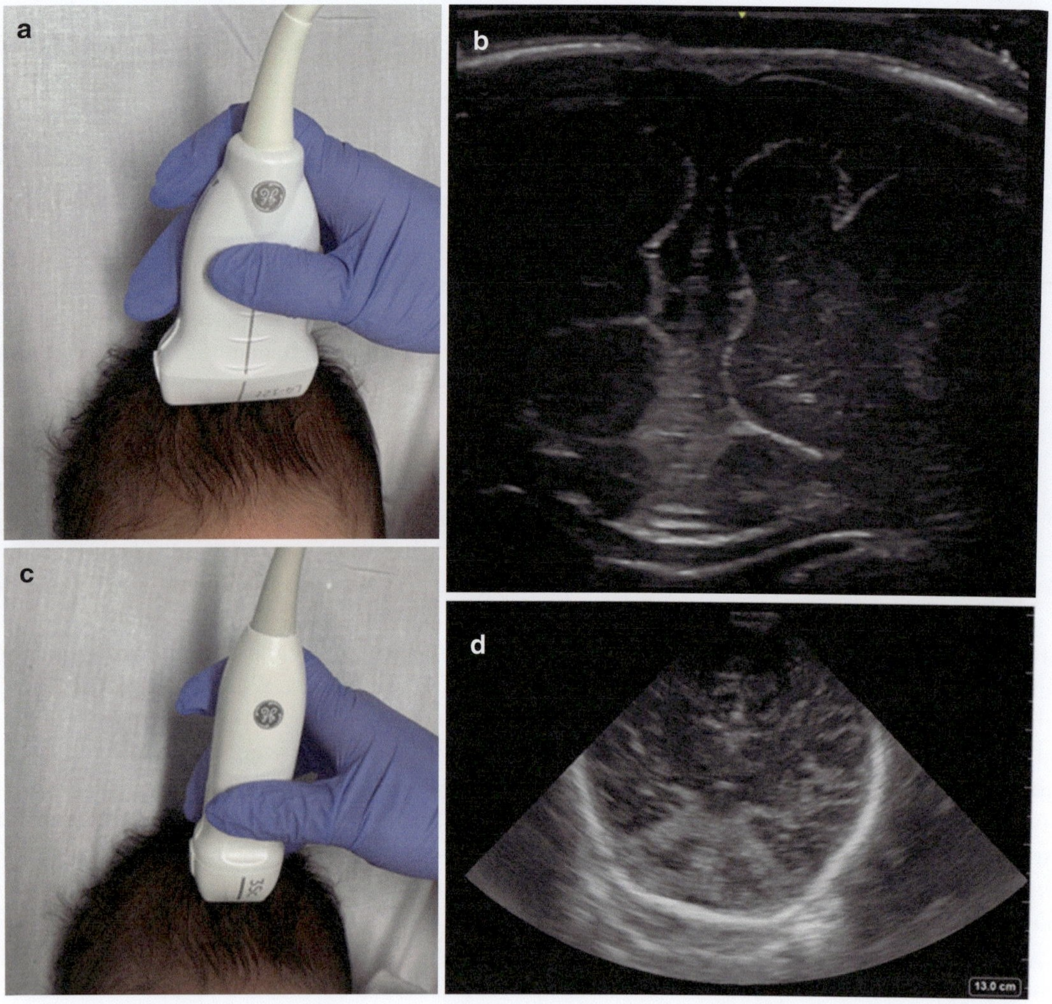

Fig. 16.22 Transfontanelle scans through the anterior fontanelle. (**a**) Linear probe over the anterior fontanelle of an infant. (**b**) Brain imaging through the anterior fontanelle using a linear probe. (**c**) Phased array probe over the anterior fontanelle of an infant. (**d**) Infant brain through the anterior fontanelle scan using a phased array probe

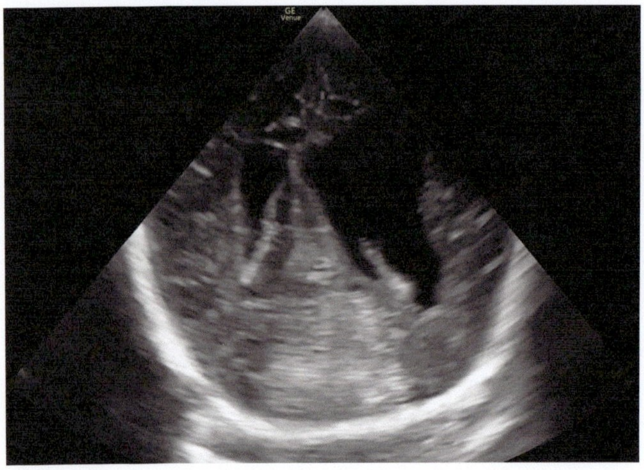

Fig. 16.23 Asymmetric ventricle sizes in an infant's brain with hydrocephalus

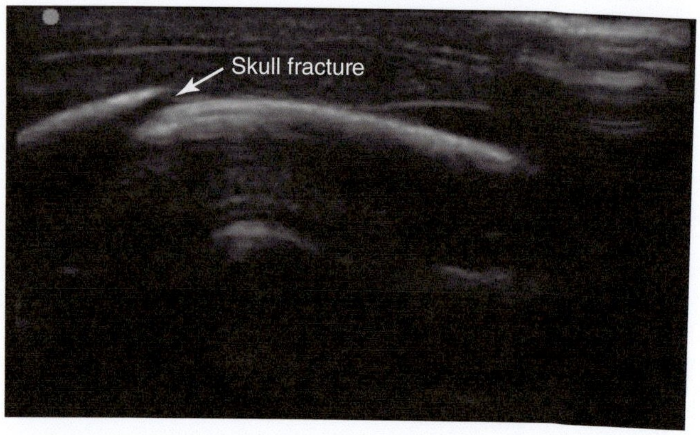

Fig. 16.24 Skull fracture in a pediatric patient. *(Image courtesy of Adriana Manikian, MD)*

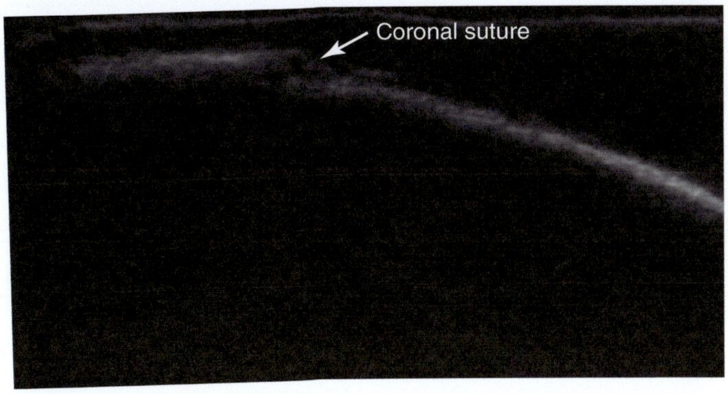

Fig. 16.25 Right coronal suture line in an infant skull. *(Image courtesy of Adriana Manikian, MD)*

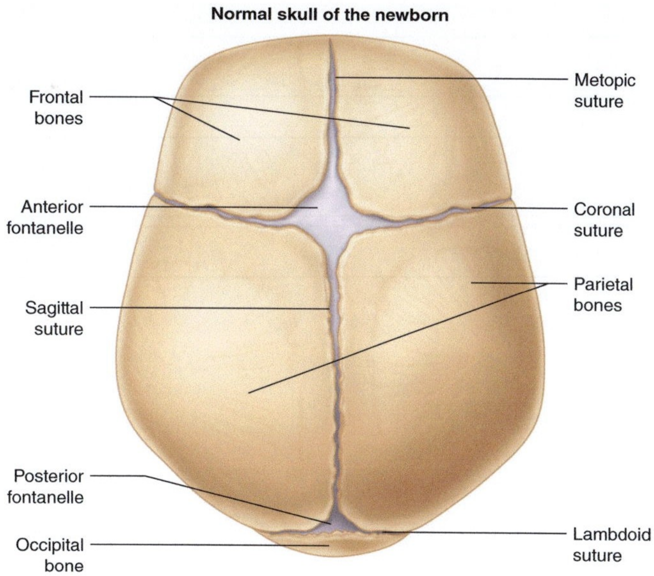

Fig. 16.26 Normal skull and suture lines in newborns

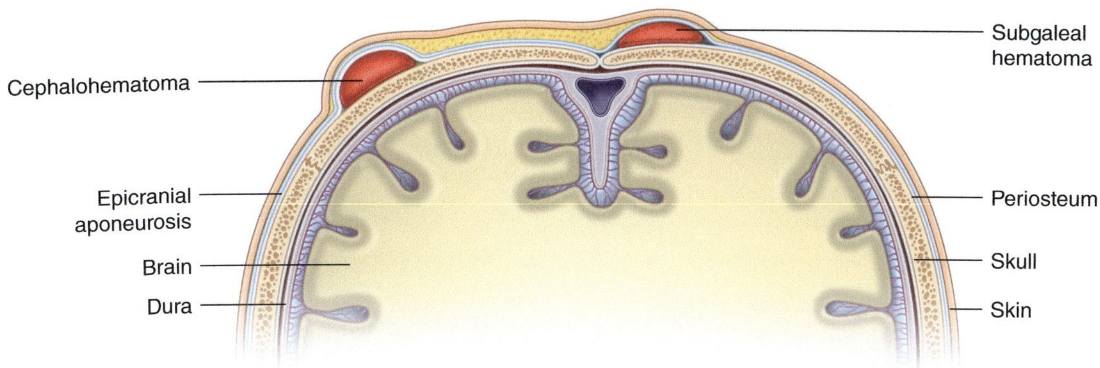

Fig. 16.27 Cranial hematoma locations

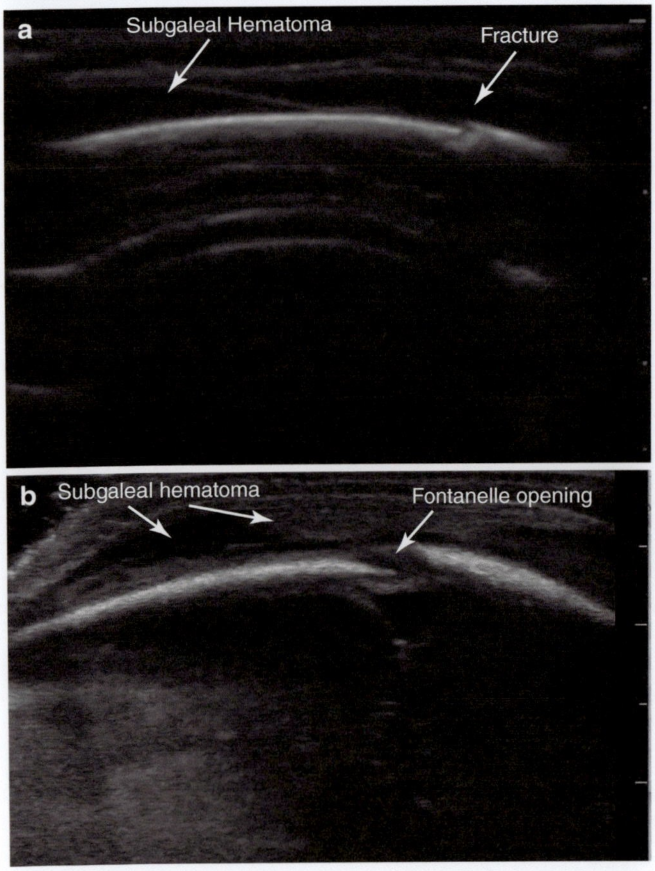

Fig. 16.28 (**a**). Skull fracture with a subgaleal hematoma. (**b**) Subgaleal hematoma crossing over suture line

Key Ultrasound Findings

Pathology	Imaging finding
Intracranial Hemorrhage	Presence of a hyperechoic area surrounded by normal brain echogenicity imaged in multiple planes to reduce the possibility of posterior enhancement artifacts creating a false positive appearance.
Extra-axial Hemorrhage	Presence of hyperechoic signals increasing the width and obscuring the inner table visibility of the contralateral skull.
Midline Shift	Discrepancy in the distance from the temporal bone to the center of the third ventricle/septum pellucidum or pineal gland as measured from both sides of the skull using the same temporal window.
Hydrocephalus	Increase in the axial dimensions of the third ventricle and lateral ventricle as compared to age-validated normal size cut-offs on axial and coronal sections. Dilatation of the lateral ventricle > 10 mm or the third ventricle on the coronal plane > 1 mm suggests hydrocephalus in pediatric patients.
Acute Ischemic Stroke	Waveform changes showing resistive waveforms that transition to post-stenotic waveforms are concerning for stenosis or occlusion. The presence of high intensity transient signals is concerning for microembolization.
Intracranial Hypertension	Presence of a high-resistance waveform throughout the brain. Serial changes showing an increase in peak systolic flow velocity with decreasing diastolic flow velocity and eventual blunting of diastolic flow. Absence of diastolic flow or oscillating waveforms with to-and-fro flow.
Ventriculoperitoneal Shunt Malfunction	Absence of flow distal to the shunt chamber when the reservoir is pressed.
Temporal Arteritis	Presence of a non-compressible temporal artery with a 'halo sign'. Enlarged superficial temporal artery intimal media thickness ranging from 0.5 to 0.9 mm.
Carotid Artery Dissection	Presence of a mobile hyperechoic dissection flap within the carotid artery. Bidirectional flow on color Doppler.
Carotid Artery Pseudoaneurysm	Presence of pseudoaneurysm sac with swirling, bidirectional, turbulent flow between the arterial lumen and the collection.
Carotid Artery Stenosis/ Plaque	Presence of an acute area of thickening (plaque) or circumferential thickening (stenosis). High-resistance waveform upstream from the stenosis with elevated peak systolic velocities and spectral broadening at the site of stenosis, followed by a *tardus et parvus* waveform downstream from the stenosis.
Cephalohematoma/ subgaleal hematomas in children (transcranial view)	Presence of a hyperechoic area between the epicranial aponeurosis and the periosteum of the skull (subgaleal heamtoma) or underneath the periosteum (cephalohematoma). Cephalohematomas do not cross suture lines. Subgaleal hematomas may cross suture lines.
Skull Fracture (transcranial view)	Area of discontinuity of bone that is not present on the other side of the skull.

Pearls and Pitfalls

- The core views include the transtemporal, submandibular, suboccipital, transorbital, and carotid views in adults and additional transfontanellar views in infants.
- POCUS, utilizing a low-frequency B-mode ultrasound, is used to assess brain topography via the temporal window to assess for intracranial pathology and midline shift.
- Transcranial color-coded duplex sonography utilizes pulsed-wave Doppler to insonate the cerebral arteries to help evaluate cerebral hemodynamics in acute ischemic stroke and intracranial hypertension.
- Giant cell arteritis may be detected using the high-frequency linear probe, evaluating the temporal arteries for a positive 'compression sign', 'halo sign', and intima-media thickening.
- Carotid artery pathology may be evaluated with a high-frequency linear probe to evaluate for the possibility of dissection flaps, pseudoaneurysm, and luminal stenosis.
- Ventriculoperitoneal shunt function may be assessed by visualizing flow distal to the shunt chamber on M-mode imaging with the high-frequency linear probe.
- Pediatric-specific POCUS is a useful adjunct to evaluate for the presence of skull fractures, hematoma formation (subgaleal and cephalohematomas), and hydrocephalus.

References

1. Mastantuono J-M, Combescure C, Elia N, Tramer MR, Lysakowski C. Transcranial Doppler in the diagnosis of cerebral vasospasm: an updated meta-analysis. Crit Care Med. 2018;46(10):1665–72.
2. Montrief T, Alerhand S, Jewell C, Scott J. Incorporation of transcranial Doppler into the ED for the neurocritical care patient. Am J Emerg Med. 2019;37(6):1144–52.
3. Rasulo FA, Calza S, Robba C, et al. Transcranial Doppler as a screening test to exclude intracranial hypertension in brain-injured patients: the IMPRESSIT-2 prospective multicenter international study. Crit Care. 2022;26(1):110.
4. Robba C, Goffi A, Geeraerts T, et al. Brain ultrasonography: methodology, basic and advanced principles and clinical applications. A narrative review. Intensive Care Med. 2019;45:913–27.
5. Robba C, Pozzebon S, Moro B, Vincent J-L, Creteur J, Taccone FS. Multimodal non-invasive assessment of intracranial hypertension: an observational study. Crit Care. 2020;24:1–10.
6. Klinzing S, Steiger P, Schüpbach R, Bèchir M, Brandi G. Competence for transcranial color-coded Duplex sonography is rapidly acquired. Minerva Anestesiol. 2014;81(3):298–304.
7. Motuel J, Biette I, Srairi M, et al. Assessment of brain midline shift using sonography in neurosurgical ICU patients. Crit Care. 2014;18:1–8.
8. Acuña J, Adhikari S. Point-of-care ultrasound to distinguish subgaleal and cephalohematoma: case report. Clin Pract Cases Emerg Med. 2021;5(2):198.
9. Dehbozorgi A, Mousavi-Roknabadi RS, Hosseini-Marvast SR, et al. Diagnosing skull fracture in children with closed head injury using point-of-care ultrasound vs. computed tomography scan. Eur J Pediatr. 2021;180:477–84.
10. Kim S, Rizvi M. Use of point of care ultrasound in the diagnosis of subgaleal hematoma following an episode of accidental pilotraction. Am J Emerg Med. 2021;45(679):e1–679. e3
11. Lau VI, Arntfield RT. Point-of-care transcranial Doppler by intensivists. Crit Ultrasound J. 2017;9:1–11.
12. Parri N, Crosby BJ, Glass C, et al. Ability of emergency ultrasonography to detect pediatric skull fractures: a prospective, observational study. J Emerg Med. 2013;44(1):135–41.
13. Parri N, Crosby BJ, Mills L, et al. Point-of-care ultrasound for the diagnosis of skull fractures in children younger than two years of age. J Pediatr. 2018;196:230–236. e2.
14. Robba C, Wong A, Poole D, et al. Basic ultrasound head-to-toe skills for intensivists in the general and neuro intensive care unit population: consensus and expert recommendations of the European Society of Intensive Care Medicine. Intensive Care Med. 2021;47:1347–67.
15. Montorfano L, Sarkissyan M, Wolfers M, Rodríguez F, Pla F, Montorfano M. POCUS and POCDUS: essential tools for the evaluation and management of carotid artery pseudoaneurysms after a gunshot wound. Ultrasound J. 2020;12:1–6.
16. Suttie R, Woo MY, Park L, Nemnom M-J, Stotts G, Perry JJ. Can emergency physicians perform carotid artery point-of-care ultrasound to detect stenosis in patients with TIA and stroke? A pilot study. West J Emerg Med. 2020;21(3):626.
17. Medicine AoE. Ultrasound guidelines: emergency, point-of-care and clinical ultrasound guidelines in medicine. Ann Emerg Med. 2023.
18. Robba C, Poole D, Citerio G, Taccone F, Rasulo F. Consensus on brain ultrasonography in critical care group. Brain ultrasonography consensus on skill recommendations and competence levels within the critical care setting. Neurocrit Care. 2020;32(2):502–11.
19. Valaikiene J, Schlachetzki F, Azevedo E, et al. Point-of-care ultrasound in neurology–report of the ean spn/esnch/ercnsono neuro-pocus working group. Ultraschall in der Medizin. 2022;43(04):354–66.
20. Purkayastha S, Sorond F. Transcranial Doppler ultrasound: technique and application. Thieme Medical Publishers; 2012. p. 411–20.
21. He L, Wu DF, Zhang JH, Zheng S, Li Y, He W. Factors affecting transtemporal window quality in transcranial sonography. Brain Behav. 2022;12(4):e2543.
22. Marinoni M, Ginanneschi A, Forleo P, Amaducci L. Technical limits in transcranial Doppler recording: Inadequate acoustic windows. Ultrasound Med Biol. 1997;23(8):1275–7.
23. Wijnhoud AD, Franckena M, Van Der Lugt A, Koudstaal PJ. Inadequate acoustical temporal bone window in patients with a transient ischemic attack or minor stroke: role of skull thickness and bone density. Ultrasound Med Biol. 2008;34(6):923–9.
24. Alexandrov AV, Sloan MA, Tegeler CH, et al. Practice standards for transcranial Doppler (TCD) ultrasound. Part II. Clinical indications and expected outcomes. J Neuroimaging. 2012;22(3):215–24.
25. Alexandrov AV, Sloan MA, Wong LK, et al. Practice standards for transcranial Doppler ultrasound: part I—test performance. J Neuroimaging. 2007;17(1):11–8.
26. Bathala L, Mehndiratta MM, Sharma VK. Transcranial doppler: Technique and common findings (Part 1). Ann Indian Acad Neurol. 2013;16(2):174–9.

27. Ivancevich NM, Pinton GF, Nicoletto HA, Bennett E, Laskowitz DT, Smith SW. Real-time 3-D contrast-enhanced transcranial ultrasound and aberration correction. Ultrasound Med Biol. 2008;34(9):1387–95.
28. Postert T, Federlein J, Przuntek H, Büttner T. Insufficient and absent acoustic temporal bone window: potential and limitations of transcranial contrast-enhanced color-coded sonography and contrast-enhanced power-based sonography. Ultrasound Med Biol. 1997;23(6):857–62.
29. Rutgers D, Blankensteijn J, Van der Grond J. Preoperative MRA flow quantification in CEA patients: flow differences between patients who develop cerebral ischemia and patients who do not develop cerebral ischemia during cross-clamping of the carotid artery. Stroke. 2000;31(12):3021–8.
30. Bellner J, Romner B, Reinstrup P, Kristiansson K-A, Ryding E, Brandt L. Transcranial Doppler sonography pulsatility index (PI) reflects intracranial pressure (ICP). Surg Neurol. 2004;62(1):45–51.
31. Wakerley BR, Sharma VK. Transcranial Doppler derived pulsatility index in the assessment of intracranial pressure: the trend is your friend. Neurosurgery. 2013;72(2):E319–20.
32. Sigman EJ, Laghari FJ, Sarwal A. Neuro POCUS. Elsevier; 2023.
33. Sarwal A, Patel Y, D'Agostino R, et al. Exploratory study to assess feasibility of intracerebral hemorrhage detection by point of care cranial ultrasound. Ultrasound J. 2022;14(1):40.
34. Seidel G, MD HC, Albers T, Meyer-Wiethe K. Transcranial sonographic monitoring of hemorrhagic transformation in patients with acute middle cerebral artery infarction. J Neuroimaging. 2005;15(4):326–30.
35. Allen BC, Kapoor S, Anzalone A, et al. Transcranial ultrasonography to detect intracranial pathology: A systematic review and meta-analysis. J Neuroimaging. 2023;33(3):333–58.
36. Matsumoto N, Kimura K, Iguchi Y, Aoki J. Evaluation of cerebral hemorrhage volume using transcranial color-coded duplex sonography. J Neuroimaging. 2011;21(4):355–8.
37. Meyer-Wiethe K, Sallustio F, Kern R. Diagnosis of intracerebral hemorrhage with transcranial ultrasound. Cerebrovasc Dis. 2009;27(Suppl. 2):40–7.
38. Xu X-M, Zhang H, Meng R-L. Cranial midline shift is a predictor of the clinical prognosis of acute cerebral infarction patients undergoing emergency endovascular treatment. Sci Rep. 2023;13(1):21037.
39. Yang W-S, Li Q, Li R, et al. Defining the optimal midline shift threshold to predict poor outcome in patients with supratentorial spontaneous intracerebral hemorrhage. Neurocrit Care. 2018;28:314–21.
40. Caldas J, Rynkowski CB, Robba C. POCUS, how can we include the brain? An overview. J Anesth Analg Crit Care. 2022;2(1):55.
41. Seidel G, Gerriets T, Kaps M, Missler U. Dislocation of the third ventricle due to space-occupying stroke evaluated by transcranial duplex sonography. J Neuroimaging. 1996;6(4):227–30.
42. Caricato A, Ioannoni E, Gelormini C. Is it really third ventricle? A pitfall in the diagnosis of hydrocephalus by brain ultrasound. Neurocrit Care. 2020;33(3):844–6.
43. Dinsmore M, Venkatraghavan L. Clinical applications of point-of-care ultrasound in brain injury: a narrative review. Anaesthesia. 2022;77:69–77.
44. Pokhrel B, Thapa A. Systematic use of point of care ultrasound in neurosurgical intensive care unit: a practical approach. Quant Imaging Med Surg. 2023;13(4):2287.
45. Vega RA, Buscher MG, Gonzalez MS, Tye GW. Sonographic localization of a nonpalpable shunt: Ultrasound-assisted ventricular shunt tap. Surg Neurol Int. 2013;4:101.
46. Sgouros S, John P, Walsh AR, Hockley AD. The value of colour Doppler imaging in assessing flow through ventriculo-peritoneal shunts. Childs Nerv Syst. 1996;12:454–9.
47. Gopalakrishnan M, Shanbhag NC, Shukla DP, Konar SK, Bhat DI, Devi BI. Complications of decompressive craniectomy. Front Neurol. 2018;9:416751.
48. Brunser AM, Lavados PM, Hoppe A, Lopez J, Valenzuela M, Rivas R. Accuracy of transcranial Doppler compared with CT angiography in diagnosing arterial obstructions in acute ischemic strokes. Stroke. 2009;40(6):2037–41.
49. Mattioni A, Cenciarelli S, Eusebi P, et al. Transcranial Doppler sonography for detecting stenosis or occlusion of intracranial arteries in people with acute ischaemic stroke. Cochrane Database Syst Rev. 2020:(2).
50. Nedelmann M, Stolz E, Gerriets T, et al. Consensus recommendations for transcranial color-coded duplex sonography for the assessment of intracranial arteries in clinical trials on acute stroke. Stroke. 2009;40(10):3238–44.
51. Zhao L, Barlinn K, Sharma VK, et al. Velocity criteria for intracranial stenosis revisited: an international multicenter study of transcranial Doppler and digital subtraction angiography. Stroke. 2011;42(12):3429–34.
52. Alexandrov AV. Extra-and intracranial waveform analysis algorithm, descriptions, classifications, and differential diagnosis. J Vasc Ultrasound. 2015;39(4):192–202.
53. Mazya MV, Ahmed N, Azevedo E, et al. Impact of transcranial Doppler ultrasound on logistics and outcomes in stroke thrombolysis: results from the SITS-ISTR. Stroke. 2018;49(7):1695–700.
54. Alexandrov AV, Tsivgoulis G, Rubiera M, et al. End-diastolic velocity increase predicts recanalization and neurological improvement in patients with ischemic stroke with proximal arterial occlusions receiving reperfusion therapies. Stroke. 2010;41(5):948–52.
55. Burgin WS, Malkoff M, Felberg RA, et al. Transcranial Doppler ultrasound criteria for recanalization after thrombolysis for middle cerebral artery stroke. Stroke. 2000;31(5):1128–32.
56. Labiche LA, Malkoff M, Alexandrov AV. Residual flow signals predict complete recanalization in stroke patients treated with TPA. J Neuroimaging. 2003;13(1):28–33.
57. Saqqur M, Tsivgoulis G, Molina CA, Demchuk AM, Shuaib A, Alexandrov AV. Residual flow at the site of intracranial occlusion on transcranial Doppler predicts response to intravenous thrombolysis: a multi-center study. Cerebrovasc Dis. 2009;27(1):5–12.
58. Saqqur M, Uchino K, Demchuk AM, et al. Site of arterial occlusion identified by transcranial Doppler predicts the response to intravenous thrombolysis for stroke. Stroke. 2007;38(3):948–54.
59. Tsivgoulis G, Ribo M, Rubiera M, et al. Real-time validation of transcranial Doppler criteria in assessing recanalization during intra-arterial procedures for acute ischemic stroke an international, multicenter study. Stroke. 2013;44(2):394–400.
60. Kim J-M, Bae J-H, Park K-Y, et al. Incidence and mechanism of early neurological deterioration after endovascular thrombectomy. J Neurol. 2019;266:609–15.
61. Baracchini C, Farina F, Palmieri A, et al. Early hemodynamic predictors of good outcome and reperfusion injury after endovascular treatment. Neurology. 2019;92(24):e2774–83.
62. Chen H, Su Y, He Y, et al. Controlling blood pressure under transcranial doppler guidance after endovascular treatment in patients with acute ischemic stroke. Cerebrovasc Dis. 2020;49(2):160–9.
63. Kneihsl M, Enzinger C, Gattringer T. Cerebral hyperperfusion syndrome after mechanical thrombectomy. J NeuroIntervent Surg. 2021;13(12):1187–8.
64. Del Brutto VJ, Sambursky JA, Krementz NA, et al. Transcranial Doppler after successful endovascular revascularization and hospitalization outcomes. Stroke. 2023;3(4):e000785.
65. Gomez J, Wolfe S, Sarwal A. Sonographic demonstration of a perfusion-dependent stroke with negative MRI and a flow-limiting stenosis. Neurocrit Care. 2020;32:883–8.
66. Kargiotis O, Psychogios K, Safouris A, et al. The role of transcranial Doppler monitoring in patients with multi-territory acute embolic strokes: a review. J Neuroimaging. 2019;29(3):309–22.
67. Cardim D, Robba C, Bohdanowicz M, et al. Non-invasive monitoring of intracranial pressure using transcranial Doppler ultrasonography: is it possible? Neurocrit Care. 2016;25:473–91.

68. Lacy A, Nelson R, Koyfman A, Long B. High risk and low prevalence diseases: Giant cell arteritis. Am J Emerg Med. 2022;58:135–40.
69. Herzberg M, Boy S, Hölscher T, et al. Prehospital stroke diagnostics based on neurological examination and transcranial ultrasound. Crit Ultrasound J. 2014;6:1–13.
70. Noumegni SR, Hoffmann C, Cornec D, Gestin S, Bressollette L, Jousse-Joulin S. Temporal artery ultrasound to diagnose giant cell arteritis: a practical guide. Ultrasound Med Biol. 2021;47(2):201–13.
71. Fernández-Fernández E, Monjo-Henry I, Bonilla G, et al. False positives in the ultrasound diagnosis of giant cell arteritis: some diseases can also show the halo sign. Rheumatology. 2020;59(9):2443–7.
72. Dejaco C, Ramiro S, Duftner C, et al. EULAR recommendations for the use of imaging in large vessel vasculitis in clinical practice. Ann Rheum Dis. 2018;77(5):636–43.
73. Schäfer VS, Chrysidis S, Dejaco C, et al. Assessing vasculitis in giant cell arteritis by ultrasound: results of OMERACT patient-based reliability exercises. J Rheumatol. 2018;45(9):1289–95.
74. Aschwanden M, Daikeler T, Kesten F, et al. Temporal artery compression sign–a novel ultrasound finding for the diagnosis of giant cell arteritis. Ultraschall in der Medizin. 2013;34(01):47–50.
75. van der Geest KSM, Borg F, Kayani A, et al. Novel ultrasonographic Halo Score for giant cell arteritis: assessment of diagnostic accuracy and association with ocular ischaemia. Ann Rheum Dis. 2020;79(3):393–9. https://doi.org/10.1136/annrheumdis-2019-216343.
76. Aranda-Valera IC, García Carazo S, Monjo Henry I, De Miguel Mendieta E. Diagnostic validity of Doppler ultrasound in giant cell arteritis. Clin Exp Rheumatol. 2017;35(Suppl 103):123–7.
77. Coath FL, Mukhtyar C. Ultrasonography in the diagnosis and follow-up of giant cell arteritis. Rheumatology. 2021;60(6):2528–36.
78. Duftner C, Dejaco C, Sepriano A, Falzon L, Schmidt WA, Ramiro S. Imaging in diagnosis, outcome prediction and monitoring of large vessel vasculitis: a systematic literature review and meta-analysis informing the EULAR recommendations. RMD Open. 2018;4(1):e000612.
79. Hernández P, Al Jalbout N, Matza M, Kohler MJ, Shokoohi H, Kohler M. Temporal artery ultrasound for the diagnosis of giant cell arteritis in the emergency department. Cureus. 2023;15(7)
80. Kirby C, Flood R, Mullan R, Murphy G, Kane D. Evolution of ultrasound in giant cell arteritis. Front Med (Lausanne). 2022;9:981659. https://doi.org/10.3389/fmed.2022.981659.
81. Drews E, Wildman-Tobriner B, Mathews A, et al. Prospective evaluation of novice-acquired three-dimensional point-of-care ultrasound for carotid stenosis. Acad Emerg Med. 2021;28(12)
82. Grant EG, Benson CB, Moneta GL, et al. Carotid artery stenosis: gray-scale and Doppler US diagnosis--Society of Radiologists in Ultrasound Consensus Conference. Radiology. 2003;229(2):340–6. https://doi.org/10.1148/radiol.2292030516.
83. AbuRahma AF, Avgerinos ED, Chang RW, et al. The Society for Vascular Surgery implementation document for management of extracranial cerebrovascular disease. J Vasc Surg. 2022;75(1):26S–98S.
84. Polak JF, Alexandrov AV. Accuracy of the Society of Radiologists in Ultrasound (SRU) Carotid Doppler velocity criteria for grading North American Symptomatic Carotid Endarterectomy Trial (NASCET) stenosis: a meta-analysis. J Ultrasound Med. 2023;42(7):1423–35.
85. Gornik HL, Rundek T, Gardener H, et al. Optimization of duplex velocity criteria for diagnosis of internal carotid artery (ICA) stenosis: A report of the Intersocietal Accreditation Commission (IAC) Vascular Testing Division Carotid Diagnostic Criteria Committee. Vasc Med. 2021;26(5):515–25.
86. Commission IA. Updated Recommendations for Carotid Stenosis Interpretation Criteria Now Available. 2024. https://intersocietal.org/vascular-testing/updated-recommendations-for-carotid-stenosis-interpretation-criteria-nov-2023/
87. Services USP. Asymptomatic Carotid Artery Stenosis: Screening. 2024. https://www.uspreventiveservicestaskforce.org/uspstf/recommendation/carotid-artery-stenosis-screening
88. Correa F, Enríquez G, Rosselló J, et al. Posterior fontanelle sonography: an acoustic window into the neonatal brain. Am J Neuroradiol. 2004;25(7):1274–82.
89. Subramaniam S, Chen AE, Khwaja A, Rempell R. Identifying infant hydrocephalus in the emergency department with transfontanellar POCUS. Am J Emerg Med. 2019;37(1):127–32.
90. Davenport SR, Fadel NB, Davila J, Barrowman N, Bijelic V, Shefrin AE. Brain point of Care Ultrasound in Young Children receiving computed tomography in the Emergency Department: a proof of Concept Study. POCUS J. 2023;8(2):165.
91. Alexandridis G, Verschuuren EW, Rosendaal AV, Kanhai DA. Evidence base for point-of-care ultrasound (POCUS) for diagnosis of skull fractures in children: a systematic review and meta-analysis. Emerg Med J. 2022;39(1):30–6.

Head and Neck Ultrasound

17

Brian Bales, Creagh Boulger, and Jeremy S. Boyd

Background

Point-of-care ultrasound (POCUS) can be utilized to rapidly identify and evaluate multiple structures and pathologies of the head and neck. These structures include the bony and soft tissues of the hypopharynx and anterior neck, epiglottis, thyroid, cricothyroid membrane (CTM), tracheal cartilages, lymphatic system, and sinuses. Because of their superficial location and differing echogenicities, these structures are well suited for sonographic assessment. POCUS can also be utilized for undifferentiated masses, painful regions, and preprocedural planning in the head and neck to better understand the underlying anatomy.

POCUS can also be used as an adjunct for airway assessment and intubation confirmation. Airway management is a critical component of emergency resuscitation, and POCUS has been increasingly adopted in the diagnosis and management of airway-related disorders [1]. POCUS is supported by the American Heart Association Adult Advanced Cardiovascular Life Support guidelines as an adjunct for the evaluation of airway placement [2]. As POCUS research and clinical applications have evolved and specialists have expanded their use of POCUS at the bedside, additional applications and techniques have increased in recent years [1].

This chapter provides a review of the sonographic assessment of key head and neck structures, as well as the following pathologies: epiglottitis, angioedema, vocal cord dysfunction, sialolithiasis, parotitis, peritonsillar abscess (PTA), sinusitis, thyroid disorders, thyroid cysts, thyroglossal duct and branchial cleft cysts, lymphadenitis, lymphadenopathy, and airway management.

Indications

Indications
- Airway management
- Dyspnea
- Dysphagia
- Dysphonia
- Inability to manage secretions
- Jaw pain/facial swelling
- Neck pain
- Neck mass

Diagnoses
- Epiglottitis
- Angioedema
- Vocal cord dysfunction
- Sialolithiasis
- Parotitis
- Peritonsillar abscess
- Sinusitis
- Thyroid dysfunction (e.g., DeQuervains, Hashimotos, Graves' Disease)
- Thyroid cysts/nodules
- Thyroglossal duct cysts
- Branchial cleft cysts
- Lymphadenitis
- Lymphadenopathy

Supplementary Information The online version contains supplementary material available at https://doi.org/10.1007/978-3-031-85308-1_17.

B. Bales
Department of Emergency Medicine, Vanderbilt University Medical Center, Nashville, TN, USA
e-mail: brian.bales@vumc.org

C. Boulger
Department of Emergency Medicine, Ohio State University, Columbus, OH, USA
e-mail: creagh.boulger@osumc.edu

J. S. Boyd (✉)
Department of Emergency Medicine, Vanderbilt University Medical Center, Nashville, TN, USA
e-mail: jeremy.s.boyd@vumc.org

M. Gottlieb, N. Panebianco (eds.), *Advanced Point-of-Care Ultrasound*, https://doi.org/10.1007/978-3-031-85308-1_17

Core Views

View	Image	Approach
Epiglottis	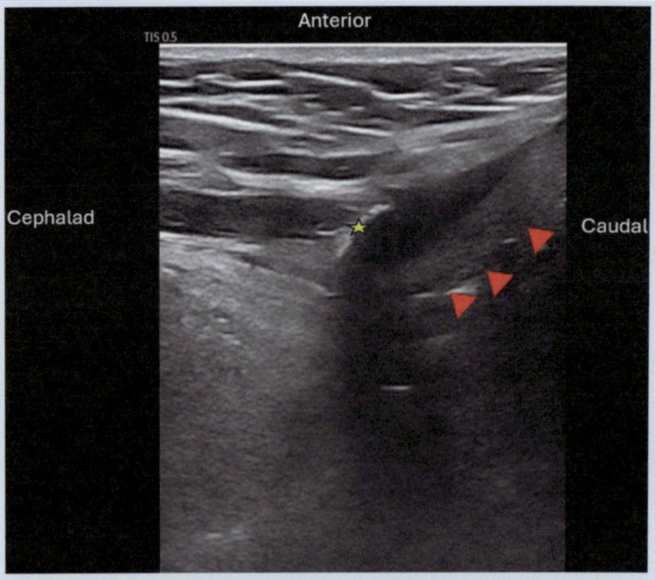 *Core View 1A. Sagittal epiglottis. Hyoid (yellow star), epiglottis (red arrowheads)* 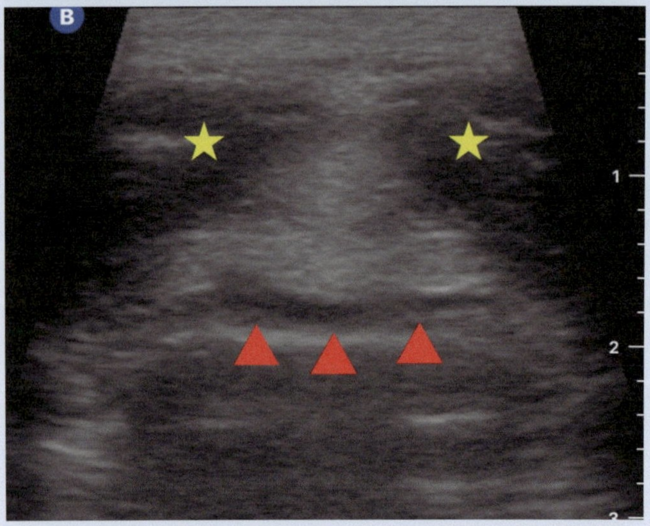 *Core View 1B. Transverse epiglottis. Strap muscles (yellow stars), epiglottis (red arrowheads)*	*Technique* Begin with the patient in the sniffing position. Place the probe on the anterior neck, inferior to the hyoid bone, and in the sagittal plane. Rotate the probe 90 degrees to the transverse plane, with the probe located between the hyoid bone superiorly and the thyroid cartilage inferiorly. The appearance of the epiglottis and strap muscles in this view resembles that of a frog or sloth face [3, 4]. *Structures visualized* Hyoid bone Thyroid cartilage Thyrohyoid membrane Strap muscles Epiglottis

View	Image	Approach
Tongue	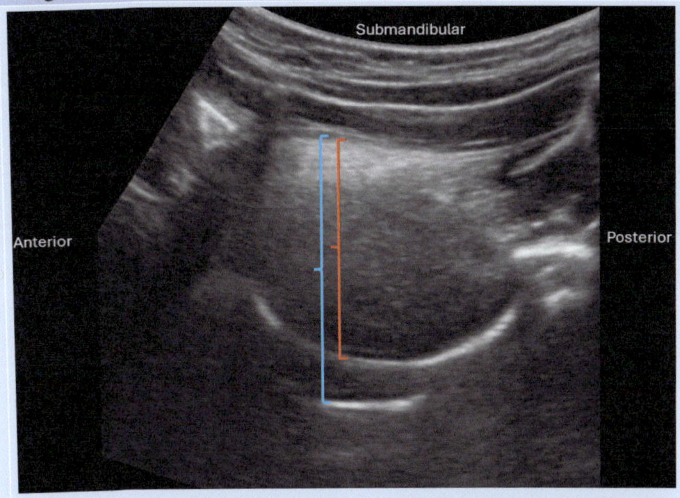 *Core View 2A. Sagittal tongue. The oral cavity is measured in blue and tongue thickness in orange* 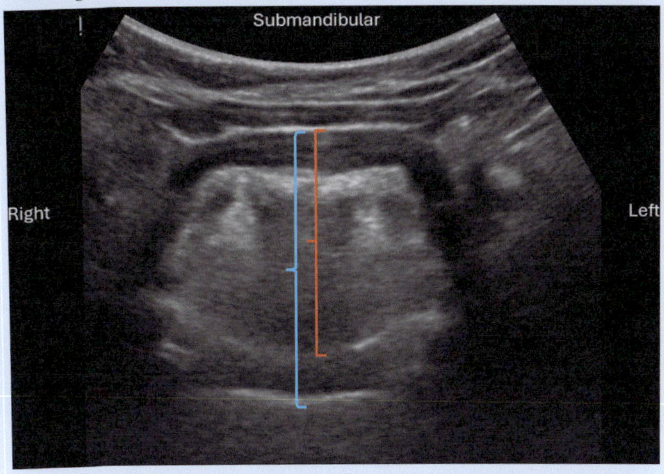 *Core View 2B. Transverse tongue. The oral cavity is measured in blue and tongue thickness in orange*	*Technique* Place a curvilinear probe in the submandibular space in the sagittal orientation. Rock and fan to center the tongue on the screen. Rotate the probe 90 degrees to the transverse plane. *Structures visualized* Lingual Arteries Tongue Palate
Vocal cords	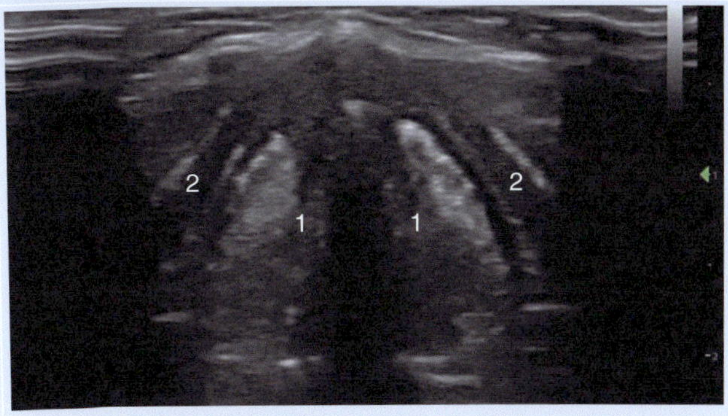 *Core View 3. Vocal cords. True vocal cords labeled with "1", thyroid cartilage labeled with "2"* Core Video 1	*Technique* The vocal cords can be best visualized in a transverse orientation starting at the level of the thyroid cartilage and moving in a caudal direction. The true vocal cords will appear as two triangular hypoechoic structures lined medially by the hyperechoic vocal ligaments. Have the patient vocalize or hum to confirm movement. *Structures visualized* True vocal cords Thyroid cartilage

View	Image	Approach
Submandibular/ sublingual glands	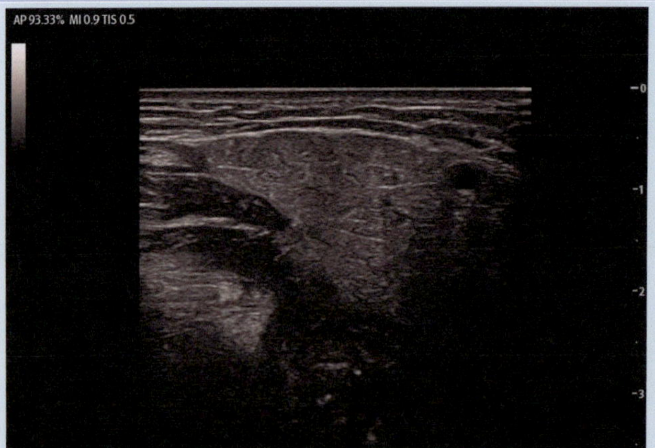 *Core View 4A. Submandibular gland* 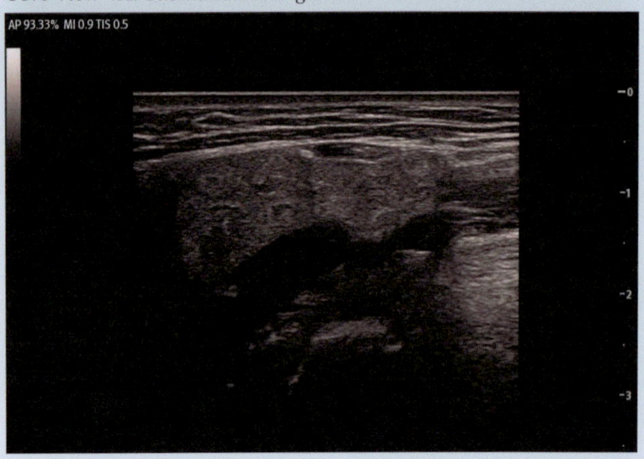 *Core View 4B. Submandibular gland*	*Technique* Place the probe under the medial aspect of the mandible in a sagittal orientation. Fan to visualize the structure, which will be hyperechoic. Add color Doppler to assess for hypervascularity. *Structures visualized* Submandibular glands Sublingual glands

View	Image	Approach
Parotid gland	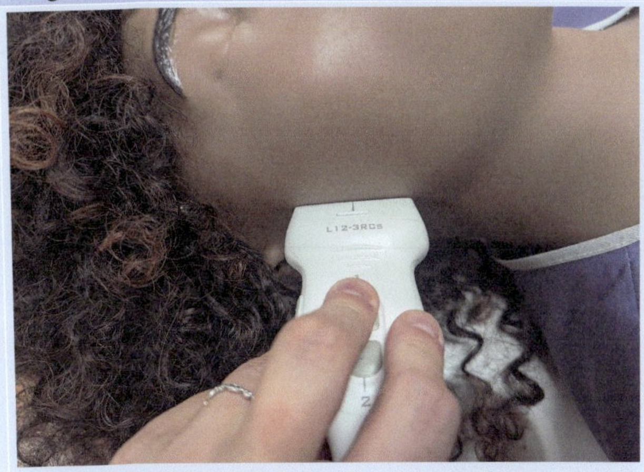 *Core View 5A. Probe positioning for the coronal plane* 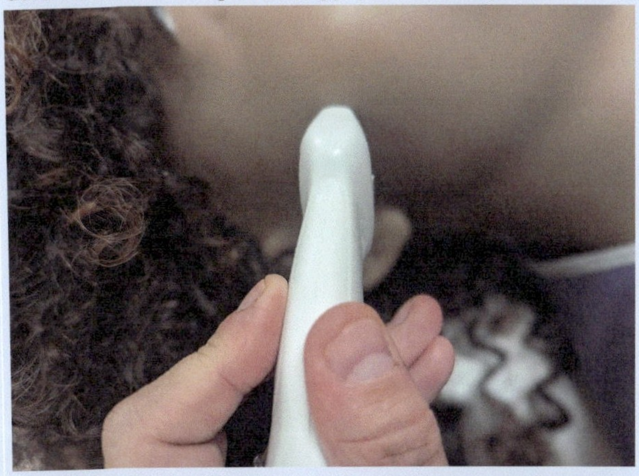 *Core View 5B. Probe positioning for the transverse plane*	*Technique* Place a linear probe in the preauricular space in a coronal orientation. The parotid gland will be a hyperechoic, superficial structure. Rotate the probe 90 degrees to visualize in the transverse plane. *Structures visualized* Parotid gland Mandible
	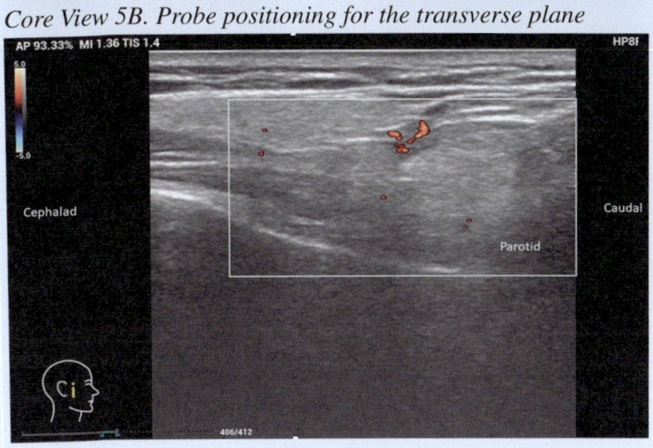 *Core View 5C. Normal parotid gland*	

View	Image	Approach
Maxillary sinuses	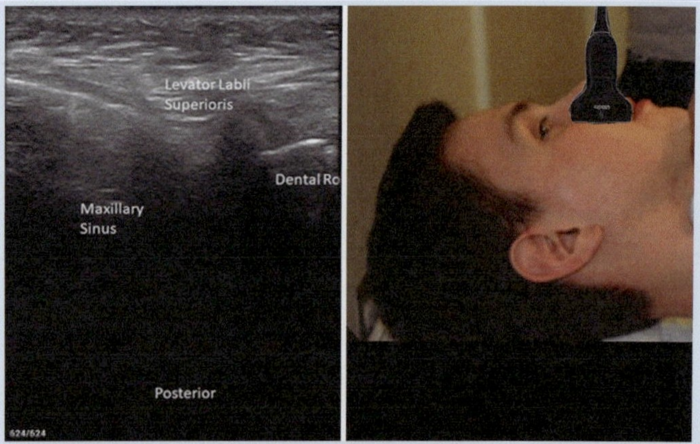 *Core View 6. Normal maxillary sinus (left) with probe positioning (right)*	*Technique* Place a linear probe on the anterior face overlying the maxilla in a sagittal orientation just inferior to the orbit. The maxillary sinus will have a thin, hyperechoic linear appearance. Rotate the probe 90 degrees to visualize in the transverse plane. *Structures visualized* Anterior and posterior walls of maxillary sinus
Thyroid	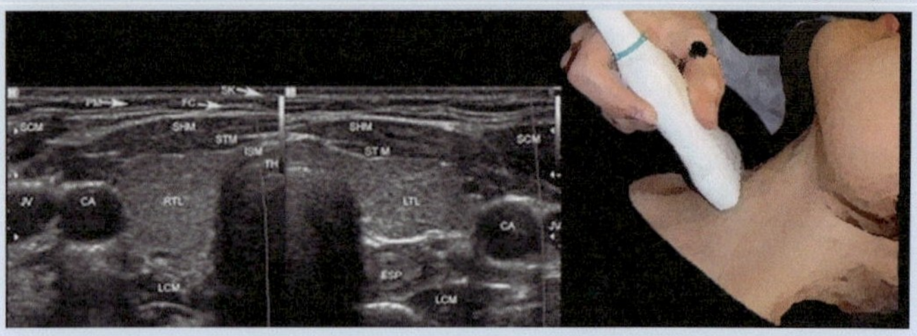 *Core View 7. Normal thyroid gland. RTL- right thyroid lobe, LTL- left thyroid lobe, SCM- stenocletomastoid muscle, CA- carotid artery, JV- jugular vein, ISM- isthmus*	*Technique* Begin with the patient supine and their neck slightly extended. Place the probe transversely across their neck just superior to the suprasternal notch and slide superiorly to visualize the thyroid gland. Rotate the probe 90 degrees and visualize each lobe. *Structures visualized* Right thyroid lobe Left thyroid lobe Sternocleidomastoid muscle Carotid artery Jugular vein Isthmus
Lymph nodes	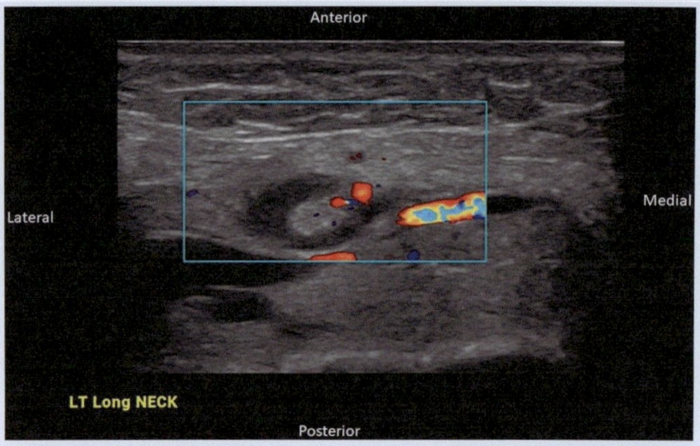 *Core View 8. Lymph node*	*Technique* Place the probe over the suspected lymph node. Rotate 90 degrees to visualize in both planes. Use color Doppler to assess for hypervascularity. *Structures visualized* Lymph Node Surrounding soft tissue structures

Core views of the structures of the head and neck are typically obtained in transverse and longitudinal planes. An oblique orientation may be needed for non-midline lateral structures such as esophagus and branchial cleft cysts. When visualizing subglottic structures, a short-axis approach may be used with the probe positioned in the submandibular region. Given the superficial location, most structures are imaged with a linear probe. If a wider field of view is needed, the extended field of view function may be enabled for the linear probe, or the curvilinear probe can be utilized.

Clinical Applications

Epiglottitis

Epiglottitis is a time-sensitive medical emergency. While this is often a clinical diagnosis, it can be challenging due to the overlap of symptoms with other diseases. Often, these patients are critically ill, limiting their ability to travel to radiology suites or to optimize their positioning to obtain high-quality radiographs or computed tomography (CT). POCUS can be a valuable diagnostic test in these patients, as it is rapid, repeatable, and readily available at the bedside without requiring manipulation of the patient.

One small study of 30 patients demonstrated a difference in the anteroposterior diameter of the epiglottis between patients with epiglottitis and healthy volunteers [5]. This difference was greatest at the lateral margins of the epiglottis, with the upper limit of the normal epiglottis being 3.2 mm, while the lower limit of those with epiglottitis was 3.6 mm. However, another study found moderate inter-rater variability between measures of epiglottic thickness when obtained across clinicians with an intraclass correlation of 0.57, so caution should be used when relying on a single measure in isolation [6]. Inter-rater reliability was greater for other measures, such as preepiglottic space.

In addition to the size thresholds, there are also notable differences in the appearance of the epiglottis when inflamed. One study described the finding known as the "alphabet P sign" [3]. The "P sign" is visualized in the sagittal plane as an edematous half circle just inferior to the shadow of the hyoid bone (Fig. 17.1).

Angioedema

Angioedema is a life-threatening condition requiring emergent endotracheal intubation in 10–34% of such patients presenting to the emergency department [7]. Determining which patients require immediate intubation is often difficult at presentation, and fiberoptic nasopharyngoscopy may not be readily available for direct visualization of the airway. There is a paucity of literature demonstrating the effectiveness of submandibular and anterior neck ultrasound in predicting the need for airway intervention in the setting of angioedema. Some observational studies and case reports suggest that quantitative measurements of the tongue, oral cavity, and tongue-to-cavity ratios may be useful predictors of airway difficulty or intubation [8–11]. However, studies have shown that the normal tongue thickness can be quite variable, with means ranging from 3.0 to 6.4 cm [10–12].

Laryngeal edema can be visualized in the transverse orientation beginning with the probe placed at the level of the thyroid cartilage and then sliding inferiorly until the vocal cords are identified, looking for asymmetry along the arytenoids and other soft tissue along the course of the airway (Fig. 17.2). This has been described in one study and may be helpful, when time allows, for predicting the need for airway intervention [9].

Vocal Cord Dysfunction

Vocal cord dysfunction can be a very challenging diagnosis and can masquerade as other life-threatening conditions. Patients often present with stridor, increased work of breathing, and respiratory distress. Vocal cord dysfunction can be readily assessed with a linear probe. This pathology is more often seen in pediatric patients and females, as well as patients who have had prior neck surgeries or trauma [13]. While fiberoptic nasopharyngoscopy is the gold standard for evaluating vocal cord paralysis, it is an invasive procedure and requires specialized equipment and training. Therefore, POCUS presents an opportunity for a noninvasive assessment of vocal cord dysfunction at the bedside [14].

With a linear probe held in a transverse orientation, the vocal cords can be visualized, which appear as triangular,

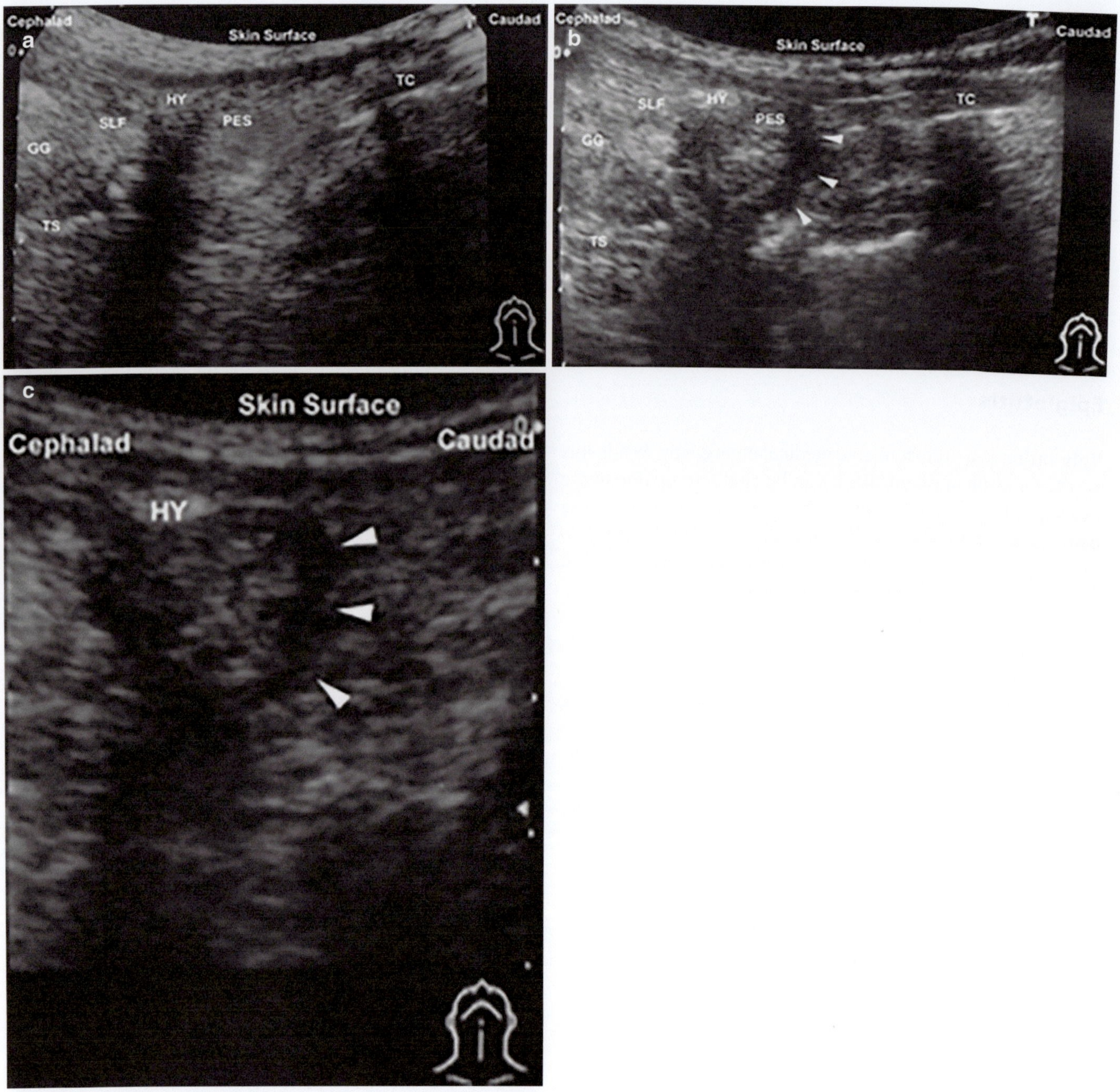

Fig. 17.1 (**a**) Normal epiglottis in the sagittal plane. (**b**) Alphabet P sign in acute epiglottitis. Note the swollen, hypoechoic region along the inferior border of the epiglottis outlined with white arrowheads. (**c**) Zoomed in view of epiglottis with appearance of a "P" from hypoechoic edema on inferior aspect (arrowheads) and hyoid bone (HY) on the superior aspect. *GG* genioglossus, *TS* tongue surface, *SLF* sublingual fat, *HY* hyoid bone, *PES* preepiglottic space, *TC* thyroid cartilage. *(Image courtesy of Hung et al.)* [3]

hypoechoic structures deep in the thyroid cartilage. Vocal cord movement can be observed during phonation by having the patient vocalize a prolonged "eeeee" and "aaaah" as well as during respiration (Videos 2, 3, and 4). Normal function should demonstrate the symmetric and coordinated motion of the vocal cords. In patients suspected of vocal cord dysfunction, findings may include a laterally displaced, shortened, or thinned vocal cord (particularly after neck or thyroid surgery); absence of movement during phonation; or displaced closure of the glottis away from the midline (Fig. 17.3) [13]. The sensitivity and specificity of ultrasound-visualized vocal cord movement may be increased by adding a lateral view of the neck with the probe in a cranial-caudal orientation to visualize the thyroid, arytenoid, and cricoid cartilages

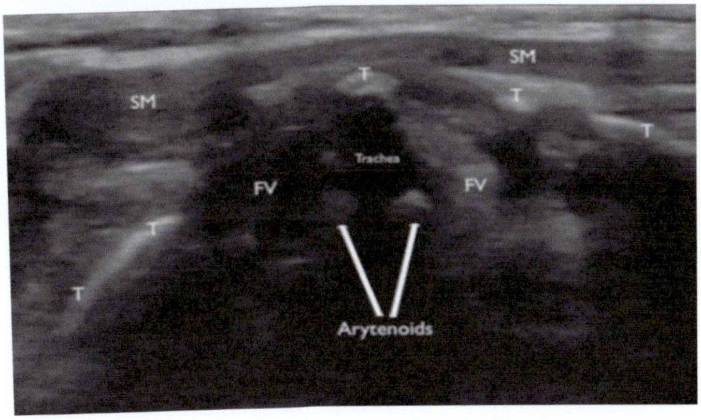

Fig. 17.2 Vocal cord edema. A transverse still image obtained just cephalad of the vocal cords and arytenoids. Asymmetry is noted by the arrow with fullness of the false vocal (FV) cord on the left side of the airway. *SM* sternocleidomastoid muscle, *T* thyroid cartilage. *(Image courtesy of Schick et al.* [9])

[15]. Another technique has also been described for paradoxical vocal cord movement. During normal respiration, the vocal cords should open. If the cords close during inspiration, this suggests paradoxical vocal cord movement. One study reported 100% accuracy by a single clinician in identifying paradoxical vocal cord motion with this approach [16].

Sialolithiasis

Sialolithiasis (i.e., salivary duct stones) is a painful condition most commonly affecting middle-aged adults, who present with neck or jaw pain with swelling that worsens with meals [17]. Diagnosis is often made on history and physical examination. However, the differential diagnosis of neck swelling

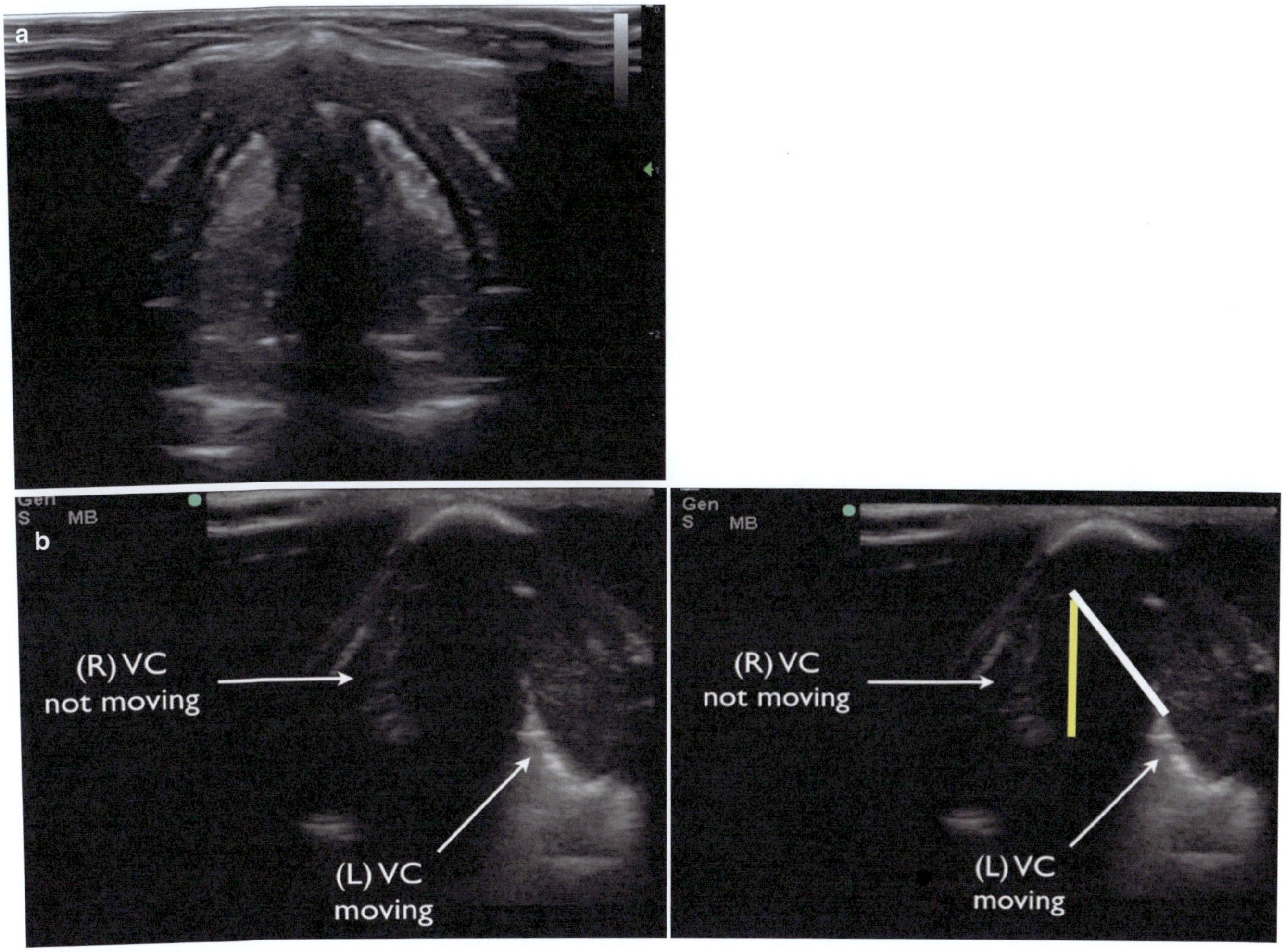

Fig. 17.3 (**a**) Normal vocal cord at rest. (*Image courtesy of Christine Prochnow, MD*). (**b**) Demonstration of the abnormal angle created when only one vocal cord is moving. (*Image courtesy of Adi Osman, MD)*

is broad and can include emergent and malignant pathology; therefore, diagnostic imaging is often obtained. While CT is the most frequently utilized imaging modality, it exposes patients to radiation, prolongs the length of stay, and increases costs. POCUS can be utilized to confirm the suspected diagnosis of sialolithiasis in a more rapid and less invasive manner. The sensitivities for POCUS for the diagnosis of sialolithiasis are best for stones ≥2 mm in diameter [18]. A 2022 systematic review reported that ultrasound was 89.9% sensitive and 96.6% specific [19]. A second study found slightly lower sensitivity and specificity, 77% and 95%, respectively, and found a drop-off in accuracy with stones <3 mm [20]. False-negative sonographic findings were associated with calculi with a diameter < 3 mm in non-dilated or dilated salivary ducts; most calculi with a diameter of ≥3 mm were correctly identified. False-positive findings were caused by ductal stenosis with wall fibrosis, which was erroneously interpreted as lithiasis. However, most of the studies were performed by otolaryngologists with significant experience in salivary gland ultrasound. There are a few case reports showing successful use of this application in other settings, such as the emergency department [21, 22].

If sialolithiasis is present, one may see hyperechoic structures or twinkling artifacts within or near the gland as well as enlargement of the gland itself (Fig. 17.4) [23]. Given that these are often acute and cause an inflammatory response, surrounding cobblestoning and hyperemia may be seen on ultrasound. Other possible associated findings that may be encountered include anechoic fluid collections representing an abscess or sialocele (Fig. 17.5).

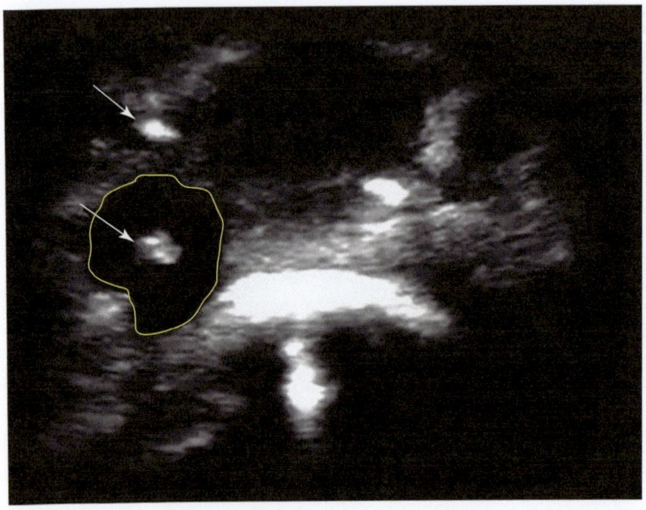

Fig. 17.4 Sialolithiasis. Arrows point to hyperechoic stones in the submandibular region. The circle outlines a dilated duct.

Parotitis

Facial swelling is a common presentation with a broad differential. Ultrasound is a feasible modality for evaluating the parotid gland for enlargement, stones, and inflammation that has been used by specialists for decades [24, 25]. The normal parotid gland, like other salivary glands, should have a homogenous echotexture with a flow similar to lymph nodes originating from the hilum. Parotid gland size varies with age and body weight. In adults, the parotid gland averages 0.7 to 3.7 cm in width and 4.6 cm in height [24]. As the parotid gland becomes inflamed, the cystic structures dilate, the gland enlarges, and the tissue becomes hyperemic (Fig. 17.6). This can give it a similar appearance to a pomegranate, prompting some to refer to this as the "pomegranate sign" [26].

Peritonsillar Abscess

Ultrasound can be utilized to evaluate the size and location of a peritonsillar abscess (PTA). The indications to assess for PTA are sore throat with the presence of swelling in the posterior oropharynx. Typically, this swelling is asymmetric,

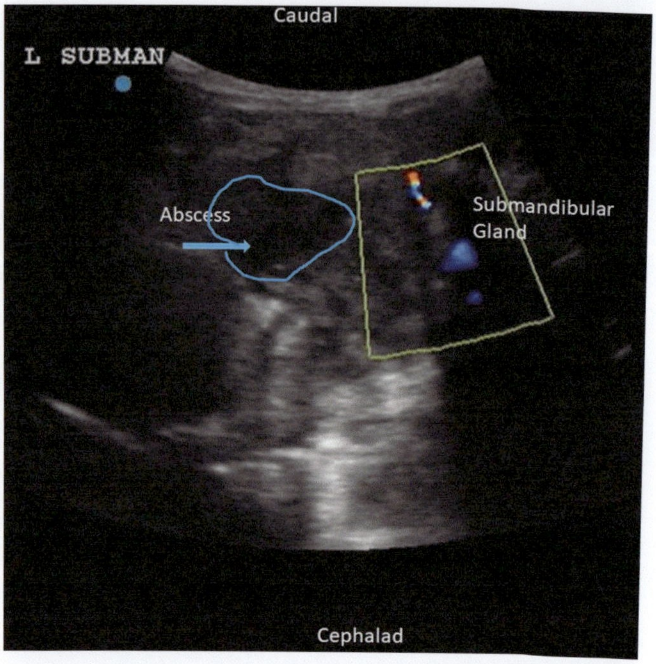

Fig. 17.5 This transmandibular approach to visualizing the left submandibular gland shows a submandibular abscess with the lingual artery highlighted with color Doppler. Twinkling artifacts can also be noted in the near field just deep to a small stone and superficial to the lingual artery.

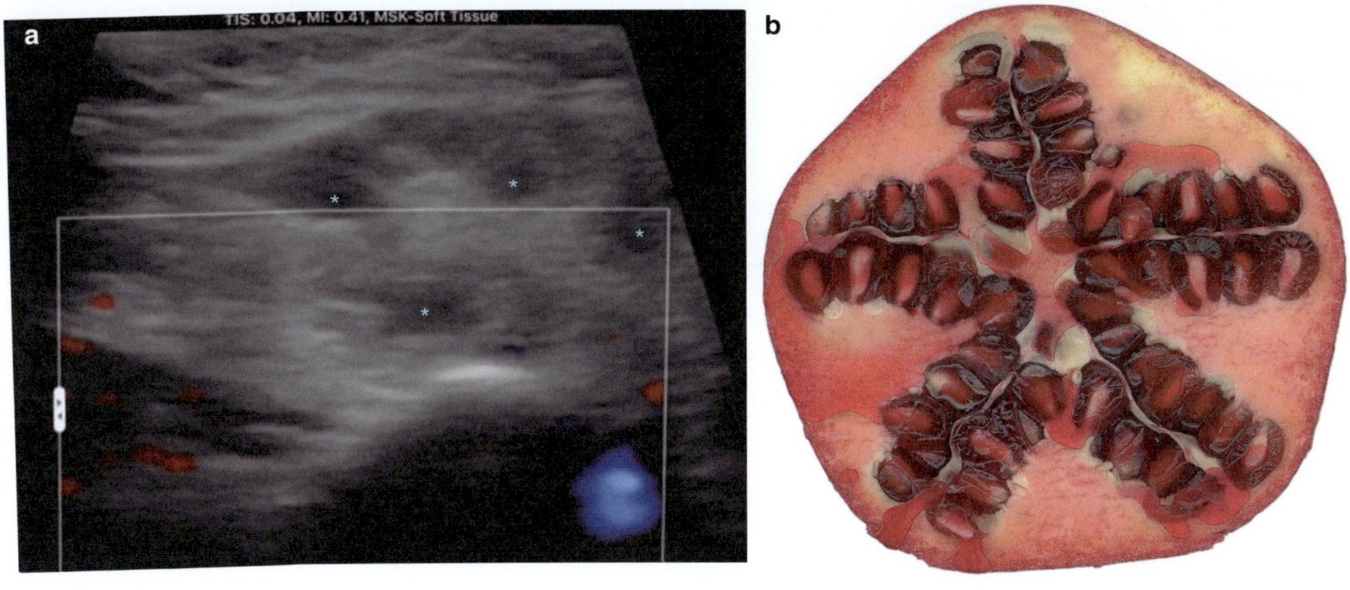

Fig. 17.6 (**a**) Parotitis. This transverse view shows an enlarged parotid gland with dilated ducts (small stars) and hyperemia. (**b**) Pomegranate image for comparison. (*Image courtesy of flutie8211.* https://pixabay.com/illustrations/pomegranate-fruit-seeds-food-7853357/)

and uvular deviation might be seen. There are two approaches that have been described for PTA: the intraoral technique and the transcervical technique.

For the intraoral approach, place a covered endocavitary probe within the oropharynx of the affected side. Identify the tonsil and any associated fluid collection (Fig. 17.7). Any potential fluid collection should be visualized in both planes, and the size should be measured. Color Doppler should also be used to identify the carotid artery and its proximity to the fluid collection. Hyperemia surrounding the fluid is common, though there should not be any color flow within the collection. Once identified, a needle can be inserted in-plane to drain the PTA under real-time guidance (Video 5).

For the transcervical approach, place a curvilinear probe in the sagittal plane just medial to the body of the mandible (Fig. 17.8). Direct the probe toward the tonsillar area by rocking or sliding the probe posteriorly. Once the view is obtained, visualize the PTA in two planes and use the color Doppler to assess proximity to the carotid artery as above. Needle drainage can also be performed using an in-plane approach with this technique (Video 6). While the transcervical technique can be slightly more challenging to align for in-plane guidance, it offers the benefit of visualizing the PTA and guiding drainage without requiring the probe to be within the oral cavity, which can be particularly challenging if trismus is present.

A systematic review found that POCUS was 74% sensitive and 79% specific for PTA when combining intraoral and transcervical techniques [27]. When comparing the two approaches, intraoral ultrasound was 91% sensitive and 75% specific, while the transcervical approach was 80% sensitive and 81% specific [27]. Similar sensitivities have been shown in a dedicated pediatric population [28]. POCUS also led to a significant reduction in the length of stay without an increase in return visits when compared to CT in pediatric patients [29]. Another study in adults found that POCUS utilization in PTA diagnosis and management improved the outcomes of bedside drainage and decreased return visits [30]. Additionally, POCUS can allow for measuring the overall size to determine the need for drainage, depth from the surface, proximity to the carotid artery, and to assess for adequacy of drainage post-procedure [31]. One case report described using POCUS to identify a postprocedural hematoma in a patient with a PTA [32].

Sinusitis

Sinusitis is often a clinical diagnosis. Recent guidelines suggest confirming a clinical diagnosis of sinusitis with objective documentation of sinus inflammation, which can be done via rhinoscopy, nasal endoscopy, or CT [33]. Ultrasound can be a viable diagnostic tool for sinusitis in the appropriate setting. Ultrasound has a sensitivity in the range of 72.7% to 96.4% for diagnosing sinusitis. However, its specificity was quite variable with values ranging from 25% to 93.2% [34–37]. One study of pediatric patients found that the sensitivity of ultrasonography for maxillary sinusitis was 64% with a specificity of 95% [38]. Another study evaluating

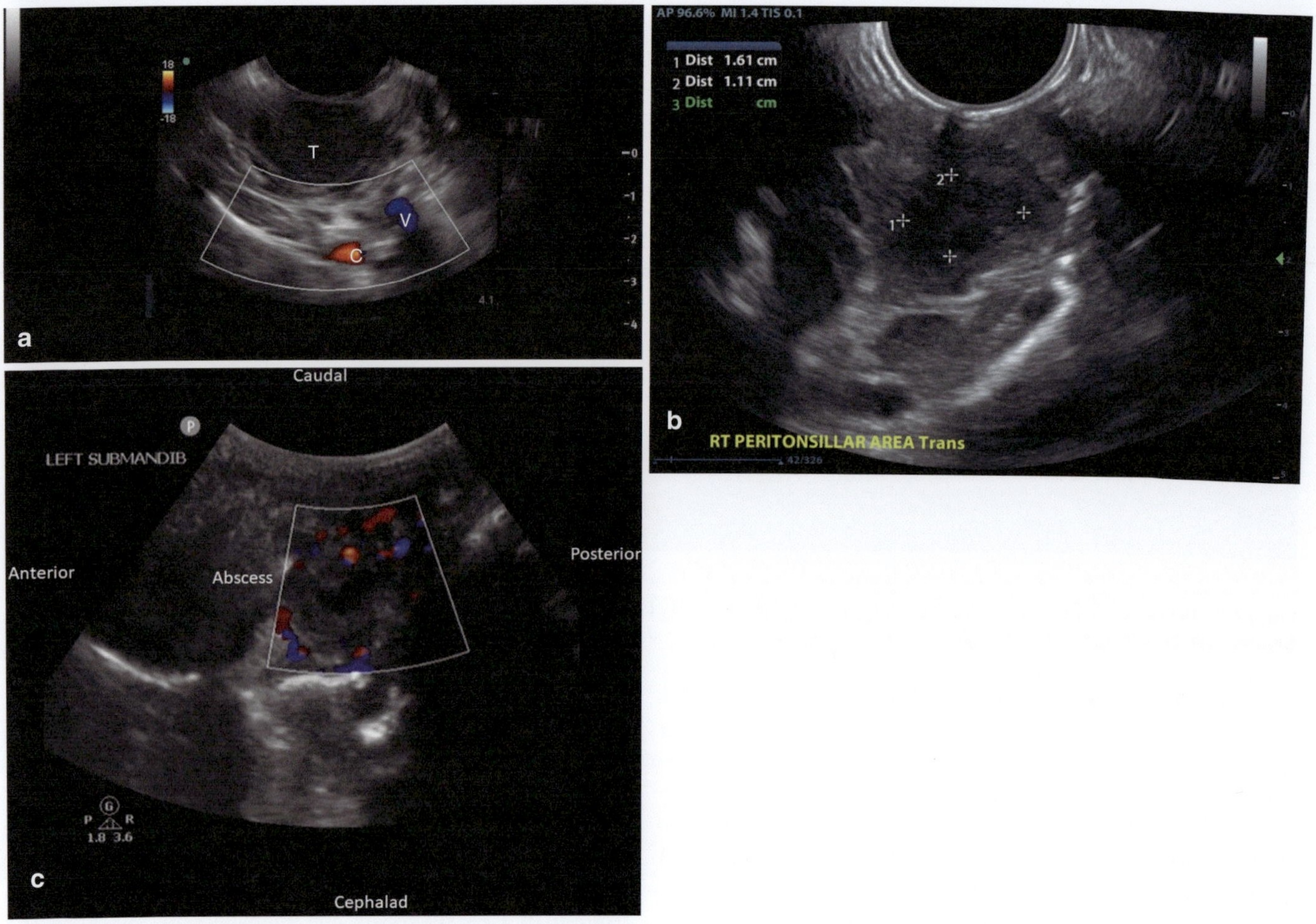

Fig. 17.7 Intraoral approach to peritonsillar abscess (PTA). (**a**) Normal tonsil appearance without PTA. Color Doppler demonstrates the proximity of the carotid artery (**c**) and internal jugular vein (V). (**b**) PTA identified with B-mode imaging with the margins measured. (*Image courtesy of Jeffrey Kramer, MD, MSc*). (**c**) Color Doppler demonstrating a PTA with surrounding hyperemia without internal vascular flow.

radiology-performed ultrasound for the same diagnosis found a sensitivity of 96.4% for diagnosing sinusitis, but the specificity was only 25% [34]. A POCUS study performed by an otolaryngologist found a sensitivity of 78.3% and a specificity of 93.1% [35]. Importantly, the majority of these studies were performed by clinicians with specific training and have been limited to maxillary sinusitis.

In order to perform this exam, the probe is placed over the sinus of interest with at least 4 cm of depth to ensure the posterior wall is within the field of view. However, the posterior wall is not usually visible unless fluid is present. The operator should assess for mucosal thickening, air-fluid levels that demonstrate mobility with position changes, or complete opacification with visualization of the posterior wall. Unilateral fluid levels that are mobile with position changes are suggestive of acute sinusitis (Fig. 17.9).

Thyroid Gland Dysfunction

Ultrasound is the mainstay of diagnostic thyroid imaging. Three commonly encountered pathologies are thyroiditis, thyroid cysts, and nodules. The normal thyroid gland will have a transverse diameter of 4–6 cm and an anteroposterior diameter of ≤ 2 cm with a volume of 10–15 mL [39]. Thyroiditis is a general inflammation of the thyroid gland from various etiologies. When scanning the thyroid, both lobes and the isthmus should be interrogated with B-mode and color Doppler.

Suppurative thyroiditis is a subset of thyroiditis most commonly found in children. If this is discovered in adults, it is typically associated with an immunocompromised state. This acute infection of the thyroid usually occurs through local spread and is rarely hematogenous. On ultrasound, the thyroid will have ill-defined borders, and an abscess can

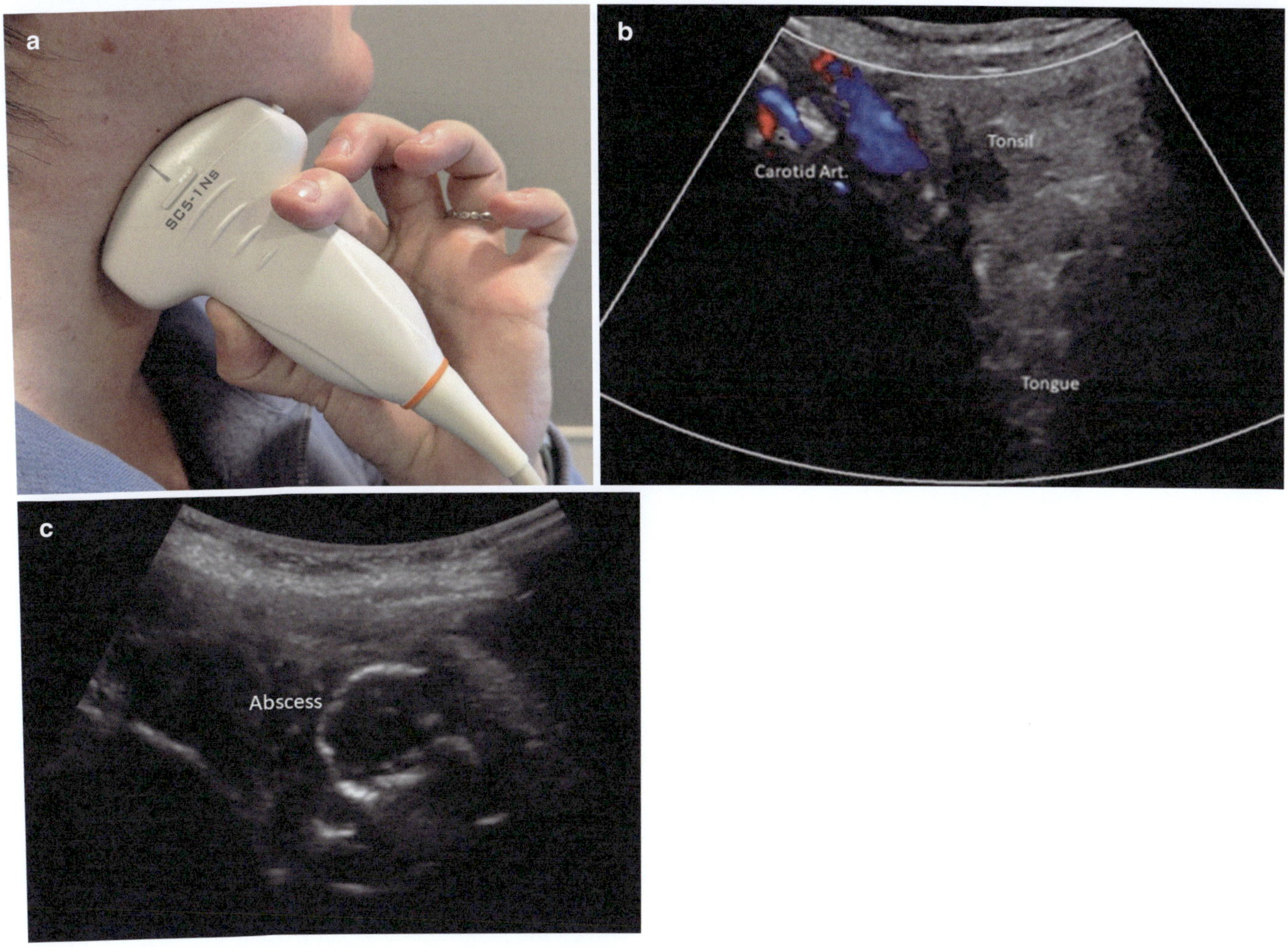

Fig. 17.8 Transcervical approach to peritonsillar abscess (PTA). (**a**) Demonstration of probe position. (**b**) Normal tonsil appearance without PTA. (**c**) PTA identified with B-mode imaging. Note the hyperechoic rim with a central hypoechoic region.

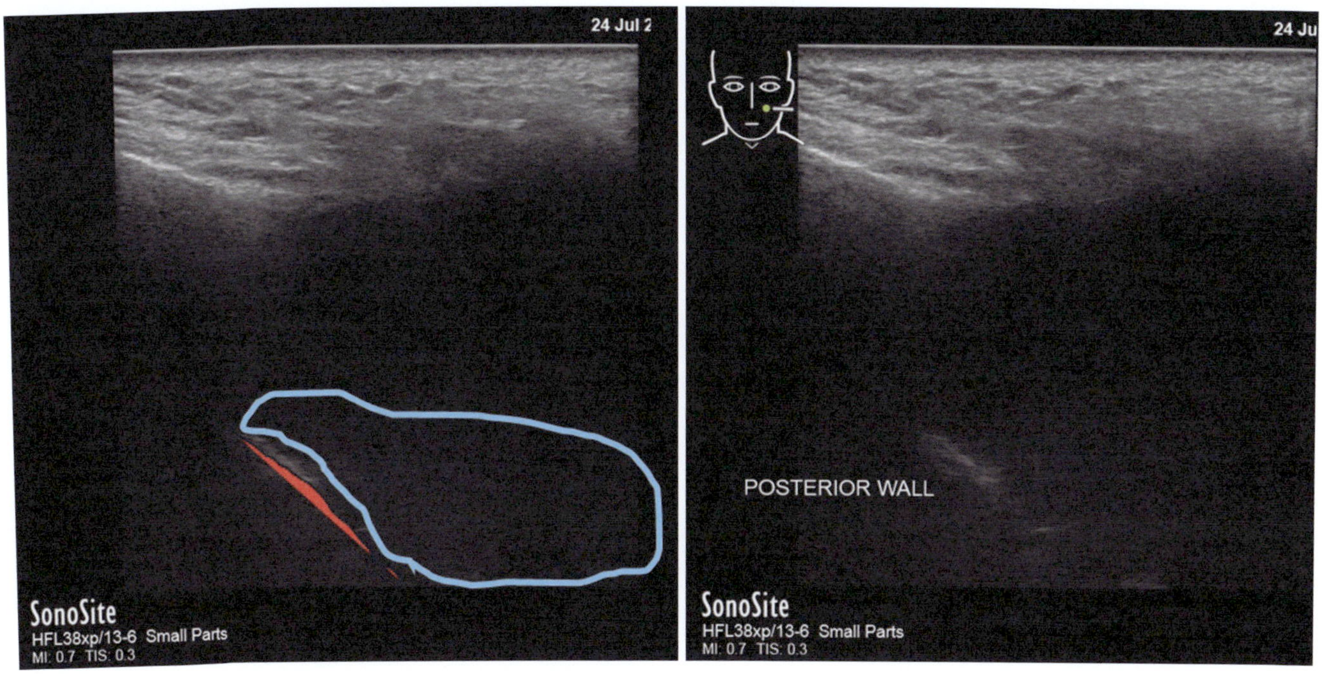

Fig. 17.9 Acute sinusitis. On the left, the hyperechoic posterior wall (red line) is outlined, with hypoechoic fluid and internal echoes outlined in blue. On the right is the corresponding image without annotations.

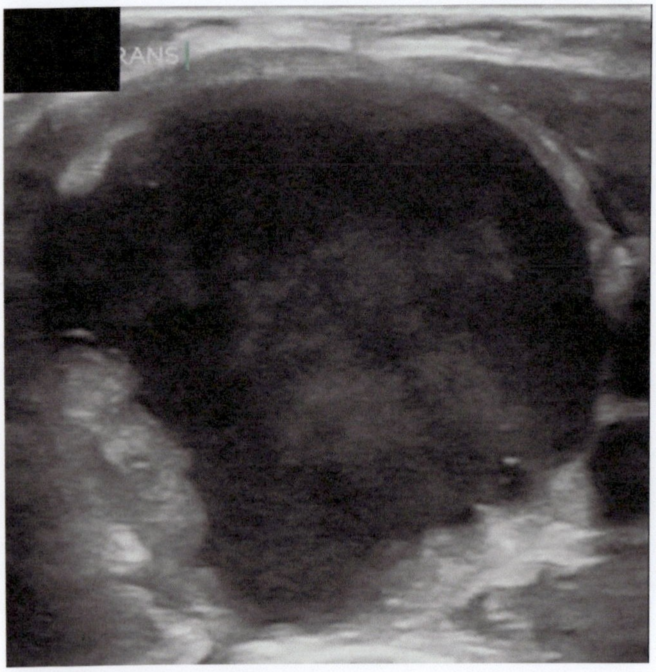

Fig. 17.10 Suppurative thyroiditis with a thyroid abscess. (*Image courtesy of Maya Lin, MD*)

often be identified within the thyroid with diffusely increased vascularity (Fig. 17.10) [40].

Hashimoto's thyroiditis is also known as chronic lymphocytic thyroiditis. Hashimoto's thyroiditis is the most common cause of hypothyroidism worldwide [41]. This is an autoimmune condition where lymphocytes infiltrate the thyroid gland. Sonographically, this will appear as hypoechogenicity with micronodules and degradation of the margins of the thyroid gland (Fig. 17.11) [42, 43].

De Quervain's thyroiditis is a subacute thyroiditis. This often occurs 1–2 weeks after a viral infection and is more common in middle-aged women. Sonographically, this will have a similar appearance to Hashimoto's thyroiditis because it is also the result of an infiltrative process. The thyroid gland will often appear enlarged, slightly hypoechoic, heterogenous, and have normal or reduced vascular flow (Fig. 17.12) [43, 44].

Graves' disease is an autoimmune-mediated thyroid disorder and the most common cause of hyperthyroidism [45, 46]. On ultrasound, the thyroid appears enlarged, typically 2–3 times the normal volume. The thyroid tissue can have mixed echogenicity and will be hypervascular on color Doppler (Fig. 17.13) [47].

Thyroid Cysts and Nodules

Thyroid nodules are common. Some studies have reported that nodules are present in approximately one-third of the general population and are often found incidentally [48, 49]. Nodules may or may not be palpated on physical examination. Ultrasound is very sensitive for the detection of these nodules but does not perform well in ruling out malignancy [50]. Fine-needle aspiration biopsy is an excellent way to assess for malignancy but is invasive.

There are several characteristics that can help stratify their risk of malignancy. The four features most commonly assessed are echogenicity, calcifications, margins, and vascularity [41, 51]. Benign lesions are typically isoechoic or hyperechoic. These lesions are often referred to as simple nodules or cysts. They often have a halo or anechoic rim, smooth margins, and peripheral vascularity (Figs. 17.14 and 17.15) [41, 52]. Suspicious nodules are usually described as hypoechoic, with irregular margins, microcalcifications, and intranodular flow. Figure 17.16 demonstrates an intermediate suspicion nodule in a patient with a multinodular goiter. Figure 17.17 demonstrates a high-suspicion nodule. Table 17.1 summarizes these lesions and their findings on ultrasound.

Thyroglossal Duct Cysts

Thyroglossal duct cysts are fluid-filled collections located between the strap muscles. They occur in about 7% of the population and are the most common congenital neck mass. They have equal prevalence in males and females [55]. These are embryological remnants from a tract resulting from the migration of the thyroid from the base of the tongue during development. These are typically discovered during childhood but may remain undiagnosed until adulthood. These are benign fluid-filled collections in the upper mid-neck adjacent to the hyoid and can move with tongue protrusion or swallowing. On ultrasound, thyroglossal duct cysts are often irregular with mixed echogenicity of the contents (Fig. 17.17).

Branchial Cleft Cysts

Branchial cleft cysts are a relatively rare congenital anomaly [56, 57]. These anomalies are often first identified on physical examinations during childhood in a patient pre-

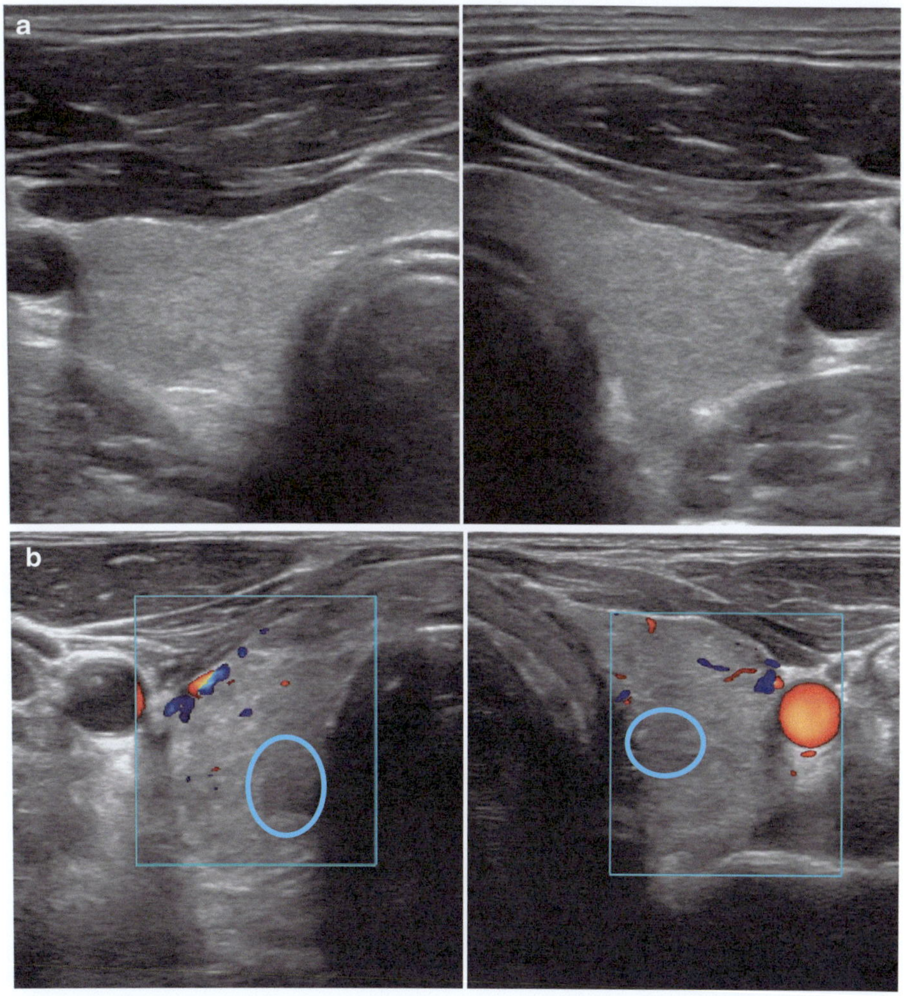

Fig. 17.11 (**a**) Transverse view of the normal thyroid gland. (**b**) Transverse view of the thyroid in a patient with Hashimoto's disease. Micronodules are highlighted by circles. There are some peripheral microcalcifications and irregular margins as compared to normal thyroid in (**a**).

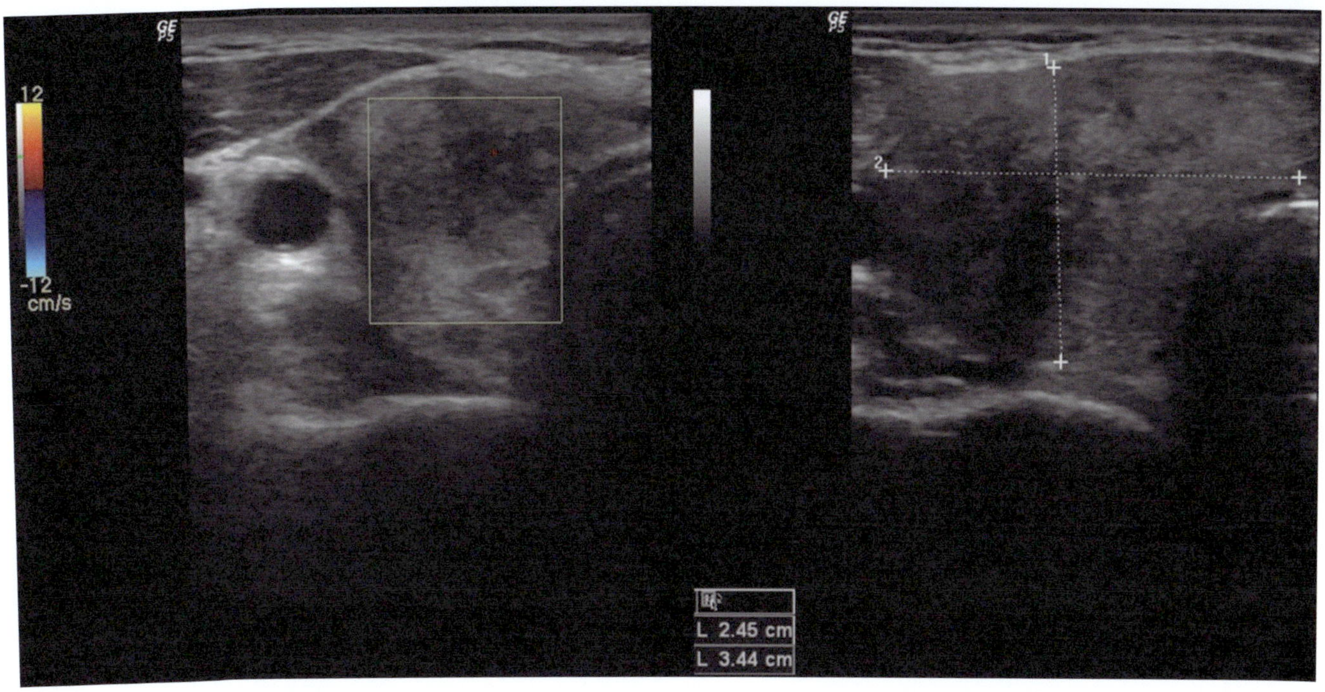

Fig. 17.12 De Quervain's thyroiditis. The thyroid is enlarged and more heterogeneously hypoechoic. When Doppler is applied, flow is markedly reduced. (*Image courtesy of Jennifer Sipos, MD*)

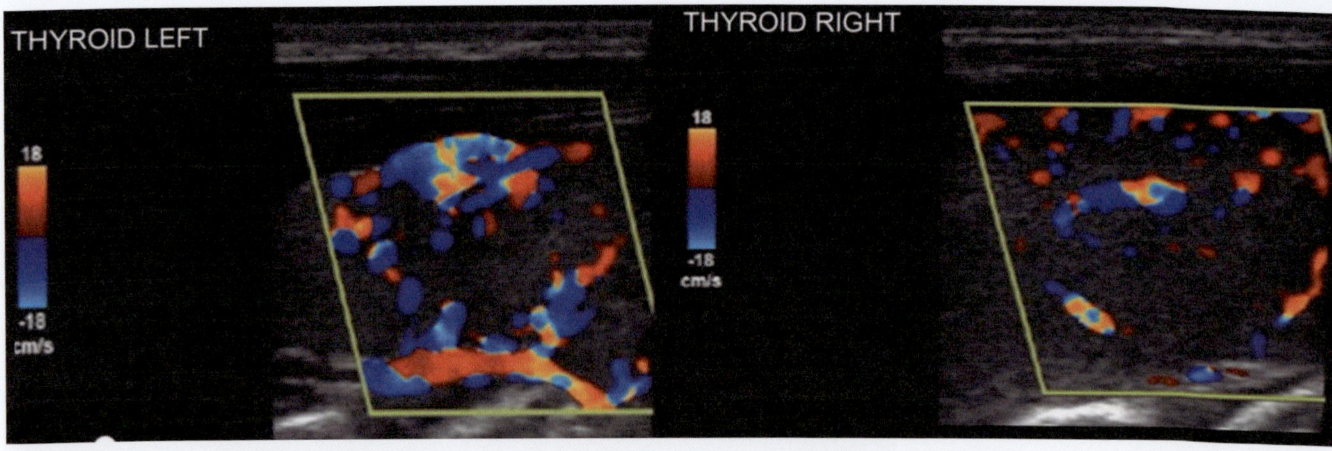

Fig. 17.13 Graves' Disease. Both lobes of the thyroid are shown in the transverse plane with hyperemic flow and homogenous thyroid echotexture.

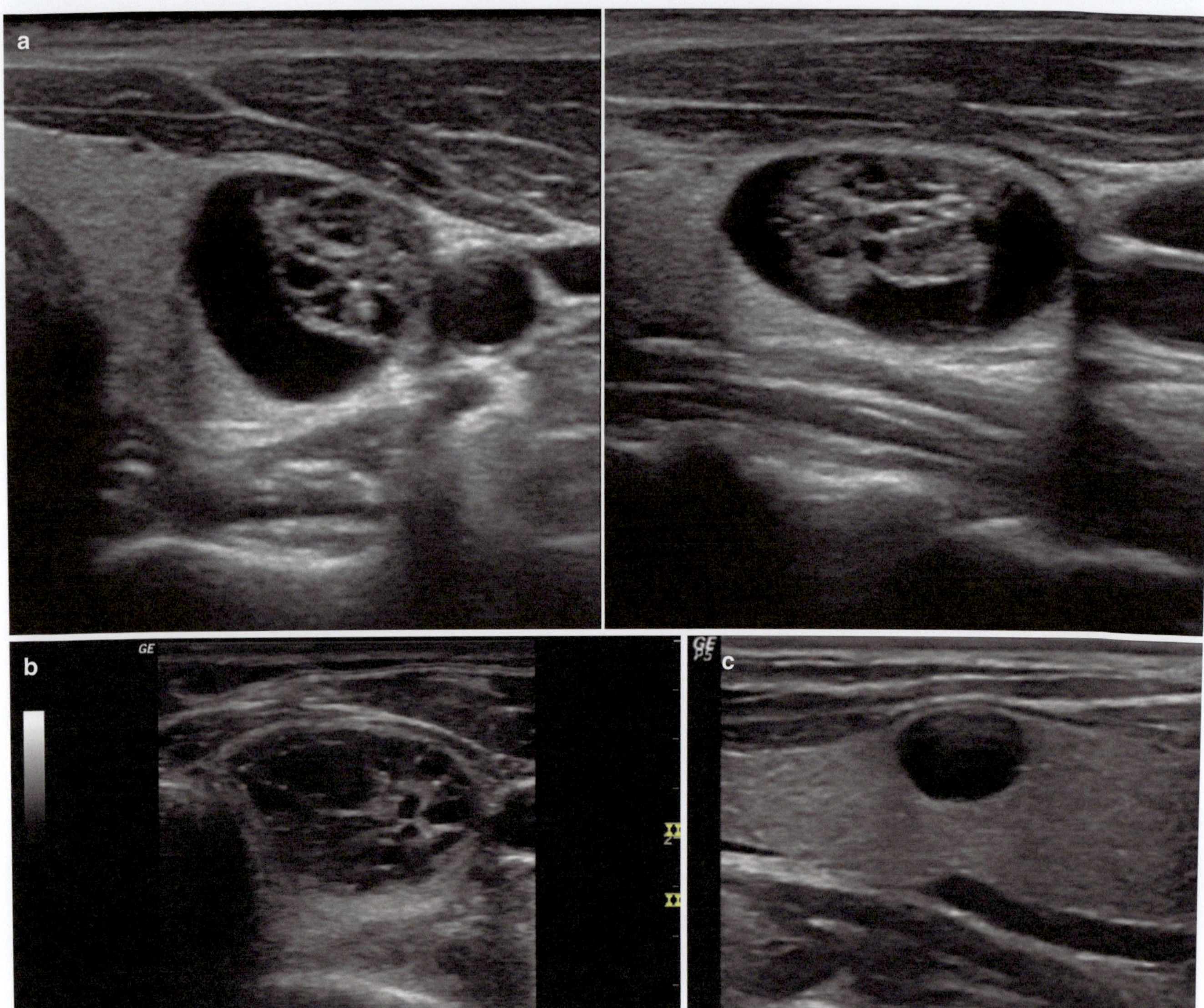

Fig. 17.14 Benign thyroid lesions. All of these lesions have smooth, clear margins. Lesions depicted in images **(a)** and **(b)** have spongiform centers, whereas image **(c)** is more homogenous. (*Images courtesy of Jennifer Sipos, MD*)

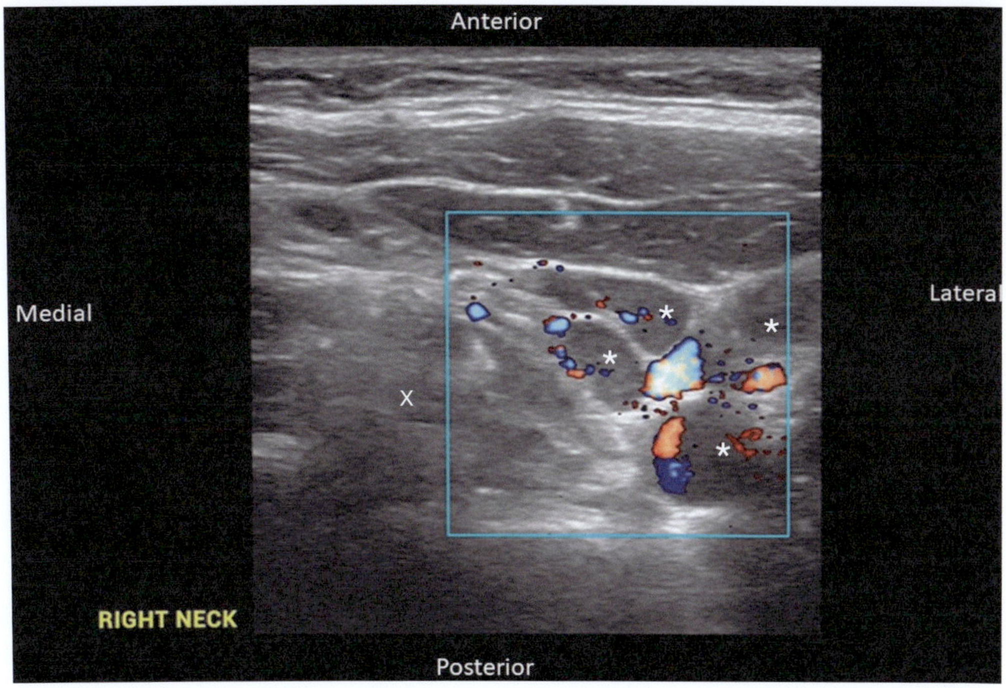

Fig. 17.15 Transverse view of the right lobe of the thyroid in a patient with a multicystic thyroid goiter. Multiple cysts are present, and hyperemia is noted. There are several hypoechoic, well-defined cystic structures (*) with surrounding hyperemia. Normal thyroid tissue for comparison is denoted by an X.

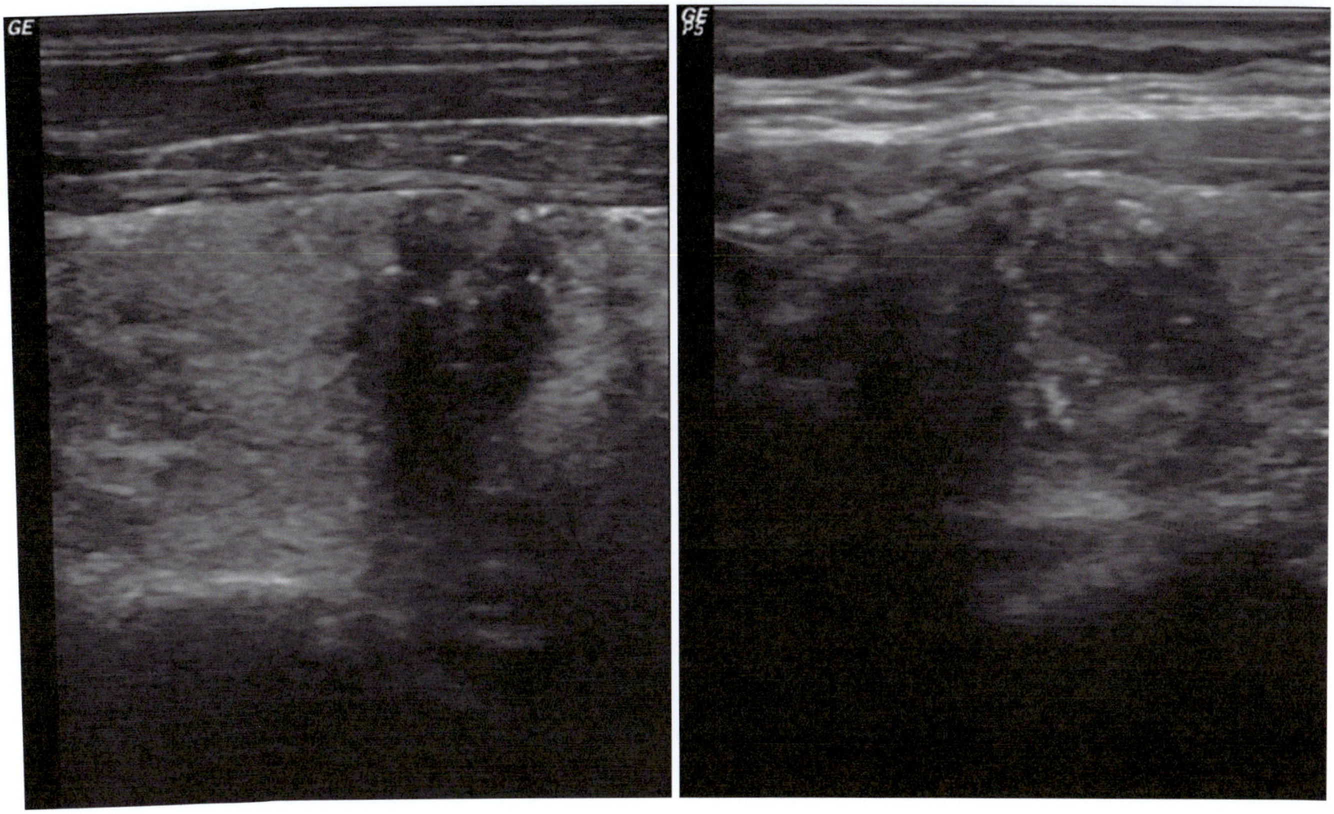

Fig. 17.16 Suspicious Nodules. These lesions have irregular margins and microcalcifications, are hypoechoic, and violate the thyroid wall. *(Images courtesy of Jennifer Sipos, MD)*

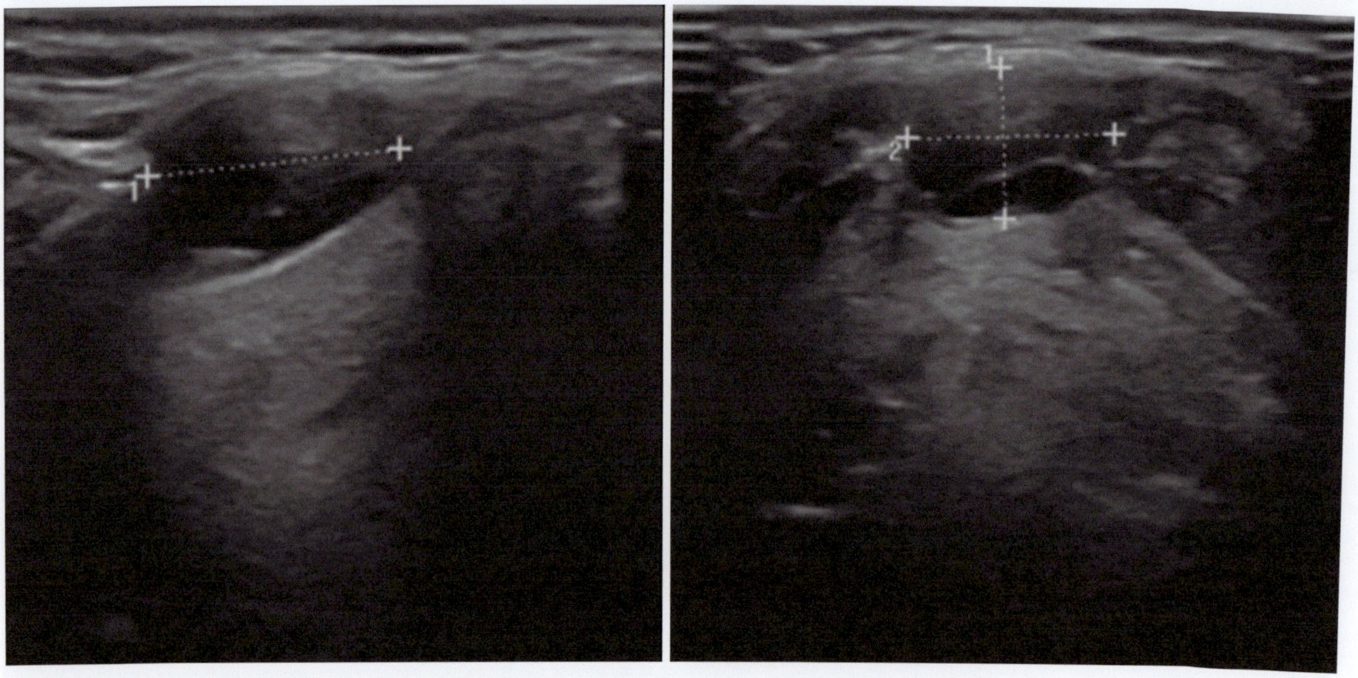

Fig. 17.17 Thyroglossal Duct Cyst. This lesion is fluid-filled and adjacent to the thyroid. Clear margins are seen with mixed internal echogenicity. (*Image courtesy of Jennifer Sipos, MD*)

Table 17.1 Thyroid nodule characteristics and malignancy risk [50, 53, 54].

Thyroid nodule malignancy likelihood	General characteristics
Benign	Simple, smooth margins, peripheral vascularity, cystic, spongiform
Low suspicion	Partially cystic, isoechoic, hyperechoic
Intermediate suspicion	Hypoechoic, solid, regular margins
High suspicion	Hypoechoic, microcalcifications, irregular, extrathyroid extension, taller than wide

senting with unilateral neck swelling [57]. Branchial cleft cysts are located more laterally than the thyroglossal duct cysts, typically along the anterior sternocleidomastoid. These too are a result of embryologic deviations. When the branchial arches separate and involute, this involution may not occur, resulting in cysts, sinuses, or fistulae. These cysts are more typical in appearance with well-defined margins and uniform anechoic fluid contents within the cyst (Fig. 17.18) [56, 57].

Lymph Nodes

Lymph nodes are the most commonly encountered neck mass [58]. The neck contains nearly half of the body's lymph nodes. Lymph nodes can be present in a multitude of conditions, including normal anatomy, infection, inflammation, and malignancy. Normal lymph nodes will measure less than 1 cm in adults and less than 2 cm in pediatric patients [59, 60]. Benign lymph nodes tend to have an oval shape. If the ratio of the long axis to the short axis is less than 2, the lymph node is more likely to be malignant [61].

Lymphadenopathy is a general term used to describe lymph node enlargement. Infection is the most common cause of cervical lymphadenopathy. Inflamed lymph nodes secondary to infection are referred to as lymphadenitis. Benign lymphadenopathy and lymphadenitis often produce midrange lymph nodes (approximately 1–2 cm in diameter) with increased flow (Fig. 17.19) [26, 58]. The sensitivities of ultrasound for detecting malignancy vary widely from 75% to 98% with specificities running from 41% to 91.5% [62, 63].

In general, lymph nodes in the neck that are immobile, matted, or greater than 1.5 cm need further evaluation for more serious pathology [58]. Cervical lymphadenopathy should raise suspicion for malignancy in patients older than 40 years when present for more than 4 weeks, if they are greater than 2 cm or enlarging, when systemic symptoms are present, or if the lymphadenopathy is diffuse [58]. The sonographic appearance of malignant lymph nodes has been described as more hypoechoic, round, and heterogeneous [63]. These nodes often also have cystic necrosis (Fig. 17.20).

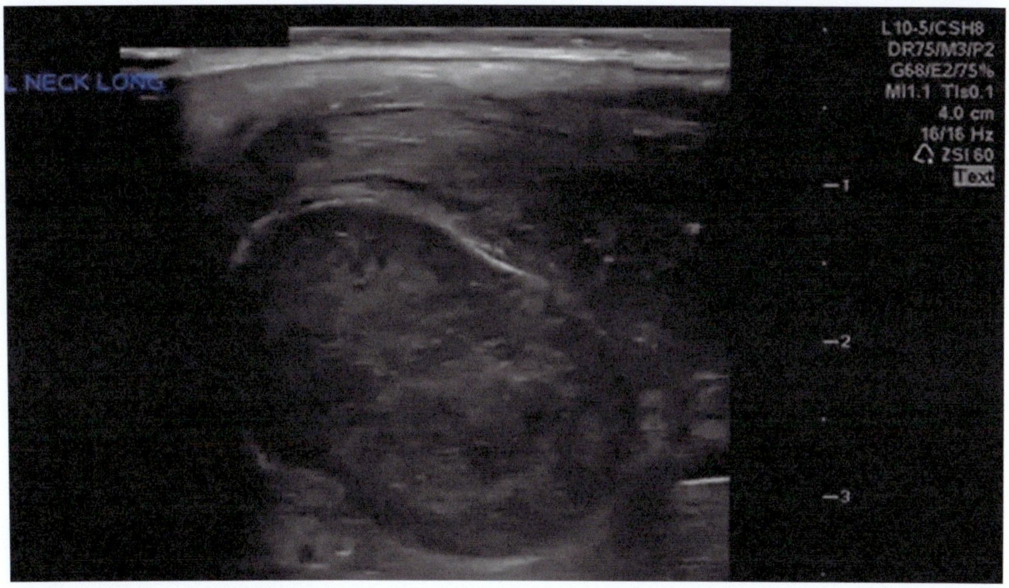

Fig. 17.18 Branchial cleft cyst. (*Image courtesy of Maya Lin, MD*)

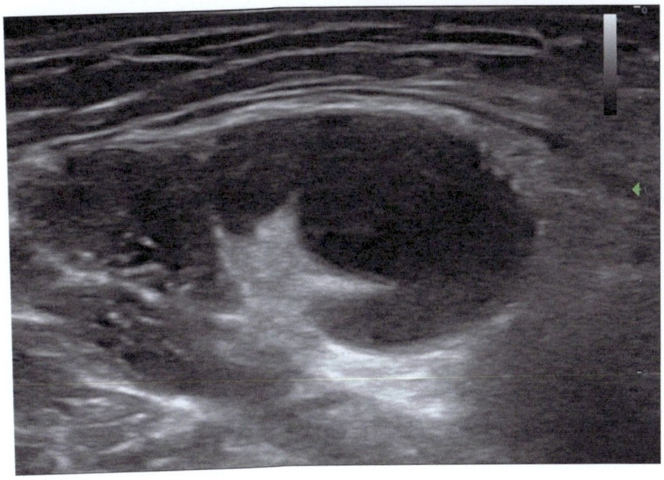

Fig. 17.19 Lymphadenopathy.

Airway Management

Emergent management of the airway is a core tenet of acute and critical care medicine both inside and outside of the operating room. Greater than 10% of emergent intubations are associated with adverse events [64, 65]. POCUS can serve as an adjunct to help predict the difficult airway, determine appropriate endotracheal tube (ETT) size, and confirm proper ETT location.

Management of the difficult airway is often unanticipated and presents a time-sensitive life threat. Numerous scoring systems and tools have been created to help predict the difficult airway with limited success [66–69]. POCUS provides a number of rapid and objective measurements such as distance from skin to the epiglottis (DSE), distance from skin to vocal cords (DSVC), hyomental distance (HMD), ratios of the HMD, and tongue thickness. Many of these measures have greater sensitivity and specificity than commonly used tools such as the modified Mallampati score or upper lip bite test [70–75].

DSE is measured on the anterior neck in transverse orientation superior to the thyroid cartilage (Fig. 17.21). The strap muscles can be visualized in the near field with the hyperechoic preepiglottic soft tissue just below the strap muscles and the hypoechoic linear or crescent-shaped epiglottis just deep to that. The distance is measured from the skin to the anterior aspect of the epiglottis. A DSE larger than 2.54 cm has been shown to have a sensitivity of 82% and specificity of 91% in predicting a difficult airway [71].

A second measurement is the skin to vocal cord distance. DSVC is obtained just below the DSE. The probe is placed in the transverse plane, and the clinician slides inferiorly to the thyroid cartilage to identify the apex of the vocal cords. The distance is measured from the skin to the anterior commissure of the vocal cords (Fig. 17.22). A systematic review and meta-analysis found that DSVC was 75% sensitive and 75% specific; however, the cutoffs used to define a difficult airway were quite broad, ranging from 0.23 cm to 1.23 cm [71].

HMD is an additional measurement that can be utilized to predict a difficult airway. This measurement is obtained in the sagittal plane with a curvilinear probe, sliding superiorly to visualize the mentum of the mandible and the hyoid bone in the same plane. With the head in neutral alignment, the distance between the mentum and hyoid is measured

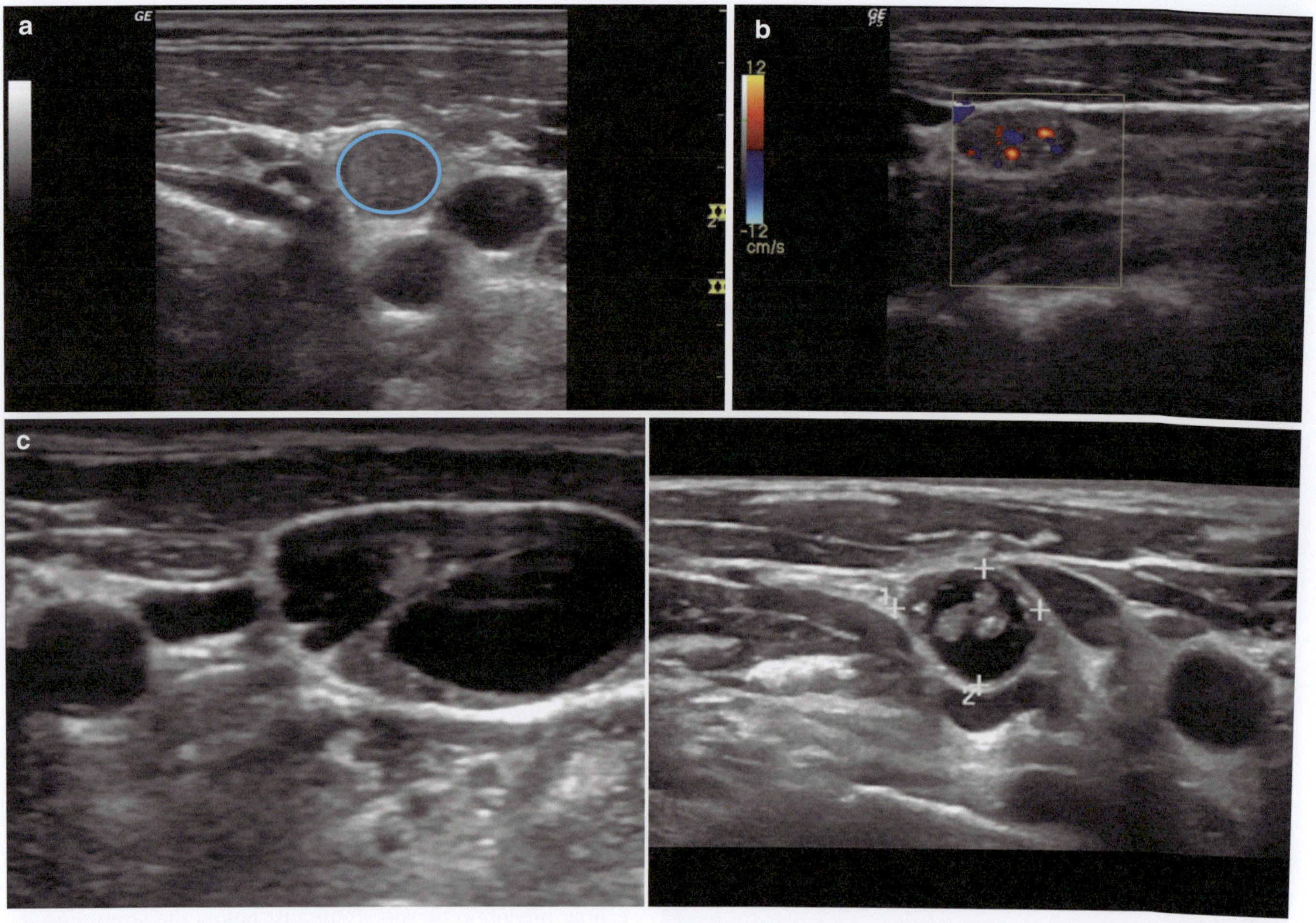

Fig. 17.20 Malignant lymph nodes. Each of these nodes is enlarged, > 2 cm. (**a**) This lymph node is more round and dense than a normal lymph node. (**b**) This lymph node has a more dense appearance and hyperemia. (**c**) These two lymph nodes have hypoechoic features, with cystic components and calcifications. (*Images courtesy of Jennifer Sipos, MD*)

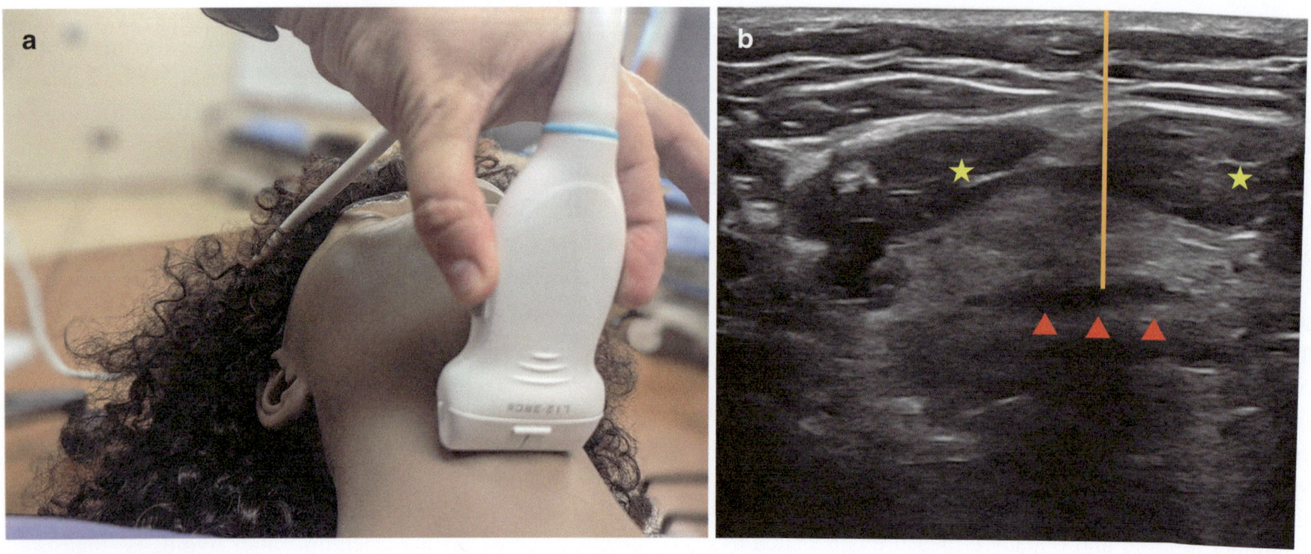

Fig. 17.21 Distance from skin to the epiglottis (DSE). (**a**) Probe positioning for measuring the DSE. (**b**) Ultrasound image depicting the DSE measurement (orange line). Yellow stars represent the strap muscle. Red arrowheads point to the hypoechoic epiglottis.

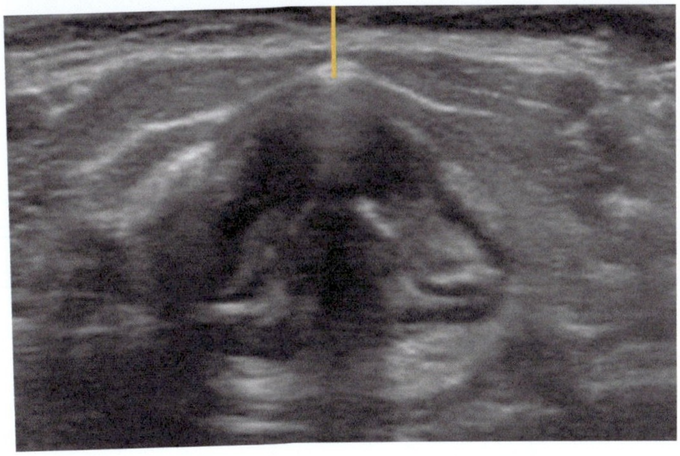

Fig. 17.22 Distance from skin to vocal cords (orange line).

(Fig. 17.23). Patients with an HMD < 4 cm are predicted to be more likely to have a difficult airway [76]. Additionally, the HMD in the neutral position can be compared to the HMD in full neck extension. Using a threshold ratio for $HMD_{extension}/HMD_{neutral}$ of 1.2, this test was found to be 100% sensitive and 90.5% specific for predicting difficult airways [73].

Tongue thickness is another measurement described in predicting difficult intubation. These images are acquired in a transverse orientation with the probe in the submandibular region (Fig. 17.24). The tongue is measured in the midline at its widest diameter. Tongue thickness greater than 6.1 cm has a sensitivity of 71% and specificity of 75% for predicting a difficult airway [74, 75].

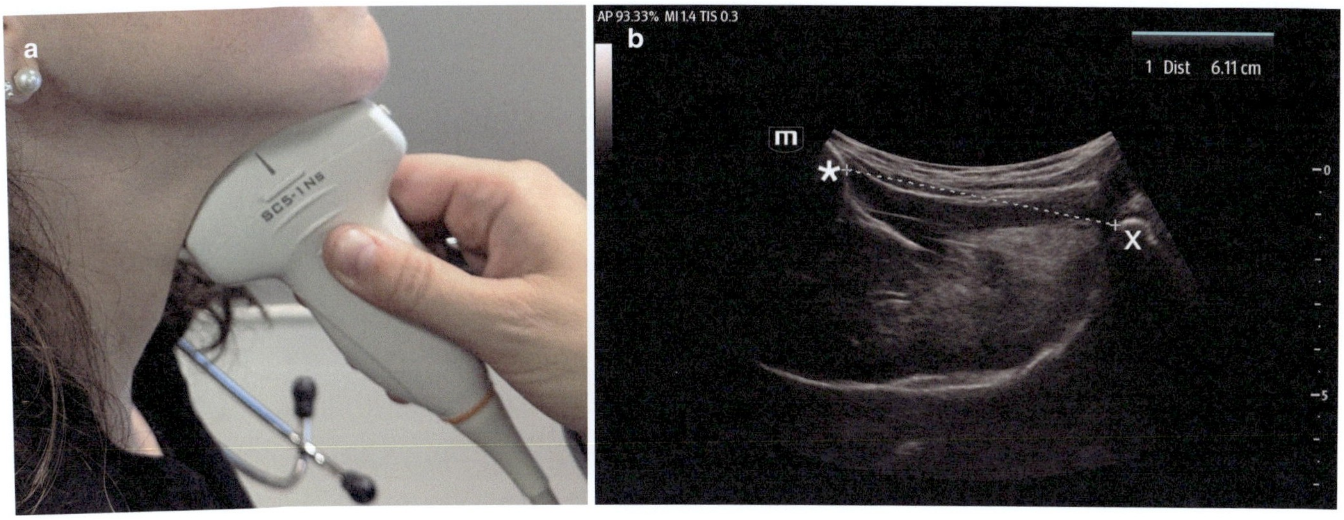

Fig. 17.23 Hyomental distance. (**a**) Probe placement for measuring hyomental distance. (**b**) Ultrasound image demonstrating the mentum of the mandible (*), hyoid bone (X), and measured hyomental distance (dotted line).

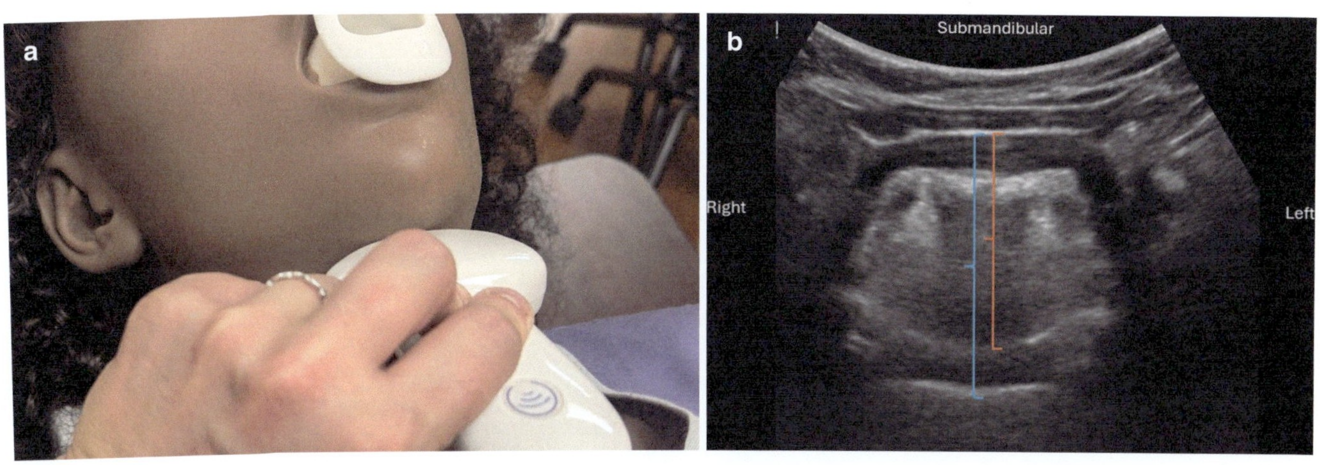

Fig. 17.24 Tongue thickness. (**a**) Probe placement for measuring transverse tongue thickness. (**b**) Ultrasound measurement of transverse tongue thickness. Orange represents tongue thickness. Blue represents oral cavity height.

Intubation Assessment

Incorrect ETT placement may occur in up to 15% of adults and 18% of children [77, 78]. While quantitative waveform capnography is highly accurate for endotracheal verification, this may not always be readily available and may have reduced accuracy in cases of low pulmonary blood flow (e.g., cardiac arrest, massive pulmonary embolism, pulmonary edema) or with hypopharyngeal placement [79, 80]. POCUS can rapidly and confidently confirm ETT placement in both adults and children with nearly 100% sensitivity and specificity [81, 82].

The ultrasound probe is placed at the suprasternal notch in a transverse plane, visualizing the tracheal rings [79, 80]. A linear or curvilinear probe can be used, though one study found that the linear probe was associated with faster time to confirmation and greater operator confidence [83]. Confirmation can be performed using a dynamic (during intubation) or static (post-intubation) technique [84–86]. For the dynamic approach, rapid, flutter-like movement would be seen as the ETT passes through the vocal cords, known as the "snowstorm sign." For the static approach, the probe is placed on the neck immediately post-intubation, and both the trachea and esophagus are evaluated. With tracheal intubation, the ETT can be seen as a second thin line immediately posterior to the trachea (Fig. 17.25). Esophageal intubation will appear as a second air-mucosa interface lateral or posterior to the trachea, referred to as the "double tract" sign. Visualization can be enhanced by gently twisting the ETT side to side to create motion artifacts or instilling saline to enhance visualization of the ETT cuff [87, 88]. Benefits of the static approach include its ability to be performed after intubation by a single clinician, as opposed to the dynamic approach which requires a second person to perform ultrasound during the intubation attempt, and avoidance of pressure on the trachea during the intubation attempt.

After the location has been confirmed, POCUS can also be used to assess ETT depth. To determine the depth, the probe is rotated 90 degrees to the sagittal orientation to visualize the second tracheal ring. Air is removed from the ETT cuff, and 5–10 mL of saline is then instilled to enhance visualization and assess the distance from the ETT cuff to the second tracheal ring (Fig. 17.26) [89]. If the anterior margin of the ETT cuff is above the second tracheal ring, the ETT is too high and needs to be advanced. If the ETT cuff is within the second to sixth tracheal rings, it is in the correct location. If the ETT cuff is below the sixth ring or not visualized, it is too deep and needs to be withdrawn. This can be assessed either statically (inflating the ETT

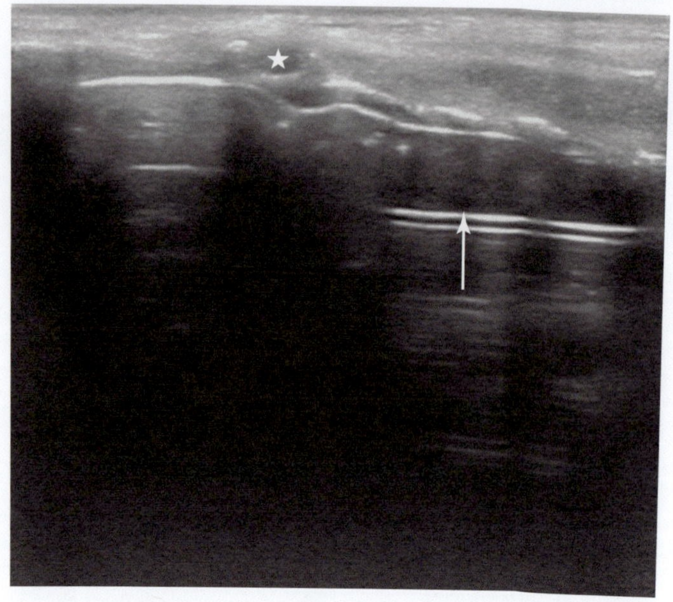

Fig. 17.26 Endotracheal tube depth. Endotracheal tube (ETT) placed at the correct depth. Posterior border of a saline-inflated ETT cuff is shown with an arrow. The cricoid ring is identified with a star. (*Image courtesy of Michael Gottlieb, MD*)

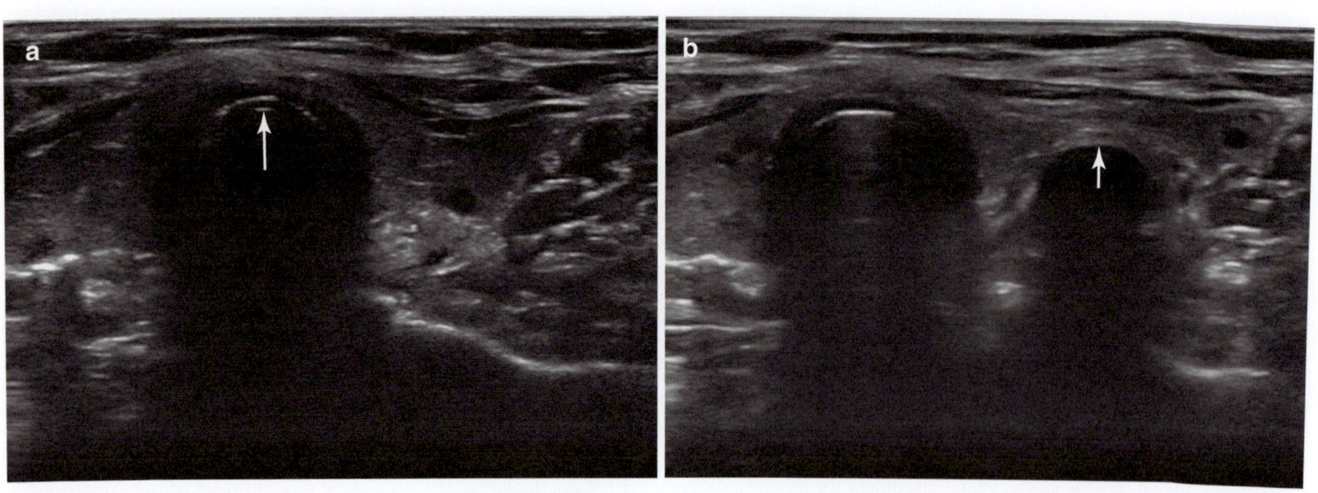

Fig. 17.25 Endotracheal intubation assessment. (**a**) Endotracheal intubation with the tube visualized within the trachea (arrow). (**b**) Esophageal intubation with an empty trachea on the left and tube visualized within the esophagus (arrow) on the right. (*Images courtesy of Michael Gottlieb, MD*)

Table 17.2 Sono-DOPES algorithm.

Potential etiology	Diagnostic assessment
Dislodged ETT	Transtracheal ultrasound to assess for ETT location and ETT depth.
Obstruction of the tube	Assess for bilateral lung sliding to demonstrate air is entering the lungs.
Pneumothorax	Assess for bilateral lung sliding in the most superior portion of the chest wall.
	If unilateral lung sliding is present, pneumothorax is suspected. Evaluate for lung pulse to differentiate single lung intubation versus pneumothorax.
Equipment malfunction	Assess for bilateral lung sliding.
	If there is no lung sliding and ETT is in the appropriate location, disconnect from the ventilator and repeat lung ultrasound with manual ventilation.
Breath stacking	Assess for bilateral lung sliding and appropriate diaphragm movement.

Adapted with permission from Gottlieb et al. [80]

cuff prior to ultrasound) or dynamically (visualizing inflation in real time). One study found that the static technique was 99% sensitive and 97% specific, while the dynamic technique was 100% sensitive and 100% specific [90].

POCUS is also useful in evaluating the deteriorating ventilated patient. The Sono-DOPES (dislodgement, obstruction, pneumothorax, equipment malfunction, stacking of breaths) approach has been proposed to describe the role of POCUS in enhancing each stage of the widely adopted clinical DOPES algorithm. This algorithm has been adapted and outlined in Table 17.2 [80].

Cricothyroidotomy

Cricothyroidotomy is an uncommon procedure that is used to secure the airway in cases of respiratory failure in which the patient cannot be intubated or ventilated. As such, it is often performed under high-acuity and high-stress conditions and requires identifying a small anatomical area in a very limited time window—which may be made additionally more difficult due to patient factors (e.g., obesity, neck masses).

Among patients with average anatomy, POCUS has been found to improve the accuracy of cricothyroid membrane (CTM) identification by up to two-fold, while POCUS improves the accuracy among patients with poorly defined anatomy by five-to-ten-fold [91–94]. Studies suggest that the technique requires minimal training and can be performed in less than 30 seconds, with comparable time to the landmark-based approach [95–99]. This approach should be considered in any patient with an anticipated difficult airway.

Prior to medication or induction, the patient should be placed in position for a cricothyroidotomy, and ultrasound should be used to evaluate for the CTM. The membrane and relevant landmarks can be noted on the skin with indelible ink prior to the start of the procedure to aid in the time and accuracy of the procedure.

To identify the CTM in the transverse plane, the probe is placed transversely on the anterior neck overlying the thyroid cartilage. We recommend using the "TACA" technique ("Thyroid cartilage-Airline-Cricoid cartilage-Airline") [95]. First, the triangular shape of the thyroid cartilage is visualized, appearing like a "taco" shell (Fig. 17.27). Then, the probe is slid caudally until the line of air at the CTM is identified with reverberation artifact deep to the hyperechoic CTM (Fig. 17.28). Third, the probe is moved further caudally to the

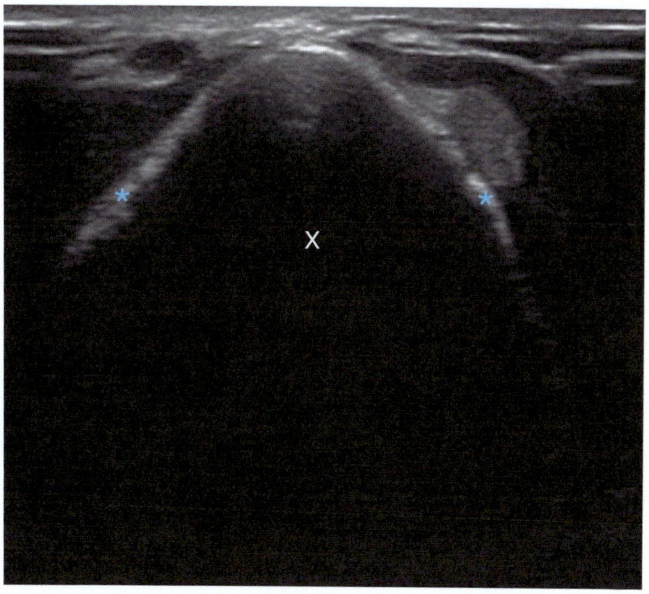

Fig. 17.27 Thyroid cartilage with a taco shell appearance.

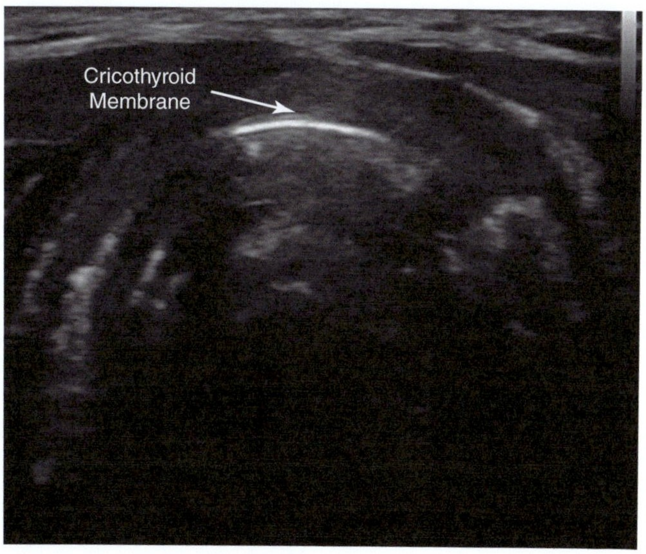

Fig. 17.28 Cricothyroid membrane visualized in the transverse plane.

cricothyroid cartilage, which appears as a hypoechoic wide ring overlying the bright hyperechoic mucosal air interface (Fig. 17.29). The final step is to return the probe back in the cranial direction to identify the approximate center of the airline or CTM, which can then be marked with a surgical pen.

The longitudinal approach to identifying the CTM starts with the probe in the sagittal plane on the central neck inferior to the thyroid cartilage. The tracheal rings can be identified as bright, hypoechoic linear rings appearing as a "string of pearls" from cranial to caudal with posterior reverberation artifacts (A-lines). Immediately cranial to this is the larger hypoechoic ring (cricoid cartilage). Immediately cranial to the cricoid cartilage is the hyperechoic linear line (cricothyroid membrane), and then superior to this is the thyroid cartilage (Fig. 17.30). The CTM should be marked with the neck in the position the procedure would be performed. Alternatively, if using POCUS to identify landmarks at the time of the procedure (not pre-marking), one may consider inserting a saline-filled needle for the Seldinger approach or as a guide for the scalpel.

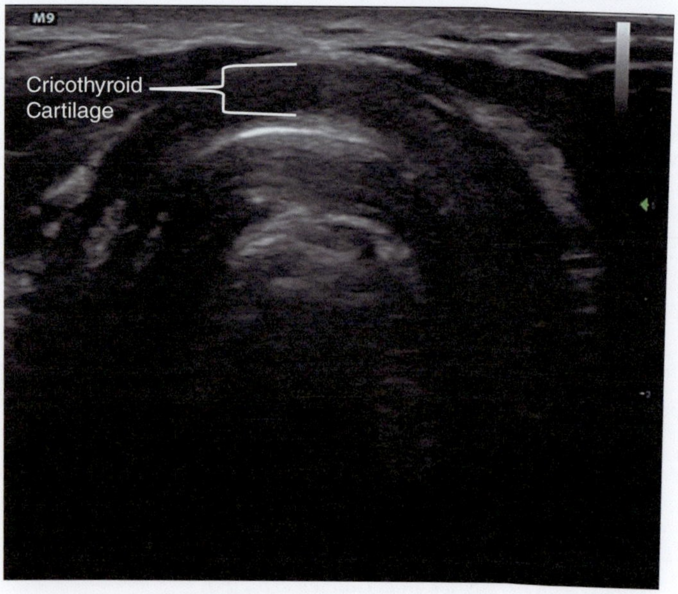

Fig. 17.29 Cricoid cartilage in the transverse plane.

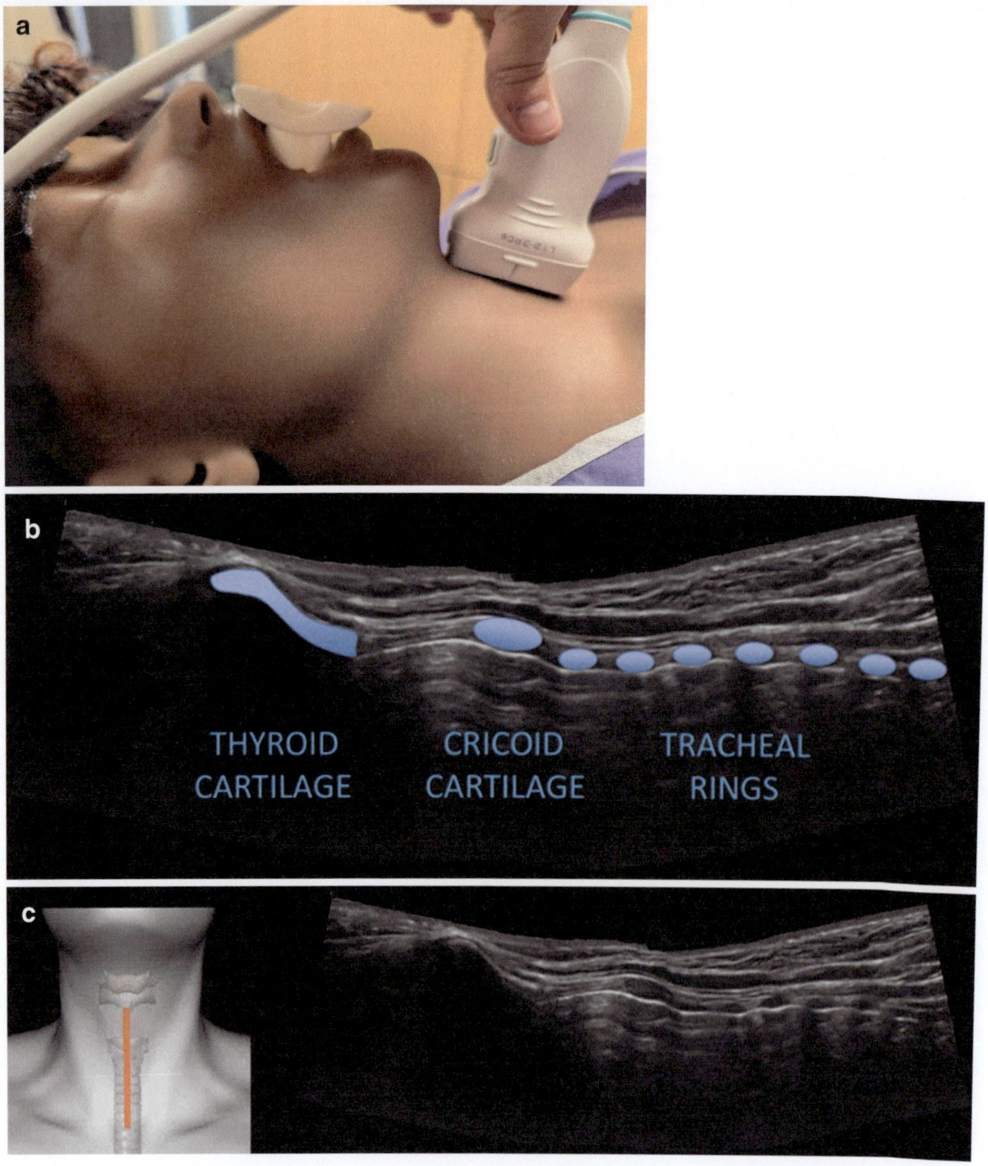

Fig. 17.30 (**a**) Probe position for the sagittal approach to cricothyroidotomy. (**b**) Sonographic image of the cricothyroid membrane. (**c**) Labeled image of the thyroid cartilage, cricoid cartilage, and tracheal rings. (*Images courtesy of Rob Ferre, MD*)

Key Ultrasound Findings

Pathology	Key ultrasound findings
Angioedema	Thickened tongue and laryngeal edema.
Vocal cord dysfunction	Absence or asymmetrical movement of vocal cords during phonation.
Sialolithiasis	Hyperechoic structures in the parotid gland or sublingual space with posterior shadowing. Lower sensitivity for stones <2 mm in diameter.
Parotitis	Dilated cystic structures within the gland, enlarged parotid gland, hyperemic.
Epiglottitis	Thickened lateral epiglottis >3.6 mm.
Peritonsillar abscess	Enlarged tonsil, typically with hyperemic flow, and an anechoic walled-off area within the tonsil that lacks flow.
Sinusitis	Mucosal thickening and air-fluid levels. Posterior wall visible.
Hashimoto's thyroiditis	Hypoechogenicity, micronodules, and degradation of the margins of the thyroid.
De Quervain's thyroiditis	Heterogeneous hypoechoic in these images and slightly enlarged. When Doppler is applied, flow is markedly reduced.
Graves' disease	Enlarged with increased flow on color Doppler.
Thyroid masses-benign	Simple, well-defined margins, peripheral flow, cystic.
Thyroid masses – malignant	Irregular margins, extrathyroid extension, central flow, microcalcifications. Taller than wide.
Thyroglossal duct cysts	Fluid-filled collections located between the strap muscles. Often irregular with mixed echogenicity of the contents.
Branchial cleft cysts	Along the anterior sternocleidomastoid. Well-defined margins and uniform anechoic fluid contents within the cyst.
Lymphadenopathy	Immobile, matted, or greater than 1.5 cm need further evaluation for more serious pathology. Abnormal when >1 cm in adults and >2 cm in pediatric patients. Malignant lymph nodes are more hypoechoic, round, and heterogeneous and may have cystic necrosis.
Endotracheal intubation	With tracheal intubation, the endotracheal tube can be seen as a second thin line immediately posterior to the trachea.
Esophageal intubation	Esophageal intubation will appear as a second air-mucosa interface lateral or posterior to the trachea, referred to as the "double tract" sign.
Cricothyroid membrane	The 'TACA' technique, Thyroid cartilage-Airline-Cricoid cartilage-Airline, can help identify the cricothyroid membrane.

Pearls and Pitfalls

- Because head and neck structures are superficial, most applications utilize the high-frequency linear probe. Care must be taken to apply the appropriate amount of pressure and anchoring to optimize imaging.
- The epiglottis is not routinely visible in the longitudinal orientation in healthy patients.
- Incidental findings may be commonly visualized while scanning the thyroid, cervical lymph nodes, and other head and neck structures. Clinicians should ensure that patients are informed of these findings and have appropriate follow-up imaging where indicated.
- If unable to perform intraoral evaluation for peritonsillar abscess due to trismus, an extraoral submandibular approach with a lower frequency probe may be used.
- Ultrasound can be used to assess ETT location and depth and to identify and manage ventilator complications.
- Assessment of endotracheal intubation has been shown to be accurate and repeatable utilizing a variety of both standard and dynamic imaging techniques. Approaches should be tailored to the clinical circumstances and resource availability.
- In anticipated difficult airways requiring endotracheal intubation, ultrasound can be used to identify the cricothyroid membrane as part of procedural preparation, in addition to providing dynamic needle or scalpel guidance during the procedure.

References

1. Gottlieb M, Olszynski P, Atkinson P. Just the facts: point-of-care ultrasound for airway management. CJEM. 2021;23(3):277–9. https://doi.org/10.1007/s43678-020-00075-7. Epub 2021 Jan 25. PMID: 33959928.
2. Link MS, Berkow LC, Kudenchuk PJ, et al. Part 7: adult advanced cardiovascular life support: 2015 American Heart Association guidelines update for cardiopulmonary resuscitation and emergency cardiovascular care. Circulation. 2015;132(18 Suppl 2) https://doi.org/10.1161/CIR.0000000000000261.
3. Hung TY, Li S, Chen PS, et al. Bedside ultrasonography as a safe and effective tool to diagnose acute epiglottitis. Am J Emerg Med. 2011;29(3):359.e1–3. https://doi.org/10.1016/j.ajem.2010.05.001.

4. Huang CY, Chang CJ, Sim SS, Ma MH, Sun JT. A practical way to use point-of-care ultrasound for the diagnosis of acute supraglottitis in the emergency department. Intern Emerg Med. 2023;18(6):1859–61. https://doi.org/10.1007/s11739-023-03269-w.
5. Ko DR, Chung YE, Park I, et al. Use of bedside sonography for diagnosing acute epiglottitis in the emergency department. J Ultrasound Med. 2012;31(1):19–22. https://doi.org/10.7863/jum.2012.31.1.19.
6. Hall EA, et al. Ultrasound evaluation of the airway in the ED: a feasibility study. Crit Ultrasound J. 2018;10:1–8.
7. Smith A, Ray M, Jain N, Zhang H, Sebelik M. The burden of angioedema on United States emergency departments: 2006-2010. Laryngoscope. 2017;127(4):828–34. https://doi.org/10.1002/lary.26336.
8. Lin DH, Meyers B, Nisar S, Heinz ER. Role of submandibular ultrasound in airway management of a patient with angioedema. Cureus. 2022;14(3):e22823. https://doi.org/10.7759/cureus.22823.
9. Schick M, Grether-Jones K. Point-of-care sonographic findings in acute upper airway edema. West J Emerg Med. 2016;17(6):822–6. https://doi.org/10.5811/westjem.2016.9.31528.
10. Lin HY, et al. Submental ultrasound is effective in predicting difficult mask ventilation but not in difficult laryngoscopy. Ultrasound Med Biol. 2021;47(8):2243–9.
11. Helbing A, et al. Utilization of submandibular ultrasound to measure oral cavity changes with interventions in routine airway management. Baylor Univ Med Cent Proc. 2022;35(1):1–12.
12. Dass C, et al. Evaluation of staging criteria for disposition and airway intervention in emergency department angioedema patients. Acute Med Surg. 2021;8(1):e704.
13. Kumar A, Sinha C, Singh AK, Bhadani UK. Vocal cord dysfunction: Ultrasonography-aided diagnosis during routine airway examination. Saudi J Anaesth. 2017;11(3):370–1. https://doi.org/10.4103/1658-354X.206811.
14. Wiltrakis SM, Gutierrez P. Use of POCUS in the diagnosis of paradoxical vocal cord movement. Pediatr Emerg Care. 2022;38(3):e1085.
15. Ruan Z, Ren R, Dong W, Ma J, Xu Z, Mao Y, Jiang L. Assessment of vocal cord movement by ultrasound in the ICU. Intensive Care Med. 2018;44(12):2145–52. https://doi.org/10.1007/s00134-018-5469-1.
16. Finnoff JT, Orbelo DM, Ekbom DC. Can ultrasound identify paradoxical vocal fold movement? A pilot study. Clin J Sport Med. 2020;30(5):e120.
17. Huoh KC, Eisele DW. Etiologic factors in sialolithiasis. Otolaryngol Head Neck Surg. 2011;145(6):935–9.
18. Jäger L, Menauer F, Holzknecht N, Scholz V, Grevers G, Reiser M. Sialolithiasis: MR sialography of the submandibular duct—an alternative to conventional sialography and US. Radiology. 2000;216:665–71.
19. Kim DH, et al. Utility of ultrasonography for diagnosis of salivary gland sialolithiasis: a meta-analysis. Laryngoscope. 2022;132(9):1785–91.
20. Terraz S, Poletti PA, Dulguerov P, et al. How reliable is sonography in the assessment of sialolithiasis? AJR Am J Roentgenol. 2013;201(1):W104. https://doi.org/10.2214/AJR.12.9383.
21. Oliveira LG, Hurst ND, Magajna PW. Bedside emergency ultrasound in a case of acute parotid duct sialolithiasis. J Emerg Med. 2014;47:e49.
22. Huang F, Caton R, Colla J. Point-of-care ultrasound diagnosis of acute sialolithiasis with sialadenitis. Clin Pract Cases Emerg Med. 2017;1:437–8.
23. Pabst G, Strobel K, Zehnder J. The value of the twinkling artefact for the diagnosis of sialolithiasis of the large salivary glands. J Laryngol Otol. 2018;132(2):162–7. https://doi.org/10.1017/S002221511700250X.
24. Katz P, Hartl DM, Guerre A. Clinical ultrasound of the salivary glands. Otolaryngol Clin N Am. 2009;42(6):973–1000.
25. Gupta A, Gupta A, Sharma K. A prospective study to assess the reliability of ultrasonography as a diagnostic aid in various salivary gland pathologies. J Evol Med Dent Sci. 2015;4:2890–7.
26. Ng C, Tupchong K, Thomas-Mohtat R. Parotitis on ultrasound: the pomegranate sign. Pediatr Emerg Care. 2020;36(4):205–7.
27. Kim DJ, et al. Test characteristics of ultrasound for the diagnosis of peritonsillar abscess: A systematic review and meta-analysis. Acad Emerg Med. 2023;30:859.
28. Fordham MT, et al. Transcervical ultrasonography in the diagnosis of pediatric peritonsillar abscess. Laryngoscope. 2015;125(12):2799–804.
29. Zhao X, et al. Impact of transcervical ultrasound for the diagnosis of pediatric peritonsillar abscesses on emergency department performance measures. J Ultrasound Med. 2020;39(4):715–20.
30. Gibbons RC, Costantino TG. Evidence-based medicine improves the emergent management of peritonsillar abscesses using point-of-care ultrasound. J Emerg Med. 2020;59(5):693–8.
31. Long B, Gottlieb M. Managing peritonsillar abscess. Ann Emerg Med. 2023;82(1):101–7. https://doi.org/10.1016/j.annemergmed.2022.10.023.
32. Floyd J, et al. Peritonsillar abscess and post-aspiration bleed identified with point-of-care ultrasound using endocavitary probe: a case report. Clin Pract Cases Emerg Med. 2024;8(2):129.
33. Rosenfeld RM, Piccirillo JF, Chandrasekhar SS, et al. Clinical practice guideline (update): adult sinusitis. Otolaryngol Head Neck Surg. 2015;152(2 Suppl):S1–S39. https://doi.org/10.1177/0194599815572097. PMID: 25832968.
34. Niazi AAK, et al. Ultrasonography: A novel diagnostic tool for maxillary sinusitis. Ann PIMS-Shaheed Zulfiqar Ali Bhutto Med Univ. 2020;16(4):219–24.
35. Neagos A, et al. Ultrasonography used in the diagnosis of chronic rhinosinusitis: From experimental imaging to clinical practice. Exp Ther Med. 2021;21(6):1–4.
36. Ho NH, et al. Combining sinus plain film and sinus ultrasound as a screening tool for maxillary fungal sinusitis. J Chin Med Assoc. 2022;85(3):375–80.
37. Valkov A, et al. The application of ultrasound examination in the treatment of Acute Sinusitis. Comparing X-ray to ultrasound of paranasal sinuses. Int Bull Otorhinolaryngol. 2021;17(1):40–1.
38. Puhakka T, et al. Validity of ultrasonography in diagnosis of acute maxillary sinusitis. Arch Otolaryngol. 2000;126(12):1482–6.
39. Viduetsky A, Herrejon C. Sonographic evaluation of thyroid size: a review of important measurement parameters. J Diagn Med Sonogr. 2019;35(3):206–10.
40. Lafontaine N, McLennan H, Kim A, et al. Suppurative thyroiditis: systematic review and clinical guidance. Clin Endocrinol. 2021;95(2):253–64.
41. Moon HJ, Lee JH, Kwak JY, et al. Diagnostic performance of gray-scale US and elastography in solid thyroid nodules. Radiology. 2012;262(3):1002–13.
42. Caturegli P, De Remigis A, Rose NR. Hashimoto thyroiditis: clinical and diagnostic criteria. Autoimmun Rev. 2014;13(4):391–7.
43. Kapici OB. Ultrasonographic findings of thyroiditis. Health Sci. 2021;2021-III:199.
44. Frates MC, Marqusee E, Benson CB, Alexander EK. Subacute granulomatous (de Quervain) thyroiditis: grayscale and color Doppler sonographic characteristics. J Ultrasound Med. 2013;32(3):505–11.
45. Wémeau JL, Klein M, Sadoul JL, Briet C, Vélayoudom-Céphise FL. Graves' disease: introduction, epidemiology, endogenous and environmental pathogenic factors. Ann Endocrinol (Paris). 2018;79(6):599–607.
46. Hussain YS, Hookham JC, Allahabadia A, Balasubramanian SP. Epidemiology, management and outcomes of Graves' disease-real life data. Endocrine. 2017;56(3):568–78.
47. Baldini M, Boni G, Boi F, et al. Relationship between the sonographic appearance of the thyroid and the clinical course and

autoimmune activity of Graves' disease. J Clin Ultrasound. 2005;33(8):381–5.
48. Guth S, Theune U, Aberle J, Galach A, Bamberger CM. Very high prevalence of thyroid nodules detected by high frequency (13 MHz) ultrasound examination. Eur J Clin Investig. 2009;39(8):699–706.
49. Haugen BR, Alexander EK, Bible KC, et al. 2015 American Thyroid Association management guidelines for adult patients with thyroid nodules and differentiated thyroid cancer: the American Thyroid Association guidelines task force on thyroid nodules and differentiated thyroid cancer. Thyroid. 2016;26(1):1–133.
50. Fresilli D, Lombardi CP, Russo E, et al. Thyroid nodule characterization: how to assess the malignancy risk. update of the literature. Diagnostics (Basel). 2021;11(8):1374.
51. Ahn SS, Kim EK, Kang DR, Lim SK, Kwak JY, Kim MJ. Biopsy of thyroid nodules: comparison of three sets of guidelines. AJR Am J Roentgenol. 2010;194(1):31–7.
52. Moon WJ, Jung SL, Lee JH, et al. Benign and malignant thyroid nodules: US differentiation—multicenter retrospective study. Radiology. 2008;247(3):762–70.
53. Durante C, Grani G, Lamartina L, Filetti S, Mandel SJ, Cooper DS. The diagnosis and management of thyroid nodules: a review. JAMA. 2018;319(9):914–24.
54. Tessler FN, Middleton WD, Grant EG, et al. ACR thyroid imaging, reporting and data system (TI-RADS): white paper of the ACR TI-RADS committee. J Am Coll Radiol. 2017;14(5):587–95.
55. Patel S, Bhatt AA. Thyroglossal duct pathology and mimics. Insights Imaging. 2019;10:1–12.
56. Wang FJ, Xu F, Xiao LH, et al. Ultrasound diagnosis and treatment of branchial cleft cyst and preoperative management. Eur Arch Otorrinolaringol. 2024;281(1):419–25. https://doi.org/10.1007/s00405-023-08209-0.
57. Delantoni A, Onder M, Orhan K. B-mode and color Doppler imaging of different types of branchial cleft cysts in children. A multicenter study and review of the literature. J Ultrasonogr. 2022;22(90):e174. https://doi.org/10.15557/jou.2022.0028.
58. Verma R, Khera S. Cervical lymphadenopathy: a review. Int J Health Sci Res. 2020;10(10):292–8.
59. Bazemore AW, Smucker DR. Lymphadenopathy and malignancy. Am Fam Physician. 2002;66(11):2103–11.
60. Sambandan T, Christeffi MR. Cervical lymphadenopathy—a review. JIADS. 2011;2(1):31–3.
61. Steinkamp HJ, Cornehl M, Hosten N, Pegios W, Vogl T, Felix R. Cervical lymphadenopathy: ratio of long- to short-axis diameter as a predictor of malignancy. Br J Radiol. 1995;68(807):266–70. https://doi.org/10.1259/0007-1285-68-807-266.
62. Ahuja AT, Ying M. Sonographic evaluation of cervical lymph nodes. AJR Am J Roentgenol. 2005;184(5):1691–9.
63. Sproll KC, Sprave T, Belka C, et al. Comparative analysis of diagnostic ultrasound and histopathology for detecting cervical lymph node metastases in head and neck cancer. J Cancer Res Clin Oncol. 2023;1–15:17319.
64. Turner JS, et al. Association of checklist use in endotracheal intubation with clinically important outcomes: a systematic review and meta-analysis. JAMA Netw Open. 2020;3(7):–e209278.
65. De Jong A, et al. Cardiac arrest and mortality related to intubation procedure in critically ill adult patients: a multicenter cohort study. Crit Care Med. 2018;46(4):532–9.
66. Alp G, Koşucu M. Which test best predicts difficult endotracheal intubation? A prospective cohort study. Turk J Trauma Emerg Surg. 2023;29(4):477.
67. Long B, Koyfman A, Gottlieb M. Factors predicting difficult endotracheal intubation. Acad Emerg Med. 2019;26(11):1294–6. https://doi.org/10.1111/acem.13824. Epub 2019 Jul 23. PMID: 31251423.
68. Karamchandani K, Wheelwright J, Yang AL, Westphal ND, Khanna AK, Myatra SN. Emergency airway management outside the operating room: current evidence and management strategies. Anesth Analg. 2021;133(3):648–62. https://doi.org/10.1213/ANE.0000000000005644. PMID: 34153007.
69. Detsky ME, Jivraj N, Adhikari NK, Friedrich JO, Pinto R, Simel DL, Wijeysundera DN, Scales DC. Will this patient be difficult to intubate?: the rational clinical examination systematic review. JAMA. 2019;321(5):493–503. https://doi.org/10.1001/jama.2018.21413. Erratum in: JAMA 2020;323(12):1194. PMID: 30721300.
70. Roth D, Pace NL, Lee A, Hovhannisyan K, Warenits AM, Arrich J, Herkner H. Airway physical examination tests for detection of difficult airway management in apparently normal adult patients. Cochrane Database Syst Rev. 2018;5(5):CD008874. https://doi.org/10.1002/14651858.CD008874.pub2. PMID: 29761867; PMCID: PMC6404686.
71. Carsetti A, Sorbello M, Adrario E, Donati A, Falcetta S. Airway ultrasound as predictor of difficult direct laryngoscopy: a systematic review and meta-analysis. Anesth Analg. 2022;134(4):740–50. https://doi.org/10.1213/ANE.0000000000005839. PMID: 34914641; PMCID: PMC8903216.
72. Wu H, Wang H. Diagnostic efficacy and clinical value of ultrasonography in difficult airway assessment: based on a prospective cohort study. Contrast Media Mol Imaging. 2022;2022:4706438. https://doi.org/10.1155/2022/4706438. PMID: 36082062; PMCID: PMC9433204.
73. Petrisor C, Szabo R, Constantinescu C, Prie A, Hagau N. Ultrasound-based assessment of hyomental distances in neutral, ramped, and maximum hyperextended positions, and derived ratios, for the prediction of difficult airway in the obese population: a pilot diagnostic accuracy study. Anaesthesiol Intens Ther. 2018;50(2):110–6. https://doi.org/10.5603/AIT.2018.0017. PMID: 29953573.
74. Yadav NK, Rudingwa P, Mishra SK, Pannerselvam S. Ultrasound measurement of anterior neck soft tissue and tongue thickness to predict difficult laryngoscopy - An observational analytical study. Indian J Anaesth. 2019;63(8):629–34. https://doi.org/10.4103/ija.IJA_270_19. PMID: 31462808; PMCID: PMC6691631.
75. Yao W, Wang B. Can tongue thickness measured by ultrasonography predict difficult tracheal intubation? Br J Anaesth. 2017;118(4):601–9. https://doi.org/10.1093/bja/aex051. PMID: 28403413.
76. Andruszkiewicz P, Wojtczak J, Sobczyk D, Stach O, Kowalik I. Effectiveness and validity of sonographic upper airway evaluation to predict difficult laryngoscopy. J Ultrasound Med. 2016;35:2243–52.
77. Men XQ, Yan XX. Tracheal ultrasound for the accurate confirmation of the endotracheal tube position in obese patients. J Ultrasound Med. 2020;39(3):509–13. https://doi.org/10.1002/jum.15127. Epub 2019 Sep 6. PMID: 31490565.
78. Harris EA, Arheart KL, Penning DH. Endotracheal tube malposition within the pediatric population: a common event despite clinical evidence of correct placement. Can J Anaesth. 2008;55(10):685–90. https://doi.org/10.1007/BF03017744. PMID: 18835966.
79. Gottlieb M, Holladay D, Burns KM, Nakitende D, Bailitz J. Ultrasound for airway management: An evidence-based review for the emergency clinician. Am J Emerg Med. 2020;38(5):1007–13. https://doi.org/10.1016/j.ajem.2019.12.019. Epub 2019 Dec 11. PMID: 31843325.
80. Gottlieb M, O'Brien JR, Ferrigno N, Sundaram T. Point-of-care ultrasound for airway management in the emergency and critical care setting Clin Exp Emerg Med. 2023. https://doi.org/10.15441/ceem.23.094. Epub ahead of print. PMID: 37620036.
81. Gottlieb M, Holladay D, Peksa GD. Ultrasonography for the confirmation of endotracheal tube intubation: a systematic review and meta-analysis. Ann Emerg Med. 2018;72(6):627–36. https://doi.org/10.1016/j.annemergmed.2018.06.024. Epub 2018 Aug 14. PMID: 30119943.
82. Long B, Koyfman A, Gottlieb M. Diagnostic accuracy of ultrasound for confirmation of endotracheal tube placement. Acad Emerg Med.

2019;26(9):1096–8. https://doi.org/10.1111/acem.13773. Epub 2019 May 23. PMID: 31046166.

83. Gottlieb M, Holladay D, Burns K, et al. Accuracy of ultrasound for endotracheal intubation between different transducer types. Am J Emerg Med. 2019;37(12):2182–5. https://doi.org/10.1016/j.ajem.2019.03.016.
84. Gottlieb M, Nakitende D, Sundaram T, Serici A, Shah S, Bailitz J. Predictive value of tracheal rapid ultrasound exam performed in the emergency department for verification of tracheal intubation. West J Emerg Med. 2018;19(2):412–6. https://doi.org/10.5811/westjem.2017.12.36714.
85. Chou HC, Tseng WP, Wang CH, Ma MH, Wang HP, Huang PC, Sim SS, Liao YC, Chen SY, Hsu CY, Yen ZS, Chang WT, Huang CH, Lien WC, Chen SC. Tracheal rapid ultrasound exam (T.R.U.E.) for confirming endotracheal tube placement during emergency intubation. Resuscitation. 2011;82(10):1279–84. https://doi.org/10.1016/j.resuscitation.2011.05.016. Epub 2011 Jun 1. PMID: 21684668.
86. Masoumi B, Azizkhani R, Emam GH, Asgarzadeh M, Kharazi BZ. Predictive value of tracheal rapid ultrasound exam performed in the emergency department for verification of tracheal intubation. Open Access Maced J Med Sci. 2017;5(5):618–23. https://doi.org/10.3889/oamjms.2017.072. PMID: 28932302; PMCID: PMC5591591.
87. Gottlieb M, Burns K, Holladay D, Chottiner M, Shah S, Gore SR. Impact of endotracheal tube twisting on the diagnostic accuracy of ultrasound for intubation confirmation. Am J Emerg Med. 2020;38(7):1332–4. https://doi.org/10.1016/j.ajem.2019.10.032.
88. Gottlieb M, Patel D, Jung C, et al. Comparison of saline versus air for identifying endotracheal intubation with ultrasound. Am J Emerg Med. 2022;58:131–4. https://doi.org/10.1016/j.ajem.2022.05.053.
89. Tessaro MO, et al. Tracheal rapid ultrasound saline test (TRUST) for confirming correct endotracheal tube depth in children. Resuscitation. 2015;89:8–12.
90. Gottlieb M, Cozzi N, Hartrich M, et al. Comparison of dynamic versus static ultrasound to confirm endotracheal tube depth. Am J Emerg Med. 2023;74:17–20. https://doi.org/10.1016/j.ajem.2023.09.014.
91. You-Ten KE, Wong DT, Ye XY, Arzola C, Zand A, Siddiqui N. Practice of ultrasound-guided palpation of neck landmarks improves accuracy of external palpation of the cricothyroid membrane. Anesth Analg. 2018;127(6):1377–82. https://doi.org/10.1213/ANE.0000000000003604. PMID: 29958219.
92. Siddiqui N, Yu E, Boulis S, You-Ten KE. Ultrasound is superior to palpation in identifying the cricothyroid membrane in subjects with poorly defined neck landmarks: A randomized clinical trial. Anesthesiology. 2018;129(6):1132–9. https://doi.org/10.1097/ALN.0000000000002454. PMID: 30260895.
93. Siddiqui N, Arzola C, Friedman Z, Guerina L, You-Ten KE. Ultrasound improves cricothyrotomy success in cadavers with poorly defined neck anatomy: A randomized
94. Cho SA, Kang P, Song IS, Ji SH, Jang YE, Lee JH, Kim JT, Kim HS, Kim EH. Performance time of anesthesiology trainees for cricothyroid membrane identification and characteristics of cricothyroid membrane in pediatric patients using ultrasonography. Paediatr Anaesth. 2022;32(7):834–42. https://doi.org/10.1111/pan.14451. Epub 2022 Apr 7. PMID: 35362653.
95. Kristensen MS, Teoh WH. Ultrasound identification of the cricothyroid membrane: the new standard in preparing for front-of-neck airway access. Br J Anaesth. 2021;126(1):22–7. https://doi.org/10.1016/j.bja.2020.10.004. Epub 2020 Oct 31. PMID: 33131758.
96. Oliveira KF, Arzola C, Ye XY, Clivatti J, Siddiqui N, You-Ten KE. Determining the amount of training needed for competency of anesthesia trainees in ultrasonographic identification of the cricothyroid membrane. BMC Anesthesiol. 2017;17(1):74. https://doi.org/10.1186/s12871-017-0366-7. PMID: 28577552; PMCID: PMC5457559.
97. Alerhand S. Ultrasound for identifying the cricothyroid membrane prior to the anticipated difficult airway. Am J Emerg Med. 2018;36(11):2078–84. https://doi.org/10.1016/j.ajem.2018.07.027. Epub 2018 Jul 12. PMID: 30025948.
98. Lavelle A, Drew T, Fennessy P, McCaul C, Shannon J. Accuracy of cricothyroid membrane identification using ultrasound and palpation techniques in obese obstetric patients: an observational study. Int J Obstet Anesth. 2021;48:103205. https://doi.org/10.1016/j.ijoa.2021.103205. Epub 2021 Jun 30. PMID: 34280884.
99. Hung KC, Chen IW, Lin CM, Sun CK. Comparison between ultrasound-guided and digital palpation techniques for identification of the cricothyroid membrane: a meta-analysis. Br J Anaesth. 2021;126(1):e9–e11. https://doi.org/10.1016/j.bja.2020.08.012. Epub 2020 Sep 28. PMID: 32896429.

Skin and Soft Tissue Ultrasound

18

David Killeen, Resa E. Lewiss, and Amy Marks

Background

Skin and soft tissue infections (SSTIs) are a common presentation, resulting in more than 6.3 million physician office visits annually, along with a high frequency of presentation to emergency care settings [1–3]. SSTIs, along with other skin pathologies, can be challenging to diagnose, largely owing to the unreliability of systemic symptoms (e.g., fever, chills) and limitations in performing a reliable and reproducible physical examination [4, 5]. Point-of-care ultrasound (POCUS) has high diagnostic accuracy in SSTIs and leads to rapid, accurate bedside management changes in more than 10% of cases [6, 7]. Furthermore, POCUS avoids the misdiagnosis of an abscess, thereby saving the patient from an incision and drainage (I&D) [7]. POCUS also limits the failure rate of abscesses treated with I&D and reduces unnecessary procedures [7]. POCUS is a suggested imaging modality in soft tissue guidelines as a means of improving diagnosis and treatment [8]. As with other POCUS applications, ultrasound is cost-efficient and safer than other imaging modalities, such as computed tomography and magnetic resonance imaging.

Beyond the clinical utility of SSTIs, POCUS also assists in the identification of neck masses, distinguishing benign soft tissue lesions from vascular malformations, and in the initial assessment of other dermatologic complaints, such as nail pathologies [9–11]. Finally, soft tissue ultrasound is easy to perform for novice users [12, 13]. This chapter discusses the role of POCUS in cellulitis, abscess, necrotizing fasciitis, foreign bodies, lymph nodes, lipomas, cysts, and nail pathology.

Indications and Diagnoses

Indications
- Soft tissue mass
- Pain
- Erythema
- Swelling
- Foreign body concern
- Crepitus
- Abnormal physical examination
- Procedural guidance

Diagnoses
- Cellulitis
- Abscess
- Necrotizing fasciitis
- Foreign body evaluation
- Lymph node assessment
- Lipoma
- Cyst evaluation
- Nail pathology

Core Views

Skin and soft tissue ultrasound is utilized to examine the skin, subcutaneous tissue, fascia, and muscle layers (Figs. 18.1, 18.2, and 18.3). The skin consists of the epidermis and dermis, layers that can be challenging to differentiate with POCUS unless a wide footprint, high-frequency probe is used. The epidermis appears as a thin, hyperechoic layer in the near field of the ultrasound screen. The dermis is hyperechoic compared to deeper tissues, yet less echogenic than the epidermis. Additionally, the dermis is thicker com-

Supplementary Information The online version contains supplementary material available at https://doi.org/10.1007/978-3-031-85308-1_18.

D. Killeen (✉)
Neighborhood Health, Alexandria, VA, USA

R. E. Lewiss
Department of Emergency Medicine, University of Alabama at Birmingham Heersink School of Medicine, Birmingham, AL, USA

A. Marks
Department of Emergency Medicine, Rush University Medical Center, Chicago, IL, USA

M. Gottlieb, N. Panebianco (eds.), *Advanced Point-of-Care Ultrasound*, https://doi.org/10.1007/978-3-031-85308-1_18

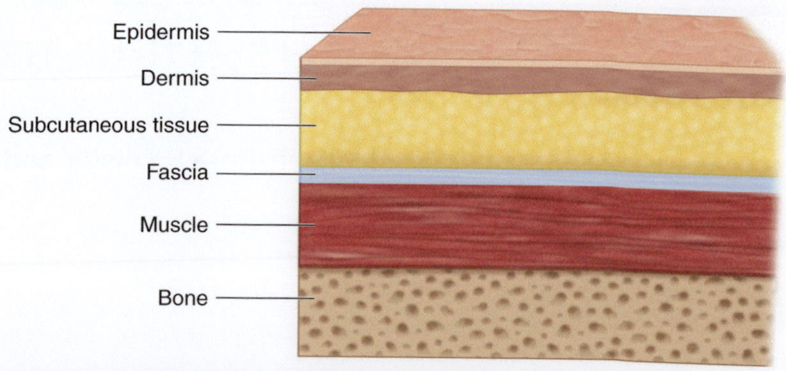

Fig. 18.1 Illustration of normal soft tissue anatomy of superficial layers

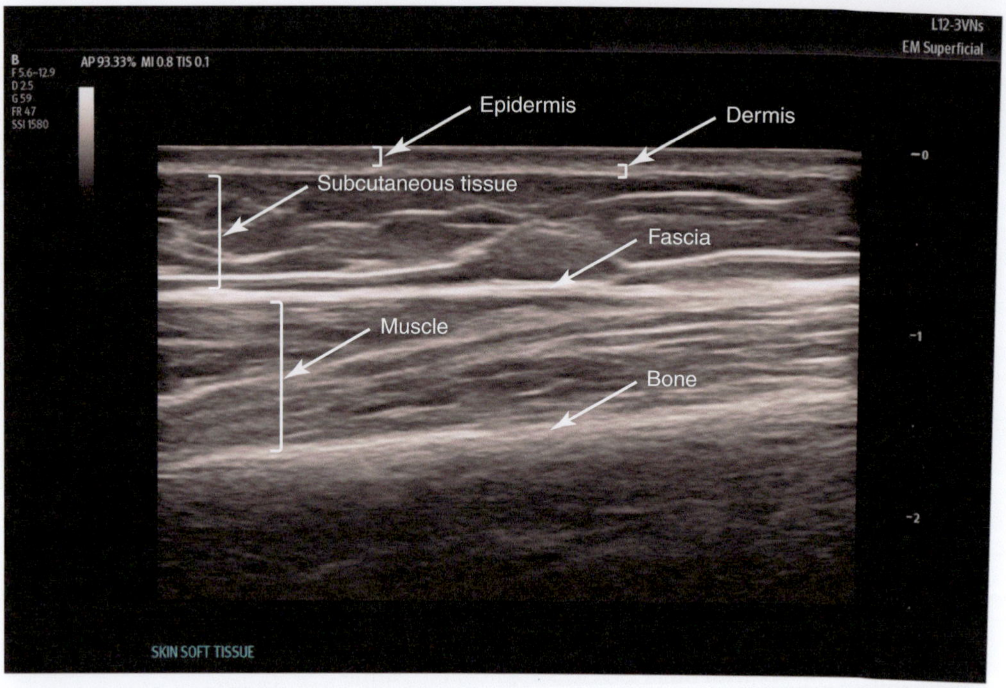

Fig. 18.2 Normal tissue observed using a high-frequency linear probe in the longitudinal axis

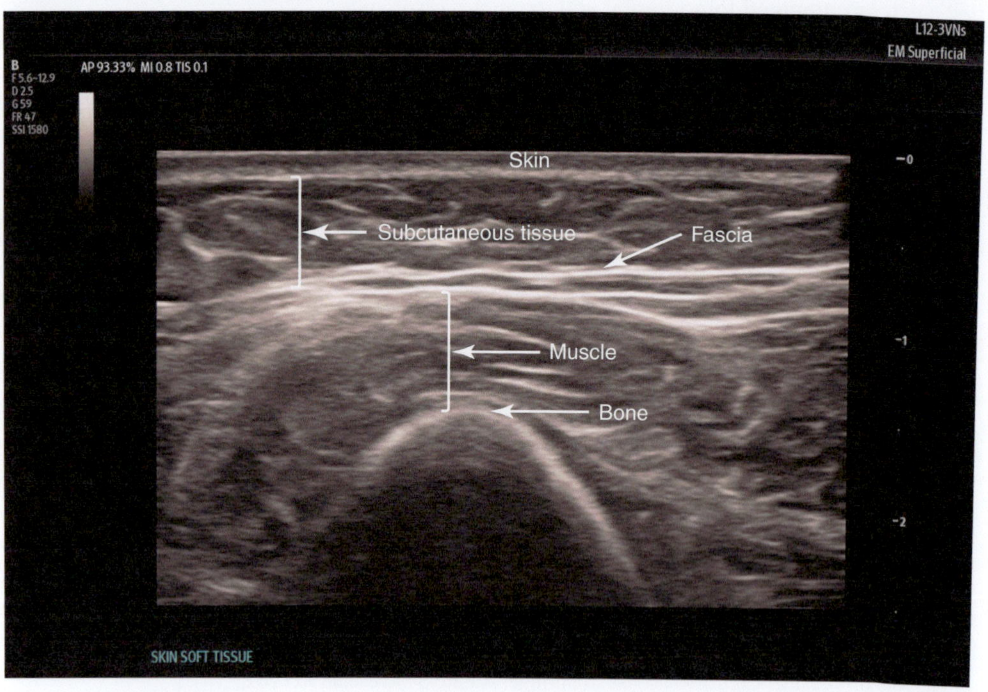

Fig. 18.3 Normal tissue observed using a high-frequency linear probe in the transverse axis

pared to the epidermis. The subcutaneous tissue, or hypodermis, contains adipose and connective tissue layers and appears hypoechoic in relation to the epidermis and the dermis. The fascia can vary in thickness depending on location and often appears hyperechoic when compared to the surrounding tissues.

A systematic approach to skin and soft tissue ultrasound is important given the variety of clinical presentations and diagnoses. The anatomic area of interest should be evaluated by obtaining images in two orthogonal planes [14]. Following B-mode image acquisition, the area can be explored with color Doppler depending on the location, area of concern, and the focused question. Three measurements can be made in two orthogonal planes to account for width, length, and depth. Whenever possible, the unaffected contralateral side of the body should be imaged for comparison.

Patient-centered care always takes into account the patient's positioning for comfort and to minimize pain. Apply minimal pressure to the affected area to reduce patient discomfort. To improve resolution, a copious amount of gel should be used when scanning superficial structures. Operators may additionally use a standoff pad or a water bath to optimize the visualization in these cases (Fig. 18.4) [15]. A lateral or modified approach can also be performed using a plastic container (Fig. 18.5) [16]. For open skin or puncture wounds, utilize water-based, single-use sterile gel and follow high-level disinfection protocols.

A linear probe should be utilized for most SSTI POCUS examinations. For improved image resolution of superficial structures (e.g., epidermal, dermal, and nail pathology), a wide footprint, high-frequency (18–20 MHz) probe can be used. In contrast, a curvilinear probe can be used for deeper structures when more depth is needed or when a finding extends out of the field of view. An endocavitary probe, if available, can also be considered because of its higher frequency and smaller footprint.

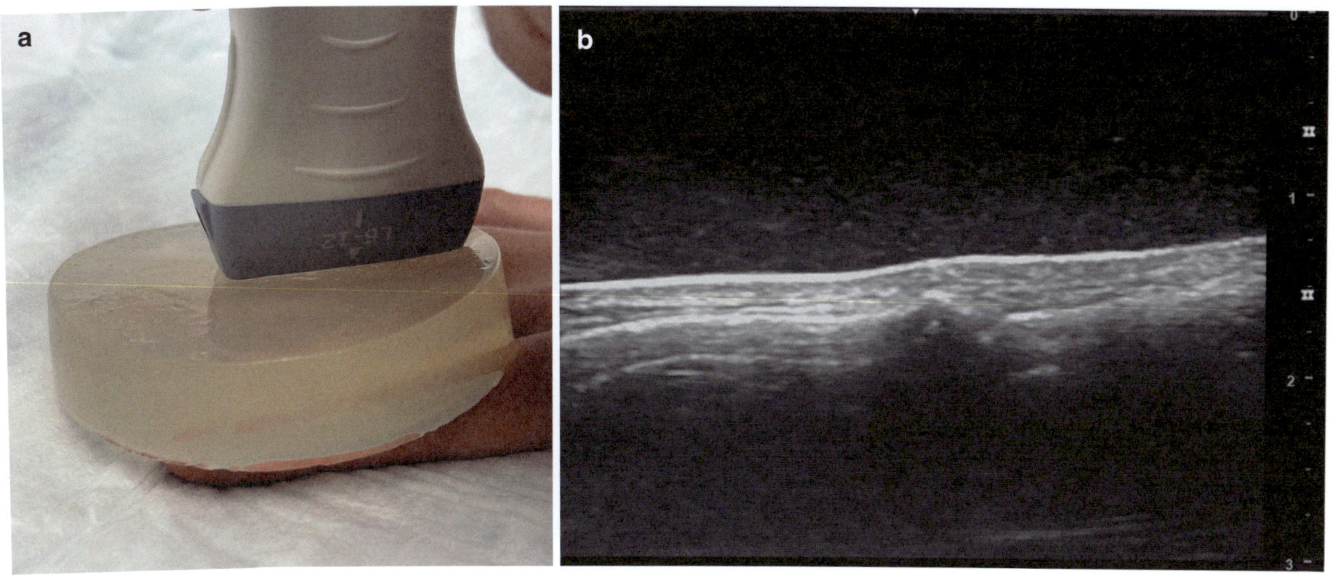

Fig. 18.4 (**a**) A commercial standoff pad being used to image a finger. Note that this standoff pad's depth is approximately 1 cm. (**b**) Corresponding ultrasound image with standoff pad

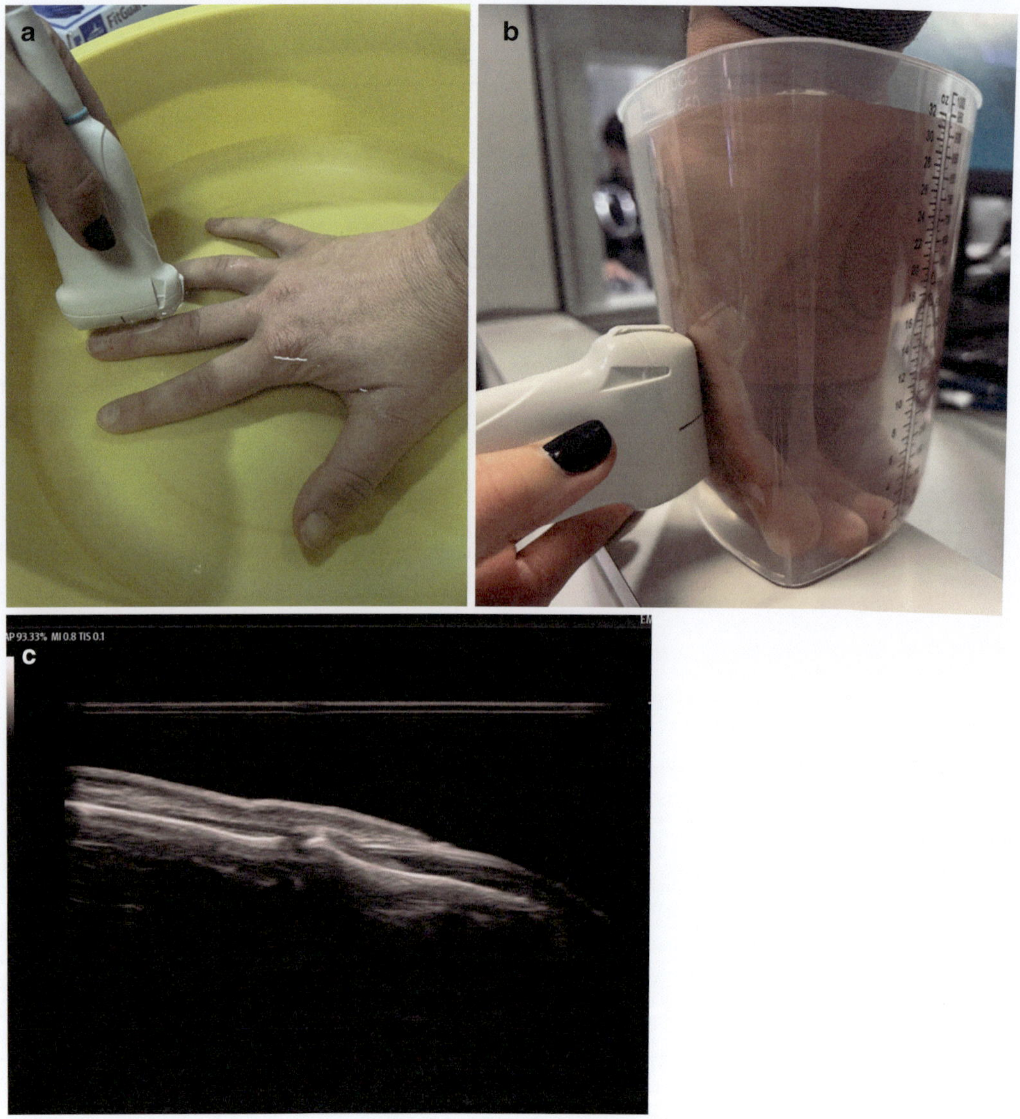

Fig. 18.5 (**a**) A water bath allows for the visualization of superficial structures. (**b**) A modified water bath utilizes a clear plastic container and gel to similarly visualize superficial structures to move the structure of interest (a finger) to the focal zone of the image, resulting in improved resolution. (**c**) Corresponding ultrasound image of the structure in **a** using the water bath technique

Clinical Applications

Cellulitis

SSTI is a common reason for patients to present to an acute care and outpatient care setting with an annual incidence ranging from 22 to 50 per 1000 persons and more than 14 million cases per year in the United States [17]. While cellulitis is typically considered a clinical diagnosis, it can overlap with other conditions, including deeper infections (e.g., abscess, necrotizing fasciitis) that may be difficult to elucidate based on history and physical examination alone. POCUS helps differentiate these conditions.

Sonographically, early findings of cellulitis include dermal thickening and increased vascularity of tissues on color Doppler [18]. Later findings include the visualization of fluid between hyperechoic fat lobules, subcutaneous fluid, and increased echogenicity of the subcutaneous tissues. This is commonly called "cobblestoning" due to its resemblance to a cobblestone street (Fig. 18.6). These POCUS findings should be interpreted in conjunction with the clinical history, physical examination, and comparison views of unaffected body parts. Cobblestoning is nonspecific and can also be seen in conditions associated with tissue edema, such as heart failure, venous stasis, lymphedema, or deep vein thrombosis.

Abscess

Differentiating cellulitis from an abscess by physical examination alone can be challenging [19]. Studies have shown poor interrater reliability for physical examination in the diagnosis of abscesses [4], highlighting the importance of

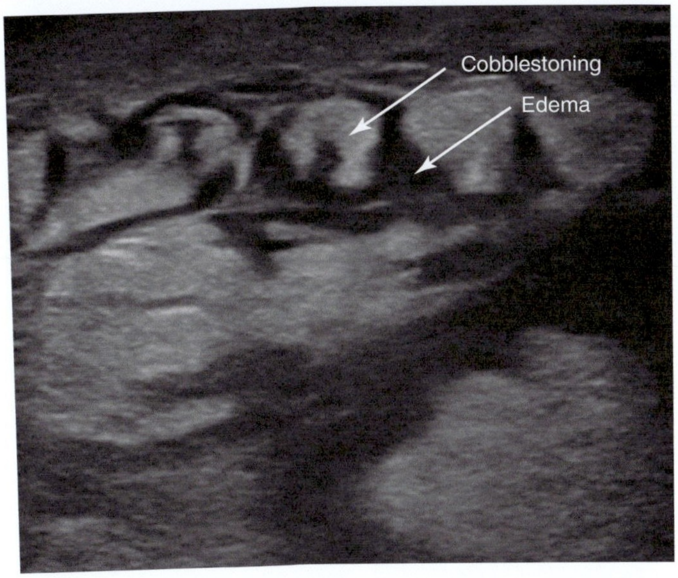

Fig. 18.6 Cellulitis with cobblestoning and thickened epidermis

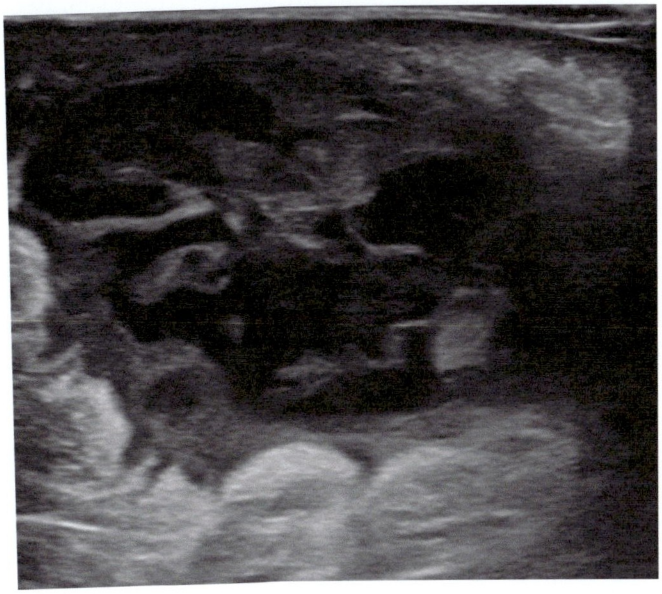

Fig. 18.7 Abscess with mixed echogenicity indicating both fluid and semisolid elements. Note the posterior acoustic enhancement deep to the fluid collection

POCUS for greater diagnostic certainty [20]. POCUS is 90% to 95% sensitive in the detection of an abscess for adult and pediatric patient populations [6, 21]. POCUS has also been shown to lead to a correct change in management in approximately 10% of cases [6].

On ultrasound, an abscess appears as an irregularly bordered soft tissue structure that can be hypoechoic or anechoic and may include echogenic internal debris (Fig. 18.7). Abscesses will have posterior acoustic enhancement deep to the collection due to the internal fluid contents, which can help identify the structure as an abscess even when it appears isoechoic to the surrounding tissue. Graded compression of the abscess is a diagnostic technique that can be useful when there is isoechoic internal debris and the diagnosis is unclear. When pressure is applied, an abscess will demonstrate dynamic swirling of the internal debris, often called the "swirl" or "squish" sign (Video 1). Gas can be present in an abscess and will appear as "dirty shadowing" with reverberation and speckled artifacts. This may be an expected finding if there is disruption to the skin barrier, such as spontaneous or instrumented drainage. In the absence of an open track to the skin, dirty shadowing should raise concern for a gas-forming infection and necrotizing SSTI in the appropriate clinical context.

Color or pulsed-wave Doppler should be used to help differentiate an abscess from other findings such as pseudoaneurysms or arteriovenous malformations. Abscesses will have surrounding hyperemia without internal flow, whereas vascular structures will have internal vascular flow (Fig. 18.8). POCUS can also play a role in determining the ideal location for an I&D procedure, as it can show the margins, depth, and the area of greatest fluctuance to determine the best incision location for open I&D or loop drainage [22, 23]. The location of surrounding vasculature and nerves can also be assessed to avoid those structures when performing an I&D. Additionally, POCUS can be used after drainage to demonstrate the adequacy of the procedure or to assess for resolution during reassessment.

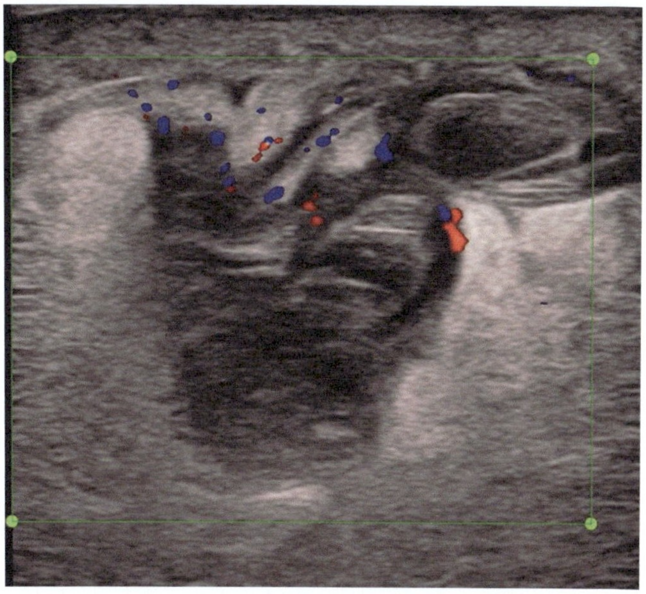

Fig. 18.8 Hyperemia noted around and within the abscess when color Doppler is used

Necrotizing Fasciitis

Patients with necrotizing fasciitis are at risk for delays in diagnosis, which can lead to significantly increased morbidity and mortality [24]. POCUS can be used to aid in a more timely diagnosis, with studies reporting a sensitivity of 85% to 100% and a specificity of 45% to 98% [25]. Moreover, POCUS can be performed at the bedside, avoiding the need to transfer unstable patients for computed tomography and allowing easily repeated examinations in unclear cases or when the patient's condition changes.

Sonographic findings suggestive of necrotizing fasciitis include thickening of the deep fascia, diffuse thickening of the overlying fatty tissue, and a fluid layer at least 4 mm in thickness along the deep fascia [26]. There is increasing specificity with each 1 mm increase in the fascial fluid diameter [27]. If a gas-producing organism is present, the presence of gas may appear as hyperechoic small rounded structures in the soft tissue or fascial plane with posterior "dirty" shadowing. The "STAFF" mnemonic (*S*ubcutaneous *T*hickening, *A*ir, and *F*ascial *F*luid) has been used to describe ultrasound findings of necrotizing fasciitis (Fig. 18.9) [28].

Some POCUS mimics of necrotizing fasciitis findings include an open or draining wound or a recently performed I&D procedure that causes air to track into the subcutaneous tissues. These findings highlight the importance of utilizing the sonographic findings in the context of the clinical picture when making this diagnosis. POCUS has not demonstrated sufficient sensitivity to adequately rule out necrotizing fasciitis. Thus, when clinical suspicion for necrotizing fasciitis exists and sonographic findings are negative, further evaluation with computed tomography or surgical consultation should be pursued.

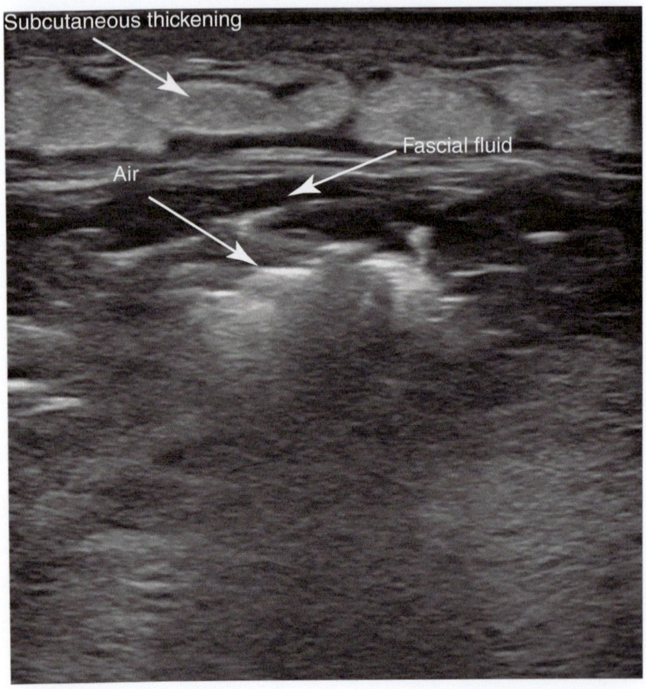

Fig. 18.9 Necrotizing fasciitis with subcutaneous thickening, air, and fascial fluid

Foreign Body

Physical examination alone fails to identify soft tissue foreign bodies in up to 38% of patients [29]. When there is a concern for a foreign body in a soft tissue wound and the foreign body is not directly visualized, further imaging should be pursued. X-rays can provide diagnostic assistance if the foreign body material is radiopaque, such as metal; however, X-rays may miss radiolucent materials like organic matter (e.g., wood), glass, or plastic [30, 31]. One study found that X-rays missed up to 25% of glass foreign bodies and 93% of organic-based foreign bodies [32]. Ultrasound is superior for diagnosing foreign bodies in the soft tissues compared to X-rays and generally identifies the majority of foreign bodies [33]. Studies have demonstrated sensitivities of 57% to 83% and specificities of 88% to 95%, though this is dependent upon the specific foreign body (Fig. 18.10) [29].

To maximize the diagnostic accuracy, scan in an organized and stepwise fashion in two planes [34]. Color Doppler can help distinguish surrounding vascular structures and identify surrounding inflammation. Foreign bodies can be difficult to detect due to their small size, complex anatomy, or sonographic artifacts; therefore, sonographers will need to scan slowly and carefully [37]. Superficial foreign bodies may be undetectable due to the limitations of the probe, proximal image resolution, and focal length. To improve visualization, the focal length can be extended by using a water bath or standoff pad. Foreign bodies appear as hyperechoic objects with variable echogenicity based on the material type, thickness, angle of insonation, and the presence of surrounding scar tissue or reactive edema (Table 18.1, Figs. 18.11, 18.12, 18.13, 18.14, and 18.15, Videos 2 and 3) [35]. Metallic foreign bodies may also demonstrate twinkling artifacts, appearing as enhanced color Doppler signals deep to the object [36]. Gaping wounds may physically impair sonographic evaluation or may introduce subcutaneous air that obscures the underlying anatomy. To address this, use copious gel or consider a water bath as described above.

Structures that can mimic a foreign body on ultrasound include sesamoid bones, scar tissue, and soft tissue calcifications. These can be differentiated based on location, sonographic appearance, and comparison to the unaffected contralateral body part. A "halo" sign can also be seen when the host response creates a fluid pocket surrounding the object. A halo sign is typically seen when a foreign body is present for over 24 hours [38].

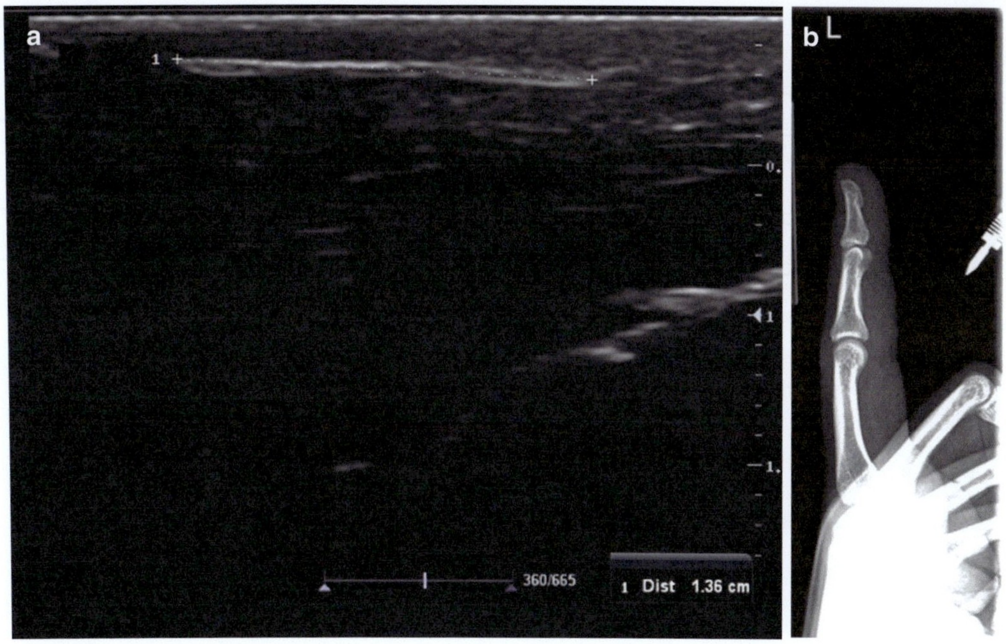

Fig. 18.10 (**a**) A wooden foreign body in an index finger seen on ultrasound in long axis as a hyperechoic line. (**b**) X-ray image of the same index finger in **a** with no foreign body noted

Table 18.1 Echogenicity and reverberation artifact based upon the foreign body material [36]

Material	Echogenicity	Reverberation	X-ray finding	Surrounding inflammation	Example image
Glass	Hyperechoic	Sometimes present	Radiodense	Present	Figure 18.11
Organic material (e.g., wood, stinger)	Hyperechoic	Posterior shadow	Radiopaque	Present	Figure 18.12 and Video 2
Metal	Hyperechoic	Comet tail	Radiodense	Present	Figure 18.13
Medical devices (e.g., catheter, contraceptive implant)	Hyperechoic	Edge shadow	Variable Radiodensity	Absent	Figure 18.14
Cosmetic filler	Variable echogenicity depending on the type of filler	Variable	Radiopaque	Absent (can be present if there is a reaction to the substance injected)	Figure 18.15 and Video 3

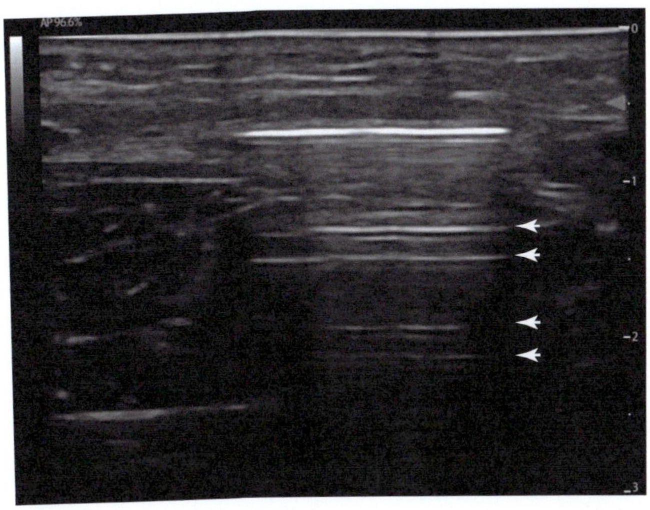

Fig. 18.11 Glass as seen on ultrasound as a hyperechoic structure with reverberation artifacts (arrows). (*Image courtesy of Benjamin C. Smith, 3rd, MD*)

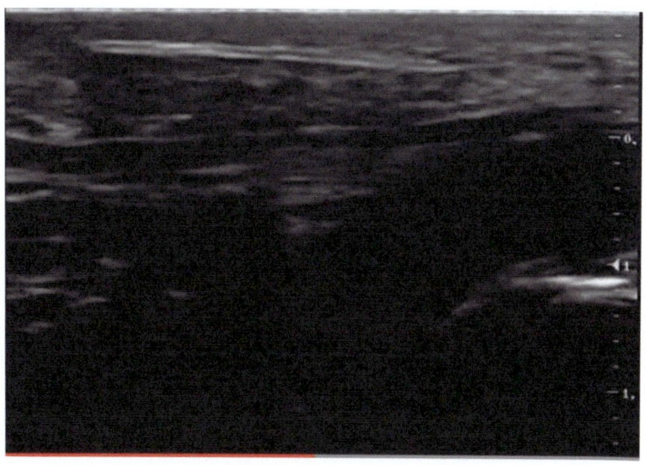

Fig. 18.12 Splinter in the subcutaneous tissue, appearing hyperechoic with posterior shadowing

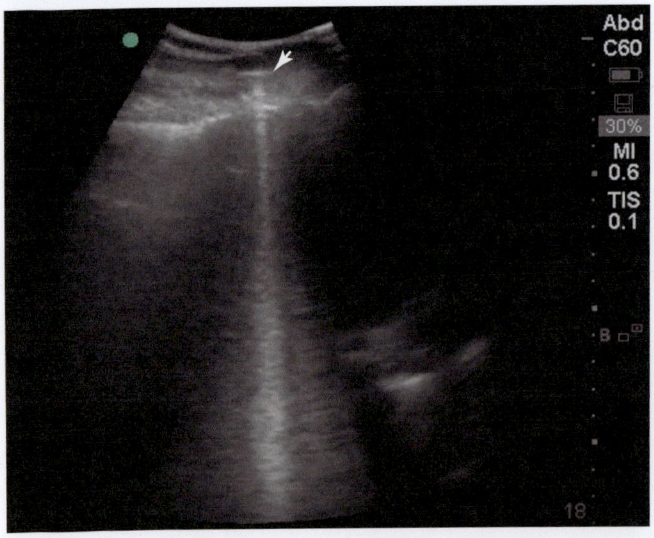

Fig. 18.13 Metal object (arrow) in the chest, appearing as a hyperechoic object with comet tail artifact. Note that the artifact is coming from the metal object and not the lung parenchyma.

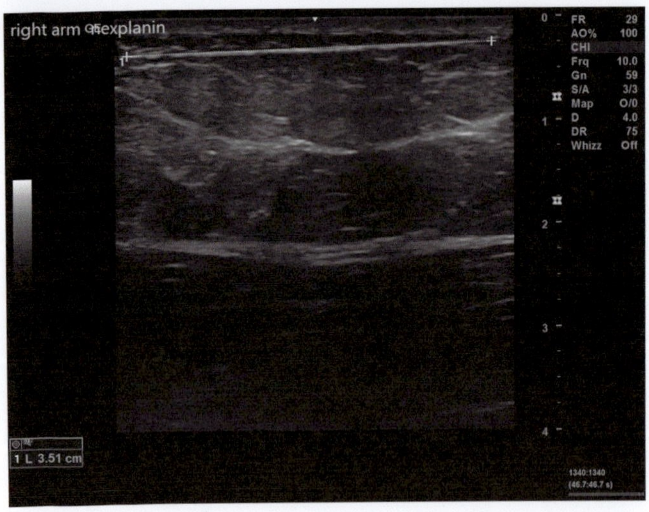

Fig. 18.14 Hyperechoic contraception implant in the subcutaneous tissue of the upper arm

Once a foreign body is encountered, POCUS can assist or directly guide the clinician in the removal of a soft tissue foreign body. For the ultrasound-assisted technique, the clinician should mark the skin for a place of entry and measure the depth at which they would expect to reach the foreign body. The foreign body can then be removed by making an incision over the marked regions without active use of the ultrasound during removal. Ultrasound can also guide the clinician in the removal of soft tissue foreign bodies in real time. In this technique, a hyperechoic object, such as a sterile needle, can be advanced in the anesthetized skin. The needle is advanced until it can be seen to make contact with the foreign body. A second needle may be placed at the other end of the foreign body. Then, make a skin incision between the two needles and use forceps for blunt dissection to the level of the foreign body to grasp the object and minimize tissue injury.

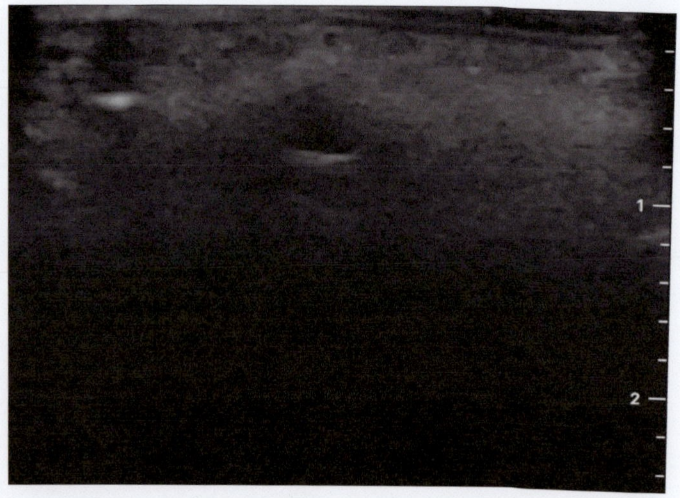

Fig. 18.15 The two areas of silicone fillers noted in the subcutaneous tissue are round and hypoechoic with some posterior acoustic enhancement

Hematoma

Hematomas are common in patients with musculoskeletal injuries occurring from sports and trauma, as well as in coagulopathic disorders (e.g., Hemophilia A and B). They can be intra- or intermuscular, intrabursal, or intra-articular. POCUS can identify hematomas and may additionally help select lesions that benefit from aspiration. A "hematocrit sign," defined as the layering of gravity-dependent cellular debris that shifts with the patient's movements, can aid in the diagnosis of a hematoma [39]. Hematomas can appear anechoic, complex, heterogeneous, or echogenic (Fig. 18.16, Video 4). Ossification of hematomas may also occur with increased chronicity.

Color Doppler can be used to look for active extravasation [40]. Dynamic needle guidance for aspiration may be pursued based on symptoms and clinical discretion in an effort to alleviate patient symptoms, allow a return to activities, and reduce potential ossification. In general, anechoic hematomas are more amenable to needle decompression as compared to echogenic hematomas [41].

Lymphadenopathy

Lymph nodes follow the lymphatic distribution of the human body and can be identified with POCUS (Fig. 18.17). Lymph nodes are classified as normal, reactive, malignant, indeterminate, or necrotic (Table 18.2). The classic lymph node

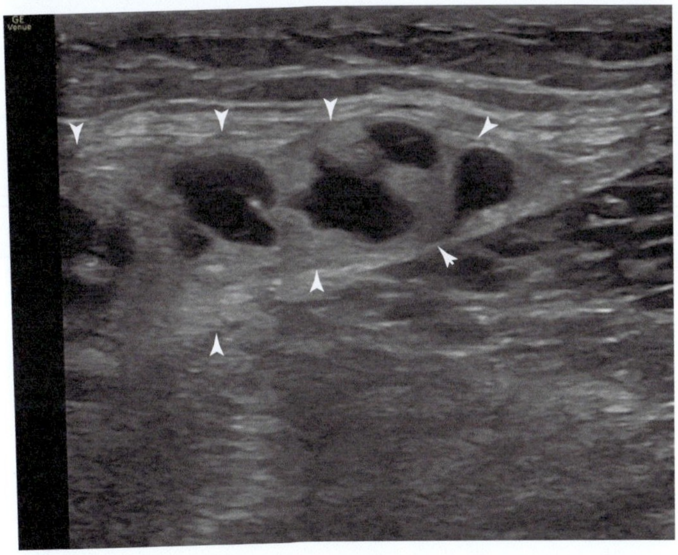

Fig. 18.16 Right groin hematoma (outlined with arrowheads) with internal septations

appearance is an oval or kidney bean-shaped mass (Fig. 18.18). POCUS findings for normal lymph nodes include a well-defined hyperechoic band in the center, surrounded by a hypoechoic cortex. Normal lymph nodes will be wider than tall and usually do not exceed a maximum measurement of 1 cm, although lymph nodes in the inguinal area can measure up to 2 cm [42].

Reactive lymph nodes can have variable but distinct appearances, including central, tree-like, vascularity, mild enlargement, and a rounder shape (Fig. 18.19). There can also be variable loss of the normal hyperechoic hilum. A patient with reactive lymph nodes should be instructed to follow up for repeat imaging to ensure resolution. Studies that examined the resolution of postvaccination reactive lymphadenopathy have typically reported a time frame of two to three months for follow-up examination to ensure resolution [43, 44].

The sonographic features associated with malignant lymph nodes include a disorganized blood flow or peripheral vascularity (referred to as the "ring of fire"), a loss of the

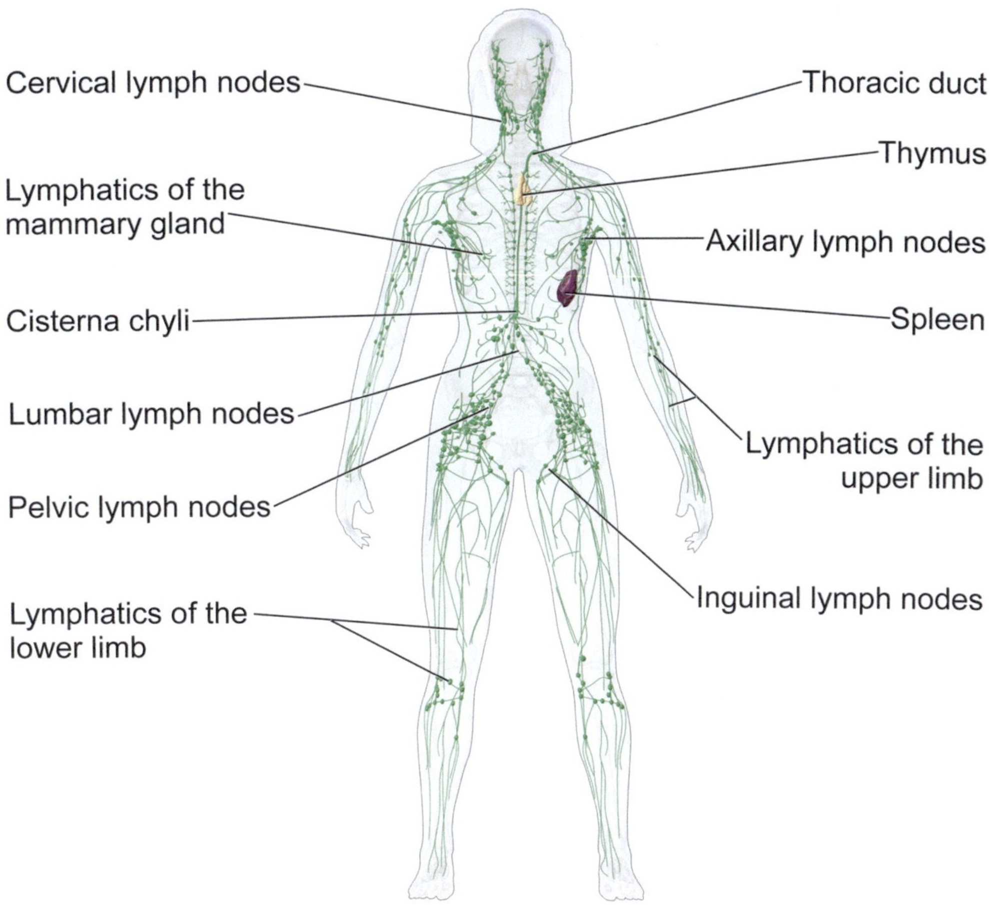

Fig. 18.17 Lymphatic system. Lymph nodes are distributed throughout the body and are connected to each other through lymphatic vessels. (*Image reference: Blausen Medical* [45]

Table 18.2 Differentiation of normal, reactive, and malignant lymph nodes.

Lymph Node Category	Vascularity	Shape	Echogenicity	Size
Normal	Avascular or minimal vascularity within the hilum	Oval	Hyperechoic hilum with hypo/anechoic interior	Most < 1 cm in diameter.
Reactive	Central Flow (i.e., tree-like)	Oval to Round	Hyperechoic hilum (variable)	Mild Enlargement
Malignant	Disorganized blood flow, peripheral (i.e., ring of fire)	Round	Loss of hyperechogenic hilum	Enlarged

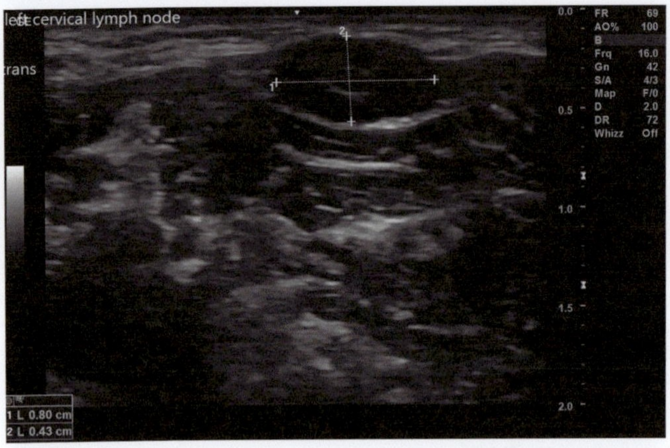

Fig. 18.18 Normal appearing lymph node with a hyperechoic hilum, width greater than height, and maximal diameter measuring less than 1 cm

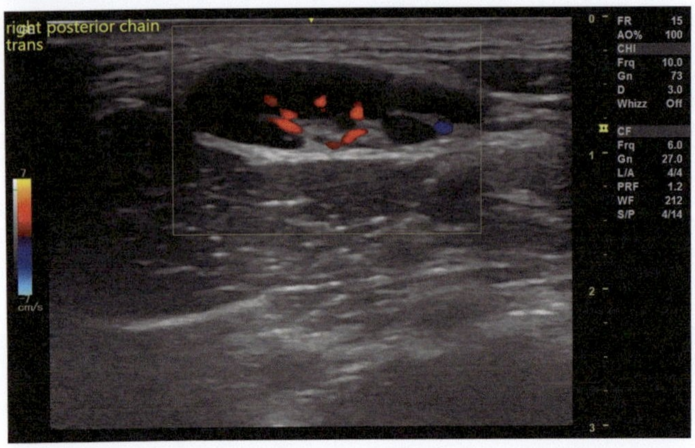

Fig. 18.19 Enlarged lymph node, measuring greater than 1 cm in diameter with increased vascularity consistent with reactive lymph node

hyperechoic hilum, an enlarged size (>1 cm), and a round shape (Fig. 18.20, Video 4) [46]. Tissue biopsy or further imaging is needed to confirm the diagnosis in a patient with lymph nodes that have malignant features or are indeterminate.

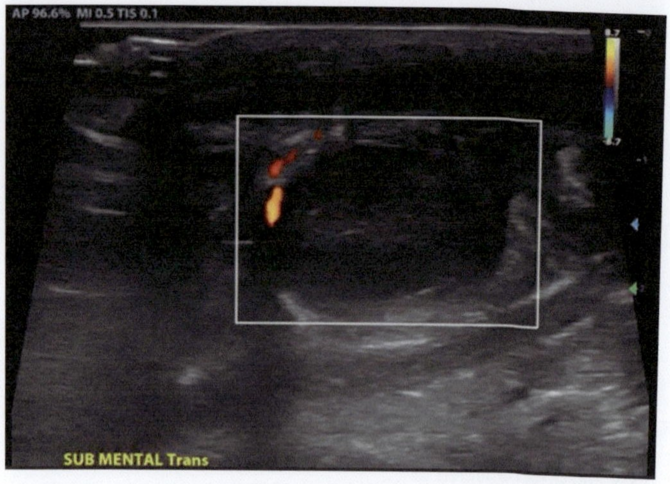

Fig. 18.20 Malignant lymph node with increase in peripheral vascularity, loss of hyperechoic hilum, and more rounded appearance

Lipoma

Lipomas are the most common benign soft tissue tumors, composed of mature adipose cells. Clinical features of lipomas include palpable masses that are generally painless, although pain can occur depending upon their relation to nearby anatomical structures such as vessels, muscles, and nerves [47]. Lipomas do not typically have any overlying skin changes. Ultrasound is considered to be the first-line imaging modality, owing to its high sensitivity (87%) and specificity (96%) [48]. The echogenicity of lipomas can vary widely; while most are isoechoic, they can also be hypoechoic or hyperechoic [48]. Lipomas can vary in size and are normally compressible (Video 6). In general, lipomas are less than 5 cm in diameter [49]. When identifying lipomas, clinicians may appreciate curved echogenic lines that are parallel to the skin on ultrasound. A thin, fibrous pseudocapsule that surrounds the lipoma may also be present (Fig. 18.21).

While lipomas are normally located in the subcutaneous tissue, they can occur in muscle. Lipomas are normally avascular. If more than minimal vascular flow is detected with color Doppler, this should raise the suspicion for an atypical

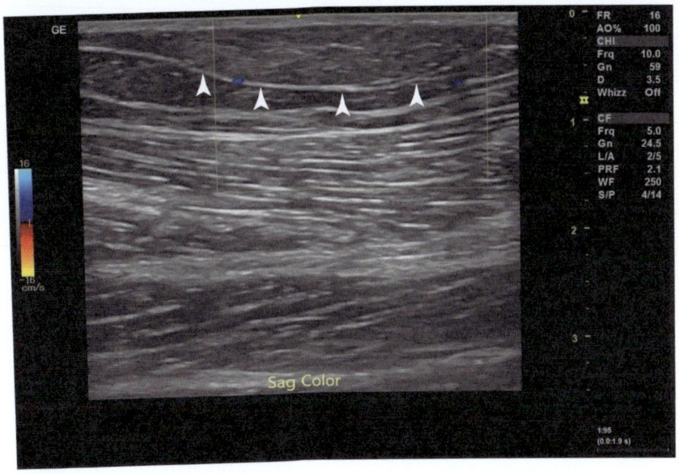

Fig. 18.21 Lipoma noted with a thin fibrous pseudocapsule (outlined with arrows), without any internal vascularity

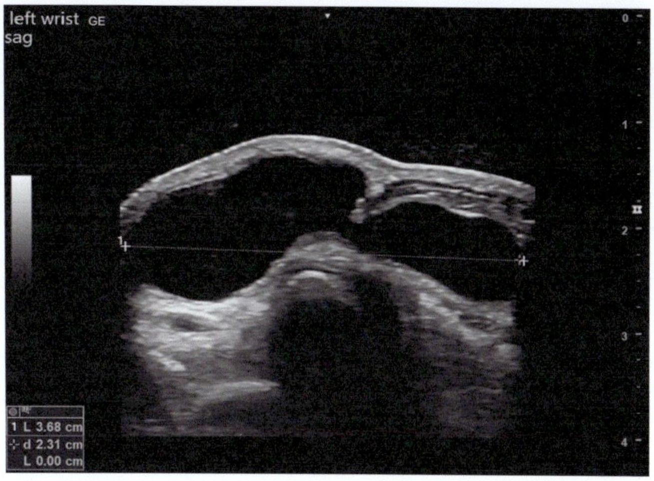

Fig. 18.22 Ganglion cyst of the wrist noted as an anechoic structure

process, such as malignancy. Other features suggesting a malignancy include a shape that is taller than wide or one that includes speculations into the surrounding tissue [50]. If atypical features are detected with ultrasound or there is clinical concern warranting further investigation, magnetic resonance imaging or appropriate consultation should be obtained. Close attention should be given to any suspicious soft tissue lesions in the thigh or gluteal region, as those have been found to have an elevated occurrence rate for malignancy [46]. Follow-up ultrasound can be performed to monitor growth and to identify those at risk of progression to a more aggressive soft tissue lesion (e.g., sarcoma). Lipomas measuring over 5 cm or with significant symptoms should be considered for excision, although most still have low malignant potential [51].

Ganglion Cysts and Synovial Cysts

Ganglion cysts (GCs) often appear near joint or tendon sheaths and are fluid-filled, hypoechoic superficial masses that sometimes have internal septations (Fig. 18.22). Oftentimes, it is possible to visualize a connection to an adjacent joint space [40]. GCs have limited compressibility when compared to other similar structures such as synovial cysts (SCs) [52]. Location can also help the clinician determine the etiology, as GCs are more commonly seen in the hand and wrist, while SCs are seen more commonly in the knee (e.g., Baker's cyst) [53]. Finally, GCs and SCs generally exhibit minimal or no flow with color Doppler. Atypical features warrant consideration of other pathologies or follow-up imaging. Making a correct diagnosis is important, as GCs and SCs are treated differently. GCs often require incision or steroid injection, while SCs require treating the underlying joint or tendon disorder.

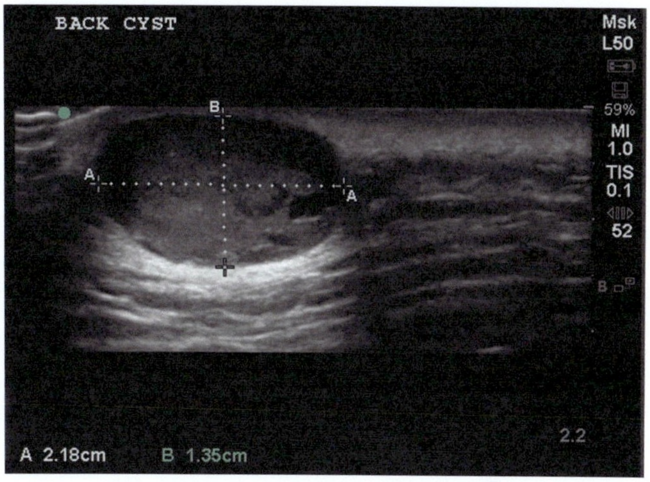

Fig. 18.23 Sebaceous cyst of the back, which is well-circumscribed, hypoechoic, and relatively homogenous in the superficial tissue layers. (*Image courtesy of Matthew Chan, MD*)

Sebaceous Cysts

Sebaceous cysts are nodules that result from the obstruction of hair follicles. On ultrasound, they are often oval-shaped and hypoechoic with a homogenous appearance also known as "pseudo-testis" (Fig. 18.23). They can also have a target or laminar appearance. The target appearance is made of a thin peripheral hypoechoic halo, which represents the stratified keratinized squamous epithelial wall. The cysts often have a visible cutaneous pore that connects to the epidermis, which is a diagnostic indicator of a sebaceous cyst [53].

Pilar (Trichilemmal) Cysts

Pilar cysts often arise from areas of dense hair follicles. They are more often found in females and are most commonly located on the scalp, followed by the face, neck, arms, and legs. On ultrasound, they most often appear hypoechoic and frequently have internal hyperechogenicity. This finding represents calcification or cholesterol crystals and usually appears as a lump-like pattern [54]. These cysts will have no flow on color Doppler and exhibit posterior acoustic enhancement (Fig. 18.24).

Epidermal Inclusion Cysts

Epidermal inclusion cysts (EICs) are typically round or oval in appearance, with a well-circumscribed capsule, and can appear similar to sebaceous cysts (Fig. 18.25). EICs have been classically described as having a punctum or "witch's hat" that can be seen as a hypoechoic extension through the epidermis, although this is seen in less than half of EICs [56]. Some EICs will have hyperechoic layers, classically referred to as an "onion" pattern [57]. EICs can become inflamed, infected, and rupture. Sonographic findings of infected or inflamed cysts include hyperemia and internal particulate movement when pressure is applied with the ultrasound probe. Performing an ultrasound prior to I&D can help to avoid rupturing an intact capsule. In these latter cases, it is best to try to remove the entire capsule at a later time when the cyst is not infected or inflamed [56].

Acne Vulgaris and Hidradenitis Suppurativa

Acne vulgaris is a common condition that impacts the pilosebaceous unit of the hair follicle and frequently impacts the chest, face, and neck. The clinical examination is important in both conditions but is limited to the superficial appearance

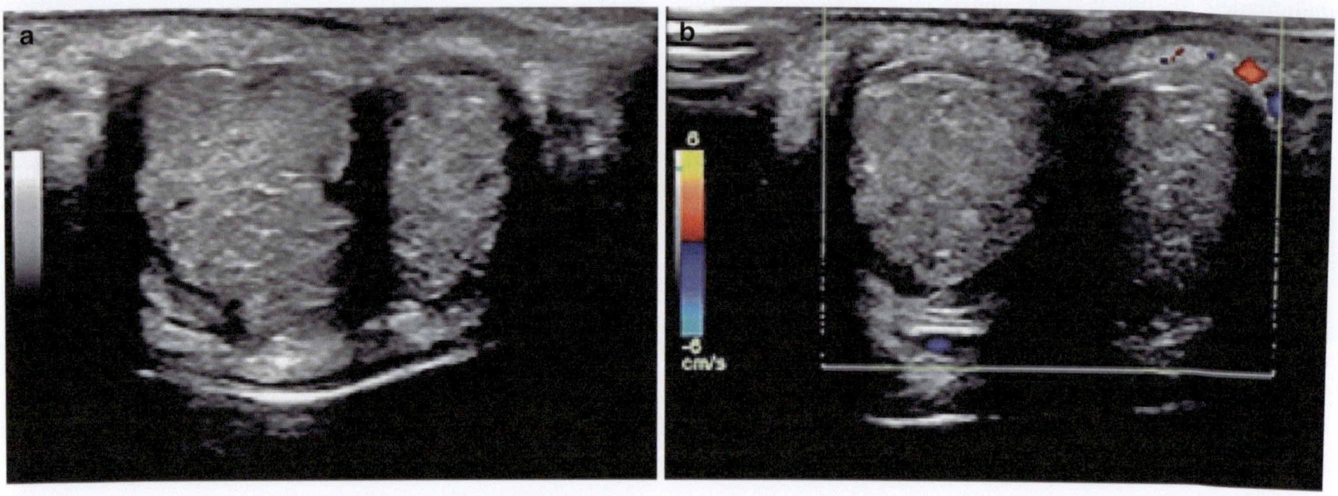

Fig. 18.24 (**a**) B-mode of trichilemmal cyst. (**b**) Color Doppler of trichilemmal cyst. (*Image reproduced with permission from Li et al.* [55])

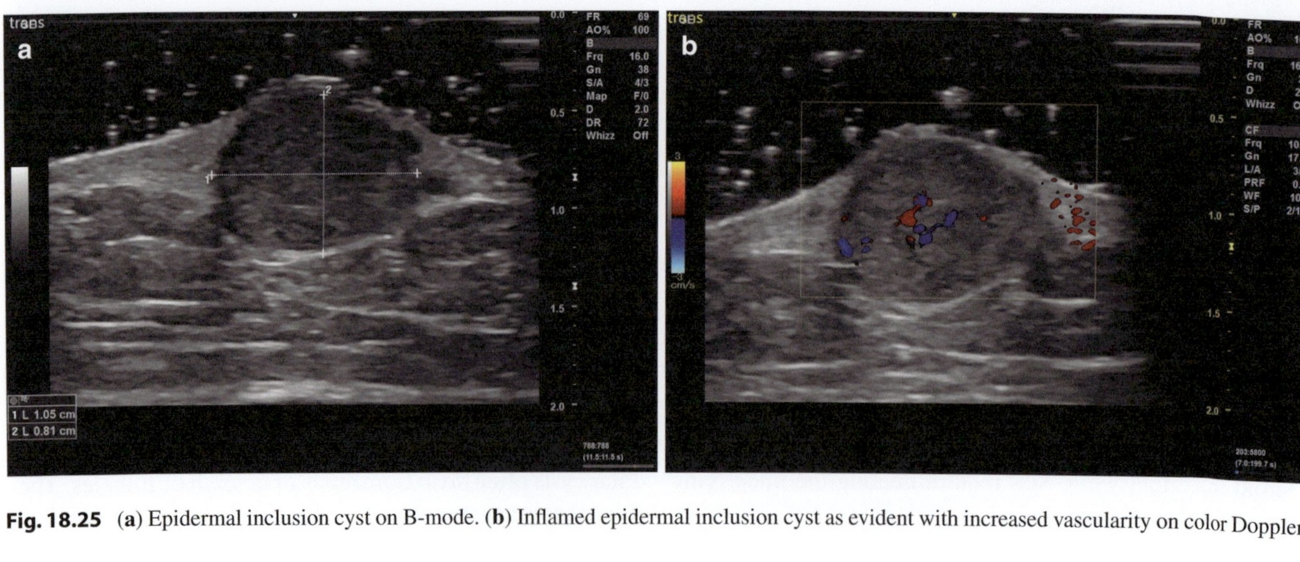

Fig. 18.25 (**a**) Epidermal inclusion cyst on B-mode. (**b**) Inflamed epidermal inclusion cyst as evident with increased vascularity on color Doppler

of the skin and can miss potentially extensive disease underlying the skin surface. Ultrasound can characterize disease burden not evident on physical examination, including pseudocysts (focal hypoechoic lesions), nodules, calcinosis (hyperechoic punctate lesions), and fistulae (horizontal hypoechoic lesions traversing dermis) (Fig. 18.26). Recent advances in ultrasound with increased availability of wideband high and ultrahigh frequency probes allow for increased applications, including in the field of dermatology [58]. Acne can be treated with topical or systemic therapies depending on disease severity. Hidradenitis suppurativa is a chronic inflammatory condition affecting the intertriginous regions of the body, which can be difficult to diagnose and treat depending on disease burden.

Severity scores have been developed and well-studied for both acne (SOS-Acne) and hidradenitis suppurativa (SOS-HS) [59, 60]. These scores characterize both the presence and number of pseudocysts along with the presence of fistulas, which clinicians can use to make the diagnosis and understand the disease burden, thereby helping patients receive appropriate treatment in a more expedited fashion. SOS-Acne grades acne as mild, moderate, or severe, with patients in the severe category benefiting from systemic therapy (Table 18.3) [59]. The SOS-HS scale grades disease severity from stage 1 up to stage 3b, with each stage having defining characteristics (Table 18.4) [60].

Nails

Ultrasound can be helpful when a patient presents with undifferentiated nail pathology. For ultrasound of the nail, it is important to use a high-frequency linear probe of at least 15 MHz. Pathologies including onychomycosis, psoriasis, glomus tumors, paronychia, abscess, and subungual hematoma can be distinguished by sonographic features [11]. Due to the superficial nature of nail pathology, use large amounts of gel, a water bath, or standoff pads to ensure adequate image resolution. Anchoring using a distal finger and "floating" the probe with minimal pressure will help ensure clear images. Nail ultrasound includes a two-plane view of the nail plate and nail bed. Normal nail anatomy includes a dorsal and ventral nail plate that appear as separated but parallel, smooth, linear, and hyperechoic structures (Fig. 18.27) [61]. There should be minimal vascularity in the nail bed. Increased vascularity on ultrasound raises the suspicion for an inflammatory or infectious process.

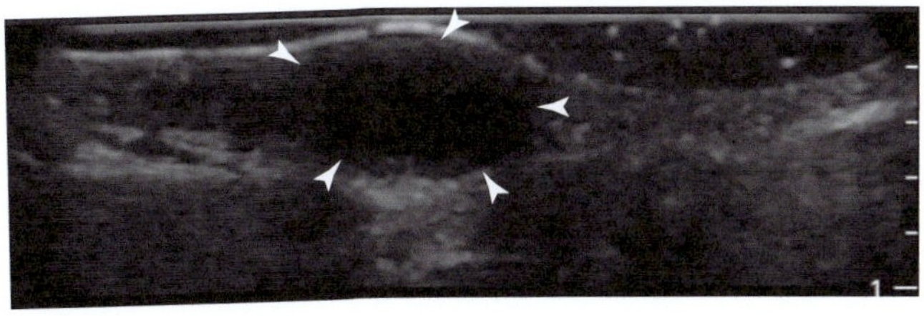

Fig. 18.26 Hypoechoic cyst (outlined by arrowheads) noted in a patient with acne vulgaris

Table 18.3 Acne vulgaris SOS-acne classification of severity (*Adapted from Wortsman et al.* [59])

Severity	Number of lesions
Mild	< 5 pseudocysts without fistulas
Moderate	5–9 pseudocysts without fistulas
Severe	≥ 10 pseudocysts with or without fistulas

Table 18.4 Sonographic Scoring of Hidradenitis Suppurativa (SOS-HS) (*Adapted from Wortsman et al.* [60])

Stage	Ultrasound findings
1	Single fluid collection and dermal changes (presence of hypo- or anechoic pseudocystic nodules, thickening of hair follicles, alterations in dermal thickness), affecting one body area (e.g., axilla, groin, breast, buttock). No presence of fistulous tracts
2	2 to 4 fluid collections or a fistulous tract, with dermal changes affecting one or two body areas
3a	≥ 5 fluid collections, 2–4 noncommunicating tunnels, or < 3 communicating tunnels
3b	≥ 5 noncommunicating tunnels or ≥3 communicating tunnels

Ultrasound has been found to have a high diagnostic utility in diagnosing nail pathology (Fig. 18.28). A study on the use of POCUS in an emergency department setting found that in patients with nail bed injuries, POCUS had a sensitivity of 93% and 100% in detecting nail bed injuries and distal phalanx fractures, respectively [62].

The majority of patients with psoriasis will have nail involvement, which commonly mimics fungal infections on physical exam [63]. Typical findings in nail psoriasis include increased vascularity of the nail bed, thickened nail plate, and loss of the ventral plate [64]. Onychomycosis will have a classic appearance with a thickened nail plate (more pronounced than in psoriasis) and loss of the ventral plate. Ultrasound can be used to follow up for improvement in treatment responses in patients with inflammatory or infectious nail conditions.

Ultrasound can be useful in the evaluation of patients with paronychia and blisters around the nail and distal digit. A simple, uncomplicated blister appears as a hypoechoic area, without internal echoes, mixed echogenicity, or vascularity. A paronychia will demonstrate increased vascularity along with surrounding tissue thickening. Infections in and around the nail bed (felons) can have similar sonographic features as an abscess, such as a squish sign and increased vascularity (Video 7). Glomus tumors are typically well-circumscribed, hypoechoic cystic structures with varying degrees of vascularity.

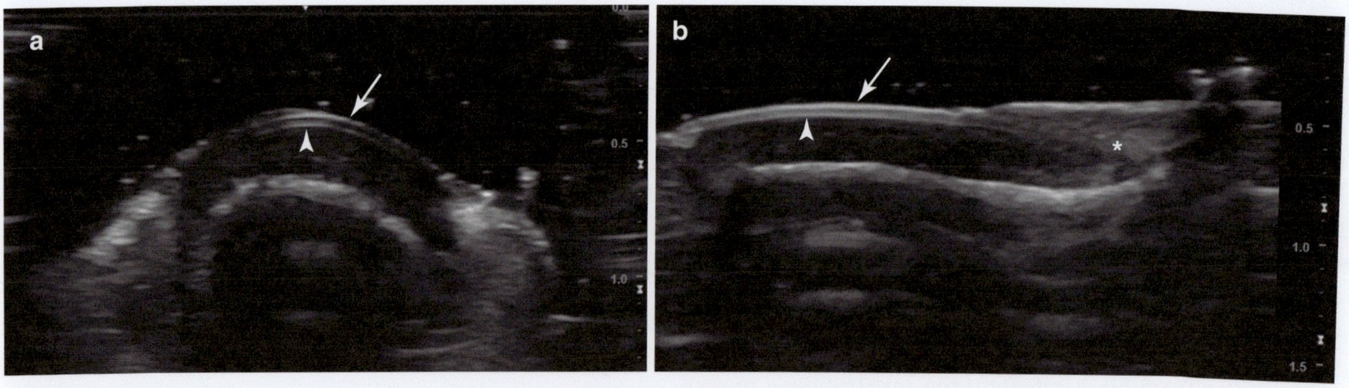

Fig. 18.27 (**a**) Short-axis view demonstrating the double-layer lamina with dorsal (arrow) and ventral (arrowhead) nail plates. (**b**) Long-axis view of the nail with a hyperechoic dorsal (arrow) and ventral (arrowhead) nail plate. The matrix is noted by an asterisk

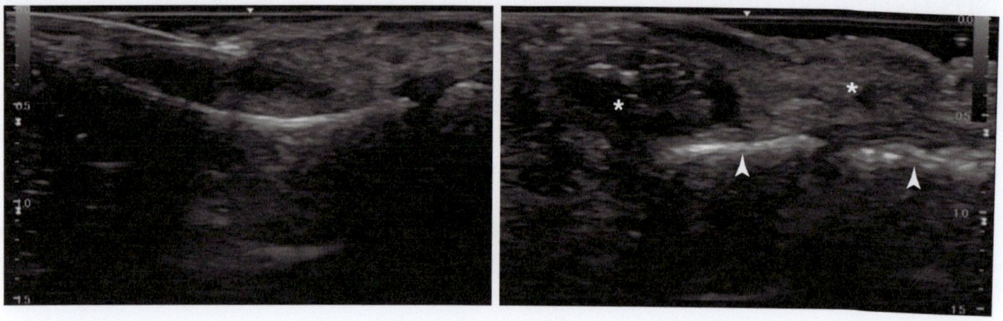

Fig. 18.28 The image on the left is the patient's unaffected contralateral nail in the long axis, while the image on the right is the affected nail with embedded nail fragments (arrow) after trauma with surrounding edema (asterisk)

Key Ultrasound Findings

Pathology	Common sonographic findings
Cellulitis	Hyperechoic fat lobules with fluid in subcutaneous tissue aka "cobblestoning".
Abscess	Irregularly bordered, hypoechoic collection with hyperechoic internal debris, posterior acoustic enhancement, lack of internal vascularity, and surrounding hyperemia.
Necrotizing fasciitis	Subcutaneous thickening, fascial fluid >4 mm, subcutaneous emphysema, and dirty shadowing.
Foreign body	Generally hyperechoic with possible reverberation and surrounding fluid.
Hematoma	Intramuscular, intermuscular, intrabursal, or intra-articular fluid collection that can be anechoic, complex, heterogenous, or echogenic in appearance.
Reactive/malignant nodes	Enlarged (>1 cm), loss of hyperechoic hilum, increased or disorganized vascularity.
Lipoma	Oval (wider than tall) with no vascularity.
Ganglion cyst	Anechoic, well-defined, limited compressibility, more common near hand and wrist.
Synovial cyst	Anechoic, well-defined, greater compressibility, more common near knee.
Sebaceous cyst	Oval-shaped, hypoechoic, homogeneous, "pseudo-testis" appearance.
Pilar (Trichilemmal) cysts	Hypoechoic with internal hyperechogenicity and no flow on color Doppler.
Epidermal inclusion cyst	Mixed echogenicity, well-defined structure with capsule; may have a punctum ("witch's hat") or hyperechoic layers ("onion" pattern).
Nails	Two well-defined plates. Limited vascularity.

Pearls and Pitfalls

- For superficial structures, use copious gel, a water bath, or a standoff pad to increase the distance between your probe and the zone of examination and enhance proximal image resolution.
- Use ultrasound to identify the abscess, surrounding vasculature, and the ideal location for I&D.
- Ultrasound has superior detection for foreign bodies compared to X-ray, especially nonmetal objects that appear as hyperechoic structures with varying reverberation artifacts.
- Artifacts can mimic pathology. Be sure to image soft tissue structures in two planes.
- As often as feasible, perform comparison views of the unaffected contralateral side.
- An absence of sonographic findings of necrotizing fasciitis does not rule out the disease, and surgical consultation should be pursued with clinical suspicion.
- Generally, masses that are taller than wide should raise clinical suspicion for a malignant process.

Disclosures/Conflicts of Interest Dr. Lewiss is a paid consultant for GE Healthcare and voluntary consultant for Médecins Sans Frontières.

References

1. Poulakou G, Lagou S, Tsiodras S. What's new in the epidemiology of skin and soft tissue infections in 2018? Curr Opin Infect Dis. 2019;32(2):77. https://doi.org/10.1097/QCO.0000000000000527.
2. Stevens DL, Bisno AL, Chambers HF, et al. Practice guidelines for the diagnosis and management of skin and soft tissue infections: 2014 update by the Infectious Diseases Society of America. Clin Infect Dis. 2014;59(2):e10–52. https://doi.org/10.1093/cid/ciu296.
3. Gottlieb M, Bernard K. Epidemiology of abscess and cellulitis among United States emergency departments from 2016 to 2023. Acad Emerg Med. Published online July 12, 2024. https://doi.org/10.1111/acem.14986
4. Giovanni JE, Dowd MD, Kennedy C, Michael JG. Interexaminer agreement in physical examination for children with suspected soft tissue abscesses. Pediatr Emerg Care. 2011;27(6):475. https://doi.org/10.1097/PEC.0b013e31821d8545.
5. Marin JR, Bilker W, Lautenbach E, Alpern ER. Reliability of clinical examinations for pediatric skin and soft-tissue infections. Pediatrics. 2010;126(5):925–30. https://doi.org/10.1542/peds.2010-1039.
6. Gottlieb M, Avila J, Chottiner M, Peksa GD. Point-of-care ultrasonography for the diagnosis of skin and soft tissue abscesses: a systematic review and meta-analysis. Ann Emerg Med. 2020;76(1):67–77. https://doi.org/10.1016/j.annemergmed.2020.01.004.
7. Gaspari RJ, Sanseverino A, Gleeson T. Abscess incision and drainage with or without ultrasonography: a randomized controlled trial. Ann Emerg Med. 2019;73(1):1–7. https://doi.org/10.1016/j.annemergmed.2018.05.014.
8. Duane TM, Huston JM, Collom M, et al. Surgical infection society 2020 updated guidelines on the management of complicated skin and soft tissue infections. Surg Infect. 2021;22(4):383–99. https://doi.org/10.1089/sur.2020.436.
9. Friedman N, Tseng F, Savic R, et al. Reliability of neck mass point-of-care ultrasound by pediatric emergency physicians. J Ultrasound Med. 2019;38(11):2893–900. https://doi.org/10.1002/jum.14993.
10. Blaivas M, Adhikari S. Unexpected findings on point-of-care superficial ultrasound imaging before incision and drainage. J Ultrasound Med. 2011;30(10):1425–30. https://doi.org/10.7863/jum.2011.30.10.1425.
11. Aluja Jaramillo F, Quiasúa Mejía DC, Martínez Ordúz HM, González Ardila C. Nail unit ultrasound: a complete guide of the nail diseases. J Ultrasound. 2017;20(3):181–92. https://doi.org/10.1007/s40477-017-0253-6.
12. Shen-Wagner J, Deutchman M. Point-of-care ultrasound: a practical guide for primary care. Fam Pract Manag. 2020;27(6):33–40.
13. Berger T, Garrido F, Green J, Lema PC, Gupta J. Bedside ultrasound performed by novices for the detection of abscess in ED patients with soft tissue infections. Am J Emerg Med. 2012;30(8):1569–73. https://doi.org/10.1016/j.ajem.2011.08.002.
14. Adhikari S, Blaivas M. Sonography first for subcutaneous abscess and cellulitis evaluation. J Ultrasound Med. 2012;31(10):1509–12. https://doi.org/10.7863/jum.2012.31.10.1509.
15. Blaivas M, Lyon M, Brannam L, Duggal S, Sierzenski P. Water bath evaluation technique for emergency ultrasound of painful superficial structures. Am J Emerg Med. 2004;22(7):589–93. https://doi.org/10.1016/j.ajem.2004.09.009.
16. Cotton J, Bahner D, Prats M. The lateral approach water bath: a novel method of ultrasound imaging of the hand. Am J Emerg Med. 2024;77:164–8. https://doi.org/10.1016/j.ajem.2023.11.005.
17. Long B, Gottlieb M. Diagnosis and management of cellulitis and abscess in the emergency department setting: an evidence-based review. J Emerg Med. 2022;62(1):16–27. https://doi.org/10.1016/j.jemermed.2021.09.015.
18. Chao HC, Lin SJ, Huang YC, Lin TY. Sonographic evaluation of cellulitis in children. J Ultrasound Med. 2000;19(11):743–9. https://doi.org/10.7863/jum.2000.19.11.743.
19. Ramirez-Schrempp D, Dorfman DH, Baker WE, Liteplo AS. Ultrasound soft-tissue applications in the pediatric emergency department: to drain or not to drain? Pediatr Emerg Care. 2009;25(1):44–8. https://doi.org/10.1097/PEC.0b013e318191d963.
20. Goulding M, Haran J, Sanseverino A, Zeoli T, Gaspari R. Clinical failure in abscess treatment: the role of ultrasound and incision and drainage. CJEM. 2022;24(1):39–43. https://doi.org/10.1007/s43678-021-00179-8.
21. Wu J, Ge L, Wang X, Jin Y. Role of point-of-care ultrasound (POCUS) in the diagnosis of an abscess in pediatric skin and soft tissue infections: a systematic review and meta-analysis. Med Ultrason. 2022;24(3):339–47. https://doi.org/10.11152/mu-3166.
22. Russell FM, Rutz M, Rood LK, McGee J, Sarmiento EJ. Abscess size and depth on ultrasound and association with treatment failure without drainage. West J Emerg Med. 2020;21(2):336–42. https://doi.org/10.5811/westjem.2019.12.41921. PMID: 32191191; PMCID: PMC7081847.
23. Gottlieb M, Schmitz G, Peksa GD. Comparison of the loop technique with incision and drainage for skin and soft tissue abscesses: a systematic review and meta-analysis. Acad Emerg Med. 2021;28(3):346–54. https://doi.org/10.1111/acem.14151. Epub 2020 Nov 9. PMID: 33037713.
24. McHenry CR, Piotrowski JJ, Petrinic D, Malangoni MA. Determinants of mortality for necrotizing soft-tissue infections. Ann Surg. 1995;221(5):558–65.

25. Marks A, Patel D, Sundaram T, Johnson J, Gottlieb M. Ultrasound for the diagnosis of necrotizing fasciitis: a systematic review of the literature. Am J Emerg Med. 2023;65:31–5. https://doi.org/10.1016/j.ajem.2022.12.037.
26. Yen ZS, Wang HP, Ma HM, Chen SC, Chen WJ. Ultrasonographic screening of clinically-suspected necrotizing fasciitis. Acad Emerg Med. 2002;9(12):1448–51. https://doi.org/10.1111/j.1553-2712.2002.tb01619.x.
27. Lin CN, Hsiao CT, Chang CP, Huang TY, Hsiao KY, Chen YC, Fann WC. The relationship between fluid accumulation in ultrasonography and the diagnosis and prognosis of patients with necrotizing fasciitis. Ultrasound Med Biol. 2019;45(7):1545–50. https://doi.org/10.1016/j.ultrasmedbio.2019.02.027. Epub 2019 Apr 26. PMID: 31031033.
28. Castleberg E, Jenson N, Dinh VA. Diagnosis of necrotizing fasciitis with bedside ultrasound: the STAFF exam. West J Emerg Med. 2014;15(1):111–3. https://doi.org/10.5811/westjem.2013.8.18303.
29. Davis J, Czerniski B, Au A, Adhikari S, Farrell I, Fields JM. Diagnostic accuracy of ultrasonography in retained soft tissue foreign bodies: a systematic review and meta-analysis. Acad Emerg Med. 2015;22(7):777–87. https://doi.org/10.1111/acem.12714. Epub 2015 Jun 25. PMID: 26111545
30. Rockett MS, Gentile SC, Gudas CJ, Brage ME, Zygmunt KH. The use of ultrasonography for the detection of retained wooden foreign bodies in the foot. J Foot Ankle Surg. 1995;34(5):478–84. https://doi.org/10.1016/S1067-2516(09)80024-0.
31. Crankson S, Oratis P, Al MG. Ultrasound in the diagnosis and treatment of wooden foreign bodies in the foot. Ann Saudi Med. 2004;24(6):480–1. https://doi.org/10.5144/0256-4947.2004.480.
32. Levine MR, Gorman SM, Young CF, Courtney DM. Clinical characteristics and management of wound foreign bodies in the ED. Am J Emerg Med. 2008;26(8):918–22. https://doi.org/10.1016/j.ajem.2007.11.026. PMID: 18926353.
33. Banerjee B, Das RK. Sonographic detection of foreign bodies of the extremities. Br J Radiol. 1991;64(758):107–12. https://doi.org/10.1259/0007-1285-64-758-107.
34. Dean AJ, Gronczewski CA, Costantino TG. Technique for emergency medicine bedside ultrasound identification of a radiolucent foreign body. J Emerg Med. 2003;24(3):303–8. https://doi.org/10.1016/s0736-4679(02)00765-5.
35. del Cura J, Aza I, Zabala R, Sarabia M, Korta I. US-guided localization and removal of soft-tissue foreign bodies. Radiographics. 2020;40:200001. https://doi.org/10.1148/rg.2020200001.
36. Marín-Díez E, Landeras Álvaro RM, Lamagrande Obregón A, Pelaz Esteban M, Gallardo Agromayor E. Ultrasonography of subcutaneous foreign bodies: differences depending on their nature, complications, and potential diagnostic errors. Radiologia. 2020;62(1):3–12. https://doi.org/10.1016/j.rx.2019.05.009.
37. Hill R, Conron R, Greissinger P, Heller M. Ultrasound for the detection of foreign bodies in human tissue. Ann Emerg Med. 1997;29(3):353–6. https://doi.org/10.1016/s0196-0644(97)70347-0.
38. Mohammadi A, Ghasemi-Rad M, Khodabakhsh M. Non-opaque soft tissue foreign body: sonographic findings. BMC Med Imaging. 2011;11(1):9. https://doi.org/10.1186/1471-2342-11-9.
39. Lam J, Montague S. Hematocrit sign elucidates cause of abdominal pain. POCUS J. 2021;6(1):8–9. https://doi.org/10.24908/pocus.v6i1.14751. PMID: 36895502; PMCID: PMC9979907
40. Wagner JM, Rebik K, Spicer PJ. Ultrasound of soft tissue masses and fluid collections. Radiol Clin North Am. 2019;57(3):657–69.
41. Yoon ES, Lin B, Miller TT. Ultrasound of musculoskeletal hematomas: relationship of sonographic appearance to age and ease of aspiration. AJR Am J Roentgenol. 2021;216(1):125–30. https://doi.org/10.2214/AJR.19.22752.
42. Mohseni S, Shojaiefard A, Khorgami Z, Alinejad S, Ghorbani A, Ghafouri A. Peripheral lymphadenopathy: approach and diagnostic tools. Iran J Med Sci. 2014;39(2 Suppl):158–70. PMID: 24753638; PMCID: PMC3993046.
43. Heaven CL, Barber L, Ahmadi O, Selvarajah K, Shetty S. COVID-19 vaccine associated cervical lymphadenopathy: a case series. ANZ J Surg. 2022;92(9):2286–91. https://doi.org/10.1111/ans.17808.
44. Ha SM, Chu AJ, Lee J, et al. US evaluation of axillary lymphadenopathy following COVID-19 vaccination: a prospective longitudinal study. Radiology. 2022;305(1):46–53. https://doi.org/10.1148/radiol.220543.
45. HaBlausen.com staff. Medical gallery of Blausen Medical 2014. WikiJournal of Medicine, August 29, 2014; 1(2). https://doi.org/10.15347/WJM/2014.010.
46. Gruber L, Gruber H, Luger AK, Glodny B, Henninger B, Loizides A. Diagnostic hierarchy of radiological features in soft tissue tumours and proposition of a simple diagnostic algorithm to estimate malignant potential of an unknown mass. Eur J Radiol. 2017;95:102–10. https://doi.org/10.1016/j.ejrad.2017.07.020.
47. Hsu YC, Shih YYI, Gao HW, Huang GS. Subcutaneous lipoma compressing the common peroneal nerve and causing palsy: sonographic diagnosis. J Clin Ultrasound. 2010;38(2):97–9. https://doi.org/10.1002/jcu.20643.
48. Rahmani G, McCarthy P, Bergin D. The diagnostic accuracy of ultrasonography for soft tissue lipomas: a systematic review. Acta Radiol Open. 2017;6(6):2058460117716704. https://doi.org/10.1177/2058460117716704.
49. Shimamori N, Kishino T, Okabe N, et al. Discrimination of well-differentiated liposarcoma from benign lipoma on sonography: an uncontrolled retrospective study. J Med Ultrasonics. 2020;47(4):617–23. https://doi.org/10.1007/s10396-020-01051-531.
50. Jacobson JA, Middleton WD, Allison SJ, et al. Ultrasonography of superficial soft-tissue masses: Society of radiologists in ultrasound consensus conference statement. Radiology. 2022;304(1):18–30. https://doi.org/10.1148/radiol.211101.
51. Styring E, Billing V, Hartman L, et al. Simple guidelines for efficient referral of soft-tissue sarcomas: a population-based evaluation of adherence to guidelines and referral patterns. J Bone Joint Surg Am. 2012;94(14):1291–6. https://doi.org/10.2106/JBJS.K.01271.
52. Giard MC, Pineda C. Ganglion cyst versus synovial cyst? Ultrasound characteristics through a review of the literature. Rheumatol Int. 2015 Apr;35(4):597–605. https://doi.org/10.1007/s00296-014-3120-1.
53. Solivetti FM, Desiderio F, Elia F, Guerrisi A, Cota C, Morrone A. Sonographic appearance of sebaceous cysts. Our experience and a review of the literature. Int J Dermatol. 2019;58(12):1353–9. https://doi.org/10.1111/ijd.14515.
54. Ren WW, Wu L, Wang Q, Shan DD, Wang LF, Chen ZT, Li L, Sun LP, Guo LH, Xu HX. The value of ultrasound for differentiating trichilemmal cysts from epidermoid cysts. J Ultrasound Med. 2023;42(9):1941–50. https://doi.org/10.1002/jum.16211.
55. Li Y, Zhao Q, Tian Q, Wu J, Pan X, Shi M. Rare Trichilemmal Cyst Localized in the Pulp of the Middle Finger. Med Ultrason. 2023;25(4):474–475.
56. Yuan WH, Hsu HC, Lai YC, Chou YH, Li AFY. Differences in sonographic features of ruptured and unruptured epidermal cysts. J Ultrasound Med. 2012;31(2):265–72. https://doi.org/10.7863/jum.2012.31.2.265.

57. Min HJ, Lee JM, Han JK, Kim YJ. Influence factor in thickness of cyst wall of epidermal cysts. J Craniofac Surg. 2017;28(4):e369–72. https://doi.org/10.1097/SCS.0000000000003687.
58. Gonzalez C, Wortsman X. How to start on dermatologic ultrasound: Basic anatomical concepts, guidelines, technical considerations, and best tips. Semin Ultrasound CT MR. Published online December 4, 2023:S0887-2171(23)00092-6. https://doi.org/10.1053/j.sult.2023.11.001
59. Wortsman X, Claveria P, Valenzuela F, Molina MT, Wortsman J. Sonography of acne vulgaris. J Ultrasound Med. 2014;33(1):93–102. https://doi.org/10.7863/ultra.33.1.93.
60. Wortsman X. Update on ultrasound diagnostic criteria and new ultrasound severity and activity scorings of hidradenitis Suppurativa: modified SOS-HS and US-HSA. J Ultrasound Med. 2024;43(1):207–13. https://doi.org/10.1002/jum.16351.
61. Wortsman X, Jemec G. Dermatologic ultrasound with clinical and histologic correlations. Springer Science & Business Media; 2013.
62. Gungor F, Akyol KC, Eken C, Kesapli M, Beydilli I, Akcimen M. The value of point-of-care ultrasound for detecting nail bed injury in ED. Am J Emerg Med. 2016;34(9):1850–4. https://doi.org/10.1016/j.ajem.2016.06.067.
63. Salomon J, Szepietowski JC, Proniewicz A. Psoriatic nails: a prospective clinical study. J Cutan Med Surg. 2003;7(4):317–21. https://doi.org/10.1007/s10227-002-0143-0.
64. Gutierrez M, Wortsman X, Filippucci E, De Angelis R, Filosa G, Grassi W. High-frequency sonography in the evaluation of psoriasis. J Ultrasound Med. 2009;28(11):1569–74. https://doi.org/10.7863/jum.2009.28.11.1569.

Musculoskeletal Ultrasound

19

Dana DiRenzo and Robert Farrow

Background

Musculoskeletal ultrasound is an important imaging modality when evaluating joint and soft tissue pathology. The field of musculoskeletal ultrasound has rapidly grown since the early 2000s and is widely utilized by radiologists, rheumatologists, internists, and emergency medicine physicians, among many other specialists. There are multiple important applications of musculoskeletal ultrasound, including the diagnosis of soft tissue injury and inflammation, tendon injury and inflammation, joint pathology, muscle pathology, identification of masses and cystic structures, and guidance for aspirations and injections [1, 2]. Musculoskeletal ultrasound is considered an imaging procedure and may be billed when accompanied by proper documentation. Rigorous training and credentialing are now offered to North American rheumatologists through the American College of Rheumatology and their European counterparts through the European Alliance of Associations for Rheumatology [3, 4]. Similarly, point-of-care ultrasound (POCUS) training and fellowships, which include dedicated musculoskeletal ultrasound education, have become widespread throughout North America [5, 6].

When approaching a musculoskeletal ultrasound study, the "bone" or "musculoskeletal" presets are helpful. For superficial and intermediate structures (hand, wrist, shoulder, knees, ankles, feet), start with higher frequencies and adjust accordingly. Suggested settings include a frequency of 12–16 MHz and a gain of 40–45 dB. Because joint and tendon synovium is considered a low or slow blood flow state, power Doppler is preferred over color Doppler. For very superficial structures, a water bath, commercial step-off pad, or homemade step-off pad (e.g., a glove full of water with air removed) may improve resolution.

With the advanced ultrasound practitioner in mind, this chapter discusses common musculoskeletal pathologies, standard ultrasound views, and key sonographic findings.

Indications and Diagnoses

Indications
- Pain
- Swelling
- Palpable deformities or masses
- Decreased range of motion
- Suspected fracture or dislocation

Diagnoses
- Myositis
- Fractures
- Effusions
- Bursitis
- Dislocations
- Tendon/ligament injuries
- Tenosynovitis
- Tendinitis

Supplementary Information The online version contains supplementary material available at https://doi.org/10.1007/978-3-031-85308-1_19.

D. DiRenzo
Division of Rheumatology, Department of Medicine, University of Pennsylvania, Philadelphia, PA, USA
e-mail: dana.direnzo@pennmedicine.upenn.edu

R. Farrow (✉)
Department of Emergency Medicine, Mount Sinai Medical Center, Miami Beach, FL, USA
e-mail: Robert.FarrowII@msmc.com

M. Gottlieb, N. Panebianco (eds.), *Advanced Point-of-Care Ultrasound*, https://doi.org/10.1007/978-3-031-85308-1_19

Core Views

View	Image	Approach
Muscle	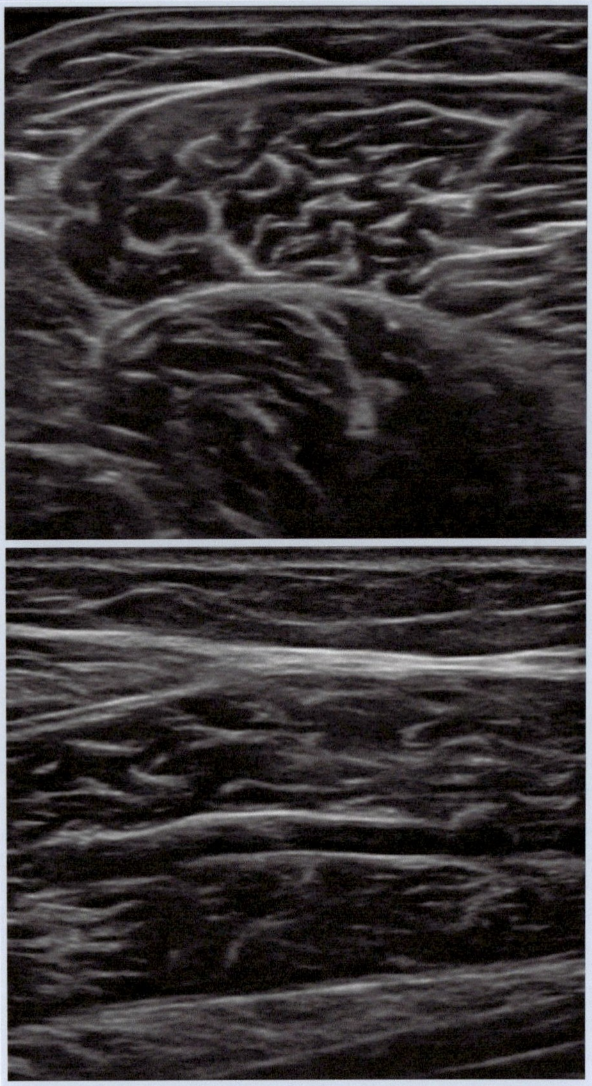 Core View 1. Normal muscle visualized in short axis (left) and long axis (right). *Images courtesy of Michael Gottlieb, MD* Core Video 1 Core Video 2	Muscles should be scanned in long- and short-axis planes. Muscles typically take on a "starry night" appearance with hyperechoic speckles scattered throughout the hypoechoic muscle fibers. Anisotropy can be common when scanning muscles, which often have curved fibers, and thus dynamic scanning is key.

View	Image	Approach
Long bones	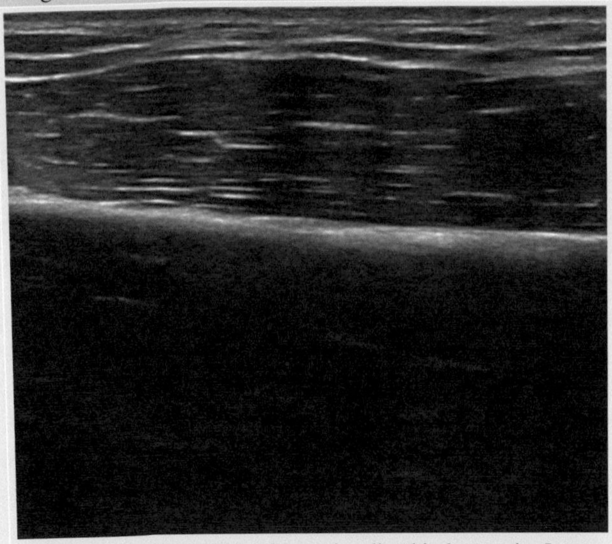 Core View 2. Normal long bone visualized in long axis. *Image courtesy of Michael Gottlieb, MD*	Due to the superficial position of most osseous structures, fractures are easily visible using a high-frequency linear probe. A curvilinear or low-frequency probe may be needed if the bone is deep. Typically, bones will appear as hyperechoic lines with clean shadowing or reverberation artifact. Occasionally, mirror artifact will also be seen below the hyperechoic line. Cortical disruption should be assessed in the long axis. Presence of secondary signs of fracture, such as hematoma, soft tissue deformation, edema, effusion, or lipohemarthrosis, should also be assessed.
Tendon	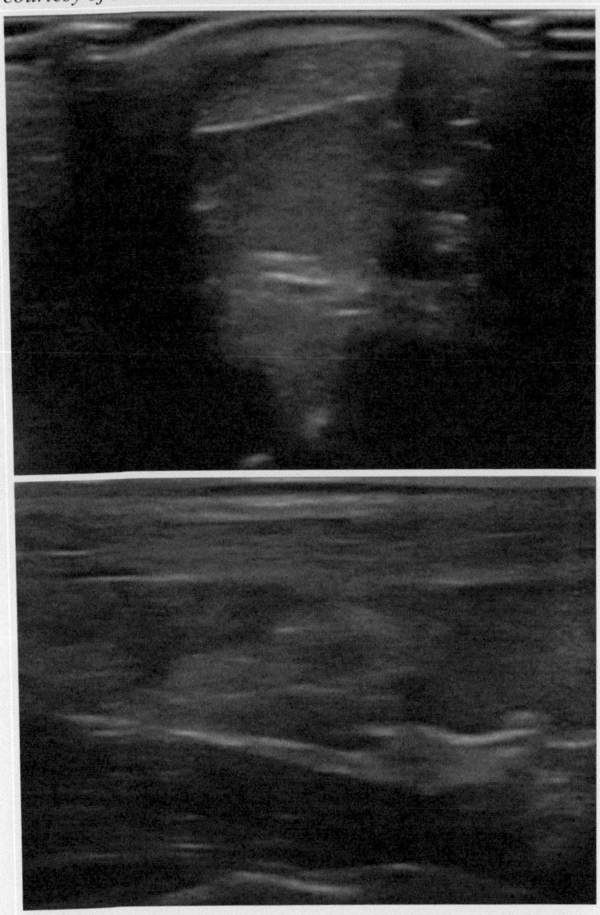 Core View 3. Normal tendon visualized in short axis (left) and long axis (right). *Images courtesy of Michael Gottlieb, MD*	Use copious ultrasound gel or a step-off pad to ensure sufficient contact with the skin. Follow the tendon along its entire length in both the short axis and long axis. As tendons can demonstrate anisotropy, it is important to keep the probe as close to perpendicular as possible. Fan the probe as needed to maximize visualization. Compression can be applied to assess for areas of fluid or thickening.

Clinical Applications

Myositis

Myositis is broadly defined as inflammation of the muscle, though it is more commonly used to refer to a grouping of systemic autoimmune and inflammatory diseases. The most common myopathies include dermatomyositis, antisynthetase syndrome, immune-mediated necrotizing myopathy, polymyositis, and inclusion body myositis [7]. There are several established imaging findings that may be useful in the diagnosis and assessment of disease activity, particularly with regard to echogenicity [8].

The sonographic findings of myositis include increased muscle echogenicity and potentially scattered hypoechoic areas, muscle hypertrophy or atrophy, increased vascularity, and fascial thickening [7] (Fig. 19.1). Additionally, one may see subcutaneous edema, especially in dermatomyositis. Soft tissue calcifications can also be found in chronic cases. For inclusion body myositis, increased echogenicity may be found within the muscles, signifying fibrosis, particularly at the flexor digitorum profundus and gastrocnemius muscles [9].

Rhabdomyolysis involves acute muscle breakdown and is characterized by hypo- and hyperechoic areas of muscle fibers, muscle strand disorganization, and increased muscle edema [10] (Video 3). Rhabdomyolysis can overlap in appearance with myositis, so it is critical to correlate the findings with the clinical history and physical examination.

Importantly, muscles look different across individuals, depending upon age, fat content of muscle, and muscle mass. In general, obese and elderly patients may have a more hypoechoic appearance to their muscles for these reasons [11]. Therefore, it is important to compare abnormal findings against a similar muscle group on the patient's contralateral side to assess their baseline appearance.

Long Bone Fractures

Ultrasound evaluation of fractures is limited primarily to the evaluation of the superficial cortex and surrounding soft tissues [12–14]. Sonography is particularly useful in cases where the diagnosis is time-sensitive, there is strong clinical suspicion for fracture with an inconclusive radiograph, or there is limited access to radiography. For example, minimally displaced fractures may not be well-visualized on radiographs, but the cortical break can be clearly seen via sonography. This is consistent with the literature, with data showing that the sensitivity for rib fractures is higher with ultrasound than with radiography (97% vs. 77%) [15].

The cortex of the bone should be evaluated for irregularities and breaches in the long axis, followed by the short axis (Fig. 19.2). Secondary signs may also point to an occult frac-

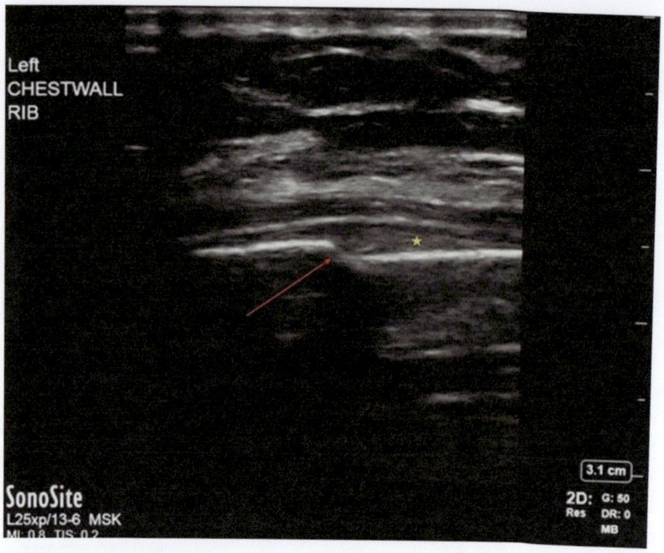

Fig. 19.2 Linear imaging of rib fracture. Yellow star denotes hematoma with elevation of the periosteal lining. Red arrow demonstrates cortical break with step-off

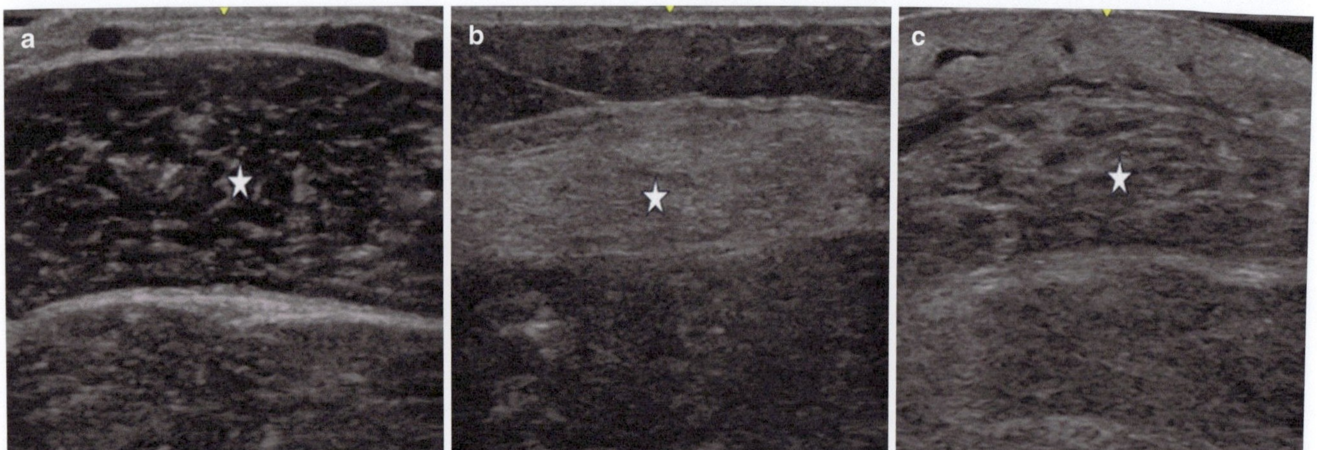

Fig. 19.1 (**a**) Normal gastrocnemius muscle. (**b**) Inclusion body myositis with markedly increased muscle echogenicity. (**c**) Dermatomyositis with patchy areas of increased muscle echogenicity with overlying subcutaneous edema. (*Images courtesy of Jemima Albayda, MD*)

ture. These signs can include tissue displacement, a surrounding hematoma, or prominent joint effusions with lipohemarthrosis (for intra-articular fractures). For example, in a patient presenting with elbow pain after sustaining a fall on an outstretched hand, the presence of an effusion in the olecranon fossa provides a sonographic parallel to the radiographic "posterior fat pad" sign, thereby suggesting an occult fracture despite the inability to directly visualize this [19]. The presence of lipohemarthrosis (i.e., the presence of blood and lipid in the joint space) has been proposed by some to be a strong independent indicator of occult fracture when the mechanism is appropriate [16–19].

Beyond triage assessment and evaluation for occult fracture, ultrasound can also be utilized to assist in fracture reduction. This modality has had some debate about the routine use in the adult population [20–22]. For example, in a study of adult patients with distal radius fracture randomized to POCUS-guided reduction vs. standard of care, there was no statistical difference in the number of patients that needed more than 1 reduction attempt (6% vs. 12%) [20].

There is stronger evidence for POCUS-guided reduction in the management of pediatric fractures [23]. POCUS use in pediatric fracture assessment follows the same general principles of evaluation seen in adult medicine, and a growing number of studies demonstrate good sensitivity, specificity, positive predictive, and negative predictive value in assessing for pediatric fractures [24]. To that end, there has recently been a concerted effort to evaluate the utility of musculoskeletal ultrasound in the primary management of nonoperative pediatric forearm fractures [25, 26].

There are some fracture patterns commonly seen in pediatric patients such as buckle (torus) and minimally displaced greenstick fractures that can be easily identified with POCUS [27–29] (Fig. 19.3). Recent literature suggests that an ultrasound-first evaluation strategy may be sufficient in pediatric patients without notable deformity, obvious fracture, or with evidence only of a buckle-type fracture on ultrasound evaluation [30].

Scaphoid Fractures

Scaphoid fractures can be readily identified on ultrasound due to the superficial position of the scaphoid in the wrist (Fig. 19.4). The clinical importance of diagnosis, limited ability of radiography, and implications of immobilization make it an ideal osseous structure for ultrasound evaluation. In one European study using a diagnostic workflow for patients with tenderness over the scaphoid on examination, by including POCUS evaluation after negative radiographs, the authors reported a sensitivity of 100% and specificity of 98% when using the criterion of cortical break [31]. Additionally, in this study, the presence of occult fracture on radiographs was 9.3% (5 out of 54), and all 5 were detected via ultrasonography with only a single false positive. In the assessment of fractures to the scaphoid, scanning techniques vary but should include both dorsal and volar wrist views [32]. Some experts have proposed incorporating sonography into cases with negative radiography using ultrasound evidence of cortical disruptions, soft tissue abnormalities, and clinical suspicion to determine the treatment approach [32]. A 2018 meta-analysis found a pooled sensitivity of 85.6% and specificity of 83.3% for the diagnosis of occult scaphoid fractures with ultrasound [33].

Osteomyelitis

While magnetic resonance imaging is the imaging modality of choice, POCUS can be used to evaluate for high-risk features associated with osteomyelitis in a similar manner to radiography. Ultrasound features suggestive of osteomyelitis include deep soft tissue fluid collections adjacent to the bone, periosteal thickening, subperiosteal fluid collection, and increased vascularity of the periosteum [34] (Fig. 19.5). Multiple case reports and studies have demonstrated an early role for POCUS, with the sensitivity ranging from 76% to 100% [34–41]. Early evaluation by ultrasound can be useful

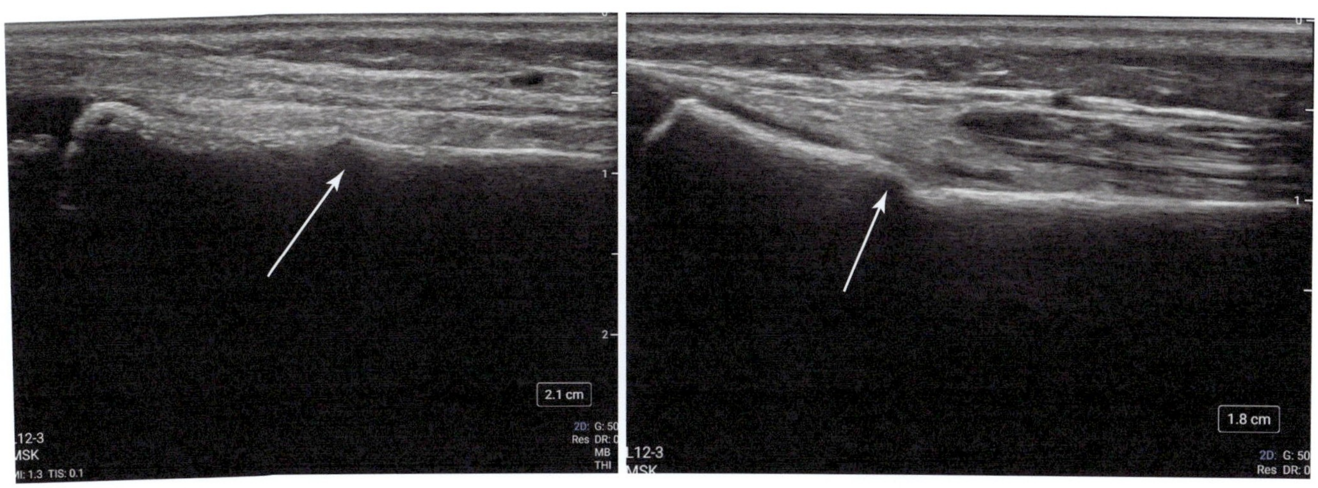

Fig. 19.3 Buckle fracture of the cortex denoted by white arrow. (*Image courtesy of Paul Khalil, MD*)

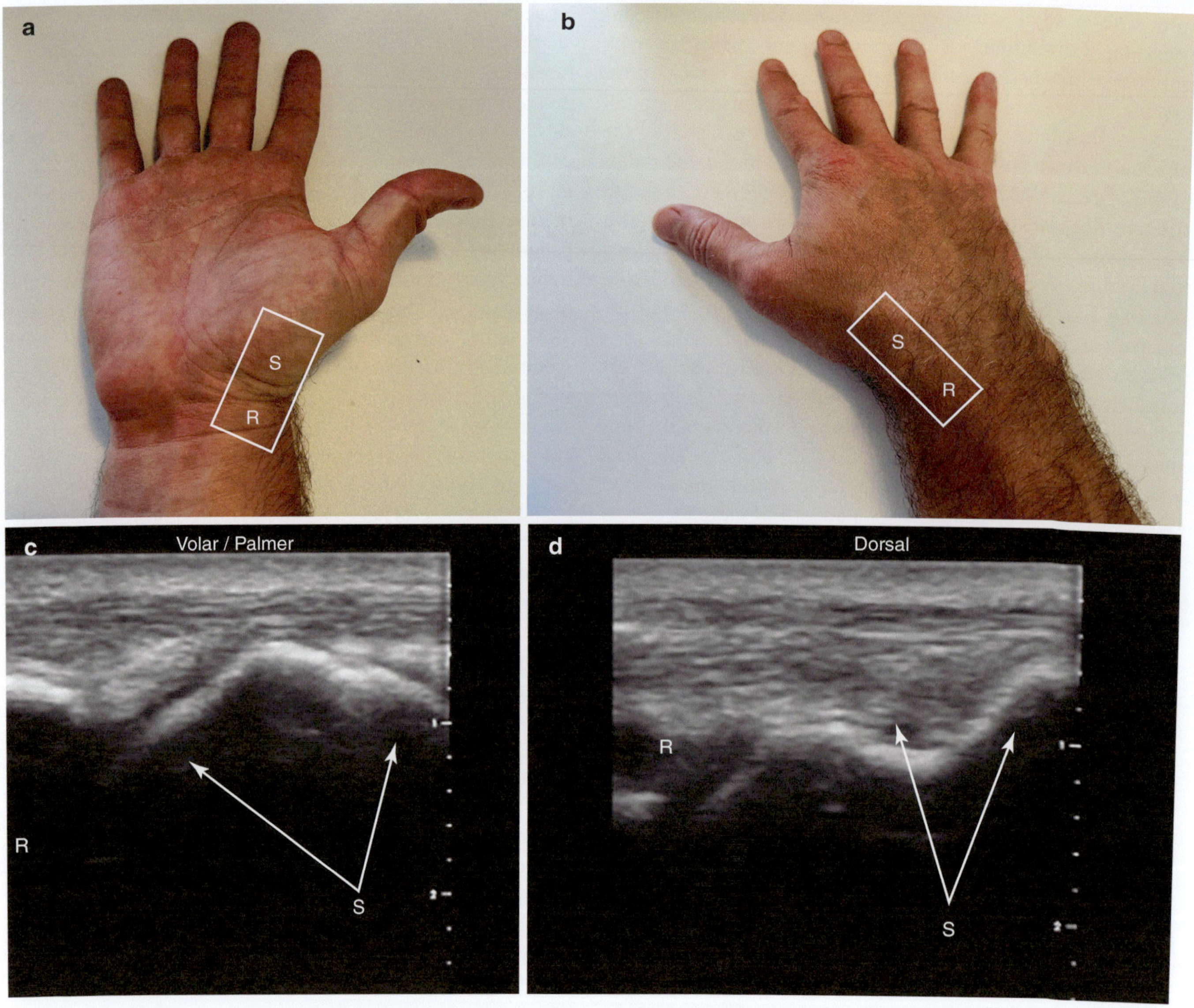

Fig. 19.4 Assessment of the scaphoid bone. Using a linear probe, visualize the volar side of the scaphoid bone in long axis with the indicator pointed towards the distal radius. Repeat this from the dorsal side. The volar scaphoid will have a peanut-shaped appearance (image **c**), whereas the dorsal scaphoid will have a pyramid-like shape with a notched appearance (image **d**). *S* scaphoid, *R* radius

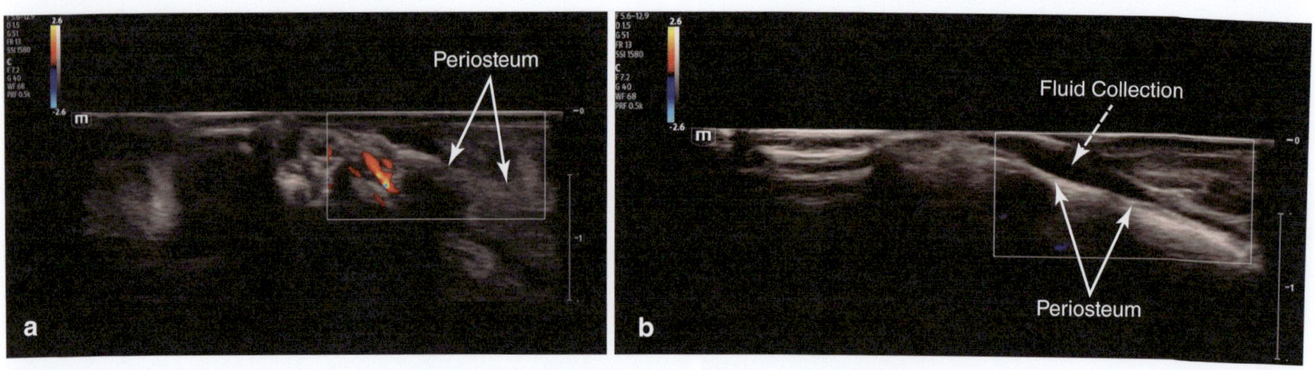

Fig. 19.5 Ultrasound imaging of osteomyelitis. (**a**) Periosteal thickening, increased vascularity of the periosteum, and surrounding soft tissue adjacent to a subperiosteal fluid collection. (**b**) A fluid collection adjacent to the periosteum

in populations where minimizing radiation is advantageous (e.g., pediatrics, obstetrics) or when frequent imaging is required to monitor treatment.

Effusions and Arthrocentesis

Joint effusions are common with a diverse range of inflammatory and noninflammatory causes. Inflammatory etiologies of joint effusion include inflammatory arthritides (e.g., rheumatoid arthritis, psoriatic arthritis, spondyloarthritis), crystalline arthritis (e.g., gout, pseudogout), or infectious/septic arthritis. Noninflammatory etiologies of joint effusions may include degenerative arthritis or injury (e.g., ligamentous injury, cartilaginous tears), hemarthrosis, or lipohemarthrosis. Ultrasound can aid in the diagnosis of joint effusion and be used to guide arthrocentesis and joint injections to facilitate analgesia or reduce inflammation.

Sonographically, effusions are typically anechoic to hypoechoic but can have mixed echogenicity if chronic or inflammatory and are compressible. In chronic and inflammatory joint effusions (e.g., rheumatoid arthritis, crystalline arthritis) that are present, the joint fluid may be loculated or display surrounding areas of "fronding" (i.e., synovial thickening). Inflamed synovial folds may have increased vascularity seen with color or power Doppler.

Additionally, there are several sonographic findings that should raise suspicion for gout due to its relatively unique sonographic appearance (Fig. 19.6). The double contour sign is a double-echogenic layer overlying cartilage which signifies the urate crystals layering on the surface and hyperechoic "clumps," typically with surrounding effusion in the acute gout flare [42]. Within the joint space or tendon, crystalline arthropathies (inclusive of both gout and pseudogout) can have speckled, hyperechoic foci (referred to as "snowstorm" appearance), which signify calcifications. Aside from crystalline arthritis, the differential for a snowstorm sign also includes rice bodies (echogenic collections of fibrin and leukocytes) as well as gas bubbles (noninfectious), which are findings of a longstanding degenerated joint [43]. Finally, tophi can be seen as heterogeneously hyperechoic structures surrounded by a hypoechoic "halo" from chronic inflammation [44]. The presence of both tophi and double contour signs in the context of hyperuricemia is highly specific for gout [45].

Before discussing specific techniques, there are a few commonalities across all ultrasound-guided injections and aspirations. First, it is important to fully identify the extent of the effusion prior to aspirating in the short and long axes. In doing so, one can identify where the fluid pocket is the largest and the most accessible (e.g., no overlying vasculature). Second, when using the in-plane technique (needle visualized longitudinally), the needle should be visualized throughout the whole course to avoid damage to surrounding vascular structures and nerves. Finally, always aspirate prior to injecting to reduce the risk of inadvertent vascular injection.

Glenohumeral Joint

The glenohumeral joint can be accessed via a posterior or anterior approach. For the posterior approach, begin by placing a linear or curvilinear probe on the posterior humerus in the transverse plane and visualize the humeral head where it articulates with the glenoid capsule. Assess for any surrounding vasculature. Then, advance the needle from the lateral direction toward the joint space (Fig. 19.7, Video 4). Depending on the depth and body habitus, a longer needle (e.g., spinal needle or echogenic nerve block needle) may be needed. While the landmark-based approach has a relatively high success rate of 75%, data show that ultrasound can substantially increase the accuracy [46–48].

For the anterior approach, begin by identifying the coracoid process and humeral head, as discussed further in the

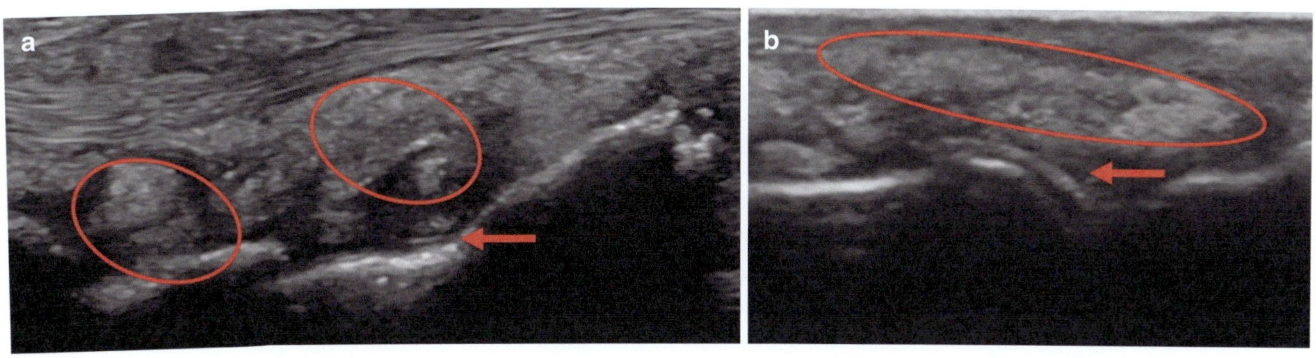

Fig. 19.6 Sonographic findings of gout. (**a**) Dorsal, longitudinal view of the wrist carpal bones with overlying tophi (circles) and a faint double contour sign (arrow). (**b**) Longitudinal view of the great toe with double contour sign (arrow) over the cartilage line and overlying tophi (circle). (*Images courtesy of Marta Bean, MD*)

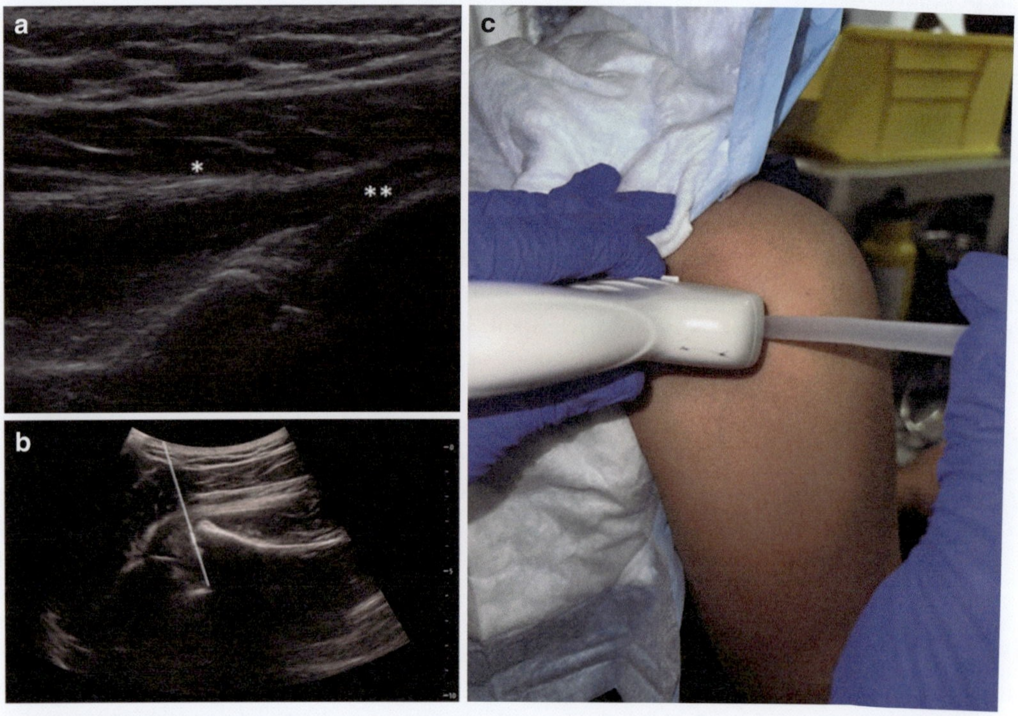

Fig. 19.7 Posterior approach to the glenohumeral joint. (**a**) Longitudinal view of a normal posterior glenohumeral joint with intact infraspinatus (*) and smooth joint capsule (**). (**b**) Posterior glenohumeral joint with degenerative arthritis changes and effusion. The white line denotes projected in-plane needle placement. (**c**) Demonstration of probe placement and needle positioning for posterior aspiration. (*Image **a** courtesy of Levon Nazarian, MD. Images **b** and **c** courtesy of Michael Gottlieb, MD*)

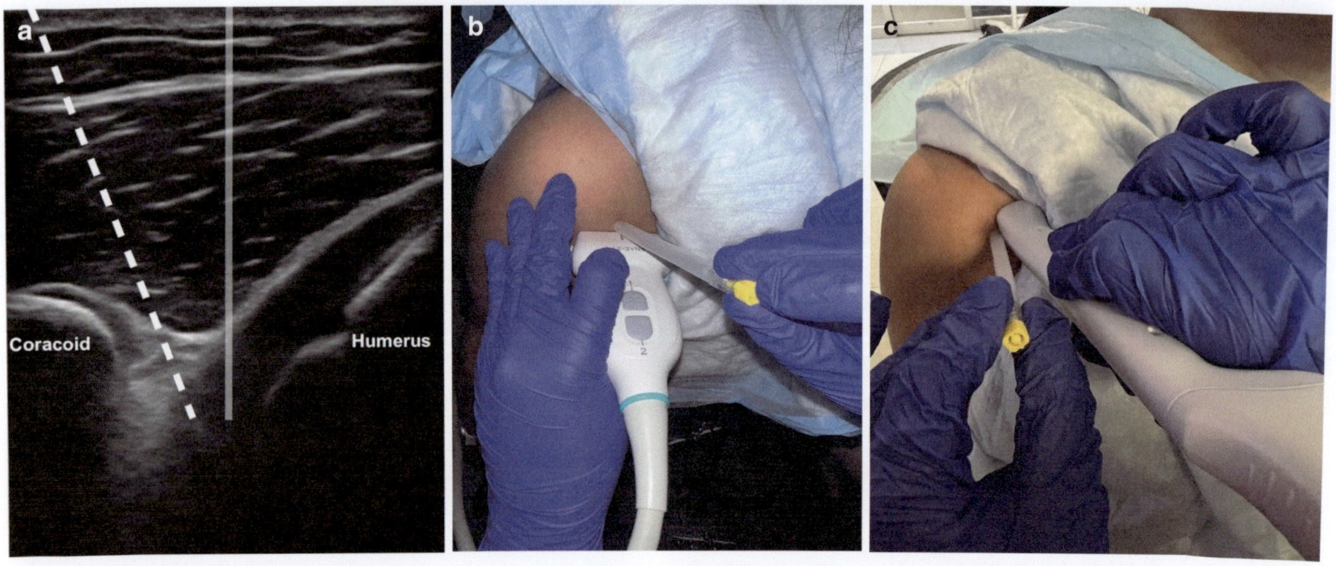

Fig. 19.8 Anterior approach to the glenohumeral joint. (**a**) Sonographic visualization of coracoid process, humeral head, and needle direction. The solid line depicts the out-of-place approach, and the dashed line demonstrates the in-plane approach. (**b**) Demonstration of probe placement and needle positioning for anterior aspiration using the out-of-plane approach with a linear probe. (**c**) Demonstration of probe placement and needle positioning for anterior aspiration using the in-plane approach with an endocavitary probe. (*Images courtesy of Michael Gottlieb, MD*)

section on shoulder dislocations. Often, a linear probe is used, though a hockey stick or endocavitary probe can also be considered, offering the benefits of enhanced image resolution with a smaller probe footprint [49]. Then, a needle is inserted in the center between the coracoid process and the humeral head (Fig. 19.8). This can be performed using either an in-plane or out-of-plane technique.

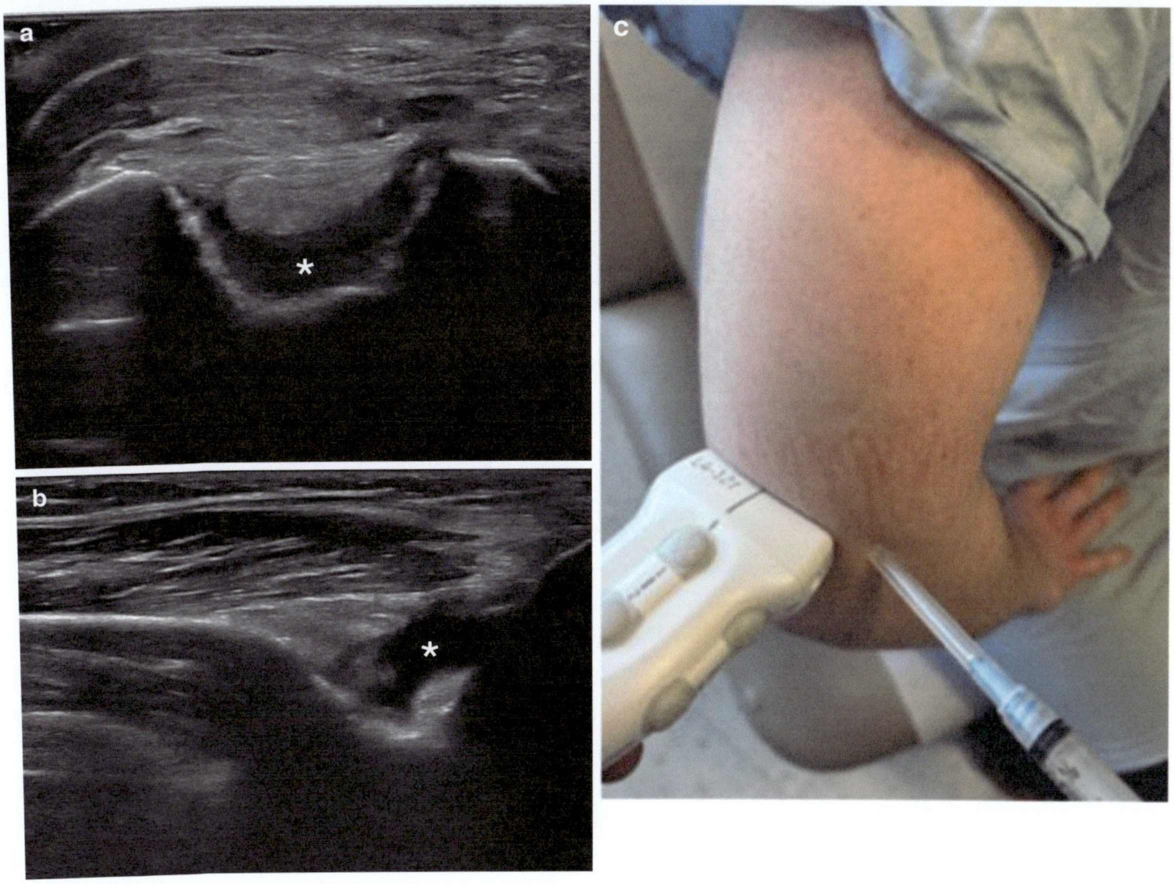

Fig. 19.9 Elbow joint effusion. (**a**) Elbow effusion (star) with fat pad elevation in the short axis. (**b**) Elbow effusion (star) with fat pad elevation in the long axis. (**c**) Demonstration of ultrasound probe placement for elbow aspiration. (*Images **a** and **b** courtesy of Michael Gottlieb, MD*)

Elbow Joint

In general, the diagnostic accuracy for aspirations/injections improves with ultrasound guidance; however, the evidence looking at accuracy for this particular joint is limited [50]. For elbow aspiration, begin by visualizing the distal humerus from the posterior side at the level of the olecranon fossa. An effusion will appear as an anechoic collection deep to the triceps tendon and fat pad (Fig. 19.9). Aspiration can be performed in-plane or out-of-plane but should be performed from the lateral side to avoid the ulnar nerve (Video 5). It is also important to ensure the trajectory is sufficiently lateral to avoid the triceps tendon.

Wrist

Ultrasound has demonstrated similar benefits over landmark-based wrist arthrocentesis [51]. The wrist is best visualized from the dorsal side, assessing for effusion surrounding the carpal bones. Similar to other effusions, this will appear as an anechoic fluid collection (Fig. 19.10). When performing fluid aspiration, start along the dorsal wrist and look for the extensor carpi radialis tendon. With the probe covering the extensor carpi radialis tendon, insert the needle from the ulnar side into the fluid pocket, being careful to avoid the tendon. This can be performed using either the in-plane or out-of-plane technique.

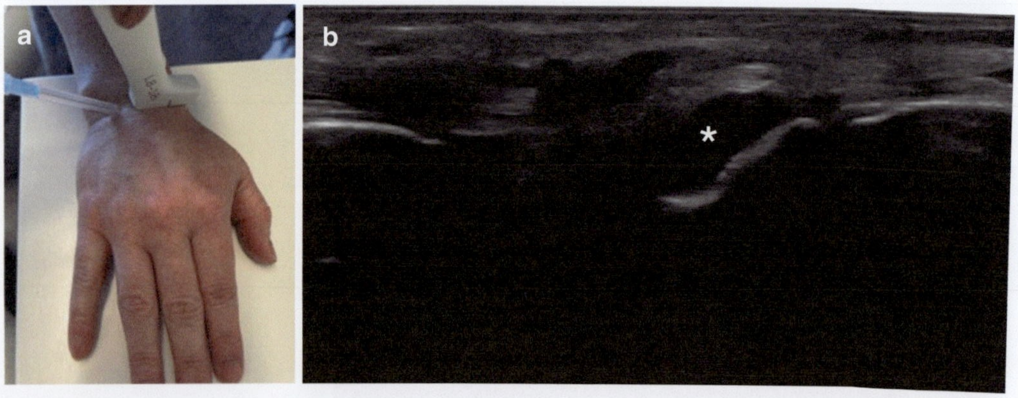

Fig. 19.10 Wrist effusion. (**a**) Demonstration of ultrasound probe placement for wrist aspiration using an in-plane technique. (**b**) Wrist effusion (star) visualized from the dorsal side. (*Image* ***b*** *courtesy of Michael Gottlieb, MD*)

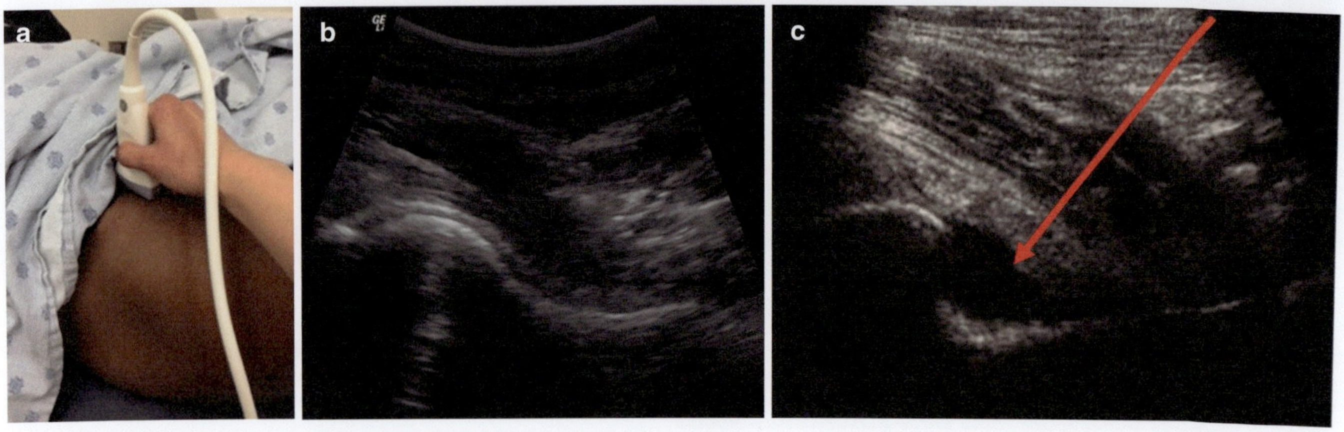

Fig. 19.11 Hip effusion. (**a**) Demonstration of ultrasound probe placement for hip assessment. (**b**) Longitudinal view of a normal hip joint showing the femoral head and neck. (**c**) Hip joint with effusion. Ared arrow denotes the projected path for in-plane needle placement if an aspiration is required. Note that it is important to identify the location of the lateral circumflex femoral artery with color Doppler when choosing the line of needle trajectory. (*Images courtesy of Levon Nazarian, MD*)

Hip Joint

Ultrasound-guided hip injections and aspirations are more accurate than the landmark technique, with a meta-analysis finding that ultrasound was 100% successful versus 72% with the landmark approach [52]. The hip joint extends anteriorly to create an outpouching anterior to the femoral neck, referred to as the anterior synovial recess. It is at this location where joint effusions are most commonly assessed and aspirated. To identify this space, begin by identifying the femoral head and neck in the inguinal fold. Then, rotate the probe so that the indicator points toward the umbilicus. The anterior synovial recess can be visualized as an anechoic, crescent-shaped structure abutting the femoral neck (Fig. 19.11). Typically, this is not well-visualized unless an effusion is present. In general, an effusion in this region is considered abnormal if it is >5 mm in diameter or >2 mm larger in diameter than the contralateral side [53]. To aspirate the effusion, a needle should be inserted using the in-plane technique from the inferior-to-superior direction. Color Doppler should be applied to identify and avoid the lateral circumflex femoral artery, which is also located in this region [54].

Knee Joint

There have been numerous studies citing improved accuracy and less pain when knee aspirations have been performed using ultrasound guidance [47, 55, 56]. For the knee ultrasound, begin in the long-axis plane on the anterior knee just superior to the patella. Using a linear or curvilinear probe, visualize the superior margin of the patella and femur in the same plane. The quadriceps tendon should be visible extending superiorly from the patella. Immediately deep to the quadriceps tendon is an oval or triangular-shaped suprapatellar fat pad, followed by the ovoid prefemoral fat pad and the femur. When an effusion is present, an anechoic pocket will appear between the suprapatellar fat pad and the prefemoral fat pad (Fig. 19.12). This should demonstrate a direct connection to the knee joint. Once this has been confirmed, rotate the probe 90 degrees to a short-axis view of the knee and revisualize the effusion, identifying the largest and most superficial fluid pocket. Insert the needle from a lateral or medial direction into the fluid pocket using an in-plane technique, ensuring that it is sufficiently far away from the quadriceps tendon located in the center.

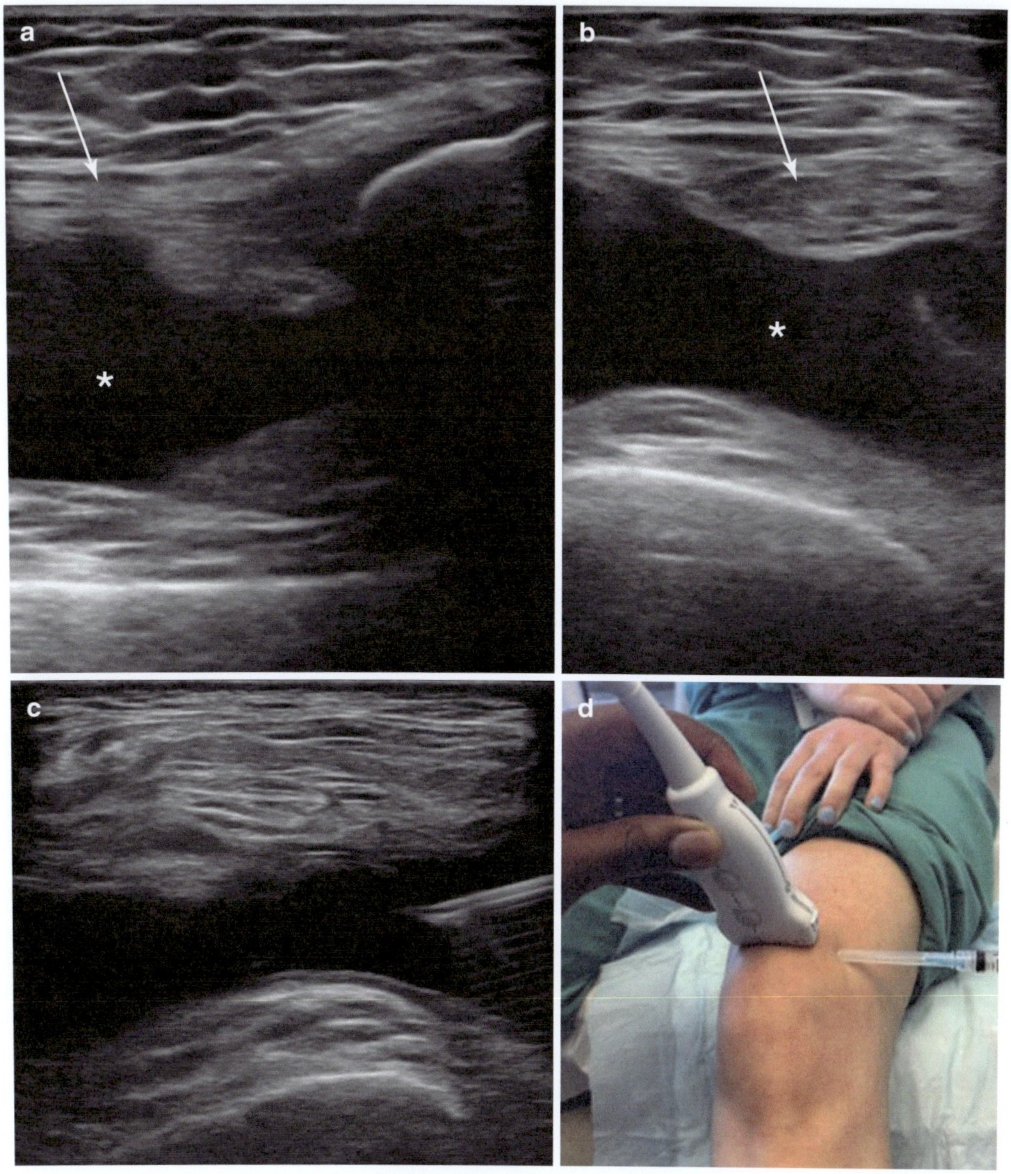

Fig. 19.12 Knee effusion. (**a**) Long-axis view demonstrating an effusion (star) and the quadriceps tendon (arrow). (**b**) Short-axis view demonstrating an effusion (star) and the quadriceps tendon (arrow). (**c**) Ultrasound-guided aspiration from the lateral side. (**d**) Probe and needle positioning for ultrasound-guided aspiration. (*Images a–c courtesy of Michael Gottlieb, MD*)

Assessment of knee pain should also include the popliteal space located posterior to the knee. Some patients can develop a focal, cystic outpouching, which can cause pain and swelling, referred to as a popliteal cyst or Baker's cyst (Fig. 19.13). Once identified, this can be treated conservatively or by ultrasound-guided aspiration in select cases.

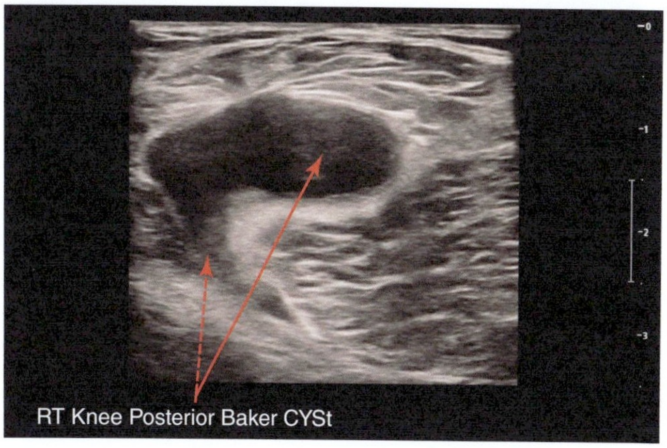

Fig. 19.13 Posterior view of the popliteal fossa of the knee showing a large Baker's cyst. The solid red arrow points to the Baker's cyst located between the medial head of gastrocnemius and the semimembranosus muscles, while the dashed red arrow highlights the pedunculated "cyst" extending posteriorly out from the synovial joint

Ankle Joint

The ankle is best visualized from the dorsal aspect in the tibio-talar articulation. To assess the ankle, begin by identifying the key landmarks, consisting of the tibialis anterior and extensor hallucis longus tendons located on the distal anterior tibia. Place the probe medial to these tendons and follow the anterior tibia inferiorly until the dome of the talus is visualized. Fluid will appear within this space with a serpiginous and triangular shape (Fig. 19.14). Once identified,

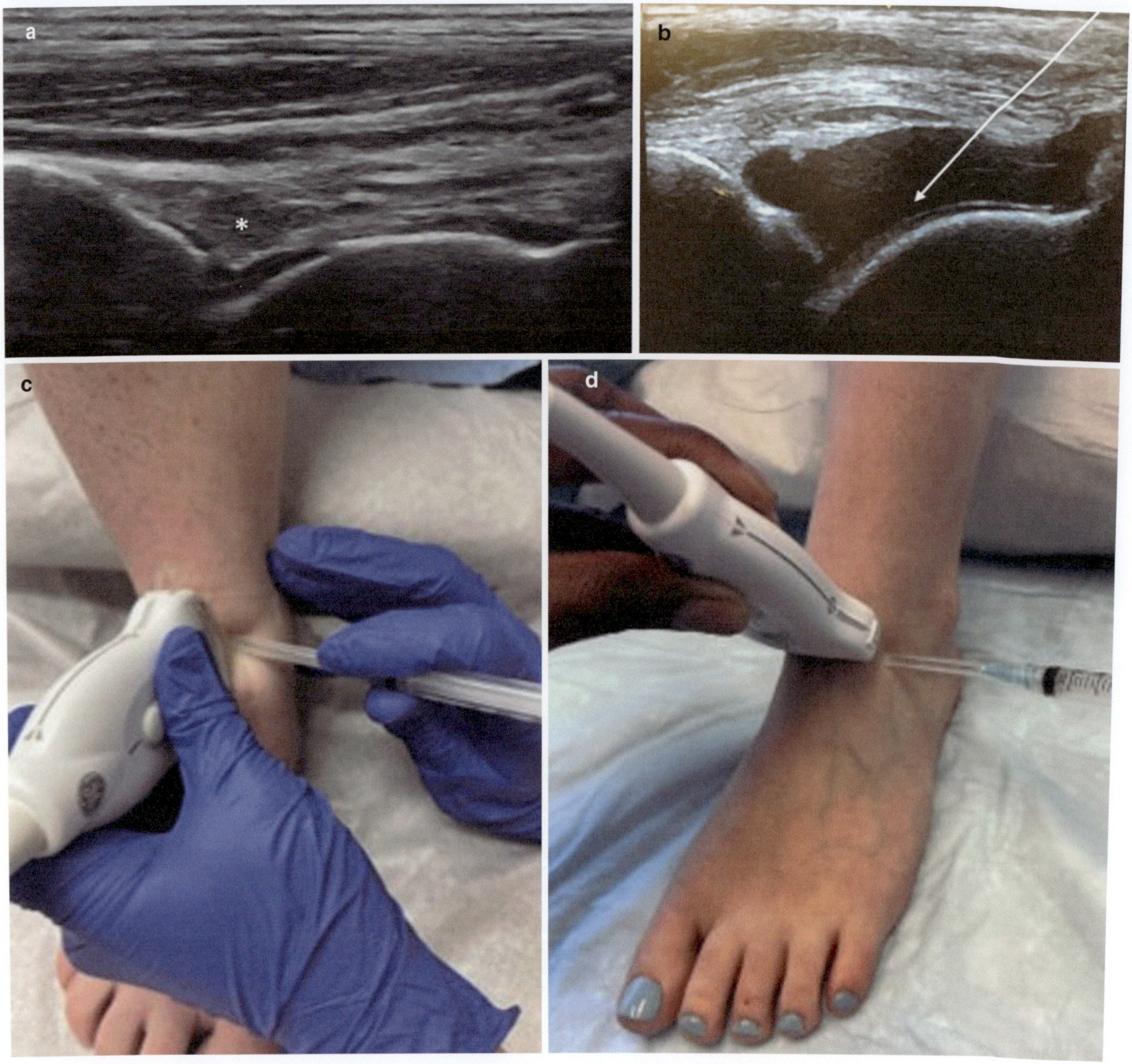

Fig. 19.14 Ankle effusion. (**a**) Longitudinal view of a normal tibiotalar joint (*) without effusion. (**b**) Tibiotalar joint with moderate effusion (arrow) and hyperechoic layering overlying the cartilage, possibly consistent with crystalline arthritis. (**c**) Probe and needle positioning for the out-of-plane technique. Note the medial position of the needle. (**d**) Probe and needle positioning for the in-plane technique. Note the lateral position of the needle

this can be aspirated using an out-of-plane technique from the medial side or an in-plane technique from the lateral side.

Bursitis

Ultrasound may be useful to diagnose inflammation of the bursa known as bursitis. The differential for bursitis is broad and depends on location but is most commonly due to repetitive or overuse injury. However, bursitis may be associated with crystalline arthritis, inflammatory arthritis, and infection. Common sites prone to the development of bursitis, which are especially amenable to ultrasound evaluation (and intra-articular steroid injection), include the subacromial bursa, the trochanteric bursa, and the olecranon bursa [57, 58].

The Outcome Measures in Rheumatology (OMERACT) Ultrasound Working Group, an international group of ultrasound researchers and clinicians, has been defining and validating ultrasonography as an outcome measurement instrument for use in clinical trials and practice. Online pic-

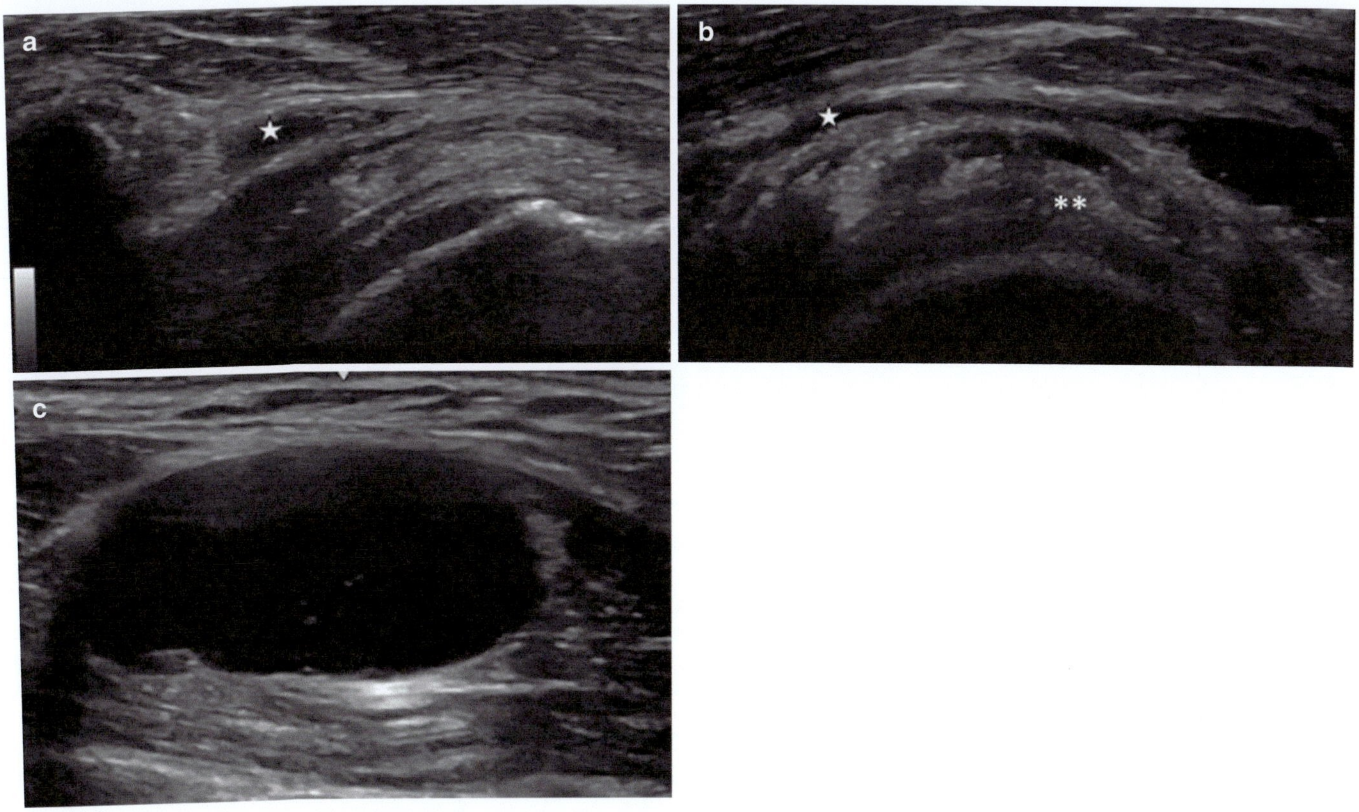

Fig. 19.15 (**a**) Subacromial bursal effusion with thickening of the bursal wall, consistent with chronic bursitis, accompanied by a small amount of tracking communication (*) to the biceps tendon sheath in transverse view. (**b**) Longitudinal view of a subacromial bursa (*) and tendinopathy with small areas of calcification and partial tears along the subscapularis tendon (**). (**c**) The subacromial bursa at its maximum size anterior and inferior to the deltoid. *(Images courtesy of Marta Bean, MD)*

torial atlases and definitions from OMERACT are easily searched online [59]. OMERACT defines bursitis as the presence of a small-to-large, anechoic, or hypoechoic collection within a bursal space that is compressible. Chronic bursitis is often associated with a thickening of the bursal wall and may have increased Doppler signal if actively inflamed. Depending on chronicity, the bursa may also contain heterogeneous and hypoechoic or hyperechoic material, especially if associated with crystalline disease.

Ultrasound findings of subacromial bursitis include fluid inferior to the deltoid muscle and superior to the supraspinatus muscle tendon (Fig. 19.15) [60]. Subacromial bursitis can be communicating or noncommunicating with the glenohumeral joint, where the former is associated with a rotator cuff tear [60]. Ultrasound-guided corticosteroid injections, compared with blind injections to the subacromial space, are associated with significantly greater improvements in shoulder function and pain [61]. Direct needle visualization via a lateral approach is typically recommended.

Ultrasound findings for trochanteric bursitis include an anechoic or hypoechoic fluid collection along the lateral aspect of the greater trochanter and inferior to the gluteus maximus [58]. While it was previously thought that pain in this vicinity was synonymous with true bursitis, it is now known that lateral hip pain is more commonly due to gluteal tendinopathy. True bursitis (presence of fluid collection with bursal wall thickening) is much less common.

Olecranon bursitis is very common. While frequently due to trauma, inflammatory causes such as crystalline arthritis may also occur. Despite the easily palpated location superficial to the olecranon process, ultrasound evaluation may be highly valuable if a gouty tophus can be visualized to aid in diagnosis [62].

Dislocations

Ultrasound can be used to diagnose and manage a variety of dislocations. While some instances of ultrasound evaluation of dislocation have been more proof-of-concept, others have become a core component of the management pathway. In this section, we will focus on three key areas: acromioclavicular (AC) joint separation, glenohumeral joint dislocation, and radial head subluxation.

AC Joint Stability and Separation

Evaluation for AC joint separation should be performed with a linear probe placed along the joint line in a longitudinal position (Figs. 19.16 and 19.17). The joint capsule can be

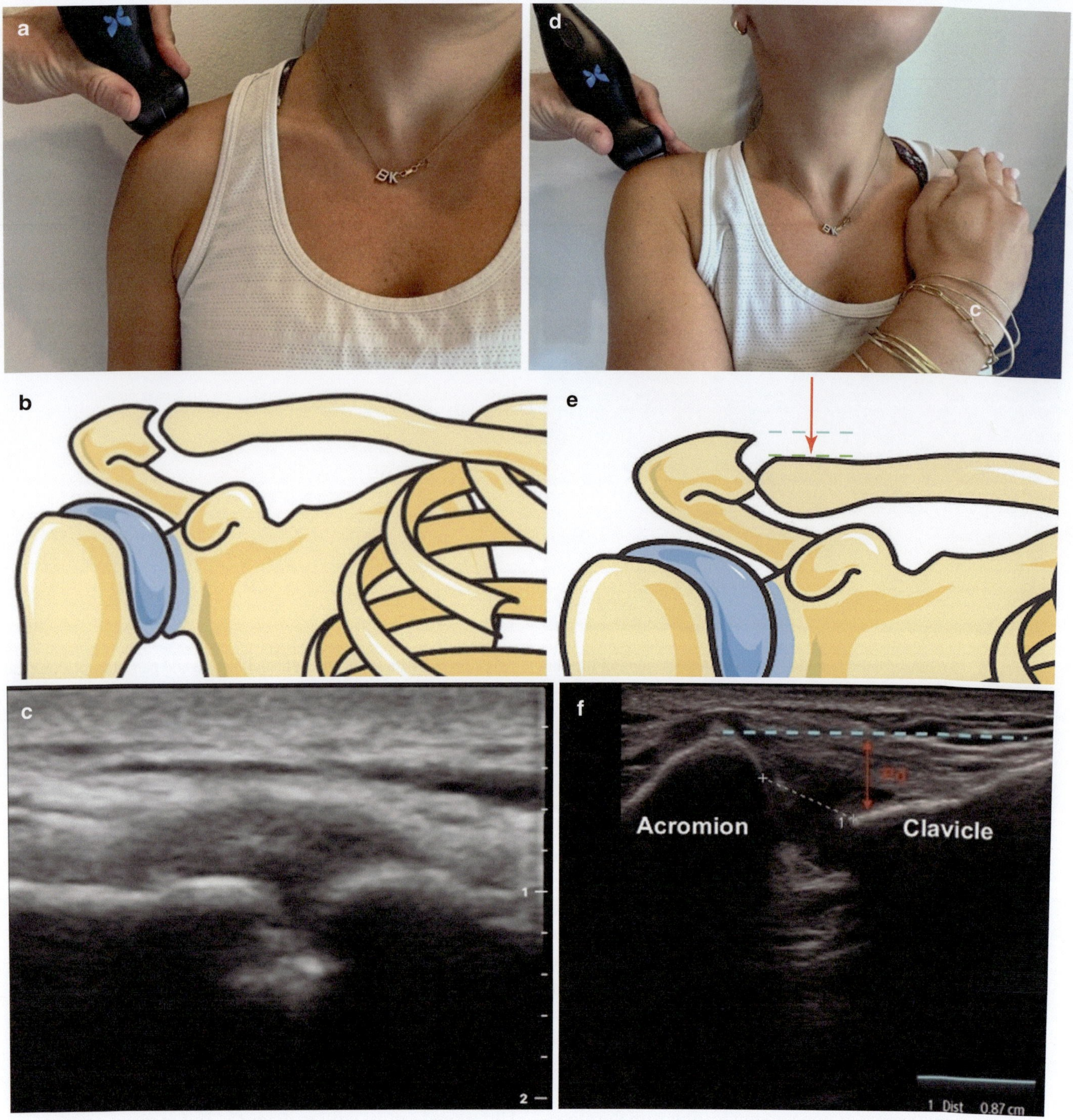

Fig. 19.16 Assessment of the acromioclavicular (AC) joint. (**a**) Initial placement of the probe for assessing the AC joint. (**b**) Normal anatomic position of the AC joint. (**c**) Normal sonographic position of the AC joint. (**d**) Dynamic assessment of the AC joint for stability. (**e**) Anatomic position of an AC joint separation. (**f**) Sonographic depiction of AC joint separation. The distance displayed by the solid red arrow represents the posterior horizontal displacement (Pd) of the clavicle in relation to the acromion when the patient is positioned as in Image (**d**). The dashed white caliper measures the lateral separation of the AC joint

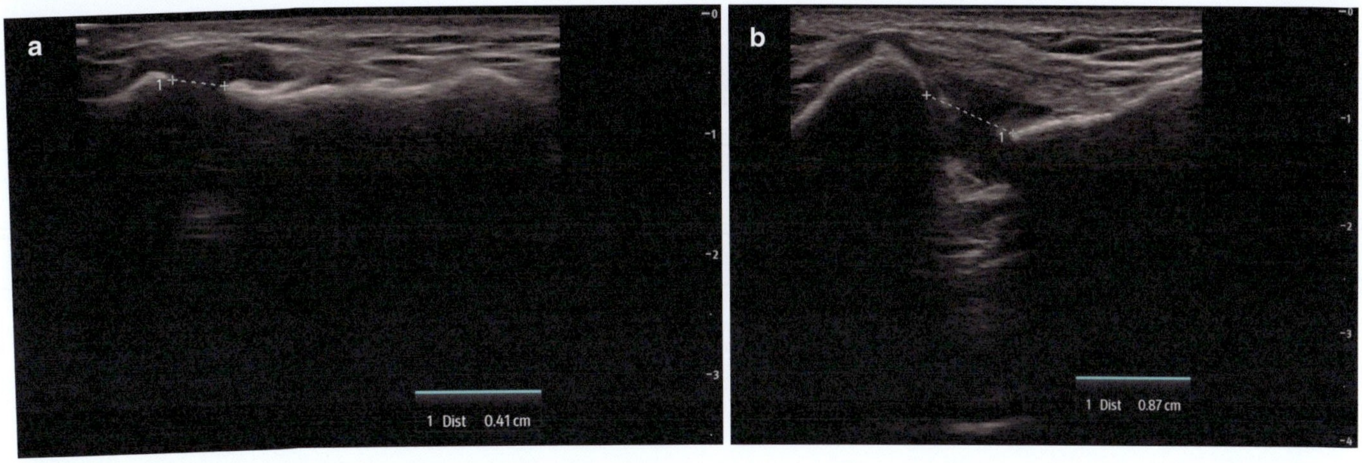

Fig. 19.17 Ultrasound images demonstrating the importance of comparing the affected side with the unaffected side when assessing for acromioclavicular (AC) joint separation. (**a**) Normal appearance of the AC joint on the unaffected side. (**b**) AC joint separation demonstrated on the affected side. (*Images courtesy of Michael Gottlieb, MD*)

evaluated and compared against the opposite shoulder. Dynamic tests can be performed by inducing traction by pulling the arm downward to enhance the separation seen on ultrasound [63]. An alternate method of dynamic evaluation of the AC joint can be performed by having the patient place the hand of the involved extremity on the opposite shoulder while assessing the AC joint from the superior position. This method evaluates the horizontal instability of the AC joint. If the clavicle moves away from the probe posteriorly, it is considered a positive finding, and the distance can be measured [64].

Glenohumeral Joint Dislocation

Approaches to evaluating for glenohumeral joint dislocations include the anterior, lateral, and posterior views, with the posterior glenohumeral view being the most commonly utilized view, with 100% sensitivity and 100% specificity [65]. The posterior glenohumeral view has demonstrated easy clinical adoption and reproducibility across multiple education levels for the diagnosis of anterior and posterior shoulder dislocations [66, 67]. To perform this view, a curvilinear or linear probe is placed along the spine of the scapula and then slid laterally until the glenoid is seen in approximation to the humeral head [68]. An alternate approach to localizing the posterior glenohumeral view is to simply trace up the posterior humerus until the glenohumeral joint comes into view [69]. In the posterior glenohumeral view, the primary anatomic landmarks are the glenoid and its position relative to the humeral head (Fig. 19.18). In this view, if the humeral head is noted to be closer to the ultrasound probe (i.e., posterior to the glenoid), it can be interpreted as a posterior dislocation. In contrast, an anterior shoulder dislocation would have the humeral head in an anterior or inferior position and further away from the transducer on the image.

An alternate approach to assessing the glenohumeral joint is the combined anterior plus lateral technique. This offers the advantage that it can be performed when the patient is in the supine position and cannot sit up to facilitate a posterior view. The anterior aspect is based on the normal horizontal proximity of the humeral head and the coracoid process. In a glenohumeral dislocation, the humeral head will appear deep to the coracoid with the anterior view, regardless of whether it is an anterior dislocation (inferiorly displaced) or a posterior dislocation (posteriorly displaced) [70] (Fig. 19.19). The lateral view utilizes the humeral head and its proximity to the acromion to determine dislocation, with a wider distance suggesting dislocation [70] (Fig. 19.20). The lateral view can be compared with the contralateral side to determine whether the degree of widening is normal for that patient.

In the case of anterior shoulder dislocations, the humeral head may also be evaluated for Hill–Sachs lesions secondary to impaction of the humeral head on the glenoid when dislocated. On ultrasound, this will appear as a sharply angulated impaction of the normally smooth humeral head (Fig. 19.21). The absence of a tendon-like structure, as well as the sharp and collapsed appearance of the cortex, will help differentiate Hill–Sachs lesions from a normal proximal bicipital groove.

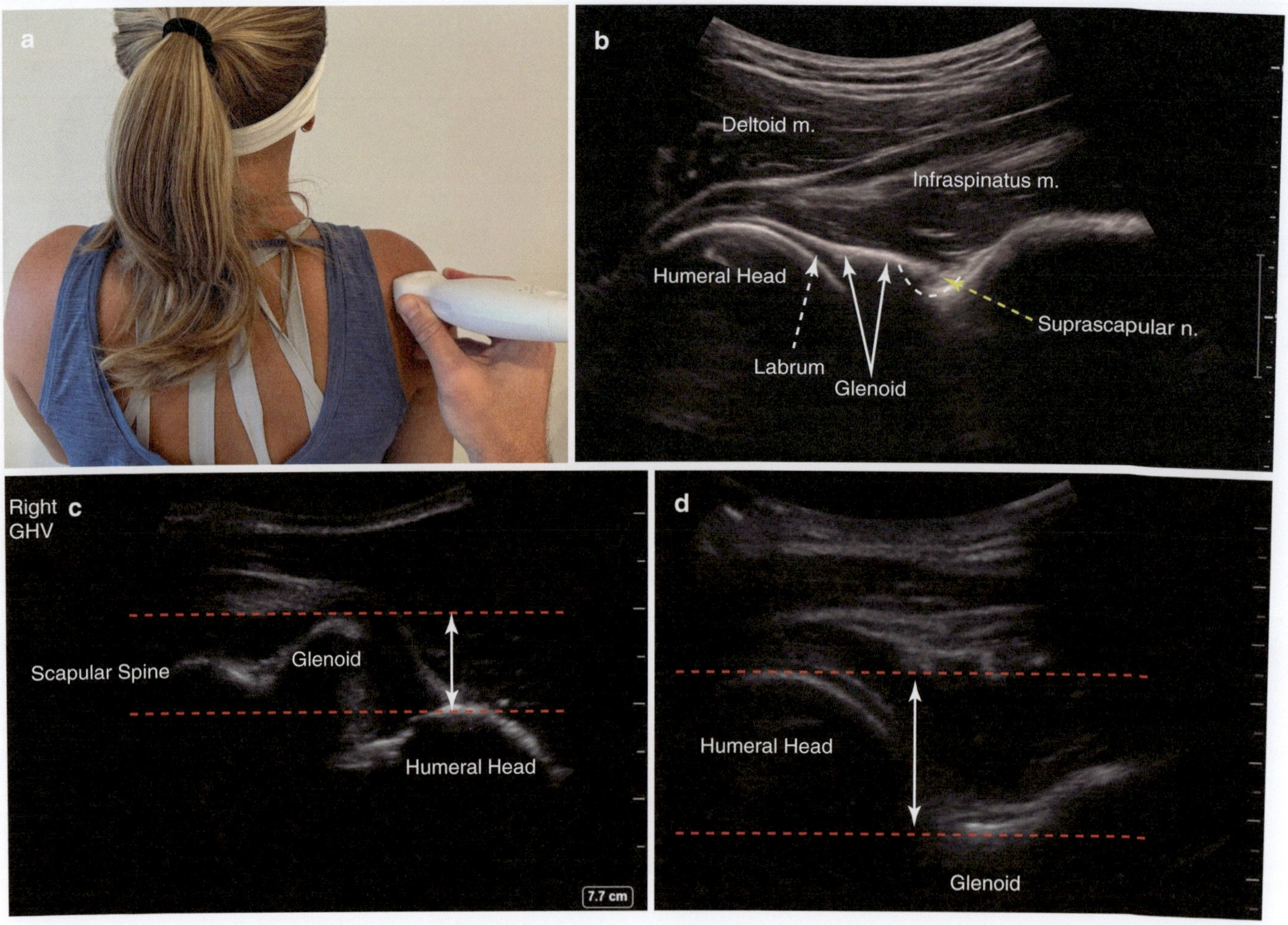

Fig. 19.18 Ultrasound imaging of posterior glenohumeral view. (**a**) Demonstration of ultrasound probe placement along the scapular spine and overlying the glenohumeral joint. (**b**) Normal sonoanatomy of the posterior glenohumeral view. The scapular notch containing the suprascapular nerve is depicted by the blue dashed line. (**c**) An anterior shoulder dislocation imaged via the posterior glenohumeral view. The humeral head is displaced away from the ultrasound probe in relation to the glenoid. (**d**) A posterior dislocation as imaged from the posterior glenohumeral view. The humeral head is displaced toward the ultrasound probe in relation to the glenoid

Radial Head Subluxation

For pediatric patients, ultrasound can be uniquely useful for the assessment of suspected radial head subluxation. In a pulled arm injury causing radial head subluxation, the annular ligament and a portion of the supinator muscle become lodged between the radial head and the capitellum. This positioning can be interpreted on ultrasound evaluation as an increased distance of the radial head and capitellum interval or even a clear lodging of the annular ligament within this space, resulting in the "hook sign" [71, 72] (Fig. 19.22). For comparison, when assessing a normal radial head with a high-resolution linear probe, the annular ligament can often be seen coursing across the radial head. Although the diagnosis is typically clinical, POCUS has demonstrated utility in cases with atypical presentation [73]. If the annular ligament is clearly seen within the radial-humeral joint space and there is clinical improvement after reduction, splinting is likely unnecessary even if an elevated posterior fat pad is noted [74].

Developmental Hip Dysplasia

POCUS has a valuable role in pediatrics for the evaluation of developmental hip dysplasia [75]. While a comprehensive ultrasound evaluation of the pediatric hip at 4–6 weeks of age remains a primary diagnostic modality when there are predisposing factors or high clinical suspicion, POCUS is

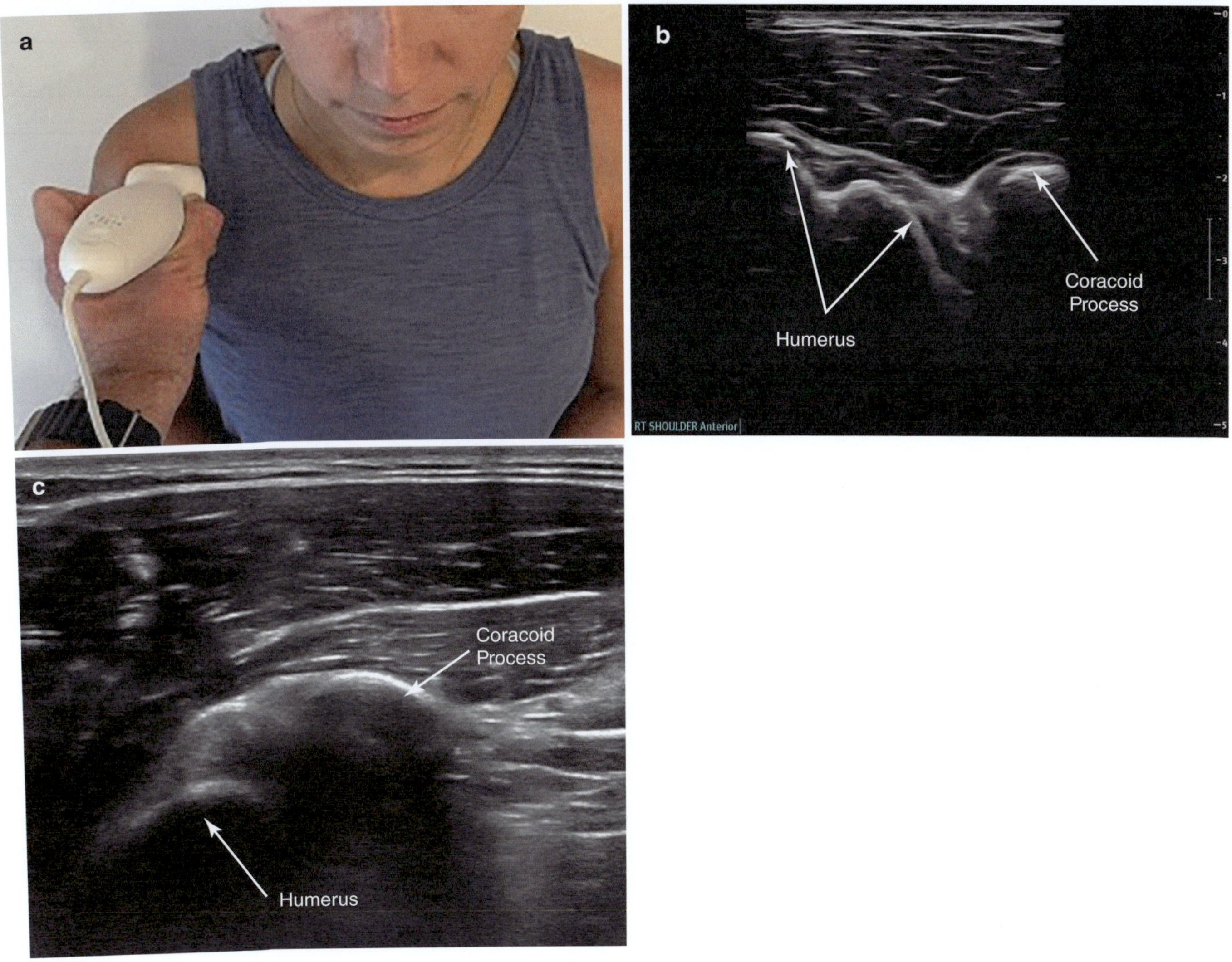

Fig. 19.19 Anterior assessment of the glenohumeral joint for dislocation. (**a**) Proper ultrasound placement for anterior evaluation. (**b**) Normal alignment of the glenohumeral joint. (**c**) Anterior shoulder dislocation with displacement of the humerus in relation to the coracoid process. (*Figure* **c** *courtesy of Michael Gottlieb, MD)*

uniquely positioned to be useful in rural or resource-limited settings [76, 77]. In evaluating for hip dysplasia, care should be taken to determine the acetabular coverage of the femoral head while in this lateral view [78]. While there is debate as to which patients are best suited for POCUS, the occult nature of hip dysplasia suggests a role for primary screening with sonography in any patient with clinical suspicion. There are inherent difficulties with broad screening programs, particularly with variations of scanning technique, the need for dynamic studies, and the timing of evaluation [79]; however, multiple studies have demonstrated that POCUS screening programs for hip dysplasia can be successfully implemented [77, 78, 80]. Recent studies have also included artificial intelligence for POCUS to screen for hip dysplasia with similar diagnostic detection rates using a simple sweep method [81, 82]. The benefit of early identification and treatment of developmental hip dysplasia and the growing prevalence of POCUS present hip dysplasia as a diagnosis that likely warrants further research [83].

When evaluating for developmental hip dysplasia, the clinician should obtain a transverse and coronal view of the hip. In the transverse view when doing the Barlow maneuver, > 5 mm translation of the femoral head is considered positive. In the coronal view of the hip, a line will be drawn along the border of the ilium through the femoral head. Another line will be drawn along the bony acetabular roof. The angle

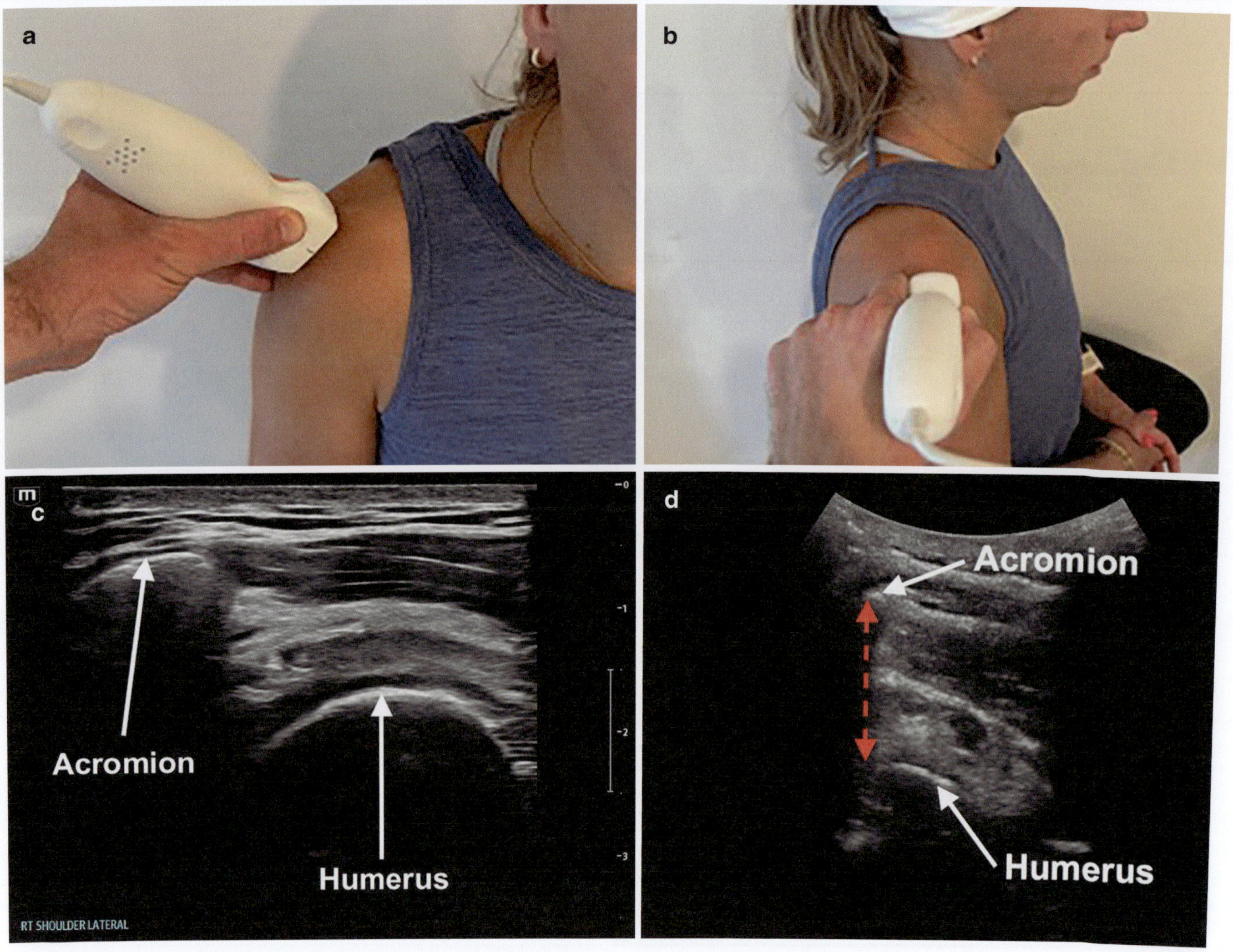

Fig. 19.20 Lateral assessment of the glenohumeral joint for dislocation. (**a**) Proper ultrasound probe placement for lateral evaluation. (**b**) Proper probe position re-demonstrated from the lateral plane. (**c**) Normal alignment of the glenohumeral joint. (**d**) An anterior shoulder dislocation with displacement of the humerus in relation to the acromion as depicted by the red dashed arrow. Note that a curvilinear probe is used in Fig. **d** due to the wider distance than in Fig. **c**. (*Figure d courtesy of Michael Gottlieb, MD)*

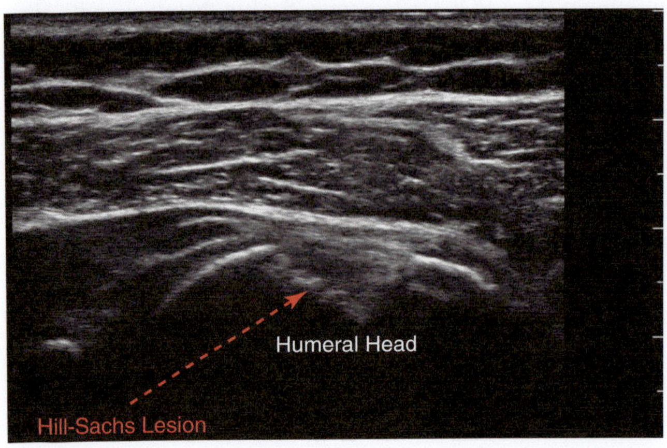

Fig. 19.21 Posterior glenohumeral view of the humeral head after reduction of anterior shoulder dislocation. A Hill–Sachs lesion is shown on the superficial surface of the humeral head as highlighted by the red dashed arrow

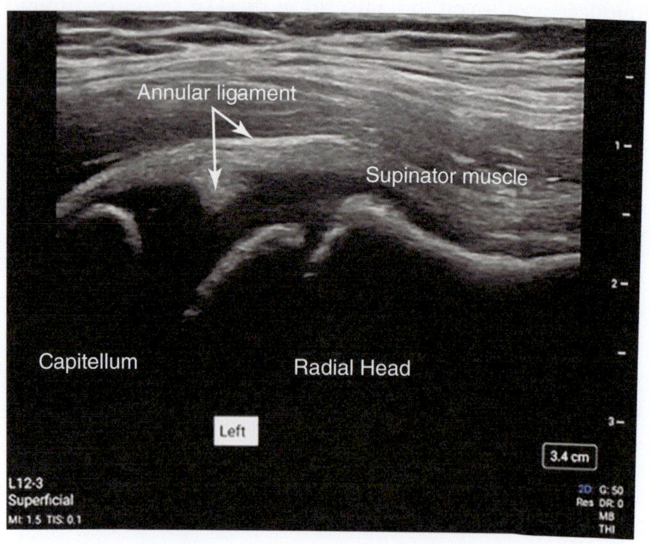

Fig. 19.22 Ultrasound imaging of radial head subluxation with "hook" sign caused by the supinator muscle being pulled into joint space by a displaced annular ligament. (*Image courtesy of Paul Khalil, MD)*

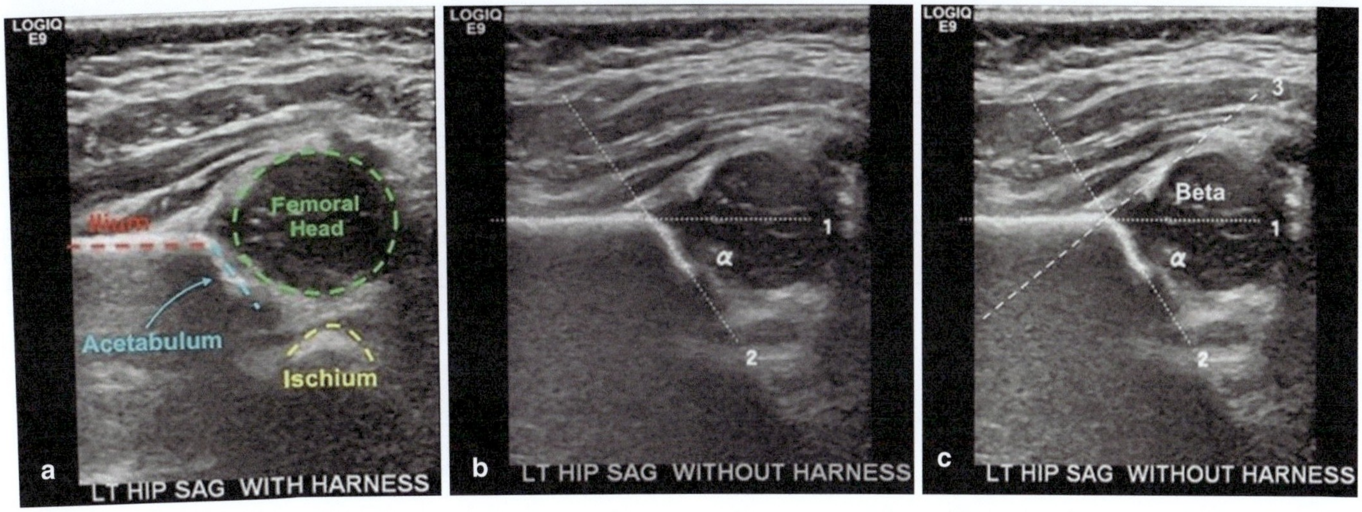

Fig. 19.23 Evaluation for developmental hip dysplasia with the lateral coronal view of the hip. (**a**) Key anatomic landmarks. (**b**) Analysis of the alpha angle (angle between the ilium and acetabular roof). (**c**) Analysis of the beta angle (angle between the ilium and labrum). (*Images courtesy of Dan Puebla, MD*)

between these two lines is referred to as the alpha angle and represents the acetabular roof angle (Fig. 19.23). This assessment is based on the Graf analysis, but a normal alpha angle is >60 degrees. Another measure that has been used, but has greater variability, is the beta angle. To measure the beta angle, the same line from the border of the ilium is used as described above. Then, a second line is drawn from the turning point to the center of the echogenic labrum. The angle between the two lines is the beta angle. The alpha angle is the primary diagnostic measure, whereas the beta angle is used for differentiated stages of developmental hip dysplasia.

Growth Plate Assessment

Assessment of pediatric fractures requires a basic understanding of growth plate locations and estimations of primary and secondary ossification centers. The natural position of a growth plate may be easily mistaken for a cortical break. A potential application for musculoskeletal ultrasound is for evaluating fractures along growth plates. Missed injuries involving the physis can potentially affect long-term growth and function. In contrast, using ultrasound to localize the growth plate and compare it to the area of pain or trauma may be able to help avoid unnecessary immobilization if not indicated [84].

One promising application of POCUS is using the fracture distance from the physis to identify significant injuries or extensions into the growth plate in the Salter-Harris II injuries. A retrospective analysis of prospectively evaluated pediatric forearm fracture assessments demonstrated that all Salter-Harris II fractures with cortical breach occurred within 1 cm of the physis [85]. While this is still an emerging application, it does demonstrate the potential utility of ultrasound evaluation to stratify patients with suspected injury to the growth plate with a cortical break.

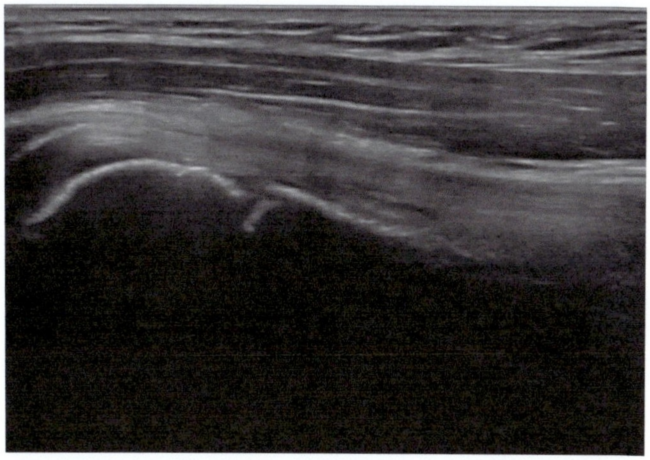

Fig. 19.24 Growth plate in a pediatric patient. (*Image courtesy of Michael Gottlieb, MD*)

Several techniques can be used to evaluate and compare a suspected fracture versus a growth plate. These include measuring the distance of a cortical break from the physis, evaluating for a surrounding hematoma or periosteal reaction along the growth plate, and comparing the physeal widening or narrowing when compared to normal ranges or the contralateral joint. When unclear, it can also be valuable to compare the growth plate with that of the contralateral extremity. One key differentiator between fractures and growth plates is that, with a suspected fracture, the cortex is often jagged and misaligned, whereas the normal growth plate has a smooth, rounded edge with alignment between both sides (Fig. 19.24).

Tendon and Ligament Injuries

Tendon and ligamentous injuries are particularly well-suited for sonographic evaluation. The appearance of acute injury to these structures will vary depending on the severity. Complete tears will have complete disruption of the organized fibular structure and architecture of the tendon with hypoechoic edema (Fig. 19.25). Acute partial tears can be more subtle and present as hypoechoic edema within the tendon or ligament, a disruption of normal architecture, or hyperemia on Doppler (Fig. 19.26). Chronic tears of ligaments may exhibit other characteristics such as calcifications, which will display as punctate hyperechoic lesions with possible acoustic shadowing within the tendon or ligament. Even if a discrete tear is not visualized, the presence of these punctate lesions and surrounding inflammation with associated pain can support a diagnosis of calcific tendinitis [86, 87].

Normally, ligaments and tendons will exhibit anisotropy due to their fibrillar structure. This artifact becomes more pronounced if the tendon is diving away from the probe, leading to a more parallel orientation to the structure. To minimize anisotropy, the ultrasound probe must be fully fanned through the area of interest, and the image must be interrogated to ensure that a suspected partial tear is not simply an artifact caused by anisotropy. In the case of anisotropy, the hypoechoic area will correct as the angle of insonation to the tendon is improved.

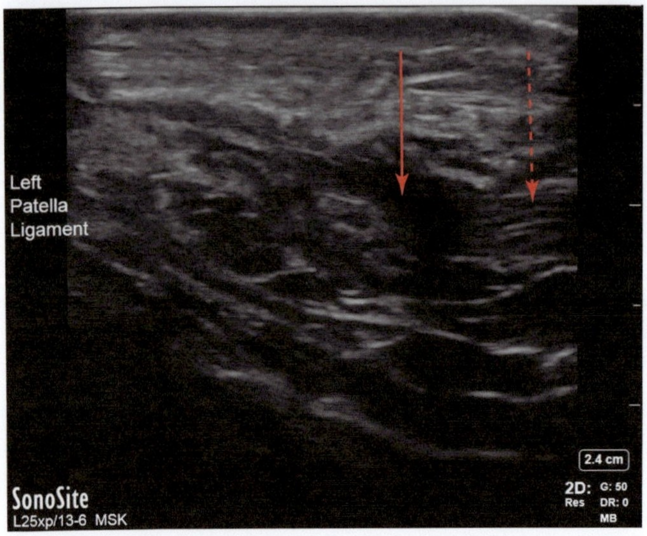

Fig. 19.25 Patellar ligament rupture. The patellar ligament is denoted by a dashed red arrow. The interrupted ligamentous architecture at the site of rupture is indicated by the solid red arrow

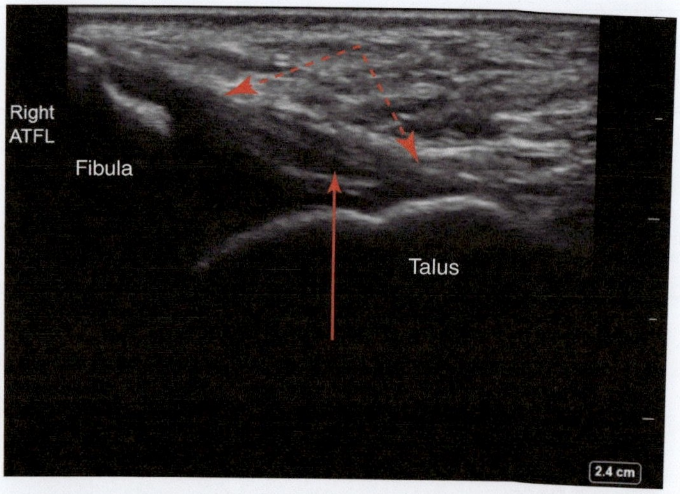

Fig. 19.26 Partial tear of the anterior talofibular ligament. The partial tear is indicated by a solid red arrow. The dashed arrows show a partially torn but intact anterior talofibular ligament

Hypoechoic edema, tendon thickening, calcifications, and bony erosion denoting inflammation may also be seen at the site of tendon insertion and are suggestive of the diagnosis of enthesitis [88]. The use of color or power Doppler can further enhance the detection of inflammation [89]. Similarly, chronic tendinopathy may be noted on ultrasound by a focal thickening of the tendon as well as possible hypervascularity on Doppler evaluation. Careful dynamic studies of suspected ligamentous injuries can be useful in assisting diagnosis by exaggerating the injury or eliciting the improper movement of the structure [90]. Dynamic ultrasound maneuvers refer to any evaluation that includes passive or active range of motion of the affected structure or external compressive pressure applied from the ultrasound probe. Dynamic maneuvers can be useful in diagnosing a variety of injuries, including subacromial shoulder impingement syndrome, snapping hip, tendon subluxations, and differentiating between partial and full-thickness tears [90]. Figures 19.27, 19.28, 19.29, and 19.30 describe focused examination techniques for tendon and ligament injuries.

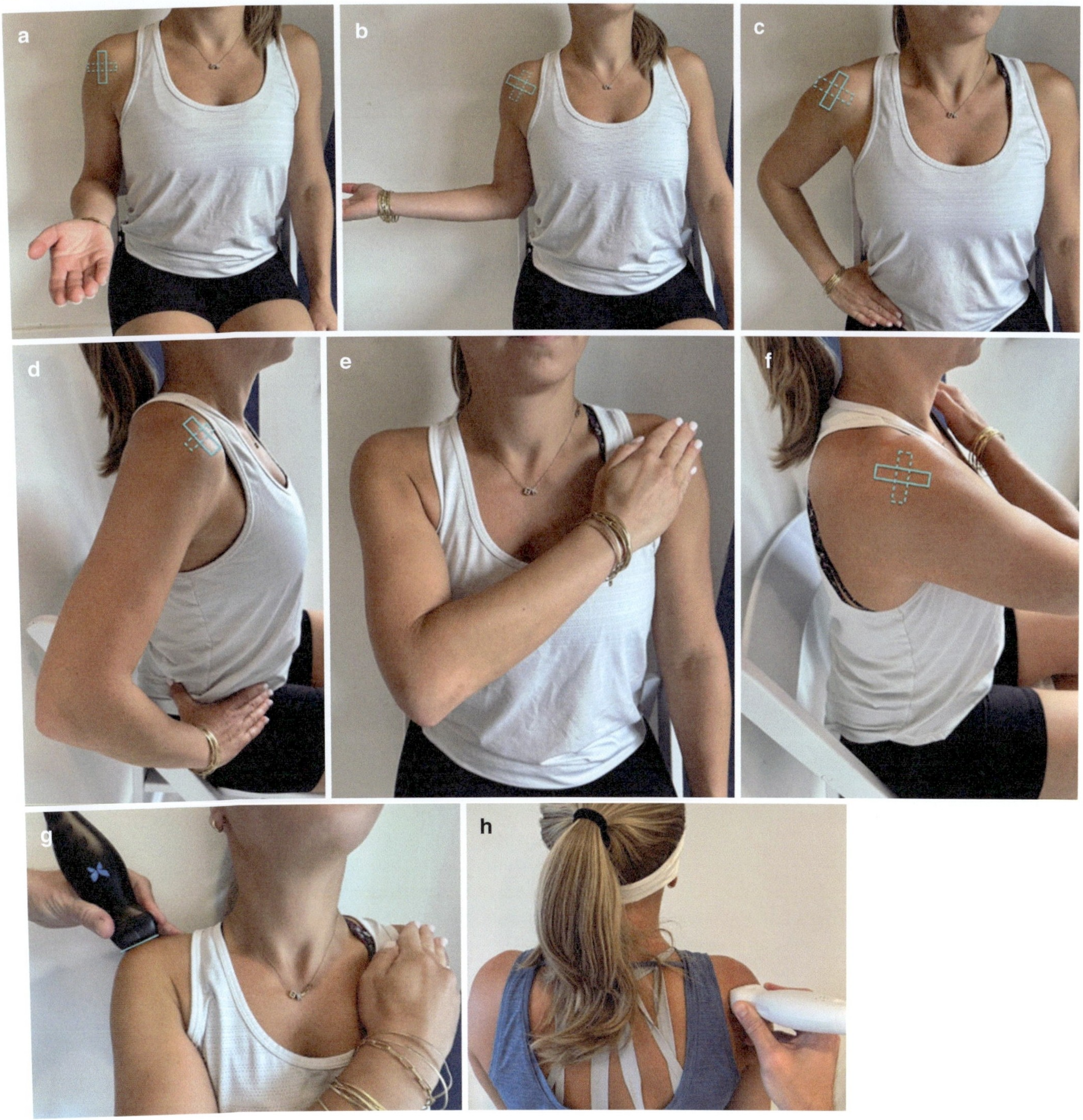

Fig. 19.27 Ultrasound probe positioning and a basic scanning protocol for a shoulder and rotator cuff evaluation. Evaluated tendons include the biceps tendon, subscapularis, supraspinatus, infraspinatus, acromioclavicular (AC) joint, and glenohumeral joint. All tendons should be imaged in the long axis (solid box) and short axis (dashed box). (**a**) Positioning for evaluating the biceps tendon. (**b**) Placement of the arm in external rotation for evaluation of the subscapularis. (**c**) Evaluation of the supraspinatus via the modified Crass position (visualized from the anterior direction). (**d**) Evaluation of the supraspinatus via the modified Crass position (visualized from the lateral direction). (**e**) Evaluation of the infraspinatus (visualized from the anterior direction). (**f**) Evaluation of the infraspinatus (visualized from the lateral direction). (**g**) Assessment of the AC joint. (**h**) Assessment of the glenohumeral joint using the posterior glenohumeral view

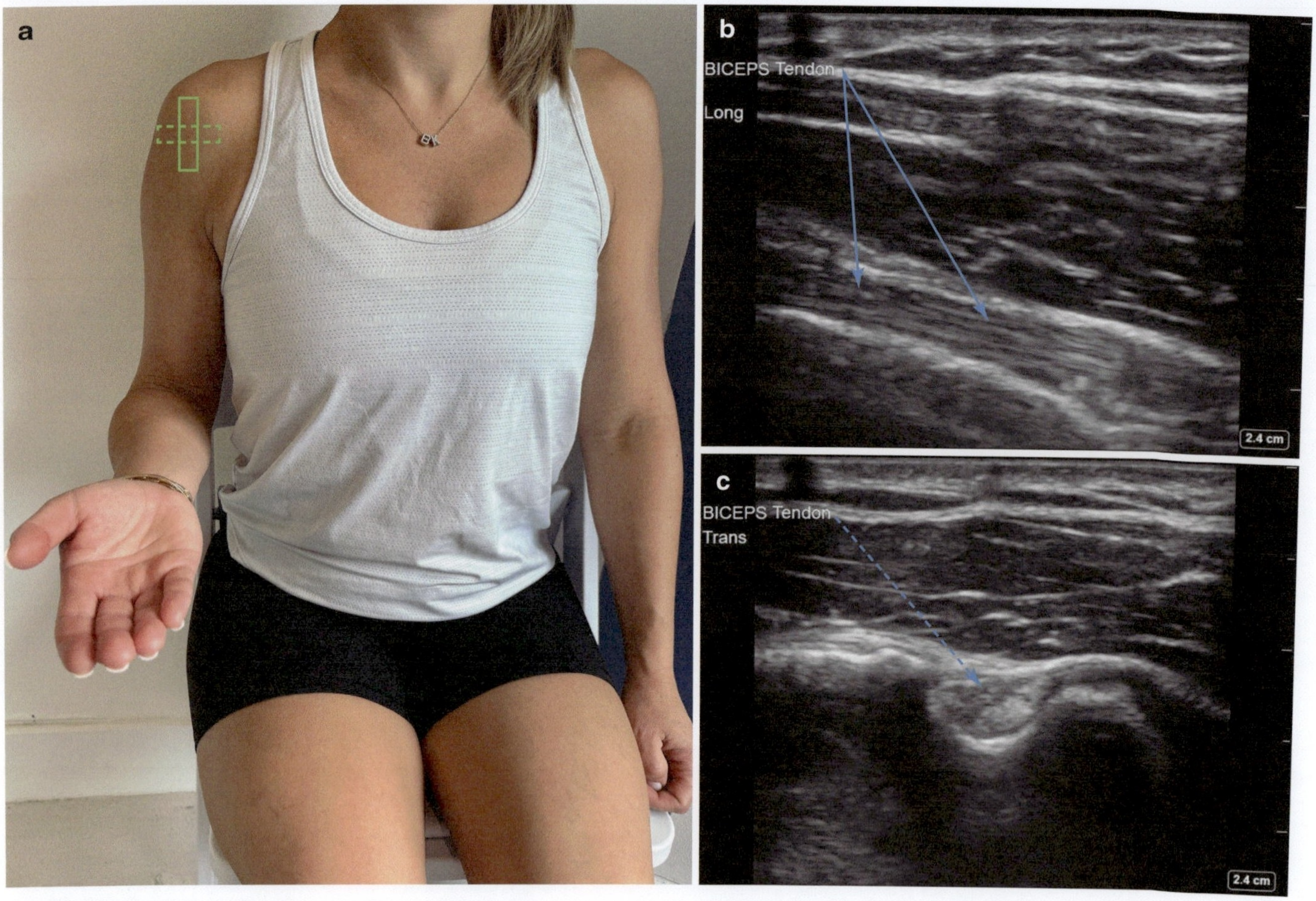

Fig. 19.28 Focused evaluation of the biceps tendon. (**a**) Probe positioning. (**b**) Long-axis view of the biceps tendon. (**c**) Short-axis view of the biceps tendon

Tenosynovitis

Tenosynovitis is inflammation of the synovial membrane that lines a tendon [91]. There are several different etiologies of tenosynovitis, including but not limited to mechanical injury, infection, crystalline arthritis (e.g., gout, pseudogout), inflammatory arthritis (e.g., rheumatoid arthritis, psoriatic arthritis, spondyloarthritis), and diabetes.

Tenosynovitis is defined by OMERACT as an "abnormal anechoic or hypoechoic (relative to tendon fibers) tendon sheath widening, which can be related both to the presence of tenosynovial abnormal fluid or hypertrophy." [92] If Doppler is performed, it should be seen in two perpendicular planes (long axis and short axis) and within the tendon sheath, thereby excluding normal vasculature. Similarly, a tendon sheath effusion is defined as a displaceable collection surrounding the tendon seen in two perpendicular planes [93]. Other supportive features include peritendinous and subcutaneous edema (Fig. 19.31).

Sonographic features of tenosynovitis may vary depending on the underlying etiology. OMERACT provided a semi-quantitative scoring rubric to grade tenosynovitis using B-mode (0–4; normal–severe) and color Doppler (0–4; normal–severe) [94]. The scoring system has been extensively used in rheumatoid arthritis, while similar algorithms have been used in other inflammatory arthritides such as psoriatic arthritis [95, 96].

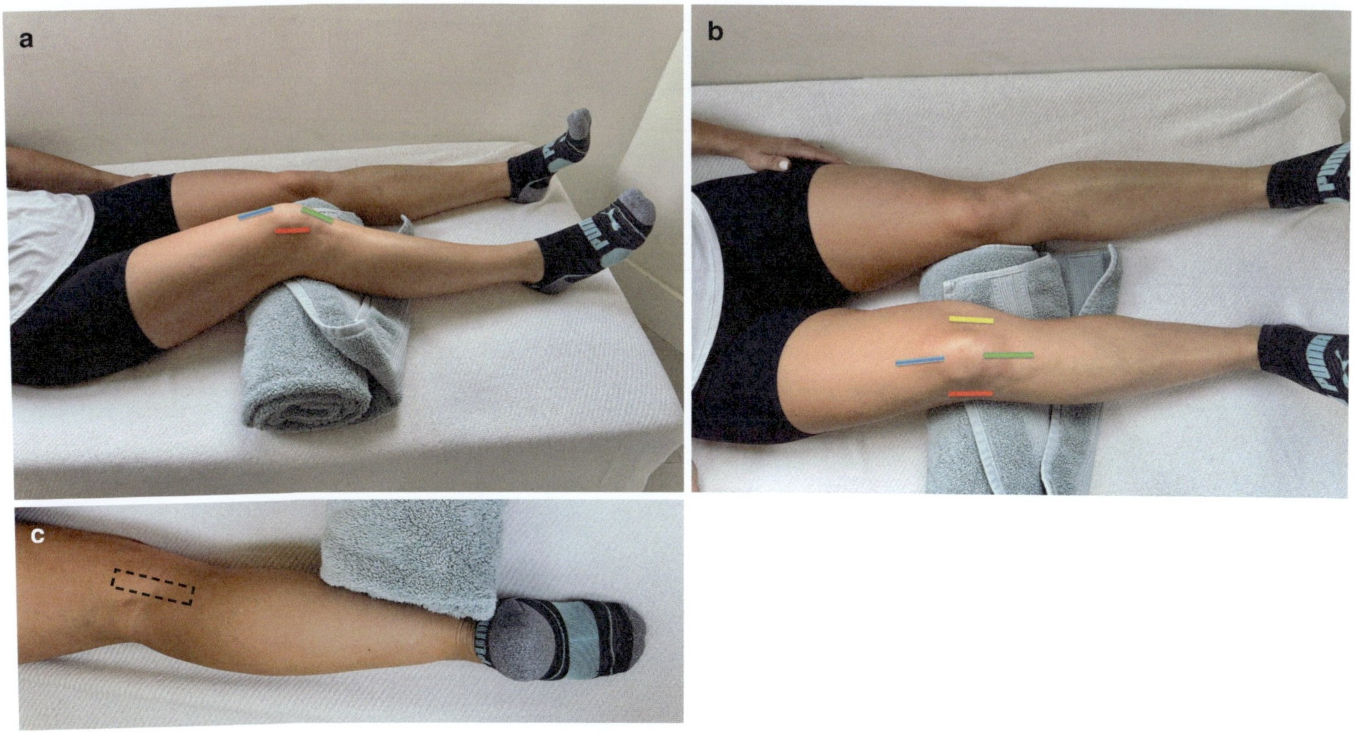

Fig. 19.29 Ultrasound probe positioning and basic scanning protocol for the knee. (**a**) Assessment of the quadriceps tendon, patellar ligament, medial collateral ligament, medial horn of the meniscus, lateral collateral ligament, and lateral horn of the meniscus (visualized from the lateral direction). (**b**) Assessment of the quadriceps tendon, patellar ligament, medial collateral ligament, medial horn of the meniscus, lateral collateral ligament, and lateral horn of the meniscus (visualized from the anterior direction). (**c**) Evaluation of the posterior fossa for Baker's cyst with the patient in the prone position

Other nuanced findings can be found in noninflammatory arthritis-associated types of tenosynovitis. In de Quervain's tenosynovitis (dorsal compartment one of the wrist), the abductor pollicis longus and extensor pollicis brevis are enlarged with a thickened intracompartmental septum [97]. In infectious tenosynovitis, such as pyogenic tenosynovitis of a digital flexor tendon, hypoechoic or dense material can sometimes be visualized within the tendon sheath, accompanied by increased Doppler signal [98]. Stenosing tenosynovitis, or "trigger finger," can be caused by overuse or mechanical injury, diabetes, or an idiopathic etiology [99]. Ultrasound findings of trigger finger include thickening of the A1 pulley, a soft tissue fiber at the base of the volar metacarpal joint, which may cause the underlying flexor tendon to become displaced or enlarged [100]. Dynamic scanning while flexing the finger may allow visualization of the tendon catching in real time. Finally, crystalline-associated tenosynovitis (e.g., gout, pseudogout) can be associated with hyperechoic deposits within or surrounding the tendon and generate an acoustic shadow [101].

Tendinitis

Tendinopathy, or tendinitis, may largely be mechanical or degenerative in nature and is generally not associated with effusion, thickened tenosynovium, or increased Doppler signal [102]. Hallmark features of tendinitis include a thickened, heterogeneous appearance to the tendon fibers with loss of fibrillar pattern and occasional hyperechoic densities consistent with calcifications [103] (Fig. 19.32).

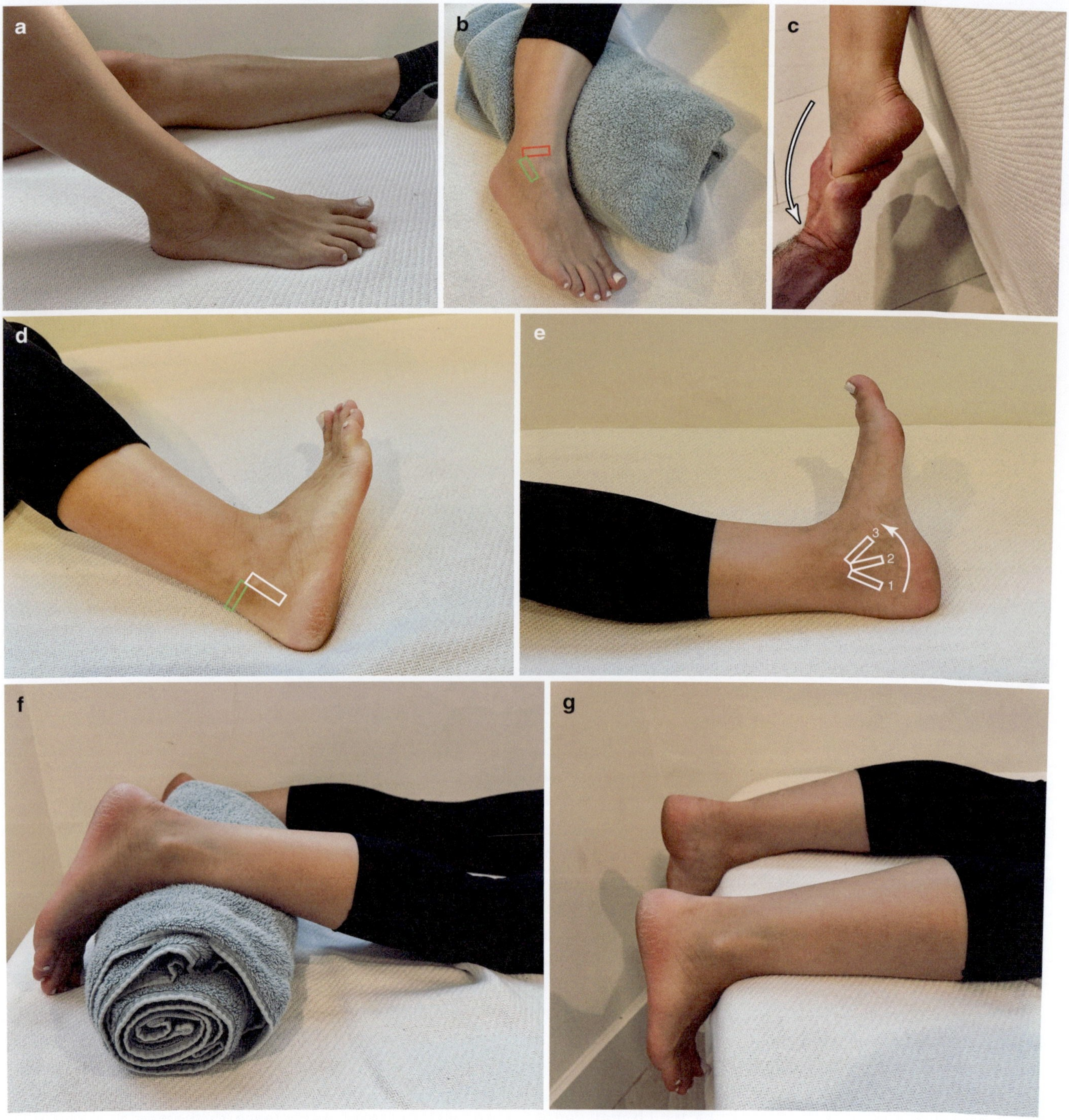

Fig. 19.30 Ultrasound probe positioning and basic scanning protocol for the ankle. (**a**) Evaluation of the talotibial space. (**b**) Evaluation of the anterior talofibular (blue box) and anterior tibiofibular (red box) ligaments. The foot should be in a plantar flexed and slightly inverted position when assessing these ligaments. (**c**) Dynamic examination of the anterior talofibular ligament by moving the foot further into plantar flexion and inversion. (**d**) Evaluation of the calcaneofibular ligament (white box) and peroneal tendons (blue box). To perform this, the foot should be placed in a dorsiflexed position. (**e**) Evaluation of the deltoid ligament. The deltoid ligament is composed of three ligaments (1 = tibiotalar, 2 = tibiocalcaneal, 3 = tibionavicular) that all originate on the medial malleolus. All three portions of the deltoid ligament can be evaluated by maintaining a relatively stationary position on the medial malleolus and moving in a sweeping motion as depicted by the arrow. (**f**) Evaluation of the Achilles tendon using a towel to elevate the ankle. (**g**) Evaluation of the Achilles tendon by allowing it to rest off the edge of the bed

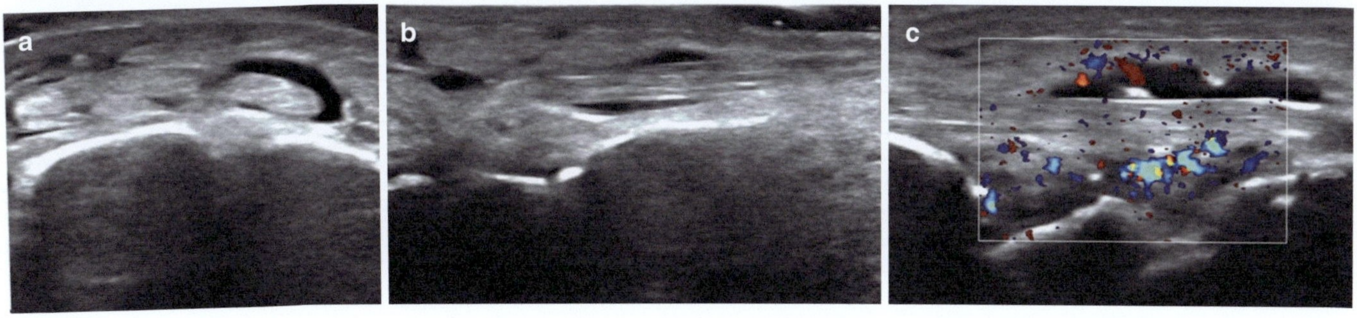

Fig. 19.31 Flexor tenosynovitis. (**a**) Short-axis view of a tendon demonstrating fluid surrounding the tendon. (**b**) Long-axis view of a tendon demonstrating fluid surrounding the tendon. (**c**) Color Doppler demonstrating associated hyperemia. (*Images courtesy of Michael Gottlieb, MD*)

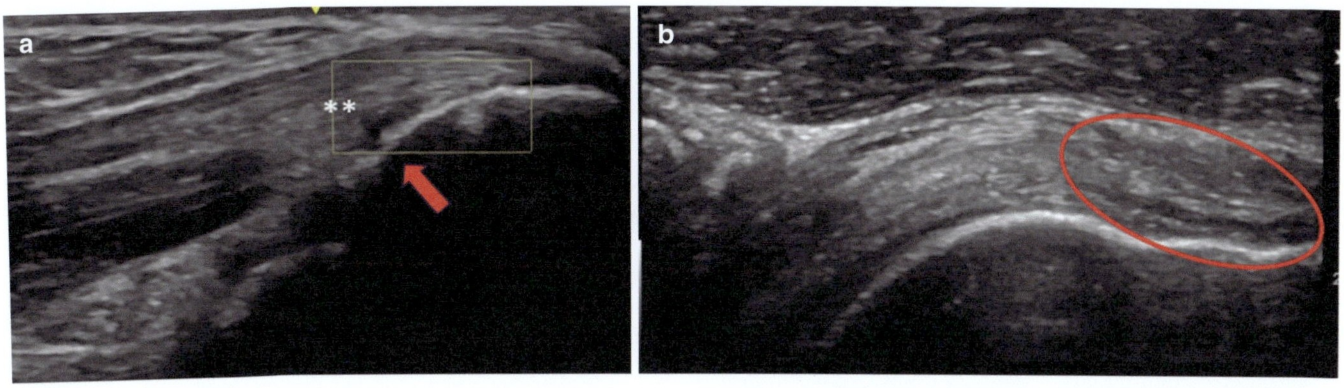

Fig. 19.32 Tendinopathy/Tendinitis. (**a**) Posterior longitudinal view of the elbow with tendinopathy/tendinitis of the triceps (**), which shows tendon fiber irregularity and patchy loss of fibrillar pattern. A bony irregularity is noted along the olecranon process with distension of the bursa underlying the triceps (arrow). (**b**) Subscapularis tendinopathy/tendinitis in which there is a heterogeneous appearance of the tendon fibers with loss of the normal fibrillar pattern and some drop out, which may additionally signal a small area of partial tear (circle)

Key Findings

Structure	Key findings
Myositis	Increased muscle echogenicity, with or without scattered hypoechoic areas. Muscle hypertrophy or atrophy. Increased vascularity. Fascial thickening.
Long bone fracture	Cortical irregularity in long axis.
Scaphoid bone fracture	Visualize in dorsal and volar planes. Volar side has peanut appearance. Dorsal side has pyramidal appearance.
Osteomyelitis	Deep soft tissue fluid collections adjacent to the bone. Periosteal thickening. Subperiosteal fluid collection. Increased vascularity of the periosteum.
Effusion	Appears as a hypoechoic or anechoic collection within the joint or recess. Visualized in two planes. Easily compressible.
Gout	Double contour sign. Snowstorm appearance of joint or tendon. Superficial tophi.
Bursitis	Small-to-large, anechoic, or hypoechoic collection within a bursal space that is compressible. Increased Doppler signal may be present depending on acuity and inflammation.

(continued)

Structure	Key findings
Acromioclavicular joint separation	Abnormal widening of alignment of the acromion process with the lateral aspect of the clavicle.
Glenohumeral joint dislocation	Anterior glenohumeral dislocations present with the humerus distal (anterior) to the probe when visualized with the posterior technique, whereas posterior dislocations are closer (posterior) to the probe. With the anterior technique, the humerus will be deep to the coracoid process. With the lateral technique, the humerus will be farther away from the acromion process than on the contralateral side.
Radial head subluxation	Widened distance between the radial head and capitellum. "Hook sign" with the annular ligament lodged within the radial head and capitellum.
Tendon or ligament injury	Complete tears: complete disruption of the organized fibular structure with hypoechoic edema. Partial tears: hypoechoic edema within the tendon or ligament, disruption of normal architecture, or hyperemia on Doppler. Chronic tears: punctate hyperechoic lesions with possible acoustic shadowing within the tendon or ligament.
Enthesitis	Hypoechoic edema, tendon thickening, calcifications, or bony erosion at the site of tendon insertion.
Tenosynovitis	Peritendinous and subcutaneous edema. Anechoic or hypoechoic tendon sheath widening. Anechoic or hypoechoic material surrounding the tendon. Increased Doppler signal.
Tendinitis	Thickened, heterogeneous appearance to the tendon fibers. Hyperechoic densities consistent with calcifications.

Pearls and Pitfalls

- When assessing musculoskeletal injuries, image the contralateral structure as an example of normal for comparison.
- Obese and elderly patients may have more hypoechoic-appearing muscles.
- When imaging tendons for pathology, be aware of anisotropy and fan through the structure to confirm pathology.
- Fanning the probe is helpful for the avoidance of anisotropy, which can be misconstrued as a ligamentous abnormality or effusion surrounding tendons or in muscle tissue.
- When aspirating an effusion, first assess your target in both the long- and short-axis planes to maximize success. The in-plane approach allows direct visualization of the needle throughout the entire procedure.
- Evaluation for musculoskeletal injury is typically performed with a high-frequency linear probe. However, at times a curvilinear probe with a lower frequency range may be needed to evaluate deep structure or in obese patients.
- Ultrasound should be considered when assessing for occult fractures.
- Cortical step-offs are seen best in the long axis.
- Shoulder dislocations can be readily identified via the posterior glenohumeral view of the shoulder. Use the spine of the scapula as a guide to ensure correct orientation while sliding the probe footprint laterally. However, the combined anterior and lateral approach is helpful when a patient is supine and there is insufficient room to place the ultrasound probe posteriorly.

References

1. Patil P, Dasgupta B. Role of diagnostic ultrasound in the assessment of musculoskeletal diseases. Ther Adv Musculoskel Dis. 2012;4(5):341–55. https://doi.org/10.1177/1759720X12442112.
2. Adhikari S, Leo M, Liu R, et al. The 2023 Core content of advanced emergency medicine ultrasonography. J Am Coll Emerg Physicians Open. 2023;4(4):e13015. https://doi.org/10.1002/emp2.13015.
3. Torralba KD, Cannella AC, Kissin EY, et al. Musculoskeletal ultrasound instruction in adult rheumatology fellowship programs. Arthritis Care Res (Hoboken). 2020;72(6):859–70. https://doi.org/10.1002/acr.23336.
4. Kane D, Grassi W, Sturrock R, Balint PV. A brief history of musculoskeletal ultrasound: 'from bats and ships to babies and hips'. Rheumatology. 2004;43(7):931–3. https://doi.org/10.1093/rheumatology/keh004.
5. Alerhand S, Situ-Lacasse E, Ramdin C, Gottlieb M. National survey of point-of-care ultrasound scholarly tracks in emergency medicine residency programs. West J Emerg Med. 2021;22(5):1095–101. https://doi.org/10.5811/westjem.2021.5.52118.
6. Goldflam K, Papanagnou D, Lewiss RE. Emergency ultrasound: a survey study of fellowship graduate characteristics and career paths. J Ultrasound Med. 2018;37(2):487–92. https://doi.org/10.1002/jum.14364.
7. Dimachkie MM, Barohn RJ, Amato AA. Idiopathic inflammatory myopathies. Neurol Clin. 2014;32(3):595–628. https://doi.org/10.1016/j.ncl.2014.04.007.
8. Albayda J, van Alfen N. Diagnostic value of muscle ultrasound for myopathies and myositis. Curr Rheumatol Rep. 2020;22(11):82. https://doi.org/10.1007/s11926-020-00947-y.
9. Abdelnaby R, Mohamed KA, Elgenidy A, et al. Muscle sonography in inclusion body myositis: a systematic review and meta-analysis of 944 measurements. Cells. 2022;11(4) https://doi.org/10.3390/cells11040600.
10. Hans PS, Ahn JS, Kim DJ. Ultrasound features of rhabdomyolysis. CJEM. 2020;22(3):386–8. https://doi.org/10.1017/cem.2020.16.
11. Nijboer-Oosterveld J, Van Alfen N, Pillen S. New normal values for quantitative muscle ultrasound: obesity increases muscle echo intensity. Muscle Nerve. 2011;43(1):142–3. https://doi.org/10.1002/mus.21866.
12. Chen KC, Lin AC, Chong CF, Wang TL. An overview of point-of-care ultrasound for soft tissue and musculoskeletal applications in

the emergency department. J Intensive Care. 2016;4:55. https://doi.org/10.1186/s40560-016-0173-0.
13. Cocco G, Ricci V, Villani M, et al. Ultrasound imaging of bone fractures. Insights Imaging. 2022;13(1):189. https://doi.org/10.1186/s13244-022-01335-z.
14. Chartier LB, Bosco L, Lapointe-Shaw L, Chenkin J. Use of point-of-care ultrasound in long bone fractures: a systematic review and meta-analysis. CJEM. 2017;19(2):131–42. https://doi.org/10.1017/cem.2016.397.
15. Ackermann O, Fischer CA, Grosser K, et al. Fracture sonography-review of literature and current recommendations. Arch Orthop Trauma Surg. 2024;144(7):3025–43. https://doi.org/10.1007/s00402-024-05396-1.
16. Rabiner JE, Khine H, Avner JR, Friedman LM, Tsung JW. Accuracy of point-of-care ultrasonography for diagnosis of elbow fractures in children. Ann Emerg Med. 2013;61(1):9–17. https://doi.org/10.1016/j.annemergmed.2012.07.112.
17. Varga M, Papp S, Kassai T, Bodzay T, Gáti N, Pintér S. Standardized sonographic examination of pediatric elbow injuries is an effective screening method and improves diagnostic efficiency. Injury. 2021;52(Suppl 1):S25–30. https://doi.org/10.1016/j.injury.2020.02.056.
18. Aponte EM, Novik JI. Identification of lipohemarthrosis with point-of-care emergency ultrasonography: case report and brief literature review. J Emerg Med. 2013;44(2):453–6. https://doi.org/10.1016/j.jemermed.2012.07.062.
19. Azizkhani R, Hosseini Yazdi Z, Heydari F. Diagnostic accuracy of ultrasonography for diagnosis of elbow fractures in children. Eur J Trauma Emerg Surg. 2022;48(5):3777–84. https://doi.org/10.1007/s00068-021-01648-6.
20. Haak SL, Borgstede MG, Stolmeijer R, et al. Point-of-care ultrasound-guided versus standard reduction of displaced distal radius fractures in the emergency department: a randomised controlled clinical trial. Emerg Med J. 2023;40(12):826–31. https://doi.org/10.1136/emermed-2023-213178.
21. Wood D, Reddy M, Postma I, et al. Ultrasound in forearm fractures: a pragmatic study assessing the utility of Point of Care Ultrasound (PoCUS) in identifying and managing distal radius fractures. Emerg Radiol. 2021;28(6):1107–12. https://doi.org/10.1007/s10140-021-01957-8.
22. Bozkurt O, Ersel M, Karbek Akarca F, Yalcinli S, Midik S, Kucuk L. The diagnostic accuracy of ultrasonography in determining the reduction success of distal radius fractures. Turk J Emerg Med. 2018;18(3):111–8. https://doi.org/10.1016/j.tjem.2018.04.001.
23. Scheier E, Balla U. Ultrasound-guided distal forearm fracture reduction by pediatric emergency physicians: a single center retrospective study. Pediatr Emerg Care. 2022;38(2):e756–60. https://doi.org/10.1097/pec.0000000000002464.
24. Caroselli C, Raffaldi I, Norbedo S, et al. Accuracy of point-of-care ultrasound in detecting fractures in children: a validation study. Ultrasound Med Biol. 2021;47(1):68–75. https://doi.org/10.1016/j.ultrasmedbio.2020.09.012.
25. Herren C, Sobottke R, Ringe MJ, et al. Ultrasound-guided diagnosis of fractures of the distal forearm in children. Orthop Traumatol Surg Res. 2015;101(4):501–5. https://doi.org/10.1016/j.otsr.2015.02.010.
26. Snelling PJ, Jones P, Moore M, et al. Describing the learning curve of novices for the diagnosis of paediatric distal forearm fractures using point-of-care ultrasound. Australas J Ultrasound Med. 2022;25(2):66–73. https://doi.org/10.1002/ajum.12291.
27. Cho KH, Lee SM, Lee YH, Suh KJ. Ultrasound diagnosis of either an occult or missed fracture of an extremity in pediatric-aged children. Korean J Radiol. 2010;11(1):84–94. https://doi.org/10.3348/kjr.2010.11.1.84.
28. Pountos I, Clegg J, Siddiqui A. Diagnosis and treatment of greenstick and torus fractures of the distal radius in children: a prospective randomised single blind study. J Child Orthop. 2010;4(4):321–6. https://doi.org/10.1007/s11832-010-0269-3.
29. Snelling PJ, Keijzers G, Ware RS. Point-of-care ultrasound pronator quadratus hematoma sign for detection of clinically non-angulated pediatric distal forearm fractures: a prospective cohort study. J Ultrasound Med. 2022;41(1):193–205. https://doi.org/10.1002/jum.15695.
30. Snelling PJ, Jones P, Bade D, et al. Ultrasonography or radiography for suspected pediatric distal forearm fractures. N Engl J Med. 2023;388(22):2049–57. https://doi.org/10.1056/NEJMoa2213883.
31. Hauger O, Bonnefoy O, Moinard M, Bersani D, Diard F. Occult fractures of the waist of the scaphoid: early diagnosis by high-spatial-resolution sonography. AJR Am J Roentgenol. 2002;178(5):1239–45. https://doi.org/10.2214/ajr.178.5.1781239.
32. Herrera Ortiz AF, Guevara SZ, Ramírez SM, et al. What is the role of ultrasonography in the early diagnosis of scaphoid fractures? Eur J Radiol Open. 2021;8:100358. https://doi.org/10.1016/j.ejro.2021.100358.
33. Kwee RM, Kwee TC. Ultrasound for diagnosing radiographically occult scaphoid fracture. Skeletal Radiol. 2018;47(9):1205–12. https://doi.org/10.1007/s00256-018-2931-7.
34. Paliwal AK, Sahdev R, Deshwal A, Ram B. Role of ultrasound in the diagnosis of paediatric acute osteomyelitis. J Ultrason. 2021;21(84):34–40. https://doi.org/10.15557/JoU.2021.0005.
35. Emiley PJ, Kendall JL, Bellows JW. Acute hematogenous osteomyelitis of the rib identified on bedside ultrasound. J Emerg Med. 2015;48(1):e15–7. https://doi.org/10.1016/j.jemermed.2014.07.031.
36. Schleifer J, Liteplo AS, Kharasch S. Point-of-care ultrasound in a child with chest wall pain and rib osteomyelitis. J Emerg Med. 2019;57(4):550–3. https://doi.org/10.1016/j.jemermed.2019.03.036. Epub 2019 Oct 4
37. Williamson SL, Seibert JJ, Glasier CM, Leithiser RE, Aronson J. Ultrasound in advanced pediatric osteomyelitis. A report of 5 cases. Pediatr Radiol. 1991;21(4):288–90. https://doi.org/10.1007/BF02018627.
38. Howard CB, Einhorn M, Dagan R, Nyska M. Ultrasound in diagnosis and management of acute haematogenous osteomyelitis in children. J Bone Joint Surg Br. 1993;75(1):79–82. https://doi.org/10.1302/0301-620X.75B1.8421042.
39. Darghouth M, Essaddam H, Ben Hamida M, et al. The value of ultrasound in acute osteomyelitis. French J Orthop Surg. 1989;3:174–80.
40. Inusa BPD, Oyewo A, Brokke F, Santhikumaran G, Jogeesvaran KH. Dilemma in differentiating between acute osteomyelitis and bone infarction in children with sickle cell disease: the role of ultrasound. PLoS One. 2013;8(6):e65001. https://doi.org/10.1371/journal.pone.0065001.
41. Ezzat T, EL-Hamid AA, Mostafa M, EL-Kady L. Early diagnosis of acute osteomyelitis in children by high-resolution and power Doppler sonography. Egypt J Radiol Nucl Med. 2011;42(2):233–42. https://doi.org/10.1016/j.ejrnm.2011.05.002.
42. Ogdie A, Taylor WJ, Neogi T, et al. Performance of ultrasound in the diagnosis of gout in a multicenter study: comparison with monosodium urate monohydrate crystal analysis as the gold standard. Arthritis Rheumatol. 2017;69(2):429–38. https://doi.org/10.1002/art.39959.
43. Persons B, Kissin EY. Scruples over speckles. J Med Ultrasound. 2020;28(3):179–80. https://doi.org/10.4103/jmu.Jmu_122_19.
44. de Ávila Fernandes E, Kubota ES, Sandim GB, Mitraud SA, Ferrari AJ, Fernandes AR. Ultrasound features of tophi in chronic tophaceous gout. Skeletal Radiol. 2011;40(3):309–15. https://doi.org/10.1007/s00256-010-1008-z.
45. Zhang Q, Gao F, Sun W, Ma J, Cheng L, Li Z. The diagnostic performance of musculoskeletal ultrasound in gout: a system-

atic review and meta-analysis. PLoS One. 2018;13(7):e0199672. https://doi.org/10.1371/journal.pone.0199672.
46. Aly AR, Rajasekaran S, Ashworth N. Ultrasound-guided shoulder girdle injections are more accurate and more effective than landmark-guided injections: a systematic review and meta-analysis. Br J Sports Med. 2015;49(16):1042–9. https://doi.org/10.1136/bjsports-2014-093573.
47. Gottlieb M, Alerhand S. Ultrasound should be considered for all arthrocentesis. Ann Emerg Med. 2020;75(2):261–2. https://doi.org/10.1016/j.annemergmed.2019.04.018.
48. Sibbitt WL, Kettwich LG, Band PA, et al. Does ultrasound guidance improve the outcomes of arthrocentesis and corticosteroid injection of the knee? Scand J Rheumatol. 2012;41(1):66–72. https://doi.org/10.3109/03009742.2011.599071.
49. Souza PM, Aguiar RO, Marchiori E, Bardoe SA. Arthrography of the shoulder: a modified ultrasound guided technique of joint injection at the rotator interval. Eur J Radiol. 2010;74(3):e29–32. https://doi.org/10.1016/j.ejrad.2009.03.020.
50. Balint PV, Kane D, Hunter J, McInnes IB, Field M, Sturrock RD. Ultrasound guided versus conventional joint and soft tissue fluid aspiration in rheumatology practice: a pilot study. J Rheumatol. 2002;29(10):2209–13.
51. Gibbons RC, Zanaboni A, Genninger J, Costantino TG. Ultrasound-versus landmark-guided medium-sized joint arthrocentesis: a randomized clinical trial. Acad Emerg Med. 2022;29(2):159–63. https://doi.org/10.1111/acem.14396.
52. Hoeber S, Aly AR, Ashworth N, Rajasekaran S. Ultrasound-guided hip joint injections are more accurate than landmark-guided injections: a systematic review and meta-analysis. Br J Sports Med. 2016;50(7):392–6. https://doi.org/10.1136/bjsports-2014-094570.
53. Kang YR, Koo J. Ultrasonography of the pediatric hip and spine. Ultrasonography. 2017;36(3):239–51. https://doi.org/10.14366/usg.16051.
54. Zhang M, Pessina MA, Higgs JB, Kissin EY. A vascular obstacle in ultrasound-guided hip joint injection. J Med Ultrasound. 2018;26(2):77–80. https://doi.org/10.4103/JMU.JMU_8_17.
55. Wu T, Dong Y, Song HX, Fu Y, Li JH. Ultrasound-guided versus landmark in knee arthrocentesis: a systematic review. Semin Arthritis Rheum. 2016;45(5):627–32. https://doi.org/10.1016/j.semarthrit.2015.10.011.
56. Wiler JL, Costantino TG, Filippone L, Satz W. Comparison of ultrasound-guided and standard landmark techniques for knee arthrocentesis. J Emerg Med. 2010;39(1):76–82. https://doi.org/10.1016/j.jemermed.2008.05.012.
57. Messina C, Banfi G, Orlandi D, et al. Ultrasound-guided interventional procedures around the shoulder. Br J Radiol. 2016;89(1057):20150372. https://doi.org/10.1259/bjr.20150372.
58. Hilligsøe M, Rathleff MS, Olesen JL. Ultrasound definitions and findings in greater trochanteric pain syndrome: a systematic review. Ultrasound Med Biol. 2020;46(7):1584–98. https://doi.org/10.1016/j.ultrasmedbio.2020.03.008.
59. Backhaus M, Burmester G-R, Gerber T, et al. Guidelines for musculoskeletal ultrasound in rheumatology. Ann Rheum Dis. 2001;60(7):641–9. https://doi.org/10.1136/ard.60.7.641.
60. Ivanoski S, Nikodinovska VV. Sonographic assessment of the anatomy and common pathologies of clinically important bursae. J Ultrason. 2019;19(78):212–21. https://doi.org/10.15557/JoU.2019.0032.
61. Wu T, Song HX, Dong Y, Li JH. Ultrasound-guided versus blind subacromial-subdeltoid bursa injection in adults with shoulder pain: a systematic review and meta-analysis. Semin Arthritis Rheum. 2015;45(3):374–8. https://doi.org/10.1016/j.semarthrit.2015.05.011.
62. Tortora S, Messina C, Albano D, et al. Ultrasound-guided musculoskeletal interventional procedures around the elbow, hand and wrist excluding carpal tunnel procedures. J Ultrason. 2021;21(85):e169–76. https://doi.org/10.15557/JoU.2021.0027.
63. Selame LAJ, Matsas B, Krauss B, Goldsmith AJ, Shokoohi H. A stepwise guide to performing shoulder ultrasound: the acromioclavicular joint, biceps, subscapularis, impingement, supraspinatus protocol. Cureus. 2021;13(9):e18354. https://doi.org/10.7759/cureus.18354.
64. Bockmann B, Venjakob AJ, Thrasyvoulidis G, Holschen M, Schulte TL, Nebelung W. Sonographic measurement of dynamic horizontal instability in acromioclavicular joint instability: description of a simple technique and correlation to radiographic parameters. J Ultrasound Med. 2022;41(2):409–15. https://doi.org/10.1002/jum.15719.
65. Gottlieb M, Patel D, Marks A, Peksa GD. Ultrasound for the diagnosis of shoulder dislocation and reduction: a systematic review and meta-analysis. Acad Emerg Med. 2022;29(8):999–1007. https://doi.org/10.1111/acem.14454.
66. Lahham S, Becker B, Chiem A, et al. Pilot study to determine accuracy of posterior approach ultrasound for shoulder dislocation by novice sonographers. West J Emerg Med. 2016;17(3):377–82. https://doi.org/10.5811/westjem.2016.2.29290.
67. Boswell B, Farrow R, Rosselli M, et al. Emergency medicine resident-driven point of care ultrasound for suspected shoulder dislocation. South Med J. 2019;112(12):605–9. https://doi.org/10.14423/smj.0000000000001046.
68. Secko MA, Reardon L, Gottlieb M, et al. Musculoskeletal ultrasonography to diagnose dislocated shoulders: a prospective cohort. Ann Emerg Med. 2020;76(2):119–28. https://doi.org/10.1016/j.annemergmed.2020.01.008.
69. Marks A, Schraft E, Gottlieb M. Skin, soft tissue, and musculoskeletal ultrasound. Emerg Med Clin North Am. 2024;42(4):863–90. https://doi.org/10.1016/j.emc.2024.05.010.
70. Abbasi S, Molaie H, Hafezimoghadam P, et al. Diagnostic accuracy of ultrasonographic examination in the management of shoulder dislocation in the emergency department. Ann Emerg Med. 2013;62(2):170–5. https://doi.org/10.1016/j.annemergmed.2013.01.022.
71. Sohn Y, Lee Y, Oh Y, Lee W. Sonographic finding of a pulled elbow: the "hook sign". Pediatr Emerg Care. 2014;30(12):919–21. https://doi.org/10.1097/pec.0000000000000299.
72. Averill LW, Kraft DB, Sabado JJ, Atanda A, Long SS, Nazarian LN. Ultrasonography of the pediatric elbow. Pediatr Radiol. 2023;53(8):1526–38. https://doi.org/10.1007/s00247-023-05623-8.
73. Güngör F, Kılıç T. Point-of-care ultrasonography to assist in the diagnosis and management of subluxation of the radial head in pediatric patients: a case series. J Emerg Med. 2017;52(5):702–6. https://doi.org/10.1016/j.jemermed.2017.01.049.
74. Lee SH, Kim SG, Kwak D, Hong SH, Lee YK, Jang WY. The usefulness of ultrasound and the posterior fat pad sign in pulled elbow. Injury. 2019;50(6):1227–31. https://doi.org/10.1016/j.injury.2019.04.026.
75. Roovers EA, Boere-Boonekamp MM, Castelein RM, Zielhuis GA, Kerkhoff TH. Effectiveness of ultrasound screening for developmental dysplasia of the hip. Arch Dis Child Fetal Neonatal Ed. 2005;90(1):F25–30. https://doi.org/10.1136/adc.2003.029496.
76. Herrero C, Colon Y, Nagapurkar A, Castañeda P. Point-of-care ultrasound reduces visit time and cost of care for infants with developmental dysplasia of the hip. Indian J Orthop. 2021;55(6):1529–34. https://doi.org/10.1007/s43465-021-00541-z.
77. Charlton SL, Schoo A, Walters L. Early dynamic ultrasound for neonatal hip instability: implications for rural Australia. BMC Pediatr. 2017;17(1):82. https://doi.org/10.1186/s12887-017-0830-z.
78. Kilsdonk I, Witbreuk M, Van Der Woude HJ. Ultrasound of the neonatal hip as a screening tool for DDH: how to screen and differences in screening programs between European countries.

J Ultrason. 2021;21(85):e147–53. https://doi.org/10.15557/JoU.2021.0024.
79. Yousefi MR, Yazdanprast M, Neshati H, Abdi R, Hasanian M, Alamdaran SA. Comparison static and dynamic ultrasound techniques of DDH: the role of the patient's position. Arch Bone Jt Surg. 2024;12(3):191–7. https://doi.org/10.22038/abjs.2023.69347.3264.
80. Inagaki-Asano A, Honda C, Matsumoto H, Yoshioka-Maeda K. Universal ultrasound screening for developmental dysplasia of the hip among infants in community settings in Japan: a scoping review. SAGE Open Nurs. 2024;10:23779608241272462. https://doi.org/10.1177/23779608241272462.
81. Jaremko JL, Hareendranathan A, Bolouri SES, Frey RF, Dulai S, Bailey AL. AI aided workflow for hip dysplasia screening using ultrasound in primary care clinics. Sci Rep. 2023;13(1):9224. https://doi.org/10.1038/s41598-023-35603-9.
82. Libon J, Ng C, Bailey A, Hareendranathan A, Joseph R, Dulai S. Remote diagnostic imaging using artificial intelligence for diagnosing hip dysplasia in infants: results from a mixed-methods feasibility pilot study. Paediatr Child Health. 2023;28(5):285–90. https://doi.org/10.1093/pch/pxad013.
83. Chen M, Cai R, Zhang A, Chi X, Qian J. The diagnostic value of artificial intelligence-assisted imaging for developmental dysplasia of the hip: a systematic review and meta-analysis. J Orthop Surg Res. 2024;19(1):522. https://doi.org/10.1186/s13018-024-05003-4.
84. Dion V, Sabhaney V, Ahn JS, Erdelyi S, Kim DJ. The physical examination is unreliable in determining the location of the distal fibular physis. Am J Emerg Med. 2021;50:97–101. https://doi.org/10.1016/j.ajem.2021.07.040.
85. Snelling PJ, Jones P, Gillespie A, Bade D, Keijzers G, Ware RS. Point-of-care ultrasound fracture-physis distance association with salter-Harris II fractures of the distal radius in children: the "POCUS 1-cm Rule". Ultrasound Med Biol. 2023;49(2):520–6. https://doi.org/10.1016/j.ultrasmedbio.2022.10.002.
86. Merolla G, Singh S, Paladini P, Porcellini G. Calcific tendinitis of the rotator cuff: state of the art in diagnosis and treatment. J Orthop Traumatol. 2016;17(1):7–14. https://doi.org/10.1007/s10195-015-0367-6.
87. Odom MJ, Grace KA, Brigido MK, Theyyunni NR, Kessler RA, Greineder CF. Shoulder pseudodislocation associated with calcific tendinitis/bursitis and diagnosed by point of care ultrasound. J Emerg Med. 2020;58(1):72–6. https://doi.org/10.1016/j.jemermed.2019.08.051.
88. Zhang H, Liang J, Qiu J, Wang F, Sun L. Ultrasonographic evaluation of enthesitis in patients with ankylosing spondylitis. J Biomed Res. 2017;31(2):162–9. https://doi.org/10.7555/jbr.31.20160088.
89. D'Agostino MA, Said-Nahal R, Hacquard-Bouder C, Brasseur JL, Dougados M, Breban M. Assessment of peripheral enthesitis in the spondylarthropathies by ultrasonography combined with power Doppler: a cross-sectional study. Arthritis Rheum. 2003;48(2):523–33. https://doi.org/10.1002/art.10812.
90. Bureau NJ, Beauchamp M, Cardinal E, Brassard P. Dynamic sonography evaluation of shoulder impingement syndrome. AJR Am J Roentgenol. 2006;187(1):216–20. https://doi.org/10.2214/ajr.05.0528.
91. Blood TD, Morrell NT, Weiss AC. Tenosynovitis of the hand and wrist: a critical analysis review. JBJS Rev. 2016;4(3) https://doi.org/10.2106/jbjs.Rvw.O.00061.
92. Bruyn GA, Iagnocco A, Naredo E, et al. OMERACT definitions for ultrasonographic pathologies and elementary lesions of rheumatic disorders 15 years On. J Rheumatol. 2019;46(10):1388–93. https://doi.org/10.3899/jrheum.181095.
93. Naredo E, D'Agostino MA, Wakefield RJ, et al. Reliability of a consensus-based ultrasound score for tenosynovitis in rheumatoid arthritis. Ann Rheum Dis. 2013;72(8):1328–34. https://doi.org/10.1136/annrheumdis-2012-202092.
94. Wakefield RJ, Balint PV, Szkudlarek M, et al. Musculoskeletal ultrasound including definitions for ultrasonographic pathology. J Rheumatol. 2005;32(12):2485–7.
95. Ammitzbøll-Danielsen M, Østergaard M, Naredo E, et al. The use of the OMERACT ultrasound tenosynovitis scoring system in multicenter clinical trials. J Rheumatol. 2018;45(2):165–9. https://doi.org/10.3899/jrheum.170501.
96. Tang Y, Cheng S, Yang Y, et al. Ultrasound assessment in psoriatic arthritis (PsA) and psoriasis vulgaris (non-PsA): which sites are most commonly involved and what features are more important in PsA? Quant Imaging Med Surg. 2020;10(1):86–95. https://doi.org/10.21037/qims.2019.08.09.
97. Morisaki S, Tsuchida S, Oda R, Takahashi K. Quantitative analysis of ultrasonography for de Quervain's disease: comparison of the affected side with the asymptomatic side. J Ultrasound Med. 2023;42(7):1437–43. https://doi.org/10.1002/jum.16152.
98. Jardin E, Delord M, Aubry S, Loisel F, Obert L. Usefulness of ultrasound for the diagnosis of pyogenic flexor tenosynovitis: a prospective single-center study of 57 cases. Hand Surg Rehabil. 2018;37(2):95–98.n. https://doi.org/10.1016/j.hansur.2017.12.004.
99. Vasiliadis AV, Itsiopoulos I. Trigger finger: an atraumatic medical phenomenon. J Hand Surg Asian Pac. 2017;22(2):188–93. https://doi.org/10.1142/s021881041750023x.
100. Bianchi S, Gitto S, Draghi F. Ultrasound features of trigger finger: review of the literature. J Ultrasound Med. 2019;38(12):3141–54. https://doi.org/10.1002/jum.15025.
101. Grassi W, Meenagh G, Pascual E, Filippucci E. "Crystal clear"-sonographic assessment of gout and calcium pyrophosphate deposition disease. Semin Arthritis Rheum. 2006;36(3):197–202. https://doi.org/10.1016/j.semarthrit.2006.08.001.
102. Canosa-Carro L, Bravo-Aguilar M, Abuín-Porras V, et al. Current understanding of the diagnosis and management of the tendinopathy: an update from the lab to the clinical practice. Dis Mon. 2022;68(10):101314. https://doi.org/10.1016/j.disamonth.2021.101314.
103. Bruno F, Palumbo P, Arrigoni F, et al. Advanced diagnostic imaging and intervention in tendon diseases. Acta Biomed. 2020;91(8-s):98–106. https://doi.org/10.23750/abm.v91i8-S.10007.

Vascular Ultrasound

20

Viveta Lobo and Christy Moore

Background

The origins of vascular ultrasound date back to 1842, when Christian Doppler described his eponymous effect, stating that the frequency of sound, light, or other waves measured by an observer depends on the relative motion between the source and the receiver [1]. This principle has been used in medicine since the late 1950s. In the mid-1970s, a group of clinicians and bioengineers at the University of Washington built a prototype duplex scanner that combined B-mode imaging and pulsed-wave Doppler flow detection in a single machine [2]. They began imaging patients with carotid disease and found that spectral waveform parameters were correlated with contrast arteriograms. This work led to the duplex criteria for carotid artery disease, which have since been widely utilized and modified [3].

In the 1980s and 1990s, the only widely utilized vascular ultrasound application was for the assessment of carotid artery intima-media thickness (IMT) and plaques [4]. In 2001, researchers began using carotid ultrasound routinely to assess the risk of stroke in elderly males. Soon after, lower extremity venous ultrasound was developed for the diagnosis of deep vein thrombosis with "economy class syndrome," or clots that were associated with air travel [5]. Next, the focus shifted to the assessment of the aorta and lower extremity arteries in arterial disease and renal artery stenosis in the setting of hypertension. The role of vascular ultrasound continued to expand into other anatomical regions and disease processes such as varicose veins, shunt placement, and management in dialysis patients. While diagnostic accuracy of vascular ultrasound may be difficult to establish in all exam types, it has been well-documented to be safe, noninvasive, and often the ideal initial diagnostic test.

Indications

Indications
- Unilateral extremity edema or pain
- Dyspnea
- Claudication
- Atherosclerosis
- Atypical chest pain
- Undifferentiated shock

Diagnoses
- Lower extremity deep venous thrombosis
- Upper extremity deep venous thrombosis
- Pseudoaneurysm
- Arteriovenous (AV) fistula
- Peripheral artery disease
- Carotid artery stenosis
- Superficial thrombophlebitis
- Lemierre's syndrome

Supplementary Information The online version contains supplementary material available at https://doi.org/10.1007/978-3-031-85308-1_20.

V. Lobo
Department of Emergency Medicine, Stanford University, Palo Alto, CA, USA
e-mail: vlobo@stanford.edu

C. Moore (✉)
Department of Emergency Medicine, University of Pennsylvania, Perelman School of Medicine, Philadelphia, PA, USA
e-mail: christy.moore@pennmedicine.upenn.edu

M. Gottlieb, N. Panebianco (eds.), *Advanced Point-of-Care Ultrasound*, https://doi.org/10.1007/978-3-031-85308-1_20

Core Views

<table>
<tr><th>View</th><th>Image</th><th>Approach</th></tr>
<tr><td colspan="3">Peripheral arterial</td></tr>
<tr><td>Peripheral artery short axis</td><td>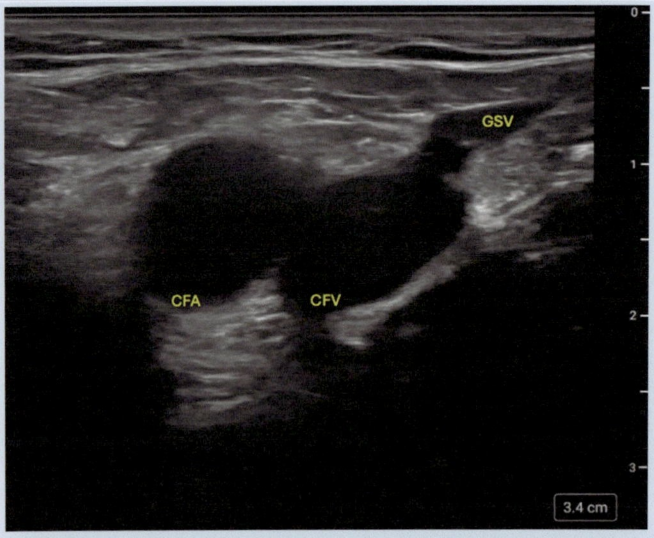

Core View 1. Normal common femoral arterial (CFA) ultrasound next to the common femoral vein (CFV) with branching off the great saphenous vein (GSV)
Core Video 1. Normal CFA adjacent to CFV with branching off of the GSV</td><td>Place the patient in the supine position, with their leg externally rotated and slightly flexed at the knee. Using a linear probe in the short-axis plane, start proximally at the inguinal canal and slide distally to locate the pulsating anechoic femoral artery located between the femoral vein and the femoral nerve. Compression of the artery can enhance pulsatility. Continue scanning distally from the common femoral artery as described above to identify the pulsating superficial and deep femoral arteries along the femoral vein. Further distal in the popliteal fossa, the popliteal artery is visualized, often deep and pulsating to the popliteal vein.</td></tr>
<tr><td>Peripheral artery long axis with color Doppler</td><td>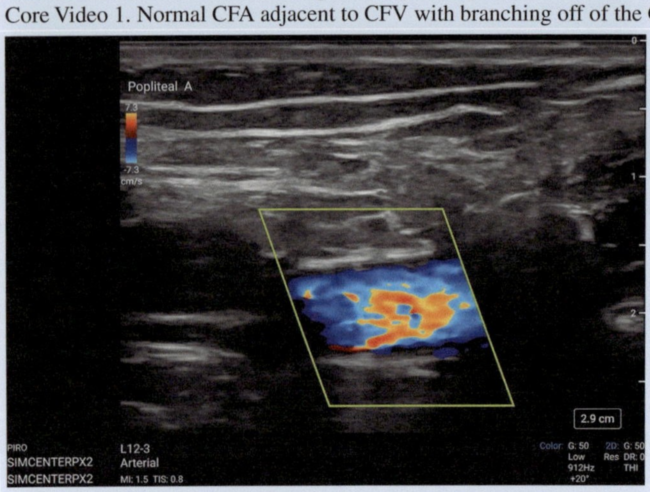

Core View 2. Normal color Doppler assessment of the popliteal artery
Core Video 2. Color Doppler assessment of popliteal artery</td><td>Rotate the probe 90 degrees to view the artery in the long axis, and use the color Doppler to evaluate for normal flow. Optimize the size of the color box, gain, and color velocity scale (or pulse repetition frequency). The box should only sample the area of interest and be as small and superficial as possible to maximize the frame rate and improve the image quality and resolution.</td></tr>
</table>

Peripheral artery long axis with pulsed-wave Doppler	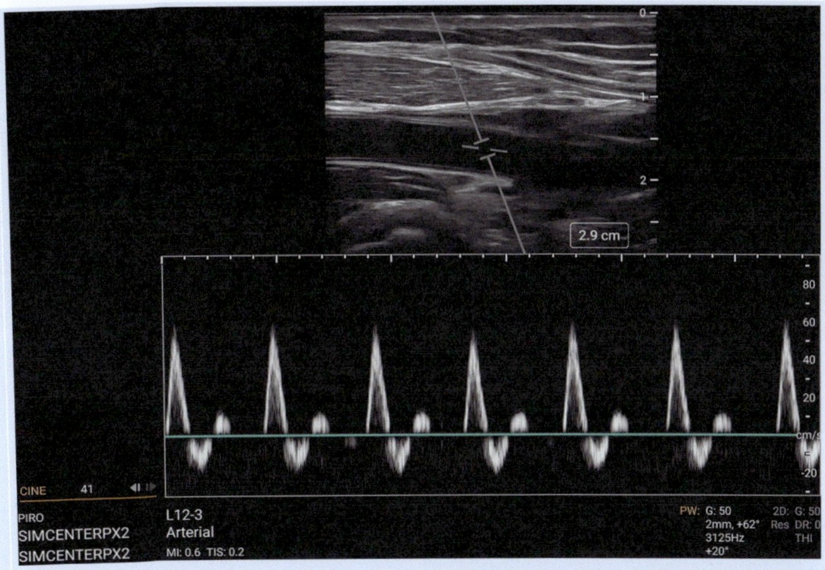 Core View 3. Pulsed-wave Doppler assessment of the popliteal artery. Note the beam is steered to align parallel to the flow of blood, indicated by the line in the center of the pulsed-wave Doppler gate	The cursor should be placed in the center of the arterial lumen, with the sample volume size set to one-third to one-half the luminal diameter. The Doppler angle and the arterial axis should be between 45 degrees and 60 degrees for optimal accuracy and to visualize the normal multiphasic pattern. A normal femoral artery should demonstrate a triphasic high-resistance flow pattern.
Venous assessment – lower extremity		
Common femoral vein	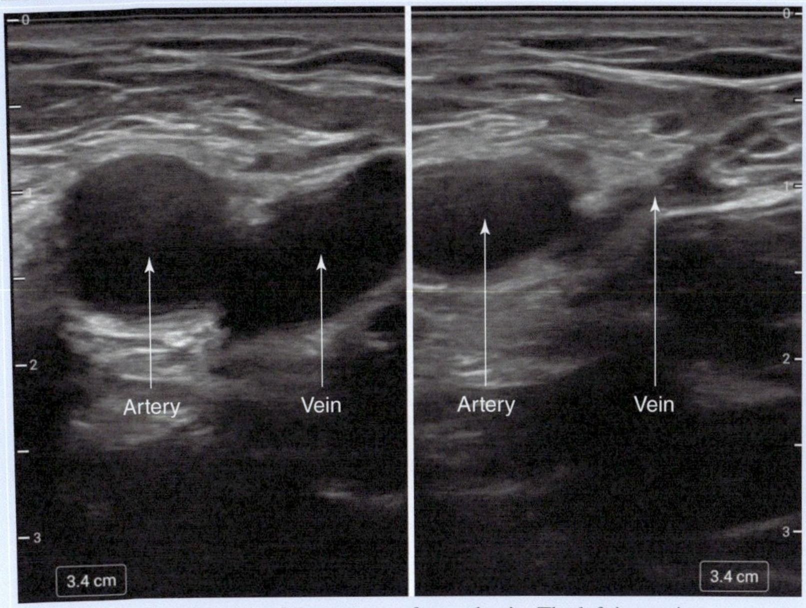 Core View 4. Compression of the common femoral vein. The left image is uncompressed, and the right image is compressed Core Video 3. Compression of the common femoral vein	Place the patient in a supine position with their leg externally rotated and slightly flexed at the knee [6, 7]. Place the probe in the short-axis plane just distal to the inguinal ligament. Compress every 1 to 2 cm along the vein while sliding the probe distally along the common femoral vein, continuing along the femoral vein to the popliteal vein. In a normal exam, the vein should compress fully under light pressure from the probe. Use the femur bone to provide counter-pressure while compressing to facilitate collapsibility.

View	Image	Approach
Popliteal vein	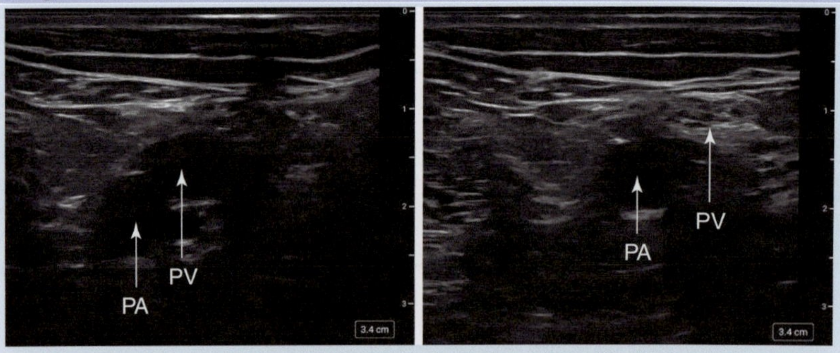 Core View 5. (Still and Video)- Ultrasound of a collapsed popliteal vein under normal compression Core Video 4. Compression of the popliteal vein	Evaluate the popliteal vein by gently placing the probe in the short-axis plane within the popliteal fossa. The popliteal vein is generally superficial to the deeper popliteal artery in the popliteal fossa. Compressions are performed every 1–2 cm distally along the vein until the trifurcation of the popliteal vein into the anterior tibial, posterior tibial, and peroneal veins. It is key to ensure the angle of insonation is perpendicular to the course of the vessel as the knee may be bent. Calf veins may be followed distally; however, these structures have not generally been included in POCUS protocols.
Venous assessment – upper extremity		
Internal jugular vein	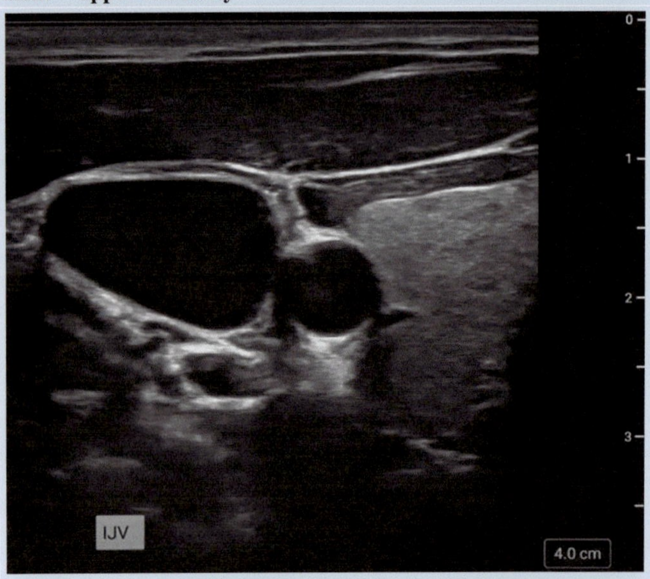 Core View 6. Normal ultrasound of the internal jugular vein (IJV) (short axis)	Place the patient in the supine position. Start with the probe just cranial to the clavicle at the level of the thyroid. Locate the internal jugular vein immediately lateral to the thyroid. Having the patient perform a Valsalva or hum may aid in recognition of the vessel when it is not readily visible. Evaluate the internal jugular vein in the short and long axes.
Subclavian vein	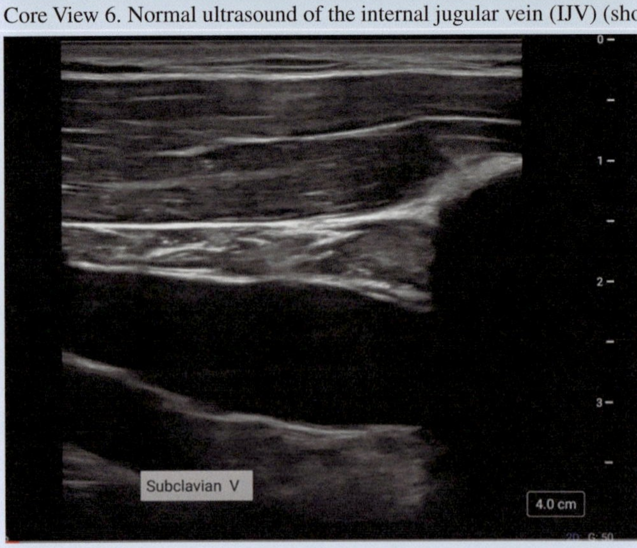 Core View 7. Normal ultrasound of the subclavian vein (long axis)	From the transverse plane at the anterolateral base of the neck, find the internal jugular vein and follow this inferiorly to the junction with the subclavian vein. Follow the subclavian vein laterally (usually beneath the clavicle) and visualize it in both the short and long axes using B-mode and color Doppler to exclude nonocclusive filling defects.

Axillary vein

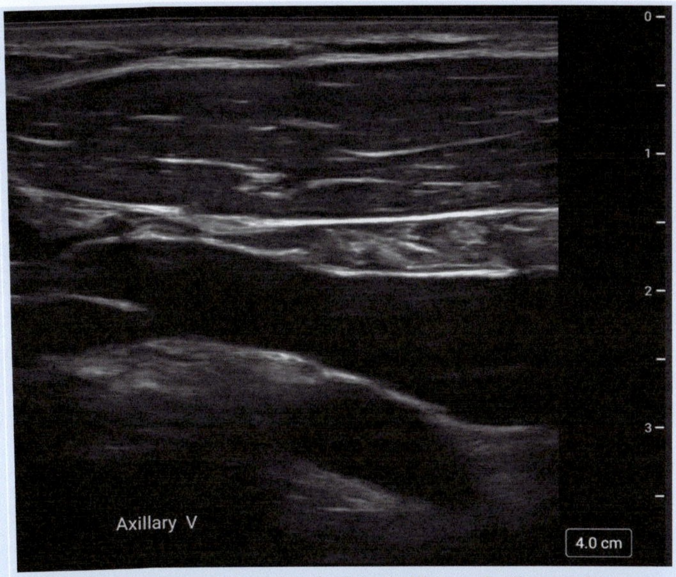

Core View 8. Normal ultrasound of the axillary vein (long axis)

Place the patient in the supine position with their ipsilateral hand over their head and elbow flexed to allow access to the axilla. Find the subclavian vein and follow this through the axilla while compressing every 1–2 cm in B-mode. Color Doppler can also be used in the long axis to help evaluate for filling defects. Upon reaching the proximal arm, the axillary vein will divide into the basilic and brachial veins.

Brachial and basilic veins

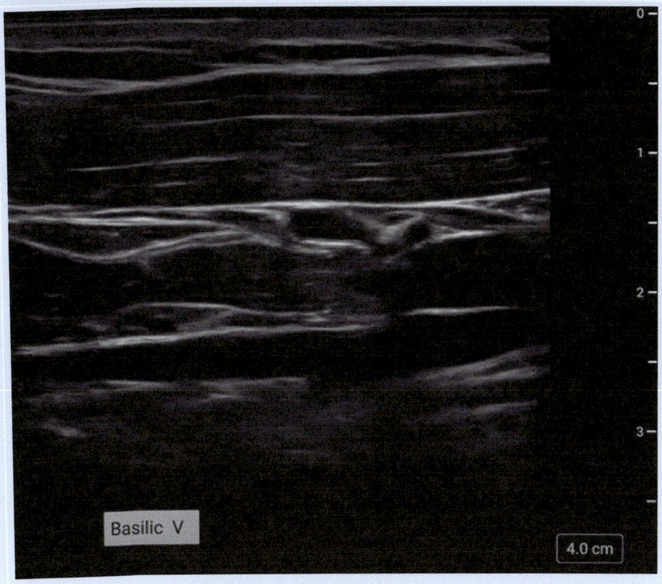

Core View 9. Normal ultrasound of the basilic vein (short axis)

Have the patient sit up on the bed with their arm supinated. The basilic vein is the largest and most superficial vein in the upper arm. Continue from the axillary vein in the short-axis plane and follow the basilic and brachial veins while compressing them every 1–2 cm along the way.

At the antecubital fossa, the brachial vein will divide into the radial and ulnar veins. Continue following these veins through the radial and ulnar veins to the wrist, confirming compressibility and flow.

Waveform Analysis

Pressure and volume have direct effects on the display of waveforms. Variations in flow patterns can show if there has been a change in volume or pressure either within the vessel or throughout the circulatory system. Arterial waveforms that occur due to a vascular bed not needing flow throughout the cardiac cycle are considered high resistance and have a sharp upstroke and brisk downstroke [8]. Arterial flow through the femoral artery at rest is an example of a high-resistance vessel (Fig. 20.1). Arterial waveforms that occur because of a vascular bed that demands constant flow throughout the cardiac cycle can be considered low resistance. These generally appear as monophasic waveforms, with a slower and gentler systolic upstroke and a prolonged downstroke [8]. Arterial flow through the internal carotid artery is an example of a low-resistance vessel (Fig. 20.2).

Venous flow is a result of the pressure from the thoracic cavity or the pressure from the heart and can be considered phasic or pulsatile. Venous flow through the common femoral vein is phasic in nature (Fig. 20.3). The closer that the interrogated vein is to the heart, the more pulsatile the flow is. Venous flow through the subclavian veins is also pulsatile (Fig. 20.4). Alternatively, pulsatile flow in vessels that are further away from the heart (e.g., the popliteal vein) means that there is a disruption of the normal hemodynamics and

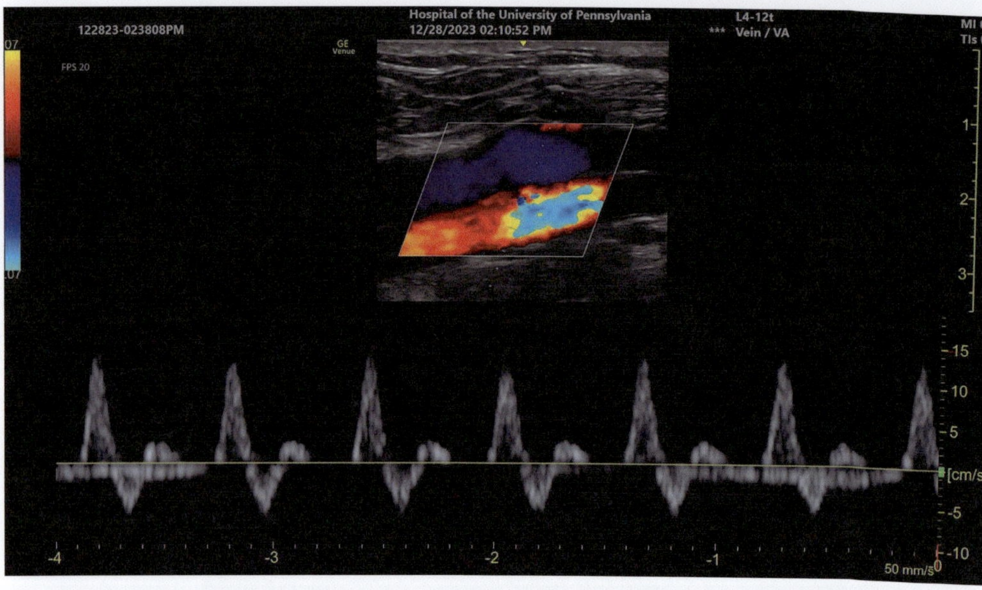

Fig. 20.1 Arterial flow through the femoral artery at rest can be considered high resistance

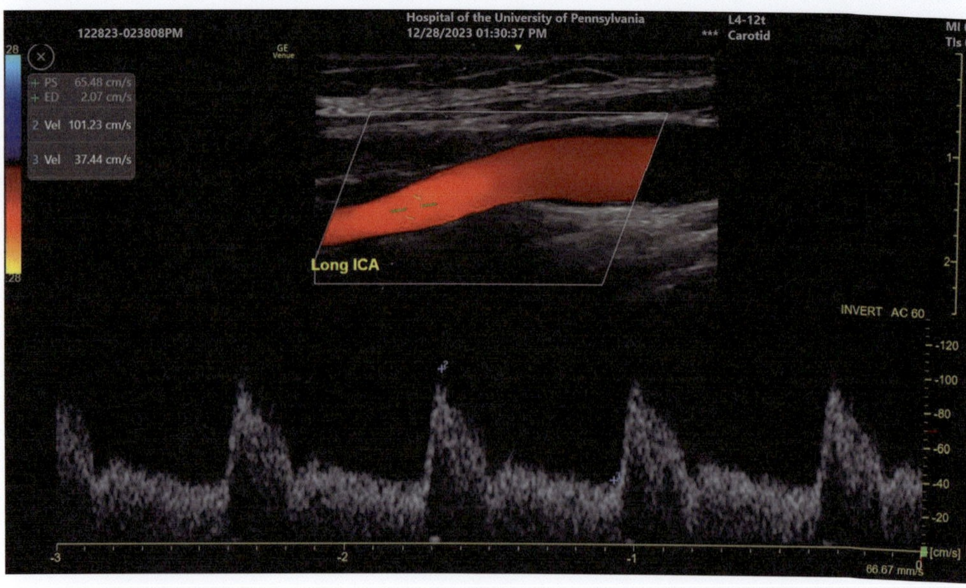

Fig. 20.2 Arterial flow through the internal carotid artery can be considered low resistance

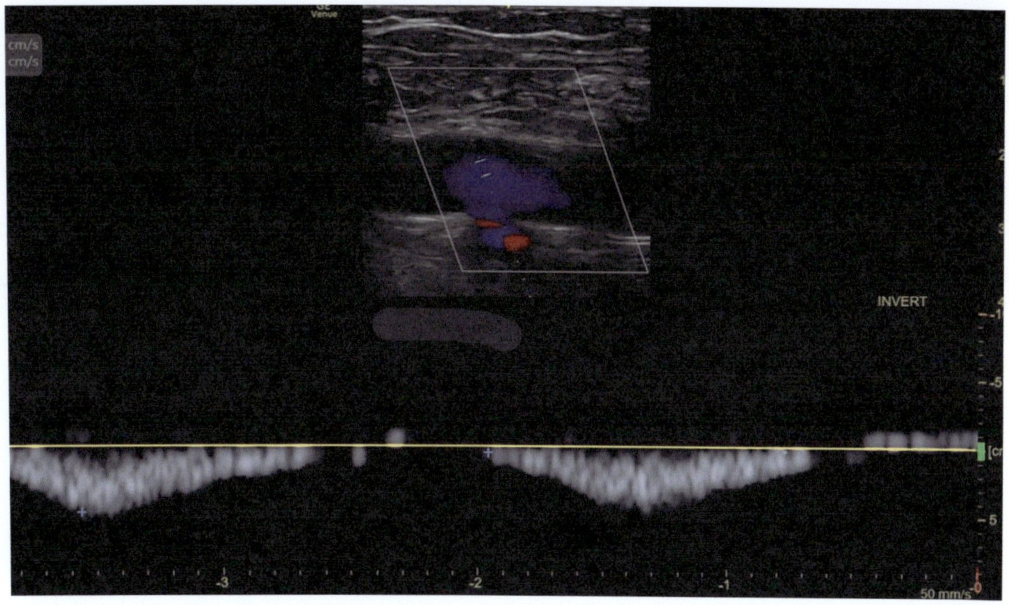

Fig. 20.3 Venous flow through the common femoral vein is phasic

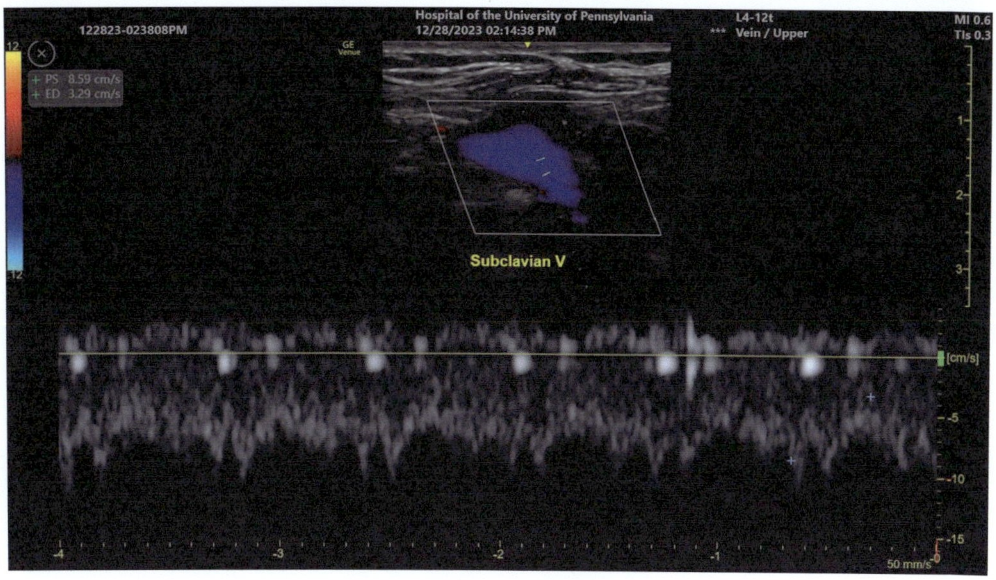

Fig. 20.4 Venous flow through the subclavian vein is pulsatile

may be a result of elevated central venous pressure. The detection of a pulsatile peripheral venous blood flow constitutes an early sign of right heart failure and is more sensitive than clinical evaluation or direct measures of central venous pressure (Fig. 20.5) [9]. In contrast, continuous or absent venous flow throughout the cardiac cycle at any interrogation point is considered abnormal and is almost always associated with a more proximal obstruction (Fig. 20.6). Other relevant equations for blood flow are included in Table 20.1.

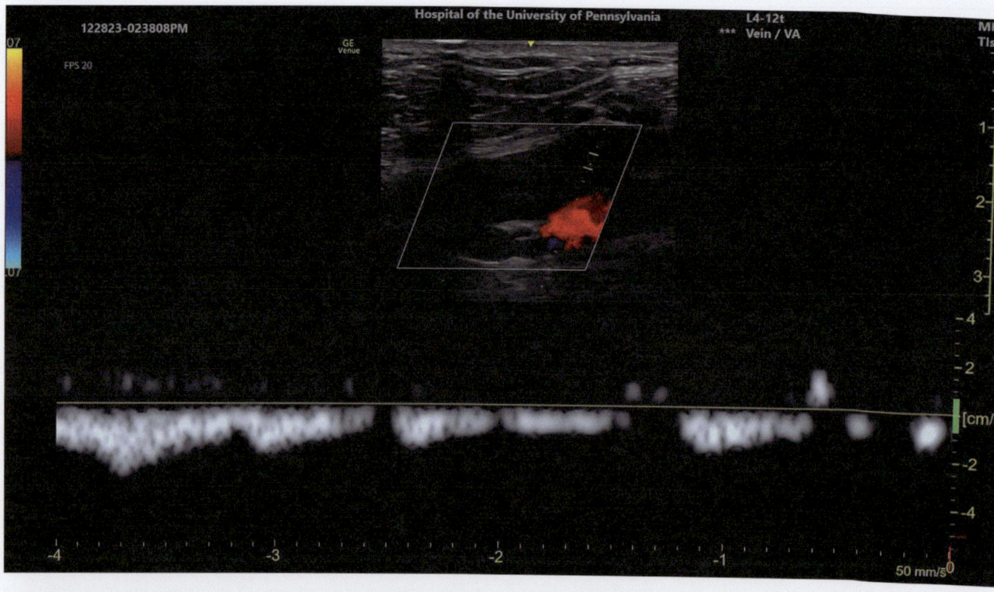

Fig. 20.5 Pulsatile flow is seen in the popliteal vein as flow below the baseline with clear phasicity. This tracing can indicate elevated central venous pressure

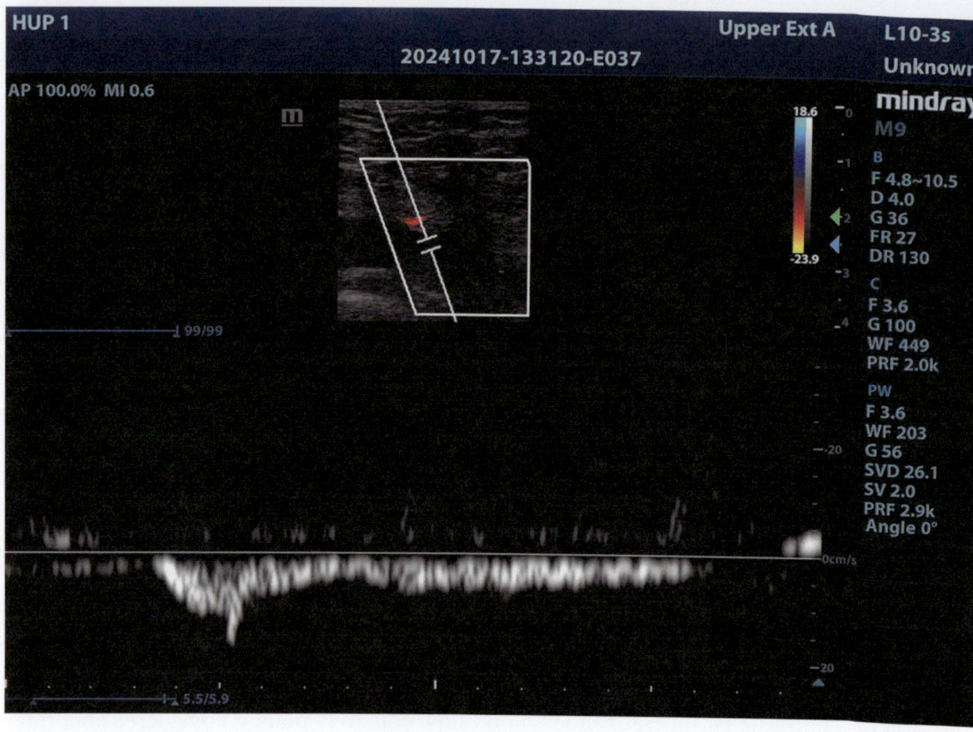

Fig. 20.6 Continuous venous flow is highly suggestive of proximal obstruction

Table 20.1 Key equations

Key term	Pathophysiological concept	Formula	Abbreviations
Bernoulli effect: Constant blood through a vessel keeps the velocity unchanged and therefore the pressure unchanged.	Stenosis will change pressures in vessels; therefore, velocity will increase with pressure increase.	$(\Delta P) = 4\left(V_2^2 - V_1^2\right)$	ΔP: Change in pressure between two chambers V_1: Velocity in chamber 1 V_2: Velocity in chamber 2
Poiseuille's law: The size of the blood vessel and the thickness of the blood cause a drop in pressure.	As fluid increases in viscosity or the size decreases (e.g., stenosis, vasospasm), pressure increases.	$q = \dfrac{\pi P r 4}{8 \eta \iota}$	q: Flow rate P: Pressure r: Radius n: Fluid viscosity l: Length of tubing

Clinical Applications

Arterial Assessment

Among approaches for evaluating peripheral arterial disease (PAD), Doppler ultrasonography offers the benefit that it does not require contrast enhancement, prolonged patient preparation, or radiation exposure. It can efficiently assess peripheral arterial diseases such as arterial stenosis and occlusions, arteriovenous (AV) fistulas, pseudoaneurysms, and carotid artery plaques. This technique can be applied as a general protocol for an entire limb or as a focused examination of a specific area of interest (Fig. 20.7).

Duplex ultrasonography refers to both the use of B-mode and spectral Doppler ultrasound, which can include color or pulsed-wave Doppler. B-mode ultrasound can visualize structural abnormalities, anatomical variations, and plaques within the artery lumen. Color Doppler can evaluate flow disturbances from stenotic or occluded vessel segments, and pulsed-wave Doppler can measure flow velocities and determine the degree of severity of the stenosis based on an analysis of the waveform.

Peripheral Arterial Disease

Peripheral arterial disease is the narrowing of the peripheral arteries, usually caused by atherosclerosis, impacting 5.6% of people, with approximately 236 million adults affected worldwide [10]. When examining a focused arterial segment, examine blood flow patterns sequentially along the artery. This is important as flow disturbances caused by arterial narrowing are propagated along the vessel for a relatively short distance (approximately only a few vessel diameters).

A normal arterial velocity waveform exhibits three phases, known as triphasic flow. When the movement of blood is consistent in speed and direction with a laminar flow pattern, it provides a multiphasic or triphasic waveform with a narrow spectral width throughout the pulse cycle. This includes a sharp upward peak during systole, a downward peak in early diastole, and a forward flow in late diastole (Fig. 20.8). The late diastolic wave will decrease or disappear when peripheral resistance is present. A biphasic arterial Doppler velocity waveform has a quick upstroke followed by a relatively fast downstroke, with flow above the baseline during all phases of the forward flow during diastole

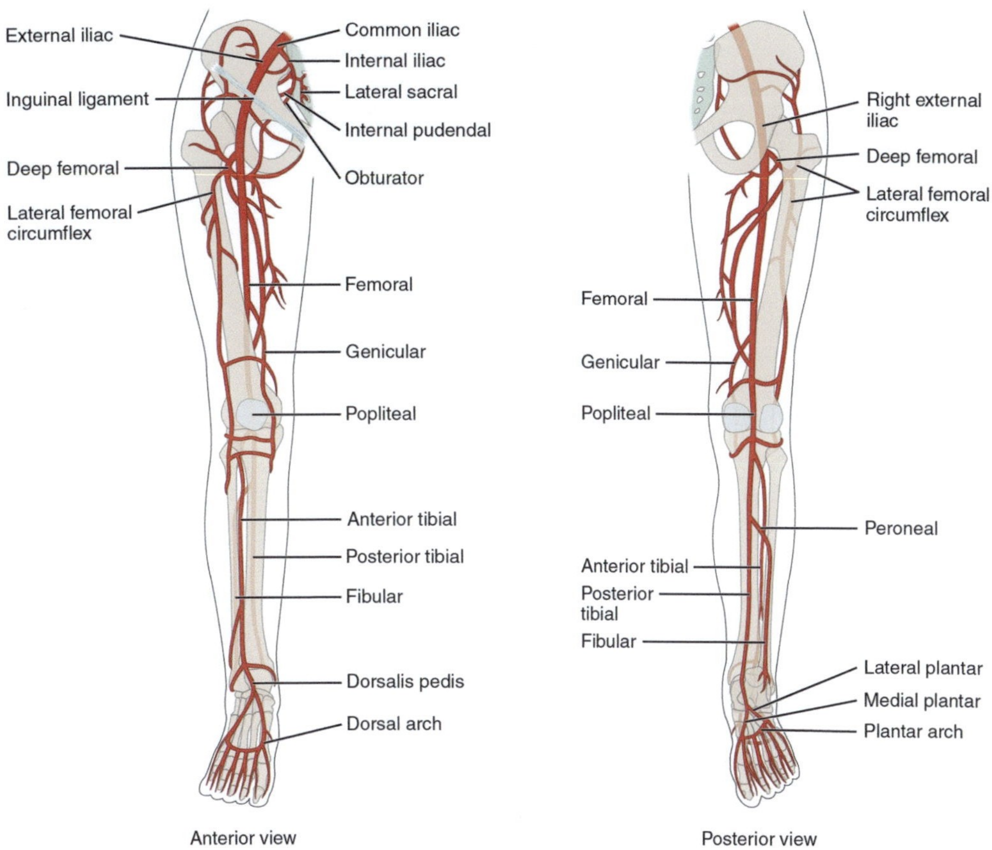

Fig. 20.7 Illustration of the anatomy of lower extremity arterial vasculature. (*Image courtesy of* AnatomyTOOL.org *by OpenStax*)

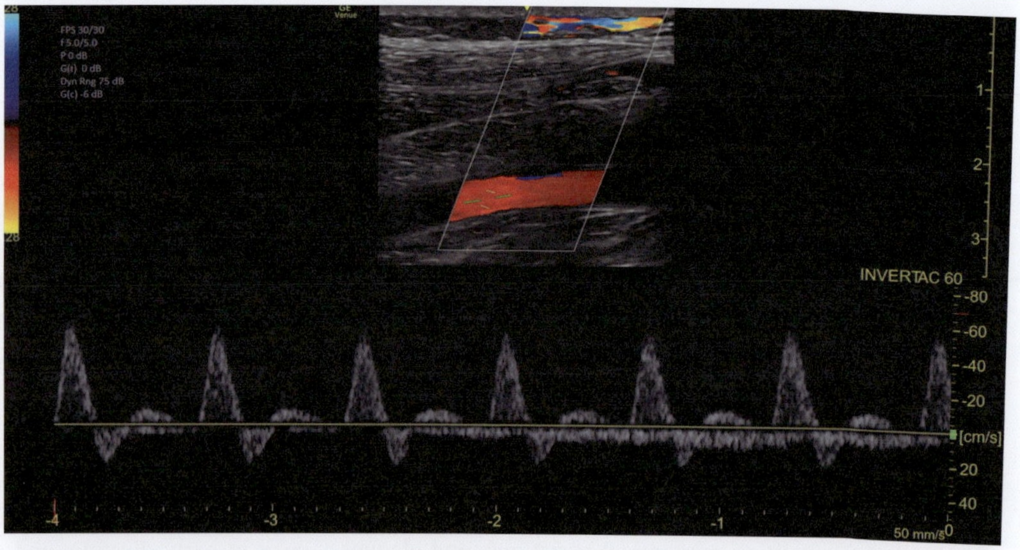

Fig. 20.8 Normal triphasic arterial waveform in pulsed-wave Doppler

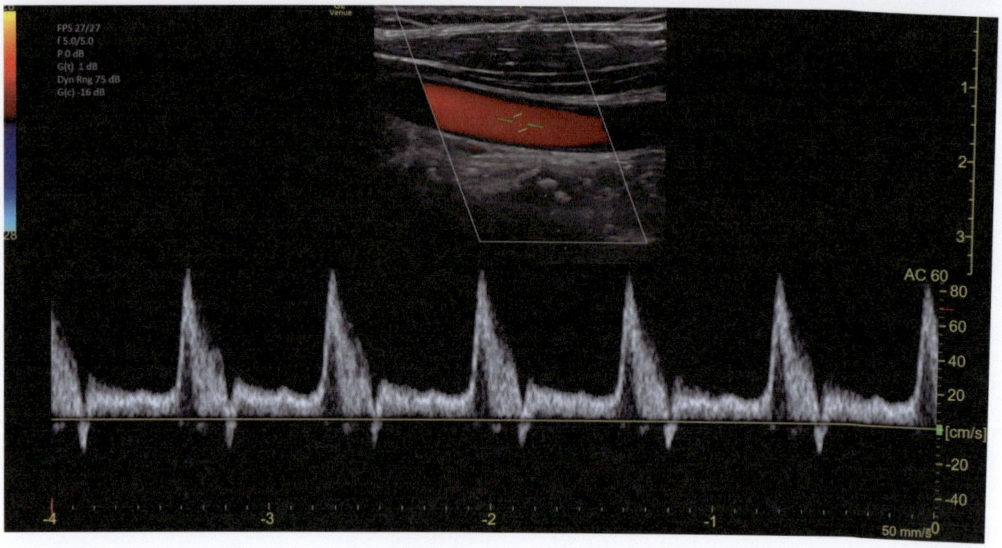

Fig. 20.9 Biphasic arterial waveform in pulsed-wave Doppler

(Fig. 20.9). Monophasic Doppler waveforms are characterized by non-sharp, rounded peaks, no flow reversal, and a faint upstroke and downstroke (Fig. 20.10). This is typically seen in multilevel obstructive arterial disease.

When peripheral arteries develop flow disturbance or stenoses, the flow inside the blood vessels becomes turbulent and causes the Doppler waveform to display spectral broadening. Spectral broadening occurs when the pulsed-wave Doppler waveform displays a wide range of velocities and is "filled in." This reflects the machine calculating the relatively high-velocity flow from the stenosis, as well as slower velocities adjacent to the vessel walls. Decreasing the sample volume and correcting the Doppler angle of insonation may reduce spectral broadening (Fig. 20.11) [11].

As PAD progresses, the normal triphasic flow is replaced by biphasic flow due to arterial fibrosis, which reduces the elastic recoil. If the disease worsens or is at the site of severe stenosis or occlusion, the early diastolic flow reversal disappears, which results in a monophasic waveform. The Bernoulli principle states that when the diameter of an artery decreases, as in arterial stenosis, the flow velocity through the stenosis should increase. However, when the stenosis severity exceeds 95%, the velocity decreases [8].

Because of its accuracy, high-quality duplex ultrasonography performed by well-trained operators represents a good alternative to computed tomographic angiography in patients with PAD [12]. When assessing for PAD, use the pulsed-wave Doppler to determine the peak systolic velocity (PSV) for the artery segment being assessed. If the PSV is abnormal, then continue the assessment by determining the PSV of the proximal non-stenotic vessel segment. To determine the degree of stenosis, calculate the PSV ratio. The PSV ratio is calculated by dividing the PSV of the stenotic lesion by the PSV of the unaffected section of the vessel (proximal to the

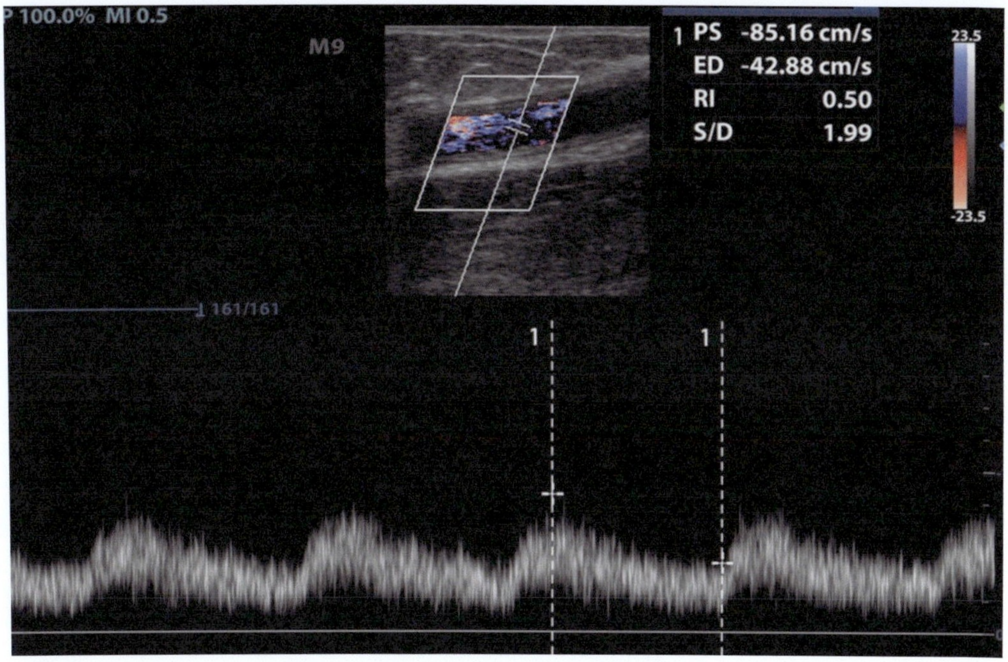

Fig. 20.10 Monophasic arterial waveform in pulsed-wave Doppler

non-stenotic area). A PSV ratio of 1.5 to 2 indicates 30–49% stenosis, a PSV ratio of 2 to 4 indicates 50–75%, and a PSV ratio greater than 4 indicates >75% stenosis. A peripheral arterial lesion is significant if it causes >50% stenosis in the presence of an atherosclerotic plaque. This ratio of PSVs provides a more accurate evaluation of peripheral arterial stenosis than absolute PSV measurements [13]. This is due to significant variability in PSV measurements between individuals. In high-grade stenosis, a *tardus et parvus* pattern may also be observed. This finding presents as a waveform that has lost its rapid systolic upstroke and has a delayed peak systole (Fig. 20.12). Mean sizes and PSV values for common arteries are included in Table 20.2.

Pseudoaneurysm

True aneurysms occur when all three layers of the arterial wall (intima, media, and adventitia) form a localized dilation, whereas pseudoaneurysms usually develop from direct arterial trauma and do not involve all three layers. In pseudoaneurysms, hematoma formation most commonly leads to dilation between the media and the adventitia or a pseudofibrous capsule outside the vessel wall [14]. Iatrogenic injury due to arterial access in percutaneous procedures is the most frequent cause of femoral and radial artery pseudoaneurysms [15]. An abnormal examination or pain at the site of an endovascular procedure should prompt sonographic evaluation for this condition.

Duplex ultrasonography is the gold standard for diagnosis and characterization of size, anatomy, and origin. Complete evaluation of pseudoaneurysms includes assessment of size, measurements of the residual lumen, and the length and width of the surrounding channel. In B-mode, a pseudoaneurysm will demonstrate an outpouching of the wall of the artery. Color Doppler may show the classic "yin-yang" sign caused by the swirling blood within the affected area (Fig. 20.13). The waveform may also display a rapid systolic upstroke, an exaggerated deceleration, and an elongated reverse flow component, referred to as the "to-and-fro" flow pattern [8]. Diagnosis of a pseudoaneurysm usually warrants comprehensive ultrasound follow-up, along with appropriate consultative evaluation.

Arteriovenous Fistula

Arteriovenous access for hemodialysis is created surgically by connecting a vein to an artery (AV fistula) or by interposing a conduit, usually of synthetic material, between an artery and a vein (AV graft). The ideal location for placement of an AV fistula in the upper arm involves transposition in the radial-cephalic, brachial-cephalic, or brachial-basilic regions. Prosthetic grafts can be used as an alternative, though they are associated with a higher complication rate [16]. Physical examination alone is insensitive for early complications of an AV fistula. Sonographic assessment can provide more detail and characterize the type of malfunction so that a treatment plan can be made expeditiously [17]. Indications for fistula or graft evaluation include pain, swelling, redness, and difficult cannulation.

The patient should be placed in a supine or semi-recumbent position with the arm externally rotated and extended from the body to about a 45-degree angle. Begin

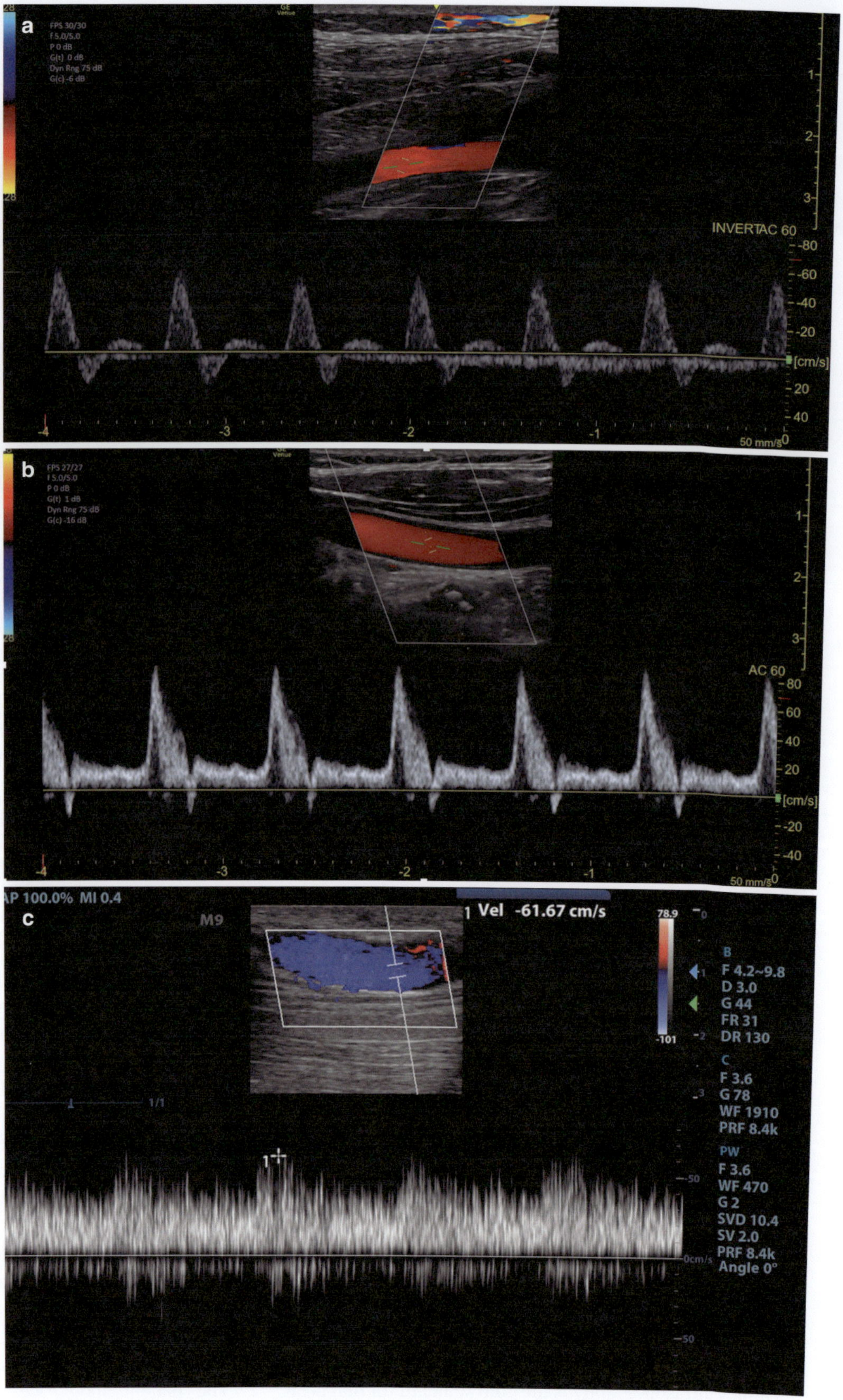

Fig. 20.11 Examples of spectral Doppler waveforms: (**a**) laminar flow pattern; (**b**) disturbed flow pattern; (**c**) turbulent flow pattern

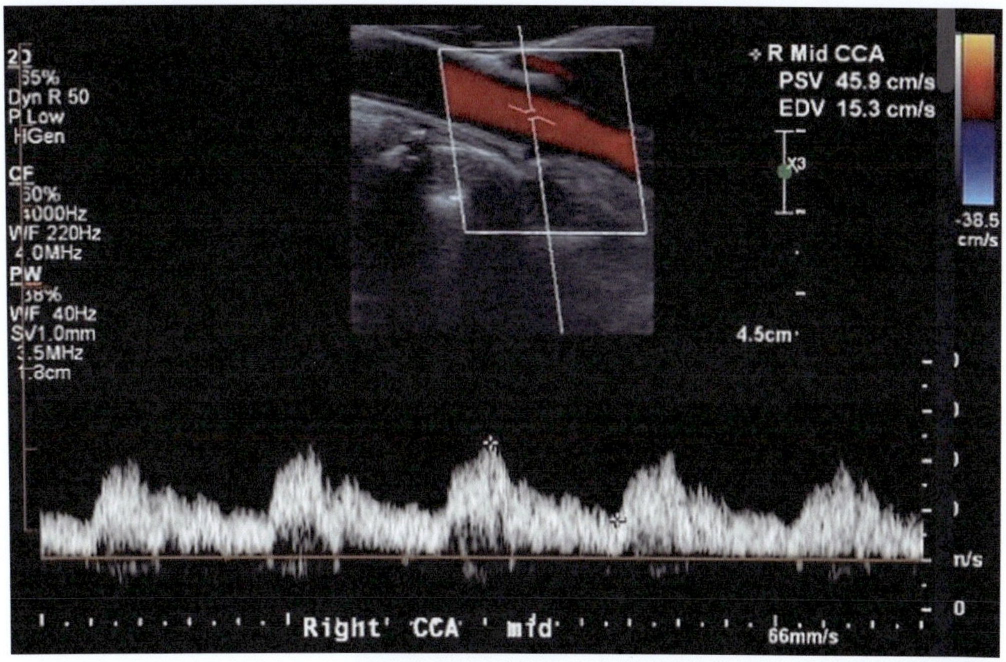

Fig. 20.12 Monophasic *tardus et parvus* waveform in pulsed-wave Doppler

Table 20.2 Mean artery diameters and peak systolic velocities in healthy subjects [13]

Artery	Mean (±SD) Diameter (cm)	Mean (±SD) Velocity (cm/s)
Infrarenal aorta	2.0 ± 0.2	55 ± 12
Common iliac	1.5 ± 0.18	70 ± 18
External iliac	0.8 ± 0.13	115 ± 21
Common femoral	0.8 ± 0.14	114 ± 24
Superior femoral	0.6 ± 11	90 ± 14
Popliteal	0.5 ± 0.1	68 ± 14
Tibial arteries	0.3 ± 0.4	55 ± 10

SD standard deviation

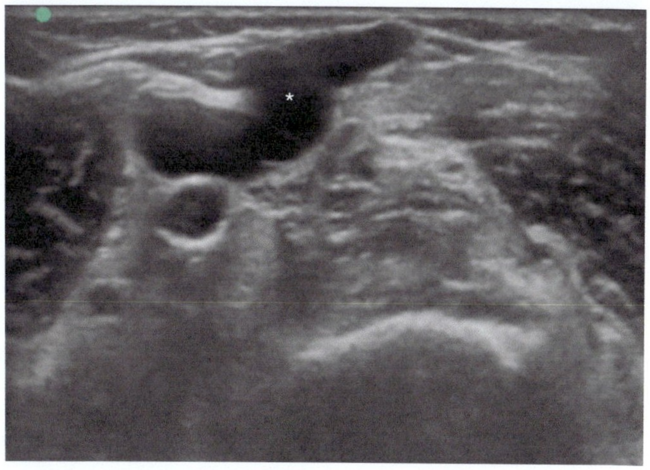

Fig. 20.14 Arteriovenous fistula with anastomosis (asterisk)

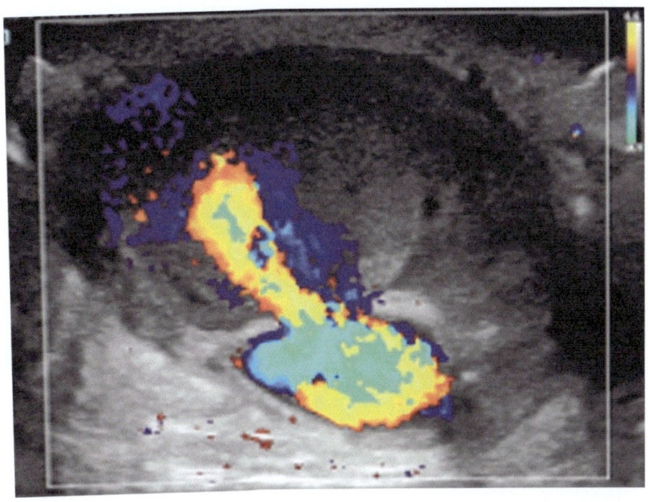

Fig. 20.13 Color Doppler image depicting the classic "yin-yang" sign of pseudoaneurysm

the scan of the graft or fistula with the evaluation of the inflow artery in the short-axis view (Fig. 20.14). The entire length of the access should be scanned in this orientation from the inflow artery to the outflow vein for an overall appreciation of anatomy. Next, return to the inflow artery and rotate the view to long axis. Examine the native arterial anastomosis sites with color Doppler and pulsed-wave Doppler (Figs. 20.15 and 20.16). As the AV fistula provides low-resistance outflow to the arterial bed, expect to see spectral broadening and diastolic flow throughout this area instead of the triphasic waveforms normally seen in peripheral arterial beds (Fig. 20.17). Continue scanning the remainder of the access in the long-axis view using color flow Doppler imaging as a guide for the placement of the pulsed-wave Doppler sample volume [18].

Patency should be assessed by visualizing the entire AV connection via color Doppler. If the flow is visualized throughout the entire vessel, then patency is confirmed (Fig. 20.18). Stenosis may be observed with color images when there is a narrowing of the lumen and turbulent flow is observed (Fig. 20.19). Pulsed-wave Doppler can help confirm this by demonstrating increased velocities (Fig. 20.20). A partial occlusion can be confirmed when color produces only a partial fill-in of the area being interrogated (Fig. 20.21). If no flow is visualized on color Doppler, this should raise concern for a complete occlusion but must be confirmed with pulsed-wave Doppler (Fig. 20.22). Evaluation should also assess for pseudoaneurysm (as described previously) (Fig. 20.23).

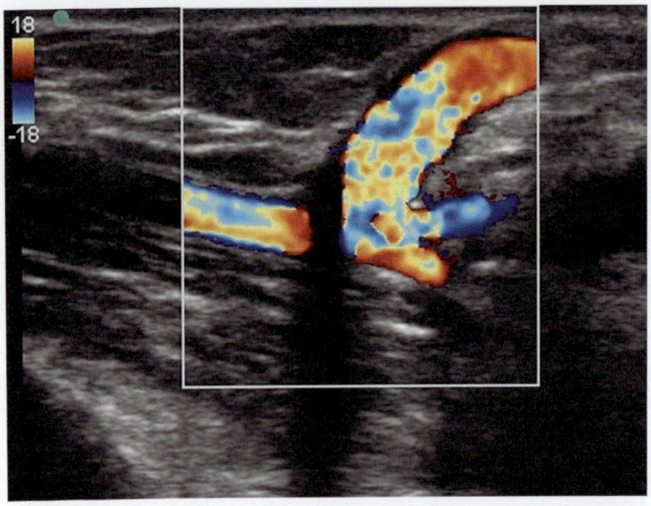

Fig. 20.15 Arteriovenous fistula anastomosis being evaluated with color Doppler and showing multidirectional flow

Carotid Artery Stenosis

Atherosclerotic carotid artery disease is a significant cause of stroke in the United States and globally [19]. Carotid artery ultrasound can be used to diagnose internal carotid artery (ICA) stenosis, detect an occluded vessel, and infer the cause of ischemic stroke [20].

Indications for carotid evaluation include stroke, concern for stenosis, intimal thickness measurement, dissection, occlusion, and plaque characterization and screening. Ultrasound has been shown to have a high level of accuracy compared to angiography for the diagnosis of severe stenosis with 85% sensitivity and 98% specificity for occlusions in the 70–99% range [21]. POCUS has been used for plaque screening to identify patients who might benefit from intensive medical therapy and has been shown to correlate with comprehensive carotid ultrasound performed in the vascular or radiology department [22].

Because of its superficial location in the anterior neck, evaluation of the carotid arteries can be performed with relative ease on most patients. The right common carotid artery (CCA) arises from the innominate artery, while the left CCA arises directly from the aortic arch. Each CCA then bifur-

Fig. 20.16 Arteriovenous fistula being evaluated with pulsed-wave Doppler and showing expected spectral broadening that occurs with turbulent flow

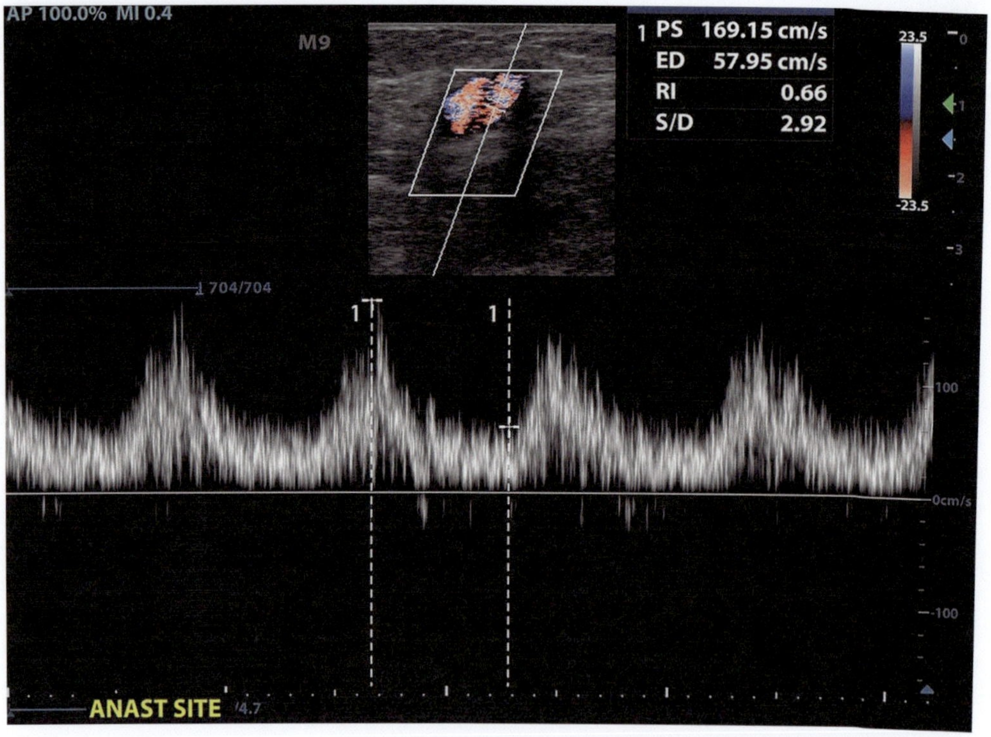

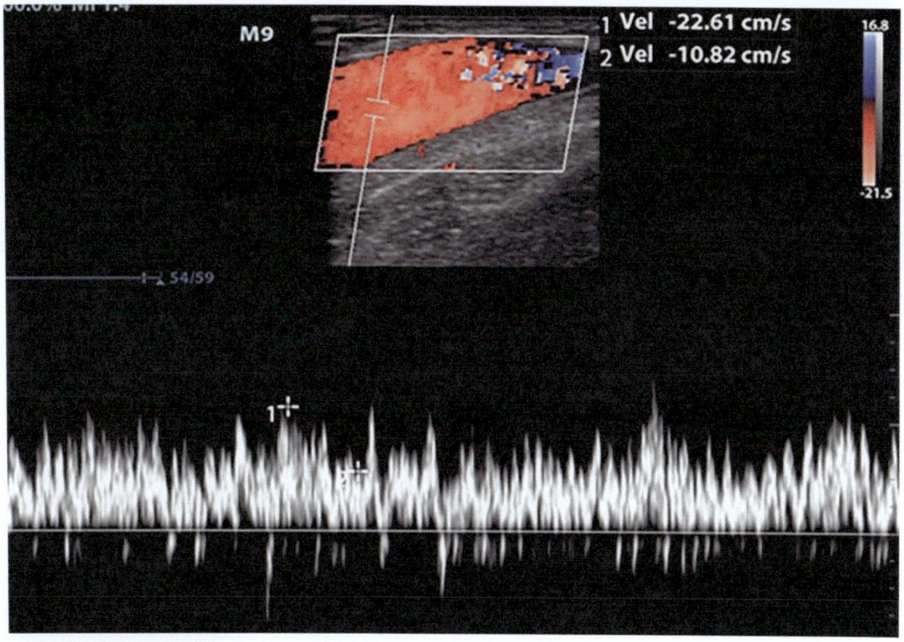

Fig. 20.17 Color and pulsed-wave Doppler of a patent arteriovenous fistula. Note the turbulent flow displayed on the spectral analysis

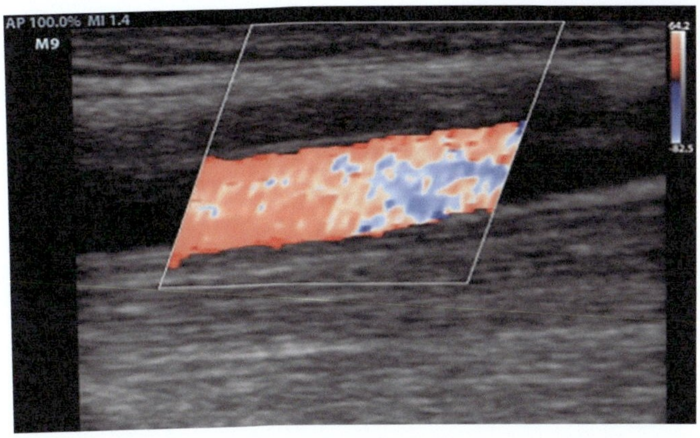

Fig. 20.18 Flow through a patent arteriovenous fistula visualized with color Doppler

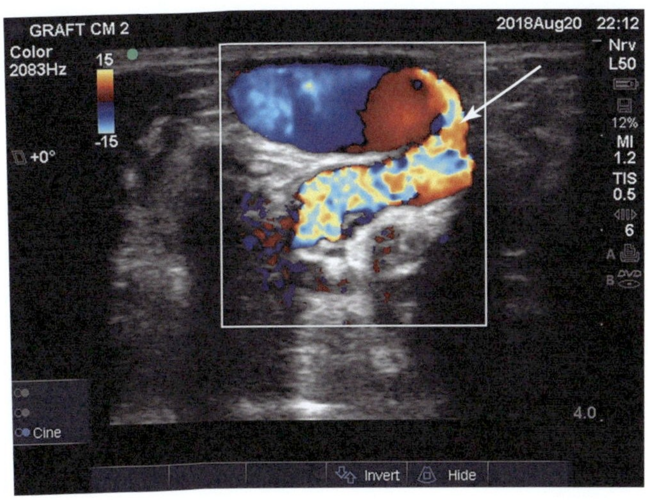

Fig. 20.19 Arteriovenous fistula with stenosis at the anastomosis (arrow)

cates into the ICA and the external carotid artery (ECA) (Fig. 20.24).

To perform the POCUS examination, patients should be positioned supine with their heads turned away from the side being interrogated. Copious amounts of ultrasound gel and a high-frequency linear probe should be used. In a complete evaluation, views of the CCA, carotid bulb, ICA, and ECA should all be obtained in the long and short axes, including color and pulsed-wave Doppler. The Doppler angle should be between 45 and 60 degrees for accurate velocity measurements.

Normal findings include smooth, plaque-free walls, an intima-media thickness (IMT) between 0.6–0.7 mm, and laminar flow on color Doppler (Figs. 20.25 and 20.26). The color scale should be set to around 35 m/sec. If the scales are set too low, a false positive for occlusion may occur due to lack of flow. If they are set too high, a false negative can occur due to color bleeding from surrounding structures. Waveforms demonstrated on spectral analysis when interrogating the extracranial vessels are either high or low resistance depending on the location. The CCA and ICA should demonstrate a low-resistance waveform with velocities not exceeding 180 cm/sec (Fig. 20.27a, b). The carotid bulb should demonstrate a turbulent waveform that is low resistance. The ECA should demonstrate a high-resistance waveform, though velocities should still not exceed 180 cm/s (Fig. 20.27c). Differentiating the ECA from the ICA can be performed by evaluating the flow pattern, as the proximity of these vessels to each other sometimes makes it difficult to differentiate between the two. The ECA should have a brisk upstroke and downstroke contrasted with the slower upstroke and prolonged downstroke of the ICA.

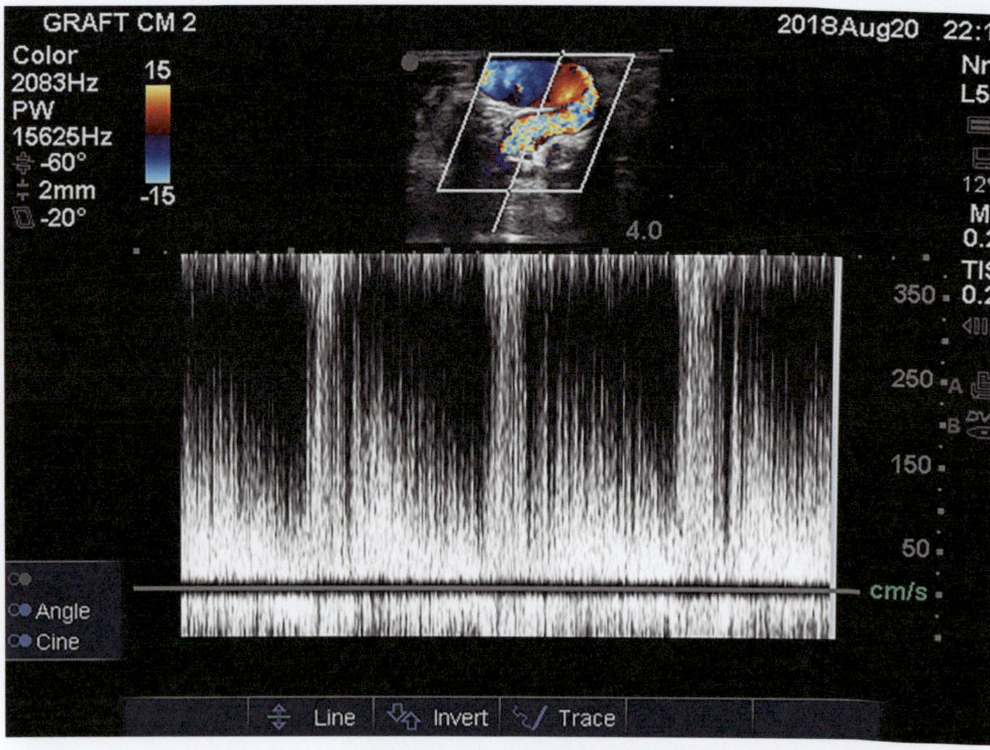

Fig. 20.20 Pulsed-wave Doppler showing stenosis at the anastomosis site

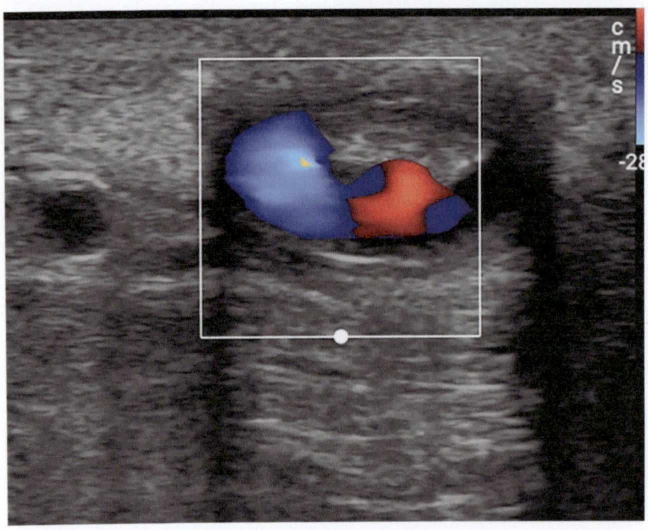

Fig. 20.21 Color flow seen surrounding echogenic thrombus in an arteriovenous fistula indicating a partial occlusion of the vessel

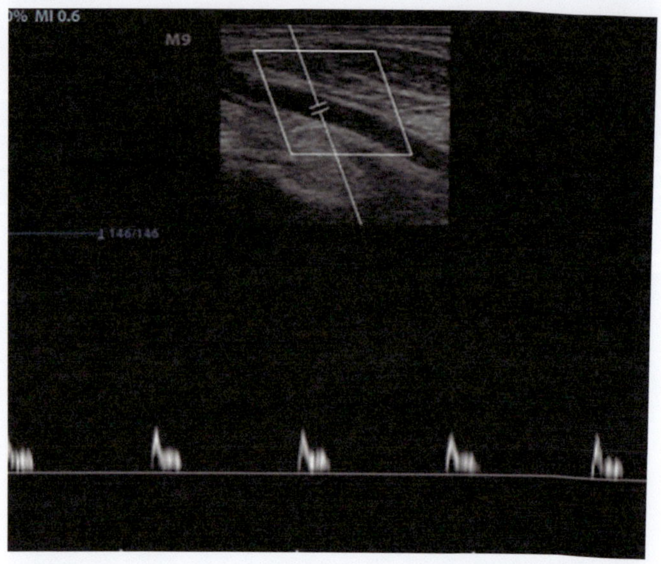

Fig. 20.22 Pulsed-wave Doppler showing significantly diminished flows in the case of an occlusive thrombus

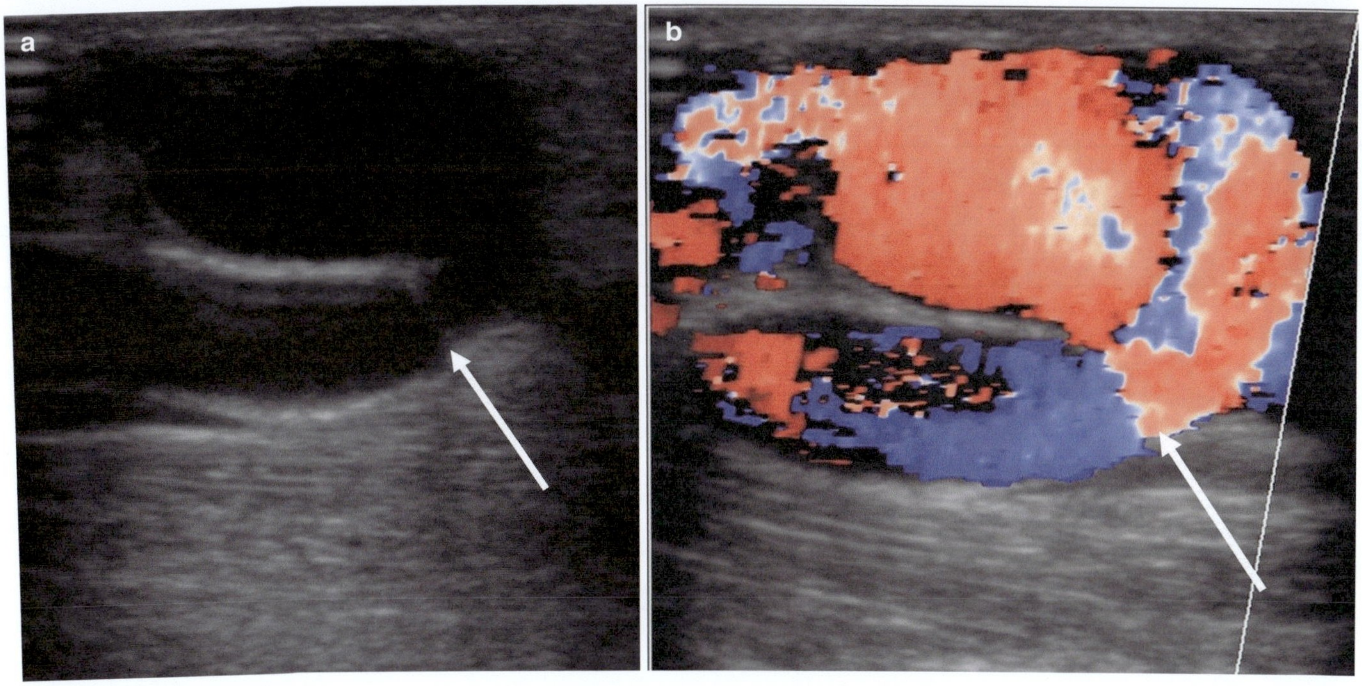

Fig. 20.23 Arteriovenous fistula aneurysm on (**a**) grayscale and (**b**) color Doppler

Fig. 20.24 Illustration of the anatomy of the vasculature of the neck

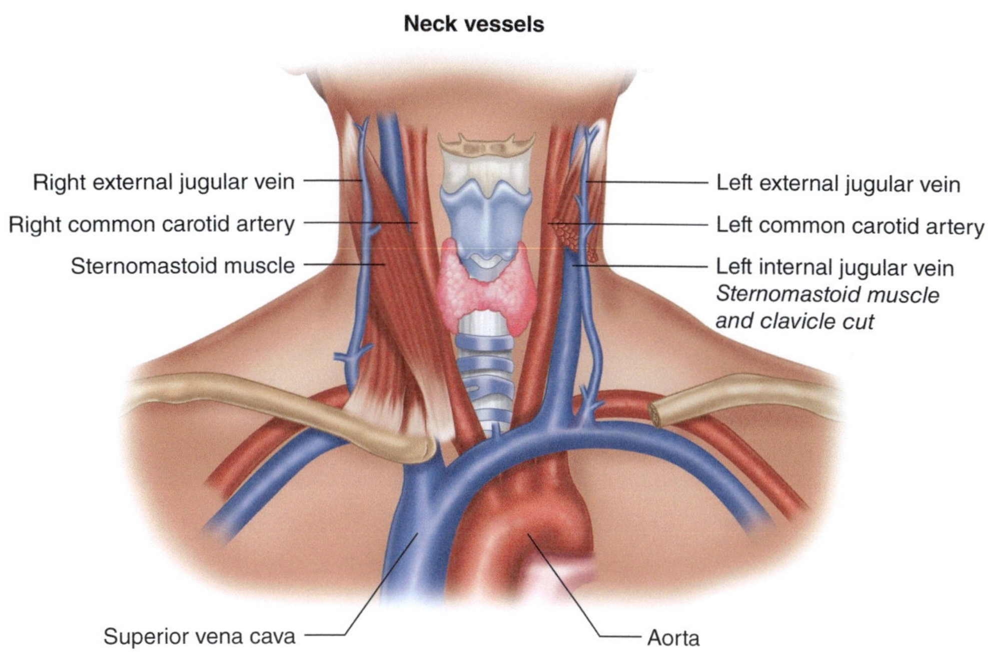

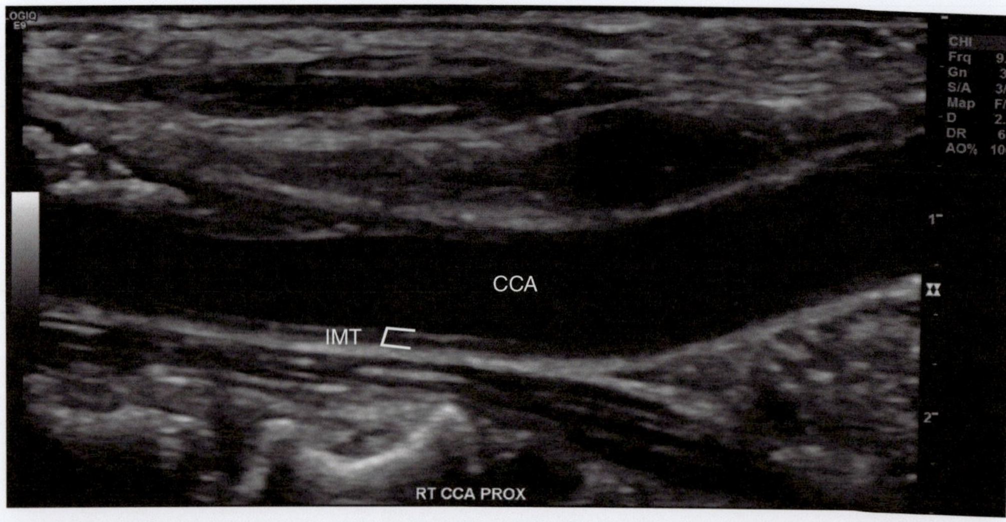

Fig. 20.25 Common carotid artery (CCA) with intima-media thickness (IMT) labeled

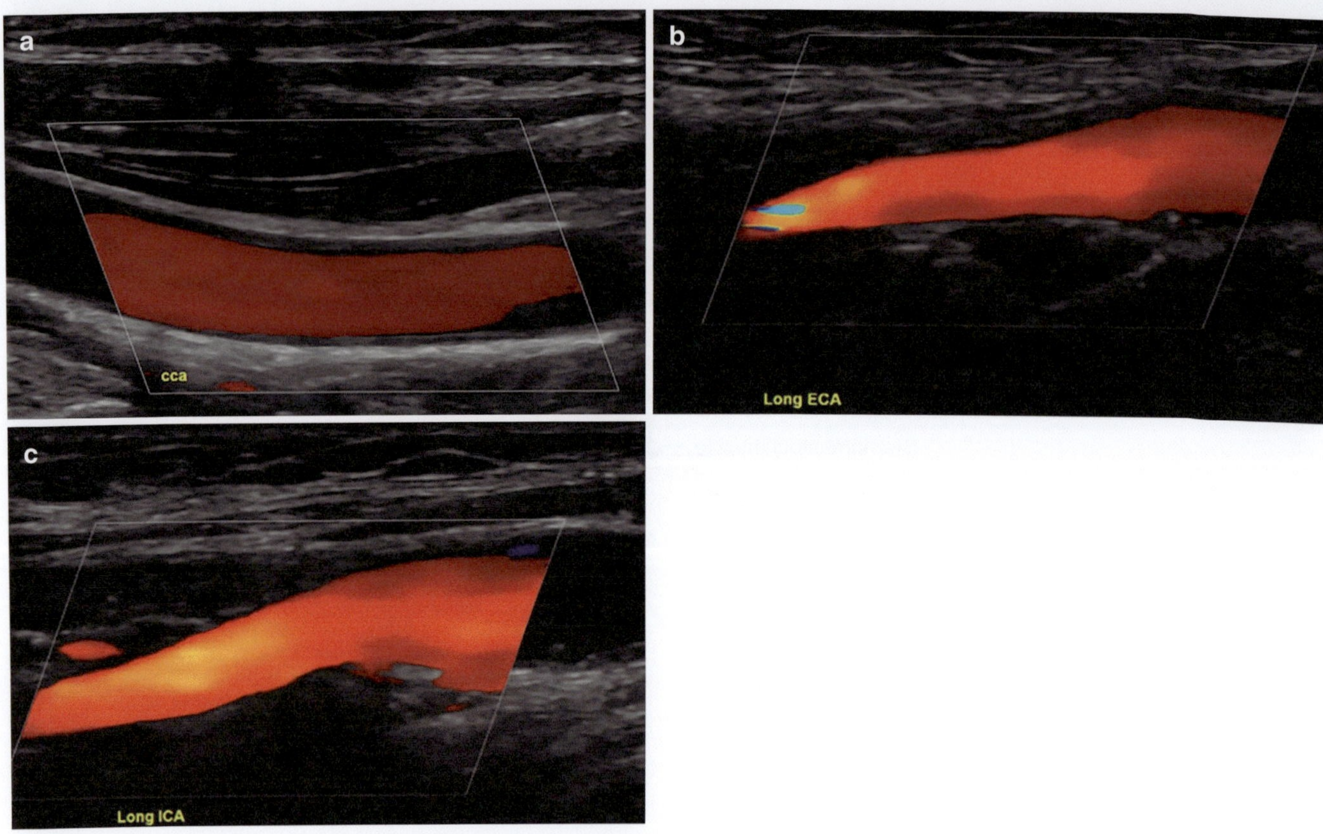

Fig. 20.26 (**a**) Long-axis view of the common carotid artery with color Doppler; (**b**) Long-axis view of the external carotid artery with color Doppler; (**c**) Long-axis view of the internal carotid artery with color Doppler

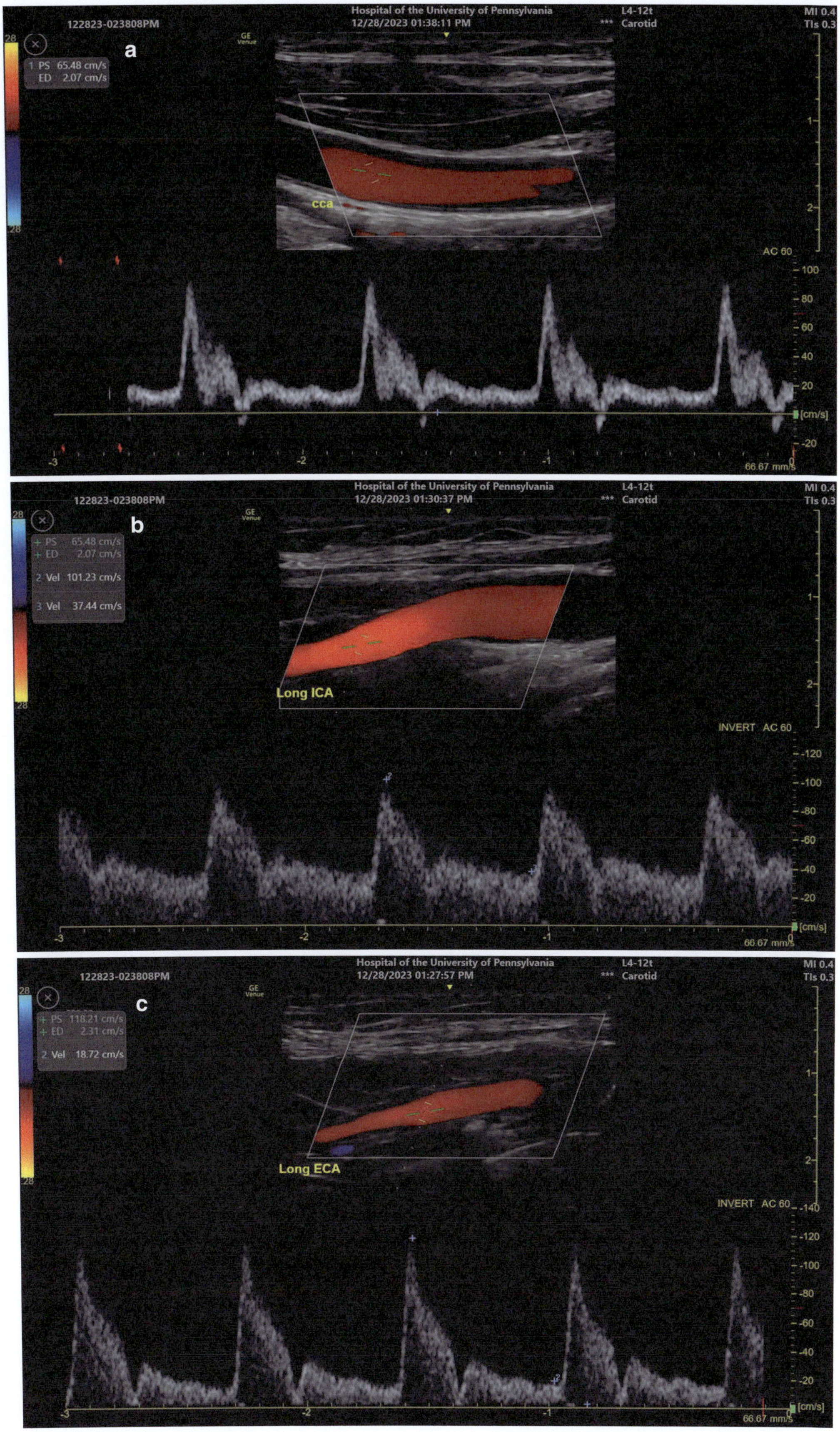

Fig. 20.27 (**a**) Pulsed-wave Doppler of the common carotid artery demonstrating a low-resistance waveform with gentle upstroke and prolonged downstroke; (**b**) Pulsed-wave Doppler of the internal carotid artery demonstrating a low-resistance waveform; (**c**) Pulsed-wave Doppler of the external carotid artery demonstrating a high-resistance waveform that has a brisk upstroke and downstroke

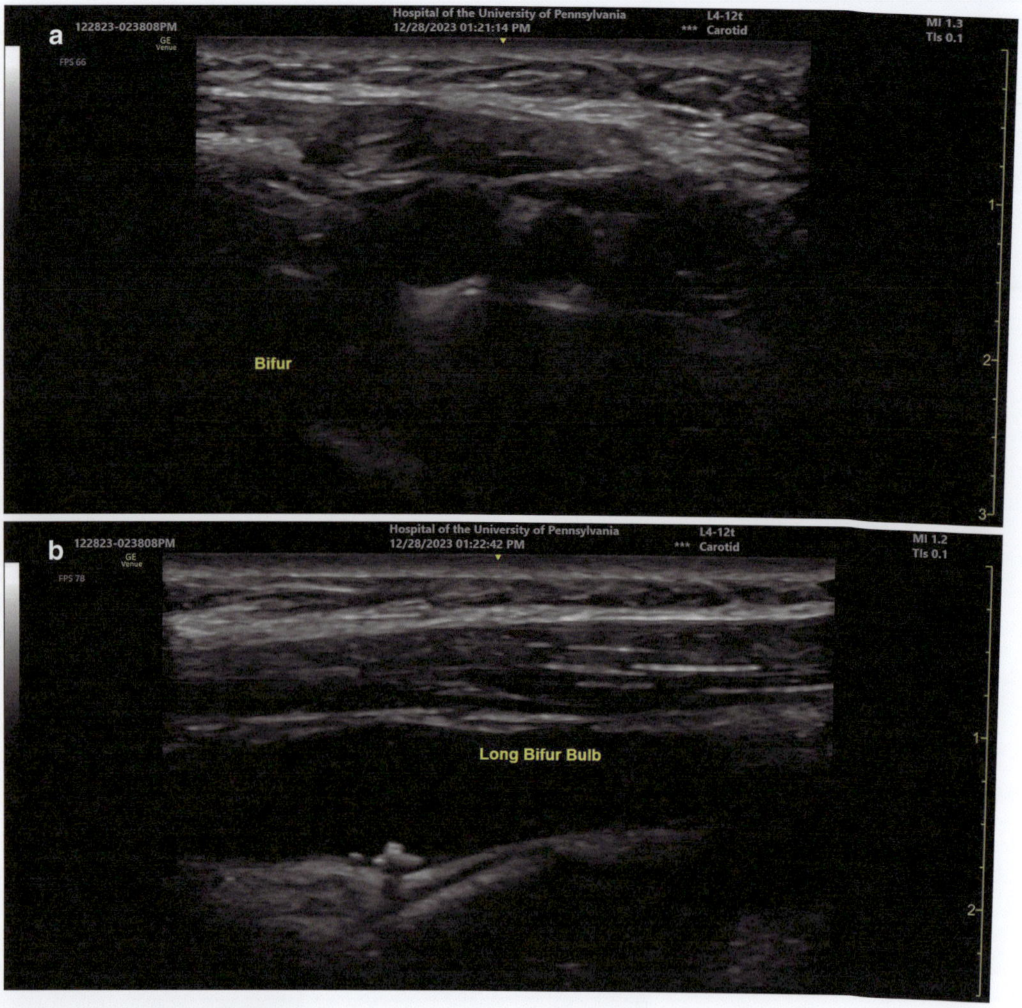

Fig. 20.28 (**a**) B-mode image of the carotid bulb and bifurcation in short axis; (**b**) B-mode images of the carotid bulb and bifurcation in long axis. Note the calcified plaque in the bulb with posterior shadowing

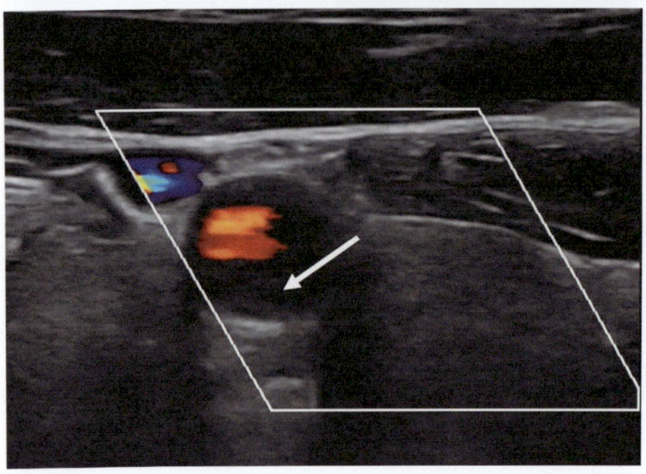

Fig. 20.29 Soft plaque seen within the common carotid indicated by the arrow. Note how there is a lack of echogenicity and shadowing, and the plaque only becomes readily apparent with the use of color Doppler

Carotid stenosis findings include narrowing of the lumen due to plaque, which may be calcified (i.e., hard) or anechoic (i.e., soft) (Figs. 20.28 and 20.29). Color Doppler images will demonstrate a turbulent string flow in the central portion of the vessel, shown with a variation of colors indicating variable velocities and directionality of flow (Fig. 20.30). On spectral Doppler analysis, velocities in the ICA exceeding 180 cm/sec along with a visual plaque estimate of >50% are consistent with a 50–69% stenosis (Fig. 20.31) [23]. Visual plaque estimates can be confirmed with a B-mode and color Doppler image showing a narrowing of 50%.

The accuracy of carotid duplex ultrasound in diagnosing total carotid occlusion has been shown to have a sensitivity of 91% and a specificity of 99% [24]. On color Doppler, the lumen will lack flow, and echogenic material may be observed in the vessel. On pulsed-wave Doppler, the lack of Doppler signal is confirmatory for an occlusion.

Carotid dissection occurs when the intimal layer tears away from the media, allowing blood to become trapped between the layers. The risk factors for dissection include trauma, connective tissue disorders, and family history. Dissection appears as a pulsating echogenic line within the lumen of the vessel. Flow should be assessed with color Doppler, which can show a string of color in the true lumen and flow in the opposite direction in the false lumen or a complete lack of flow in the false lumen due to thrombosis (Fig. 20.32).

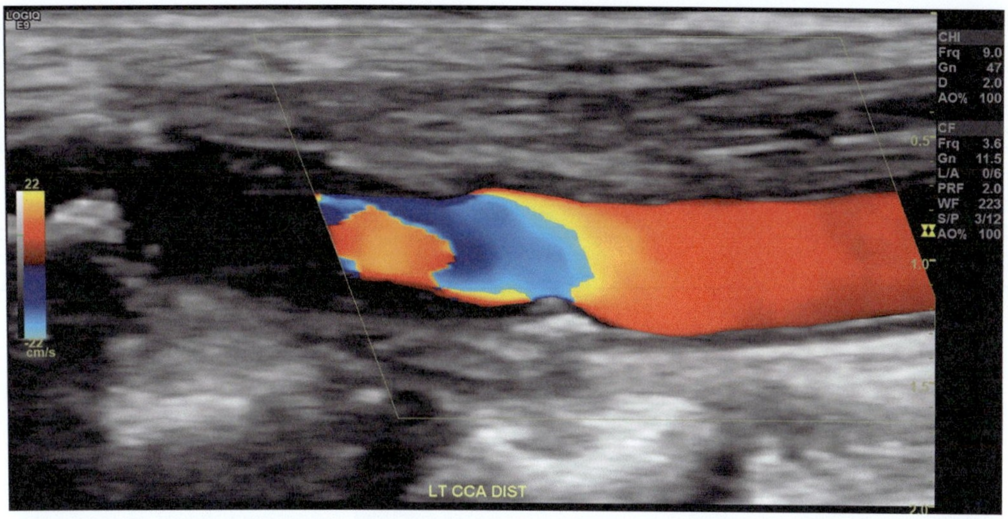

Fig. 20.30 Color Doppler showing stenosis with luminal narrowing and turbulence of flow

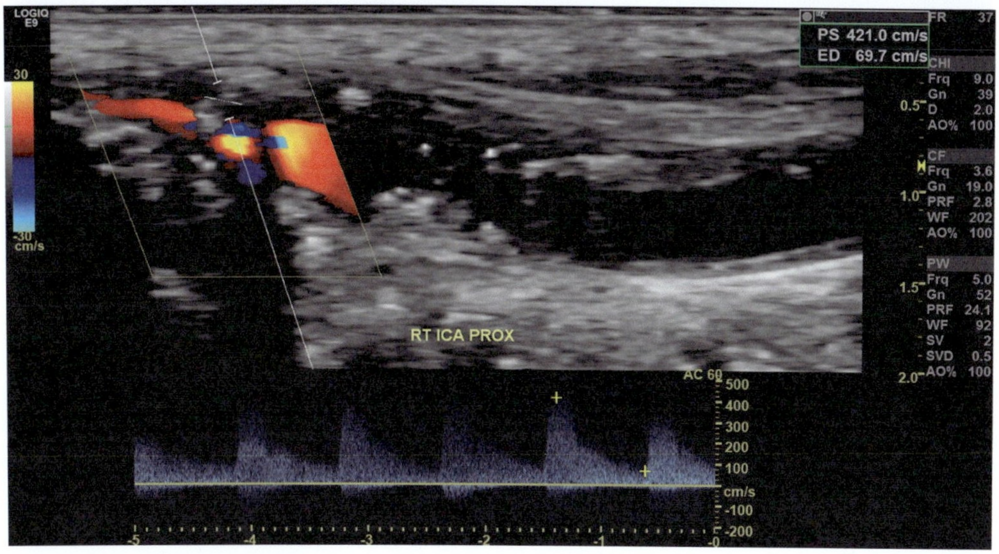

Fig. 20.31 Pulsed-wave Doppler demonstrating stenosis of the internal carotid artery showing peak velocities of nearly 400 cm/s and loss of the internal carotid artery's typical low-resistance waveform

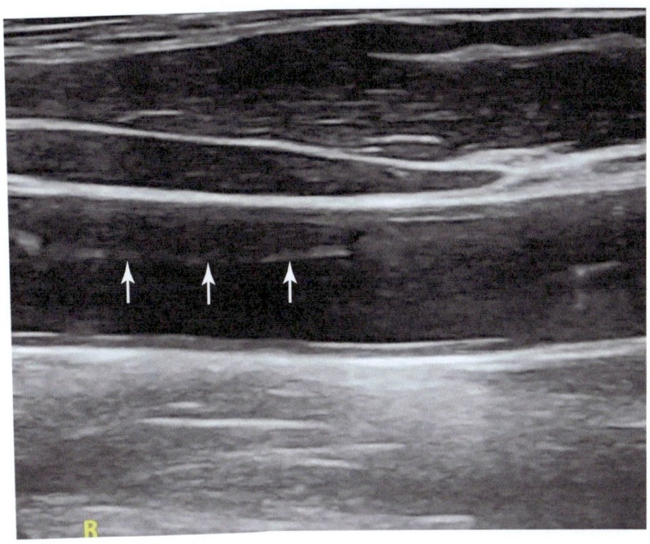

Fig. 20.32 Dissection of the carotid artery with the arrows marking the flap

Venous Assessment

Doppler ultrasound is a noninvasive diagnostic test capable of providing an anatomic and hemodynamic map for the venous circulation in real time and is often the gold standard test for assessing venous disease including deep venous thrombosis (DVT) [25]. Sonographically, vasculature appears as well-defined, anechoic circular structures in a transverse view. Arteries tend to be thicker-walled, pulsatile, rounder, and more difficult to compress. In contrast, veins have thinner walls, are nonpulsatile, and are easier to compress (Fig. 20.33). Importantly, both veins and arteries can be compressed, particularly in the hypotensive patient, so reliance on compression in isolation should not be used to differentiate these structures. We recommend applying partial pressure to distort the walls and assessing for pulsatility to differentiate artery from vein. Color or pulsed-wave Doppler assessment can also help to differentiate the pulsatile waveform in arteries from the low steady flow state of veins. The majority of Doppler ultrasound venous assessments are performed using B-mode ultrasound; however, color and pulsed-wave Doppler may be used to further characterize pathology as part of a duplex ultrasound examination.

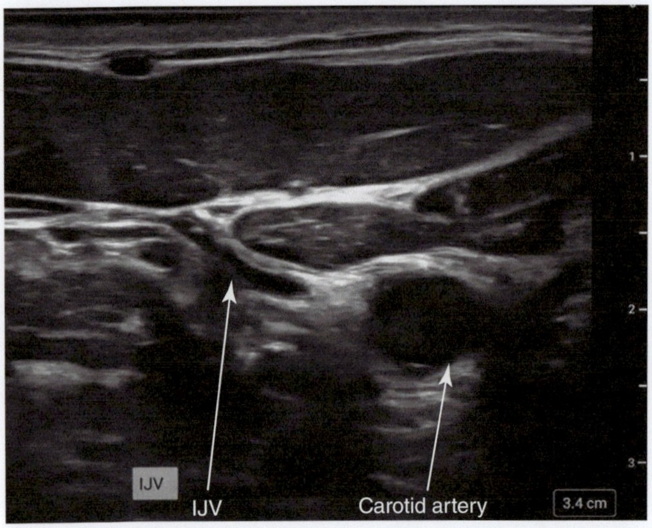

Fig. 20.33 Collapsing internal jugular vein (IJV) and non-compressed carotid artery under pressure from ultrasound probe

Lower Extremity Deep Venous Thrombosis

POCUS is an easy and efficient diagnostic tool for DVT. With adequate training, physicians can perform lower extremity compression ultrasonography exams rapidly and with high diagnostic accuracy to detect a DVT [26]. A meta-analysis of 15 studies showed that POCUS can accurately diagnose lower extremity DVT with a pooled sensitivity of 90% and specificity of 95%, with improved accuracy seen among more experienced users [27].

Classic vascular studies performed by radiology use a combination of B-mode imaging with compression and the use of color and/or spectral Doppler ultrasound. Recent literature in emergency medicine and critical care has demonstrated that B-mode compression ultrasound exams alone yield similar accuracy as radiology-performed vascular studies [28]. Fig. 20.34 shows the anatomy of the lower extremity venous vasculature, along with normal venous structures in grayscale.

Fig. 20.34 Illustration of the anatomy of lower extremity venous vasculature

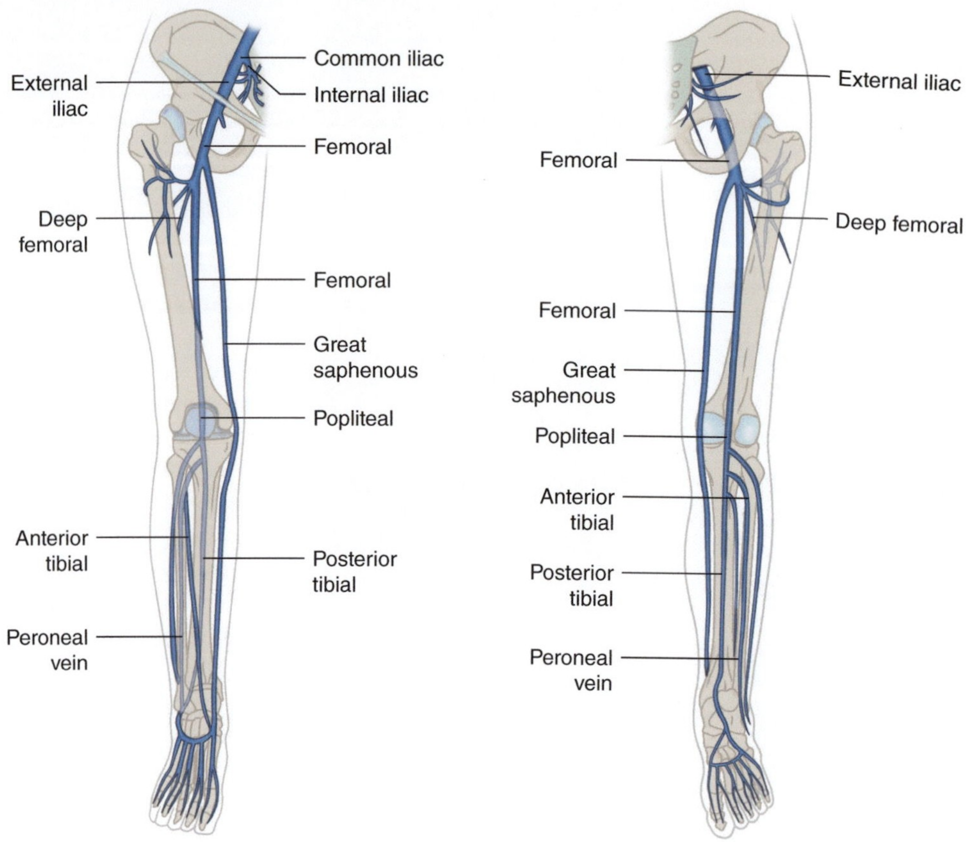

There are different approaches when performing this application: two region, three region, and comprehensive [29]. Two-region ultrasound refers to a focused assessment of only the common femoral vein and popliteal vein, with these two sites being selected because they are two of the higher-risk areas of the lower extremity for DVT [30]. Importantly, while this is commonly referred to as two-point ultrasound in the literature, it is more appropriately considered two region, as it involves compression of the femoral veins 1–2 cm above and below the saphenofemoral junction and compression of the popliteal vein extending through the confluence of the calf veins [31]. Three-region ultrasound (also known as extended compression ultrasound) includes the two regions previously mentioned, as well as the femoral vein (previously referred to as the superficial femoral vein) (Fig. 20.35). Compression of the femoral vein should occur every 1–2 cm down the length of the leg as it transitions to the popliteal vein [31]. The two-region technique offers the advantage of being faster to perform and avoiding the challenges of tracking the femoral vein distally. When a normal D-dimer blood test is used in combination with the two-region technique, this strategy performs with comparable accuracy to whole-leg ultrasound [32].

While some literature had suggested that the two-region and three-region techniques had nearly equivalent diagnostic accuracy [33], other studies have reported that up to 5.5% of all DVTs may be isolated to the femoral vein [30]. Therefore, a three-region technique may have a lower risk of missing DVTs and is generally favored when there is reasonable concern for the pathology. The comprehensive approach is generally considered to be outside of the scope of POCUS and is usually limited to radiology settings. It includes scanning the

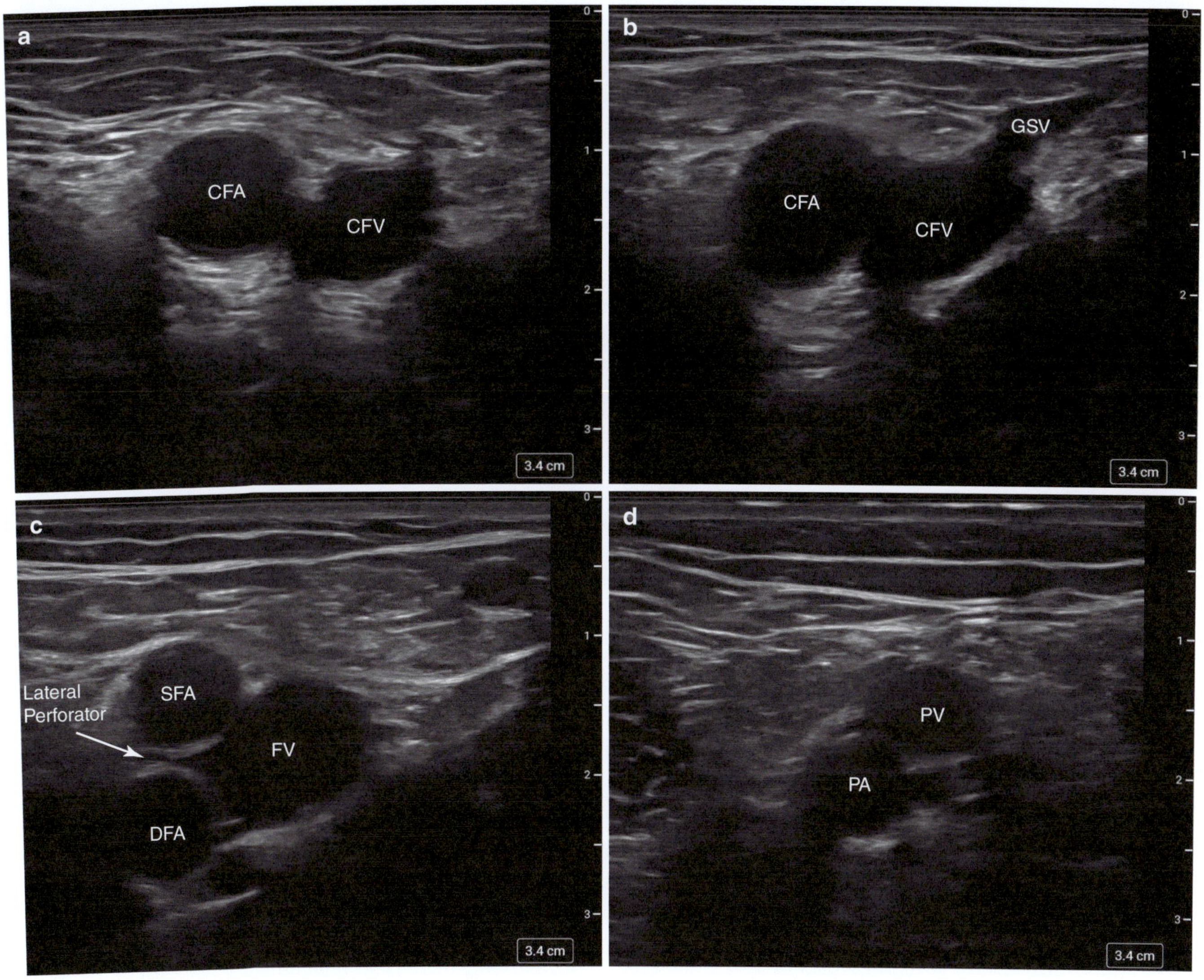

Fig. 20.35 (**a**) Common femoral vein just distal to the inguinal canal; (**b**) Common femoral vein at the saphenofemoral junction; (**c**) Femoral vein adjacent to the superficial and deep femoral artery. Note the lateral perforator vein (arrow) traversing the bifurcated artery; (**d**) Popliteal vein at the level of the popliteal crease

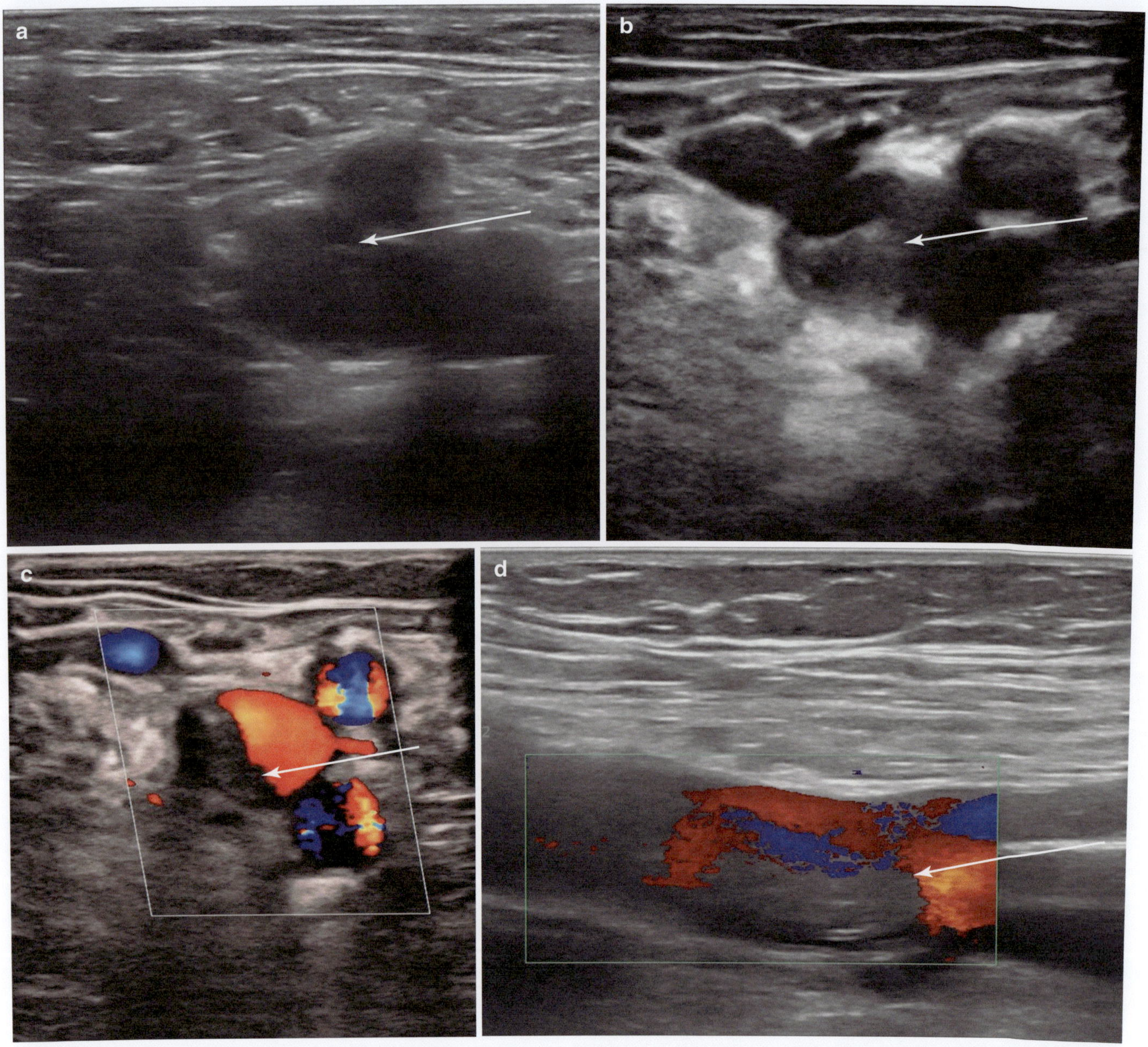

Fig. 20.36 (**a**) Acute deep venous thrombosis (arrow) found in the common femoral vein at the saphenofemoral junction. Note the hypoechoic appearance suggesting an acute deep venous thrombosis; (**b**) Subacute deep venous thrombosis (arrow) found in the common femoral vein at the saphenofemoral junction. Note the more hyperechoic appearance suggesting greater chronicity; (**c**) Deep venous thrombosis with filling defect (arrow) seen on color Doppler in short axis in this same patient as (**b**). (**d**) Deep venous thrombosis with filling defect (arrow) seen on color Doppler in long axis. (*Images courtesy of Michael Gottlieb, MD)*

entire lower extremity from the common femoral veins through to the calf veins.

Normal veins should fully compress with opposing walls completely collapsing under light pressure. The inability to completely compress the venous lumen is the main criterion for diagnosing an acute DVT. Most DVT develops around valve sinuses, especially at the bifurcations where there is decreased blood flow and turbulence, so it is particularly important to thoroughly assess these regions (e.g., saphenofemoral junction, popliteal trifurcation). The sonographic appearance of venous thrombi varies based on age, extent, and location. Acute DVTs appear anechoic or hypoechoic and cause greater venous distention than chronic thrombi (Fig. 20.36a, Video 5). Subacute or chronic thrombi are more echogenic due to fibrin deposition and can often be seen without compression (Fig. 20.36b, Video 6). At times, after a DVT episode, there is an inflammatory response in the vein wall and in the thrombus itself, leading to a dynamic process in which the thrombus regresses due to recanalization (return of blood flow to a venous segment that had previously been

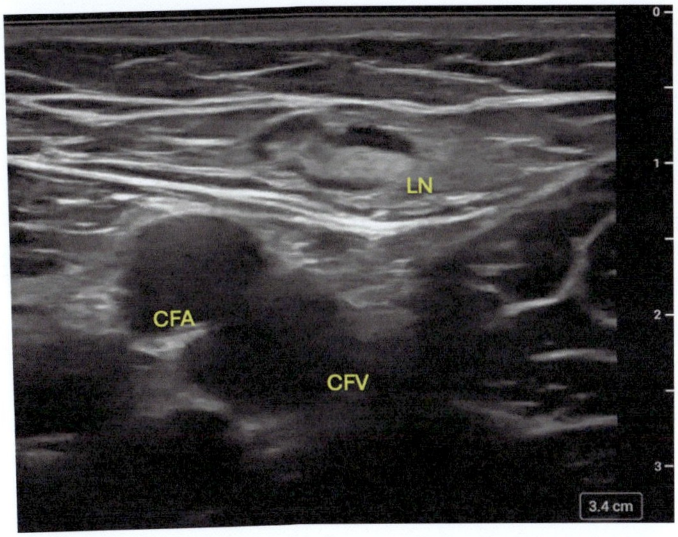

Fig. 20.37 Ultrasound image of an inguinal lymph node (LN) next to the common femoral artery (CFA) and common femoral vein (CFV)

occluded), resulting in partial compressibility of the lumen [34]. Knowledge of the location of the previous DVT may be helpful when determining acute clots from chronic inflammation.

Inguinal lymph nodes (LNs) can be mistaken for DVTs due to their similar appearance and non-compressibility. It is important to recognize that lymph nodes have a hypoechoic appearance and are ovoid structures (Fig. 20.37). Additionally, they are generally more superficial, do not have an adjacent arterial structure, and cannot be tracked proximally or distally along the limb.

Color Doppler can be used to further assess the vein or to confirm a diagnosis when B-mode is nondiagnostic or if one has concerns for a possible anechoic DVT. Fanning the ultrasound beam toward the patient's heart will cause venous blood flow to appear blue (the direction of flow is away from the probe). In a normal exam, color fills the entire venous lumen. This technique should be performed in both planes (Fig. 20.36c, d, Video 7).

Color Doppler assessment can further be enhanced by using augmentation. Augmentation is a technique where the probe is placed proximally on the leg, typically at the popliteal vein, while in color or pulsed-wave Doppler mode. The calf is then squeezed or compressed along the venous system in order to increase venous return (Fig. 20.38). In theory, if no DVT is present, there will be an increase in flow velocity noted once the blood flow passes the area of the ultrasound probe. A lack of increased flow may suggest an occlusive or partially occlusive thrombus between the two points. However, augmentation has largely fallen out of favor in vascular labs as it rarely provides additional information in the diagnosis of DVT and can present a false negative finding if there is sufficient collateral blood flow [35]. Therefore, single-point augmentation does not add to the standard compression ultrasound examination for suspected DVT and should not be routinely performed.

Use of respiratory phasicity can also provide indirect venous assessment of the adjacent vein segments and should be performed to confirm or further investigate a suspected positive study. Respiratory phasicity assessment involves placing the ultrasound probe along the common femoral vein and using the pulsed-wave Doppler mode. Flow velocity in the deep venous structures should vary with a normal respiratory and cardiac cycle. A lack of variation in flow may be suggestive of an obstructive process such as a thrombus along the venous system between the inferior vena cava and the location of the ultrasound probe (Fig. 20.39) [36].

Upper Extremity DVT

Upper extremity DVT accounts for approximately 5 to 10 percent of all cases of DVT [37]. In the upper extremity, the deep veins include the radial, ulnar, brachial, axillary, and subclavian veins. The most common site of upper extremity DVT involves the axillary and subclavian veins; however, the more distal brachial vein may also be involved [38]. Catheter-associated upper extremity DVT is the most common etiology and accounts for the increasing incidences of upper extremity DVTs [37]. Other risk factors include malignancy, recent surgery or trauma, use of hormone therapy, hereditary or acquired thrombophilia, strenuous muscular effort, and anatomical abnormalities including an enlarged costoclavicular ligament [39].

Comprehensive duplex examination has high accuracy for the detection of upper extremity DVTs and is the screening technique of choice with a sensitivity ranging from 78% to 100% and specificity of 82% to 100% [40]. Upper extremity DVT assessment has not been well-studied in the point-of-care setting; therefore, diagnostic accuracies have been abstracted from radiology literature. There are sonographic limitations, as false negative results may occur with small nonobstructive thrombi that cannot be directly assessed with compression techniques because of overlying bones. In addition, segments of the subclavian vein, the brachiocephalic vein, and their confluence with the superficial vena cava may be difficult to visualize in some patients. Therefore, contrast-enhanced computed tomographic or magnetic venography may be needed in select cases [41].

The venous anatomy of the upper extremity is illustrated in Fig. 20.40. The general ultrasound protocol for the assessment of upper extremity DVT includes the interrogation of the internal jugular, brachiocephalic, subclavian, axillary, brachial, and basilic veins of the symptomatic upper extremity. Evaluation of the cephalic vein at its confluence with the subclavian vein should also be performed, although this may

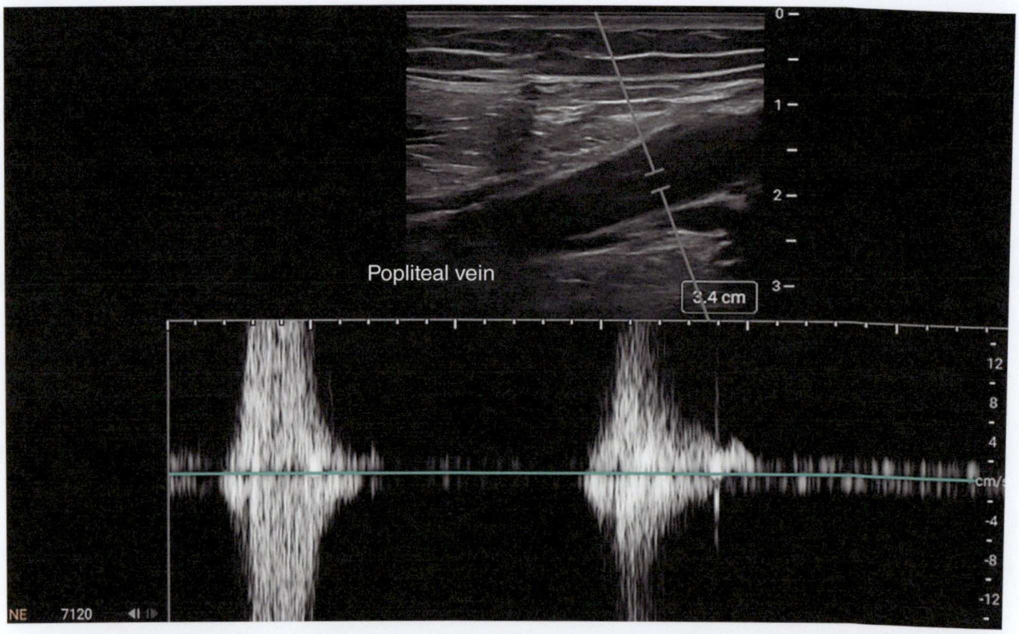

Fig. 20.38 Pulsed-wave Doppler demonstrating increased venous return with augmentation of the popliteal vein

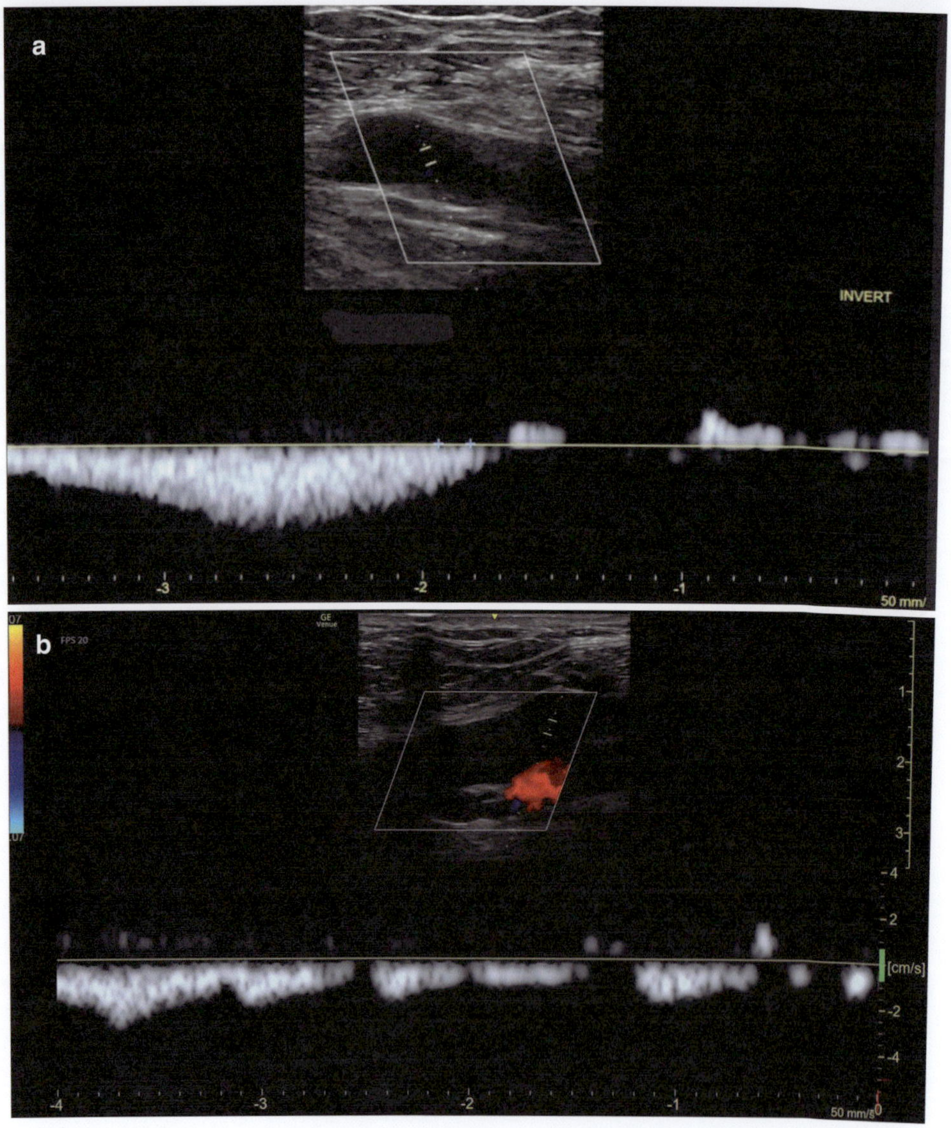

Fig. 20.39 (**a**) Normal common femoral vein waveforms with pulsed-wave Doppler; (**b**) Abnormal common femoral vein waveforms with pulsed-wave Doppler

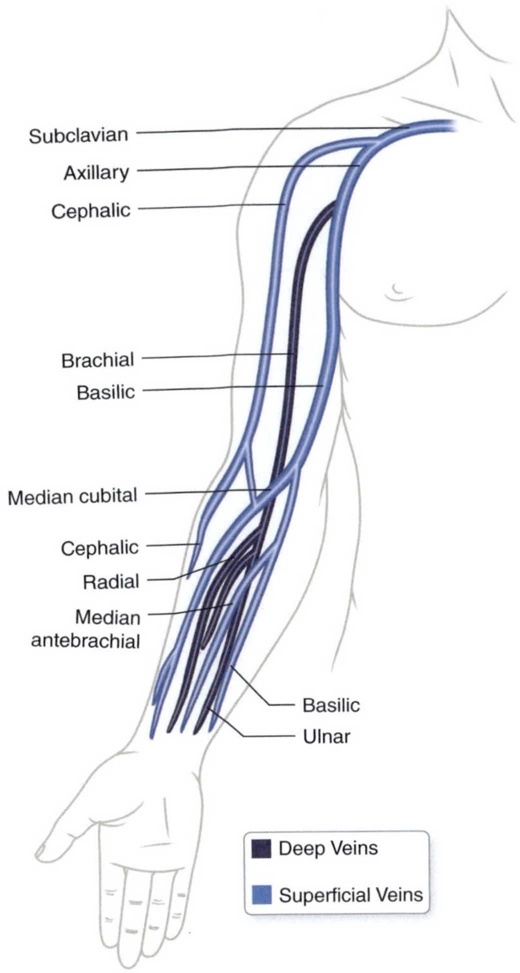

Fig. 20.40 Illustration of the anatomy of upper extremity venous vasculature

be difficult to visualize in some patients. The radial and ulnar veins may be interrogated when there are specific symptoms referable to these regions. Duplex Doppler sonography of the contralateral asymptomatic limb is also typically performed because waveform asymmetry may indicate a more central obstruction that is difficult to visualize directly. When possible and accessible, a transverse compression technique should always be used primarily. Color Doppler, as well as pulsed-wave Doppler, imaging may be used as an adjunct or for further investigation when direction compression is not possible (Fig. 20.41).

The patient should be placed in the supine position with the arm to be examined comfortably extended to approximately 60° from the chest. Hyperextension should be avoided as it inhibits normal flow and may create the appearance of an abnormal waveform. Use a high-frequency linear array probe. Curvilinear probes may be preferred in the axillary areas or in larger individuals because of better depth penetration. Place the probe gently over the mid-portion of the inner aspect of the upper arm in a transverse plane and identify the

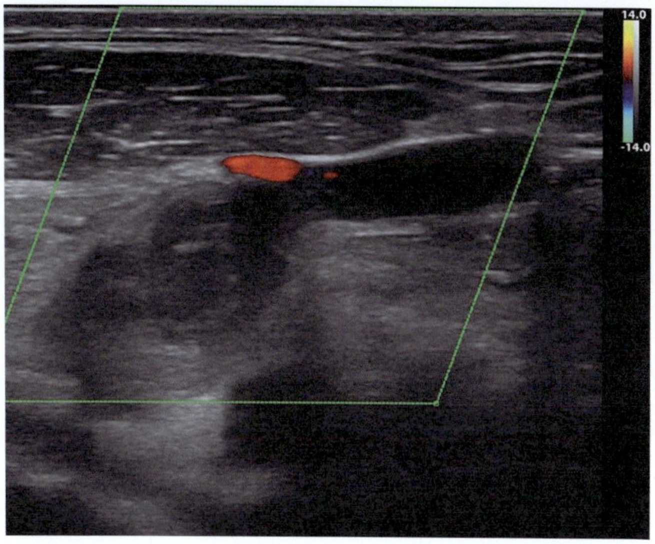

Fig. 20.41 Ultrasound of a subclavian vein DVT with color Doppler

brachial artery. The artery can be differentiated from the veins by its pulsatility and direction. The brachial veins, which are often paired, are generally close to the artery. Superficial to this area, the basilic vein is identified, which is often larger than the deep brachial veins, despite being part of the superficial venous system. The basilic vein can develop significant clot burden; hence, it is important to assess it during the exam. Once the veins of the arm are interrogated, move the probe proximal toward the axillary vein, which lies beneath the pectoralis minor. Over the chest wall, angle the probe cephalad and slide medially beneath the clavicle to identify part of the subclavian vein. When viewed from beneath the clavicle, the vein lies superficial and caudal to the adjacent artery. Complete the exam by evaluating the internal jugular vein.

Superficial Thrombophlebitis

Superficial thrombophlebitis occurs when there is a thrombosis or inflammation of the superficial veins. Most commonly, this occurs in varicose veins, specifically in the great saphenous vein [42]. While a comprehensive evaluation may include starting from the proximal entry of the great saphenous vein into the femoral vein or the small saphenous vein into the popliteal vein, this can be time-consuming and technically challenging. More frequently, the clinician performs a focused examination at the site of the symptoms. Findings that are common in DVT (non-compressibility of the vein) are also present in superficial thrombophlebitis, along with surrounding inflammation, or cobblestoning, of the surrounding tissues (Fig. 20.42). When performing an initial survey of the underlying anatomical structures, the operator should take care not to obscure the vessel due to pressure from the probe, as this can lead to a nondiagnostic scan. To avoid this, place the fifth finger of the hand holding the probe at a distant site to reduce pressure and use copious ultrasound gel.

Lemierre's Syndrome

Lemierre's syndrome is a rare but serious complication of oropharyngeal infections. It is characterized by the penetration of the primary infection into the lateral pharyngeal space, suppurative thrombophlebitis of the internal jugular vein, and metastatic infections from septic emboli. While the gold standard imaging choice remains a contrast-enhanced computed tomography of the neck, ultrasound can assess for the presence of a DVT involving the internal jugular and deep upper extremity veins. Multiple case reports have described extensive clot burden of the internal jugular vein extending into the axillary vein through to the basilic vein (Fig. 20.43) [43, 44].

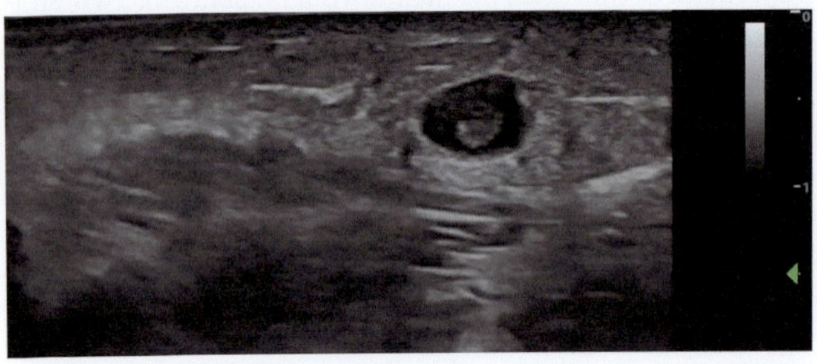

Fig. 20.42 Superficial thrombophlebitis

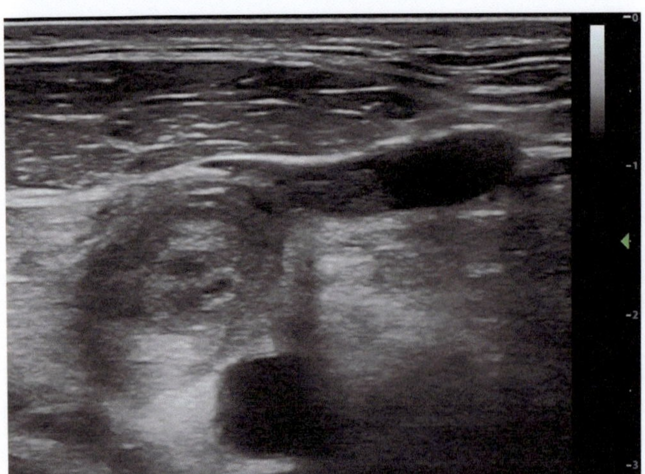

Fig. 20.43 Thrombophlebitis of the internal jugular vein (IJV) with clot burden extension into the axillary and basilic vein

Key Ultrasound Findings

Diagnosis	Diagnostic criteria
Peripheral arterial disease	Plaque or arterial structure abnormality in B-mode. Flow pattern and direction in color Doppler mode. Flow waveform and peak systolic velocity in pulsed-wave Doppler mode. Peak systolic velocity ratios.
Pseudoaneurysm	Measurement of their size, residual lumen, and length and width in B-mode. Identifying the neck of the lesion. Visualizing the classic "yin-yang" sign. Visualizing the "to-and-fro" pattern of blood flow in femoral pseudoaneurysm.
Arteriovenous fistula patency	B-mode: Smooth walls, uniform in size throughout, no echogenic material present in the lumen. Color Doppler: Laminar flow throughout, minimal color aliasing at the anastomosis sites.
Carotid artery stenosis	B-mode: Visible plaque in the internal carotid artery. Color Doppler: Decreased flow in the lumen (usually in the area where the plaque is present); no flow in areas of complete occlusion.
Deep venous thrombosis (lower and upper)	Incomplete compression of the vein. Visualizing clot or structural abnormality in B-mode. The clot may be anechoic if more acute. Filling defects using color Doppler. Changes in normal respiratory phasicity.
Superficial thrombophlebitis	Non-compressibility of a superficial vessel. Cobblestoning.
Lemierre's syndrome	Visualizing the internal jugular vein for abnormalities and clot burden (seen as echogenic material within the lumen). Incomplete compression of the deep venous veins in the neck and upper extremity including the subclavian, axillary, brachial, and basilic veins. Filling defects using color Doppler of the internal jugular vein and other deep veins. Changes in normal respiratory phasicity using spectral Doppler.

Pearls and Pitfalls

- When using duplex ultrasonography for arterial assessment, enhance the image by optimizing color gain and pulse repetition frequency to easily see flow abnormalities, ensuring the vessel sample size is small and fits in the lumen to avoid extra noise and artifacts, and the angle is corrected to the direction of blood flow at 60 degrees or less.

(continued)

- When assessing arterial disease in the lower extremity, consider extending the exam to include the aorta when a central cause is suspected, particularly with a positive bilateral lower extremity arterial exam.
- A detailed knowledge of vascular anatomy for a given region, including branches and bifurcation points, is important, as these are the most common places for thrombosis to occur.
- Compression for lower extremity DVT assessment should begin immediately distal to the inguinal canal at the level of the external iliac vein, and complete compression of veins under light pressure should be visualized in normal veins.

References

1. Katsi V, Felekos I, Kallikazaros I. Christian Andreas Doppler: a legendary man inspired by the dazzling light of the stars. Hippokratia. 2013;17(2):113–4.
2. Zierler RE. From Doppler to duplex: a personal early history of the vascular laboratory. Vasc Med. 2021;26(3):338–45. https://doi.org/10.1177/1358863X211002644.
3. Strandness DE, McCutcheon EP, Rushmer RF. Application of a transcutaneous Doppler flowmeter in evaluation of occlusive arterial disease. Surg Gynecol Obstet. 1966;122(5):1039–45.
4. Iannuzzi A, Rubba P, Gentile M, et al. Carotid atherosclerosis, ultrasound and lipoproteins. Biomedicines. 2021;9(5):521. https://doi.org/10.3390/biomedicines9050521.
5. Anderson FA, Spencer FA. Risk factors for venous thromboembolism. Circulation. 2003;107(23_suppl_1):1–9. https://doi.org/10.1161/01.CIR.0000078469.07362.E6.
6. Read H, Holdgate A, Watkins S. Simple external rotation of the leg increases the size and accessibility of the femoral vein. Emerg Med Australas. 2012;24(4):408–13. https://doi.org/10.1111/j.1742-6723.2012.01568.x.
7. Randall C, Schmeiser E, Fiers E, Little A, Dogbey G, Richardson G. Ultrasound investigation of leg position to enhance femoral vein exposure for cannulation. J Emerg Med. 2014;47(2):176–81. https://doi.org/10.1016/j.jemermed.2014.02.001.
8. Kim ES, Sharma AM, Scissons R, et al. Interpretation of peripheral arterial and venous Doppler waveforms: a consensus statement from the Society for Vascular Medicine and Society for vascular ultrasound. Vasc Med. 2020;25(5):484–506. https://doi.org/10.1177/1358863X20937665.
9. Krahenbuhl B, Restellini A, Frangos A. Peripheral venous pulsatility detected by Doppler method for diagnosis of right heart failure. Cardiology. 2008;71(4):173–6. https://doi.org/10.1159/000173661.
10. Aday AW, Matsushita K. Epidemiology of peripheral artery disease and polyvascular disease: Aday—epidemiology of PAD. Circ Res. 2021;128(12):1818. https://doi.org/10.1161/CIRCRESAHA.121.318535.
11. Guidi G, Licciardello C, Falteri S. Intrinsic spectral broadening (ISB) in ultrasound Doppler as a combination of transit time and local geometrical broadening. Ultrasound Med Biol. 2000;26(5):853–62. https://doi.org/10.1016/S0301-5629(00)00218-0.
12. Martinelli O, Alunno A, Drudi FM, Malaj A, Irace L. Duplex ultrasound versus CT angiography for the treatment planning of lower-limb arterial disease. J Ultrasound. 2020;24(4):471–9. https://doi.org/10.1007/s40477-020-00534-y.
13. Hodgkiss-Harlow KD, Bandyk DF. Interpretation of arterial duplex testing of lower-extremity arteries and interventions. Semin Vasc Surg. 2013;26(2):95–104. https://doi.org/10.1053/j.semvascsurg.2013.11.002.
14. Stolt M, Braun-Dullaeus R, Herold J. Do not underestimate the femoral pseudoaneurysm. Vasa. 2018;47(3):177–86. https://doi.org/10.1024/0301-1526/a000691.
15. Scheer BV, Perel A, Pfeiffer UJ. Clinical review: complications and risk factors of peripheral arterial catheters used for haemodynamic monitoring in anaesthesia and intensive care medicine. Crit Care. 2002;6(3):199–204.
16. Al-Jaishi AA, Liu AR, Lok CE, Zhang JC, Moist LM. Complications of the arteriovenous fistula: a systematic review. J Am Soc Nephrol. 2017;28(6):1839. https://doi.org/10.1681/ASN.2016040412.
17. Zamboli P, Fiorini F, D'Amelio A, Fatuzzo P, Granata A. Color Doppler ultrasound and arteriovenous fistulas for hemodialysis. J Ultrasound. 2014;17(4):253–63. https://doi.org/10.1007/s40477-014-0113-6.
18. Teodorescu V, Gustavson S, Schanzer H. Duplex ultrasound evaluation of Hemodialysis access: a detailed protocol. Int J Nephrol. 2012;2012:508956. https://doi.org/10.1155/2012/508956.
19. Randrianarisoa E, Rietig R, Jacob S, et al. Normal values for intima-media thickness of the common carotid artery - an update following a novel risk factor profiling. Vasa. 2015;44(6):444–50. https://doi.org/10.1024/0301-1526/a000467.
20. Dossabhoy S, Arya S. Epidemiology of atherosclerotic carotid artery disease. Semin Vasc Surg. 2021;34(1):3–9. https://doi.org/10.1053/j.semvascsurg.2021.02.013.
21. Cassola N, Baptista-Silva JC, Nakano LC, et al. Duplex ultrasound for diagnosing symptomatic carotid stenosis in the extracranial segments. Cochrane Database Syst Rev. 2022;2022(7):CD013172. https://doi.org/10.1002/14651858.CD013172.pub2.
22. Chang WL, Chen PY, Hsu PJ, Lin SK. Validity and reliability of point-of-care ultrasound for detecting moderate- or high-grade carotid atherosclerosis in an outpatient department. Diagnostics. 2023;13(11):1952. https://doi.org/10.3390/diagnostics13111952.
23. Grant EG, Benson CB, Moneta GL, et al. Carotid artery stenosis: Gray-scale and Doppler US diagnosis—Society of Radiologists in Ultrasound Consensus Conference. Radiology. 2003;229(2):340–6. https://doi.org/10.1148/radiol.2292030516.
24. AbuRahma AF, Pollack JA, Robinson PA, Mullins D. The reliability of color duplex ultrasound in diagnosing total carotid artery occlusion. Am J Surg. 1997;174(2):185–7. https://doi.org/10.1016/S0002-9610(97)90080-9.
25. Khilnani NM, Min RJ. Imaging of venous insufficiency. Semin Interv Radiol. 2005;22(3):178–84. https://doi.org/10.1055/s-2005-921950.
26. Kline JA, O'Malley PM, Tayal VS, Snead GR, Mitchell AM. Emergency clinician–performed compression ultrasonography for deep venous thrombosis of the lower extremity. Ann Emerg Med. 2008;52(4):437–45. https://doi.org/10.1016/j.annemergmed.2008.05.023.
27. Hercz D, Mechanic OJ, Varella M, Fajardo F, Levine RL. Ultrasound performed by emergency physicians for deep vein thrombosis: a systematic review. West J Emerg Med. 2024;25(2):282–90. https://doi.org/10.5811/westjem.18125.
28. Farahmand S, Farnia M, Shahriaran S, Khashayar P. The accuracy of limited B-mode compression technique in diagnosing deep venous thrombosis in lower extremities. Am J Emerg Med. 2011;29(6):687–90. https://doi.org/10.1016/j.ajem.2010.11.028.
29. Gottlieb M, Johnson J, Van Diepen K, Atkinson P. Just the facts: POCUS assessment for deep venous thrombosis. Can J Emerg Med. 2023;25(4):291–3. https://doi.org/10.1007/s43678-022-00410-0.

30. Adhikari S, Zeger W, Thom C, Fields JM. Isolated deep venous thrombosis: implications for 2-point compression ultrasonography of the lower extremity. Ann Emerg Med. 2015;66(3):262–6. https://doi.org/10.1016/j.annemergmed.2014.10.032.
31. Needleman L, Cronan JJ, Lilly MP, et al. Ultrasound for lower extremity deep venous thrombosis. Circulation. 2018;137(14):1505–15. https://doi.org/10.1161/CIRCULATIONAHA.117.030687.
32. Bernardi E, Camporese G, Büller HR, et al. Serial 2-point ultrasonography plus D-dimer vs whole-leg color-coded Doppler ultrasonography for diagnosing suspected symptomatic deep vein thrombosis: a randomized controlled trial. JAMA. 2008;300(14):1653–9. https://doi.org/10.1001/jama.300.14.1653.
33. Lee JH, Lee SH, Yun SJ. Comparison of 2-point and 3-point point-of-care ultrasound techniques for deep vein thrombosis at the emergency department. Medicine (Baltimore). 2019;98(22):e15791. https://doi.org/10.1097/MD.0000000000015791.
34. van Ramshorst B, van Bemmelen PS, Hoeneveld H, Faber JA, Eikelboom BC. Thrombus regression in deep venous thrombosis. Quantification of spontaneous thrombolysis with duplex scanning. Circulation. 1992;86(2):414–9. https://doi.org/10.1161/01.CIR.86.2.414.
35. Lockhart ME, Sheldon HI, Robbin ML. Augmentation in lower extremity sonography for the detection of deep venous thrombosis. Am J Roentgenol. 2005;184(2):419–22. https://doi.org/10.2214/ajr.184.2.01840419.
36. Lin EP, Bhatt S, Rubens D, Dogra VS. The importance of monophasic Doppler waveforms in the common femoral vein. J Ultrasound Med. 2007;26(7):885–91. https://doi.org/10.7863/jum.2007.26.7.885.
37. Muñoz FJ, Mismetti P, Poggio R, et al. Clinical outcome of patients with upper-extremity deep vein thrombosis: results from the RIETE registry†. Chest. 2008;133(1):143–8. https://doi.org/10.1378/chest.07-1432.
38. Bleker SM, van Es N, Kleinjan A, et al. Current management strategies and long-term clinical outcomes of upper extremity venous thrombosis. J Thromb Haemost. 2016;14(5):973–81. https://doi.org/10.1111/jth.13291.
39. Isma N, Svensson PJ, Gottsäter A, Lindblad B. Upper extremity deep venous thrombosis in the population-based Malmö thrombophilia study (MATS). Epidemiology, risk factors, recurrence risk, and mortality. Thromb Res. 2010;125(6):e335–8. https://doi.org/10.1016/j.thromres.2010.03.005.
40. Baarslag HJ, van Beek EJR, Koopman MMW, Reekers JA. Prospective study of color duplex ultrasonography compared with contrast venography in patients suspected of having deep venous thrombosis of the upper extremities. Ann Intern Med. 2002;136(12):865–72. https://doi.org/10.7326/0003-4819-136-12-200206180-00007.
41. Chin EE, Zimmerman PT, Grant EG. Sonographic evaluation of upper extremity deep venous thrombosis. J Ultrasound Med. 2005;24(6):829–38. https://doi.org/10.7863/jum.2005.24.6.829.
42. Décousus H, Bertoletti L, Frappé P. Spontaneous acute superficial vein thrombosis of the legs: do we really need to treat? J Thromb Haemost. 2015;13:S230–7. https://doi.org/10.1111/jth.12925.
43. Castro-Marín F, Kendall JL. Diagnosis of Lemierre syndrome by bedside emergency department ultrasound. J Emerg Med. 2010;39(4):436–9. https://doi.org/10.1016/j.jemermed.2007.10.044.
44. Craven P, End B, Griffin P. Emergency department point-of-care ultrasound identification of suspected Lemierre's syndrome: a case report. Clin Pract Cases Emerg Med. 2023;7(3):172. https://doi.org/10.5811/cpcem.1245.

Ultrasound-Guided Procedures

21

Tiffany Fong, Lawrence Haines, and Manpreet Singh

Introduction

The use of ultrasound (US) guidance improves procedural outcomes and healthcare quality. It increases overall procedural success rates while reducing the number of attempts required, time to complete the procedure, and risk of complications [1]. The most extensive body of literature exists for US-guided central venous access, for which US is considered the standard of care [2–5]; however, continually expanding evidence supports the superiority of US over landmark-based techniques for the performance of many other fundamental procedures.

Many proceduralists first developed proficiency in US guidance through vascular access. The core skills from this procedure are highly transferable to an array of other applications. For high-risk, infrequently performed procedures that might provoke apprehension, the ability to apply familiar US guidance techniques may promote a sense of greater comfort, manageability, and ultimately proficiency. This chapter begins with a brief summary of core principles for US guidance, followed by a discussion of US for vascular access, pericardiocentesis, pacemaker placement, thoracentesis, tube thoracostomy, paracentesis, nasogastric (NG) and orogastric (OG) tube placement, lumbar puncture (LP), and hematoma blocks.

Supplementary Information The online version contains supplementary material available at https://doi.org/10.1007/978-3-031-85308-1_21.

T. Fong (✉)
Department of Emergency Medicine, Johns Hopkins University School of Medicine, Baltimore, MD, USA
e-mail: tfong3@jhmi.edu

L. Haines
Department of Emergency Medicine, SUNY Downstate/Maimonides Medical Center, Brooklyn, NY, USA
e-mail: haines@maimonidesmed.org

M. Singh
Department of Emergency Medicine, Harbor-UCLA Medical Center, Torrance, CA, USA
e-mail: MaSingh@dhs.lacounty.gov

Principles of Ultrasound Procedural Guidance

Static Versus Dynamic Ultrasound Guidance

Static guidance techniques (also referred to as US-assisted) involve the use of US to identify target structures and define surrounding anatomy prior to performing the procedure, which is then completed without direct, real-time US visualization. While dynamic US guidance is preferred for most procedures, static US guidance may be useful for select procedures where real-time guidance may be unnecessary or more challenging (e.g., large volume paracentesis, lumbar puncture, cricothyroidotomy). A major limitation of the static guidance technique is that it requires the patient not to move or be repositioned between the time that structures are visualized and the procedure is performed.

Dynamic guidance techniques (also referred to as real-time or US-guided) employ US to continuously visualize the needle moving toward the target structure while avoiding important surrounding structures. In general, this technique is preferred as it permits adjustment and redirection to enhance procedural success and avoid complications.

Imaging Planes for Ultrasound-Guided Procedures

Four imaging planes for US procedural guidance have been described (Fig. 21.1): out-of-plane (also referred to as short axis), in-plane (also referred to as long axis), bi-plane (also referred to as x-plane or cross-plane), and oblique. The choice of scanning planes depends on the procedure being performed, patient-specific factors, operator experience, and

M. Gottlieb, N. Panebianco (eds.), *Advanced Point-of-Care Ultrasound*, https://doi.org/10.1007/978-3-031-85308-1_21

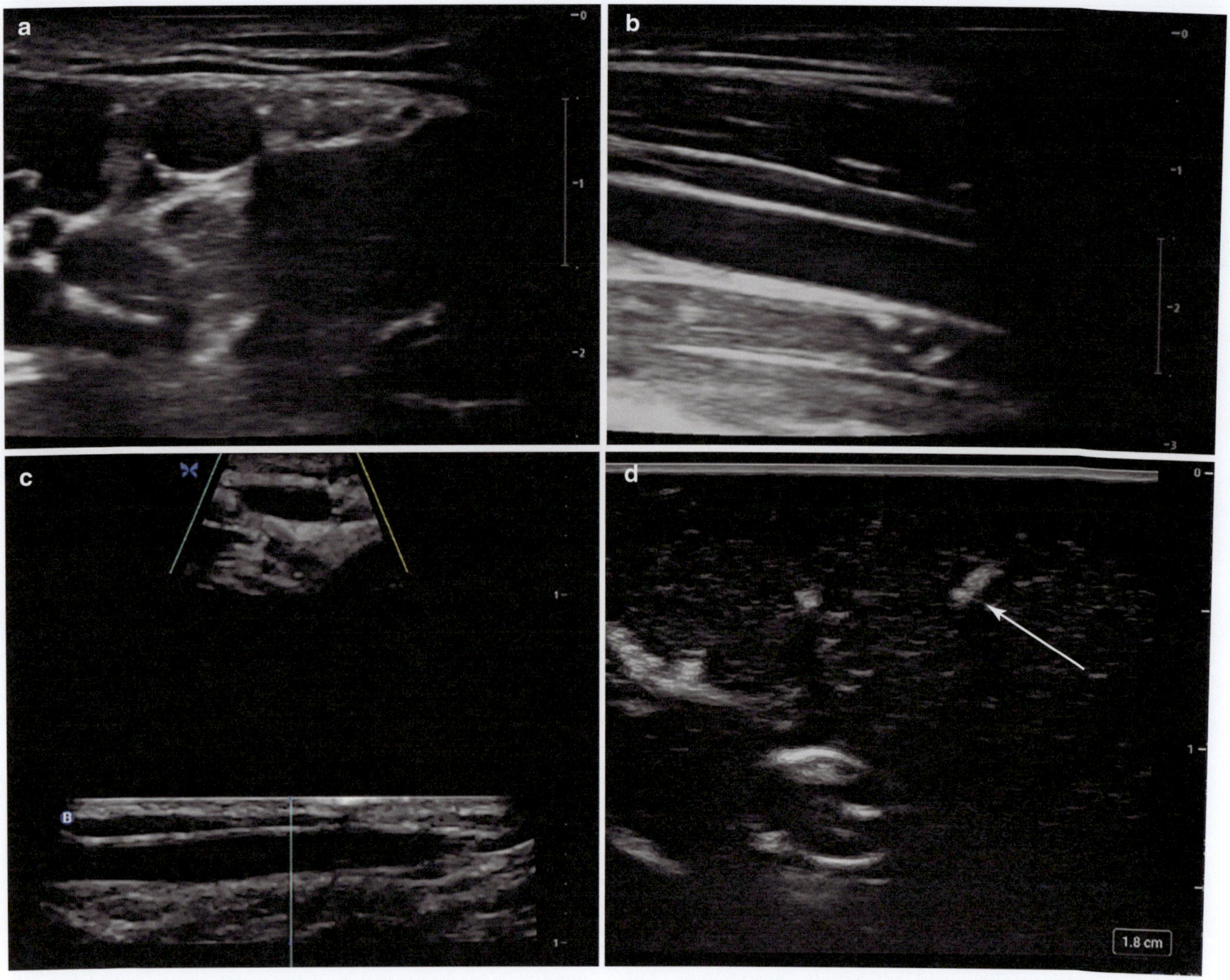

Fig. 21.1 Ultrasound imaging planes for procedural guidance. (**a**) Out-of-plane technique with the vessel seen in the short axis. (**b**) In-plane technique with the vessel seen in the long axis. (**c**) Bi-plane with simultaneous visualization of the vessel in short axis (above) and long axis (below). (**d**) Oblique plane, with the vessel visualized at 45-degree rotation, such that it midway between long axis and short axis. Note that with the oblique plane, the needle tip (arrow) is still visualized in the long axis, while only the vessel is oblique

available equipment and technologies. A summary of each plane along with the advantages and disadvantages is included in Table 21.1.

Optimization of Needle Visualization

Continuous visualization of the needle tip, particularly during needle advancement or manipulation, is key to achieving procedural success and minimizing the risk of injury to adjacent structures. There are several strategies to enhance needle visualization.

First, select an appropriate probe and imaging preset for the procedure. While image resolution for procedural guidance is usually best with a linear probe, a curvilinear probe may be needed for deeper structures. When possible, adjust the frequency to a higher frequency during the procedure to enhance proximal resolution. If limited by a small procedural space, consider an endocavitary probe (which offers a wider field of view and high proximal image resolution) or a hockey stick probe.

Many machines have presets for vascular access or procedures that optimize depth, gain, and other factors to enhance needle visualization. Further adjusting the dynamic range and centering the focal zone on the structure of interest can also enhance visualization. *Electronic beam steering* permits the direction of the transmitted US beam at an angle that strikes the needle as close to 90° as possible, maximizing reflection back to the transducer. *Spatial compound imaging* uses electronic beam steering to transmit and receive multiple US beams at different angles of incidence, then combines this sonographic data to create a single composite image; this

Table 21.1 Imaging planes for ultrasound-guided procedures

Approach	Technique	Advantages	Disadvantages
Out-of-plane	Ultrasound probe is positioned perpendicular to the course of the vessel or target structure, such that the target is viewed in cross-section. Needle enters perpendicular to the long axis of the probe.	Less technically challenging to keep target structure in view. Target structure and surrounding structures are visualized simultaneously.	Limited view of the needle, potentially causing uncertainty about whether the needle tip or needle shaft is being visualized. Risk of over-advancement of needle causing unintended puncture of deep structures (e.g., posterior vessel wall, lung, bowel).
In-plane	Ultrasound probe is positioned parallel to the course of the vessel or target structure, such that the target is viewed in a long-axis plane. In select cases (e.g., nerve blocks), the structure remains in the short axis, while only the needle is visualized in the long axis. Needle enters parallel to the long axis of the probe.	Easier identification of the needle tip and its precise position and trajectory relative to target.	Technically challenging to maintain needle and target structure in the same plane as US beam (only 1–2 mm wide). More limited view of surrounding structures. Difficult in certain anatomic locations (e.g., patients with short necks).
Bi-plane	An imaging technique that utilizes a matrix array probe to create simultaneous ultrasound displays of both the short and long axes of the needle, target structure, and surrounding anatomy-needle entry may take place in-plane or out-of-plane.	Permits advantages of both out-of-plane and in-plane techniques without the requirement of probe rotation.	Technology is not universally available.
Oblique plane	Hybrid of in-plane and out-of-plane approaches. Obtained by visualizing the target structure in the short axis, then rotating to a position midway between short- and long-axis planes to create an elongated, oblique view. Needle entry may take place in-plane or out-of-plane, though most commonly in-plane is used.	Improved visualization of both needle tip and shaft compared with an out-of-plane approach. Improved visualization of surrounding anatomy compared with an in-plane approach.	Can be more challenging to track the needle and vessel given the nonconventional orientation.

enhances visualization of the target, surrounding tissue, and needle while reducing artifact [6].

Next, patient, operator, and equipment positioning should be arranged to maximize patient comfort and operator ergonomics (Fig. 21.2). When advancing the needle, the US probe, needle, and target structure should remain aligned in the same imaging plane throughout the procedure. This can be facilitated by keeping the hand and forearm holding the needle pointed directly toward the US machine.

The angle of needle insertion will impact its sonographic appearance. The trajectory of the needle should be as perpendicular as possible to the trajectory of the US beam to maximize echoes reflected from the needle and detected by the probe. When using in-plane guidance, a *"heel-in"* maneuver allows the US beam to strike the needle more perpendicularly to enhance visualization (Fig. 21.3) [7]. Gently tapping the needle forward can create tissue artifacts and help improve visualization. However, care should be taken to use minimal movement and avoid side-to-side movement, which can damage surrounding structures. *Hydrolocalization*, a technique where a small amount of fluid is injected and visualized as a dynamically appearing anechoic focus on the screen, may help localize a difficult-to-see needle tip. Serial injections allow tracking of the needle course to the target [8]. However, be mindful that injection of agitated saline or inadvertent injection of air will create artifacts that hinder needle visualization.

Other commercially available technologies are available as procedural adjuncts that may improve procedural accuracy and time to completion. *Echogenic needles* are engineered to enhance the visualization of the needle. Some are created with irregularities in the needle surface that scatter US waves, producing a brighter signal across a spectrum of angles relative to the US beam. Other designs include encasement in polymers that generate microbubbles on the surface of the needle, which increase acoustic impedance and thus the reflection of the US beam [9]. *Needle guides* applied directly to the US probe assist in stabilizing the needle in line with the axis of the probe and the US beam. Particularly for less experienced operators they may increase needle visibility and lead to a shorter time to complete the procedure [10, 11]. However, needle guides can impede needle redirection, which is often required during US-guided procedures. *Electromagnetic needle positioning sensors*, mounted or embedded into a US probe, can detect a magnetized or sensor-embedded needle tip to provide the operator with real-time spatial information about the exact position and trajectory of the needle relative to the probe [12, 13].

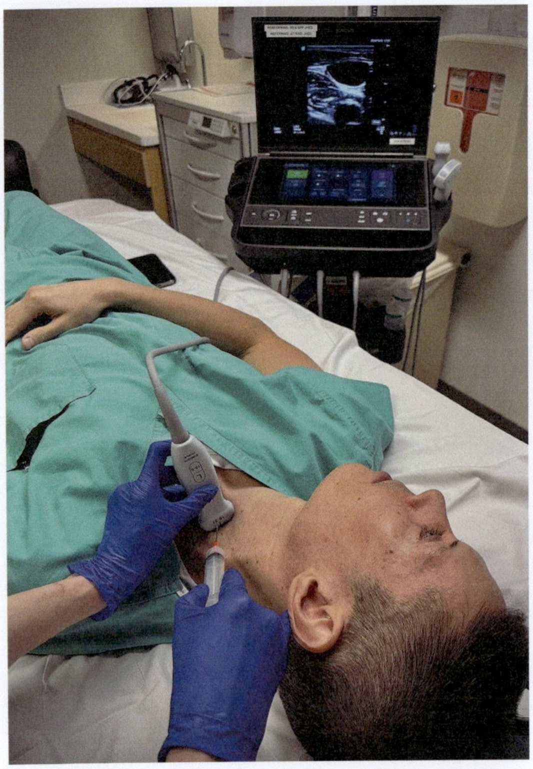

Fig. 21.2 Optimal positioning of operator, patient, and equipment for ultrasound-guided procedures. The needle, patient anatomic areas undergoing the procedure, and ultrasound machine should all lie within the same line of sight for the operator. This at times requires the ultrasound machine to be on the opposite side of the bed

Vascular Access

The advantage of US for procedural guidance was first demonstrated with central venous access, and the literature overwhelmingly showed that US guidance increased success rates and decreased mechanical complications of this procedure [14–17]. Consequently, in 2001, the Agency for Healthcare Research and Quality formally recommended the use of real-time US guidance during central line insertion to prevent complications [2]. This, coupled with increasing evidence of benefit, contributed to the widespread use of US guidance. In this section, we will discuss US guidance for central venous catheter, peripheral intravenous catheter, and arterial catheter placement.

Central Venous Access

Central venous catheter (CVC) placement is common in the critical care setting, with over five million placed annually in the United States [18]. CVCs are indicated for invasive hemodynamic monitoring, as well as delivery of medications, fluids, and nutritional support that cannot be achieved via peripheral access. However, insertion-related complications can occur in up to 3% of CVCs placed [19]. One meta-analysis found that US guidance decreased placement failure by 68%, multiple placement attempts by 40%, and complications (e.g., arterial puncture, hematoma, pneumothorax,

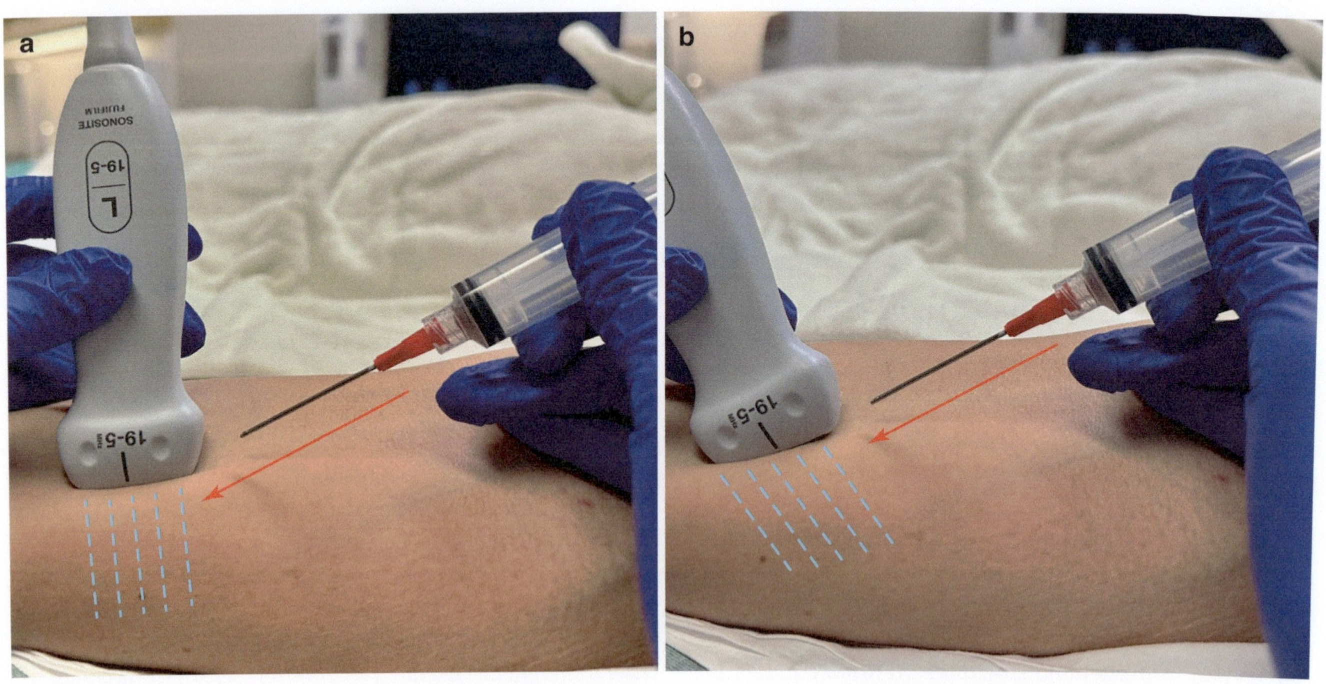

Fig. 21.3 Heel-in maneuver. To optimize needle visualization, rock the ultrasound probe from (a) a position perpendicular to the skin to (b) a heel-in position, tilting the end of the probe farthest from the needle into the soft tissue. This allows the ultrasound beam (dashed lines) to strike the needle (trajectory indicated by red arrow) at a more perpendicular angle and maximizes the reflection of echoes. While demonstrated using a long-axis approach here, a similar effect may be achieved in the short axis by fanning the probe toward the needle

hemothorax) by 78% when compared with landmark-based techniques [20]. There are three main sites for CVC access: the internal jugular, subclavian, and femoral veins.

Internal Jugular Vein

The internal jugular vein (IJV) is located deep to the sternocleidomastoid muscle and lateral to the carotid artery. Compared with the subclavian site, CVC insertion in the IJV has the advantage of a decreased incidence of pneumothorax and permits compression in the event of inadvertent arterial puncture [21]. While early studies suggested an advantage of lower catheter-related bloodstream infection rates than femoral catheterization [22], more recent data have suggested no difference in infection rates between the IJV, subclavian, and femoral sites [23]. Due to the ease of visualization of the IJV by US, this location has been increasingly used for CVC [24].

Technique

Begin by placing the patient in the Trendelenburg position. Tilting the head of the bed 5–10° is ideal, as >10° is unlikely to increase IJV size [25]. Asking the patient to perform a Valsalva maneuver can also help to increase IJV diameter. Scan the neck with the high-frequency linear probe to visualize the carotid artery and IJV on both sides. Choose the more favorable location, factoring in vessel size and proximity to key structures. The right IJV is generally preferred, especially for large bore sheath introducers or hemodialysis catheters, because the path to the cavo-atrial junction is a relatively straight one. Compress the IJV completely to verify that there are no clots within the vein and to clearly delineate the vein (thin-walled, compressible) from the artery (thick-walled, noncompressible, pulsatile). If there is doubt, Doppler modalities can be employed to distinguish the vein and artery.

Appropriately position the patient and US equipment (Fig. 21.4). Scan up and down the neck to identify a location where the IJV sits lateral to the carotid artery. This will reduce the chance of arterial puncture if the needle inadvertently penetrates the back wall of the vein [14, 26, 27]. The insertion site should also be sufficiently cephalad to avoid lung injury and to allow for sufficient space for the probe movement needed for real-time needle tracking. Once the ideal site has been located, the operator should don appropriate sterile attire, the patient should be prepared and draped, and the US probe should be covered with a sterile cover.

To start the IJV cannulation using out-of-plane US guidance, hold the probe in the nondominant hand and center the vein on the screen. Care should be taken to avoid compressing the vein by stabilizing the hand with the operator's fifth finger. Assess the depth to the middle of the vessel. The needle should enter the skin at the same distance away from the probe as the vessel is deep. If the angle of the needle trajectory is at a 45-degree angle, then the needle tip should reach the center of the vessel at the desired location (Fig. 21.5). The insertion distance should be modified if a shallower or steeper angle of insertion is desired.

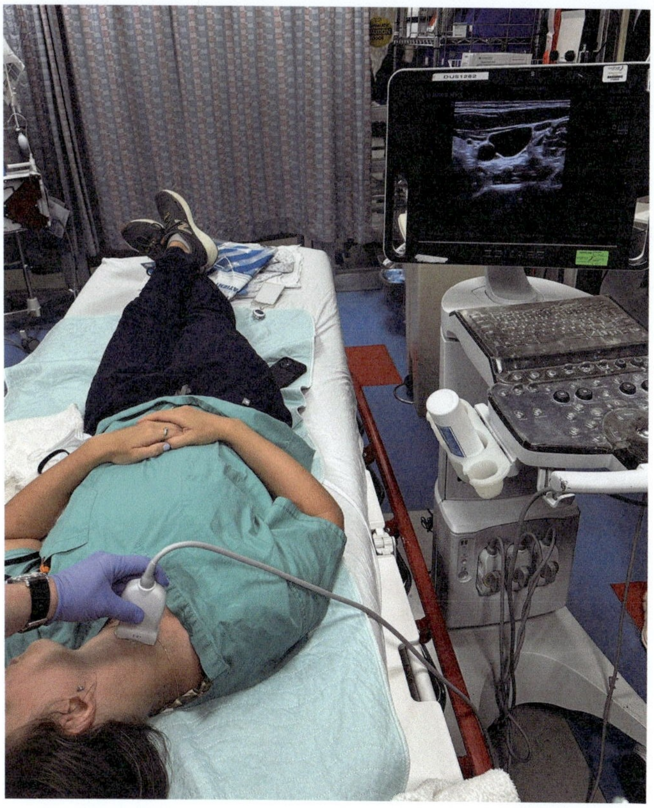

Fig. 21.4 Procedural setup for an US-guided internal jugular central venous catheterization (sterile preparation not demonstrated). Turn the head to the contralateral side of the selected vein and place the US machine next to the bed on the ipsilateral side, with the screen facing the operator at the head of the bed

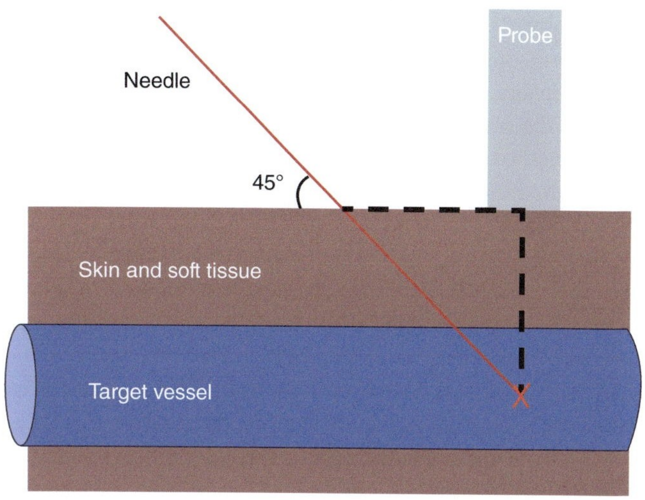

Fig. 21.5 Triangulation of the needle pathway (red line) to the center of the target vessel (red X)

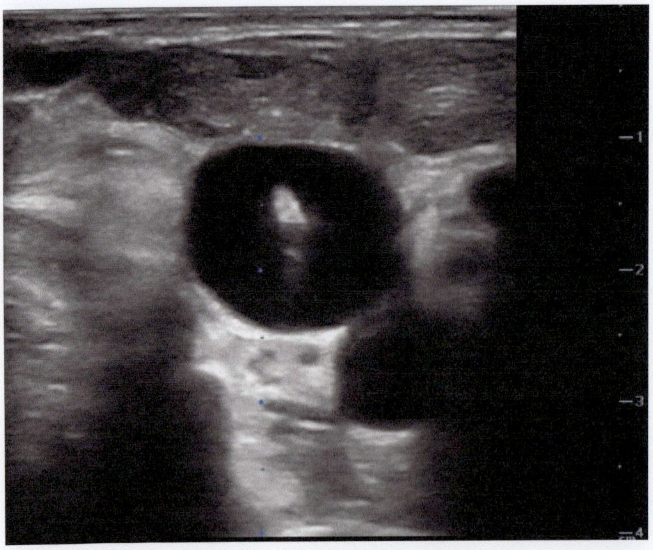

Fig. 21.6 Internal jugular central venous catheterization performed using an out-of-plane ultrasound-guided technique. The vein is seen in a transverse orientation, with an echogenic needle tip visible within the vessel lumen

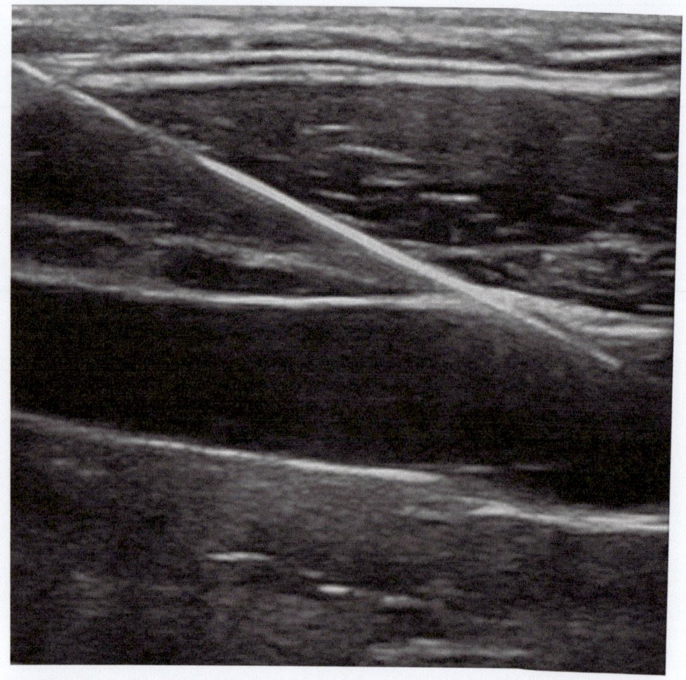

Fig. 21.7 Internal jugular central venous catheterization with confirmation of guidewire position within the vessel lumen seen in the long-axis view

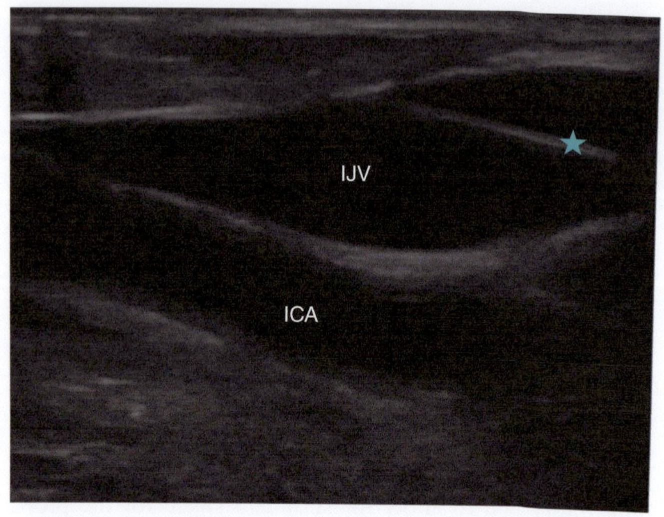

Fig. 21.8 Long-axis view of the internal jugular vein (IJV) and the internal carotid artery (ICA). The needle (star) is visualized in the lumen of the IJV

Alternatively, a "walking-in" technique can be used to guide the needle tip into the vessel. Puncture the skin directed toward the center of the probe and stop. Slide the probe toward the needle until the needle tip is seen, appearing as an echogenic dot, sometimes with a ring-down artifact (Fig. 21.6). Then, slide the probe away from the needle until the bright needle tip disappears from view. With the probe now held still, slowly advance the needle until the echogenic needle tip reappears on the screen, this time slightly deeper than before. Once the needle tip is seen, stop advancing the needle and again advance the probe forward until the needle tip disappears. Continue this process of alternating advancement of the probe with the advancement of the needle until the needle tip is seen in the lumen of the IJV (Video 21.1). At this point, venous blood should be able to be aspirated into the syringe.

Next, flatten the angle of the needle and continue "walking" the needle 1–2 cm into the lumen of the vessel, being careful to avoid the back wall of the vessel. The probe can now be placed onto the sterile field, and the remainder of the catheter placement is completed using a Seldinger technique. When the wire is in the vessel and prior to dilation, the location of the wire in the lumen can be confirmed using US (Fig. 21.7) [28].

Alternate approaches include the in-plane and oblique approaches. For the in-plane approach, first visualize the vessel in the short axis as described above. Then, rotate 90° to visualize the long axis of the vessel. The needle is inserted in-plane, parallel to the long axis of the probe. This approach offers the benefit of visualizing the entire length of the needle to ensure that the angle is sufficiently shallow to allow the wire to be advanced and to avoid injury to the posterior wall of the vessel (Fig. 21.8) [28–30]. In the oblique approach, the vessel is first identified in a short-axis view, then rotated to a position halfway toward the long-axis view, with the vessel now seen as an oval [31]. Compared to the out-of-plane approach, the oblique approach may allow better needle visualization but can take longer to perform [32].

Subclavian Vein

One advantage of inserting a subclavian vein (SCV) CVC is that it does not require Trendelenburg positioning, which may not be tolerated by some patients. However, the SCV site has the highest risk of pneumothorax and is not a compressible site if there is an inadvertent arterial puncture [19, 33]. US guidance has been shown to decrease the incidence of these mechanical complications [34–37]. Two approaches have been described: supraclavicular and infraclavicular.

Technique

Because the US beam cannot pass through the clavicle, the SCV can only be seen from above or below this structure. For the *supraclavicular approach*, begin by locating the IJV and tracking this inferiorly until the IJV joins the SCV, occurring superior and posterior to the clavicle. Then rotate the probe along the long axis of the SCV (Fig. 21.9). While this procedure is often performed with a linear probe, a small-footprint probe such as an endocavitary or hockey stick probe may be advantageous in this constrained space [38]. Once this view is obtained, introduce the needle using an in-plane technique, similar to that described above for the IJV.

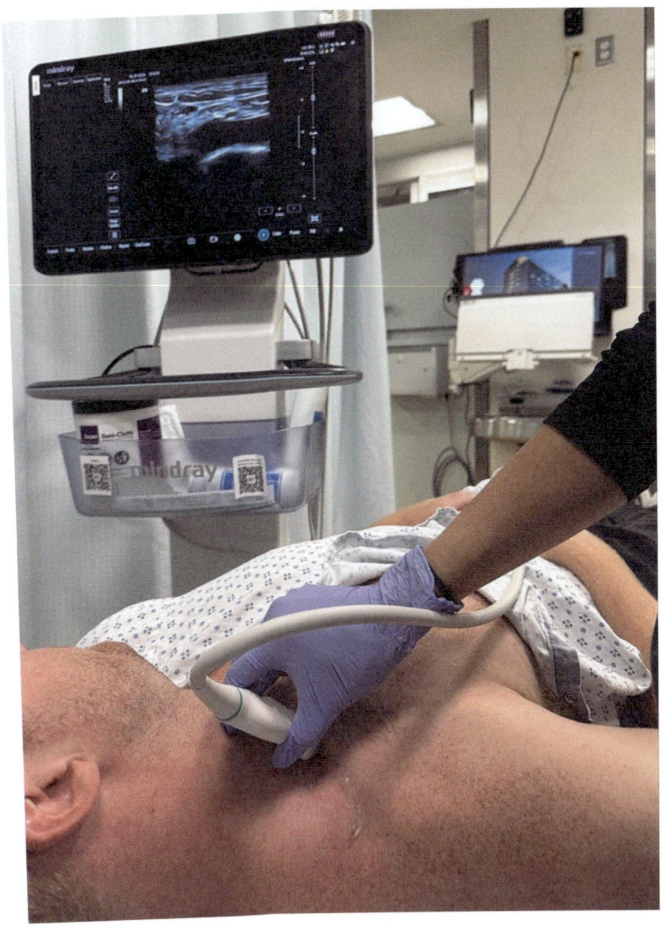

Fig. 21.9 Probe positioning for ultrasound-guided subclavian central venous catheterization using the supraclavicular approach (sterile preparation not demonstrated). A linear probe is placed superior and posterior to the clavicle, and the needle is introduced in-plane

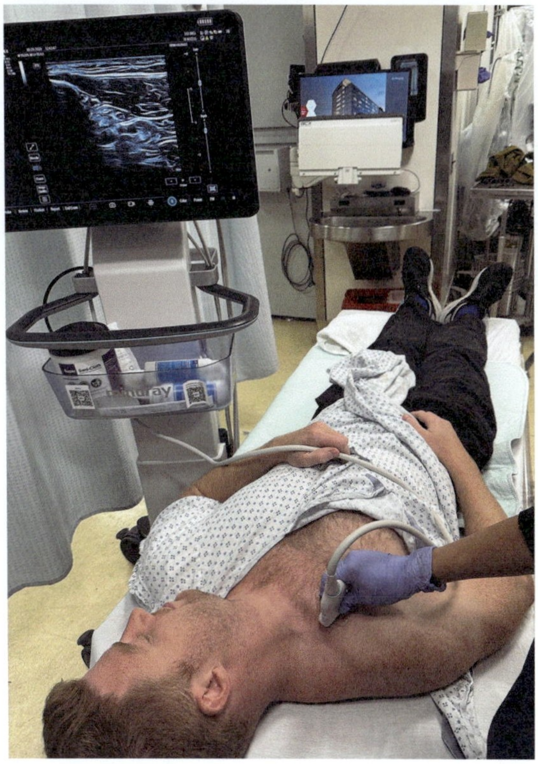

Fig. 21.10 Procedural setup for ultrasound-guided infraclavicular central venous catheterization (sterile preparation not demonstrated). The probe is placed inferior to the clavicle with the indicator toward the patient's head for an out-of-plane approach

For the *infraclavicular approach* (also known as the axillary vein approach), begin by scanning just inferior to the proximal third of the clavicle until the SCV is seen as it emerges from under the bone (Fig. 21.10). Note the positions of the subclavian artery and pleural line, which both normally lie just deep to the SCV (Fig. 21.11). When unclear, color flow or pulsed-wave Doppler can be used to identify the vein and artery. Evaluate both the left and right SCV to determine which appears favorable, factoring vessel size and proximity to vital structures. The left SCV is generally preferred as the path of the vessel entering the superior vena cava (SVC) has a shallower trajectory than on the right. This procedure can be performed using either an in-plane or out-of-plane approach depending on the comfort and skill level of the operator. However, the literature suggests a lower rate of complications and higher success rates with the out-of-plane approach [39].

Femoral Vein

The femoral vein has the advantages of being a compressible site and accessible when there is limited access to the head and neck (e.g., cervical collar) or other procedures being

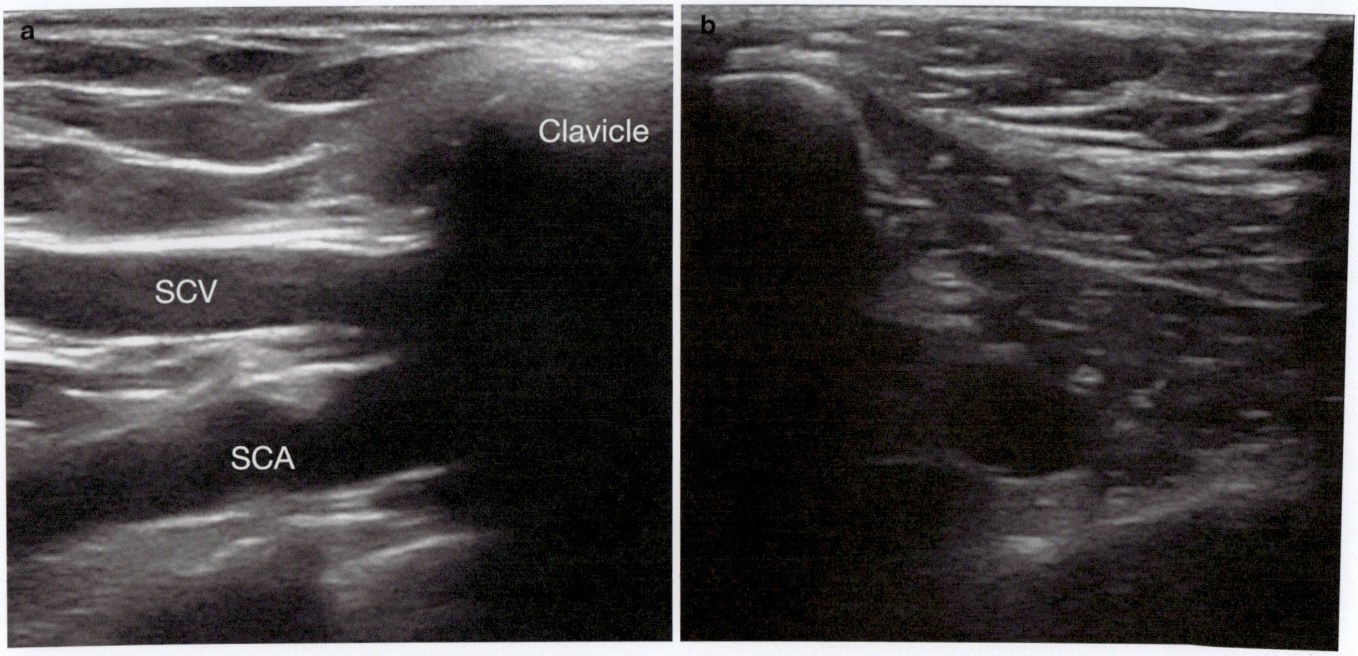

Fig. 21.11 The subclavian vein (SCV) emerges from under the clavicle and becomes the axillary vein. The SCV is located superior and anterior to the subclavian artery (SCA). (**a**) Long-axis orientation of the SCV for in-plane technique. (**b**) Short-axis view for out-of-plane technique

performed in that area (e.g., intubation). The femoral vein is located within the femoral triangle, bordered by the inguinal ligament superiorly, the adductor longus muscle medially, and the sartorius muscle laterally. The structures contained here (from laterally to medially) are the femoral nerve, femoral artery, femoral vein, empty space (femoral canal), and lymphatics, recalled by the mnemonic "NAVEL" (Fig. 21.12).

Technique

Place the patient in reverse Trendelenburg with the leg externally rotated, which serves to increase the diameter of the vein and decrease the degree of overlap between the femoral artery and vein (Fig. 21.13) [40–42]. Identify the femoral vein and trace it superiorly until the femoral artery moves laterally to the vein while remaining inferior to the inguinal ligament and cephalic to where the greater saphenous vein joins the common femoral vein. Note that the inguinal ligament is located several centimeters superior to the inguinal crease. Once the sonographic view is obtained, the femoral vein can be accessed using either the in-plane or out-of-plane approach, following similar steps to those described earlier (Fig. 21.14).

CVC Placement Confirmation

Following completion of CVC placement, US can be used to exclude complications and confirm appropriate venous position. First, lung US can rule out pneumothorax. Next, catheter malposition can be assessed by visualizing the catheter in the vein and tracing it toward the heart. Finally, a subxiphoid long-axis or apical four-chamber view of the heart can be performed to visualize the right atrium (RA). Then, agitated saline can be rapidly pushed through the CVC, observing for the rapid appearance of bubbles in the right atrium. These

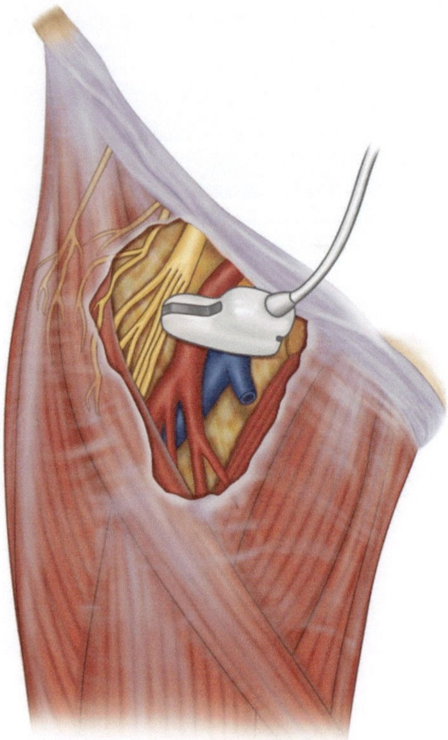

Fig. 21.12 Anatomy of the proximal thigh showing the contents of the femoral triangle and ideal ultrasound probe positioning

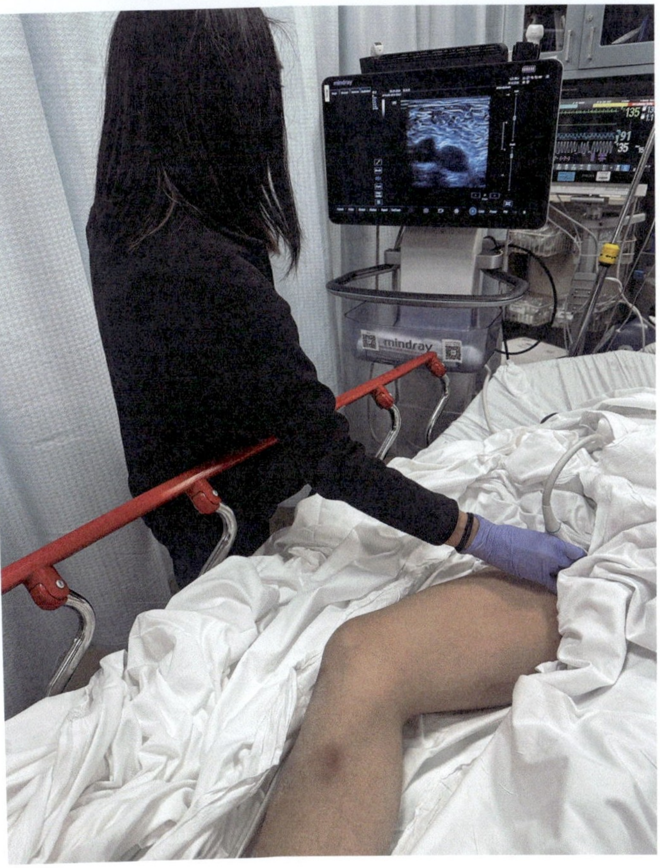

Fig. 21.13 Procedural setup for ultrasound-guided femoral central venous catheterization with the patient placed in reverse Trendelenburg and hip externally rotated (sterile preparation not demonstrated)

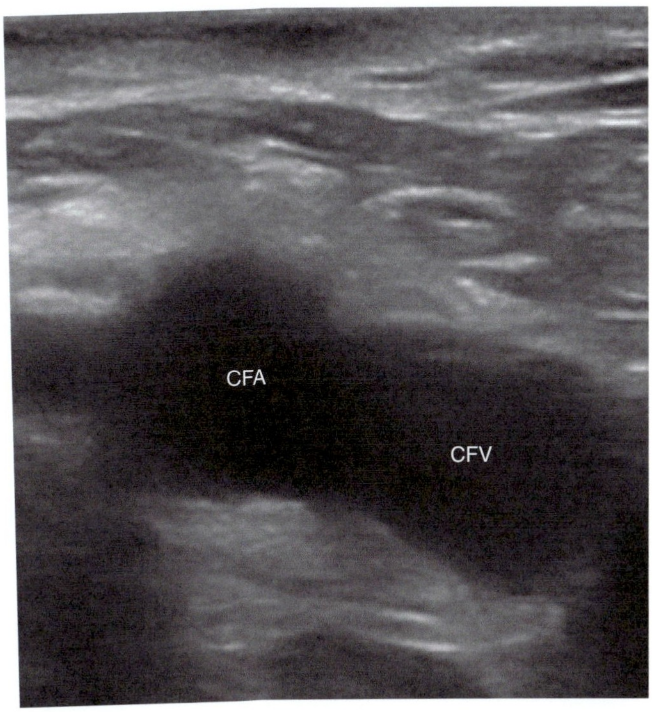

Fig. 21.14 Transverse ultrasound view of the femoral vessels, with the right common femoral artery (CFA) lying lateral to the common femoral vein (CFV)

findings have a pooled sensitivity of 82% and a specificity of 98% for catheter malposition and can lead to a significant reduction in time to confirmation [43].

Peripheral Intravenous Access

US-guided peripheral intravenous access (USGPIV) increases the chance of first-pass success in patients with difficult vascular access by up to threefold in adults and by 12% in children, compared with traditional, landmark-based techniques [44, 45]. USGPIV also reduces the number of attempts required in patients with more difficult vascular access when compared with the landmark-based approach [46–48]. Moreover, data have shown that initiation of a USGPIV program can reduce the number of CVCs placed in the emergency department by up to 85% [49, 50]. Studies have demonstrated no increase in infection rates with USGPIV when proper aseptic techniques are followed [51].

While USGIV placement can be performed using traditional length intravenous catheters, we generally recommend using longer peripheral intravenous catheters (2.5 inches) or midline catheters because the target vessel is usually deeper than those accessed by palpation [52]. A longer catheter is also less likely to dislodge or infiltrate because more catheter length will reside within the vessel [53]. When comparing the in-plane and out-of-plane techniques, limited data suggest the out-of-plane technique is associated with a higher success rate [54, 55]. However, this may depend on the skill and comfort level of the operator, as well as patient-specific characteristics (e.g., size and tortuosity of the vein).

Indications and Contraindications

Any patient who historically has had difficulty obtaining vascular access or one who has suffered multiple failed attempts is a good candidate for USGPIV. While there are no absolute contraindications, the literature suggests that USGPIV may not be advantageous in patients who are anticipated to have easy access [56]. This may reflect inadvertent compression of the vein with the ultrasound probe or the requirement for a very shallow trajectory for superficial veins that may be better approached with a landmark-based technique.

Technique

Choosing the optimal vein is paramount to success. The largest and most superficial vein is generally the most ideal one to access. A vein >1.6 cm deep is more technically difficult to access because of limitations in catheter length and the requirement for a steeper angle of insertion, with data suggesting it is more likely to infiltrate [57, 58]. Small-diameter vessels (≤3 mm wide) can lead to difficulty cannulating and advancing the catheter [57].

The antecubital fossa and forearm are the most common sites for USGPIV placement and are acceptable locations for the power injection of intravenous contrast agents for imag-

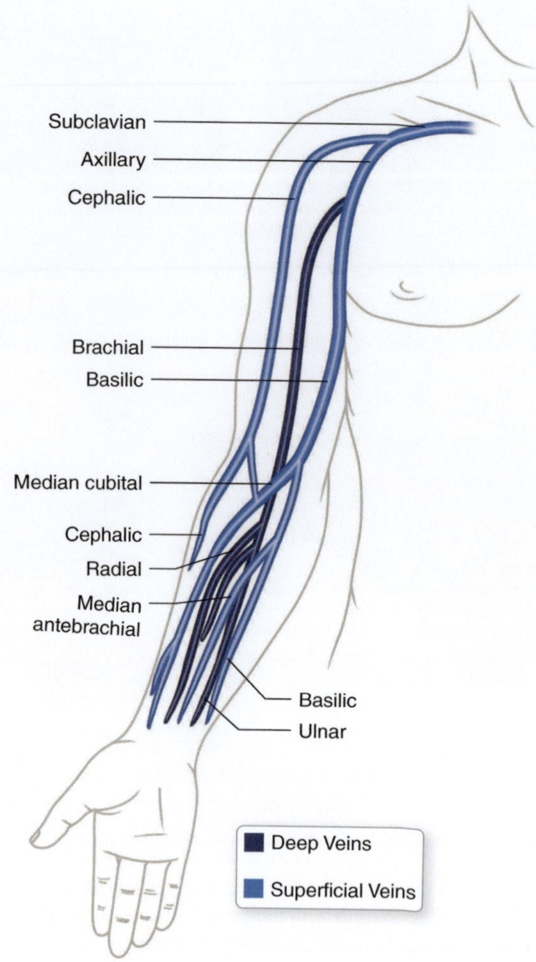

Fig. 21.15 Anatomy of the veins of the arm. The cephalic and basilic veins travel alone, whereas the brachial vein is paired with the brachial artery

ing studies [59]. However, the lower extremities may also be used for access. In the upper arm, the cephalic, basilic, and brachial veins are all typical locations for catheter placement (Fig. 21.15). The cephalic vein (coursing over the biceps muscle) and the basilic vein (coursing down the posteromedial arm) are advantageous because they are not closely paired with an artery. The deep brachial vein is also commonly used because it is superficial and large in size; however, there may be a lower success rate and higher failure rate when USGPIV is performed at this site [60, 61].

At the start of the procedure, place a tourniquet on the limb proximal to the areas that will be accessed. After a vein has been selected, a "walking-in" needle tip tracking technique (described above for CVC) may be used. An important distinction between USGPIV and CVC insertion is that the former does not typically use a Seldinger technique. As a result, it is important to visualize the needle and catheter within the center of the vessel. Relying upon blood in the catheter tubing alone can risk advancing the catheter before it is fully within the vessel and is a common source of error with this procedure [52].

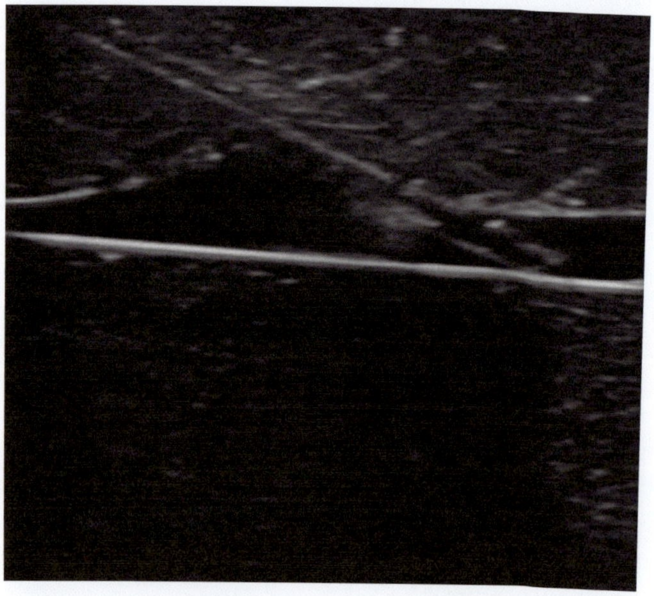

Fig. 21.16 Long axis ultrasound view of intravenous catheter entering a peripheral vein, confirming intraluminal placement

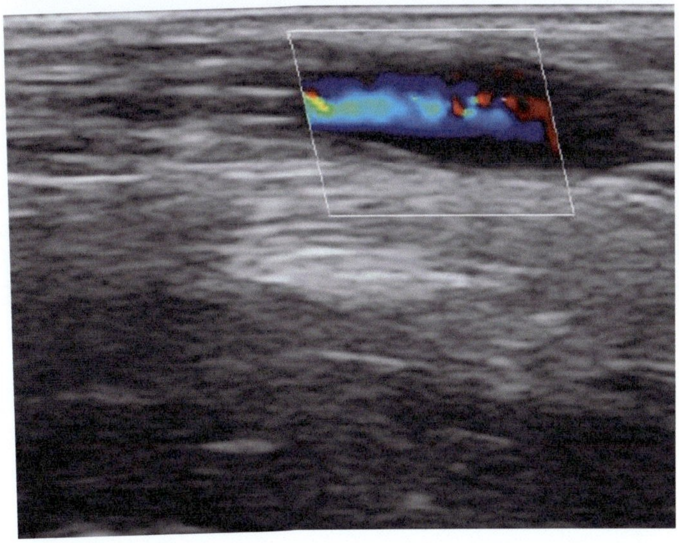

Fig. 21.17 Color Doppler visualization of a saline flush within a peripheral vein, confirming intravascular placement

Additionally, it is important to avoid using too steep of an angle (>60° from the skin) during needle puncture and advancement and to lower the angle of the needle as one approaches the vessel to avoid injuring the back wall of the vessel or kinking the catheter. Finally, operators can directly confirm placement and patency of the USGPIV at the bedside by visualizing the catheter in long axis or by injecting saline and assessing for swirling on B-mode or color Doppler (Figs. 21.16 and 21.17) [52].

Arterial Catheter Placement

Placing an arterial catheter by palpation of the pulse alone can be challenging, especially in a hypotensive patient. US guidance has been shown to increase first-pass success and reduce the time to insertion and the number of attempts [62, 63]. While this procedure can be performed in-plane or out-of-plane, data suggest the out-of-plane technique has a higher rate of posterior wall puncture and hematoma with no difference in success rate [64].

Technique

This procedure follows a similar technique as described above for needle tracking. Because many arterial catheterization kits include a needle and catheter with a wire within, the entire procedure can be performed without removing the needle. If an assistant is present, the wire can be advanced and confirmed with US in real time to avoid inadvertent placement within the soft tissue.

Pericardiocentesis

Cardiac tamponade is an imminently life-threatening condition that demands the performance of a pericardiocentesis to reverse obstructive shock. As the sonographic findings of cardiac tamponade precede hemodynamic decompensation, assessment with US enables procedural preparation prior to full depletion of the physiologic reserve. The sonographic findings and pathophysiology of pericardial effusion and cardiac tamponade are described in Chap. 4.

Notably, while pericardial effusions sufficient to produce cardiac tamponade are usually circumferential, fluid may not always distribute uniformly around the heart, with loculation present in up to one-third of nontraumatic effusions [65, 66]. Furthermore, several important structures lie within proximity of the pericardium, including the lung, diaphragm, intra-abdominal structures, internal thoracic vessels, and the heart itself. For these reasons, pericardiocentesis should be performed using real-time US guidance. For experienced operators, success rates of US-guided pericardiocentesis are high in both adults (97–99%) and children (99%), and complication rates are low (adults, 0.7–1.2% major and 3.0–3.5% minor complications; children, 1% major and 3% minor complications) [65, 67, 68].

Indications and Contraindications

Pericardiocentesis is indicated for all patients with cardiac tamponade causing hemodynamic compromise. Patients with active intrapericardial bleeding and expected re-accumulation of effusion (e.g., trauma, iatrogenic injury, myocardial rupture, aortic dissection) will require surgical intervention, with pericardiocentesis serving as a stabilizing maneuver prior to definitive management.

No contraindications exist for unstable patients with cardiac tamponade. For patients with coagulopathy, pericardiocentesis still carries only a small bleeding risk, which can be mitigated with US guidance. A review of 1196 pericardiocentesis procedures performed by experienced operators identified a low rate of bleeding complications (<1%) even in patients with INR ≥2.0 and platelets <50,000 [69].

Technique

A phased array probe is typically used to diagnose pericardial effusion; however, any probe may be used for pericardiocentesis depending upon the distance to the pericardium

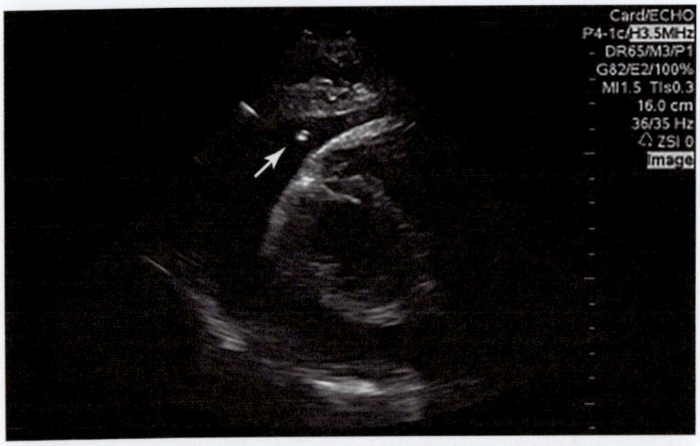

Fig. 21.18 Ultrasound-guided pericardiocentesis performed from a subxiphoid approach under real-time guidance. Needle tip (arrow) is seen entering the pericardial space from the left side of the screen

and available space on the chest wall for the probe. Because fluid may be unevenly distributed, multiple views should be performed to identify the optimal fluid pocket and needle trajectory. As tolerated, place the patient in a semi-upright or left lateral decubitus position to shift fluid away from the less accessible posterior position. Selecting the deepest available fluid pocket will reduce the risk of cardiac puncture.

Ultrasound guidance permits successful pericardiocentesis from multiple approaches. The subxiphoid approach, historically used for a landmark-based pericardiocentesis, has the greatest skin-to-pericardial fluid distance (mean 5.6 cm compared to 2.7 cm for parasternal and 2.5 cm for apical) and the highest predicted complication rate [65, 70]. Therefore, access from the apical or parasternal positions may be more favorable [70–72]. It is incumbent on the clinician to select the optimal approach by weighing several factors: the size of pericardial fluid collection, the distance from skin to fluid collection, the presence of vital structures in the needle trajectory, US image quality, and needle visualization.

Regardless of the anatomic approach, US guidance should generally be performed in-plane, with real-time localization of the needle tip (Fig. 21.18, Video 21.2). The use of a high-frequency probe may facilitate real-time visualization of the needle, in addition to providing high-resolution images of the pleura and nearby vessels. If using a low-frequency probe, needle visualization can be augmented through the use of a curvilinear rather than phased array probe (provided there is adequate space). The differential firing and steering of the ultrasound beam used to optimize cardiac imaging reduces the echoes reaching the needle and returning to the probe. Operators should also decrease the depth of the imaging field to view the target and important adjacent structures, rather than the entire heart. This depth adjustment will improve temporal resolution by increasing pulse repetition frequency and frame rate [73].

Parasternal Approach

Because of the more superficial location of the heart, a linear probe is typically preferred for the parasternal region. Begin by placing the probe in a longitudinal position and visualizing the deepest pocket of fluid. Identify and avoid the internal thoracic (mammary) vessels (Fig. 21.19) [74]. Needle puncture may take place from either the left or right parasternal chest and take either a lateral-to-medial or medial-to-lateral trajectory [75–77]. The exact technique will depend on patient-specific factors that influence the size and accessibility of the fluid pocket and the ability to visualize the needle. Approach the pericardium using a steeper needle angle (>45°) to avoid traversing the closely adjoining vital structures (e.g., pleura, lung, great vessels, internal thoracic vessels). Ensure that the needle enters at the superior border of the rib to avoid injury to the neurovascular bundle that lies at the inferior rib border.

Apical Approach

If an apical approach is selected, the patient may be placed in an upright, left lateral oblique, or lateral decubitus position, as tolerated, to maximize the size of the fluid pocket at the apex. Again, ensure that the needle enters at the superior border of the rib to avoid injury to the neurovascular bundle. The apical location has a theoretical benefit of smaller cardiac vessel size near the cardiac apex and a relatively thicker left ventricle wall that may more easily self-seal if punctured.

Subxiphoid Approach

For clinicians with experience with landmark-based pericardiocentesis, the subxiphoid approach may be more comfortable. The subxiphoid view of the heart may also be the easiest to obtain, particularly in patients with lung hyperinflation. However, needle visualization may prove more difficult, and the risk of injury to adjacent structures (e.g., lung, liver, bowel) may be higher with this technique [70].

Confirmation of Needle Position and Fluid Drainage

Aspiration of fluid or blood during pericardiocentesis may indicate procedural success but may also be seen with pleural, peritoneal, or intracardiac needle positions. Correct positioning is suggested by visualization of the needle within the pericardial space in multiple cardiac windows. Other methods of confirmation include injection of agitated saline or advancement of a guidewire, with observation of bubbles or the wire, respectively, within the pericardial space (Fig. 21.20). Hemodynamic improvement after fluid aspiration is also indicative of pericardial positioning and ultimately procedural success. A repeat ultrasound may show decreased effusion size and improved cardiac filling.

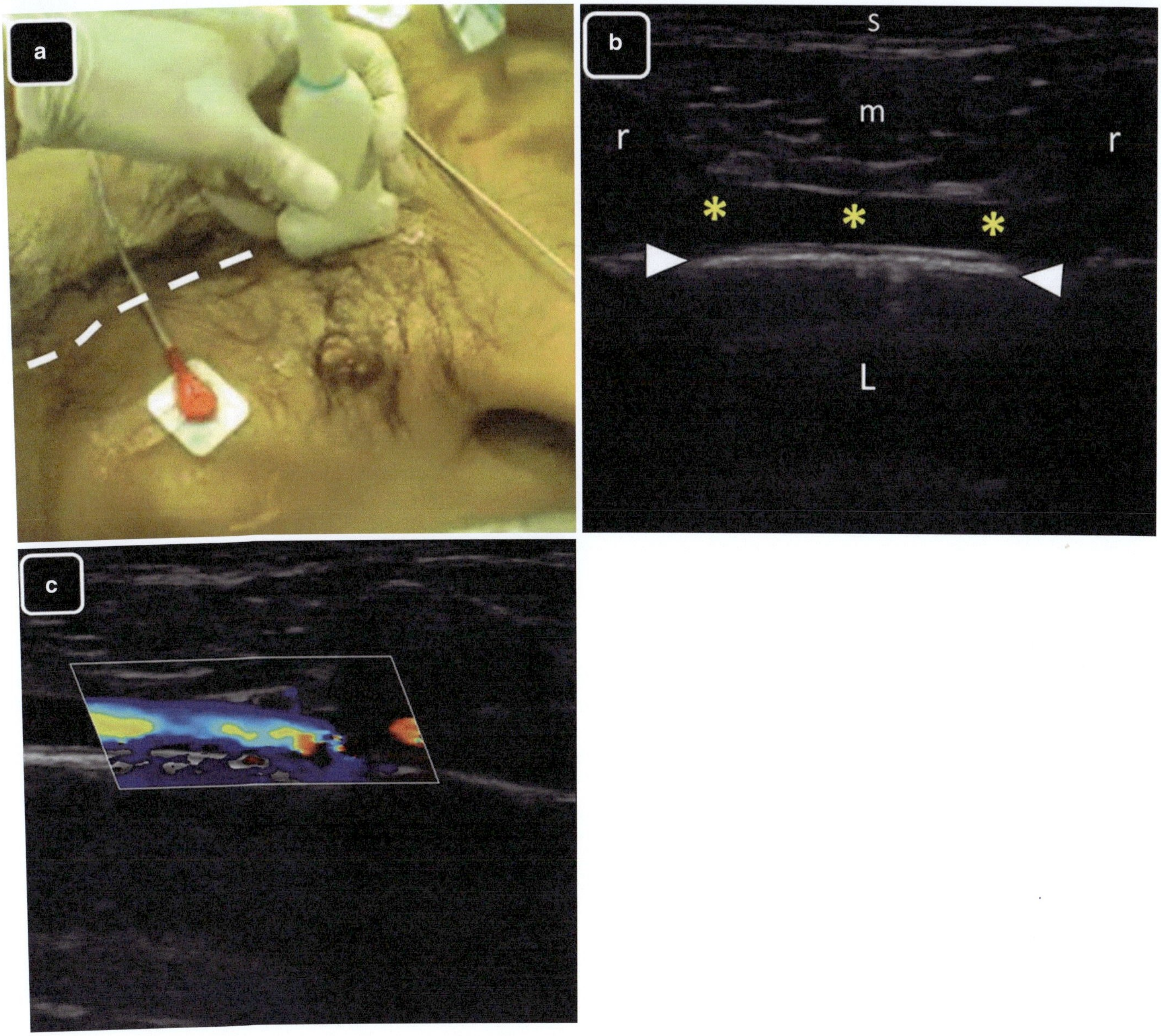

Fig. 21.19 Internal thoracic vessels. (**a**) Place a high-frequency linear probe on the anterior chest in the sagittal plane, 1–3 centimeters lateral to the sternal border. The dashed line corresponds to the location of the internal thoracic vessels. (**b**) The anechoic internal thoracic artery (*) can be visualized sonographically, lying deep to the ribs (r) and pectoralis and intercostal muscles (m), and superficial to the pleural line (arrowheads) and lung (L). (**c**) Color Doppler evaluation demonstrates vascular flow from the internal thoracic artery. (*Images courtesy of Blanco et al.* [74])

For cases of pericardial effusion where re-accumulation or the need for serial aspirations is anticipated, a pericardial catheter can be placed. In this case, once the pericardial space has been entered, only the amount of fluid needed to regain hemodynamic stability should initially be removed. Removing the entire pericardial effusion can reduce the potential space for guidewire and pericardial catheter insertion. After the initial volume of fluid has been removed, the catheter can then be inserted using the Seldinger technique, and subsequent fluid can be removed as appropriate through the pericardial catheter. Rapid removal of large fluid volumes (>500 mL) should be avoided due to the risk of pericardial decompression syndrome, associated with ventricular failure and cardiogenic pulmonary edema [78, 79]. In general, drainage should be performed until hemodynamic improvement is seen and be followed by a more gradual decompression as needed.

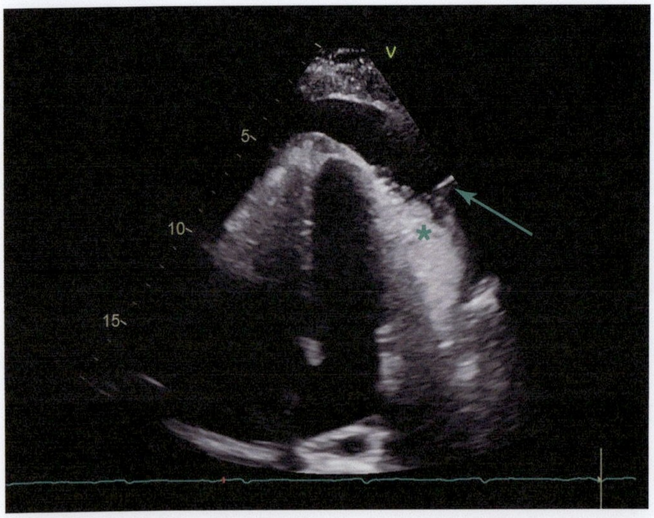

Fig. 21.20 Agitated saline injection with intrapericardial bubbles (*) visualized adjacent to the left ventricle, confirming the appropriate placement of needle tip (arrow) during apical approach for pericardiocentesis

Transvenous Pacemaker Placement

Placement of a temporary transvenous cardiac pacemaker is a potentially life-saving procedure in patients with unstable dysrhythmias. Ultrasound can facilitate the successful placement of a pacing catheter in the right ventricular (RV) apex and assess for procedural complications.

Indications and Contraindications

Transvenous pacing is indicated in hemodynamically unstable patients with severe bradycardia, tachycardia requiring overdrive pacing, or failure of transcutaneous pacing. It is contraindicated in asystole and hypothermia. Known structural cardiac abnormalities, including a prosthetic tricuspid valve, are relative contraindications. Dysrhythmias with a clear underlying cause (e.g., hypothermia, hyperkalemia, acidemia, myxedema coma, and drug toxicity such as beta blocker, calcium channel blocker, and digoxin) should be medically managed prior to pacing.

Technique

This procedure takes place in three stages: (1) insertion of a central venous introducer sheath; (2) guidance of a pacing catheter into the RV apex and achieving electromechanical capture; and (3) programming the pacing generator to address the patient's underlying pathophysiology [80].

Placement of Introducer Sheath

A dedicated transvenous pacing kit may include its own introducer sheath. However, if a separate Cordis or other large bore catheter is used, it is important to ensure an appropriate diameter is selected. Most pacing catheters (also referred to as pacing wire) are 3F to 5F in size; a 5F pacing catheter will fit through a 5F or larger introducer sheath. The use of an introducer sheath that is too large (e.g., 7F to 8.5F Cordis catheters commonly available in emergency settings) can lead to ongoing bleeding around the diaphragm of the catheter.

Ensure the patient is on a cardiac monitor and sterilely place a central venous introducer sheath. The right IJV access site is preferred for its most direct trajectory into the RV. The left SCV site is an alternative with a favorable anatomic course to reach the heart but should be avoided if possible, as it is the typical site selected for a permanent pacemaker.

Transvenous Pacing Setup

The operator in sterile attire should test the balloon at the end of the pacing catheter by inflating it using the air-filled syringe included in the kit. The syringe allows a maximum volume of 1.5 mL to prevent balloon rupture. Immerse the inflated balloon in sterile saline and ensure no bubbles are observed, which would indicate an air leak. Then, thread the pacing catheter through the sterile sheath, taking care to verify correct directionality, with the wire exiting at the end that will attach to the central venous introducer sheath. The sheath is critical to ensure that the catheter remains sterile and can be adjusted post-procedure as needed. (Fig. 21.21).

The non-sterile pacing generator (often referred to as the "box") is managed by an assistant, who has no requirement for sterile attire. The assistant should connect the cable to the ventricular output of the box, then help the operator connect the pacing catheter, via adaptor pins, to the negative and positive terminals of the pacing generator. The positive port of the generator connects to the proximal lead of the pacing catheter ("P-to-P") and the negative port connects to the distal lead [80]. The assistant may then set the pacing specifications (Fig. 21.22, Table 21.2).

Placement of the Pacing Catheter

Insert the pacing catheter through the central venous introducer sheath. To facilitate a trajectory into the RA, the curve of the wire should be oriented to midline if using the IJV or caudally if using the left SCV. After the pacing catheter is advanced beyond the tip of the introducer sheath (approximately 15–20 cm), inflate and lock the balloon, and turn on the pacing generator. The balloon acts as a sail to allow the wire to "float" with the flow of blood from the SVC into the

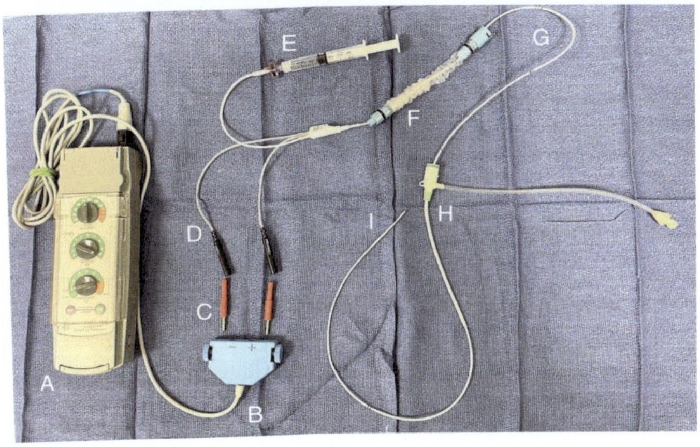

Fig. 21.21 Temporary transvenous pacemaker setup. The pacing generator (**a**) and connecting cable (**b**) are joined via adapter pins (**c**) to the positive and negative transvenous pacing catheter electrodes (**d**). An air-filled syringe (**e**) inflates the balloon and may be locked in position. During setup, a sterile sheath (**f**) must be placed over the pacing catheter (**g**). The pacing catheter can then be threaded through an introducer sheath or Cordis catheter (**h**) already placed in the right internal jugular or left subclavian vein. After it passes through the length of the introducer sheath, the balloon tip (**i**) of the pacing catheter can be inflated

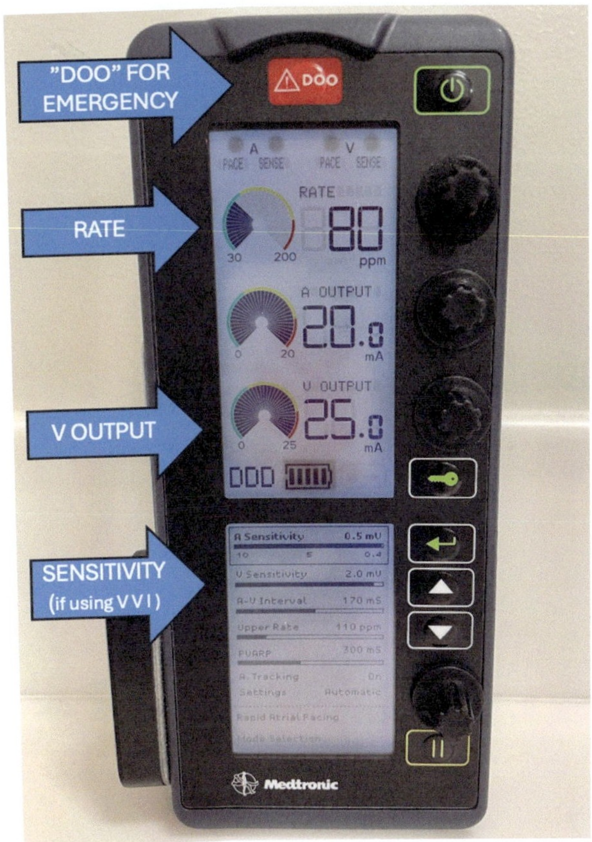

Fig. 21.22 Dual-chamber pacing generator. Basic transvenous pacing settings include manipulation of rate, ventricular output, and sensitivity. An emergency pacing mode can be initiated by pressing the "DOO" key. This initiates asynchronous pacing independent of intrinsic rhythm, with maximal atrial and ventricular outputs

Table 21.2 Pacemaker generator settings

For emergent pacing, start with the "DOO" setting, 25 mA ventricular output, and a rate of 80 bpm	
Output	Amplitude of electrical current delivered by pacemaker (range: 0.1 to 25 mA). Typically, start at 25 mA to assure capture. After capture, identify the pacing threshold by decreasing the current until capture is lost. The output is then set at two to three times the pacing threshold, typically 2–3 mA (an ideal threshold is <1 mA).
Rate	Start at a ventricular rate of 80 bpm, or 20–30 bpm above the intrinsic rate.
Sensitivity	Minimum detected intrinsic electrical signal from the heart at which the output from the pacemaker generator is suppressed (range: 0.5 to 25 mV). Set to minimum sensitivity (corresponding to the *highest* number of mV). This allows asynchronous pacing, with pacemaker firing independent of underlying cardiac rhythm.

bpm beats per minute

RA and the RV. Positioning within the RV and subsequent capture may be anticipated near an insertion depth of 35–40 cm. When the RV is reached, the balloon is deflated to prevent ongoing passage into the pulmonary artery. The traditional method of localizing a pacing wire location involves placing an alligator clip connected to lead V1 on the pacing wire and observing classic waveforms as the wire advances.

Transthoracic or transesophageal echocardiography can facilitate real-time guidance of the wire into the appropriate location [81, 82]. Once the pacing catheter has entered the SVC, the assistant obtains an apical four-chamber or subxiphoid long-axis view, which permits visualization of the right heart while avoiding the sterile procedural field. If a transesophageal echocardiography probe is already in place, a mid-esophageal four-chamber view may be used instead. The echogenic pacing wire is observed advancing through the RA, tricuspid valve, RV, and abutting the myocardium in the RV apex (Fig. 21.23). While not required to guide the procedure, a subcostal bicaval view may be obtained, ideally demonstrating catheter advancement from the SVC into the RA, or conversely into the inferior vena cava (IVC) (Fig. 21.24) [83]. A return to the subxiphoid long-axis or apical four-chamber views allows continued visualization of catheter advancement from the RA through the tricuspid valve to the RV.

Ultrasound may also identify and facilitate troubleshooting of catheter malposition within the IVC or coiling in the RA [84]. In these cases, the balloon should be deflated, and the wire should be withdrawn, rotated, or repositioned. After this manipulation, the balloon can be reinflated, and the catheter readvanced.

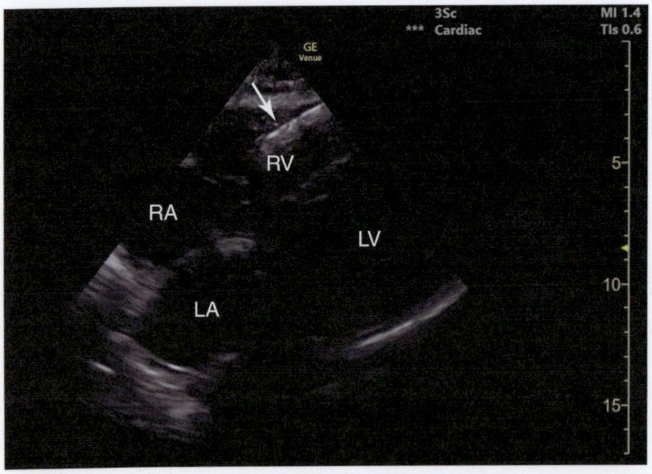

Fig. 21.23 Subxiphoid ultrasound view of the heart demonstrating an echogenic, linear pacing catheter (arrow) terminating in the RV. As the catheter will not generally lie in a single plane, tilting the probe may be required to visualize its full course

Confirming Capture

When the RV wall is reached, electrical capture may be appreciated on the cardiac monitor through the appearance of pacing spikes followed by a wide-complex left bundle branch block pattern in V1. Mechanical capture is verified through the presence of a waveform on pulse oximetry or arterial line, palpation of a pulse, or myocardial contraction on ultrasound. These should all match the rate set by the generator.

After electromechanical capture is confirmed, the operator deflates the balloon, pulls the sterile sheath over the pacing catheter and connects it to the central venous introducer sheath, tightens the plastic locking cap at the opposite end of the sterile sheath to secure the it to the pacing catheter, and finally secures the introducer sheath and pacing catheter to the chest wall. The assistant should adjust the generator settings, decreasing output current until capture is lost, then selecting an output with mA that is two to three times this threshold to maintain pacing.

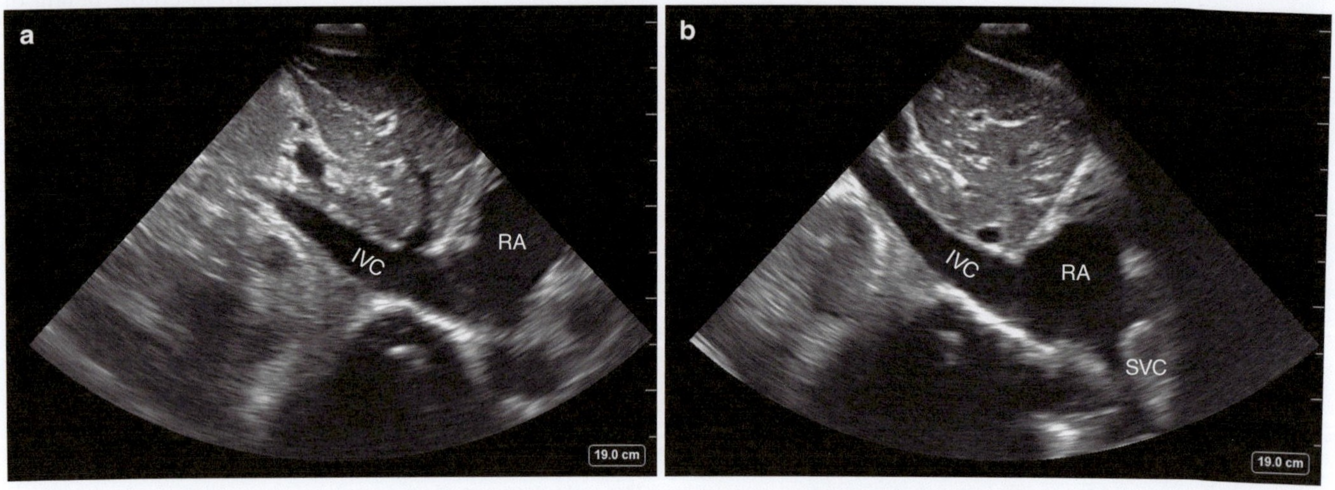

Fig. 21.24 Bicaval view from a subcostal approach, allowing visualization of the inferior vena cava (IVC), right atrium (RA), and superior vena cava (SVC). First, acquire (**a**) a conventional subcostal long axis view of the IVC and cavoatrial junction, then rock the probe cephalad and fan slightly rightward as needed to generate (**b**) a bicaval view.

Thoracentesis

Overview

The accuracy and safety of thoracentesis are enhanced by US guidance [85]. Unlike traditional approaches that rely solely on anatomical landmarks, US guidance permits real-time visualization of the pleural space and precise needle placement, especially into small pockets or windows. This enables adjustments to be made dynamically during the procedure to optimize patient outcomes. This may be especially true in patients with obesity in whom identifying bone versus intercostal space may be challenging without US [86]. The success rate for obtaining pleural fluid is 99% with real-time US guidance, compared with 88% without real-time guidance [87]. The use of US minimizes the risk of complications such as inadvertent puncture of vital structures (e.g., pneumothorax, liver injury) and ensures the successful aspiration of fluid or air from the pleural cavity [88, 89]. Another benefit of US-guided thoracentesis is to predict procedural complexity. By visualizing the pleural space, US can help identify the presence of loculated fluid collections, pleural thickening, or other abnormalities that may alter the approach to the procedure (e.g., patient with rib fractures and/or plating) [90]. Unlike X-ray, US can distinguish pleural effusion from other conditions, such as lung consolidation or masses, which require alternative diagnostic or therapeutic interventions. Finally, US can visualize vasculature and allow avoidance of aberrant intercostal vessels that are not in the typical location in the costal groove beneath the rib.

Indications and Contraindications

Thoracentesis is generally indicated for diagnostic assessment when encountering a pleural effusion of unclear etiology and therapeutic purposes when the effusion is causing respiratory difficulty. There are no absolute contraindications. Relative contraindications include coagulopathy, chest wall cellulitis, or effusions that cannot be safely accessed due to size or location.

Technique

Place the patient in a seated, forward-leaning position with arms and head supported by a table. If this position cannot be tolerated, a lateral decubitus position with the arm raised over the head can be used. A linear or curvilinear probe can be selected, depending on patient habitus. With the indicator facing cephalad, place the probe on the posterior or lateral chest wall and identify an accessible underlying fluid collection, depending on provider experience and comfort. A safely accessed pocket typically ranges from 2 to 10 cm. It is important to recognize and avoid vital structures, including the lung, diaphragm, liver, and spleen. When selecting an ideal location, ensure that these structures do not cross the needle insertion site throughout the entire respiratory cycle, as both the diaphragm and liver move superiorly during expiration.

Once the pleural fluid pocket is identified, a dynamic or static technique can be used to access the fluid. For the static technique, the location of the target collection is marked, and a needle is subsequently inserted without direct US visualization. In contrast, the dynamic approach allows for real-time US visualization of the needle during both processes of anesthetizing the parietal pleura and entering the pleural space. The dynamic approach can be performed out-of-plane or in-plane. For the out-of-plane technique, orient the probe sagittally and insert the needle at the center of the probe, observing the needle tip enter the thoracic cavity. For the in-plane technique, rotate the probe within the intercostal space in an orientation parallel to the ribs and insert the needle near the edge of the probe (Fig. 21.25, Video 21.3). In either approach, ensure the needle is inserted at the superior border of the rib to avoid injuring the neurovascular bundle.

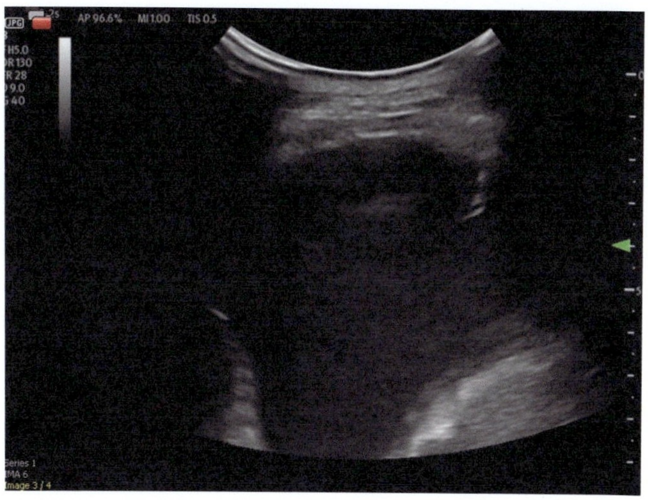

Fig. 21.25 Dynamic in-plane ultrasound-guided thoracentesis showing a needle (right side of image) entering the pleural space

Chest Tube Placement

Overview

Tube thoracostomy is a common procedure performed in the acute and critical care setting. Using a landmark-based approach, complications can occur in up to 30% of cases, including tube malposition, bleeding, and organ injury (e.g., liver, spleen, diaphragm) [91]. Studies have shown that using landmarks alone, junior physicians were only able to properly identify the correct thoracostomy site in 36–44% of cases, with the most common error being the selection of a position too low in the thoracic cavity [92, 93]. In a head-to-head study of US versus landmark-based identification of a correct thoracostomy site, US was significantly more accurate (91% vs 48%) [93]. In addition, US can be used post-placement to visualize the thoracostomy tube and confirm its position in the pleural space (sensitivity 100%, specificity 96–100%) [94, 95].

Indications and Contraindications

Chest tubes are generally placed for therapeutic reasons in order to drain larger volumes of fluid or air causing patient symptoms. The contraindications are similar to those outlined for thoracentesis above.

Technique

Place the patient in a recumbent position with the arm abducted and over the head to allow for palpation of chest wall anatomy. Consider performing an erector spinae plane block or serratus anterior plane block prior to the procedure for analgesia. Using a linear or curvilinear probe with the indicator placed cephalad, identify the diaphragm and slide the probe up at least two rib spaces superiorly. Ensure that the diaphragm and intra-abdominal structures do not cross the imaging plane during respirations. Place the probe centered on the intercostal space, such that there is a rib above and a rib below with intercostal space in between. The puncture location should be superior to the rib border in order to avoid damage to the neurovascular bundle. The puncture location can be marked by a skin impression using a syringe or with a skin marker, or performed under direct guidance with a Seldinger technique for smaller thoracic drains (e.g., pigtail catheter). It is important to note the depth of the thoracic wall from skin to parietal pleura, as well as skin to lung, to help guide catheter insertion.

Post-insertion Confirmation

After the chest tube has been placed, the ultrasound probe can track the chest tube to confirm that it has entered the thoracic space by following the length of the tube between two rib spaces (Fig. 21.26). This can be performed in either the short axis or long axis orientation. If the chest tube is visualized coursing below the rib, this can be confirmed as intrathoracic (Video 21.4). If the chest tube disappears in the soft tissue prior to entering the thoracic cavity, this can be confirmed as extrathoracic (Video 21.5). Improvement in the pneumothorax or hemothorax can also be assessed with serial thoracic ultrasound examinations.

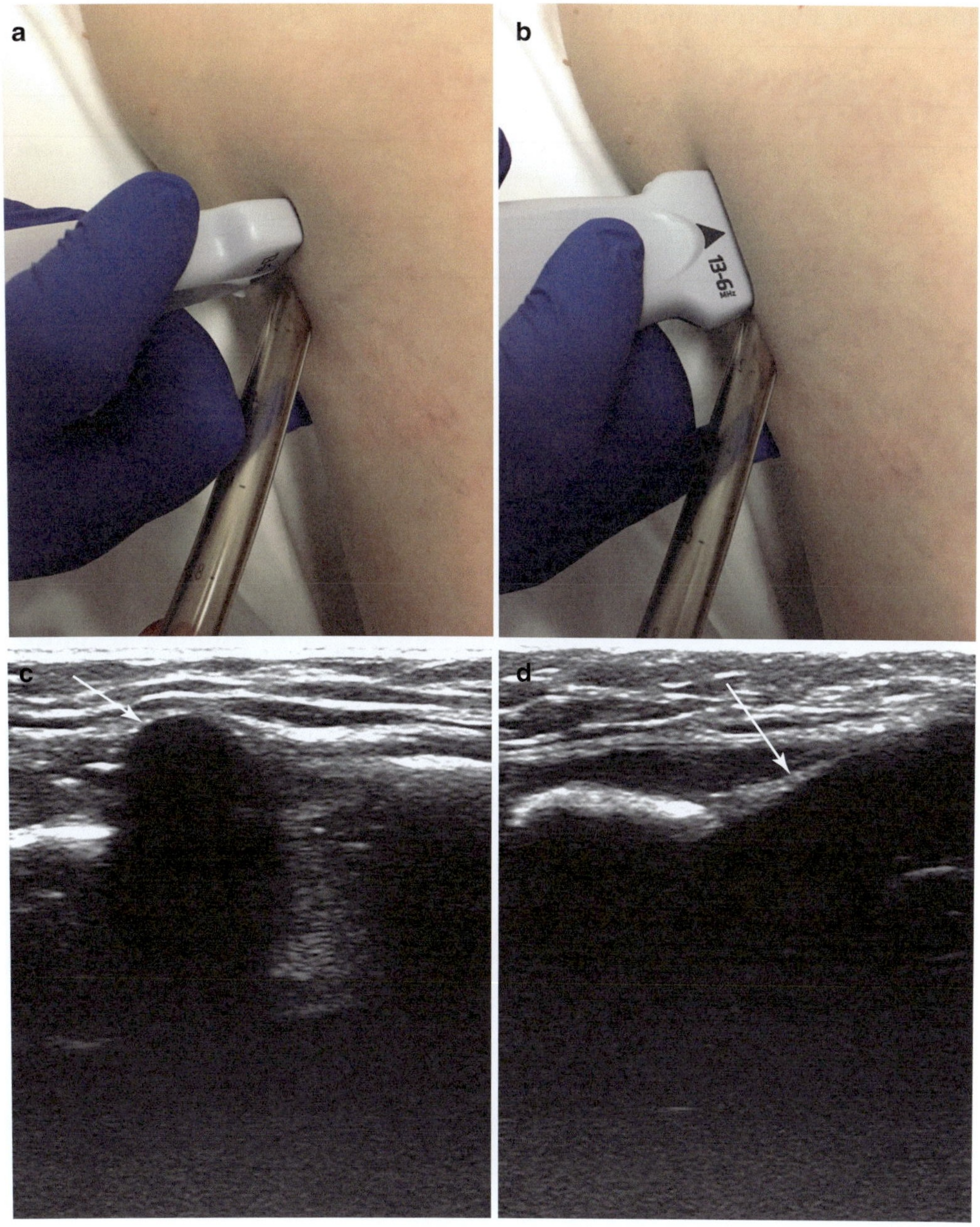

Fig. 21.26 Chest tube confirmation. (**a**) Probe positioning for short-axis approach. (**b**) Probe positioning for long-axis approach. (**c**) Chest tube (arrow) entering the thoracic cavity between two ribs in short axis. (**d**) Chest tube (arrow) entering the thoracic cavity between two ribs in long axis. (*Images courtesy of Michael Gottlieb, MD*)

Paracentesis

Overview

US-assisted or US-guided paracentesis offers several benefits that make it a preferred method over the landmark-based approach. With multiple potential needle insertion site options in the abdomen, a primary advantage of US is the ability to identify the largest fluid collection. Dynamic US guidance specifically permits precise needle direction, increasing the likelihood of successful removal of even small fluid collections for diagnostic sampling. While the success rate with landmark-based paracentesis is high at baseline, US guidance can further improve the success rate and serve as a rescue technique for failed landmark-based paracentesis [96, 97]. Another benefit of US is that it provides dynamic visualization of the needle to anesthetize the parietal peritoneum to reduce pain during the procedure. Real-time tracking of the needle's trajectory also allows avoidance of vital structures, such as peritoneal carcinomatosis, bowel, and abdominal wall vessels (e.g., prominent inferior epigastric vessels or varices in patients with cirrhosis) [98, 99].

Indications and Contraindications

Paracentesis is indicated for diagnostic assessment when encountering ascites of unclear etiology or to rule out spontaneous bacterial peritonitis. It may also be used for therapeutic purposes when larger volumes of ascites result in significant discomfort or respiratory distress. There are no absolute contraindications. Relative contraindications include coagulopathy, abdominal wall cellulitis, massive bowel distention, or ascites volume that is too small to safely access.

Technique

The patient should be in a supine, semi-recumbent position to allow fluid to pool dependently in the lower abdominal quadrants. Use a curvilinear probe to identify the largest fluid pocket, which is also a safe distance from the liver, spleen, kidneys, bladder, and bowel. Doppler ultrasound should also be used to assess for the inferior epigastric vessels [100]. The distances from skin to fluid collection and skin to underlying bowel should both be noted. Anesthetization of the parietal peritoneum should be done with in-plane visualization of the needle to provide optimal comfort. Next, advance the needle into the ascites pocket while aspirating until there is fluid return (Fig. 21.27, Video 21.6). Skin traction should be performed with the ulnar aspect of the hand or fifth finger of the ultrasound hand to produce a noncontiguous track between the dermis and peritoneum ("Z-track technique") to reduce the risk of persistent ascites leak.

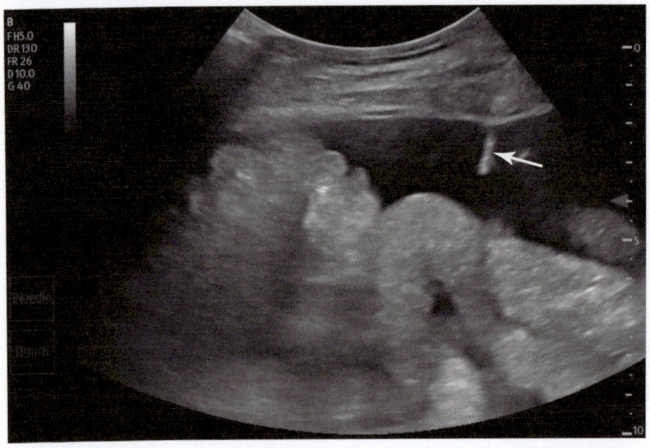

Fig. 21.27 Paracentesis performed under real-time ultrasound guidance. The needle (arrow) is seen in-plane entering the peritoneal space and avoiding mobile loops of bowel

Orogastric and Nasogastric Tube Placement

Overview

Blind insertion of orogastric (OG) and nasogastric (NG) tubes has a baseline failure rate of 50–66% and can lead to various complications such as nosebleeds, sore throat, tracheal placement, entanglement, and dislodgement—especially with repeated attempts [101]. Studies demonstrate that the use of US guidance is associated with higher success rates, fewer complications, and improved patient comfort [102, 103]. An NG tube can be visualized in the esophagus during insertion over 90% of the time [104]. In addition, compared to X-ray imaging, the accuracy of US in confirming tube placement is high (sensitivity 95–96%, specificity 91–100%) [105–107]. US can also reduce time to confirmation and reduce radiation exposure for pediatric patients [103, 108].

Indications and Contraindications

NG and OG tubes have a variety of uses, including feedings, medication administration, and removal of contents from the stomach for decompression. Relative contraindications include facial fractures.

Technique

To confirm tube position, two areas are assessed: the cervical esophagus and the stomach. Using a high-frequency linear probe, begin by scanning in a transverse plane at the anterolateral neck just superior to the suprasternal notch; this technique is similar to that for confirmation of endotracheal tube placement. Identify the esophagus, which will appear posterolateral to the trachea (most often to the left) as a flattened oval with muscular layers. Once insertion of the NG or OG tube has begun, look for a small, curved echogenic structure entering the esophageal lumen (Fig. 21.28). Rotating to a sagittal plane may demonstrate the tube as two parallel echogenic lines traversing through the esophagus.

Next, switch to a curvilinear probe and place it over the epigastrium. Visualize the stomach in the oblique and sagittal planes to observe the tube coursing through the gastric fundus and terminating in the antrum, confirming correct placement. Commonly, air in the stomach may make it difficult to directly visualize the tube. In these cases, injection of air or agitated saline through the tube can be useful for localization [109].

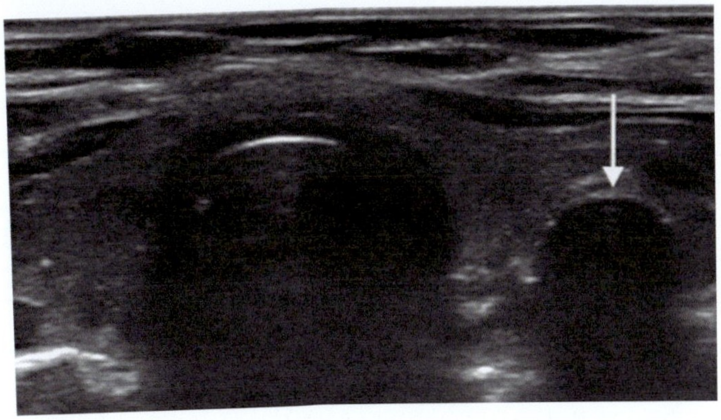

Fig. 21.28 Orogastric tube (arrow) in the esophagus in an intubated patient visualized on ultrasound in the short-axis plane

Lumbar Puncture

Overview

The performance of a lumbar puncture (LP) traditionally relies on the palpation of bony landmarks of the iliac crest and the spinous processes. This may be difficult due to body habitus, anatomic variations, or the inability to properly position a patient. Palpation-guided LP has a reported failure rate of 28% and a 17% incidence of traumatic tap [110, 111]. While the rate of performance of most emergency department procedures has remained stable over time, LP performance rates have been decreasing [112, 113], possibly due to changes in clinical guidelines and pathways. This may lead to skill atrophy and even lower success rates among those performing limited numbers of LPs during training [114]. Compared with the landmark-based approach, US-assisted LP is associated with higher success rates, fewer traumatic LPs, shorter time to successful LP, fewer needle passes, and lower patient pain scores [115, 116].

Indications and Contraindications

LP is indicated when there is suspicion of meningitis, subarachnoid hemorrhage, idiopathic intracranial hypertension, or other neurologic emergencies. While all patients may benefit from a US-assisted LP, the largest benefit may be in those with landmarks that are more challenging to palpate or in whom there may be spinal abnormalities (e.g., scoliosis). Contraindications include coagulopathy, skin infection at the site of needle insertion, concern for epidural abscess, or suspicion of increased intracranial pressure with risk for cerebral herniation.

Technique

Begin by placing the patient in a sitting or a lateral decubitus position with the spine flexed as much as possible to open the posterior vertebral spaces (Fig. 21.29). The high-frequency linear probe is preferred, but the low-frequency curvilinear probe may be necessary for larger patients to visualize the bones under several centimeters of adipose tissue.

US guidance may either be static or dynamic [117]. For the static approach, first place the probe at the top of the gluteal fold in a transverse orientation to visualize the sacrum. Moving the probe superiorly, identify the midline by visualizing and marking the spinous processes (Fig. 21.30). Once the midline is identified, rotate the probe 90° to a longitudinal orientation with the probe marker toward the patient's head. The probe is moved in a cephalad fashion in the middle of the spine. The first break in the bony cortex is the L5-S1 intervertebral space. The L5 spinous process then appears as a convex, hyperechoic line and should correspond to the same depth as the spinous process noted in the transverse image. Moving the probe superiorly, the L4 and L3 spinous

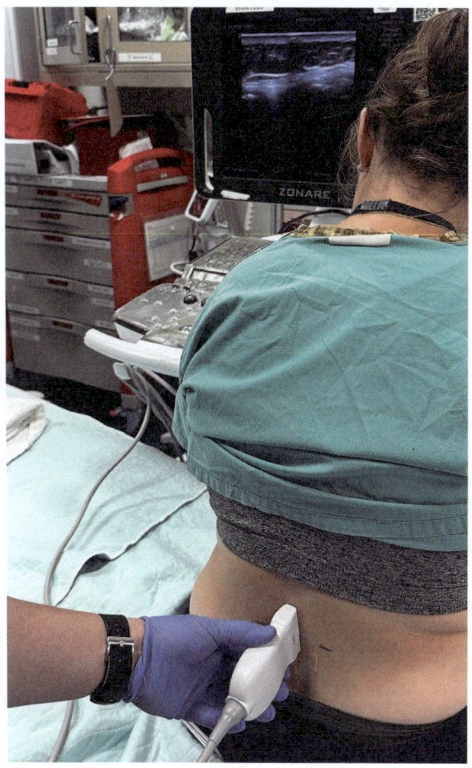

Fig. 21.29 Procedural setup for US-assisted lumbar puncture (sterile preparation not demonstrated)

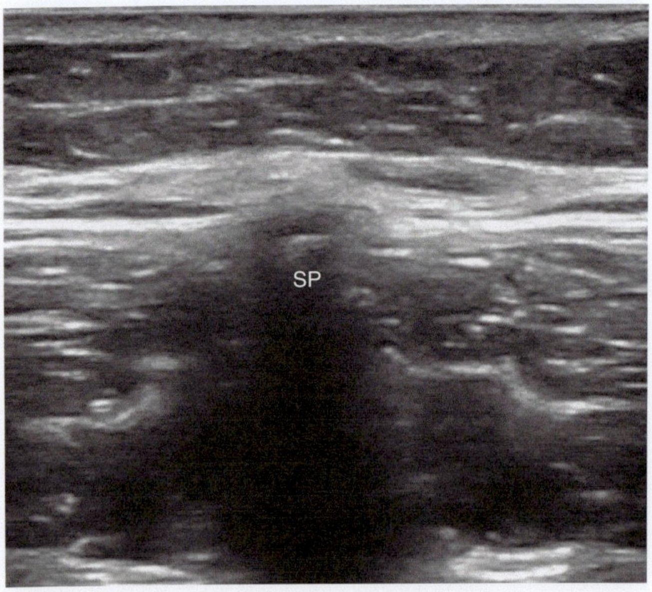

Fig. 21.30 A hyperechoic spinous process (SP) with posterior shadowing is seen after the placement of the ultrasound probe in a transverse orientation in the spinal midline

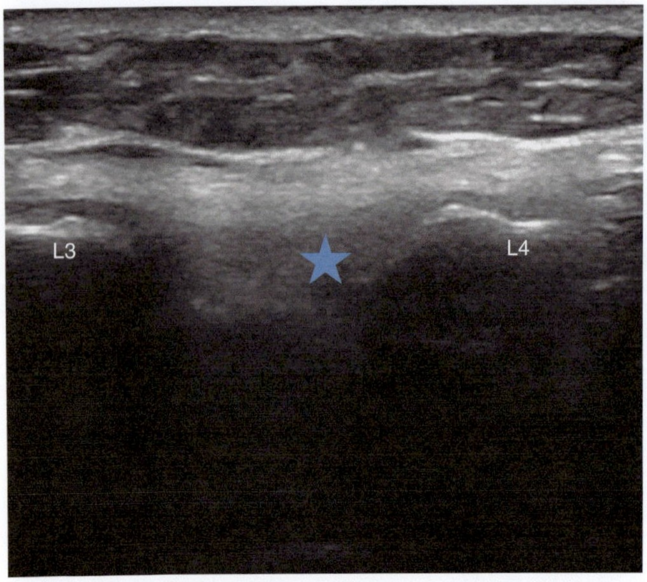

Fig. 21.31 Placing the ultrasound probe in a sagittal orientation in the spinal midline with the marker cephalad, the L3 and L4 spinous processes appear as hyperechoic lines with posterior shadowing. The star represents the target interspinous space between them

processes can be visualized (Fig. 21.31). The desired interspinous space(s) are also marked.

Either the L5-S1, L4-L5, or the L3-L4 spaces may be used. Place the middle of the target intervertebral space in the center of the screen and mark a line on the skin with a surgical marker in the middle of the probe. Ensure that the marker used will not be wiped away during the skin preparation process. The crosshairs marked on the skin (at the intersection of spinal midline and desired interspinous space) is the optimal place to introduce the needle (Fig. 21.32). An alternative approach to marking the site of needle insertion is to mark both the lower border of the superior spinous process and the superior border of the inferior spinous process to demonstrate the extent of the intervertebral space. Using either approach, we recommend marking two spaces so that if the initial attempt is not successful, an alternate site is available. The LP can then proceed in the traditional manner using the markings instead of the bony landmarks as a guide. Care must be taken that the patient does not move between the marking of the site and the performance of the procedure.

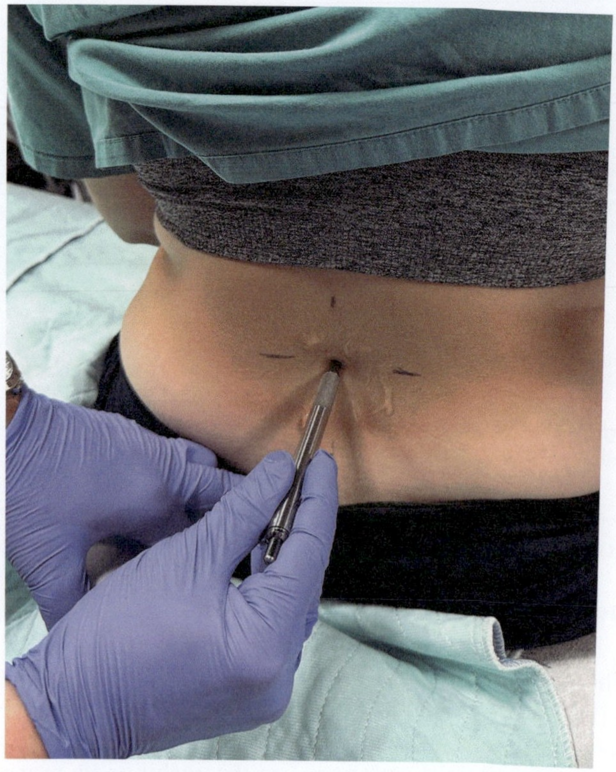

Fig. 21.32 The intersection of the marked spinal midline and the targeted interspinous space denotes the site of needle insertion. After the gel is removed, use the marking pen to connect the hatch marks

Hematoma Block

Overview

Hematoma blocks involve injecting local anesthetic into the hematoma at the site of a displaced fracture to mitigate the pain that is associated with manual reduction of the fracture. Traditionally, a fracture is first identified on radiographs, localized via palpation, and injection is performed at the site of the hematoma. This can be difficult if there is significant soft tissue swelling or if there are multiple fractures. US guidance allows visualization of the fracture line and precise guidance of the needle tip to the fracture site, allowing for accurate placement of the local anesthetic. US-guided hematoma blocks have been shown to be as effective as procedural sedation for the reduction of distal radius fractures and are associated with a significantly decreased length of stay [118, 119].

Indications and Contraindications

Hematoma blocks are indicated in any displaced or angulated fracture site where manual reduction will be required. They may also be used for fractures that will not be reduced but cause significant pain (e.g., humerus fracture, isolated distal fibular fracture). Contraindications are allergy to the local anesthetic or a location directly adjacent to a vessel where intravascular injection is likely.

Technique

To perform this block, place a high-frequency linear probe on the fracture site parallel to the long axis of the bone. A curvilinear probe may be needed for bones that underlie a significant distance of soft tissue (e.g., femur). The cortex of the bone appears as a hyperechoic, bright white line. A displaced fracture will be visualized as a break in the continuity of this hyperechoic line with a step-off. The needle is introduced in an in-plane fashion, aiming to position the needle tip at the site of the fracture (Fig. 21.33). Small test aliquots of local anesthetic can be used to help localize the needle tip and ensure that the local anesthetic is being placed at the fracture site. When the anesthetic solution is injected into the correct location, the fracture site will appear slightly widened, and fluid will be seen swirling within the hematoma [120]. To prevent local anesthetic systemic toxicity, a safe dose of local anesthetic should be calculated in advance, and care should be taken not to exceed this dose.

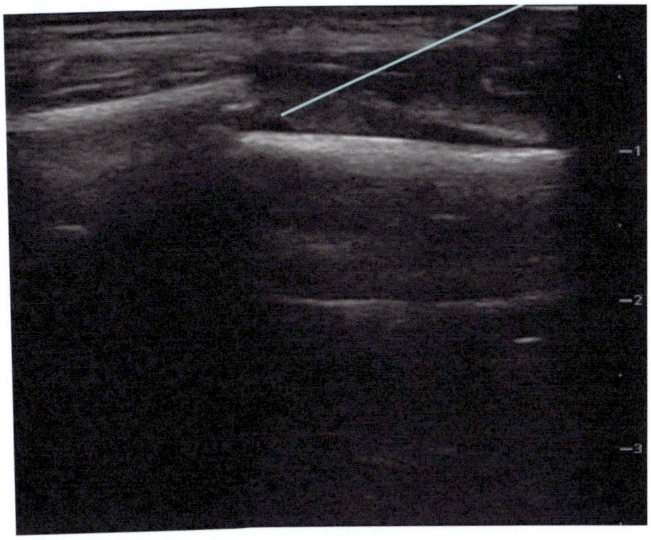

Fig. 21.33 Target site for hematoma block. A displaced fracture of the radius is seen as a discontinuity and step-off of the hyperechoic bony cortex. The trajectory of the needle is depicted (blue line) with the needle tip positioned within the hypoechoic hematoma. Local anesthetic should be injected into this space

Pearls and Pitfalls

- Refining various techniques to maximize needle visualization and developing comfort with both out-of-plane and in-plane guidance techniques will lead to performance benefits for all US-guided procedures.
- US guidance reduces the mechanical complications from all vascular access procedures. Make sure to always know where the needle tip is when performing this procedure and never advance the needle if uncertain as to the needle tip's location. If unsure, stop moving the needle and move the probe to find the needle tip before advancing the needle.
- During real-time guidance of pericardiocentesis, decreasing depth to focus on the target fluid pocket or the use of a high-frequency linear probe will facilitate needle visualization. Aspiration of fluid or blood is not sufficient for confirmation of intrapericardial needle placement.
- If uncertain about pacemaker settings, use the emergency pacing mode ("DOO" key), which initiates asynchronous pacing independent of intrinsic rhythm, with maximal atrial and ventricular outputs.
- Make sure to account for the dynamic anatomy of the thoracic cavity. During thoracentesis, use US to ensure the pleural fluid collection remains accessible and critical structures (lung, diaphragm, spleen, liver) remain distant from the needle insertion site throughout the respiratory cycle.
- Inadvertent puncture of bowel is a risk during static US guidance of paracentesis. Ensure distances from skin to fluid collection and skin to the nearest bowel loop are measured to both anticipate the depth of needle insertion when fluid should be aspirated and the maximal depth a needle should be advanced.
- Avoid malposition of an NG or OG tube during placement by visualizing it in the esophagus at the level of the neck, above the sternal notch. Actively observe the trachea for evidence of an echogenic foreign body or movement suggesting malposition.
- Ensure the articular processes are not misidentified as spinous processes during LP by sliding to visualize the most superficial portion and ensuring the depth is the same on both short- and long-axis views.

References

1. Brass P, Hellmich M, Kolodziej L, Schick G, Smith AF. Ultrasound guidance versus anatomical landmarks for internal jugular vein catheterization. Cochrane Database Syst Rev. 2015;2017(6) https://doi.org/10.1002/14651858.CD006962.PUB2/MEDIA/CDSR/CD006962/IMAGE_T/TCD006962-CMP-003-06.XXX.
2. Making Health Care Safer: A Critical Analysis of Patient Safety Practices. Accessed 10 Mar 2024. https://archive.ahrq.gov/clinic/ptsafety/
3. Corporation R, HealthSystem Consortium U. AHRQ Quality Indicators Toolkit Selected Best Practices and Suggestions for Improvement PSI 7: Central Venous Catheter (CVC)-Related Bloodstream Infections (BSIs) Why Focus on Central Line-Related Bloodstream Infections (CLABSIs)?
4. Guidance on the use of ultrasound locating devices for placing central venous catheters. Published online 2002. Accessed 3 Oct 2024. www.nice.org.uk/guidance/ta49
5. Franco-Sadud R, Schnobrich D, Mathews BK, et al. Recommendations on the use of Ultrasound guidance for central and peripheral vascular access in adults: a position statement of the Society of Hospital Medicine. J Hosp Med. 2019;14(9):E1. https://doi.org/10.12788/JHM.3287.
6. Reusz G, Sarkany P, Gal J, Csomos A. Needle-related ultrasound artifacts and their importance in anaesthetic practice. Br J Anaesth. 2014;112(5):794–802. https://doi.org/10.1093/BJA/AET585.
7. Smith J, Finnoff JT, Fitzgerald J, et al. AIUM practice parameter for the performance of selected ultrasound-guided procedures. J Ultrasound Med. 2016;35(9):1–40. https://doi.org/10.7863/JUM.2016.35.9.5.
8. Garnier T, Bloc S, Mercadal L, Ecoffey C, Dhonneur G. Hydrolocalization during ultrasound-guided regional anesthesia. Anesthesiology. 2007;107:A639.
9. Wiesmann T, Bornträger A, Zoremba M, Neff M, Wulf H, Steinfeldt T. Compound imaging technology and echogenic needle design: effects on needle visibility and tissue imaging. Reg Anesth Pain Med. 2013;38(5):452–5. https://doi.org/10.1097/AAP.0B013E31829730D5.
10. Gupta RK, Lane J, Allen B, Shi Y, Schildcrout JS. Improving needle visualization by novice residents during an in-plane ultrasound nerve block simulation using an in-plane multiangle needle guide. Pain Med. 2013;14(10):1600–7. https://doi.org/10.1111/PME.12160.
11. Raft J, Dupanloup D, Clerc-Urmès I, Baumann C, Richebé P, Bouaziz H. Training novice in ultrasound-guided venipuncture: A randomized controlled trial comparing out-of-plane needle-guided versus free-hand ultrasound techniques on a simulator. J Vasc Access. 2021;22(6):898–904. https://doi.org/10.1177/1129729820962916.
12. England JR, Fischbeck T, Tchelepi H. The value of needle-guidance Technology in Ultrasound-Guided Percutaneous Procedures Performed by radiology residents: A comparison of freehand, in-plane, fixed-angle, and electromagnetic needle tracking techniques. J Ultrasound Med. 2019;38(2):399–405. https://doi.org/10.1002/JUM.14701.
13. Johnson AN, Peiffer JS, Halmann N, Delaney L, Owen CA, Hersh J. Ultrasound-guided needle technique accuracy: prospective comparison of passive magnetic tracking versus unassisted echogenic needle localization. Reg Anesth Pain Med. 2017;42(2):223–32. https://doi.org/10.1097/AAP.0000000000000549.
14. Slama M, Novara A, Safavian A, Ossart M, Safar M, Fagon JY. Improvement of internal jugular vein cannulation using an ultrasound-guided technique. Intensive Care Med. 1997;23(8):916–9. https://doi.org/10.1007/s001340050432.
15. Hilty WM, Hudson PA, Levitt MA, Hall JB. Real-time ultrasound-guided femoral vein catheterization during cardiopulmonary resuscitation. Ann Emerg Med. 1997;29(3):331–336; discussion 337. https://doi.org/10.1016/s0196-0644(97)70344-5.
16. Theodoro D, Bausano B, Lewis L, Evanoff B, Marin K. A descriptive comparison of ultrasound-guided central venous cannulation of the internal jugular vein to landmark-based subclavian vein cannulation. Acad Emerg Med. 2010;17(4):416–22. https://doi.org/10.1111/J.1553-2712.2010.00703.X.
17. Miller AH, Roth BA, Mills TJ, Woody JR, Longmoor CE, Foster B. Ultrasound guidance versus the landmark technique for the placement of central venous catheters in the emergency department. Acad Emerg Med. 2002;9(8):800–5. https://doi.org/10.1111/J.1553-2712.2002.TB02168.X.
18. DeFrances CJ, Hall MJ. National hospital discharge survey. Adv Data. 2005;2007(385):1–19.
19. McGee DC, Gould MK. Preventing complications of central venous catheterization. N Engl J Med. 2003;348(12):1123–33. https://doi.org/10.1056/NEJMRA011883.
20. Randolph AG, Cook DJ, Gonzales CA, Pribble CG. Ultrasound guidance for placement of central venous catheters: a meta-analysis of the literature. Crit Care Med. 1996;24(12):2053–8. https://doi.org/10.1097/00003246-199612000-00020.
21. Parienti JJ, Mongardon N, Mégarbane B, et al. Intravascular complications of central venous catheterization by insertion site. N Engl J Med. 2015;373(13):1220–9. https://doi.org/10.1056/NEJMOA1500964.
22. Timsit JF. What is the best site for central venous catheter insertion in critically ill patients? Crit Care. 2003;7(6):397–9. https://doi.org/10.1186/CC2179.
23. Marik PE, Flemmer M, Harrison W. The risk of catheter-related bloodstream infection with femoral venous catheters as compared to subclavian and internal jugular venous catheters: a systematic review of the literature and meta-analysis. Crit Care Med. 2012;40(8):2479–85. https://doi.org/10.1097/CCM.0B013E318255D9BC.
24. Tolbert TN, Haines LE, Terentiev V, et al. An ultrasound training program's effect on central venous catheter locations and complications. Am J Emerg Med. 2014;32(10):1290–3. https://doi.org/10.1016/J.AJEM.2014.07.025.
25. Garcia-Leal M, Guzman-Lopez S, Verdines-Perez AM, et al. Trendelenburg position for internal jugular vein catheterization: a systematic review and meta-analysis. J Vasc Access. 2023;24(2):338–47. https://doi.org/10.1177/11297298211031339.
26. Denys BG, Uretsky BF, Reddy PS. Ultrasound-assisted cannulation of the internal jugular vein. A prospective comparison to the external landmark-guided technique. Circulation. 1993;87(5):1557–62. https://doi.org/10.1161/01.CIR.87.5.1557.
27. Hrics P, Wilber S, Blanda MP, Gallo U. Ultrasound-assisted internal jugular vein catheterization in the ED. Am J Emerg Med. 1998;16(4):401–3. https://doi.org/10.1016/S0735-6757(98)90140-1.
28. Stone MB, Moon C, Sutijono D, Blaivas M. Needle tip visualization during ultrasound-guided vascular access: short-axis vs long-axis approach. Am J Emerg Med. 2010;28(3):343–7. https://doi.org/10.1016/J.AJEM.2008.11.022.
29. Stone MB, Nagdev A, Murphy MC, Sisson CA. Ultrasound detection of guidewire position during central venous catheterization. Am J Emerg Med. 2010;28(1):82–4. https://doi.org/10.1016/J.AJEM.2008.09.019.
30. Blaivas M. Video analysis of accidental arterial cannulation with dynamic ultrasound guidance for central venous access. J Ultrasound Med. 2009;28(9):1239–44. https://doi.org/10.7863/JUM.2009.28.9.1239.

31. Phelan M, Hagerty D. The oblique view: an alternative approach for ultrasound-guided central line placement. J Emerg Med. 2009;37(4):403–8. https://doi.org/10.1016/J.JEMERMED.2008.02.061.
32. Balaban O, Aydin T, Musmul A. Lateral oblique approach for internal jugular vein catheterization: randomized comparison of oblique and short-axis view of ultrasound-guided technique. North Clin Istanb. 2019;7(1) https://doi.org/10.14744/NCI.2019.86658.
33. Lorente L, Henry C, Martín MM, Jiménez A, Mora ML. Central venous catheter-related infection in a prospective and observational study of 2,595 catheters. Crit Care. 2005;9(6):R631. https://doi.org/10.1186/CC3824.
34. Subramony R, Spann R, Medak A, Campbell C. Ultrasound-Guided vs. Landmark method for subclavian vein catheterization in an academic emergency department. J Emerg Med. 2022;62(6):760–8. https://doi.org/10.1016/J.JEMERMED.2021.11.002.
35. Lalu MM, Fayad A, Ahmed O, et al. Ultrasound-Guided subclavian vein catheterization: A systematic review and meta-analysis. Crit Care Med. 2015;43(7):1498–507. https://doi.org/10.1097/CCM.0000000000000973.
36. Fragou M, Gravvanis A, Dimitriou V, et al. Real-time ultrasound-guided subclavian vein cannulation versus the landmark method in critical care patients: a prospective randomized study. Crit Care Med. 2011;39(7):1607–12. https://doi.org/10.1097/CCM.0B013E318218A1AE.
37. Sidoti A, Brogi E, Biancofiore G, et al. Ultrasound- versus landmark-guided subclavian vein catheterization: a prospective observational study from a tertiary referral hospital. Sci Rep. 2019;9(1):12248. https://doi.org/10.1038/S41598-019-48766-1.
38. Mallin M, Louis H, Madsen T. A novel technique for ultrasound-guided supraclavicular subclavian cannulation. Am J Emerg Med. 2010;28(8):966–9. https://doi.org/10.1016/J.AJEM.2009.07.019.
39. Vezzani A, Manca T, Brusasco C, et al. A randomized clinical trial of ultrasound-guided infra-clavicular cannulation of the subclavian vein in cardiac surgical patients: short-axis versus long-axis approach. Intensive Care Med. 2017;43(11):1594–601. https://doi.org/10.1007/S00134-017-4756-6.
40. Randall C, Schmeiser E, Fiers E, Little A, Dogbey G, Richardson G. Ultrasound investigation of leg position to enhance femoral vein exposure for cannulation. J Emerg Med. 2014;47(2):176–81. https://doi.org/10.1016/J.JEMERMED.2014.02.001.
41. Read H, Holdgate A, Watkins S. Simple external rotation of the leg increases the size and accessibility of the femoral vein. Emerg Med Australas. 2012;24(4):408–13. https://doi.org/10.1111/J.1742-6723.2012.01568.X.
42. Werner SL, Jones RA, Emerman CL. Effect of hip abduction and external rotation on femoral vein exposure for possible cannulation. J Emerg Med. 2008;35(1):73–5. https://doi.org/10.1016/J.JEMERMED.2007.03.023.
43. Ablordeppey EA, Drewry AM, Beyer AB, et al. Diagnostic accuracy of central venous catheter confirmation by bedside ultrasound versus chest radiography in critically ill patients: a systematic review and meta-analysis. Crit Care Med. 2017;45(4):715. https://doi.org/10.1097/CCM.0000000000002188.
44. Poulsen E, Aagaard R, Bisgaard J, Sørensen HT, Juhl-Olsen P. The effects of ultrasound guidance on first-attempt success for difficult peripheral intravenous catheterization: a systematic review and meta-analysis. Eur J Emerg Med. 2023;30(2):70–7. https://doi.org/10.1097/MEJ.0000000000000993.
45. Mitchell EO, Jones P, Snelling PJ. Ultrasound for pediatric peripheral intravenous catheter insertion: a systematic review. Pediatrics. 2022;149(5) https://doi.org/10.1542/PEDS.2021-055523.
46. Costantino TG, Parikh AK, Satz WA, Fojtik JP. Ultrasonography-guided peripheral intravenous access versus traditional approaches in patients with difficult intravenous access. Ann Emerg Med. 2005;46(5):456–61. https://doi.org/10.1016/J.ANNEMERGMED.2004.12.026.
47. Juvin P, Blarel A, Bruno F, Desmonts JM. Is peripheral line placement more difficult in obese than in lean patients? Anesth Analg. 2003;96(4):1218. https://doi.org/10.1213/01.ANE.0000050570.85195.29.
48. Dargin JM, Rebholz CM, Lowenstein RA, Mitchell PM, Feldman JA. Ultrasonography-guided peripheral intravenous catheter survival in ED patients with difficult access. Am J Emerg Med. 2010;28(1):1–7. https://doi.org/10.1016/J.AJEM.2008.09.001.
49. Au AK, Rotte MJ, Grzybowski RJ, Ku BS, Fields JM. Decrease in central venous catheter placement due to use of ultrasound guidance for peripheral intravenous catheters. Am J Emerg Med. 2012;30(9):1950–4. https://doi.org/10.1016/J.AJEM.2012.04.016.
50. Shokoohi H, Boniface K, McCarthy M, et al. Ultrasound-guided peripheral intravenous access program is associated with a marked reduction in central venous catheter use in noncritically ill emergency department patients. Ann Emerg Med. 2013;61(2):198–203. https://doi.org/10.1016/J.ANNEMERGMED.2012.09.016.
51. Adhikari S, Blaivas M, Morrison D, Lander L. Comparison of infection rates among ultrasound-guided versus traditionally placed peripheral intravenous lines. J Ultrasound Med. 2010;29(5):741–7. https://doi.org/10.7863/JUM.2010.29.5.741.
52. Gottlieb M, Sundaram T, Holladay D, Nakitende D. Ultrasound-Guided peripheral intravenous line placement: a narrative review of evidence-based best practices. West J Emerg Med. 2017;18(6):1047–54. https://doi.org/10.5811/WESTJEM.2017.7.34610.
53. Elia F, Ferrari G, Molino P, et al. Standard-length catheters vs long catheters in ultrasound-guided peripheral vein cannulation. Am J Emerg Med. 2012;30(5):712–6. https://doi.org/10.1016/J.AJEM.2011.04.019.
54. Mahler SA, Wang H, Lester C, Skinner J, Arnold TC, Conrad SA. Short- vs long-axis approach to ultrasound-guided peripheral intravenous access: a prospective randomized study. Am J Emerg Med. 2011;29(9):1194–7. https://doi.org/10.1016/J.AJEM.2010.07.015.
55. Gottlieb M, Holladay D, Peksa GD. Comparison of short- vs Long-axis technique for Ultrasound-guided peripheral line placement: a systematic review and meta-analysis. Cureus. 2018;10(5):e2718. https://doi.org/10.7759/CUREUS.2718.
56. McCarthy ML, Shokoohi H, Boniface KS, et al. Ultrasonography versus landmark for peripheral intravenous cannulation: a randomized controlled trial. Ann Emerg Med. 2016;68(1):10–8. https://doi.org/10.1016/J.ANNEMERGMED.2015.09.009.
57. Panebianco NL, Fredette JM, Szyld D, Sagalyn EB, Pines JM, Dean AJ. What you see (sonographically) is what you get: vein and patient characteristics associated with successful ultrasound-guided peripheral intravenous placement in patients with difficult access. Acad Emerg Med. 2009;16(12):1298–303. https://doi.org/10.1111/j.1553-2712.2009.00520.x.
58. Fields JM, Dean AJ, Todman RW, et al. The effect of vessel depth, diameter, and location on ultrasound-guided peripheral intravenous catheter longevity. Am J Emerg Med. 2012;30(7):1134–40. https://doi.org/10.1016/J.AJEM.2011.07.027.
59. ACR-NASCI-SPR Practice Parameter for the Performance and Interpretation of Cardiac Computed Tomography (CT) | Enhanced Reader. Available at: https://www.acr.org/-/media/ACR/Files/Practice-Parameters/Quant-CardiacCT-MR.pdf
60. Chinnock B, Thornton S, Hendey GW. Predictors of success in nurse-performed ultrasound-guided cannulation. J

Emerg Med. 2007;33(4):401–5. https://doi.org/10.1016/J.JEMERMED.2007.02.027.
61. Hardie AD, Kereshi B. Incidence of intravenous contrast extravasation: increased risk for patients with deep brachial catheter placement from the emergency department. Emerg Radiol. 2014;21(3):235–8. https://doi.org/10.1007/S10140-013-1185-X.
62. Flumignan RLG, Trevisani VFM, Lopes RD, Baptista-Silva JCC, Flumignan CDQ, Nakano LCU. Ultrasound guidance for arterial (other than femoral) catheterisation in adults. Cochrane Database Syst Rev. 2021;10(10):CD013585. https://doi.org/10.1002/14651858.CD013585.PUB2.
63. Raphael CK, El Hage Chehade NA, Khabsa J, Akl EA, Aouad-Maroun M, Kaddoum R. Ultrasound-guided arterial cannulation in the paediatric population. Cochrane Database Syst Rev. 2023;3(3):CD011364. https://doi.org/10.1002/14651858.CD011364.PUB3.
64. Cao L, Tan Y, Wei T, Li H. Comparison between the long-axis in-plane and short-axis out-of-plane approaches for ultrasound-guided arterial cannulation: a meta-analysis and systematic review. BMC Anesthesiol. 2023;23(1):120. https://doi.org/10.1186/S12871-023-02076-2.
65. Tsang TSM, Enriquez-Sarano M, Freeman WK, et al. Consecutive 1127 therapeutic echocardiographically guided pericardiocenteses: clinical profile, practice patterns, and outcomes spanning 21 years. Mayo Clin Proc. 2002;77(5):429–36. https://doi.org/10.4065/77.5.429.
66. Cooper JP, Oliver RM, Currie P, Walker JM, Swanton RH. How do the clinical findings in patients with pericardial effusions influence the success of aspiration? Br Heart J. 1995;73(4):351. https://doi.org/10.1136/HRT.73.4.351.
67. Cho BC, Kang SM, Kim DH, et al. Clinical and echocardiographic characteristics of pericardial effusion in patients who underwent echocardiographically guided pericardiocentesis: Yonsei Cardiovascular Center experience, 1993–2003. Yonsei Med J. 2004;45(3):462–8. https://doi.org/10.3349/YMJ.2004.45.3.462.
68. Tsang TSM, El-Najdawi EK, Seward JB, Hagler DJ, Freeman WK, O'Leary PW. Percutaneous echocardiographically guided pericardiocentesis in pediatric patients: evaluation of safety and efficacy. J Am Soc Echocardiogr. 1998;11(11):1072–7. https://doi.org/10.1016/S0894-7317(98)70159-2.
69. Ryu AJ, Kane GC, Pislaru SV, et al. Bleeding complications of Ultrasound-Guided Pericardiocentesis in the presence of coagulopathy or thrombocytopenia. J Am Soc Echocardiogr. 2020;33(3):399–401. https://doi.org/10.1016/j.echo.2019.11.006.
70. Stolz L, Situ-Lacasse E, Acuña J, et al. What is the ideal approach for emergent pericardiocentesis using point-of-care ultrasound guidance? World J Emerg Med. 2021;12(3):169–73. https://doi.org/10.5847/wjem.j.1920-8642.2021.03.001.
71. Fields JM, Paziana K, Vuljaj N, Fischer J, Ku BS. Emergency Ultrasound-guided Pericardiocentesis using a high-frequency linear Array transducer to improve needle tip visualization. Acad Emerg Med. 2012;19(5):e16. https://doi.org/10.1111/J.1553-2712.2012.01344.X.
72. Zhang L, Zhang XF, Liu Z, et al. High frequency ultrasound-guided pericardiocentesis performed in the sitting position: a novel apical approach. Clin Cardiol. 2021;44(8):1106. https://doi.org/10.1002/CLC.23657.
73. Alerhand S, Adrian RJ, Long B, Avila J. Pericardial tamponade: a comprehensive emergency medicine and echocardiography review. Am J Emerg Med. 2022;58:159–74. https://doi.org/10.1016/J.AJEM.2022.05.001.
74. Blanco P, Volpicelli G. Looking a bit superficial to the pleura. Crit Ultrasound J. 2014;6(1):13. https://doi.org/10.1186/S13089-014-0013-1.
75. Mohammed NA, Al-zubairi TA, Al-soumai MH. A case report on ultrasound-guided pericardiocentesis with a right parasternal approach: a novel in-plane lateral-to-medial technique. Int J Emerg Med. 2024;17(1):1–8. https://doi.org/10.1186/S12245-024-00592-7/FIGURES/3.
76. Ferro B, Vegnuti L, Santonocito O, Roncucci P. Ultrasound emergency lateral-to-medial parasternal pericardiocentesis with high frequency probe in COVID-19: a case report. Eur Heart J Case Rep. 2022;6(5) https://doi.org/10.1093/EHJCR/YTAC203.
77. Osman A, Wan Chuan T, Ab Rahman J, Via G, Tavazzi G. Ultrasound-guided pericardiocentesis: a novel parasternal approach. Eur J Emerg Med. 2018;25(5):322. https://doi.org/10.1097/MEJ.0000000000000471.
78. Adler Y, Charron P, Imazio M, et al. 2015 ESC guidelines for the diagnosis and management of pericardial diseases: the task force for the diagnosis and Management of Pericardial Diseases of the European Society of Cardiology (ESC)Endorsed by: the European Association for Cardio-Thoracic Surgery (EACTS). Eur Heart J. 2015;36(42):2921–64. https://doi.org/10.1093/EURHEARTJ/EHV318.
79. Pradhan R, Okabe T, Yoshida K, Angouras DC, DeCaro MV, Marhefka GD. Patient characteristics and predictors of mortality associated with pericardial decompression syndrome: a comprehensive analysis of published cases. Eur Heart J Acute Cardiovasc Care. 2015;4(2):113–20. https://doi.org/10.1177/2048872614547975.
80. Long B, Bridwell RE, DeVivo A, Gottlieb M. Transvenous pacemaker placement: a review for emergency clinicians. J Emerg Med. 2024;66(4):e492–502. https://doi.org/10.1016/J.JEMERMED.2023.11.018.
81. Lerner RP, Haaland A, Lin J. Temporary transvenous pacer placement under transesophageal echocardiogram guidance in the Emergency Department. Am J Emerg Med. 2020;38(5):1044.e3–4. https://doi.org/10.1016/J.AJEM.2019.12.027.
82. Tabak B, Elliott CL, Mahnke CB, Tanaka LY, Ogino MT. Transthoracic echocardiography visualization of bicaval dual lumen catheters for veno-venous extracorporeal membrane oxygenation. J Clin Ultrasound. 2012;40(3):183–6. https://doi.org/10.1002/JCU.21873.
83. Sjaus A, Fayad A. The use of subcostal echocardiographic views to guide the insertion of a right ventricular temporary Transvenous pacemaker—description of the technique. J Cardiothorac Vasc Anesth. 2019;33(10):2797–803. https://doi.org/10.1053/j.jvca.2019.01.033.
84. Aguilera PA, Durham BA, Riley DC. Emergency transvenous cardiac pacing placement using ultrasound guidance. Ann Emerg Med. 2000;36(3):224–7. https://doi.org/10.1067/MEM.2000.108654.
85. Rodriguez Lima DR, Yepes AF, Birchenall Jiménez CI, Mercado Díaz MA, Pinilla Rojas DI. Real-time ultrasound-guided thoracentesis in the intensive care unit: prevalence of mechanical complications. Ultrasound J. 2020;12(1):25. https://doi.org/10.1186/s13089-020-00172-9.
86. Sperandeo M, Quarato CMI, Squatrito R, et al. Effectiveness and safety of real-time transthoracic ultrasound-Guided thoracentesis. Diagnostics. 2022;12(3):725. https://doi.org/10.3390/diagnostics12030725.
87. Stevic R, Colic N, Bascarevic S, et al. Sonographic indicators for treatment choice and follow-up in patients with pleural effusion. Can Respir J. 2018;2018(1):9761583. https://doi.org/10.1155/2018/9761583.
88. Cantey EP, Walter JM, Corbridge T, Barsuk JH. Complications of thoracentesis: incidence, risk factors, and strategies for prevention. Curr Opin Pulm Med. 2016;22(4):378–85. https://doi.org/10.1097/MCP.0000000000000285.

89. Cavanna L, Mordenti P, Bertè R, et al. Ultrasound guidance reduces pneumothorax rate and improves safety of thoracentesis in malignant pleural effusion: report on 445 consecutive patients with advanced cancer. World J Surg Oncol. 2014;12(1):139. https://doi.org/10.1186/1477-7819-12-139.
90. Feller-Kopman D. Ultrasound-Guided thoracentesis. Chest. 2006;129(6):1709–14. https://doi.org/10.1378/chest.129.6.1709.
91. Hernandez MC, El Khatib M, Prokop L, Zielinski MD, Aho JM. Complications in tube thoracostomy: systematic review and meta-analysis. J Trauma Acute Care Surg. 2018;85(2):413–9. https://doi.org/10.1097/TA.0000000000001840.
92. Kwiatt M, Tarbox A, MarkJ S, et al. Thoracostomy tubes: a comprehensive review of complications and related topics. Int J Crit Illn Inj Sci. 2014;4(2):143. https://doi.org/10.4103/2229-5151.134182.
93. Taylor LA, Vitto MJ, Joyce M, Tozer J, Evans DP. Ultrasound-guided thoracostomy site identification in healthy volunteers. Crit Ultrasound J. 2018;10(1):1–5. https://doi.org/10.1186/S13089-018-0108-1/FIGURES/4.
94. Nakitende D, Gottlieb M, Ruskis J, Kimball D, Christian E, Bailitz J. Ultrasound for confirmation of thoracostomy tube placement by emergency medicine residents. Trauma. 2017;19(1):35–8. https://doi.org/10.1177/1460408616649218.
95. Jenkins JA, Gharahbaghian L, Doniger SJ, et al. Sonographic identification of tube Thoracostomy study (SITTS): confirmation of intrathoracic placement. West J Emerg Med. 2012;13(4):305–11. https://doi.org/10.5811/WESTJEM.2011.10.6680.
96. Cho J, Jensen TP, Reierson K, et al. Recommendations on the use of Ultrasound guidance for adult abdominal paracentesis: a position statement of the Society of Hospital Medicine. J Hosp Med. 2019;14:E7. https://doi.org/10.12788/JHM.3095.
97. Nazeer SR, Dewbre H, Miller AH. Ultrasound-assisted paracentesis performed by emergency physicians vs the traditional technique: a prospective, randomized study. Am J Emerg Med. 2005;23(3):363–7. https://doi.org/10.1016/j.ajem.2004.11.001.
98. Sekiguchi H, Suzuki J, Daniels CE. Making paracentesis safer. Chest. 2013;143(4):1136–9. https://doi.org/10.1378/chest.12-0871.
99. Stone JC, Moak JH. Feasibility of sonographic localization of the inferior epigastric artery before ultrasound-guided paracentesis. Am J Emerg Med. 2015;33(12):1795–8. https://doi.org/10.1016/j.ajem.2015.06.067.
100. Barsuk JH, Rosen BT, Cohen ER, Feinglass J, Ault MJ. Vascular ultrasonography: a novel method to reduce paracentesis related major bleeding. J Hosp Med. 2018;13(1):30–3. https://doi.org/10.12788/JHM.2863.
101. Jonnavithula N, Padhy S, Ravula R, Alekhya G. Comparison of ease of insertion of nasogastric tube in standard sniffing position and in additional flexion of the neck: a randomized control trial. Trends Anaesthesia Crit Care. 2019;26-27:48–51. https://doi.org/10.1016/J.TACC.2019.03.002.
102. Hernández-Socorro CR, Marin J, Ruiz-Santana S, Santana L, Manzano JL. Bedside sonographic-guided versus blind nasoenteric feeding tube placement in critically ill patients. Crit Care Med. 1996;24(10):1690–4. https://doi.org/10.1097/00003246-199610000-00015.
103. Yaseen M, Kumar A, Bhoi S, et al. Point-of-care ultrasonography-assisted nasogastric tube placement in the emergency department: a randomized controlled trial. Eur J Emerg Med. 2022;29(6):431–6. https://doi.org/10.1097/MEJ.0000000000000962.
104. Gok F, Kilicaslan A, Yosunkaya A. Ultrasound-guided nasogastric feeding tube placement in critical care patients. Nutr Clin Pract. 2015;30(2):257–60. https://doi.org/10.1177/0884533614567714.
105. Peng J, Tang M, Liu LL, Chen WT, Ye QH. Diagnostic accuracy of ultrasonography for detecting gastric tube placement: an updated meta-analysis. Eur Rev Med Pharmacol Sci. 2022;26(17):6328–39. https://doi.org/10.26355/EURREV_202209_29657.
106. Yıldırım Ç, Coşkun S, Gökhan Ş, Pamukçu Günaydın G, Özhasenekler A, Özkula U. Verifying the placement of nasogastric tubes at an emergency center: comparison of Ultrasound with chest radiograph. Emerg Med Int. 2018;2018:1–6. https://doi.org/10.1155/2018/2370426.
107. Lin T, Gifford W, Lan Y, et al. Diagnostic accuracy of ultrasonography for detecting nasogastric tube (NGT) placement in adults: a systematic review and meta analysis. Int J Nurs Stud. 2017;71:80–8. https://doi.org/10.1016/j.ijnurstu.2017.03.005.
108. Mori T, Takei H, Ihara T, Hagiwara Y, Nomura O. Ultrasound-guided nasogastric tube placement in a pediatric emergency department. J Clin Ultrasound. 2021;49(2):106–9. https://doi.org/10.1002/jcu.22958.
109. Zatelli M, Vezzali N. 4-Point ultrasonography to confirm the correct position of the nasogastric tube in 114 critically ill patients. J Ultrasound. 2016;20(1):53–8. https://doi.org/10.1007/s40477--016-0219-0. Published 2016 Oct 28
110. Williams P, Tait G, Wijeratne T. Success rate of elective lumbar puncture at a major Melbourne neurology unit. Surg Neurol Int. 2018;9(1):12. https://doi.org/10.4103/SNI.SNI_426_17.
111. Sievänen H, Kari J, Eskola V, Huurre A, Soukka H, Palmu S. Incidence of traumatic lumbar punctures in adults: the impact of a patient's first procedure. Clin Med (Lond). 2023;23(1):31–7. https://doi.org/10.7861/CLINMED.2022-0169.
112. Shappell E, Dutta S, Sakaria S, McEvoy DS, Egan DJ. Variability in emergency department procedure rates and distributions in a regional health system: A cross-sectional observational study. Ann Emerg Med. 2023;81(5):624–9. https://doi.org/10.1016/J.ANNEMERGMED.2022.12.016.
113. Gottlieb M, Jordan J, Krzyzaniak S, et al. Trends in emergency medicine resident procedural reporting over a 10-year period. AEM Educ Train. 2023;7(1) https://doi.org/10.1002/AET2.10841.
114. Lammers RL, Temple KJ, Wagner MJ, Ray D. Competence of new emergency medicine residents in the performance of lumbar punctures. Acad Emerg Med. 2005;12(7):622–8. https://doi.org/10.1197/J.AEM.2005.01.014.
115. Nomura JT, Leech SJ, Shenbagamurthi S, et al. A randomized controlled trial of ultrasound-assisted lumbar puncture. J Ultrasound Med. 2007;26(10):1341–8. https://doi.org/10.7863/JUM.2007.26.10.1341.
116. Gottlieb M, Holladay D, Peksa GD. Ultrasound-assisted lumbar punctures: a systematic review and meta-analysis. Acad Emerg Med. 2019;26(1):85–96. https://doi.org/10.1111/ACEM.13558.
117. Gottlieb M, Kravchuk K, O'Brien JR. Ultrasound-guided paramedian approach: a novel technique for lumbar puncture in the emergency department. Am J Emerg Med. 2024;81:124–6. https://doi.org/10.1016/J.AJEM.2024.04.054.
118. Myderrizi N, Mema B. The hematoma block an effective alternative for fracture reduction in distal radius fractures. Med Arh. 2011;65(4):239–42. https://doi.org/10.5455/MEDARH.2011.65.239-242.
119. Fathi M, Moezzi M, Abbasi S, Farsi D, Zare MA, Hafezimoghadam P. Ultrasound-guided hematoma block in distal radial fracture reduction: a randomised clinical trial. Emerg Med J. 2015;32(6):474–7. https://doi.org/10.1136/EMERMED-2013-202485.
120. Gottlieb M, Cosby K. Ultrasound-guided hematoma block for distal radial and ulnar fractures. J Emerg Med. 2015;48(3):310–2. https://doi.org/10.1016/J.JEMERMED.2014.09.063.

Ultrasound-Guided Nerve Blocks

22

Mikaela Chilstrom, Andrew Goldsmith, Joseph Stegeman, Carlos Mikell, and Arun Nagdev

Introduction

Ultrasound-guided nerve blocks (UGNBs) are a vital part of the multimodal approach to acute pain management. The classic mono-modal approach that relies on opioids can lead to undesired complications (e.g., hypotension, apnea, delirium) and increased opioid use downstream [1, 2]. Integration of both didactic education and hands-on practice will allow clinicians to offer an optimal patient-centered approach to pain management. As with any procedure, it is essential to consider the necessary steps to safely and effectively perform a nerve block, anticipate complications, and know how to manage adverse events.

Supplementary Information The online version contains supplementary material available at https://doi.org/10.1007/978-3-031-85308-1_22.

M. Chilstrom (✉)
Department of Emergency Medicine, Los Angeles General Medical Center, Los Angeles, CA, USA
e-mail: mbaker@dhs.lacounty.gov

A. Goldsmith
Department of Emergency Medicine, Lahey Clinic/University of Massachusetts Burlington, Burlington, MA, USA
e-mail: andrew.goldsmith@lahey.org

J. Stegeman
Department of Emergency Medicine, Highland Hospital/Alameda Hospital System, San Francisco, CA, USA

C. Mikell
Department of Emergency Medicine, UC Davis Medical Center, Davis, CA, USA

A. Nagdev
Department of Emergency Medicine, Alameda Health System/ University of California, San Francisco, CA, USA

General Considerations for Ultrasound-Guided Nerve Blocks

Before performing an UGNB, the operator should identify the desired region of analgesia and relative exclusion criteria, which include coagulopathy, allergy to local anesthetics (LA), infection overlying the injection site, concern for compartment syndrome, altered mental status, or a history of pre-existing peripheral neuropathies. It is critical to calculate the weight-based maximum dose of LA and use lean body weight when there are comorbid conditions or other patient factors that can influence dosing amounts (e.g., pregnancy, advanced end-organ dysfunction, extremes of age, morbid obesity).

The risks and benefits should be discussed with the patient, including the signs and symptoms of local anesthetic systemic toxicity (LAST). A focused neurologic exam should be performed prior to the procedure, documenting both the motor and sensory function of the nerves that will be blocked. If a surgical intervention may be needed, discussion with the consultant may be warranted per institutional policy. The extremity and location of the block should be marked, and the anesthetic dose should be confirmed via two-person verification. Hand hygiene and field sterility should be performed per institutional standards. Before starting, perform and document a time-out.

As with most procedures, attention to setup impacts the likelihood of success. If the patient will receive a large-volume block (> 10 mL) or a block in a region with high vascularity, secure intravenous access and place the patient on cardiac telemetry to monitor for signs of LAST. In most cases, a two-person technique in which one operator advances the needle under ultrasound guidance and the other controls the syringe is ideal. Ergonomically, ensure the patient is in a position they can maintain throughout the procedure and that the ultrasound screen location and height of the bed are optimized for the operator.

Once the needle tip is visualized in the desired location, gentle hydrodissection with normal saline can open targeted

M. Gottlieb, N. Panebianco (eds.), *Advanced Point-of-Care Ultrasound*, https://doi.org/10.1007/978-3-031-85308-1_22

Table 22.1 Commonly used anesthetics in the emergency setting (*recreated courtesy of Highland Ultrasound https://highlandultrasound.com/med-guide*)

Commonly used local anesthetics in the emergency setting			
Anesthetic	Max Weight-based Dose (mg/kg)	Max Total Dose (mg)	Max Total Volume (mL)
Lidocaine 1%	4	300	30
Lidocaine 1% with epinephrine	7	500	50
Bupivacaine 0.5%	2	175	35
Ropivacaine 1%	3	300	30
Chloroprocaine 3%	11	1000	33
Mepivacaine 1.5%	4	300	20

fascial planes as well as improve needle tip localization (referred to as hydrolocalization). When the correct fascial plane is opened and the needle tip is clearly visualized within it, the operator with the syringe can switch syringes to inject anesthetic safely in the ideal location. This is best performed by using a three-way stopcock with both syringes attached to reduce the need to physically switch syringes. We recommend using blunt-tipped ultrasound-guided nerve block needles, which are scored to enhance sonographic visibility. These specialized nerve block needles have less risk of nerve injury if they contact the nerve and can optimize visualization and needle tracking [3–5]. If a nerve block needle is unavailable, a blunt-tipped spinal needle can be used instead.

Until one is familiar with dosing of LA, we advocate referring to readily available weight-based dosing charts for commonly used LA over a range of patient weights (Table 22.1). There are also a number of free resources available, including MDCalc (https://www.mdcalc.com/), the Safe Local app (https://apps.apple.com/tc/app/safelocal/id1440999841), and the Highland Ultrasound website (https://highlandultrasound.com/). After calculating a weight-based maximum dose, use the lowest possible dose to achieve the desired effect in order to decrease the risk of toxicity. If a prolonged block is desired and there are no clear contraindications, we suggest adding 4–10 mg of dexamethasone to LA.

When depositing LA, low-pressure 2–3 mL injections should alternate with gentle aspirations to ensure a lack of inadvertent vascular puncture. Clinicians should always monitor for symptoms of LAST, both during and 30–60 min after the procedure. Clinicians performing UGNBs must be familiar with early signs and symptoms of LAST and have lipid emulsion (20%) readily available to treat this rare, but life-threatening, complication.

Nerve Block Adverse Effects

Although adverse events are infrequent, each nerve block carries the risk of infection, hematoma, peripheral nerve injury, and LAST. Individual blocks may have additional risks.

Peripheral nerve injury is an uncommon event defined as persistent motor deficit, sensory deficit, or pain after a nerve block; its incidence ranges from 0.5% to 1% [6]. The mechanism of injury is not well understood, but may be a result of direct needle trauma, increased intrafascicular pressures from the injection, direct cytotoxic effects of LA, or nerve ischemia from the metabolic stress of LA. For these reasons, we recommend three steps to reduce the risk of peripheral nerve injury. First, place the needle tip close to, but not in, the nerve fascicle. Second, perform slow, low-pressure injections, pausing the procedure if the patient experiences new pain or paresthesias. Finally, avoid nerve blocks in patients with underlying peripheral neuropathy or an inability to communicate pain (e.g., intoxication, altered mental status).

Patients may develop LAST from direct vascular injection or systemic absorption. The clinical presentation is highly variable, and the onset of symptoms may be immediate or delayed 30–60 min post-block. General symptoms can include nausea, vomiting, and dizziness. Patients can present initially with neurologic or cardiovascular symptoms before progressing to cardiac arrest. Early neurologic symptoms can be nonspecific (e.g., tinnitus, perioral numbness, metallic taste, vision changes, dysarthria) or excitatory (e.g., anxiety, confusion, agitation, seizures) followed by central nervous system depression (e.g., somnolence, coma, respiratory depression) [7]. Early signs of cardiovascular instability include hypertension and tachycardia, which can ultimately progress to hypotension, bradycardia, dysrhythmias, and cardiac arrest. Treatment of LAST includes benzodiazepines for seizures, Advanced Cardiac Life Support (ACLS) for arrhythmias and cardiac arrest, and intravenous lipid emulsion, which is thought to bind and inactivate lipophilic LA. Intravenous lipid emulsion (20% solution) is given as a 1.5 mL/kg bolus (based on lean body mass) over 1 min, which can be repeated if the patient continues to demonstrate hemodynamic instability; otherwise, it should be followed by an infusion at 0.25–0.50 mL/kg/min. Note that the management of arrhythmias and cardiac arrest due to LAST has some modifications from standard ACLS including lower doses of epinephrine (start with $\leq$ 1 mcg/kg) and avoiding lidocaine, procainamide, vasopressin, calcium channel blockers, and beta blockers [7].

Post-block Evaluation and Monitoring

Evaluation and monitoring should be performed after any UGNB. A post-block neurologic examination, total anesthetic dose given, time of administration, location of the UGNB, and any complications should be documented in a procedure note. Because of the possibility of delayed onset LAST from systemic absorption, for large-volume blocks and those performed in highly vascular regions, we recommend continuous cardiac monitoring for at least 60 min post-block [8].

Ultrasound-Guided Nerve Blocks

Although there is a wide variety of nerve blocks used by anesthesiologists and pain management specialists, this chapter focuses on a core group of blocks commonly performed in the acute care setting (Table 22.2). Each of the blocks listed below can be performed using the same systematic approach described above.

Tibial Nerve Block

Indications

The tibial nerve supplies sensation to the sole of the foot and the majority of the internal structures of the foot (Fig. 22.1). The tibial nerve block provides analgesia for plantar lacerations, plantar foreign body removal, and calcaneal fractures.

Technique

The patient should be either supine in a "frog-leg" position or in the lateral decubitus position to expose the medial aspect of the affected ankle. A high-frequency linear probe should be placed proximal and posterior to the medial malleolus in a transverse orientation. The tibial artery should be located as a pulsatile structure adjacent to the medial malleolus. The tibial nerve will be seen as a hyperechoic structure typically running just posterior to the artery (Fig. 22.2).

Table 22.2 Commonly performed ultrasound-guided nerve blocks and their indications

Ultrasound-guided regional nerve blocks	
Nerve block	Indications
Lower extremities	
Tibial nerve	Calcaneal fracture, foreign body/laceration to the plantar aspect of the foot
Distal sciatic nerve in the popliteal fossa	Ankle dislocation, Achilles tendon rupture
Fascia iliaca plane or femoral nerve	Hip/femur/proximal tibia fracture, patellar subluxation, anteromedial thigh abscess/laceration
Pericapsular nerve group (PENG)	Acetabular/pubic rami/hip fractures
Upper extremities	
Forearm nerves (radial, median, ulnar nerves)	Hand injury or infection
Supraclavicular brachial plexus	Elbow or wrist dislocation
Interscalene brachial plexus	Proximal humeral fracture, shoulder dislocation, shoulder laceration/abscess
Retroclavicular approach to the infraclavicular region (RAPTIR)	Distal radius/humerus fracture, shoulder/elbow dislocation
Head/Neck	
Greater occipital nerve	Laceration to the posterior half of the scalp, occipital neuralgia and other headaches
Superficial cervical plexus	Clavicle fracture, internal jugular/subclavian vein central line placement, submandibular abscess, lateral neck/earlobe laceration or abscess
Stellate ganglion	Cardiac sympathectomy for refractory ventricular tachycardia or ventricular fibrillation
Trunk	
Serratus anterior plane	Anterior and lateral rib fractures, burn/ laceration/contusion/ herpes zoster/ postherpetic neuralgia of the anterolateral chest wall, axillary abscess, chest tube insertion/analgesia
Erector spinae plane	Posterior rib fractures, burn/ laceration/ contusion/ herpes zoster/ postherpetic neuralgia of the posterior thorax, vertebral pain, renal colic, pancreatitis, appendicitis
Interpectoral (PECS I) and pectoserratus (PECS II)	Breast/axillary abscess, cellulitis, or laceration
Transversus abdominis plane	Abdominal wall abscess, hernia, appendicitis

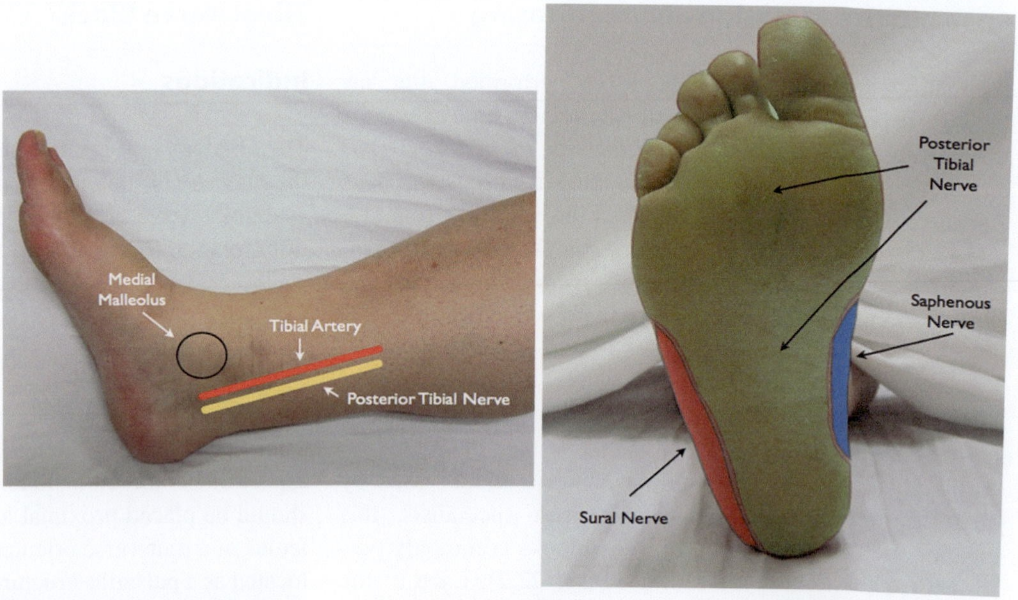

Fig. 22.1 Anatomy and sensory innervation of the tibial nerve. The tibial nerve innervates most of the plantar surface and internal structures of the foot but spares the very medial and lateral portions, which are supplied by the saphenous and sural nerves, respectively

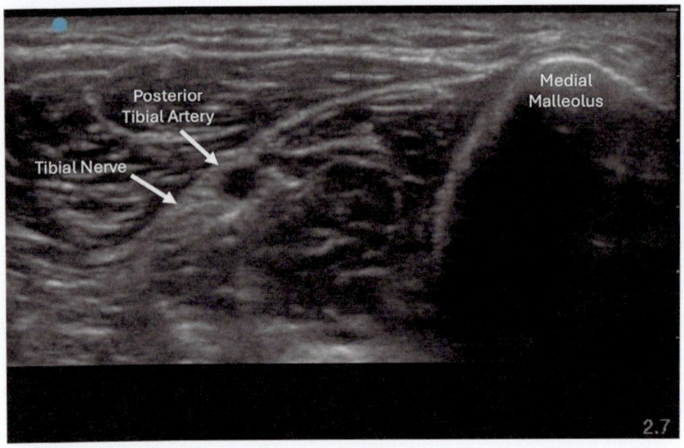

Fig. 22.2 Performing the tibial nerve block. The tibial nerve is identified posterior to the posterior tibial artery. The needle tip is advanced, using either in-plane or out-of-plane technique, until the needle tip is immediately posterior to the nerve. After negative aspiration, 5–10 mL of local anesthetic is injected, surrounding the nerve

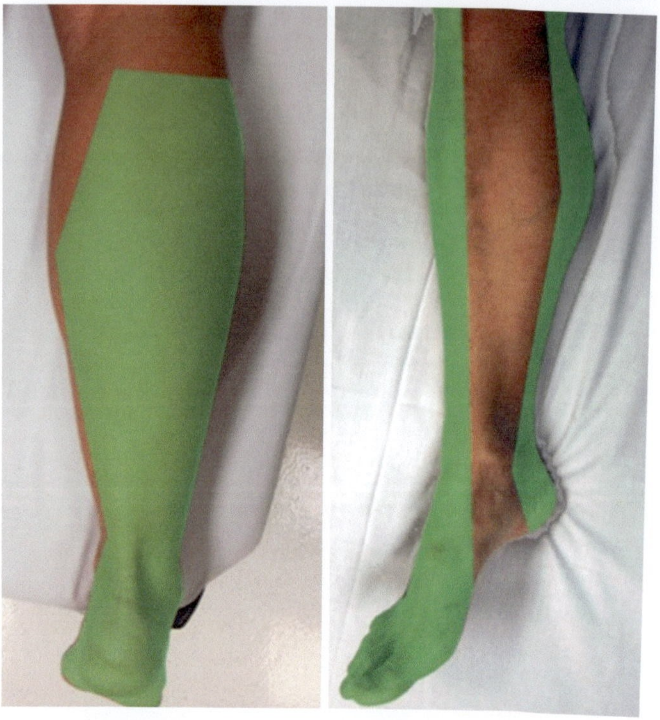

Fig. 22.3 Sensory distribution of the sciatic nerve block at the popliteal fossa. The sciatic nerve at this region supplies sensation to the majority of the lower extremity below the knee, except the medial aspect of the lower leg

Distal Sciatic Nerve Block

Indications

The distal sciatic nerve supplies sensation to most of the lower extremity below the knee, except the medial aspect of the lower leg (Fig. 22.3). The primary indications for the distal sciatic nerve block are large lateral leg lacerations, burns, abscesses, and ankle fractures.

Technique

The sciatic nerve initially runs deep in the posterior thigh before becoming superficial in the popliteal fossa. The sciatic nerve bifurcates into the tibial and common peroneal nerves within 10 cm of the popliteal fossa (Fig. 22.4). With the patient in a prone position using a high-frequency linear probe, identify the popliteal vessels in the popliteal crease. The tibial nerve is commonly superficial to the popliteal vessels. Trace the tibial nerve proximally until it joins with the common peroneal nerve (Video 22.1) to form the sciatic nerve (Fig. 22.5). Insert the needle at the lateral distal thigh to approach the nerve with a flat angle. Advance the needle and position it adjacent to the sciatic nerve just proximal to the bifurcation. Hydrodissect the nerve from the surrounding

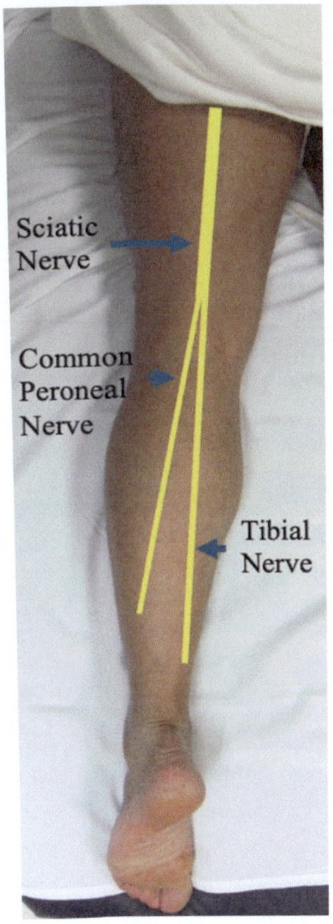

Fig. 22.4 Sciatic nerve anatomy. The sciatic nerve lies in the coronal plane of the thigh prior to dividing into the common peroneal and tibial nerve bundles superficial to the popliteal vessels

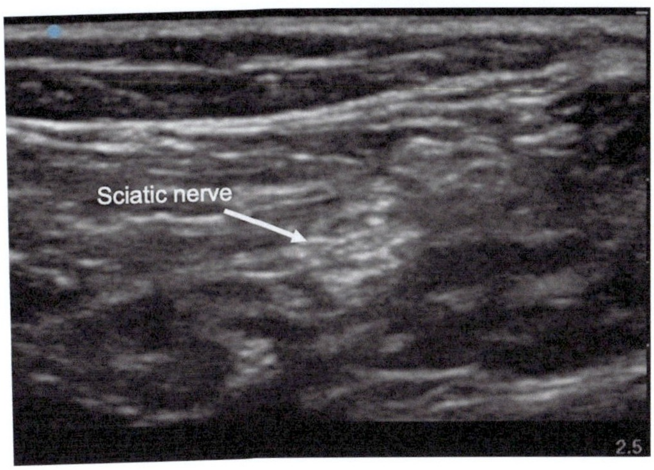

Fig. 22.5 Sonographic anatomy of the sciatic nerve in the popliteal fossa. The tibial nerve is commonly located superficial to the popliteal vessels and appears as a honeycomb structure. Once identified, follow the nerve proximally until it joins with the common peroneal nerve to form the sciatic nerve, as shown in this ultrasound image

tissue using small aliquots of normal saline to ensure that fluid is within the perineural sheath that surrounds the two nerves after the bifurcation. Once the location is confirmed, aspirate to ensure no inadvertent vessel puncture, then inject 10–15 mL of local anesthetic. Local anesthetic should track circumferentially around the nerve.

Infrainguinal Fascia Iliaca Plane Block

Indications

The primary target for the infrainguinal fascia iliaca plane block is the femoral nerve, which lies underneath the fascia iliaca in the thigh and pelvis. In addition, the fascia iliaca block also blocks the lateral femoral cutaneous nerve (which innervates the lateral aspect of the thigh). The obturator nerve (which innervates the proximal inner aspect of the medial thigh) has variable coverage with this approach. Therefore, the infrainguinal fascia iliaca plane block provides analgesia to the anterior and medial thigh, proximal lateral thigh, parts of the hip joint, and medial side of the lower leg (Fig. 22.6). The primary indications include hip and femur fractures, patella fractures, and anterior thigh lacerations or abscesses. This block is unlikely to provide adequate coverage for acetabular or pubic rami fractures. When compared to the pericapsular nerve group (PENG) block, the fascia iliaca block has motor deficits (i.e., quadriceps muscle weakness) that do not occur with the PENG block.

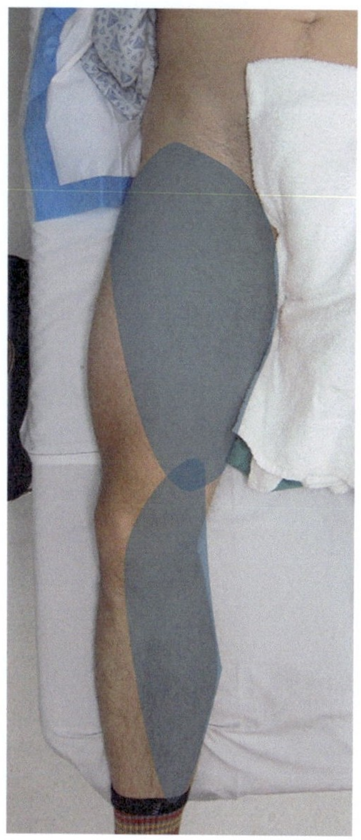

Fig. 22.6 Sensory distribution of the fascia iliaca plane block with the infrainguinal approach. The femoral and lateral femoral cutaneous nerves together supply sensation to the anterior and medial thigh, proximal lateral thigh, hip joint, and the medial side of the leg from the knee to the foot, highlighted in blue

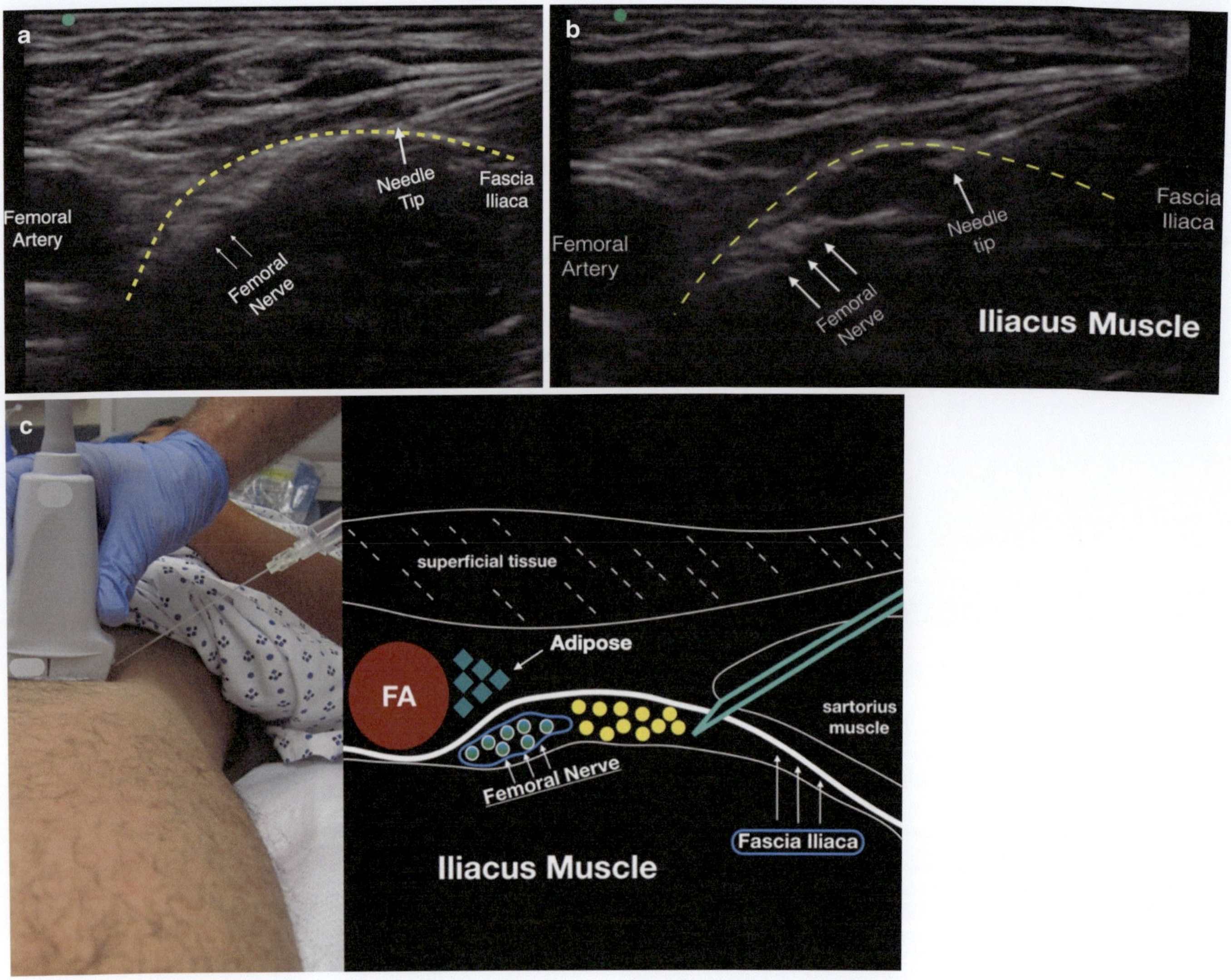

Fig. 22.7 Sonographic anatomy and probe placement for the infrainguinal fascia iliaca plane block. (**a**) Using an in-plane technique, the needle should be inserted from lateral to medial, through the fascia iliaca (yellow dashed line). (**b**) The operator may feel a "pop" when inserting the needle through the fascia lata and fascia iliaca (yellow dashed line). The needle tip should be far from the femoral nerve but under the fascia iliaca. Once through, hydrodissection will cause the fascia iliaca to move superiorly. Aspirate to confirm the needle tip is extravascular, then inject 30–40 mL of local anesthetic in 5 mL increments. Repeat aspirations every 5–10 mL to avoid inadvertent vascular injection. (**c**) Probe positioning and anatomical drawing of the infrainguinal fascia iliaca plane block where local anesthetic deposition is marked by yellow circles

Technique

Place the linear probe parallel and inferior to the inguinal crease, about one-third of the distance from the anterior superior iliac spine (ASIS) to the pubic symphysis. The iliacus muscle should be identified lateral to the femoral artery and nerve. The fascia iliaca lies on top of (anterior to) the iliacus muscle (Fig. 22.7, Video 22.2).

Suprainguinal Fascia Iliaca Plane Block

Indications

The suprainguinal fascia iliaca (SIFI) plane block targets the same fascial plane as the infrainguinal approach, but at a more proximal level with the probe and needle oriented superiorly toward the umbilicus. Compared with the infrainguinal approach, the SIFI has been shown to have a more complete sensory block of the medial, anterior, and lateral thigh [9, 10].

Technique

With the patient lying supine, palpate the ASIS. Place the linear probe directly over the ASIS, oriented obliquely so that it aims toward the umbilicus (Fig. 22.8). Identify the superficial bony contour of the ASIS, then slide the probe inferomedially, following the ilium down to the anterior inferior iliac spine (AIIS). The iliacus muscle drapes over the AIIS, while the fascia iliaca forms the superficial border of the iliacus (Fig. 22.9). The sartorius (laterally) and inferior oblique (medially) overlie the fascia iliaca in a characteristic "bow-tie" configuration. As the iliacus tracks medially and deep to the internal oblique, the deep circumflex iliac artery and vein can be visualized with color Doppler to identify the correct plane and ensure safe needle positioning.

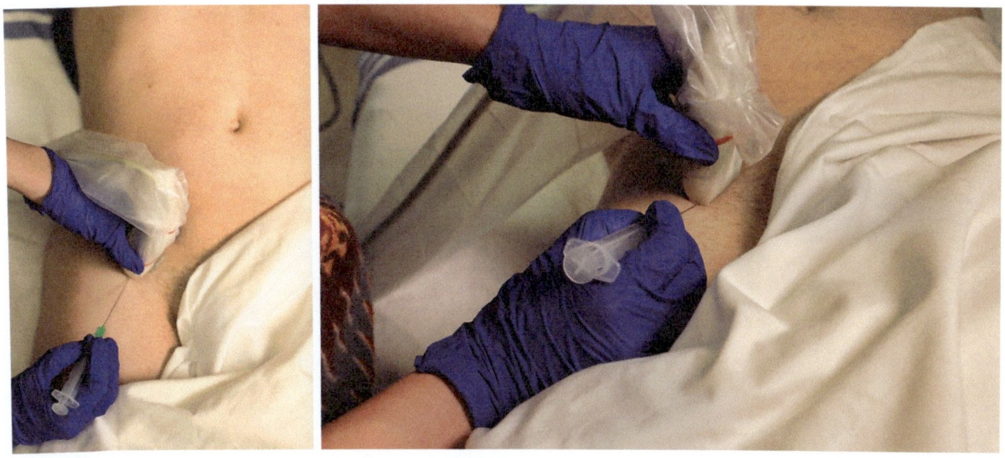

Fig. 22.8 Probe positioning and needle placement for the suprainguinal fascia iliaca plane block. The probe is positioned over the anterior superior iliac spine and aimed toward the umbilicus. Slide the probe inferomedially to identify the anterior inferior iliac spine, the overlying iliacus muscle, and the "bow-tie" appearance of the sartorius and inferior oblique muscles. The needle should be inserted from the inferior direction using an in-plane technique. (*Photos courtesy of John Barrett, DNP*)

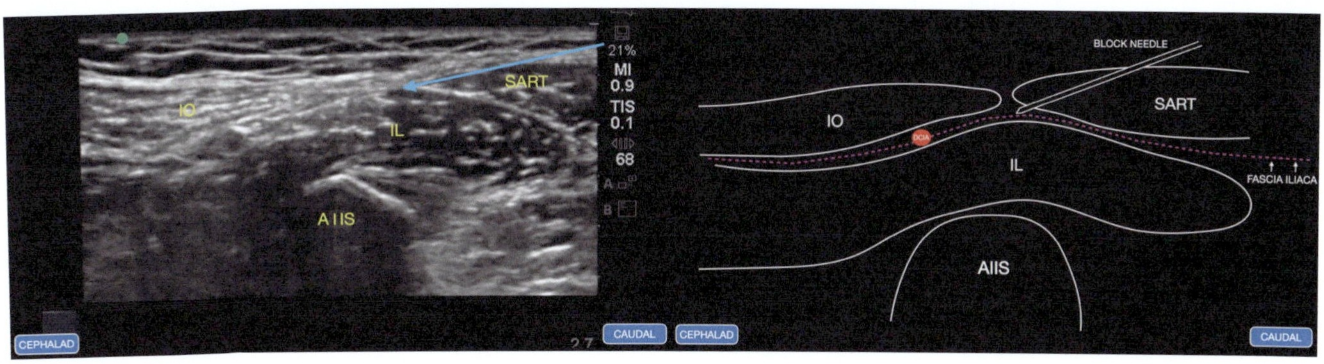

Fig. 22.9 Performing the suprainguinal fascia iliaca plane block. Prior to performing the block, identify the deep circumflex iliac vessels (red circle) with color Doppler to avoid them during injection. The needle is introduced in-plane from lateral to medial (caudal to cephalad), aimed toward the umbilicus at a shallow angle. The tip of the needle pierces the fascia iliaca near the middle of the "bow-tie" and then will need to be retracted slightly so that it lies in the fascial plane rather than within the iliacus muscle. Use hydrodissection to confirm the correct needle placement. If placed correctly, the saline will track medially in between the iliacus (IL) and internal oblique (IO) muscles, running just deep to the previously identified deep circumflex iliac vessels. After negative aspiration, incrementally inject 30–40 mL of local anesthetic into the fascial plane. *SART* sartorius muscle, *AIIS* anterior inferior iliac spine, *DCIA* deep circumflex iliac artery. (*Images courtesy of Anne Mao, MD and Tiffany S. Huang, MD*)

Pericapsular Nerve Group Block

Indications

The pericapsular nerve group (PENG) consists of the articular branches of the femoral nerve, the obturator nerve, and the accessory obturator nerves as they run deep to the psoas muscle on their way to the hip joint. These sensory-only branches innervate the intracapsular portion of the femoral head and neck, along with the acetabulum and the pubic rami, and thus can be used for proximal femur fractures or pelvic fractures. At low anesthetic volumes (15–20 mL), this block is unlikely to produce any motor effect from LA spread to the femoral or obturator nerves, so it is ideal for patients who are able to safely bear weight on the affected extremity. This is a deep, poorly compressible site, so the block should be avoided in anticoagulated patients.

Technique

With the patient lying supine, place the curvilinear probe along the course of the inguinal ligament. In thin patients, the linear probe may provide adequate depth. The femoral vessels should be identified medially, with the iliopsoas muscle lying deep and lateral to them. To determine the ideal location, image the femoral head and then slowly slide the probe proximal to locate the AIIS, psoas tendon, and iliopubic eminence (Fig. 22.10). The objective is to place the needle tip onto the ilium just deep and lateral to the hyperechoic psoas tendon (Fig. 22.11).

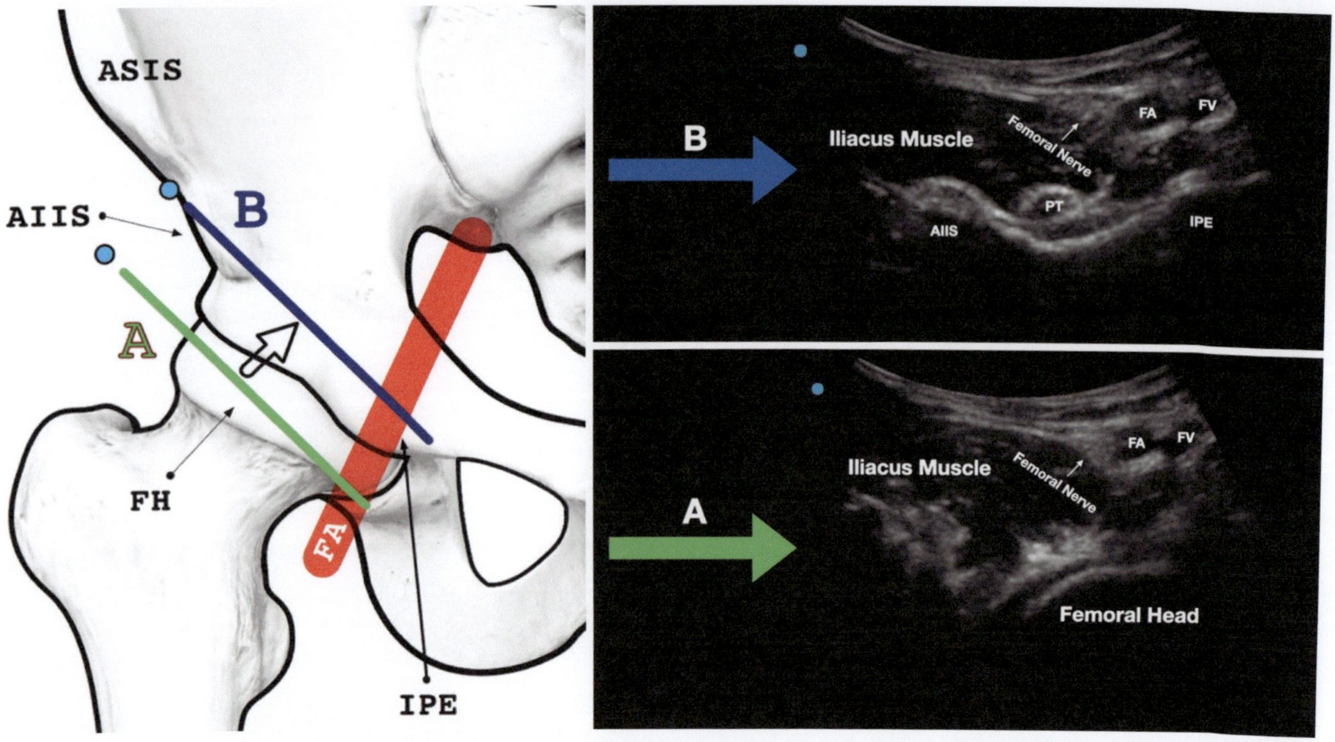

Fig. 22.10 Anatomy of the PENG block. The anatomical drawing shows probe placement over the femoral head (FH) (**a**) and ilium (**b**). (**a**) Ultrasound image generated with the probe positioned over the femoral head, slightly inferior to where the block is performed. (**b**) Ultrasound image generated with the probe positioned slightly superior, along the inguinal ligament, showing the concave-up surface of the ilium. *AIIS* anterior inferior iliac spine, *ASIS* anterior superior iliac spine, *IPE* iliopubic eminence, *FA* femoral artery, *FV* femoral vein, *PT* psoas tendon

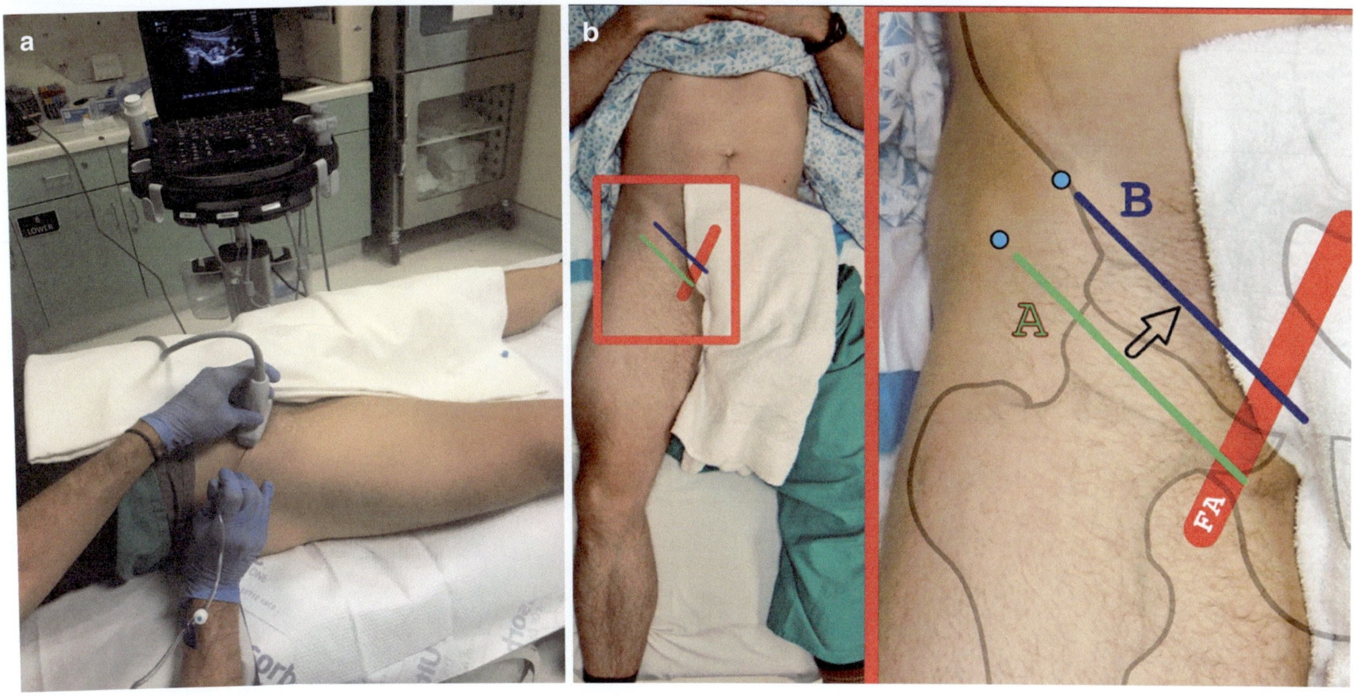

Fig. 22.11 **Performing the PENG block**. (**a**) The needle is inserted in-plane from lateral to medial at a 60-degree angle, taking care to stay lateral of the femoral vessels and nerve. The goal is to position the needle tip onto the ilium just deep and lateral to the psoas tendon (without piercing the hyperechoic tendon itself). If the needle is correctly positioned, the psoas tendon will lift up off of the ilium when a normal saline flush is injected for confirmation. After negative aspiration, incrementally inject 15–20 mL of local anesthetic. (**b**) Anatomical positioning of the ultrasound probe in comparison to bony anatomy and the femoral artery (FA)

Forearm Nerves

Indications

Forearm nerve blocks provide analgesia to the hand in a dermatomal distribution and are useful to relieve pain from hand injuries or infections. Prior to performing, it is important to review the dermatomes to ensure the nerve(s) selected match the desired region of anesthesia (Fig. 22.12).

Technique

Locate all three nerves in the short axis. For the median nerve, place the probe transversely in the mid-forearm and identify it between the muscle bellies of flexor digitorum superficialis and flexor digitorum profundus (Figs. 22.13 and 22.14). For the radial and ulnar nerves, locate the respective arteries in the wrist (Figs. 22.15 and 22.16). The nerves will be on the outside of their corresponding artery. Once identified, track the nerve proximally in the arm to find an optimal location to perform the procedure to maximize the distance between the vessel and its corresponding nerve. In general, the proximal half of the forearm will provide the best region for the nerves to be blocked. Once identified, use an in-plane technique with the needle entering on the side contralateral to the vessel (Fig. 22.17).

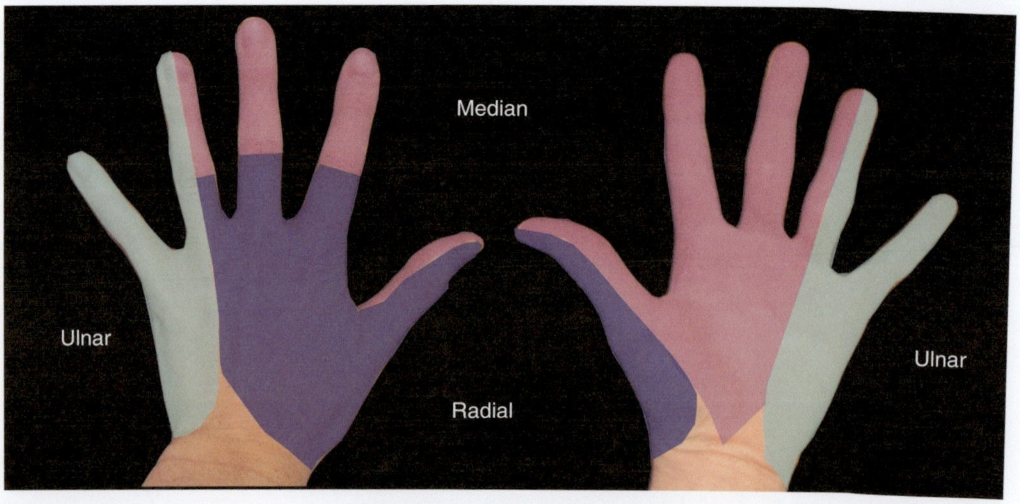

Fig. 22.12 **Sensory innervation of the left hand**. Dorsal hand on the left and palmar aspect on the right with the ulnar, median, and radial nerve innervation highlighted in green, pink, and purple, respectively. Injuries or infections often cross dermatomal lines and may require more than one nerve block

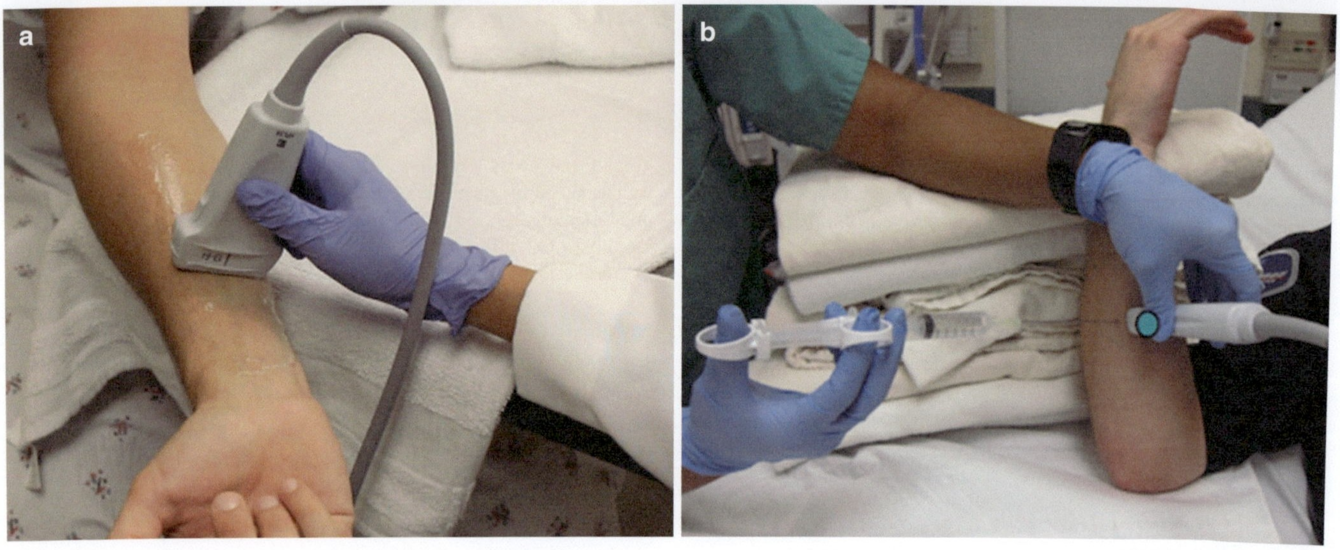

Fig. 22.13 **Positioning for the forearm nerve blocks.** (**a**) The patient should be positioned in a comfortable position (seated or supine) with the arm extended and slightly abducted with the palm up. (**b**) For the ulnar nerve, it may be easier to have the patient flex the arm at the elbow and place the arm upright or over their head (if supine) to access the ulnar aspect of the arm

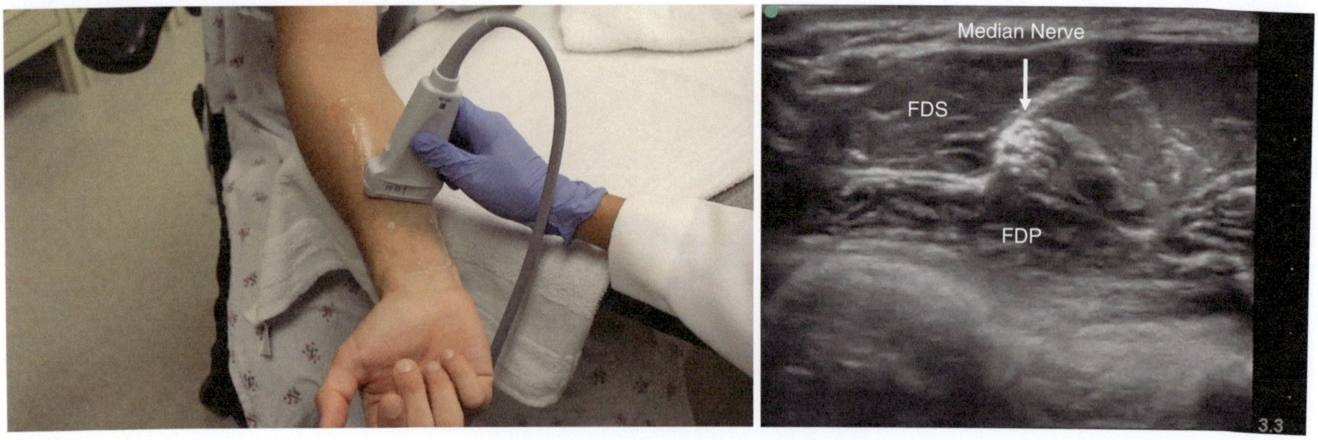

Fig. 22.14 **Probe position and sonographic anatomy of the median nerve.** The median nerve lies in the fascial plane between the muscle bellies of flexor digitorum superficialis (FDS) and flexor digitorum profundus (FDP)

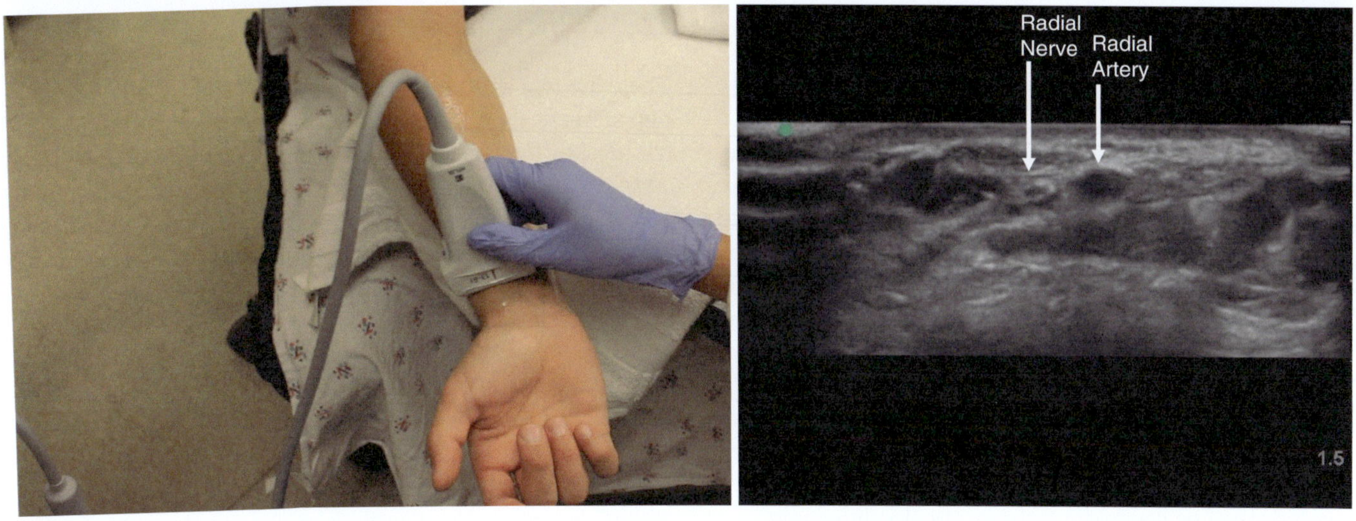

Fig. 22.15 **Probe position and sonographic anatomy of the right radial nerve.** The radial nerve is radial to the radial artery

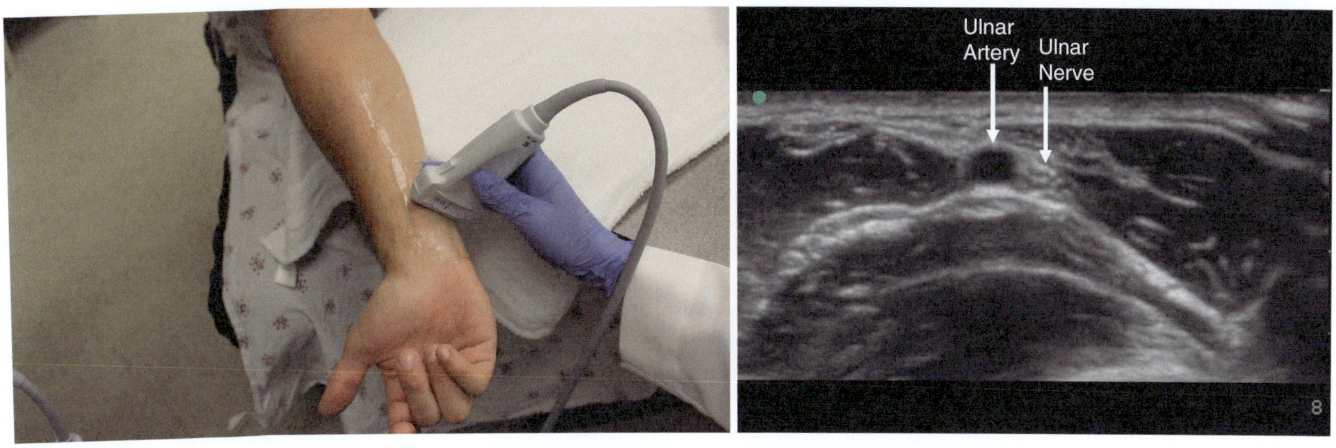

Fig. 22.16 **Probe position and sonographic anatomy of the right ulnar nerve.** The ulnar nerve is ulnar to the ulnar artery

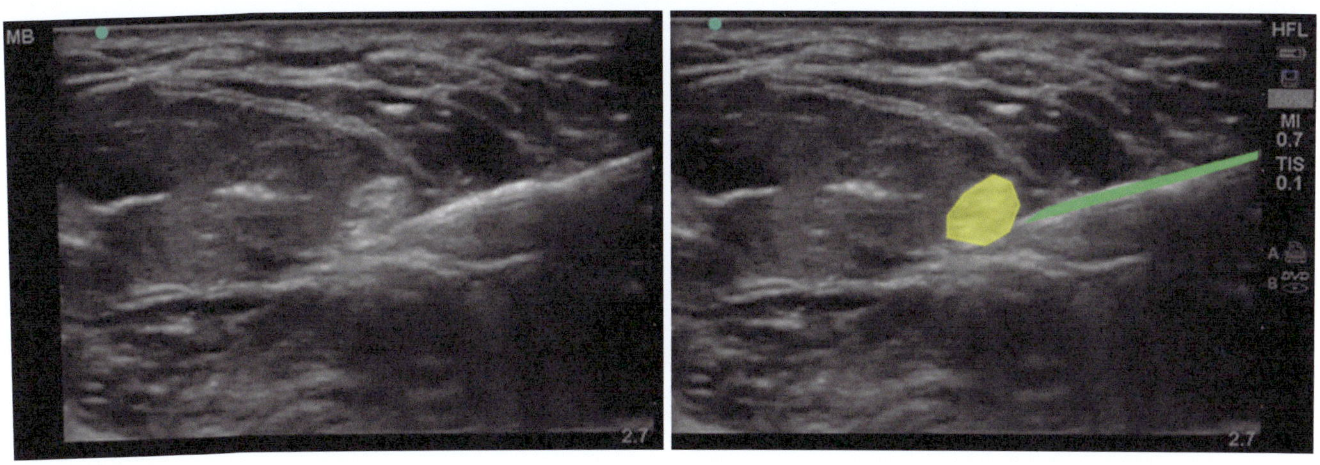

Fig. 22.17 **Performing a forearm nerve block.** Insert the needle (green) in-plane toward the base of the target nerve (yellow), into the fascial plane where the nerve lies. Inject 3–5 mL of local anesthetic to form a crescent around the target nerve. If the patient reports paresthesias or high pressures are encountered, the needle is too close to the nerve; stop injecting and withdraw the needle slightly before injecting further. These images show the approach for the median nerve. For the radial and ulnar nerves, the needle should enter the radial and ulnar aspects of the probe, respectively, to avoid the corresponding artery

Interscalene Brachial Plexus Block

Indications

The interscalene brachial plexus block provides regional anesthesia to the lateral clavicle, acromioclavicular joint, proximal humerus, and elbow, in addition to causing paresis of the shoulder muscles. In the acute care setting, the interscalene block is useful to treat pain from proximal humeral fractures, shoulder dislocations, shoulder abscesses, and lacerations. The interscalene approach has a lower risk of pneumothorax than the supraclavicular approach, as the needle enters higher on the neck (Fig. 22.18). However, the interscalene approach is more likely to cause phrenic nerve paralysis as LA tracks around the anterior scalene muscle. The risk of phrenic nerve paralysis may be decreased by using small-volume injections [11–13]. Since there is no clear evidence suggesting that phrenic nerve paralysis can be reliably avoided, this block is not recommended for patients with known low pulmonary reserve (e.g., chronic obstructive pulmonary disease) patients with known vocal cord paralysis given the rare, but potential, blockade of the recurrent laryngeal nerve.

Technique

There are two approaches to finding the interscalene groove. For the first approach, begin with the probe transversely at the level of the larynx. Identify the internal jugular vein and carotid artery and slide posteriorly until reaching the border of the clavicular head of the sternocleidomastoid muscle. The interscalene groove is located between the anterior and middle scalene muscles (Fig. 22.19). The C5, C6, and C7 nerves are arranged vertically on top of one another and appear as a "traffic light." For the alternate approach, identify the brachial plexus, which will appear as a hyperechoic "cluster of grapes," adjacent to the subclavian artery at the level of the supraclavicular fossa. Follow these hypoechoic structures cephalad until they form the "traffic light" sign within the interscalene groove at the level of the larynx. Once these are identified, insert the needle from the posterior direction using an in-plane technique (Fig. 22.20).

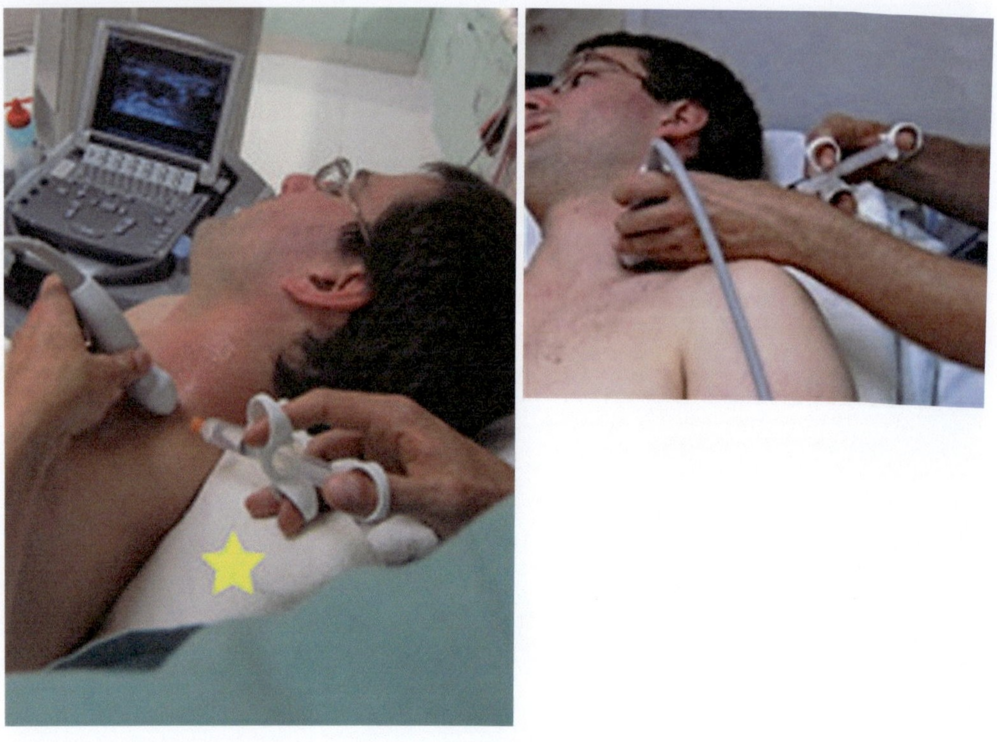

Fig. 22.18 Positioning for the interscalene block of the neck. The patient should be supine in a semi-reclining position with the head rotated 30–45° away from the side of the injury. A blanket (star) can be used to prop the patient's head up

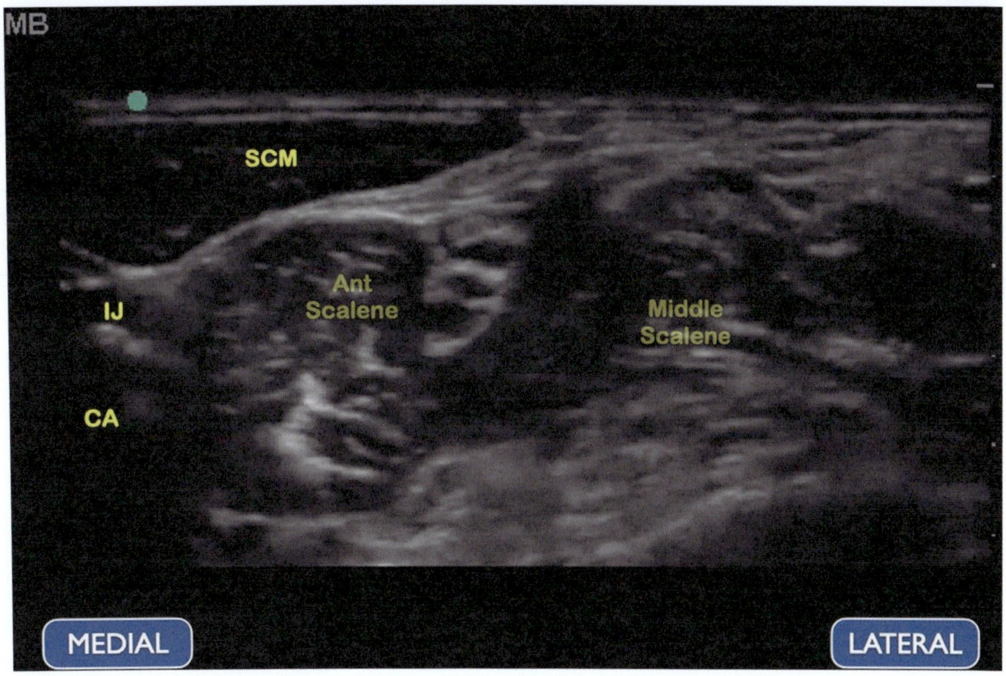

Fig. 22.19 Sonographic anatomy of the interscalene block of the left neck. The sternocleidomastoid (SCM) is located superficially, with the internal jugular vein (IJ) and carotid artery (CA) located deeper. The interscalene groove is located between the anterior and middle scalene muscles. The medial/lateral orientation of this image will reverse when scanning the contralateral side

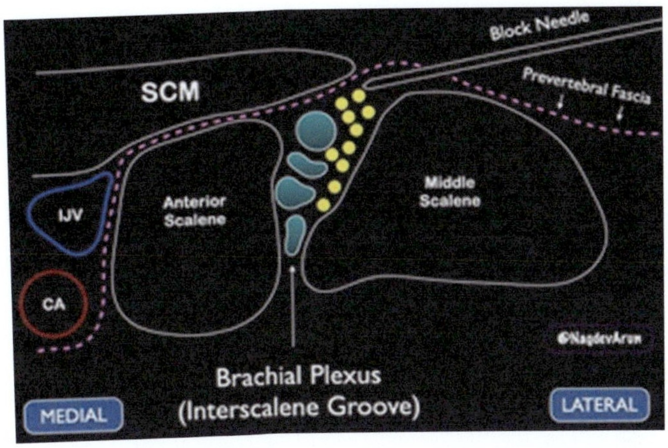

Fig. 22.20 Performing the interscalene block. The needle tip is advanced under the prevertebral fascia so that fluid (represented by yellow circles) can track along the border between the middle scalene muscle and interscalene groove. Inject 5–10 mL of local anesthetic into the potential space between the middle scalene muscle and the brachial plexus sheath. To ensure safety, the needle should never contact the brachial plexus directly

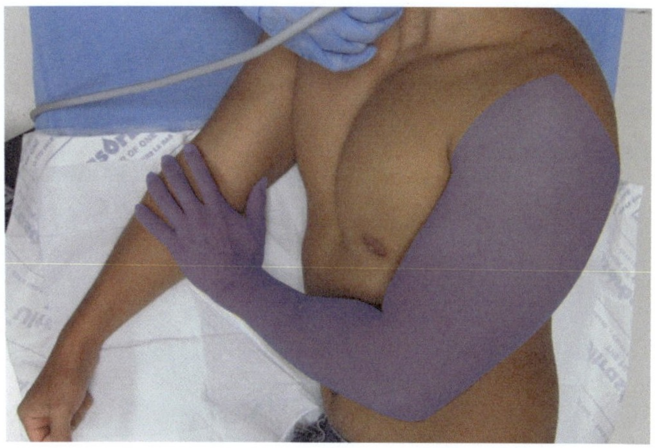

Fig. 22.21 Sensory distribution of the supraclavicular brachial plexus block

Supraclavicular Brachial Plexus Block

Indications

The supraclavicular brachial plexus block provides anesthesia to the radial, median, ulnar, musculocutaneous, and axillary nerve distributions of the arm, providing almost complete anesthesia of the arm, with the exception of the shoulder joint and the medial side of the upper arm (Fig. 22.21). The block is useful for humeral, elbow, and wrist injuries, as well as lacerations and abscesses in these regions. Notably, interscalene blocks are favored for acute shoulder injuries, as they have more reliable coverage of that region. In contrast, the supraclavicular brachial plexus block is believed to have improved analgesia to the C8-T1 nerve roots and slightly reduced concern for phrenic nerve paralysis due to its inferior location [14, 15].

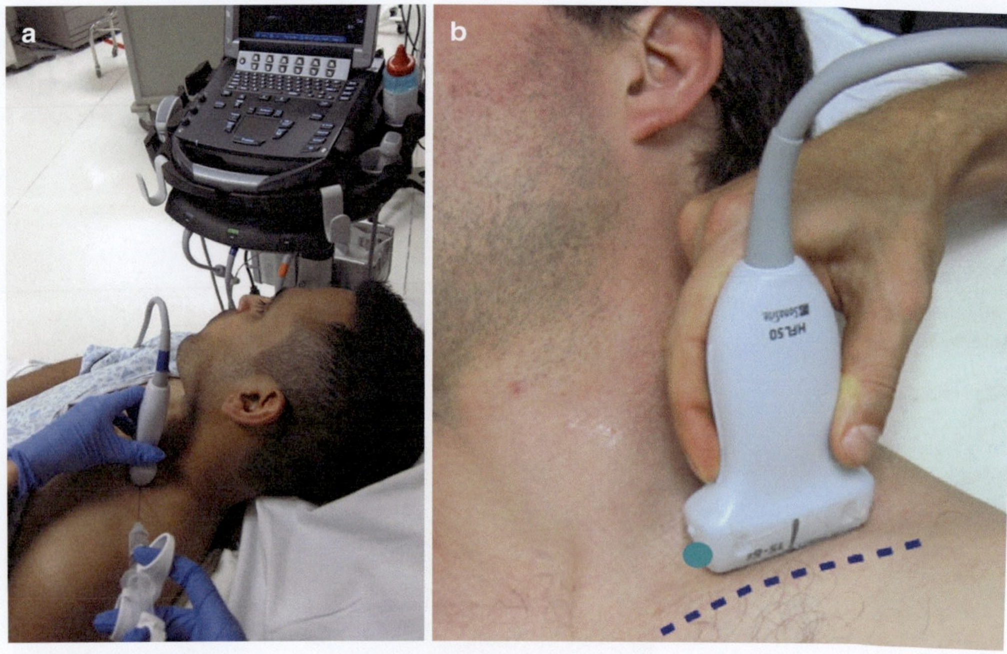

Fig. 22.22 **Positioning for the supraclavicular brachial plexus block.** (**a**) The patient should be in a semi-reclined position with the head rotated 30–45° away from the side of the block. Placing either a pillow or roll of blankets beneath the ipsilateral shoulder may improve block ergonomics. (**b**) Place the probe parallel to the clavicle (blue dashed line) to image the supraclavicular fossa

Technique

With the patient's ipsilateral shoulder slightly elevated and the head turned contralaterally, place the linear probe along the posterior border of the mid-to-lateral clavicle in a coronal or slightly oblique plane with the beam aimed inferior into the chest (Fig. 22.22). Slide the probe slightly medially or laterally to identify the round, pulsatile subclavian artery as it runs over the top of the first rib, which appears as a hyperechoic line with acoustic shadowing deep to it (Fig. 22.23). This rib will help to protect against injury to the lung, which is seen slightly deeper with characteristic pleural sliding. The brachial plexus is immediately superior and lateral to the artery and often appears similar to a "cluster of grapes." Slight oblique rotation of the probe enhances the visualization of the plexus and can bring the first rib into position underneath the plexus and artery (Fig. 22.24). Color Doppler should be utilized to ensure a safe needle path, as the transverse cervical and dorsal scapular arteries both cross the plexus at the base of the neck.

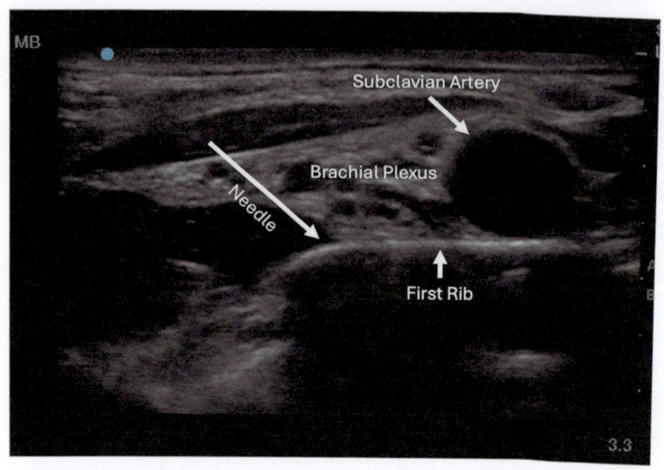

Fig. 22.23 **Sonographic anatomy of the supraclavicular brachial plexus block.** The subclavian artery is visualized in cross-section as it crosses the first rib. Pleural sliding is seen below. The brachial plexus appears as a "cluster of grapes" extending superolaterally from the artery

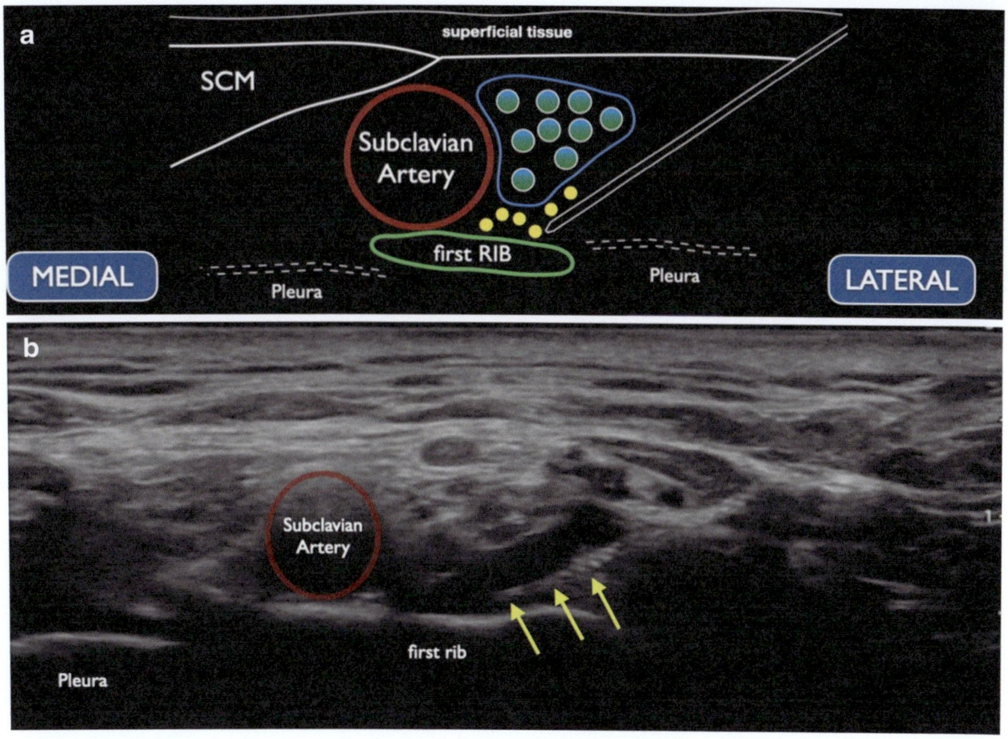

Fig. 22.24 Performing the supraclavicular brachial plexus block. After placing a skin wheal at the lateral aspect of the probe, the block needle is inserted in-plane from lateral to medial, taking care to avoid traversing the plexus itself, until the needle touches the first rib. Injection of a small amount of normal saline will ensure proper spread of fluid (yellow circles), lifting the nerve bundle (blue-green circles enclosed by a blue line) away from the first rib. After negative aspiration, local anesthetic is injected using slow incremental aliquots of 3–5 mL every 15–30 s until a total of 10–15 mL of local anesthetic is deposited

Retroclavicular Approach to the Infraclavicular Region

Indications

The retroclavicular approach to the infraclavicular region (RAPTIR) block is an alternative approach to the infraclavicular brachial plexus block and provides circumferential sensory and motor blockade from the mid-humerus to the hand. It can be used for fracture reduction, large abscess drainage, or complex laceration repairs. In the traditional infraclavicular brachial plexus block approach, the needle is inserted just inferior to the clavicle at a very steep angle to reach the plexus, as the medial, lateral, and posterior cords are positioned around the axillary artery. That steep angle frequently leads to poor needle visualization. In the retroclavicular approach, this is remedied by introducing the needle from a position slightly superior and posterior to the clavicle. This allows a trajectory parallel to the probe for improved needle visualization, but has the trade-off of not being able to visualize the needle as it passes underneath the clavicle. Consequently, this is an advanced block that should only be performed by operators with significant experience with in-plane needle guidance.

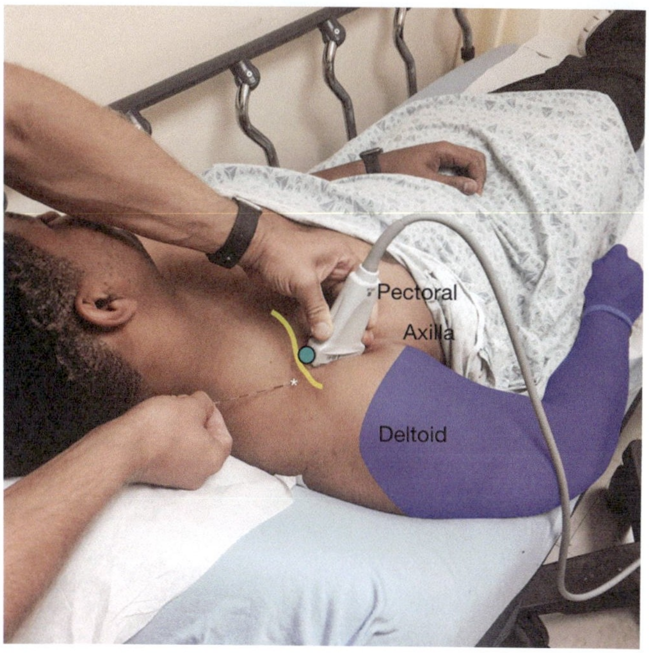

Fig. 22.25 Positioning for the RAPTIR block. The patient is positioned supine with the operator at the head of the bed. The probe is positioned at the inferior aspect of the lateral clavicle (yellow line) in a plane tangential to the thoracic cage. The corresponding region of anesthesia is outlined in purple. The green dot marks the directional indicator on the probe and the asterisk is the needle insertion site

Technique

With the patient in the supine position and the affected arm at their side, the probe is placed in a parasagittal plane over the lateral third of the clavicle (Fig. 22.25). By sliding the

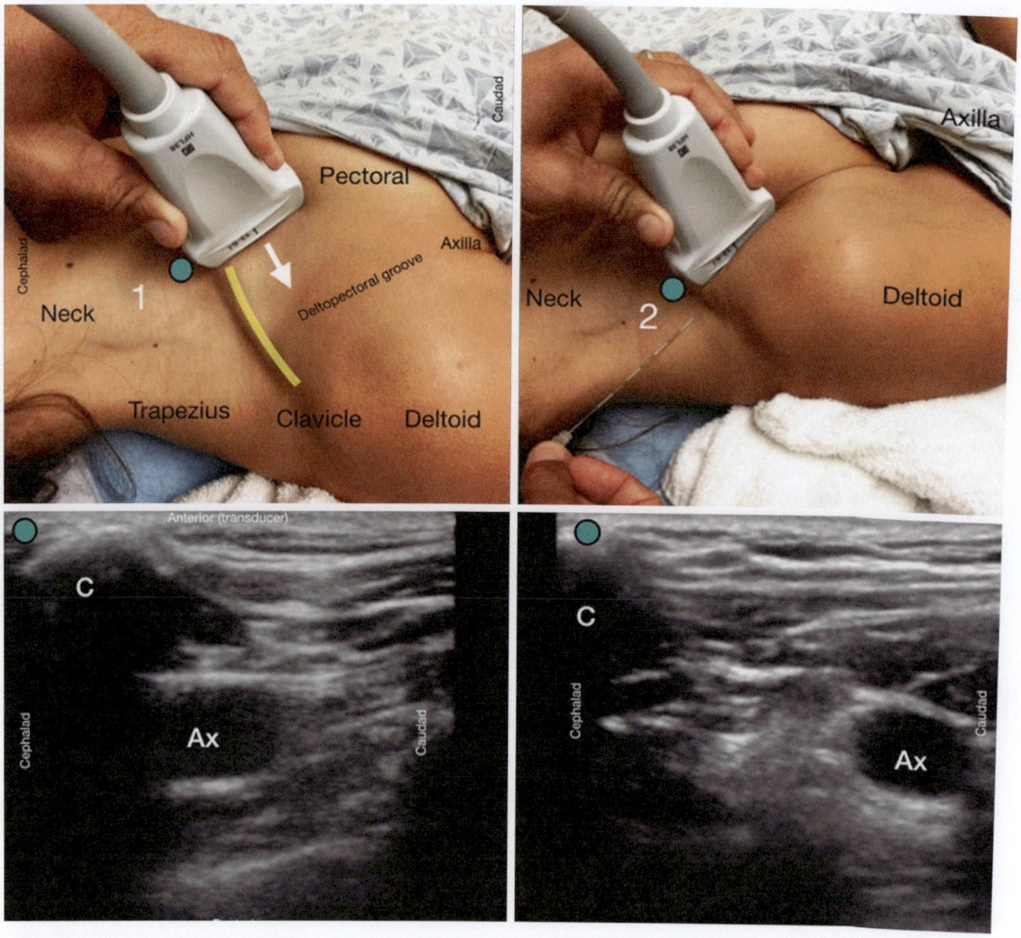

Fig. 22.26 Sonographic anatomy of the RAPTIR block. The clavicle (C) is positioned in the corner of the screen so that the needle can be visualized as it advances out from under the bone. The view is optimized to visualize the cords of the brachial plexus by sliding laterally. The axillary artery (Ax) is seen in cross-section with the cords positioned around the artery

probe slightly inferior, the axillary artery and vein will be identified deep to the pectoralis major and minor muscles. When sliding, the clavicle should be kept in view in the corner of the screen. The medial, posterior, and lateral cords are identified as hyperechoic bundles positioned around the axillary artery at the 3 o'clock, 6 o'clock, and 9 o'clock positions, respectively, but can be difficult to definitively visualize (Fig. 22.26). Once identified, the needle is inserted in-plane from superior to the clavicle in a near-horizontal position (Fig. 22.27).

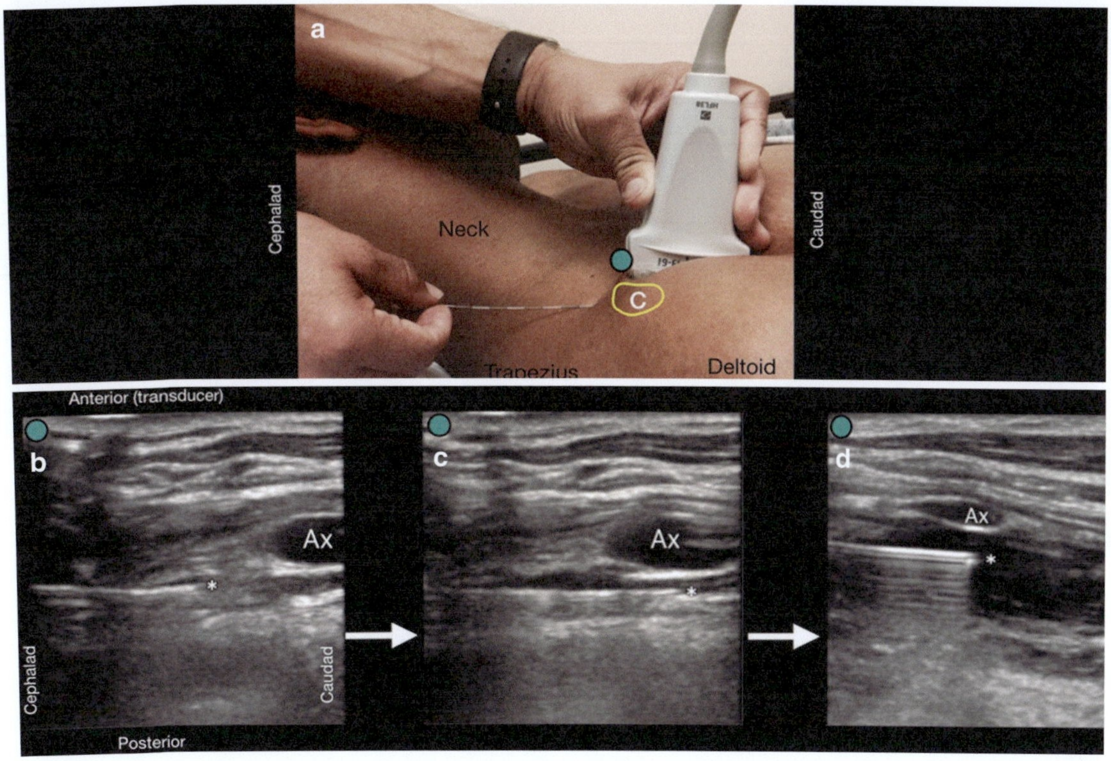

Fig. 22.27 **Performing the RAPTIR block.** The needle (star) is introduced horizontally, approximately 2 cm cephalad to the clavicle (C) and parallel to the probe face. It is slowly advanced under the clavicle and carefully aimed toward the plane of the ultrasound image until it is visualized emerging from underneath the clavicle. Trajectory changes are made to direct the needle tip to the 6 o'clock position under the axillary artery (Ax). Gentle saline hydrodissection while advancing can help avoid inadvertent arterial or nerve injury. Once in position, a normal saline flush confirms the correct needle location by spreading to the medial cord on the opposite side of the artery. After negative aspiration, 20–30 mL of local anesthetic is incrementally injected. The needle may need to be retracted slightly to ensure the local anesthetic spreads around both the medial and lateral cords. Image A demonstrates the needle position. Images B–D demonstrate the progression of the needle toward the axillary artery

Interpectoral and Pectoserratus Plane Blocks

Indications

The interpectoral (PECS 1) plane block targets the medial and lateral pectoral nerves, which innervate the pectoralis major and minor muscles. The pectoserratus (PECS 2) plane block targets the anterior and lateral cutaneous branches of the thoracic intercostal nerves T2-T6 and intercostobrachial nerves, providing anesthesia for the skin and soft tissue of the chest. In practice, PECS 1 refers to the interpectoral block, while PECS 2 refers to either the pectoserratus block in isolation or combined with PECS 1. These blocks are useful for analgesia for breast and axillary abscesses, cellulitis, or lacerations.

Technique

The PECS 1 block is performed by injecting local anesthetic into the fascial plane between the pectoralis major and minor muscles (Fig. 22.28). With the patient in a supine position and their ipsilateral arm abducted, place the ultrasound probe in the sagittal plane at the midclavicular line, where the clavicle, pectoralis major, pectoralis minor, and axillary vessels are visualized. Slide the probe caudally and laterally, toward the axilla, to the level of the second and third ribs.

For the PECS 2 block, the probe is slid further caudally and laterally with slight medial rotation of the superior portion of the probe to the level of the third and fourth ribs (Fig. 22.29). At this level, the serratus anterior muscle can be identified lying between pectoralis minor and the ribs. The pectoral branch of the thoracoacromial artery can be identified between pectoralis major and minor. If performing both blocks, do the PECS 2 block first to prevent injecting air bubbles that may obscure deeper anatomy.

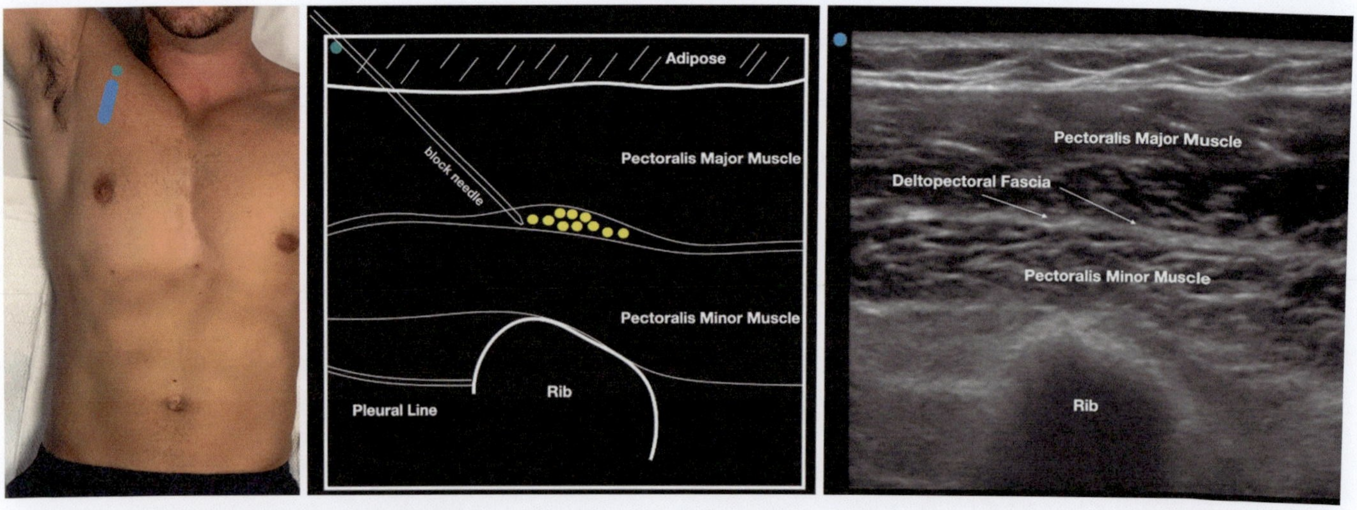

Fig. 22.28 **Performing the PECS 1 block.** With the patient in supine position and their arm abducted over their head, place the probe just lateral to the midclavicular line at the level of the second and third ribs. Advance the needle in-plane from cranial to caudal. Inject 15 mL of local anesthetic (yellow circles) in the fascial plane (deltopectoral fascia) between the pectoralis major and minor muscles

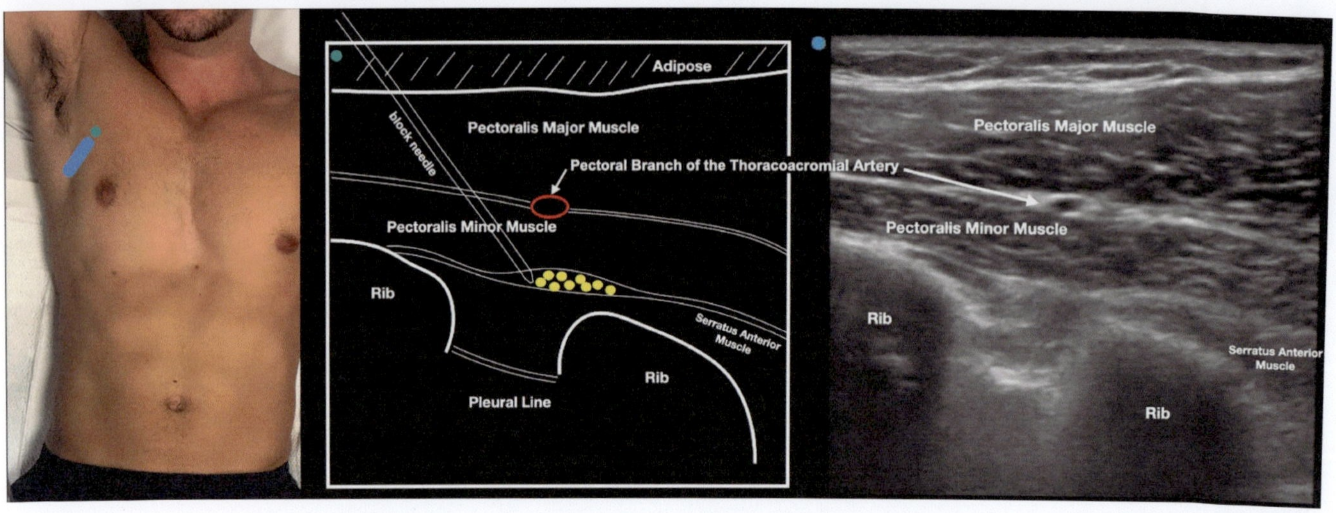

Fig. 22.29 **Performing the PECS 2 block.** The probe is slid further caudally and laterally with slight rotation (inferior aspect of the probe rotated laterally). The probe marker is directed cephalad, and the non-marker side is caudal. The pectoral branch of the thoracoacromial artery and serratus anterior muscle should be visualized at this level. Use color Doppler to identify and avoid the artery. Advance the needle in-plane from cranial to caudal, placing the needle tip between pectoralis minor and serratus anterior. Inject 15 mL of local anesthetic (yellow circles) into the fascial plane

Serratus Anterior Plane Block

Indications

The serratus anterior plane block provides thoracic analgesia to the anterior and lateral chest wall. This includes the lateral cutaneous branches of the T2–T9 intercostal nerves, the intercostobrachial nerve (which provides sensation to the axilla and upper medial aspect of the arm), the long thoracic nerve (which innervates the serratus anterior muscle), and the thoracodorsal nerve (which provides motor function to latissimus dorsi muscle). It is clinically useful for anterior and lateral rib fractures, burns, lacerations, contusions, herpes zoster, and postherpetic neuralgia of the anterolateral chest wall. It can also provide analgesia for patients receiving chest tubes or those with axillary abscesses requiring incision and drainage.

Technique

The serratus anterior fascial plane lies between the serratus anterior and latissimus dorsi muscles (Fig. 22.30). Place a linear probe transversely on the lateral chest wall at the level of the fifth rib (Fig. 22.31). Visualize the rib, pleural line, serratus anterior, and latissimus dorsi (Fig. 22.32). Using an in-plane technique, advance the needle toward the potential space between the serratus anterior and latissimus dorsi muscles (Fig. 22.33). This procedure can be performed by inject-

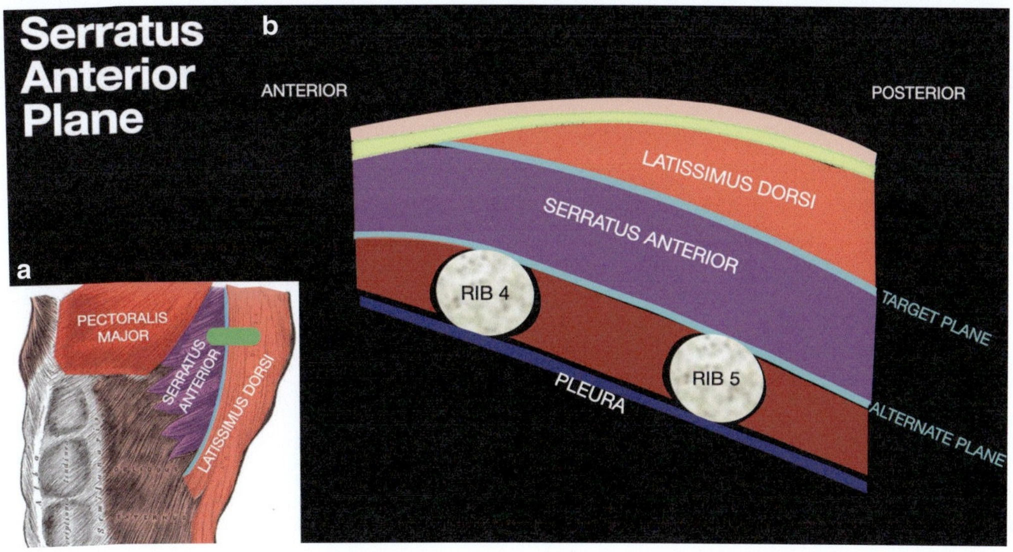

Fig. 22.30 **The serratus anterior plane block.** (**a**) There are three main muscles of the anterior and lateral chest wall: the pectoralis major, serratus anterior, and latissimus dorsi. The serratus anterior plane is the fascial plane lying between the serratus anterior and latissimus dorsi muscles, highlighted in turquoise. The probe (indicated in green) is placed transversely on the lateral chest wall. (**b**) The cross-sectional image generated in this location shows the skin (peach) and subcutaneous fat (yellow) at the top of the display screen. Beneath this are the latissimus dorsi (orange) and serratus anterior (purple) muscles, with the ribs and intercostal muscles (red) deep to the serratus anterior. The target plane for injection is highlighted in turquoise labeled "target plane." Alternatively, the injection may be placed deep to the serratus anterior muscle highlighted in turquoise labeled "alternate plane"

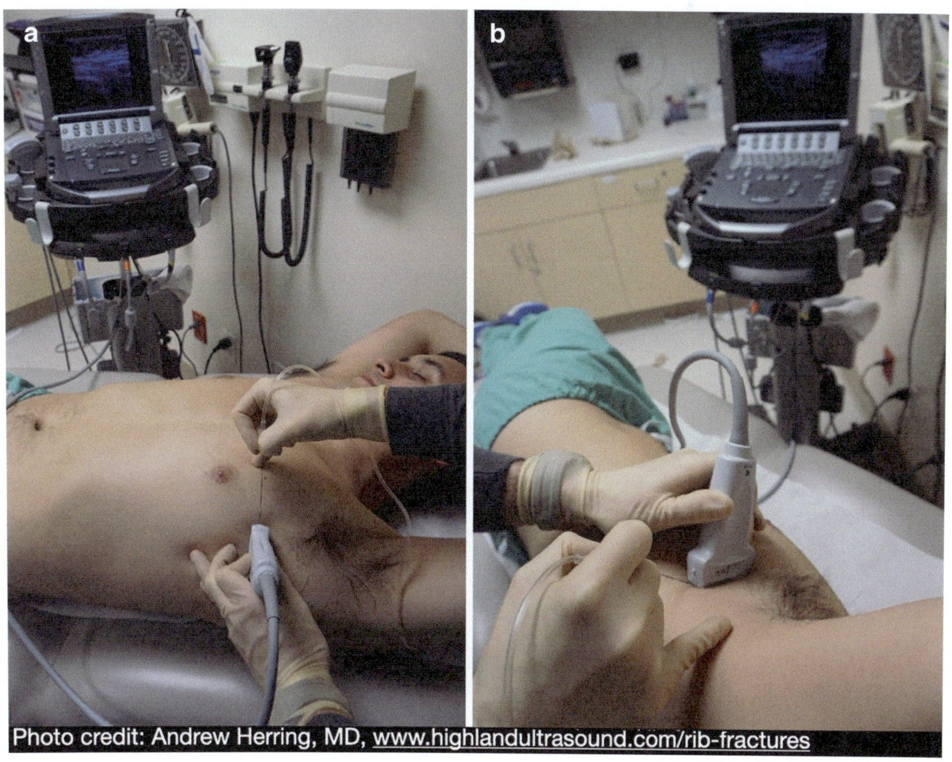

Fig. 22.31 **Patient positioning for the serratus anterior plane block.** The patient can be either supine (**a**) or in the lateral decubitus position with the affected side up (**b**). In both positions, the arm should be abducted at least 90° to allow for proper probe positioning. The operator can be located on either side of the injury depending on their preference. The probe is placed on the lateral chest wall at the level of the fifth rib in approximately the mid-axillary line. The fifth rib is located at the level of the nipple, but the ribs can also be counted by palpation or sonographically to identify the level. (*Photos Courtesy of Andrew Herring, MD*)

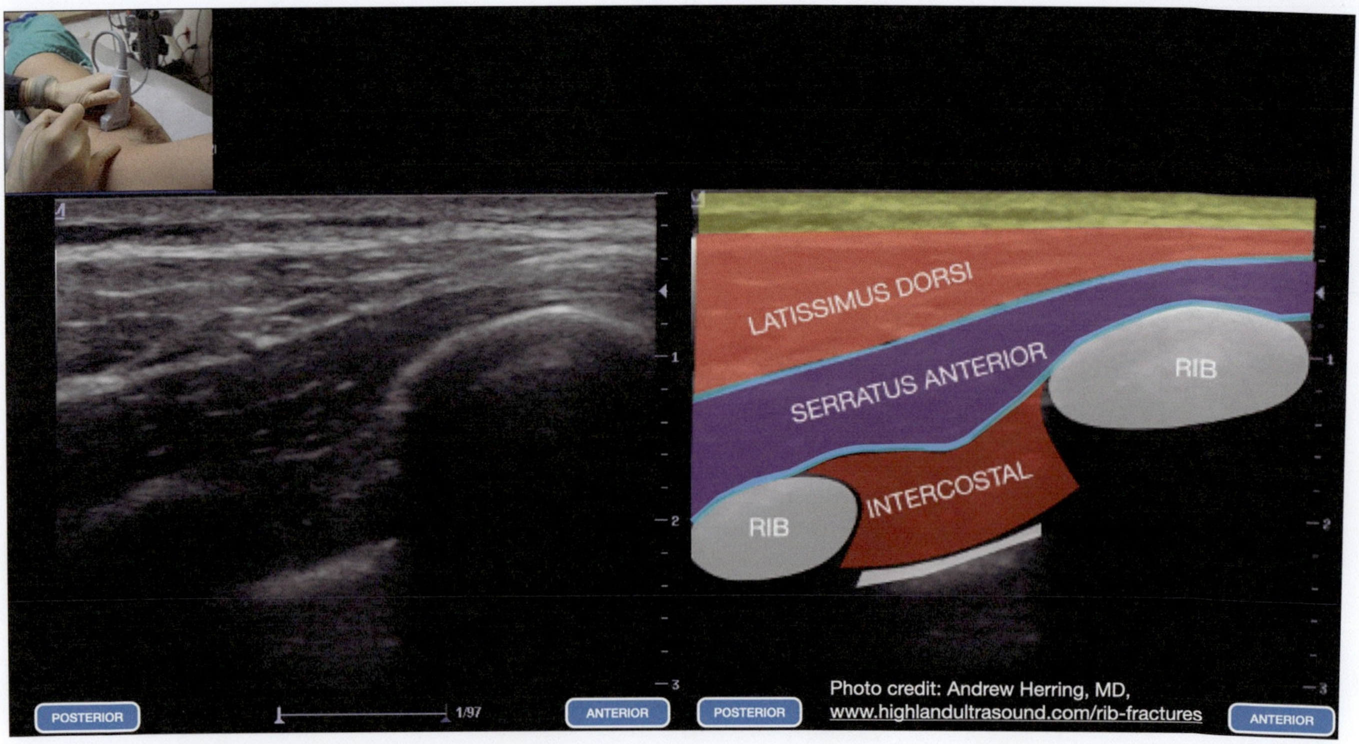

Fig. 22.32 **Sonographic anatomy of the serratus anterior plane block.** Identify the hyperechoic ribs and pleural sliding (white line) deep to the ribs and intercostal muscles (red). Beneath the skin and subcutaneous fat (yellow) is the latissimus dorsi muscle. Deep to this muscle, above the ribs, is the serratus anterior muscle. The fascial planes (turquoise lines) between the latissimus dorsi (orange) and serratus anterior (purple) muscles or between the serratus anterior muscle and the ribs are the possible targets for the injection. Sliding the probe posteriorly will bring the latissimus dorsi into view if there is difficulty visualizing it. (*Photos courtesy of Andrew Herring, MD*)

ing local anesthetic using either a superficial (between the serratus anterior and latissimus dorsi) or deep (between the serratus anterior and rib) technique. The superficial technique offers the advantage of using a shallower angle and having a greater distance between the needle and lung, whereas the deep technique allows the operator to use the rib as a backstop, facilitating separation of the fascial planes while still avoiding lung tissue.

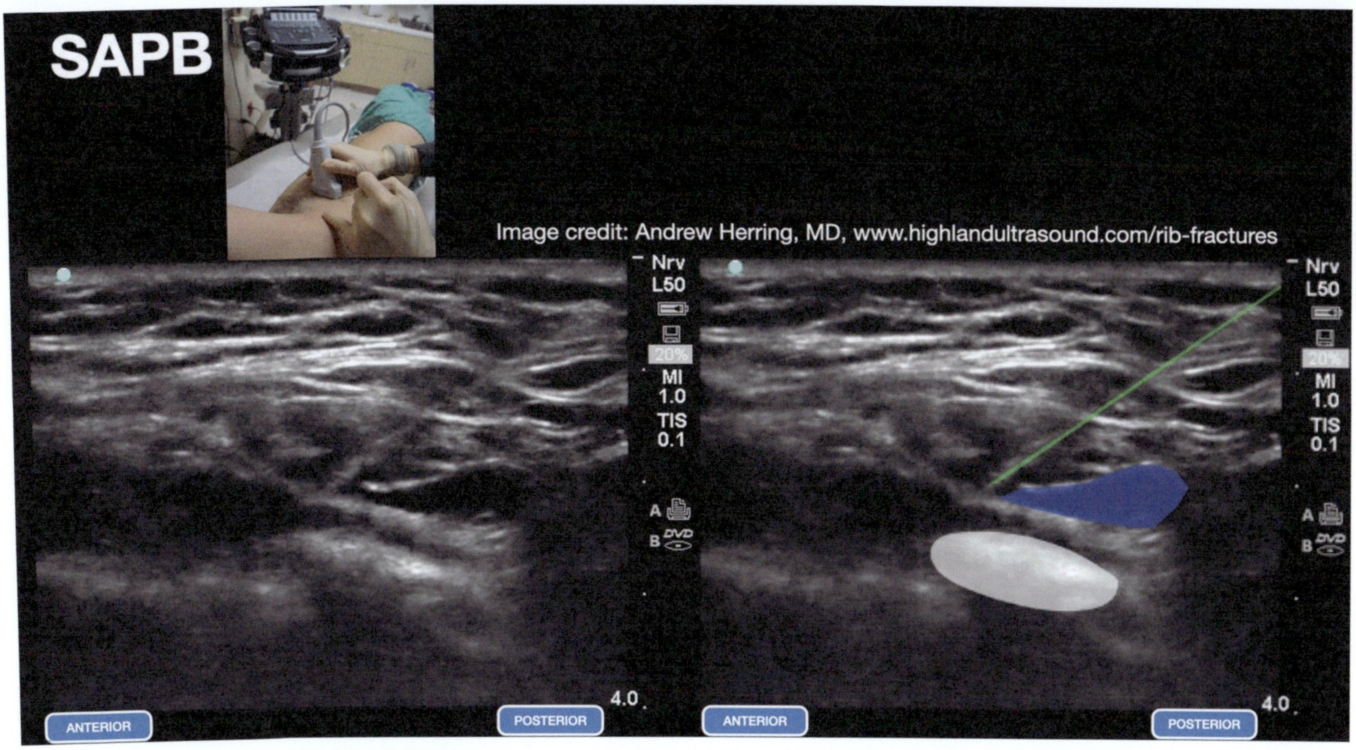

Fig. 22.33 Performing the serratus anterior plane block (SAPB). The needle (green) is advanced through the latissimus dorsi muscle toward the rib to reach the target plane. Aiming toward the rib reduces the risk of inadvertent pleural puncture. Once the needle has reached the target fascial plane, aspirate to confirm the needle is not in a vessel. Inject a small amount of normal saline (blue) to open the fascial plane, creating a fusiform anechoic fluid collection. If there is resistance or fluid remains in the muscle, the needle tip should be repositioned into the correct fascial plane. Once confirmed, inject local anesthetic using a slow incremental injection in aliquots of 2–3 mL at a time, pausing between injections, until a total of 20–40 mL of local anesthetic has been deposited in the interfascial space. (*Images courtesy of Andrew Herring, MD*)

Erector Spinae Plane Block

Indications

The erector spinae plane block (ESPB) provides analgesia to the anterior, lateral, and posterior chest walls. It is clinically useful for rib fractures, burns, lacerations, contusions, herpes zoster, and postherpetic neuralgia of the posterior thorax. This block is particularly useful for posterior rib fractures, as the serratus anterior plane block may not provide as robust anesthesia for this region. Visceral afferent nerves also arise from the region where the somatic nerves (dorsal and ventral rami) emerge from the spinal canal. Because of this, the ESPB may be effective in mitigating visceral pain from renal colic, pancreatitis, and appendicitis.

Technique

The erector spinae plane is the fascial plane located between the transverse processes of the vertebrae and the erector spinae muscle (Figs. 22.34 and 22.35). Position the patient and identify the target thoracic vertebra by first identifying the corresponding rib (Figs. 22.36 and 22.37). Slowly slide the probe medially from the rib toward the midline of the spine to bring the flat, blunt transverse process into view (Fig. 22.38). Advance the block needle toward the edge of the target transverse process (Fig. 22.39).

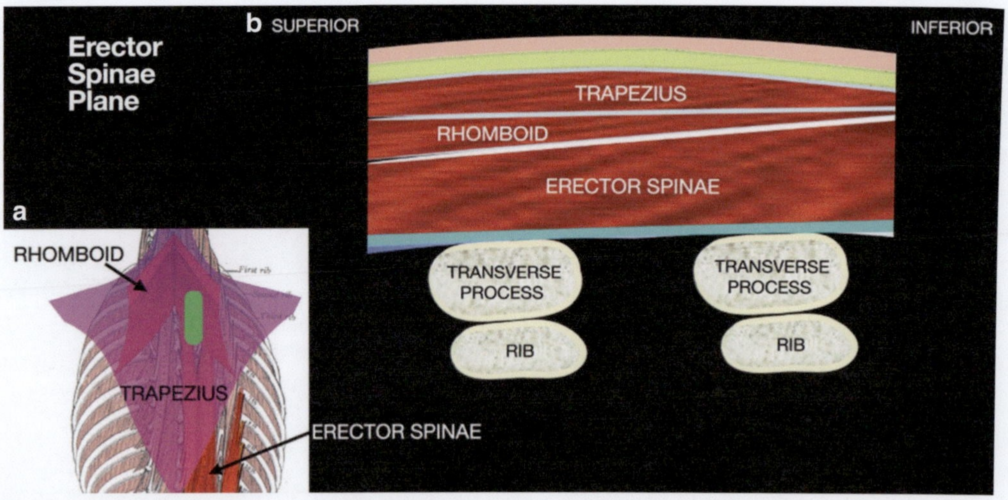

Fig. 22.34 **The erector spinae plane.** (**a**) The erector spinae muscle lies adjacent to the midline of the spine and is superficial to the laminae and the transverse processes of the vertebrae. The erector spinae plane is the fascial plane located between the transverse processes of the vertebrae and the erector spinae muscle. The rhomboid and trapezius muscles lie superficial to the erector spinae muscle. The probe (green) is placed in a parasagittal plane lateral to the spinous processes. (**b**) The cross-sectional image generated in this position shows the skin (peach) and subcutaneous fat (yellow) at the top of the display screen. Beneath this are the trapezius, rhomboid, and erector spinae muscles (red), with the transverse processes deep to the muscles. The target plane for injection (turquoise) is the fascial plane between the erector spinae muscles and the transverse processes

Fig. 22.35 **Anatomy of the erector spinae plane block.** After exiting the spinal canal, the spinal nerves bifurcate into the dorsal and ventral rami and provide innervation to the muscles in the back. The dorsal ramus travels in the erector spinae plane into the muscle itself. When high volumes of local anesthetic (blue) are deposited under the erector spinae muscle in the erector spinae plane, analgesia to the skin, muscles, and periosteum of the spine can be achieved. Deposition of local anesthetic in the erector spinae plane may also spread (turquoise) to anesthetize the spinal nerve, allowing for visceral pain relief

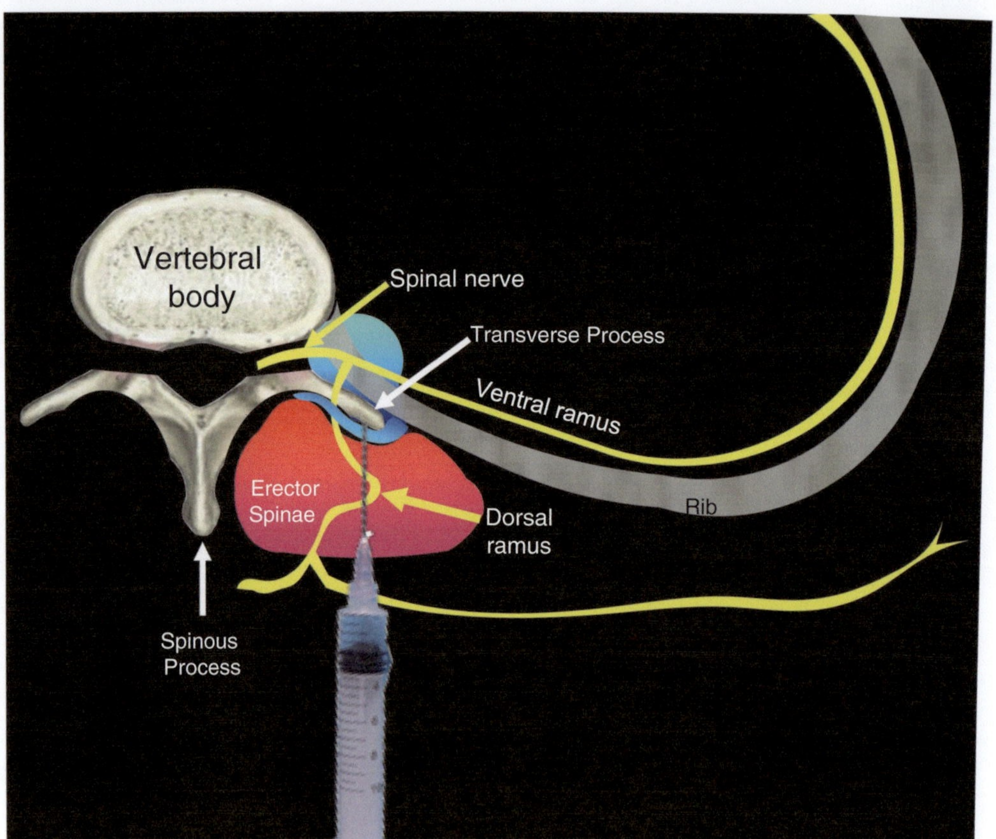

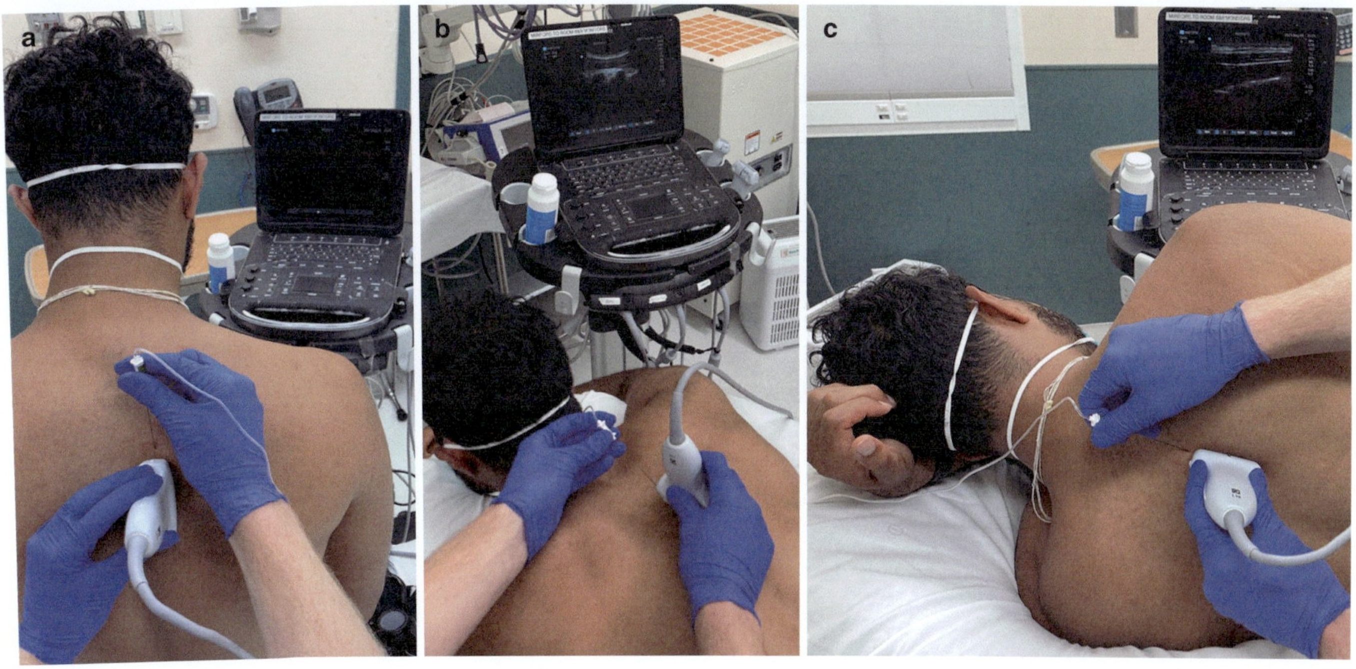

Fig. 22.36 Patient positioning for the erector spinae plane block (ESPB). The patient can be (**a**) seated, (**b**) prone, or (**c**) in the lateral decubitus position with the target side up. The ESPB can be performed at different spinal levels to achieve the desired effect. If the block is being performed for multiple rib fractures, the target should be at the middle spinal level, with the understanding that the anesthetic will spread several levels above and below the site of injection. If the block is being performed for visceral pain, the levels described are T7 for pancreatitis, T8 for renal colic, and T10 to L1 for appendicitis [16–18]. For most thoracic ESPBs, the linear probe is appropriate. In the lumbar region or in patients with a larger body habitus, the curvilinear probe may be necessary to achieve the adequate depth needed to visualize the landmarks

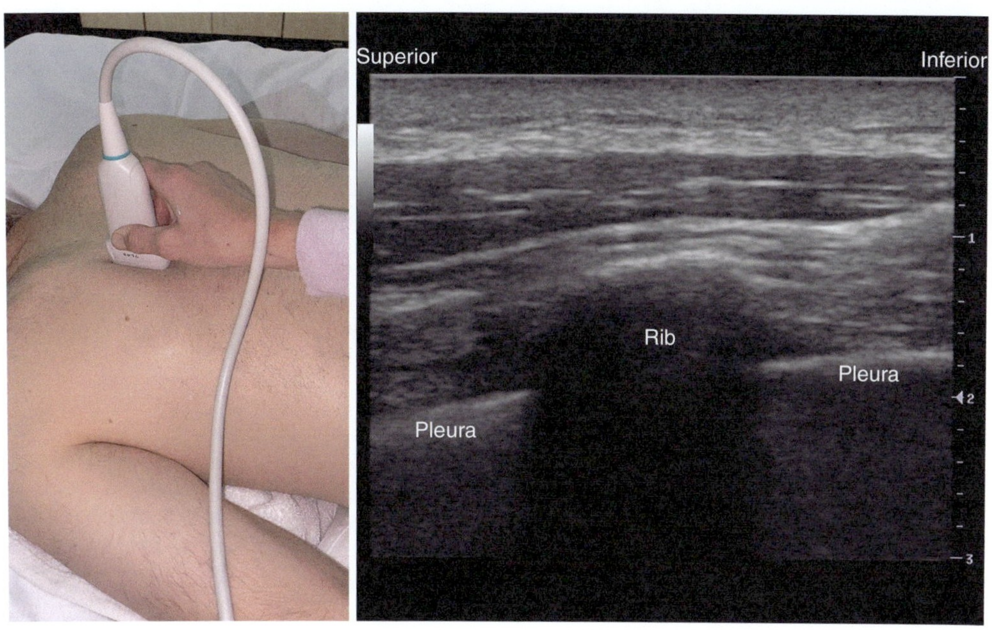

Fig. 22.37 Identify the target spinal level. Locate the target thoracic vertebra by first identifying the corresponding rib. Obtain a parasagittal image of the posterior first rib with the linear probe several inches lateral to the spine. Slide the probe inferiorly, counting ribs until the target level is reached. The pleura should be visible just deep to the ribs

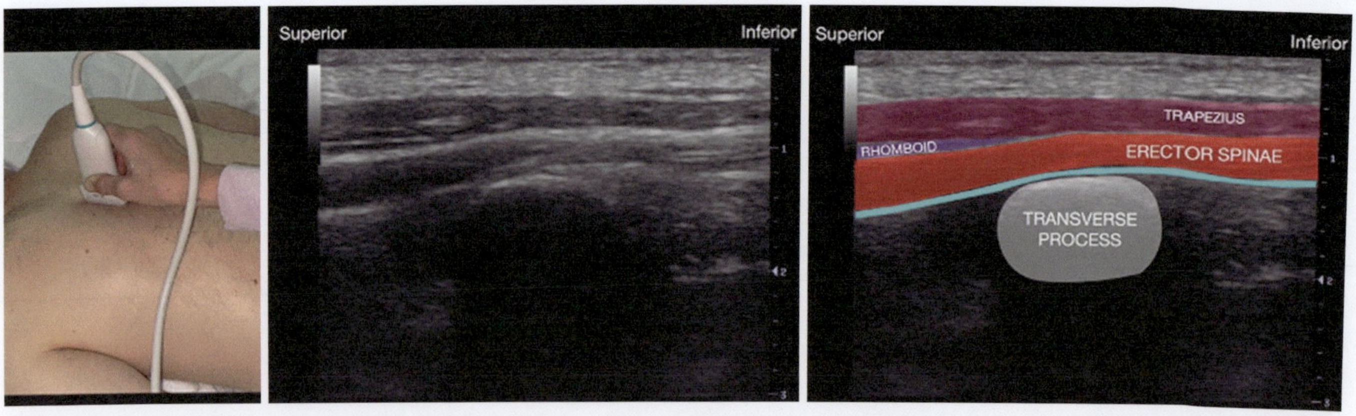

Fig. 22.38 **Identify the transverse process.** Slide the probe medially from the rib toward the midline of the spine. There is a distinct transition where the curved rib is replaced by the flat, blunt shape of the transverse process. Above the transverse process lie three defined muscle layers: the trapezius, the tail end of the rhomboid, and the erector spinae. The rhomboid muscle originates at the spinous processes of T2-T5, so it may not be visualized inferior to T5. The target plane for injection (turquoise) is the fascia separating the erector spinae muscle from the transverse process

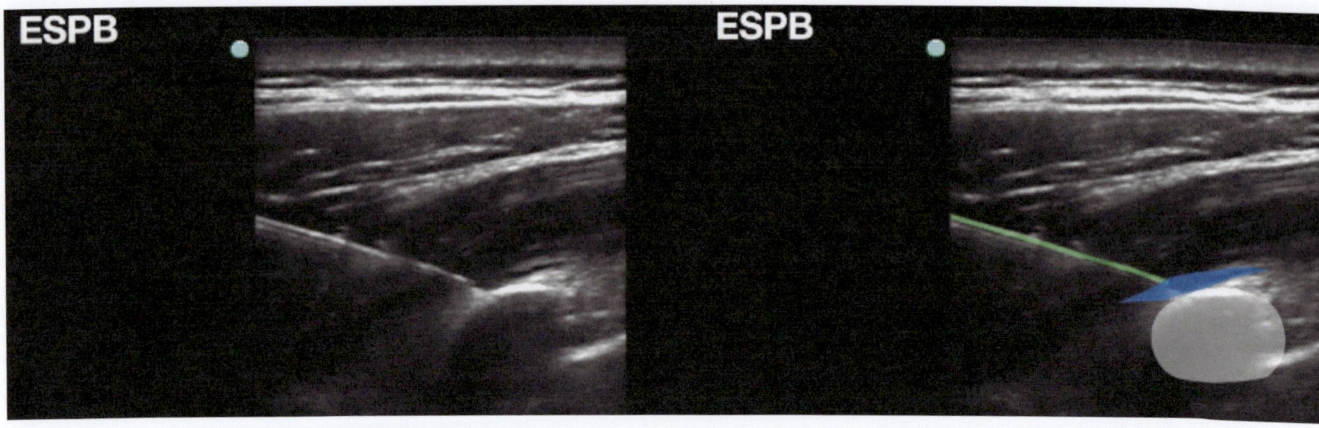

Fig. 22.39 **Performing the erector spinae plane block.** Advance the needle (green) toward the target transverse process (white). It is helpful to aim the needle toward the edge of the transverse process, not the middle, as the fascial plane of the thick erector spinae muscle lifts off more easily at this location. Once the needle reaches the target fascial plane and aspiration shows no blood, inject a small amount of saline (blue) to confirm the needle tip location. The saline should lift the erector spinae muscle off the transverse process and spread cephalad and caudal. After this, inject local anesthetic under ultrasound guidance using slow incremental injection in aliquots of 2–3 mL at a time, until a total of 20–40 mL of local anesthetic is deposited in the interfascial space. (*Images courtesy of Andrew Herring, MD*)

Greater Occipital Nerve Block

Indications

The greater occipital nerve (GON) is a sensory branch of the C2 spinal nerve that provides sensation to the skin of the occipital region. The GON block can be useful in conditions isolated to the GON, such as occipital neuralgia, as well as other types of headaches, including migraines, cluster headaches, cervicogenic headaches, and post-dural headaches [19]. The mechanism is thought to be due to the modulation of interactions between the occipital and trigeminal nerves in the trigeminocervical complex [20].

Technique

With the patient positioned prone, seated, or in lateral decubitus, start by placing a linear probe in a transverse orientation over the occipital protuberance to locate the occipital bone (Fig. 22.40a). Move the probe caudally to identify the posterior tubercle and arch of the atlas, which characteristically lacks a spinous process (Fig. 22.40b). Continue moving the probe caudad to identify the spinous process of the axis, which usually appears bifid (Fig. 22.40c). Shift the probe laterally to visualize the obliquus capitis inferior muscle (OCIM), which is located on top of the axis lamina and inserts into the transverse process of the atlas. Superficial to the OCIM lies the semispinalis capitis muscle. The GON typically appears as a hypoechoic structure within the fascial plane between the OCIM and the semispinalis capitis muscle (Fig. 22.41). Employing a lateral-to-medial in-plane approach, advance the needle into the fascial plane near the GON. Following negative aspiration, inject 10 mL of local anesthetic in 2–3 mL aliquots.

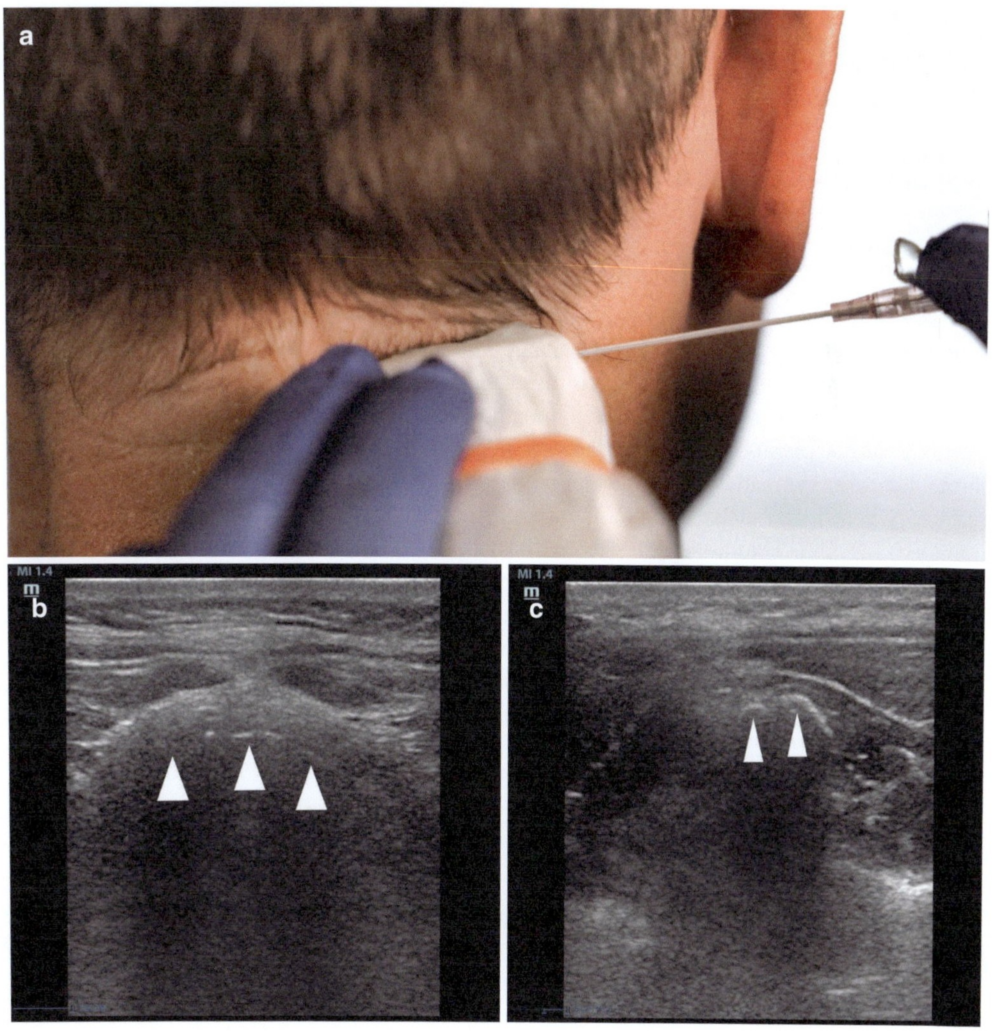

Fig. 22.40 Positioning for greater occipital nerve block. (**a**) External position for the ultrasound probe and needle. (**b**) Identify the occipital bone in the midline, then sweep the probe caudad to locate the posterior arch of the atlas (white arrowheads). (**c**) Continue sliding inferiorly to locate the bifid spinous process of the axis (white arrowheads). Once identified, slide the probe laterally to identify the obliquus capitis inferior muscle and semispinalis capitis muscle, which may require slight rotation of the probe. (*Images courtesy of Jeffrey A. Kramer, MD, MSc and John Barrett, DNP*)

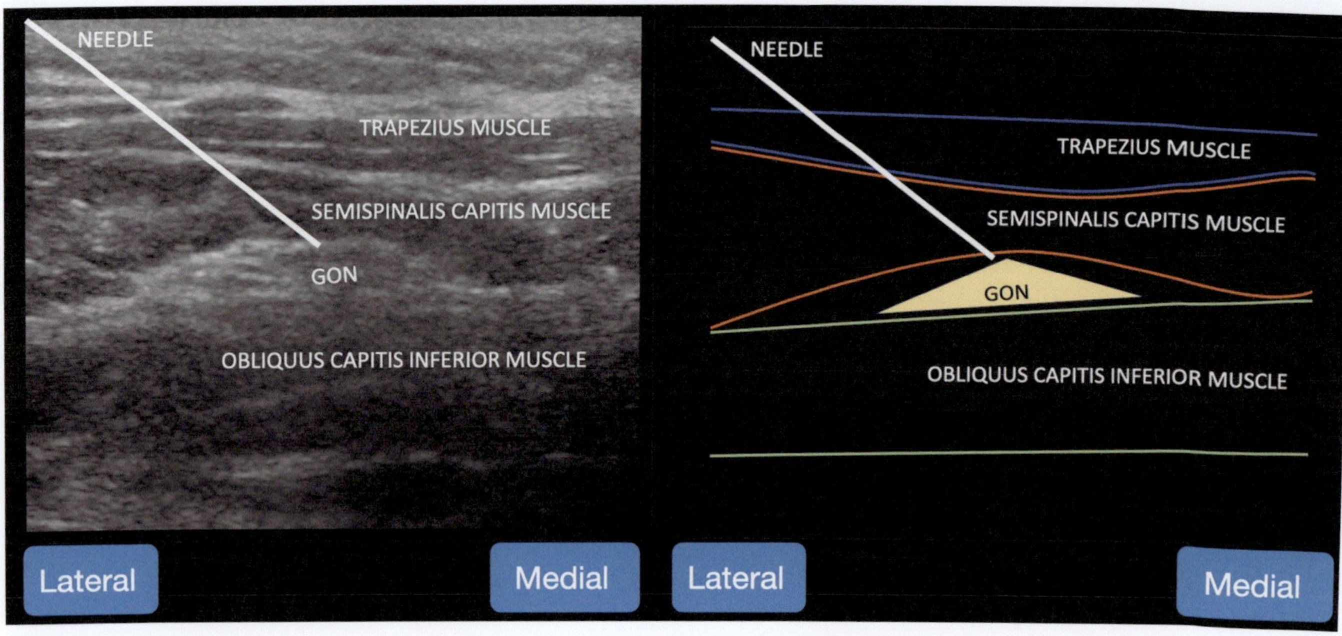

Fig. 22.41 Sonographic anatomy of the greater occipital nerve (GON) block. The obliquus capitis inferior muscle (OCIM) is located on top of the lamina of the axis. Superficial to the OCIM is the semispinalis capitis muscle. The GON typically appears as a hypoechoic oval structure situated between the OCIM and semispinalis capitis muscle. The needle should be advanced from lateral to medial using an in-plane approach. (*Images courtesy of Kyle Flattery, MD*)

Stellate Ganglion Block

Indications

The stellate ganglion block is unique among the blocks presented in this chapter, as the goal is not analgesia but rather a physiologic effect. The stellate ganglion forms the base of the cervical sympathetic chain and sends sympathetic output to the deep cardiac plexus. Blockade of the stellate ganglion produces a cardiac sympathectomy that can be used for cases of refractory ventricular tachycardia (VT) or ventricular fibrillation (VF) [21, 22]. Traditionally, this block has been reserved for regional anesthesiologists and performed on intubated patients in critical care units who have had ventricular storm refractory to medical management. However, with emergency physicians becoming increasingly facile in regional blocks, there are now case series data suggesting its efficacy in refractory VT or VF in the emergency department setting [23–25].

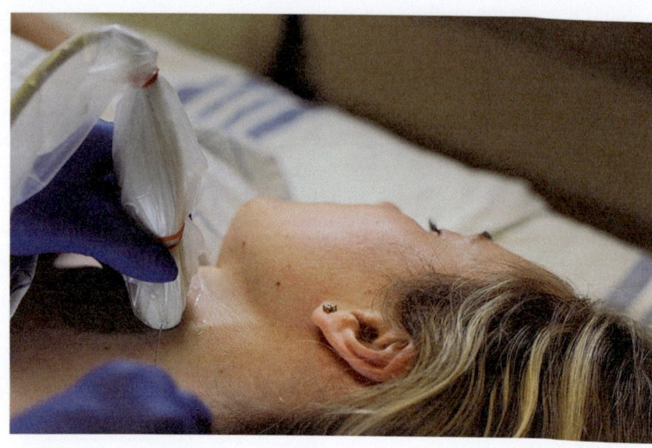

Fig. 22.42 Positioning for the stellate ganglion block. The patient should be supine with the head turned 30° to the right. The operator stands on the left side of the patient. The cricoid can be palpated or directly visualized with ultrasound. The probe is placed over the cricoid ring and then swept laterally to visualize the transverse process of C6. (*Image courtesy of John Barrett, DNP*)

Technique

Due to asymmetric sympathetic innervation and hemodynamic effects, the left stellate ganglion is preferred over the right [26]. The head should be turned approximately 30° to the right (away from the side of the block). Place the linear probe transversely over the left neck at the level of the cricoid cartilage (C6) (Fig. 22.42). The stellate ganglion is located at C7-T1, but due to the proximity of the lung and the vertebral artery, the block is typically performed at the C6 level. The characteristic anterior tubercle of the transverse process of C6 helps to identify the correct level. The ganglion itself is located posterior to the common carotid artery, along the anterior aspect of the longus colli muscle, which overlies the transverse process (Fig. 22.43). The procedure is performed using the in-plane technique with the needle inserted from the lateral to medial direction (Fig. 22.44).

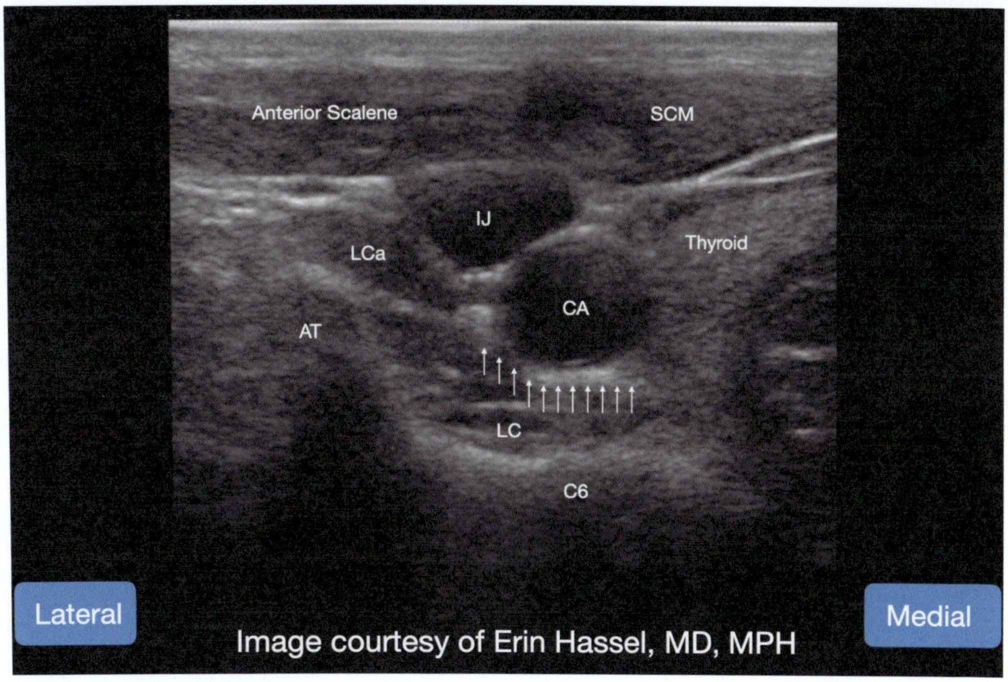

Fig. 22.43 Sonographic anatomy of the stellate ganglion block. The correct level is identified by finding the prominent anterior tubercle of the C6 transverse process (AT). Here, the carotid artery (CA) and internal jugular (IJ) vein overlay the longus colli (LC) muscle. The cervical sympathetic ganglia (identified by arrows) are located posterior to the carotid, deep to the prevertebral fascia, and just anterior to LC. Sternocleidomastoid (SCM) muscle, anterior scalene muscle, and longus capitis (LCa) muscle are labeled for context. (*Image courtesy of Erin Hassel, MD, MPH*)

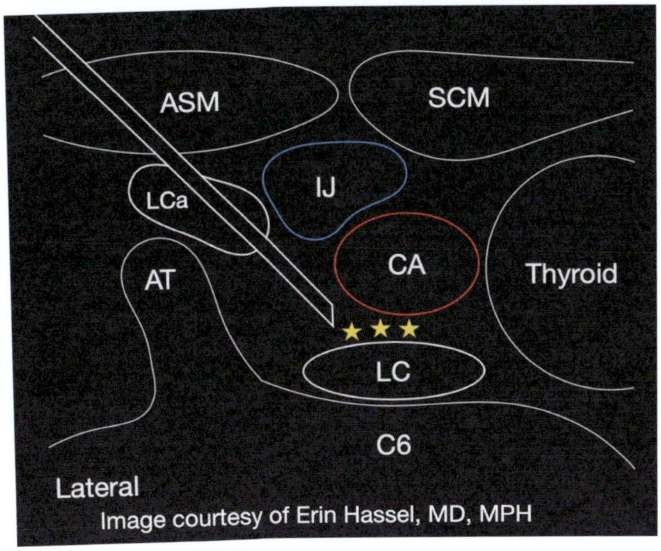

Fig. 22.44 Performing the left stellate ganglion block. Insert the needle from lateral to medial using an in-plane technique. Care should be taken to avoid the internal jugular (IJ) vein and the carotid artery (CA) as the needle is advanced slightly past the anterior tubercle of C6 (AT), deep to the carotid artery, anterior to longus colli (LC) muscle. After negative aspiration, inject 10 mL of 1% lidocaine in the region of the cervical sympathetic ganglion (yellow stars). Attempts may need to be timed with pulse checks to improve needle visualization, especially if manual compressions are being performed. *ASM* anterior scalene muscle, *SCM* sternocleidomastoid muscle, *LCa* longus capitis muscle. (*Image courtesy of Erin Hassel, MD, MPH*)

Disclosures/Conflicts of Interest

Andrew Goldsmith: Medical Director, Ultrasight Inc.
Joseph Stegeman: Consultant for Exo Inc.
Arun Nagdev: VP of Clinical, Exo Inc.

References

1. Jones CMP, Langford A, Maher CG, Abdel Shaheed C, Day R, Lin CWC. Opioids for acute musculoskeletal pain: a systematic review with meta-analysis. Drugs. 2024;84(3):305–17.
2. Gottlieb M, Nagdev A. Sound decisions: rethinking the role of ultrasound-guided regional analgesia in the emergency department. Ann Emerg Med. 2024;83(6):539–41.
3. Steinfeldt T, Poeschl S, Nimphius W, et al. Forced needle advancement during needle-nerve contact in a porcine model: histological outcome. Anesth Analg. 2011;113(2):417–20.
4. Hadzic A, Dilberovic F, Shah S, et al. Combination of intraneural injection and high injection pressure leads to fascicular injury and neurologic deficits in dogs. Reg Anesth Pain Med. 2004;29(5):417–23.
5. Neal JM, Bernards CM, Hadzic A, et al. ASRA practice advisory on neurologic complications in regional anesthesia and pain medicine. Reg Anesth Pain Med. 2008;33(5):404–15.
6. Lemke E, Johnston DF, Behrens MB, et al. Neurological injury following peripheral nerve blocks: a narrative review of estimates of risks and the influence of ultrasound guidance. Reg Anesth Pain Med. 2024;49(2):122–32.
7. Long B, Chavez S, Gottlieb M, Montrief T, Brady WJ. Local anesthetic systemic toxicity: a narrative review for emergency clinicians. Am J Emerg Med. 2022;59:42–8.

8. Brown JR, Goldsmith AJ, Lapietra A, et al. Ultrasound-guided nerve blocks: suggested procedural guidelines for emergency physicians. POCUS J. 2022;7(2):253–61.
9. Bansal K, Sharma N, Singh MR, Sharma A, Roy R, Sethi S. Comparison of suprainguinal approach with infrainguinal approach of fascia iliaca compartment block for postoperative analgesia. Indian J Anaesth. 2022;66(Suppl 6):S294–9.
10. Vermeylen K, Desmet M, Leunen I, et al. Supra-inguinal injection for fascia iliaca compartment block results in more consistent spread towards the lumbar plexus than an infra-inguinal injection: a volunteer study. Reg Anesth Pain Med. 2019; https://doi.org/10.1136/rapm-2018-100092.
11. Riazi S, Carmichael N, Awad I, Holtby RM, McCartney CJL. Effect of local anaesthetic volume (20 vs 5 ml) on the efficacy and respiratory consequences of ultrasound-guided interscalene brachial plexus block. Br J Anaesth. 2008;101(4):549–56.
12. Renes SH, Rettig HC, Gielen MJ, Wilder-Smith OH, van Geffen GJ. Ultrasound-guided low-dose interscalene brachial plexus block reduces the incidence of hemidiaphragmatic paresis. Reg Anesth Pain Med. 2009;34(5):498–502.
13. Stundner O, Meissnitzer M, Brummett CM, et al. Comparison of tissue distribution, phrenic nerve involvement, and epidural spread in standard- vs low-volume ultrasound-guided interscalene plexus block using contrast magnetic resonance imaging: a randomized, controlled trial. Br J Anaesth. 2016;116(3):405–12.
14. Bharti N, Bhardawaj N, Wig J. Comparison of ultrasound-guided supraclavicular, infraclavicular and below-C6 interscalene brachial plexus block for upper limb surgery: a randomised, observer-blinded study. Anaesth Intensive Care. 2015;43(4):468–72.
15. Ryu T, Kil BT, Kim JH. Comparison between ultrasound-guided supraclavicular and interscalene brachial plexus blocks in patients undergoing arthroscopic shoulder surgery: a prospective, randomized, parallel study. Medicine. 2015;94(40):e1726.
16. Aydin ME, Tekin E, Ahiskalioglu EO, et al. Erector spinae plane block vs non-steroidal anti-inflammatory drugs for severe renal colic pain: a pilot clinical feasibility study. Int J Clin Pract. 2021;75(3):e13789.
17. Parsons-Moss D, Martin D, Condori M, Dreyfuss A. Erector spinae plane block performed in the emergency department for abdominal pain: a case series. Clin Pract Cases Emerg Med. 2023;7(3):132–5.
18. Mantuani D, Luftig J, Herring A, Dreyfuss A, Nagdev A. A novel technique to reduce reliance on opioids for analgesia from acute appendicitis: the ultrasound-guided erector spinae plane block. Clin Pract Cases Emerg Med. 2019;3(3):248–51.
19. Zhang H, Yang X, Lin Y, Chen L, Ye H. The efficacy of greater occipital nerve block for the treatment of migraine: a systematic review and meta-analysis. Clin Neurol Neurosurg. 2018;165:129–33.
20. Hoffmann J, Mehnert J, Koo EM, May A. Greater occipital nerve block modulates nociceptive signals within the trigeminocervical complex. J Neurol Neurosurg Psychiatry. 2021;92(12):1335–40.
21. Gottlieb M, Dyer S, Peksa GD. Beta-blockade for the treatment of cardiac arrest due to ventricular fibrillation or pulseless ventricular tachycardia: a systematic review and meta-analysis. Resuscitation. 2020;146:118–25.
22. Dyer S, Mogni B, Gottlieb M. Electrical storm: a focused review for the emergency physician. Am J Emerg Med. 2020;38(7):1481–7.
23. Margus C, Correa A, Cheung W, et al. Stellate ganglion nerve block by point-of-care ultrasonography for treatment of refractory infarction-induced ventricular fibrillation. Ann Emerg Med. 2020;75(2):257–60.
24. Callipari C, Stone M, John D, Keceli M, Giles RA. Intra-cardiac arrest use of stellate ganglion block for refractory ventricular tachycardia. J Emerg Med. 2023;64(5):628–34.
25. Nair A, Bhoi S, Choudhary Y. Cease the storm – successful stellate ganglion block in terminating refractory electrical storm. Am J Emerg Med. 2024;81:160.e3–7.
26. Ganesh A, Qadri YJ, Boortz-Marx RL, et al. Stellate ganglion blockade: an intervention for the management of ventricular arrhythmias. Curr Hypertens Rep. 2020;22(12):100.

Resuscitative Ultrasound

23

Robert James Adrian, Adi Osman, and Josie Acuña

Background

Resuscitative ultrasound utilizes the diagnostic, therapeutic, treatment monitoring, hemodynamic optimization, and procedural safety aspects of point-of-care ultrasound (POCUS) to care for critically ill patients. Resuscitative ultrasound has been performed since the 1970s [1–3]. Systematic use began in the 1990s with the evolution of protocolized scanning [4, 5]. These protocols can diagnose etiologies and complications of cardiac arrest or shock from cardiac, thoracic, abdominal, vascular, and airway sources [6]. In addition to encouraging an organized approach, POCUS may be beneficial in undifferentiated shock for distinguishing the shock type and management strategies [7–16]. POCUS can also be used for diagnostics, fluid management, and hemodynamic optimization in patients with undifferentiated and septic shock [17–21].

This chapter begins with POCUS in cardiac arrest, including protocols and strategies for use. The chapter continues with POCUS in undifferentiated shock and a discussion of the hemodynamic evaluation and management of hypotensive patients. Finally, the chapter concludes with POCUS in sepsis and septic shock, including protocols, hemodynamic monitoring through cluster evaluation, volume status assessments, and source identification.

Supplementary Information The online version contains supplementary material available at https://doi.org/10.1007/978-3-031-85308-1_23.

R. J. Adrian (✉)
Department of Emergency Medicine, Christchurch Hospital, Christchurch, New Zealand

A. Osman
Emergency and Trauma Department, Hospital Raja Permaisuri Bainun, Ipoh, Perak, Malaysia

J. Acuña
Department of Emergency Medicine, University of Arizona, Tucson, AZ, USA
e-mail: jacuna1@arizona.edu

POCUS in Cardiac Arrest

POCUS can identify reversible causes of cardiac arrest and guide management [6]. When the etiology of the arrest can be identified, there is a significant survival benefit [22–24]. Various protocols exist for utilizing POCUS during cardiac arrest (Table 23.1) [5, 6, 8, 25–38]. These protocols all attempt to identify reversible etiologies and provide resuscitation guidance [6]. Specifically, POCUS can evaluate for cardiac tamponade, pulmonary embolism (PE), deep venous thrombosis (DVT), ventricular fibrillation (VF), pulseless electrical activity (PEA), asystole, aortic dissection, abdominal aortic aneurysm (AAA), hemothorax, pneumothorax, endotracheal tube (ETT) placement, intra-abdominal free fluid, hypovolemia, and has the potential to aid with pulse checks and prognosis.

Nevertheless, despite the potential benefit of ultrasound, possible harms should be considered [39]. An important consideration is that POCUS should not cause delays in high-quality chest compressions [39–43]. To minimize potential pitfalls, experts recommend several pearls (Table 23.2) [6].

Cardiac Tamponade

In a large prospective emergency department (ED) study, pericardial effusion was found in 4% of cardiac arrest patients [45]. Those who received pericardiocentesis (Fig. 23.1, Video 23.1a) had a higher rate of survival-to-discharge than those who did not (15% versus 1%) [45]. In cases of traumatic cardiac arrest, approximately 10% may be due to cardiac tamponade [46]. Emergency physicians evaluating PEA in cardiac arrest patients showed they could identify pericardial effusions with high positive predictive values [47, 48]. However, the echocardiographic findings of cardiac tamponade (e.g., right atrial systolic collapse, right ventricular diastolic collapse) are unreliable in the cardiac arrest patient due to the absence of normal blood flow and cardiovascular pressures (Fig. 23.2, Video 23.2a) [49].

M. Gottlieb, N. Panebianco (eds.), *Advanced Point-of-Care Ultrasound*, https://doi.org/10.1007/978-3-031-85308-1_23

Table 23.1 Protocols for utilizing ultrasound during cardiac arrest

Protocol	Components
Rapid Cardiac POCUS in Pulmonary-Epigastric-Abdominal Arrest [5]	Cardiac (contractility, pericardial effusion, right ventricular dilation with the small dynamic left ventricle, underfilled right ventricle with the small dynamic left ventricle)
Focused Echocardiographic Evaluation in Resuscitation (FEER) [25]	Cardiac (cardiac activity, pericardial effusion/cardiac tamponade, hypovolemia, and massive PE)
Cardiac Arrest Ultrasound Examination (CAUSE) [26]	Cardiac (cardiac tamponade, hypovolemia, and massive PE) Lung (pneumothorax)
Pulseless Electrical Activity or Pulmonary-Epigastric-Abdominal (PEA) [27]	Cardiac (pericardial effusion, cardiac activity, left ventricular size/hypertrophy/contractility, right ventricular size/contractility, and IVC filling) Lung (pneumothorax, pleural effusion, and pulmonary edema) Abdomen and other (thoracic and abdominal aortic aneurysm or dissection, peritoneal effusion, bowel obstruction or perforation, and DVT)
Focused Echocardiographic Evaluation in Life Support (FEEL) [28]	Cardiac (cardiac activity, ventricular function, right ventricular dilatation, and pericardial effusion)
Sequential Emergency Scanning Assessing Mechanical or Origin of Shock of Indistinct Cause (SESAME) [29, 30]	Lung (pulmonary edema and pneumothorax) DVT Abdomen (peritoneal effusion) Cardiac (cardiac tamponade, contractility, right ventricular dilatation, and ventricular fibrillation)
Sonography in Hypotension and Cardiac Arrest (SHoC) [8, 31, 32]	Cardiac (cardiac tamponade, right ventricular dysfunction, cardiac activity, and ventricular size) Lung (pneumothorax and pleural effusion) IVC (diameter and respiratory variation) Airway (ETT confirmation) DVT Abdomen (AAA and peritoneal effusion)
Ultrasound Circulation-Airway-Breathing (US-CAB) [33, 34]	Cardiac (contractility, cardiac tamponade, right ventricular dilatation, septal dyskinesia, and right-sided chamber flattening suggestive of hypovolemia) IVC (diameter and respirophasic collapsibility) Trachea (ETT confirmation) Lung (pneumothorax and single lung intubation)
Cardiac Arrest Sonographic Assessment (CASA) [35]	Cardiac (cardiac tamponade, right-heart strain, cardiac activity) Lung (pneumothorax) FAST
Reversible Cause in Cardiovascular Collapse at the Emergency Department Using Ultrasonography (REVIVE-US) [36]	Cardiac (cardiac activity and cardiac tamponade) FAST Aorta (dissection or aneurysm) DVT Lung (pneumothorax) Post-ROSC cardiac (contractility, right ventricular dilation, and regional wall motion abnormalities)
Point-of-Care Ultrasound in Cardiorespiratory Arrest (POCUS-CA) [37]	Cardiac (cardiac activity, chest compression efficacy, pericardial effusion/cardiac tamponade, and PE) Lung (pneumothorax) Abdominal (peritoneal effusion and AAA) Femoral (DVT)
Core Ultrasound in Resuscitation (CURE) [38]	Noncardiac (FAST, AAA, DVT, confirm ETT position, and pneumothorax) Cardiac TTE (cardiac contractility, ventricular arrhythmia, aortic emergency, intracardiac thrombus, maximal compression site, and hypovolemia) Post-ROSC transesophageal echocardiography (preload, cardiac and valvular function, procedural guidance)

Adapted with permission from Gottlieb et al. [6]

AAA abdominal aortic aneurysm, *DVT* deep venous thrombosis, *ETT* endotracheal tube, *FAST* focused assessment with sonography in trauma, *IVC* inferior vena cava, *PE* pulmonary embolism, *ROSC* return of spontaneous circulation

Table 23.2 Strategies for minimizing pauses in chest compressions when using point-of-care ultrasound

Most experienced sonographer performs the scan
Scan performed by non-team leader
Perform noncardiac evaluations (e.g., thoracic, ETT, DVT) during ongoing chest compressions
Pre-scan to identify the optimal cardiac window prior to pausing compressions (Note: parasternal long-axis may be superior to subxiphoid view [44])
Record the clip during the pause, then analyze it once compressions have resumed
Use a nearby towel to immediately wipe off ultrasound gel
Designate a person to count down from 10 s
Initiate early transesophageal echocardiography

Adapted with permission from Gottlieb et al. [6]
ETT endotracheal tube, *DVT* deep venous thrombosis

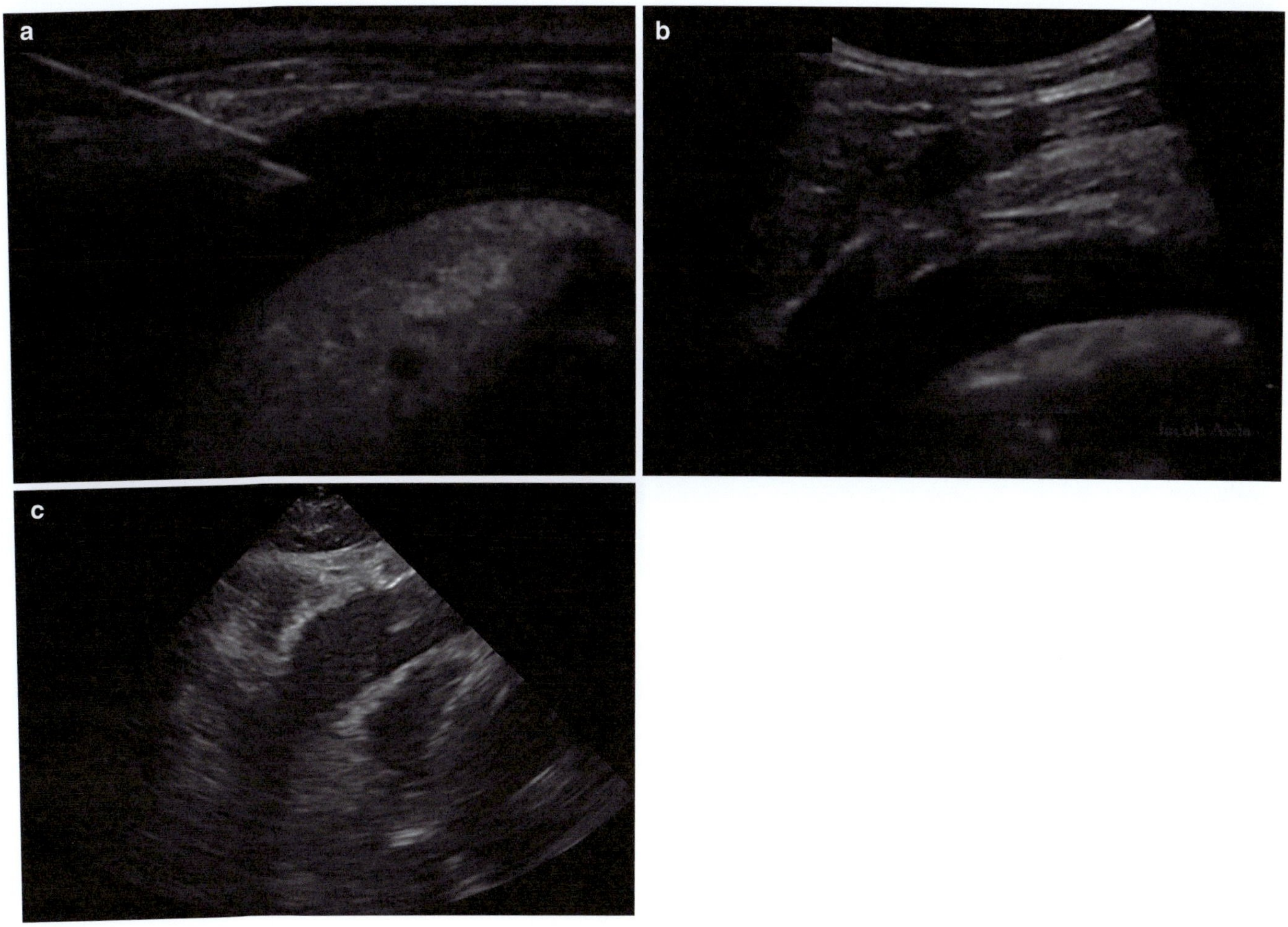

Fig. 23.1 Pericardiocentesis performed with the linear (**a**), curvilinear (**b**), and phased array probes (**c**) in cardiac tamponade. (*Images courtesy of Jailyn Avila, MD*)

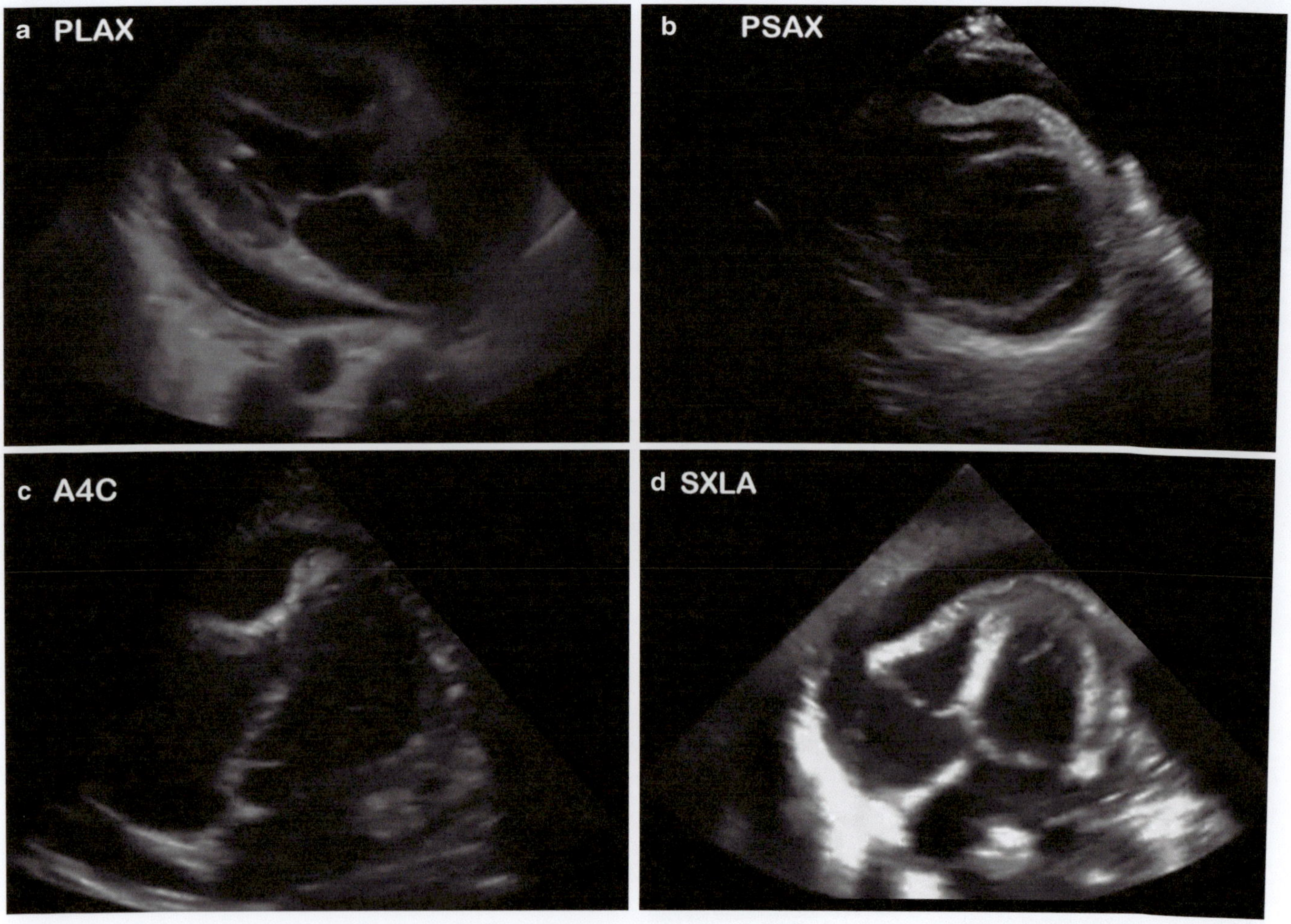

Fig. 23.2 Diastolic right ventricular collapse in cardiac tamponade. (**a**) Parasternal long-axis; (**b**) Parasternal short-axis; (**c**) Apical 4-chamber; (**d**) Subxiphoid long-axis. (*Images courtesy of Stephen Alerhand, MD and Lauren Ann J. Selame, MD*)

When evaluating pericardial effusions during arrest, larger effusions are more likely to cause tamponade [50, 51]; however, cardiac tamponade can also occur with small, rapidly accumulating effusions [49, 52]. Therefore, pericardial effusions in the cardiac arrest patient should raise concern for cardiac tamponade, and pericardiocentesis should be performed in the appropriate clinical context. The optimal location for pericardiocentesis is the largest, most superficial fluid pocket without overlying vital structures [49]. In traumatic cardiac arrest, trauma society guidelines do not discuss ultrasound in the decision to perform resuscitative thoracotomy [53]. However, less than 1% of patients survive after a resuscitative thoracotomy [53], and data show patients with cardiac etiologies have the highest survival, suggesting a clear role for early identification with POCUS [54]. Patients with traumatic cardiac arrest and a pericardial effusion require surgical management (e.g., resuscitative thoracotomy, pericardial window) in the appropriate clinical context [53–56]. However, one study found that those in traumatic cardiac arrest without cardiac motion or pericardial effusion on the focused assessment with sonography in trauma (FAST) examination had zero likelihood of survival and likely do not warrant the risk and resource burden of resuscitative thoracotomy [55].

Pulmonary Embolism

Pulmonary embolism is a major cause of cardiac arrest, with data suggesting this may be the primary etiology in 2–13% of cases [57–60]. Identification of signs of right ventricular (RV) dysfunction on cardiac POCUS (e.g., enlarged RV, septal dyskinesia, clot-in-transit) just prior to cardiac arrest is most helpful for diagnosing PE (Fig. 23.3, Video 23.3a) [6]. Once arrest has commenced, RV dilation can occur quickly due to hypovolemia, hyperkalemia, arrhythmia, and hypoxia [6]. Moreover, because new thrombus formation can occur in a median of 6 minutes into the arrest, RV assessment should be performed early (Fig. 23.4, Video 23.4a) [6, 61]. An enlarged RV can also be seen when chronic pulmonary

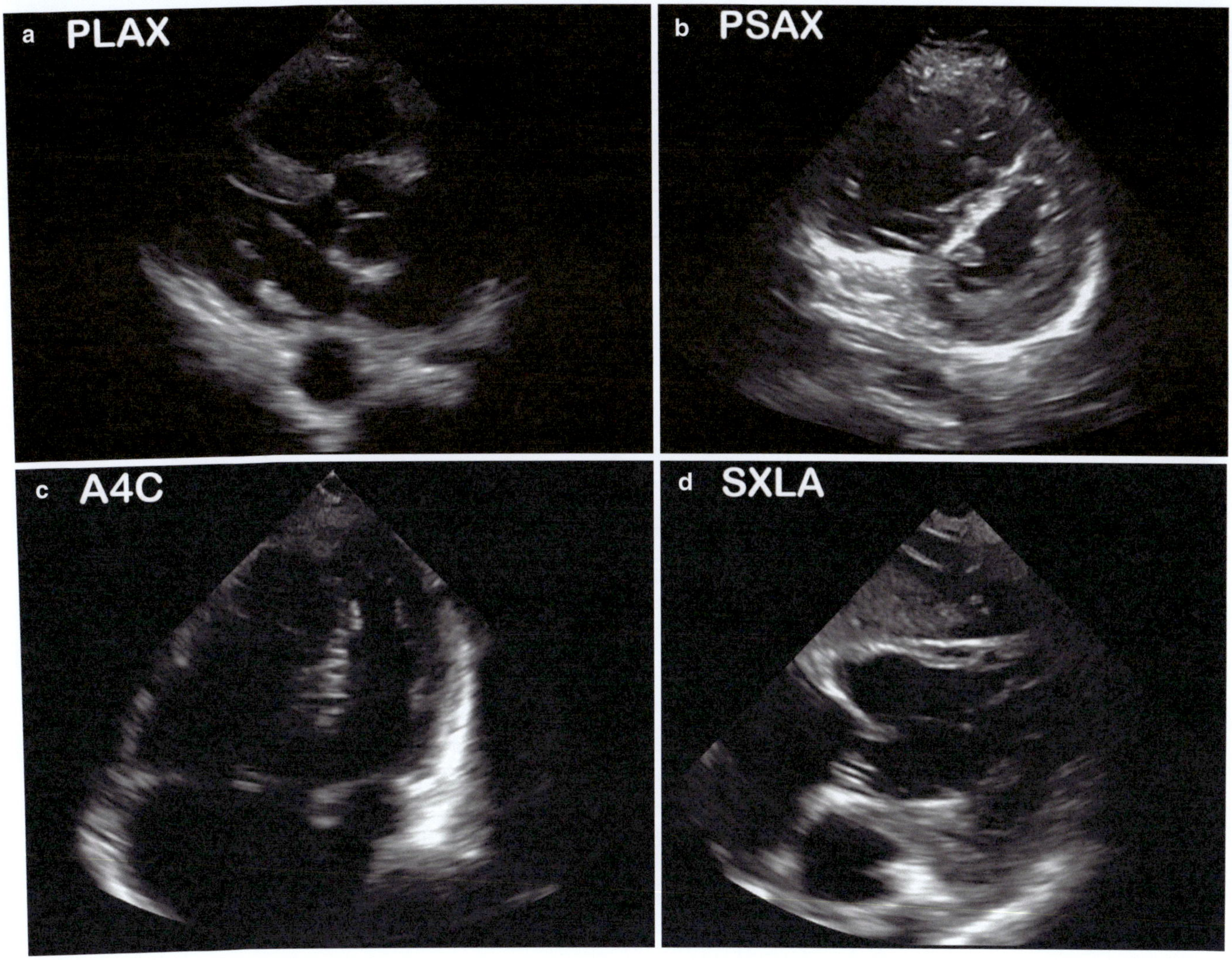

Fig. 23.3 Enlarged right ventricle in pulmonary embolism. (**a**) Parasternal long-axis; (**b**) Parasternal short-axis; (**c**) Apical 4-chamber; (**d**) Subxiphoid long-axis. (*Images courtesy of Peter Alsharif, MD*)

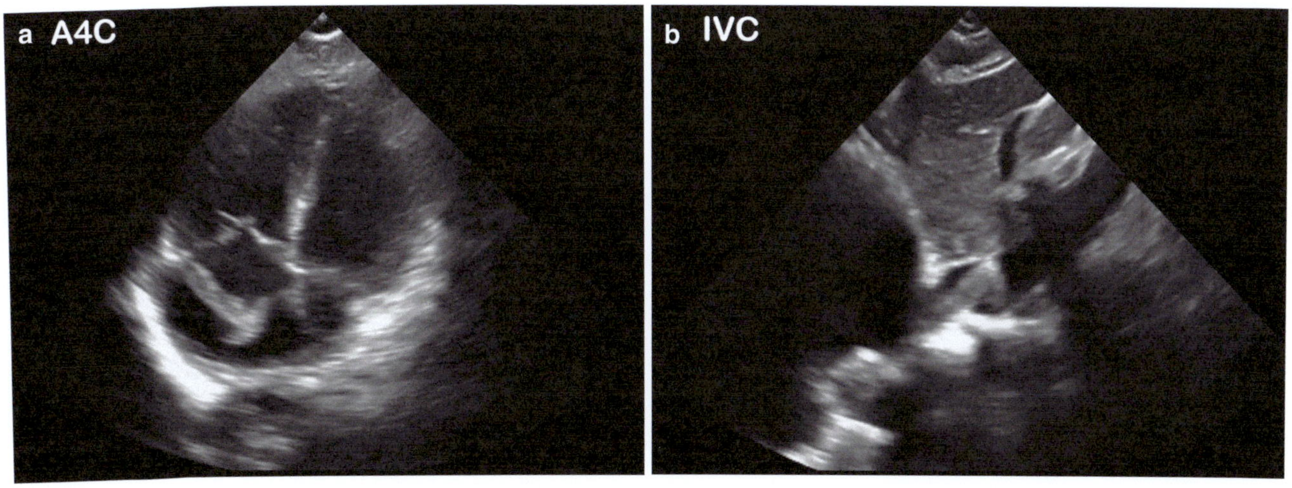

Fig. 23.4 Clot-in-transit. (**a**) Apical 4-chamber; (**b**) Inferior vena cava. (*Images courtesy of Stephen Alerhand, MD*)

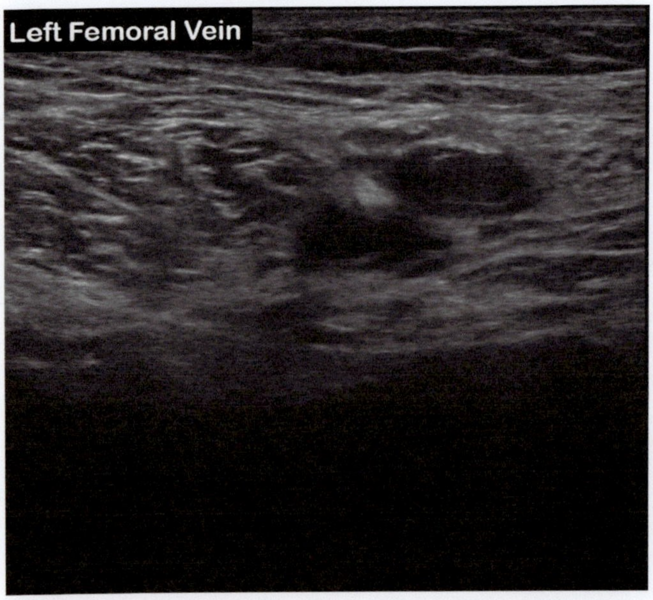

Fig. 23.5 Deep venous thrombosis of the left femoral vein with partial compression of the femoral artery during lower extremity venous ultrasonography

hypertension is present. While patients with pulmonary hypertension can still experience PE, a thickened RV-free wall (>5 mm) suggests chronic hypertrophy [62]. In contrast, an acutely dilated RV with a thin free wall in a patient for whom POCUS was performed early in the arrest would be suggestive of PE in the appropriate clinical context. Another way to assess for PE is to evaluate for DVT (Fig. 23.5, Video 23.5) [31, 38]. Compression ultrasonography of the lower extremities is particularly conducive to intra-arrest sonography, as it is not inhibited by defibrillation pads, chest compression, or other obstacles and cephalad procedures [6]. Ultimately, assessment of PE in cardiac arrest requires a thorough understanding of the nuances of the findings; however, ultrasound findings of PE combined with an appropriate clinical setting should prompt thrombolysis in the cardiac arrest patient. If available, extracorporeal membrane oxygenation (ECMO) may also be considered [63, 64].

Ventricular Fibrillation

In a systematic review of 67 prospective studies, ventricular fibrillation (VF) was reported in 27% of out-of-hospital cardiac arrests (OHCAs) [65]. Fine VF can be indistinguishable from asystole on the cardiac monitor but may be visualized using POCUS (Fig. 23.6, Video 23.6a) [66, 67]. Because patients with cardiac arrest due to VF have significantly improved outcomes compared with non-VF arrests, it is critical to make this distinction [68]. Evidence suggests improved outcomes for fine VF as well [66, 69]. Therefore, POCUS may be able to identify fine VF, prompting early defibrillation in patients who would otherwise be treated for a non-shockable rhythm without POCUS.

Pulseless Electrical Activity and Asystole

In a consolidation of large datasets, PEA occurred in approximately 22% of OHCAs and 11% of in-hospital cardiac arrests (IHCAs) [70]. The same data reported asystole in 52% of OHCAs and 79% of IHCAs (Fig. 23.7, Video 23.7) [70]. However, in electrocardiographic PEA, 6–58% of patients may demonstrate cardiac movement [28, 66, 67, 69, 71]. In electrocardiographic asystole, 4–12% of patients may have cardiac movement [66, 67, 69, 72, 73]. Cardiac activity on ultrasound during arrest has been associated with positive outcomes (e.g., return of spontaneous circulation [ROSC], survival-to-hospitalization, and survival-to-discharge) [28, 69–71, 73]. Therefore, POCUS may be able to identify cases of pseudo-PEA or pseudo-asystole and guide appropriate treatment.

Aortic Dissection

A meta-analysis reported an incidence of acute aortic dissection causing OHCA in up to 4% of patients with a mortality of 100% [74]. POCUS has been reported to have a positive predictive value of 100% for aortic dissection in cardiac

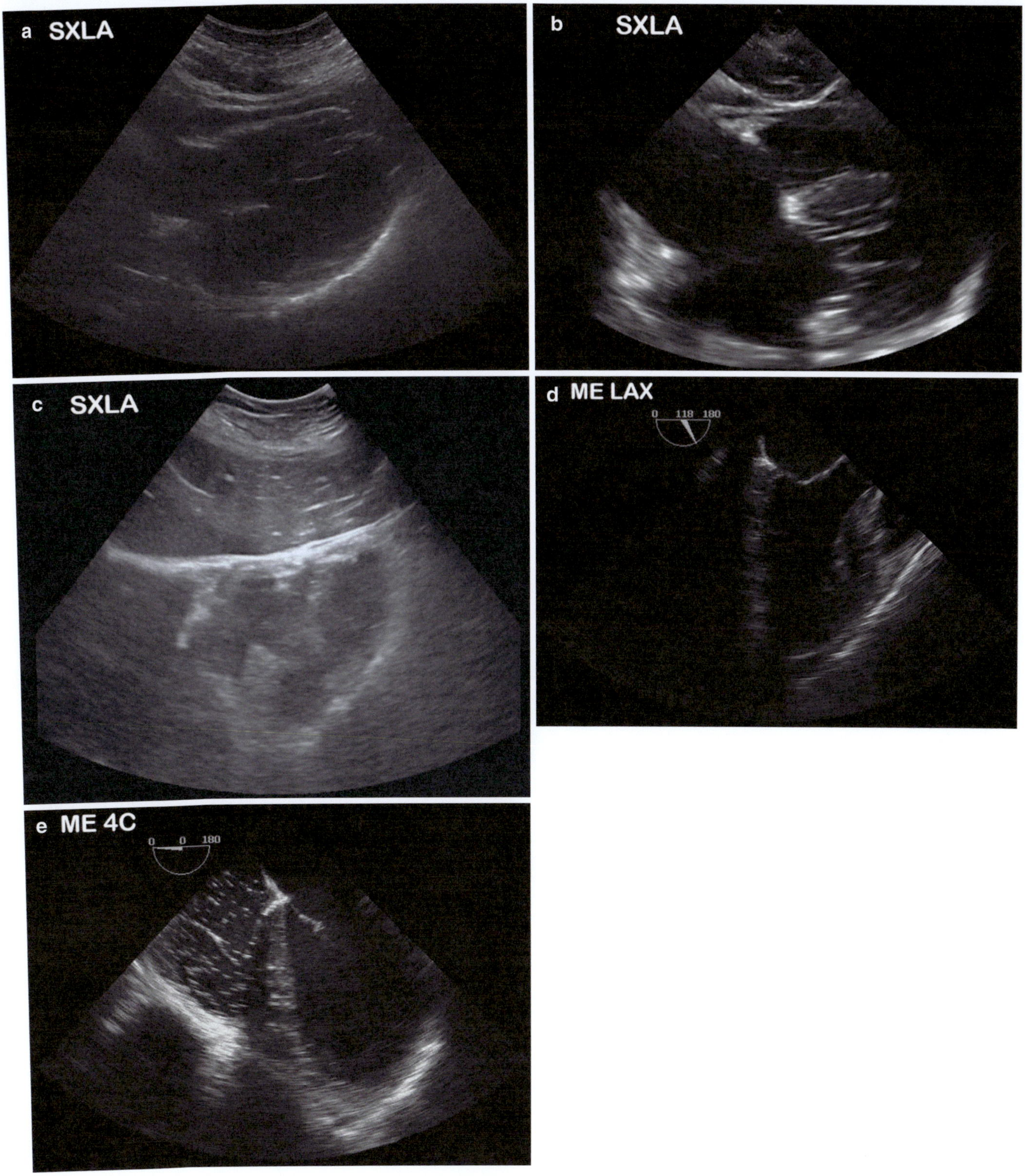

Fig. 23.6 Ventricular fibrillation in cardiac arrest via subxiphoid long-axis (**a–c**), midesophageal long-axis via transesophageal echocardiography (**d**), and midesophageal 4-chamber via transesophageal echocardiography (**e**). (*Images courtesy of Rajiv Thavanathan, MD, Ilya Ostrovsky, MD, and Stephen Alerhand, MD*)

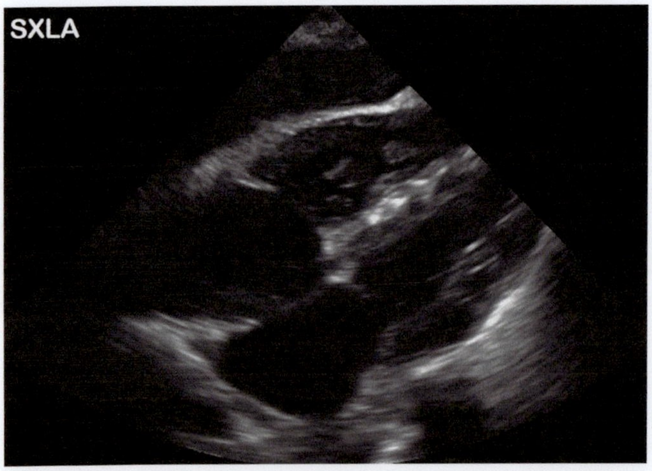

Fig. 23.7 Asystole in the subxiphoid long-axis in cardiac arrest. (*Image courtesy of Ilya Ostrovsky, MD*)

arrest [48]. Assessment for dissection should involve multiple views (often beginning with the parasternal long-axis view), evaluating for an intimal flap or indirect evidence such as aortic root enlargement, aortic regurgitation, and pericardial effusion (Fig. 23.8, Video 23.8a) [75–80]. The abdominal aorta can be evaluated for an intimal flap as well; however, evidence is limited in the setting of cardiac arrest. Therefore, it is still reasonable to assess for evidence of aortic dissection using POCUS to guide surgical intervention if ROSC is achieved and to avoid harmful interventions (e.g., thrombolysis).

Ruptured Abdominal Aortic Aneurysm

One systematic review of patients with ruptured AAA (Fig. 23.9, Video 23.9) found that 13% suffered preoperative cardiac arrest [81]. When cardiac arrest occurs from a ruptured AAA, there is a high mortality rate (49–100%) [81]; however, identification of a ruptured AAA on POCUS in cardiac arrest should not prevent vascular surgery consideration. Some evidence has reported that select patients can still achieve good long-term functional outcomes after preoperative cardiac arrest from ruptured AAA [81, 82]. The size of the AAA is also associated with the risk of rupture, with autopsy data demonstrating that 13% of AAAs <5 cm were ruptured, 40% of AAAs >5 cm were ruptured, and 60% of AAAs between 7 and 10 cm were ruptured [83]. Although the sensitivity and specificity of POCUS for ruptured AAA have been reported as >90%, test characteristics in cardiac arrest remain unknown [84, 85]. Therefore, diagnosing ruptured AAA in cardiac arrest should consider the patient's clinical presentation prior to the arrest in combination with findings of AAA on POCUS.

Pneumothorax

Although exact frequencies of pneumothorax causing cardiac arrest are not established, intensive care unit data suggest that the rate may be 1–4% [86], while a single trauma center reviewing its traumatic arrests over 1 year found that 13% of the cases were due to tension pneumothorax (Fig. 23.10, Video 23.10) [46]. In the largest Cochrane meta-analysis evaluating chest imaging, lung ultrasound in the non-arrest, supine, trauma patient was found to be 91% sensitive and 99% specific for pneumothorax (although probe selection and definitions varied per study) [87]. Lung ultrasound is also recommended by the Advanced Trauma Life Support and multiple societal guidelines [88, 89]. False positives include massive atelectasis, bullae, blebs, pleural adherence, pleurodesis, fibrosis, phrenic nerve injury, and apnea [90]. In the setting of cardiac arrest, an important false positive, especially if seen on the left lung fields, is right mainstem intubation. This can be distinguished from pneumothorax by the presence of a lung pulse, which will only be present in mainstem intubation [91]. In the appropriate clinical setting (particularly in cardiac arrest), ultrasound findings of pneumothorax (e.g., absence of lung sliding, presence of a lung point) should prompt thoracostomy [87, 90].

Endotracheal Tube Placement

POCUS can be used to evaluate the trachea and esophagus to confirm ETT placement (Fig. 23.11, Videos 23.11 and 23.12) [6, 92–94]. In cardiac arrest, end-tidal capnography may not be able to adequately distinguish between factors intrinsic to the arrest (e.g., low cardiac output, reduced pulmonary blood flow,

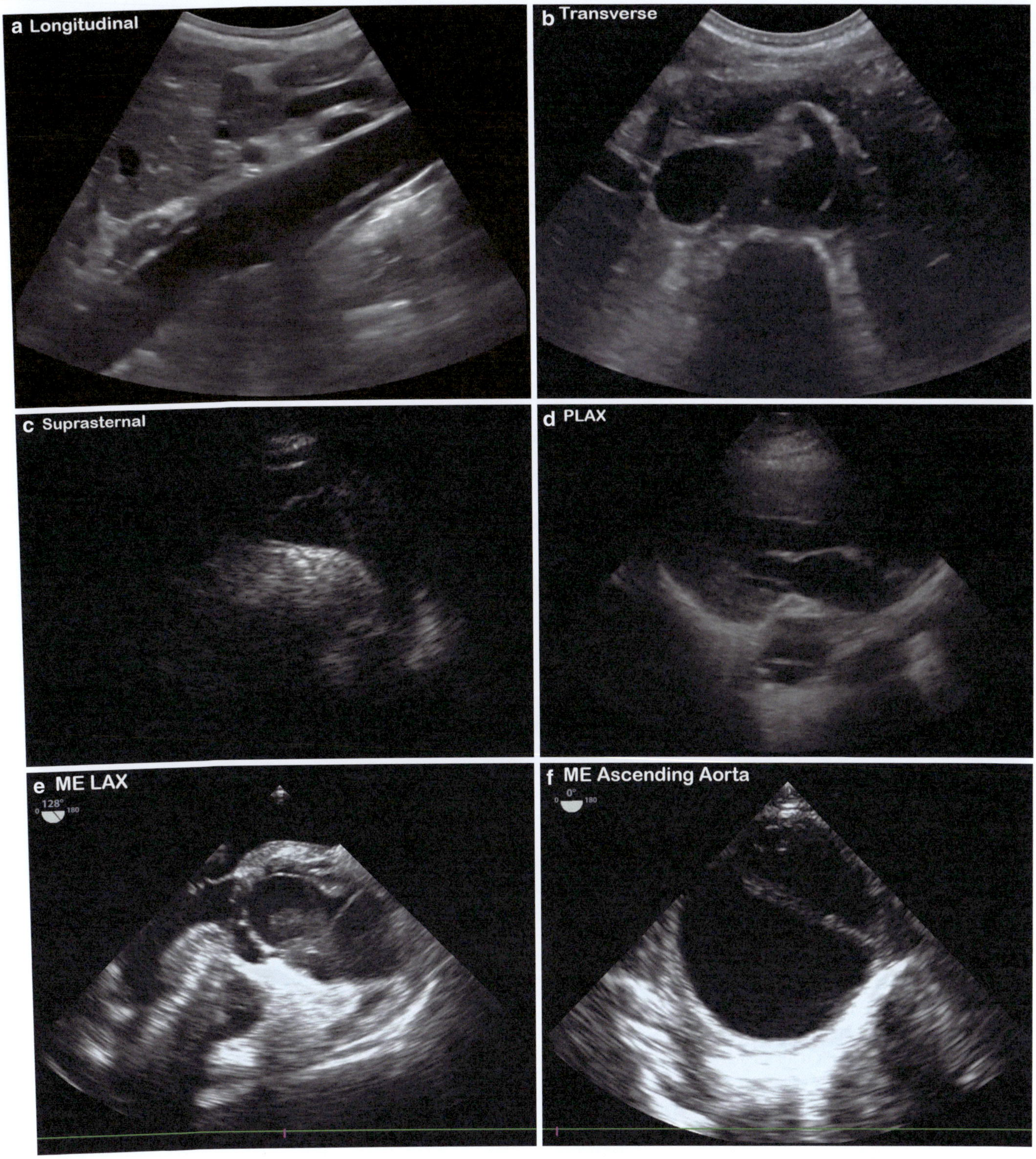

Fig. 23.8 Aortic dissection. (**a**) Abdominal aorta in long axis; (**b**) Abdominal aorta in short axis; (**c**) Suprasternal aortic arch; (**d**) Parasternal long-axis; (**e**) Midesophageal long-axis via transesophageal echocardiography; (**f**) Midesophageal ascending aorta short-axis via transesophageal echocardiography. (*Images courtesy of Stephen Alerhand, MD and Hamid Shokoohi, MD, MPH*)

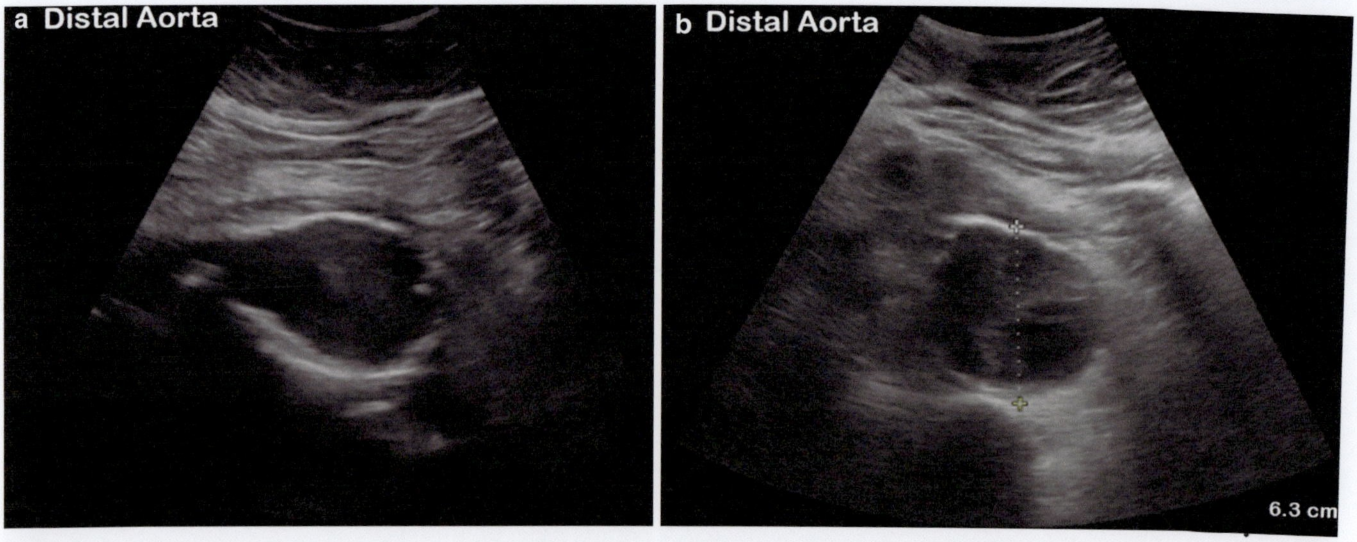

Fig. 23.9 (**a**) Ruptured abdominal aortic aneurysm identified during cardiac arrest; (**b**) Aortic aneurysm measured at a maximal diameter of 6.3 cm

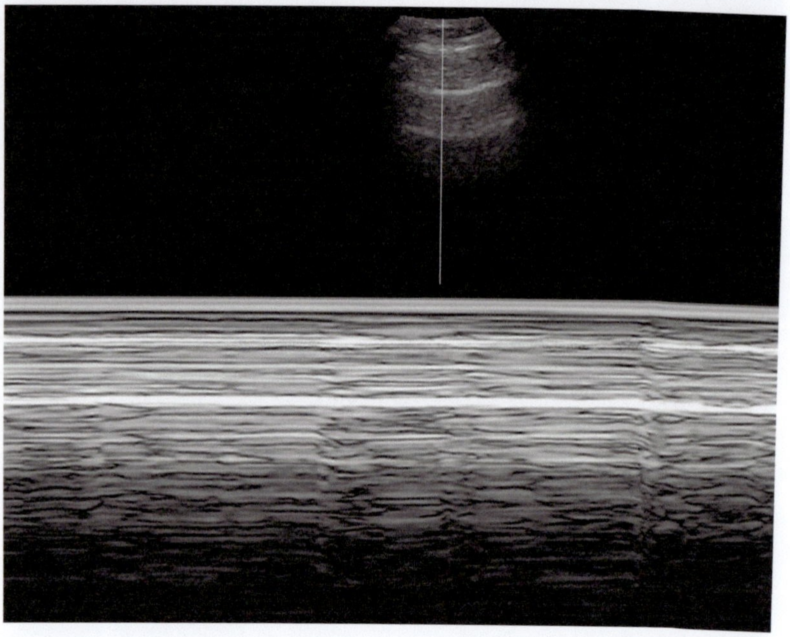

Fig. 23.10 Pneumothorax on M-mode. (*Image courtesy of Michael Gottlieb, MD*)

administration of vasopressors, prolonged arrest time, hypothermia, ventilation/perfusion mismatch) and factors related to misplaced ETT (e.g., CO_2 insufflated during bagging, dislodgement) [6]. A meta-analysis of cardiac arrest and non-arrest patients reported 99% sensitivity and 97% specificity when using POCUS to confirm tracheal versus esophageal placement of the ETT [92]. Additionally, POCUS does not require "breaths" (or gastric insufflations when incorrectly placed) for ETT confirmation and can occur simultaneously with compressions [95]. Moreover, POCUS can also assess for ETT depth to identify hypopharyngeal or mainstem placement [96, 97]. POCUS should be considered as an accurate and valuable adjunct for ETT confirmation in cardiac arrest.

Intra-Abdominal Pathology

Identifying free fluid in the abdominopelvic cavity in a cardiac arrest patient can be helpful in the correct clinical context. For example, free fluid in a person of childbearing age with a uterus can represent a ruptured ectopic pregnancy (Fig. 23.12, Video 23.13a). Free fluid in the abdomen may also suggest other acute pathology, such as organ injury in the context of trauma (Fig. 23.13, Video 23.14a). While free fluid is generally considered to be blood, an important false positive is ascites. The distinction between the two is largely clinical, although sonographic features of liver cirrhosis (e.g., small size, surface nodularity, coarse parenchyma, cau-

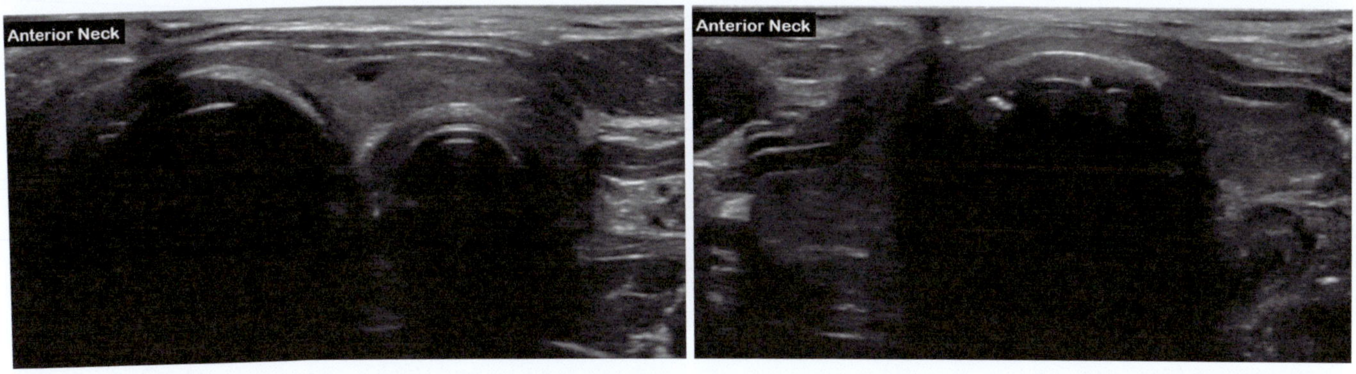

Fig. 23.11 Transtracheal ultrasound demonstrating esophageal intubation (left image), tracheal intubation (right image). (*Images courtesy of Michael Gottlieb, MD*)

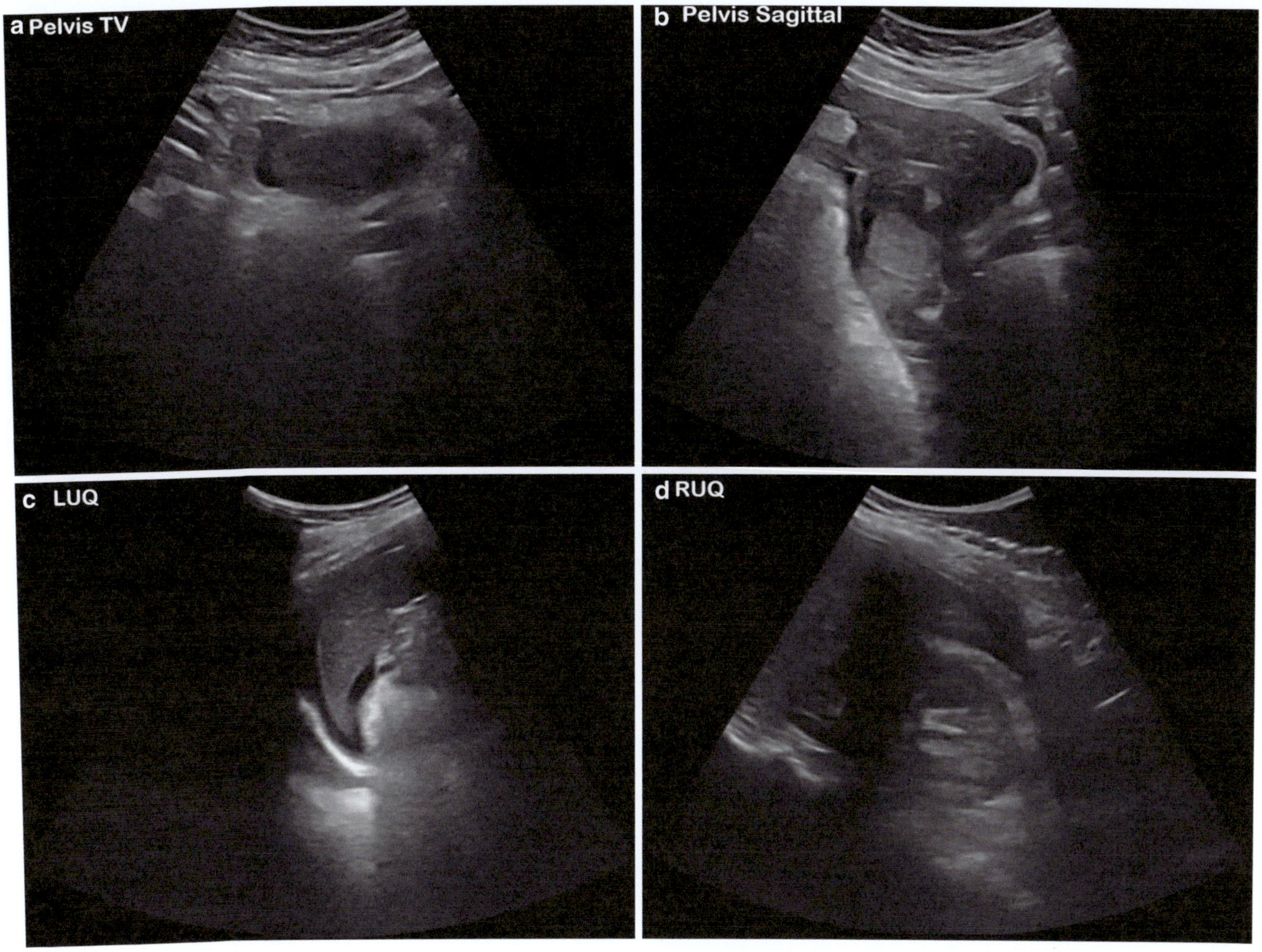

Fig. 23.12 Free fluid due to ruptured ectopic pregnancy. (**a**) Pelvis transverse view; (**b**) Pelvis sagittal view; (**c**) Left upper quadrant view; (**d**) Right upper quadrant view

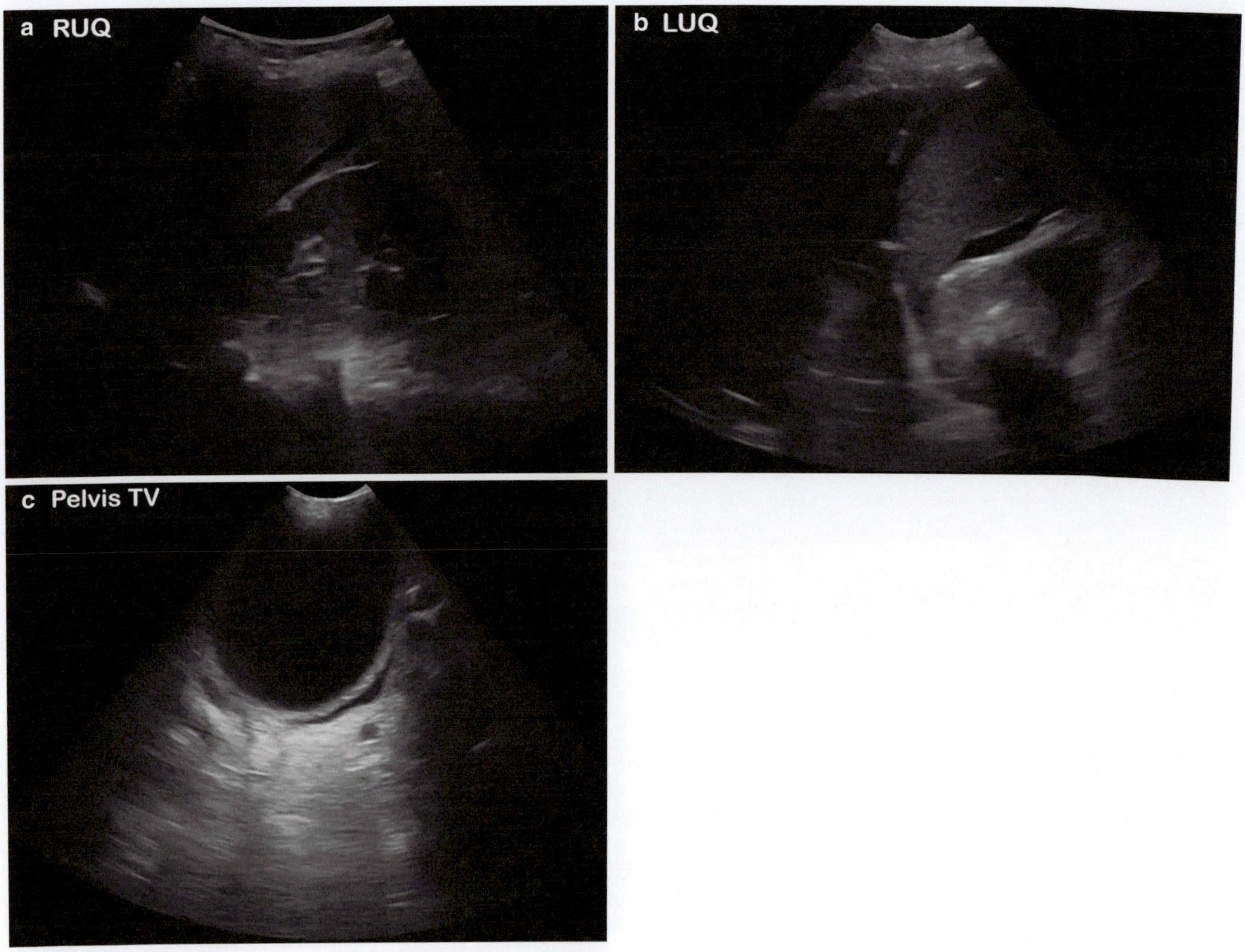

Fig. 23.13 Free fluid during a focused assessment with sonography in trauma examination. (**a**) Right upper quadrant view; (**b**) Left upper quadrant view; (**c**) Pelvis transverse view. (*Images courtesy of Mass General Brigham Emergency Ultrasound Fellowship Program and Harvard Sono*)

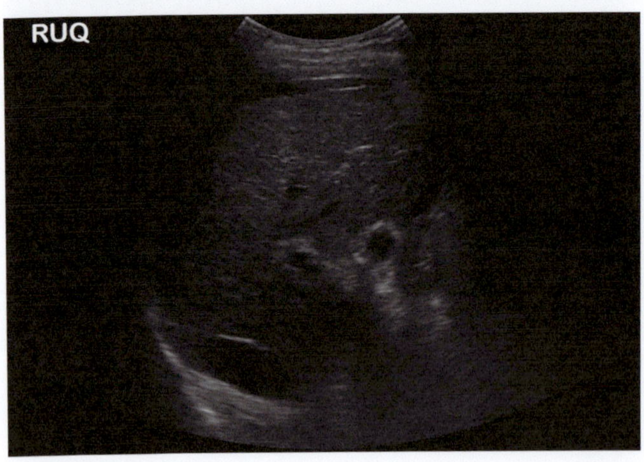

Fig. 23.14 Liver cirrhosis

date lobe hypertrophy) may be helpful (Fig. 23.14, Video 23.15) [98, 99]. POCUS may help indicate cardiac arrest etiology and guide treatment (e.g., blood transfusion, need for surgical intervention), especially if ROSC is achieved.

Hypovolemia

A systematic review found that POCUS had a positive predictive value of 100% for identifying hypovolemia as the cause of cardiac arrest [48]. This can be suggested by underfilled cardiac chambers with low end-diastolic ventricular volume (Fig. 23.15, Video 23.16) [6, 48]. However, caution is needed in relying upon the inferior vena cava (IVC) alone to make interpretations regarding volume sta-

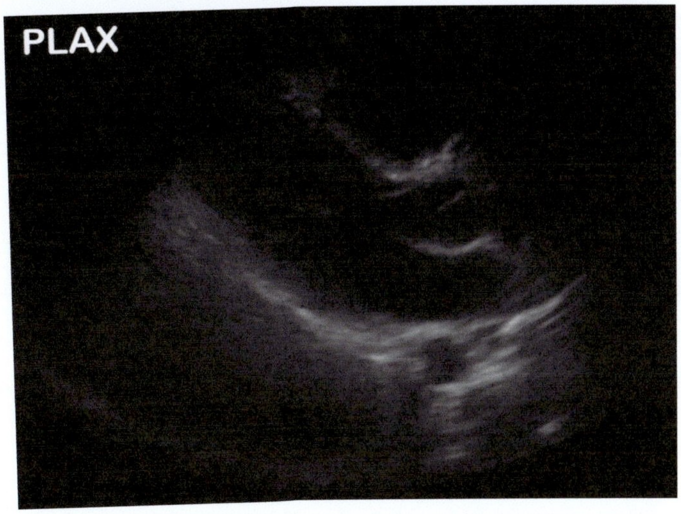

Fig. 23.15 Underfilled, hyperdynamic left ventricle. Parasternal long-axis. (*Image courtesy of Cameron Baston, MD*)

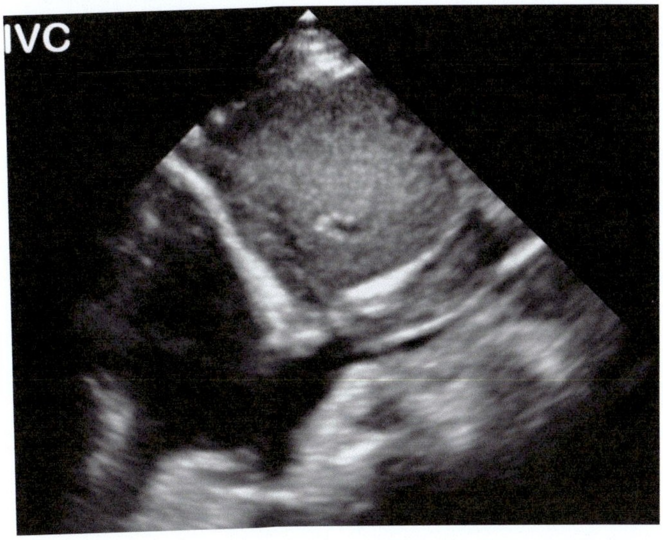

Fig. 23.16 Collapsed, thin inferior vena cava

tus. The IVC is typically dilated as a result of ongoing positive pressure ventilation [31], and is therefore of minimal diagnostic utility unless it is very small (<1 cm) with a high degree of collapsibility (>50%) (Fig. 23.16, Video 23.17) [6, 31, 48].

POCUS Pulse Checks

Evidence has demonstrated that manual pulse checks lack sufficient accuracy [100–102]. In contrast, evidence supports the use of B-mode and color Doppler to more rapidly and accurately identify the presence and absence of a pulse compared with manual palpation (Fig. 23.17, Video 23.18) [6, 103]. While data remain limited regarding the role of a sono-

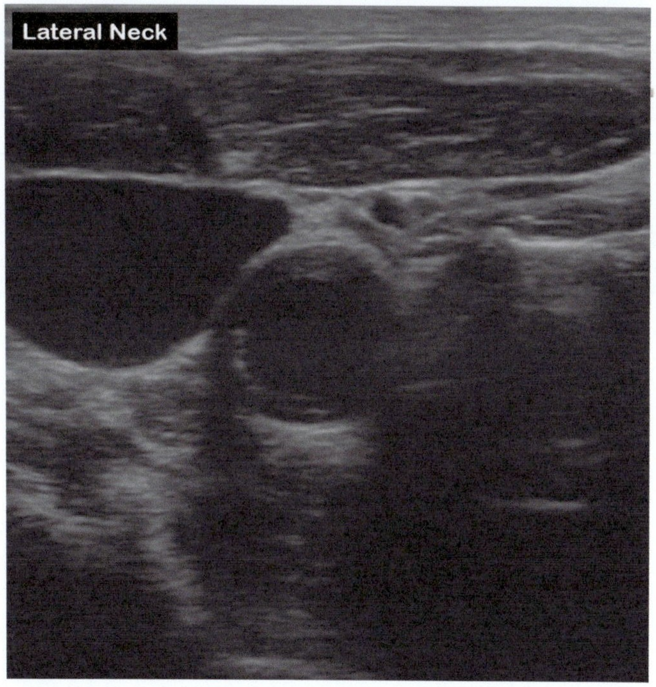

Fig. 23.17 POCUS pulse check

graphically visible pulse in the absence of a manually palpable pulse, one study found that a peak systolic velocity >20 cm/s was correlated with systolic blood pressure ≥60 mmHg [104]. Therefore, POCUS may play a role in identifying profound shock states that require vasopressors (e.g., pseudo-PEA) [105, 106].

Prognosis

POCUS may also have a role in prognostication. For non-traumatic, non-shockable cardiac arrest, a meta-analysis found that cardiac activity visualized by POCUS was 60% sensitive and 92% specific for ROSC [107]. Cardiac activity was associated with an odds ratio of 8.0 for survival-to-discharge when compared with no activity [107]. For traumatic arrest, a separate meta-analysis found that cardiac activity visualized by POCUS was 98% specific for ROSC, whereas cardiac standstill was 90% sensitive for not achieving ROSC [108]. However, the interrater reliability of identifying cardiac standstill has been shown to be only moderate among different clinicians [109]. Cardiac activity on POCUS was associated with positive outcomes (e.g., ROSC, survival-to-hospitalization, survival-to-hospital-discharge) 40–45% more often for electrocardiographic PEA (versus true PEA) and 57% more often for electrocardiographic asystole (versus true asystole) [28, 69, 71]. In the appropriate clinical setting, visualizing cardiac movement on POCUS can help prognosticate cardiac arrest outcomes.

Ultrasound in Undifferentiated Shock

Ultrasound Protocols

Many ultrasound examination protocols have been proposed for the management of patients with undifferentiated shock (Table 23.3). These protocols systematically evaluate various etiologies of shock, integrating cardiac, pulmonary, abdominal, and vascular POCUS examinations [110, 111]. The Rapid Ultrasound for Shock and Hypotension (RUSH) examination is one of the most well-known protocols and consists of a three-part framework: the "pump" (heart), "tanks" (IVC, pleura, and peritoneal cavities), and "pipes" (aorta and deep veins) [111, 112]. Some use the acronym "HI-MAP" to refer to the major areas evaluated in the RUSH exam: heart, IVC, Morison's pouch (reflecting the FAST examination), aorta, and pneumothorax. In contrast, an international consensus statement suggested organizing by core views (e.g., subxiphoid and parasternal cardiac, lung, IVC), supplementary views (e.g., other cardiac views), and additional views (proximal leg veins, ETT placement, AAA evaluation, FAST, pelvis/intrauterine pregnancy) [31].

A systematic review and meta-analysis reported 87% sensitivity and 98% specificity for identifying the type of shock using the RUSH exam [7]. However, in randomized control trials evaluating patients with undifferentiated shock (after excluding patients with a "clear mechanism" of shock or for whom POCUS was considered immediately needed [e.g., ectopic pregnancy, AAA]), POCUS in the initial stage of resuscitation has not shown a clinically meaningful difference in outcomes [8–10]. Nonetheless, observational studies support improved diagnostics and high rates of pathology identification, which may still help to tailor therapy and enhance cognitive offloading for clinicians [11–15].

The cardiac component of the RUSH examination (i.e., the "pump") primarily evaluates the left ventricle (e.g., hypodynamic, hyperdynamic), right ventricle (e.g., enlargement suggestive of PE), and the pericardium (e.g., pericardial effusion, cardiac tamponade). When the patient's type of shock is completely undifferentiated, clinicians should consider starting with the heart, as the literature suggests that the highest rates of abnormalities are identified in the cardiac portion of the RUSH examination [14, 113].

The "tank" portion of the RUSH examination involves assessment of the IVC, pleura, and peritoneal cavities. The IVC is evaluated by its diameter and respiratory collapsibility in spontaneously breathing patients or distensibility in mechanically ventilated patients. A dilated IVC with minimal collapsibility may indicate increased right atrial pressure (RAP), suggesting an obstructive or cardiogenic etiology [114]. In a *post hoc* analysis of a randomized control trial of POCUS in spontaneously breathing patients with undifferentiated hypotension, a dilated IVC with minimal collapsibility was 86% sensitive and 86% specific for

Table 23.3 Protocols utilizing ultrasound in shock

Protocol	Components
Rapid Ultrasound for Shock and Hypotension (RUSH) [110, 111]	HI-MAP and "Pump, Tank, Pipes" Heart, IVC, Morison's pouch/abdominopelvic cavity, aorta/DVT, pulmonary evaluation
Focus Assessed Transthoracic Echocardiography (FATE) [115]	Basic FATE: cardiac (subcostal, apical four-chamber, parasternal long-axis, parasternal short-axis views), pleural scanning Extended FATE: subcostal IVC, apical two-chamber, apical-three chamber, parasternal short-axis mitral plane, parasternal aortic short-axis views Advanced FATE: hemodynamics, Doppler, diastolic dysfunction, valvular disease
Focused Ultrasound in Surgical Anesthesia (FUSA) [116]	Perioperative shock (acute cor pulmonale, left ventricular dysfunction, cardiac tamponade, and hypovolemia) Acute respiratory failure (pneumothorax, acute pulmonary edema, large pleural effusion, major atelectasis, and consolidation)
Subcostal to Apical, Respiratory to ParaSternal (STARS) [117]	Subcostal (subcostal four-chamber and IVC) Apical-respiratory (apical four-chamber, right ventricle-focused, LVOT VTI, apical two-chamber, apical-three chamber, respiratory-diaphragmatic-lung interfaces) ParaSternal (parasternal long and short axes, RV inflow, anterior lung ultrasound)
Focused Echocardiographic Evaluation in Resuscitation (FEER) [25]	Cardiac (cardiac activity, pericardial effusion/cardiac tamponade, hypovolemia, and massive PE)
Focused Echocardiographic Evaluation in Life Support (FEEL) [28]	Cardiac (cardiac activity, ventricular function, dilatation, and pericardial effusion)
Sonography in Hypotension and Cardiac Arrest (SHoC) [9, 10, 14]	Cardiac (cardiac tamponade, RV dysfunction, cardiac activity, and ventricular size) Lung (pneumothorax and pleural effusion) IVC (diameter and respiratory variation) Airway (ETT confirmation) DVT Abdomen (AAA and peritoneal effusion)

HI-MAP heart, inferior vena cava, Morison's pouch/abdominopelvic cavity, aorta, pulmonary evaluations, *IVC* inferior vena cava, *DVT* deep venous thrombosis, *LVOT VTI* left ventricular outflow tract velocity time integral, *RV* right ventricle, *AAA* abdominal aortic aneurysm volume overload [114]. Moreover, in a prospective study evaluating undifferentiated shock patients using POCUS, 27% had IVC abnormalities [14]. The pleural evaluation should assess for both pneumothorax and pleural fluid (e.g., pleural effusion, hemothorax). In one prospective study evaluating undifferentiated shock patients using POCUS, 8% had pleural fluid [14]. The abdominopelvic cavity is evaluated using the FAST exam for free fluid (e.g., trauma, ectopic pregnancy), and if positive, indicate hemorrhagic shock. In a prospective study evaluating undifferentiated shock patients using POCUS, 5% had abdominal free fluid [14].

The third component of the RUSH examination is the "pipes," which consists of an evaluation of the aorta and deep veins. The aorta is evaluated for the presence of a dissection or aneurysm, while the lower extremities are evaluated for DVT.

Sonographic Phenotypes in Hypotensive Patients

POCUS can also be used to guide hemodynamic management. Moreover, classification schemes have been proposed based on Diamond-Forrester phenotypes (Fig. 23.18) [17–19, 118]. These profiles include (1) warm & dry, (2) warm & wet, (3) cold & dry, and (4) cold & wet (Table 23.4). These subsets initially used Swan-Ganz catheters to determine cardiac index (CI; CI = cardiac output/body surface area) using thermodilution and preload using pulmonary artery occlusion pressure (PAOP) (Fig. 23.19) [118]. More recently, POCUS has been used to estimate stroke volume as a surrogate for cardiac output (i.e., "flow") using left ventricular outflow tract velocity time integral (LVOT VTI) (Fig. 23.20) and estimating cardiac filling (i.e., "congestion") using venous excess ultrasound score (VExUS) [19]. Thresholds are based upon values for CI (normal: $\geq$2.2 L/min/m^2), PAOP (high: E/e′ $\geq$14), "flow" (normal: LVOT VTI $\geq$18 cm), and "congestion" (low: VExUS 0 or 1) [19]. Identifying the hemodynamic profile has diagnostic, therapeutic, and prognostic potential. In a retrospective review of over 4000 patients admitted to the cardiac ICU, the in-hospital mortality was 2.9%, 7.3%, 7.1%, and 14% for profiles 1–4, respectively [19].

Venous Excess Ultrasound Score

Traditional tools for hemodynamic assessments, such as history (e.g., diarrhea, weight gain, urine output), physical examination (e.g., blood pressure, mentation), laboratory testing (e.g., blood lactate, brain natriuretic peptide), central venous pressure, right-heart catheterization, Swan–Ganz catheter, pulse pressure variation, passive leg raise, and chest X-ray, can be invasive or insensitive for organ-level congestion [120, 121]. Using POCUS, a plethoric IVC and pulmonary edema can be helpful but both have limitations (e.g., valvulopathy, pulmonary hypertension, athletes, interstitial lung disease) as surrogates for venous congestion of encapsulated organs [120]. In response, VExUS was introduced to

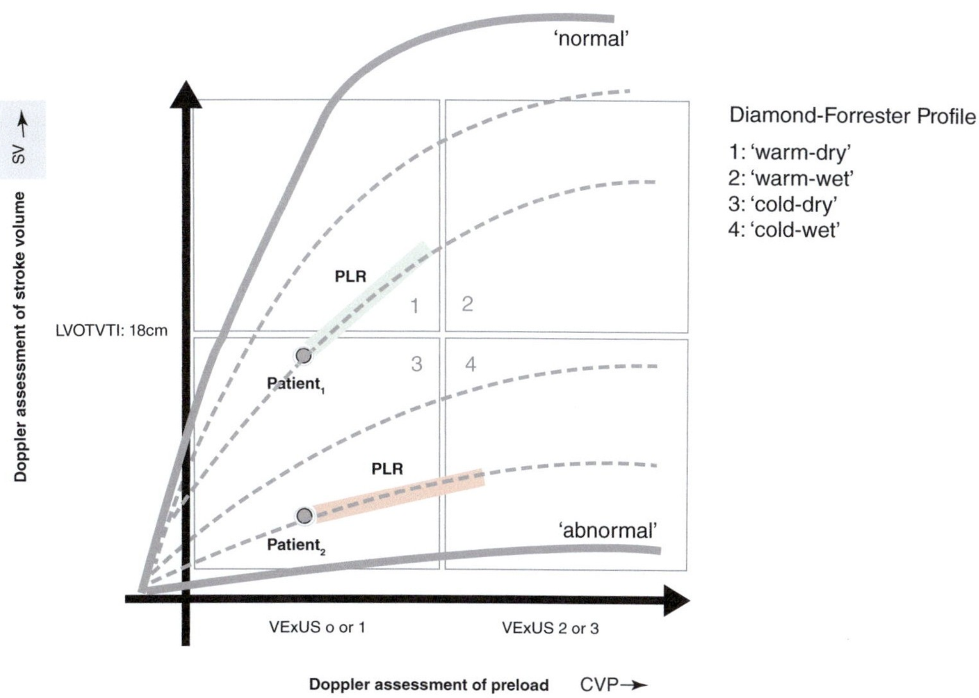

Fig. 23.18 Diamond–Forrester hemodynamic profiles. *PLR* passive leg raise, *CVP* central venous pressure, *LVOT VTI* left ventricular outflow tract velocity time interval, *SV* stroke volume. (*Adapted from Kenny et al.* [19])

Table 23.4 Approach to hypotensive patients using Diamond-Forrester hemodynamic profiles

Profile	CI	PAOP	LVOT VTI ("Flow")	VExUS ("Congestion")	Etiology	Treatment
1. Warm & dry	Normal	Low	Normal	Low	Arterial vasodilation	Vasopressor (e.g., norepinephrine)
2. Warm & wet	Normal	High	Normal	High	Peripheral vasodilation	Vasopressor (e.g., norepinephrine) Consider diuresis after dynamic assessment
3. Cold & dry	Low	Low	Low	Low	Hypovolemia or early sepsis-induced venodilation and diastolic dysfunction	May benefit from IV fluids, dynamic assessment, and prompt vasopressors (e.g., norepinephrine)
4. Cold & wet	Low	High	Low	High	Cardiac dysfunction	Inotropes, consider diuresis after dynamic assessment

Adapted from Kenny et al. [19] *Weingart* [119]

Threshold values: Normal CI is ≥2.2 L/min/m² vs low CI is <2.2 L/min/m². High PAOP is E/e′ ≥14 vs low PAOP is E/e′ <14. Normal "flow" is LVOT VTI ≥18 cm vs low "flow" is LVOT VTI <18 cm. Low "congestion" is VExUS 0-1 vs high "congestion" is VExUS 2-3.

CI cardiac index, *PAOP* pulmonary artery occlusion pressure, *LVOT VTI* left ventricular outflow tract velocity time integral, *VExUS* venous excess ultrasound score, *IV* intravenous

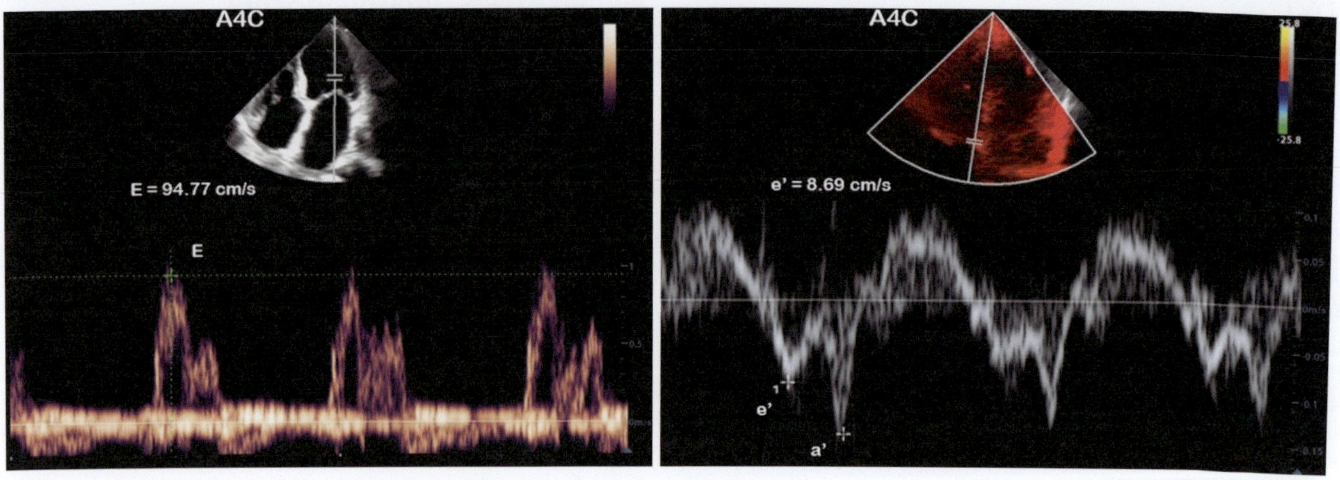

Fig. 23.19 E and e′ waves for determining the E/e′ ratio. *A4C*, apical 4-chamber. (*Image courtesy of Ilya Ostrovsky, MD*)

Fig. 23.20 Left ventricular outflow tract velocity time integral. *PLAX* parasternal long-axis, *A5C* apical 5-chamber, *VTI* velocity time integral. (*Image courtesy of Nour Al Jalbout, MD*)

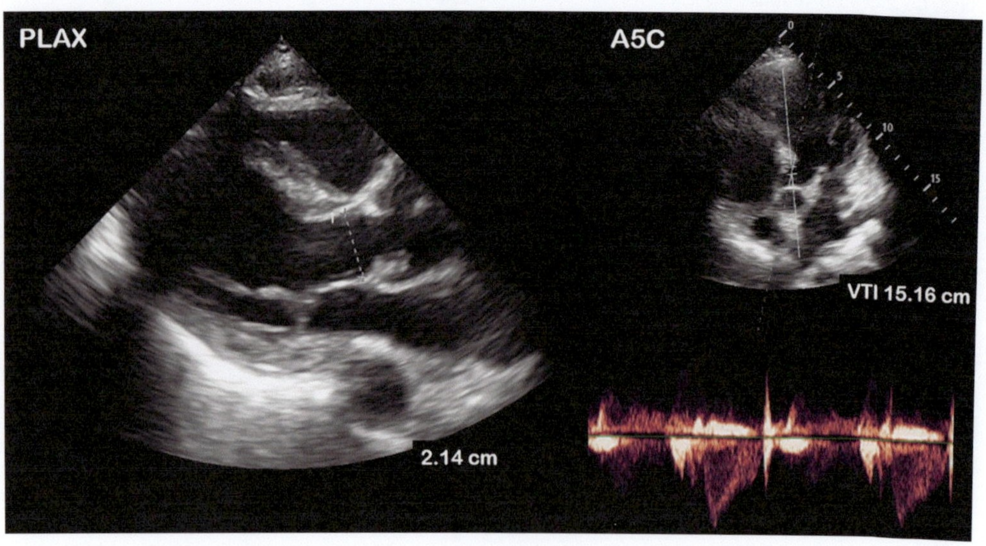

help grade organ-level venous congestion. VExUS combined examinations of the IVC and Doppler evaluations of the hepatic, portal, and intrarenal veins to provide a more complete picture of venous congestion.

The original 2020 study developed VExUS from several prototypes using the outcome of acute kidney injury (AKI) in non-critically ill adults undergoing cardiac surgery [120]. The best prototype (i.e., VExUS) found that a grade of severe congestion was 96% specific and 27% sensitive to predict AKI [120]. Since then, studies have reported VExUS as feasible [122, 123], capable of risk stratifying patients with heart failure [124] and cardiorenal syndrome [125], correlated with elevated right atrial pressure [126], mortality and AKI [123, 127], identifying AKI subtypes [128], and AKI in children [129]. In the only randomized trial, there was no significant difference between the VExUS and control groups for kidney function recovery, mortality, or days of hospitalization [130]. VExUS did significantly improve the odds of achieving decongestion, days to decongestion, and the odds of decreasing brain natriuretic peptide levels [130].

Broadly, the clinical applications for VExUS include any patient undergoing hemodynamic resuscitation (i.e., eligible for fluid resuscitation, diuresis, or vasopressor support) [131]. Prior literature and expert opinion posit that patients with heart failure, AKI, and shock are potential candidates to benefit from VExUS-guided resuscitation. In heart failure patients for whom diuresis is clearly indicated, VExUS has the potential to identify when to terminate diuresis. In patients with AKI, VExUS can help avoid the assumption that all AKI is prerenal and is treated with fluid resuscitation. In hypotensive patients, VExUS can support decisions for fluid resuscitation. It can also identify signs of congestion where vasopressors should be continued or initiated, and in cases of severe congestion, consider combination diuresis. Therefore, VExUS presents another valuable tool for the hemodynamic resuscitation of patients.

Venous congestion can be identified by initially evaluating the IVC. As RAP increases, the IVC distends, decreases respiratory collapsibility, and becomes plethoric. VExUS uses a ≥2 cm IVC diameter cutoff, considering <2 cm not congested (Fig. 23.21, Video 23.19a) [120]. Limitations to this assumption (e.g., body size, endurance athletes, increased abdominal pressure, and mechanically ventilated patients) are not incorporated into VExUS [131].

As RAP continues to increase, the IVC reaches maximum venous compliance with further congestion continuing into the hepatic vein. The normal hepatic vein Doppler waveform is multiphasic, displaying antegrade systolic (S) wave and diastolic (D) waves with the S wave larger than the D wave. With mild hepatic vein congestion, the S wave becomes

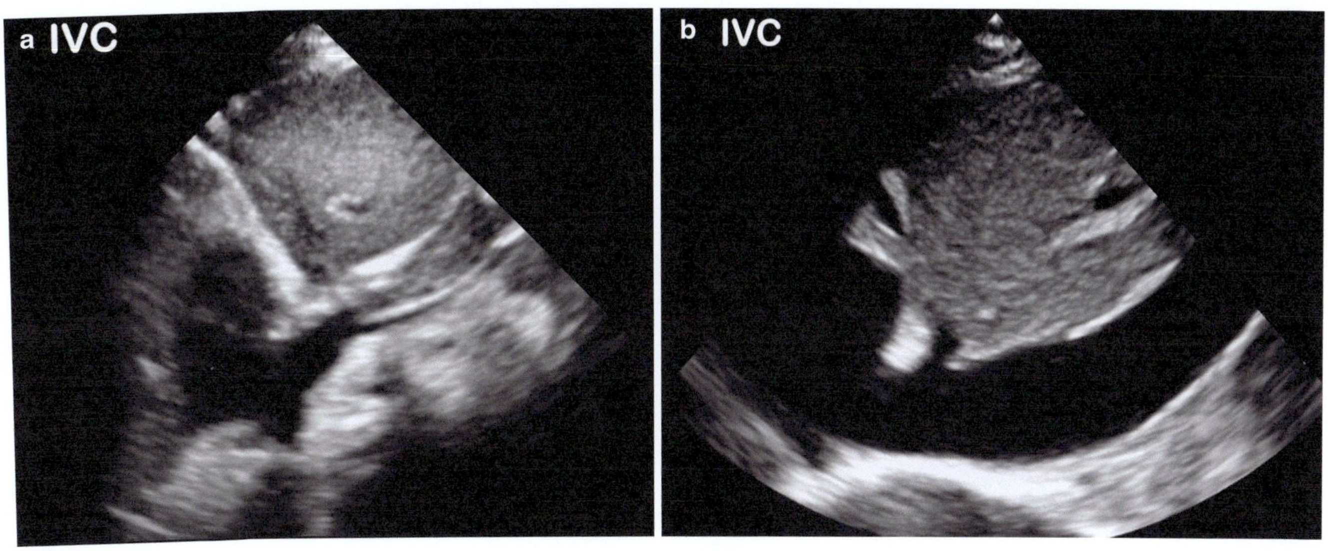

Fig. 23.21 Inferior vena cava in the extremes. (**a**) Collapsed (<2 cm) inferior vena cava (IVC); (**b**) Plethoric (≥2 cm) inferior vena cava with minimal to no respiratory variation

smaller than the D wave. Severe hepatic congestion causes S wave reversal with retrograde flow. Similarly, increased congestion affects the portal vein. Normal portal vein Doppler waveforms appear monophasic with minimal pulsatility on the pulsatility index, $(V_{max} - V_{min})/V_{max}$. Normal portal vein Doppler shows <30% on the pulsatility index, mild portal vein congestion has 30–49%, and severe congestion has ≥50%. The intrarenal veins (i.e., interlobar renal veins) normally appear as a continuous monophasic waveform on Doppler. With increasing congestion, there is dampening of the systolic component, causing a biphasic Doppler waveform with distinguishable S and D waves. Severe congestion causes further dampening of systolic flow with only the D waveform apparent using Doppler. Acquisition of the Doppler waveforms can be seen in Fig. 23.22. As the interlobar arteries run adjacent to the interlobar veins, an arterial waveform is also generated, but VExUS does not incorporate the changes in the arterial waveform. Tips for VExUS acquisition are shown in Table 23.5. Importantly, especially for hepatic vein assessment, it is advised to match the Doppler waveform to the cardiac cycle using electrocardiogram (ECG) leads when possible to avoid misidentifying flow reversal (Fig. 23.23).

Potential limitations of VExUS include liver cirrhosis, liver disease (e.g., steatosis), renal disease (e.g., chronic kidney disease, interstitial fibrosis, tubular atrophy), obstructive uropathy, severe tricuspid regurgitation, structural heart disease, hyperdynamic ejection fraction, constrictive pericarditis, increased intra-abdominal pressure (i.e., tense ascites), hepatic/portal/renal vein thrombosis, stenosis, and arrhythmia [120, 131]. Although these limitations are not absolute contraindications, VExUS has not been studied in these populations and should be interpreted with caution.

VExUS Grading

VExUS is scored on a 0–4 scale (Fig. 23.24). Grade 0 (i.e., no congestion) occurs when the IVC is <2 cm; no other Doppler evaluations are needed in this case. Grade 1 (i.e., mild congestion) occurs when the IVC ≥2 cm and Doppler evaluations display normal or mild congestion patterns. Grade 2 (i.e., moderate congestion) occurs when the IVC ≥2 cm and there is one severely congested pattern on Doppler waveforms. Grade 3 (i.e., severe congestion) occurs when the IVC ≥2 cm and there are at least two severely congested patterns on Doppler waveforms.

Table 23.5 Pearls for VExUS acquisition

Use the curvilinear probe
Measure the maximum IVC diameter 2 cm from the junction of the HV
Select the middle or right HV, main PV, and right intrarenal interlobar veins, considering patient factors (e.g., comfort, bowel gas, body habitus)
Place the pulsed-wave Doppler gate parallel to the direction of flow
Power Doppler is preferred over color Doppler for low-flow vessel identification
Use a Doppler scale of 40 cm/s for PV and HV and 20 cm/s for interlobar renal veins
Use a Doppler sweep speed of 50–66.67 mm/s
Use simultaneous ECG (if unavailable using the curvilinear probe, use a phased array probe with low wall filter)
Measure in end-expiration over several cycles

Adapted from Koratala et al. [131]
IVC inferior vena cava, *PV* portal vein, *HV* hepatic vein, *ECG* electrocardiogram

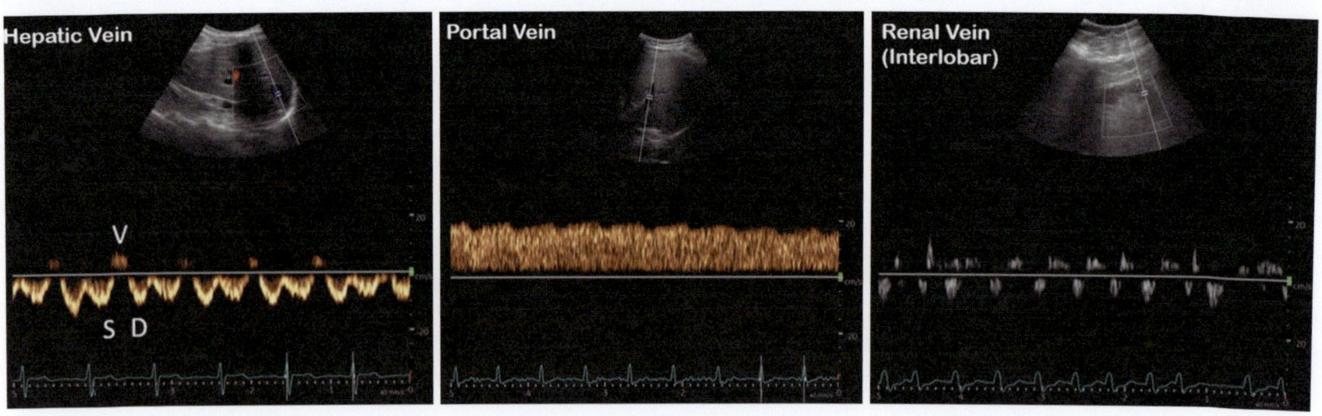

Fig. 23.22 Acquisition of Doppler waveforms for the venous excess ultrasound score (VExUS). *S* ventricular systole, *D* ventricular diastole, *V* atrial overfilling. (*Images courtesy of Abhilash Koratala, MD*)

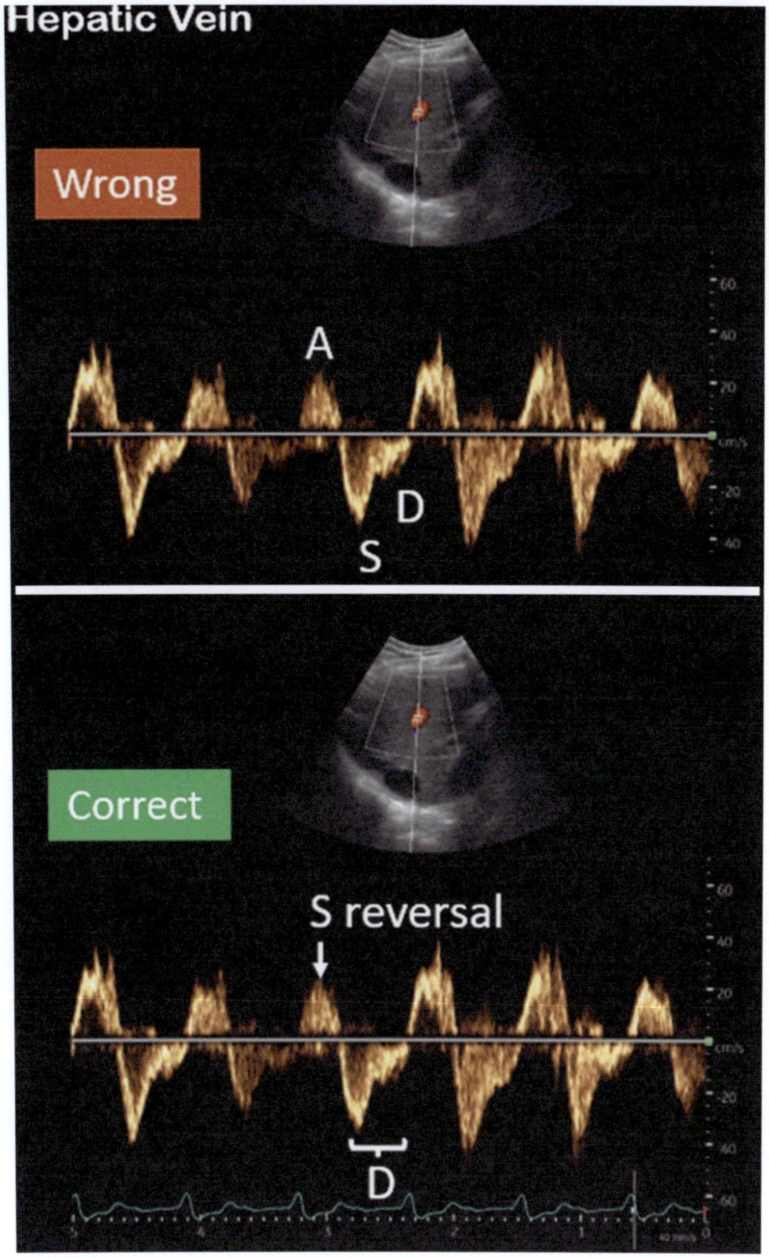

Fig. 23.23 Simultaneous ECG use in VExUS. Without simultaneous ECG, the waveform can be misidentified using morphology alone (top image). With the simultaneous ECG establishing systole, the S wave can be identified as the retrograde wave instead of an A wave (bottom image). *S* ventricular systole, *D* ventricular diastole, *A* atrial contraction, *ECG* electrocardiogram, *VExUS* venous excess ultrasound score. (*Images courtesy of Abhilash Koratala, MD*)

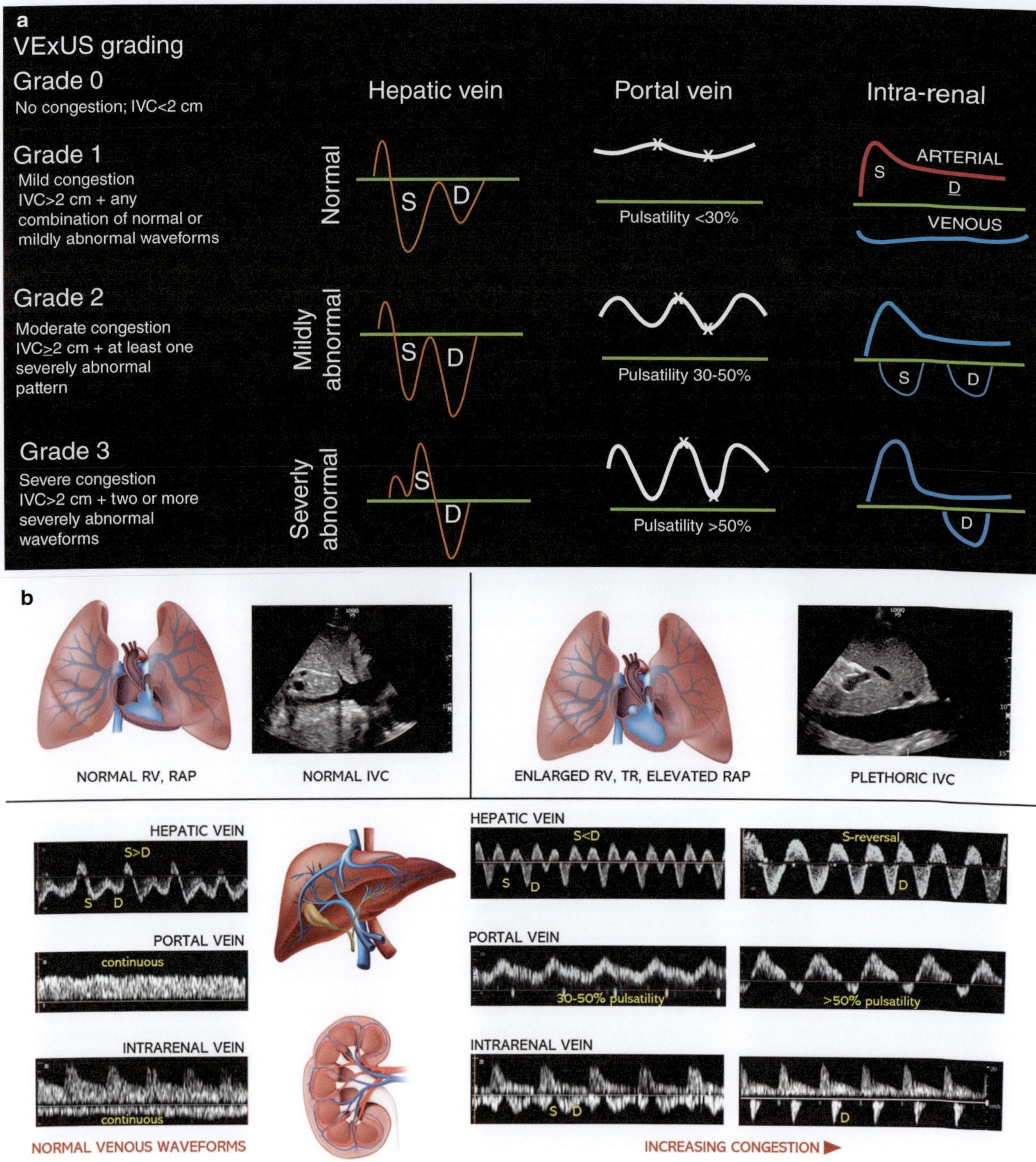

Fig. 23.24 VExUS grading. (**a**) Schematic of VExUS grading criteria. (**b**) VExUS waveform examples across increasing degrees of congestion. VExUS venous excess ultrasound score. (*Adapted from Kortala et al.* [131] *and Beaubien-Souligny et al.* [120])

Ultrasound in Sepsis and Septic Shock

Sepsis can pose a diagnostic and therapeutic challenge. POCUS may assist in identifying sepsis phenotypes and help to tailor the management. Accordingly, POCUS has been increasingly adopted in the management of sepsis, with one study reporting that POCUS was used in 21% of such encounters [132].

Sepsis-induced shock includes four primary pathophysiological processes: (1) infection-induced dysregulation, leading to the collapse of systemic vascular resistance; (2) loss of volume, resulting in depleted venous return; (3) myocardial dysfunction, due to reduced contractility or arrhythmia; and (4) potential obstructive etiologies [133]. These elements can overlap, varying the severity and complicating the clinical depiction.

POCUS can help detect infection sources promptly and accurately. As early as the 1990s, a prospective study found POCUS changed management in 22% of the patients, uncovered the sepsis source in 15%, and was 91% accurate [4]. A more recent study demonstrated that POCUS bolstered emergency physicians' ability to determine sepsis causes by 25% compared to clinical evaluation alone [134]. POCUS can also hasten diagnosis with a 73% sensitivity and 95% specificity within 10 min [134]. Other research has shown that POCUS can enhance decision-making certainty by 71% and lead to treatment plan alterations in 53% of cases [135]. This integrated POCUS approach provides a faster, more precise sepsis source identification, allowing for early initiation of appropriate antimicrobial therapies and source control strategies.

Beyond diagnostics, POCUS can be valuable for guiding clinicians in fine-tuning treatments to optimize patient hemodynamics. Treatment plans for patients with ventricular dysfunction from preexisting or sepsis-induced cardiomyopathy differ from septic patients primarily suffering from vasodilatory shock with preserved cardiac function. Several POCUS protocols have been developed to expedite hemodynamic assessments, guiding shock diagnosis and treatment, as described earlier in the chapter. These protocols leverage pattern recognition techniques to ascertain the type of shock (e.g., hypovolemic, distributive, obstructive, cardiogenic, or mixed). While these approaches share many common principles, their divergence lies predominantly in their exam sequence priority and complexity, spanning from rapid qualitative assessments to more complex quantitative measurements.

Hemodynamic Monitoring in Sepsis and Septic Shock

While septic shock is usually characterized by vasodilatory physiology with conserved or hyperdynamic left ventricular systolic function, a subset of patients exhibits a reduced ejection fraction, potentially with right ventricular dysfunction, due to sepsis-induced cardiomyopathy. The prevalence of sepsis-induced cardiomyopathy has been reported between 7% and 83%, contingent upon the definition used [136, 137]. Nonetheless, sepsis may encompass variable degrees of hypovolemia and myocardial dysfunction, highlighting the value of a comprehensive assessment to ensure diagnostic accuracy and precision in treatment [138].

Septic patients can be organized into three core hemodynamic clusters based on a three-step POCUS approach involving the subxiphoid long-axis, IVC, and lung views (Fig. 23.25) [20, 21]. Cluster 1 includes a phenotype of patients with normal or hyperdynamic ventricular systolic function; Cluster 2 comprises phenotypes with left ventricular systolic dysfunction, potentially accompanied by right ventricular dysfunction; Cluster 3 encompasses phenotypes with isolated right ventricular dysfunction (which could be acute, chronic, or acute-on-chronic) [20, 21]. Accordingly, hemodynamic management strategies can then be tailored to the patient's cluster classification. Other classification schemes include hemodynamic profiles based on the Diamond-Forrester phenotypes described earlier.

In Cluster 1, patient resuscitation begins with fluid repletion, gradually shifting toward vasoactive medications as the volume is restored and signs of systemic congestion start to arise. Conversely, Cluster 2 patients could benefit from small, calculated fluid boluses of 2.5–5 mL/kg, with the primary treatment typically involving vasoactive medications and occasionally inotropic agents when end-organ perfusion is jeopardized. These recommendations defer to the patient's volume responsiveness indicators [20]. Cluster 3 patients present unique challenges, necessitating an assessment of septal shift (i.e., septal bowing into the left ventricle during diastole, thereby inhibiting left ventricular filling) and right ventricular contractility to ascertain whether right ventricular function is compromised. If the function is indeed compensating appropriately, small fluid boluses of 2.5 mL/kg can be administered, shifting to fluid offloading measures like diuresis or renal-replacement therapy when right ventricular function decompensates. The cornerstone of treatment for these patients combines maintaining systemic blood pressure with vasoactive medications and inotropic support, minimizing pulmonary pressure increases by avoiding hypoxemia, hypercapnia, and high intrathoracic pressure with mechanical ventilation, as well as potentially incorporating pulmonary vasodilators [139].

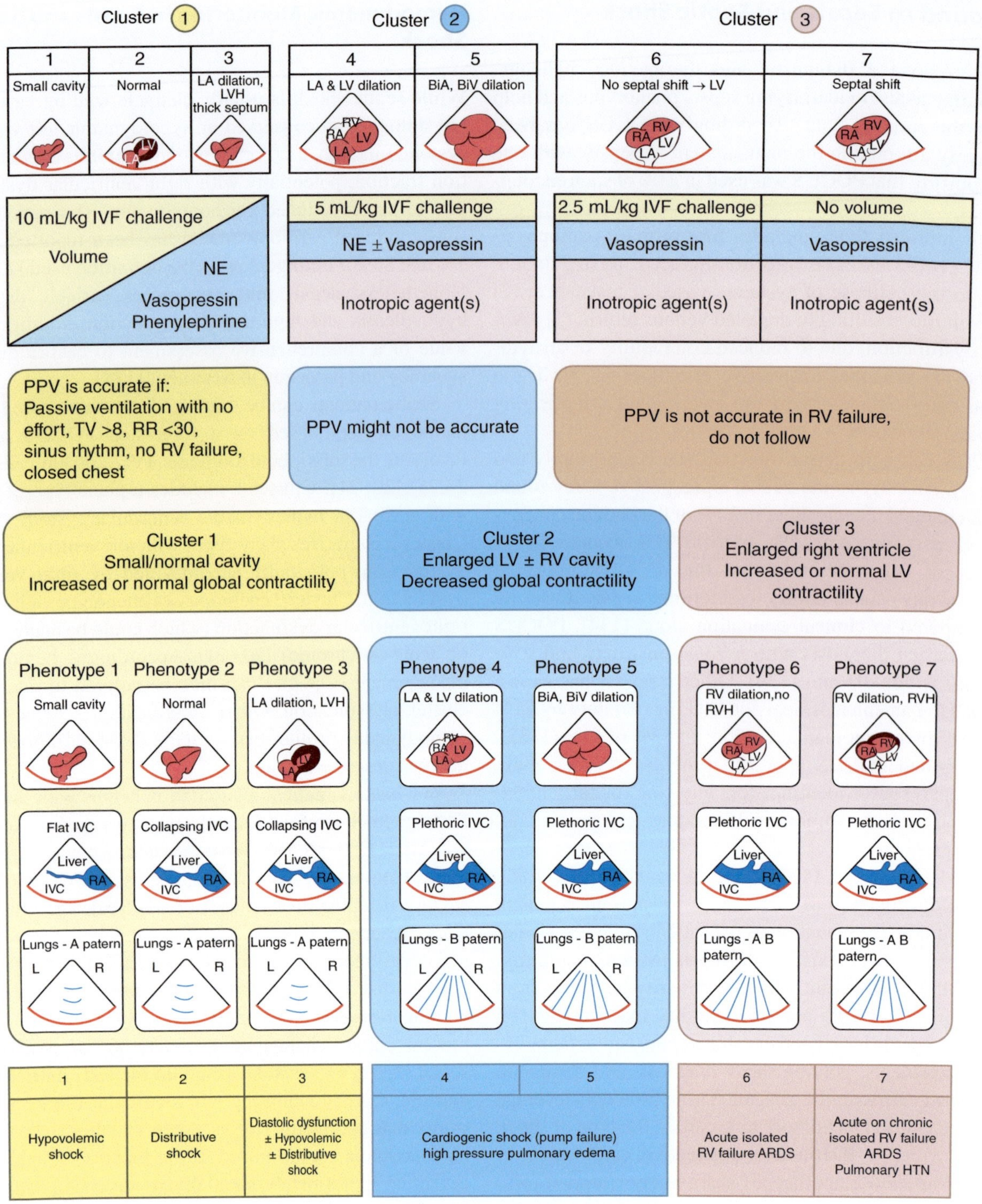

Fig. 23.25 Systematic approach to cluster identification and patient treatment using POCUS. *IVF* intravenous fluid, *NE* norepinephrine, *PPV* pulse pressure variation, *RV* right ventricle, *HTN* hypertension, *ARDS* acute respiratory distress syndrome. (*Adapted from Bughrara et al.* [20, 21])

Septic patients may also benefit from POCUS assessments to detect nonischemic stress-induced cardiomyopathy (i.e., Takotsubo cardiomyopathy) (Fig. 23.26, Video 23.20a) and dynamic left ventricular outflow tract obstruction (LVOTO) (Fig. 23.27) [140]. Takotsubo cardiomyopathy is often characterized by apical ballooning, though anatomical variations do occur. Although POCUS can be suggestive of Takotsubo cardiomyopathy, coronary artery imaging is needed to exclude ischemic heart disease. In dynamic LVOTO, a defining feature is high-speed, late-peaking, "dagger-shaped" waveforms on continuous-wave Doppler across the LV outflow tract with a velocity exceeding 3.5 m/s [140]. The presence of dynamic LVOTO demands a distinct management strategy, requiring fluid loading in hypovolemic patients, employing primarily vasoconstrictors [141], reducing the dosage of inotropic medications, and potentially introducing beta-blockers [142, 143].

Volume Status Assessment with POCUS

Due to septic patients' vasodilatory state, fluids are often initially administered to restore intravascular volume, increase cardiac output and oxygen delivery, and enhance tissue oxygenation [144]. However, a delicate balance must be achieved when administering fluids to these patients. Too little fluid resuscitation can lead to tissue hypoperfusion and aggravate organ dysfunction, while an excessive amount can cause complications (e.g., delirium, cardiac arrhythmias, pulmonary edema, prolonged ileus, hepatic congestion, AKI, impaired wound healing) [145] and elevated mortality rates [146].

Fluid Responsiveness

Early assessment of fluid responsiveness with POCUS can help correctly optimize the patient's volume status. Fluid responsiveness relies on the interaction between cardiac preload, contractility, and stroke volume (i.e., the Frank–Starling mechanism). Fluid responsiveness is defined as a cardiac output increase by more than 10–15% in response to a fluid challenge. This assumes the patient is still on the steep end of the Frank–Starling curve, where an increase in cardiac preload will result in increased stroke volume [147]. POCUS enhances the ability to anticipate fluid responsiveness in clinical settings by dynamically evaluating the components of this mechanism [148].

Dynamic indices using POCUS have been shown to be more accurate in determining fluid responsiveness compared to static markers [149]. These tests involve evaluating cardiac output after inducing temporary changes in cardiac preload through heart-lung interactions, passive leg raise, or the infusion of small volumes of fluid [150]. Passive leg raise mobilizes approximately 300 mL of blood from the lower limbs [151]. The transient preload may increase stroke volume [152]. To assess changes in cardiac output, echocardiographic parameters such as respiratory variations in maximal aortic blood flow velocity ($\Delta V_{max}Ao$), LVOT VTI, collapsibility indices of the superior vena cava (SVC) and IVC, and changes in stroke volume can be used [153]. The $\Delta V_{max}Ao$ has been shown to be the most sensitive (79%) for predicting fluid responsiveness, while the SVC collapsibility index had the best specificity (84%) [153]. In order to measure fluid responsiveness using respiratory variation in heart-lung interactions alone, the patient needs to be passively ventilated, receiving a tidal volume of at least 8 mL/kg, with no arrhythmias or significant right ventricular dysfunction [154]. If these conditions cannot be met, other maneuvers

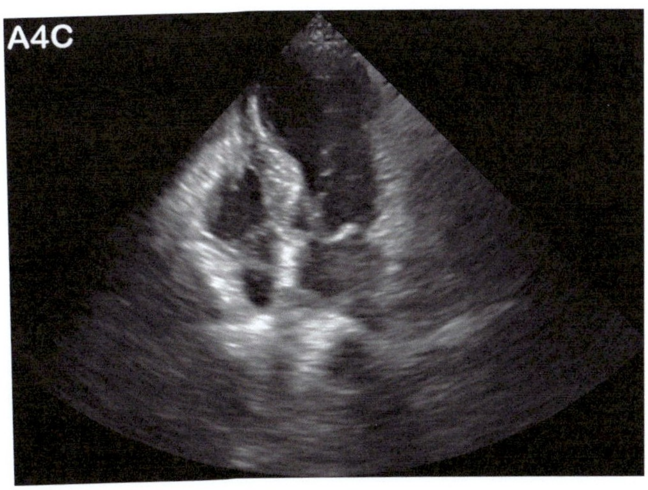

Fig. 23.26 Takotsubo cardiomyopathy in the apical 4-chamber view

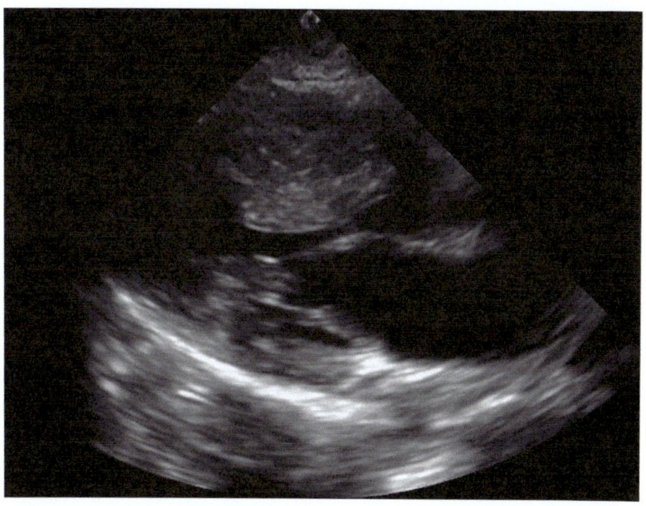

Fig. 23.27 Left ventricular outflow tract obstruction due to hypertrophic cardiomyopathy. (*Image courtesy of Ilya Ostrovsky, MD*)

like passive leg raise, end-expiratory occlusion tests, and mini-fluid challenges can be performed to assess fluid responsiveness.

In a prospective, observational study of mechanically ventilated, critically ill patients, a change ≥10% in subaortic VTI after a one-minute infusion of 100 mL colloid accurately predicted fluid responsiveness with 95% sensitivity and 75% specificity [155]. In another prospective study of critically ill patients with hypovolemic or septic shock, even smaller volume infusions (50 mL crystalloid solution given over 10 seconds), using subaortic VTI change ≥9%, predicted fluid responsiveness with 74% sensitivity and 95% specificity [156].

Fluid Tolerance

Fluid tolerance refers to the body's capacity to receive an infusion of fluids without worsening organ dysfunction. It is crucial to evaluate fluid tolerance in both the left and right-heart compartments: assessing the left-heart filling pressures and degree of pulmonary congestion, as well as the right-heart chambers' filling pressures and the severity of fluid overload in the systemic venous compartment. POCUS can be valuable in assessing fluid tolerance by estimating extravascular lung water (e.g., pulmonary edema), left ventricular filling pressures (e.g., transmitral E/A ratio, E/e′ ratio), LVOT VTI, and VExUS [120, 157, 158]. The patient's hemodynamic profile can help determine the most appropriate pathway for resuscitation (Table 23.6).

Fluid responsiveness is considered present if, after a fluid challenge (typically 500 mL of crystalloid in 10–15 min), stroke volume increases by 10–15%. Using POCUS, stroke volume can be measured using LVOT VTI. Fluid tolerance is a clinical construct that is considered absent if the patient cannot receive more fluid without worsening organ dysfunction. In the correct clinical context, pulmonary edema, a plethoric IVC, and a higher VExUS score may suggest absent fluid tolerance.

POCUS to Identify the Infection Source

The primary sources of infection in patients with sepsis and septic shock are typically the respiratory tract, urinary tract, and intra-abdominal sources [20]. Less common causes include skin and soft tissue infections, endocarditis, meningitis, and infections associated with indwelling catheters. POCUS can be useful for quickly identifying the source of infection at the patient's bedside when other imaging modalities such as radiography and computed tomography may be delayed (Table 23.7).

Table 23.6 Management based on hemodynamic profiles of fluid responsiveness and fluid tolerance

Fluid responsiveness	Fluid tolerance	Hemodynamic management
Present	Present	Volume expansion
Absent	Present	Conservative fluid management
Absent	Absent	Resuscitation: iuretics and ultrafiltration
Present	Absent	Early use of vasopressors

Adapted from Melo et al. [159]

Table 23.7 Ultrasound findings that support a sepsis-associated etiology in the appropriate clinical context

Source	Ultrasound findings
Pneumonia	Presence of consolidated lung Subpleural consolidation Focal B-lines distribution Dynamic air bronchograms Fluid bronchogram Shred sign Consolidated lung vascularity on Doppler Complex effusion or empyema (e.g., echogenic debris, septations, fibrin stranding, discrete abscess)
Pyelonephritis	Debris in the bladder Power Doppler with reduced areas of renal cortex vascularity Hypoechoic/hyperechoic regions in the renal parenchyma Renal mass Hydronephrosis Renal abscess Renal infarction Perinephric collections
Cholecystitis/ Choledocholithiasis	Sonographic murphy sign Thickened anterior gallbladder wall >3 mm Pericholecystic fluid Gallstones Dilated common bile duct >6 mm (+1 mm for every decade >60)

(continued)

Table 23.7 (continued)

Source	Ultrasound findings
Liver abscess	Semicircular mixed echogenicity
Appendicitis	Blind-ended, noncompressible, >6 mm structure
Diverticulitis	Thickness of colonic wall >4 mm Intramural air Fat stranding
Septic joint	Joint effusion Echogenic debris Septations Color Doppler may show increased vascularity
Abscess	Anechoic or hypoechoic fluid in a poorly defined or bordered capsule with septations, sediment, or gas Swirling or movement of the fluid with sonographic palpation Surrounding cobblestoning
Necrotizing soft tissue infection	Soft tissue gas appearing as dirty shadowing Distorted and thickened deep fascial planes Fascial fluid collection
Endocarditis	Vegetation(s) with similar echogenicity as cardiac tissue displaying independent movement, often on the lower pressure side of valves and associated with valve regurgitation

LV left ventricle, *IVC* inferior vena cava

Application of POCUS in Sepsis and Septic Shock

Currently, there is a lack of a unified POCUS protocol designed for systematically evaluating septic patients [160]. However, protocols developed for undifferentiated shock can be modified and incorporated into a sepsis POCUS protocol. A potential approach, with the benefits of POCUS in sepsis and septic shock, is summarized in Table 23.8.

Table 23.8 Approach for utilizing POCUS in sepsis and septic shock

1. Shock evaluation protocols	RUSH, FATE, FUSA, STARS
2. Hemodynamic monitoring	Cardiac (LVOT VTI, E/e'), lung, fluid responsiveness, fluid tolerance, VExUS
3. Diagnosis of etiology	Cardiac, lung, abdominal, skin/soft tissue
4. Dynamic monitoring	Repeat hemodynamic assessments
5. Ultrasound-guided procedures	Vascular access, thoracentesis, paracentesis, lumbar puncture, abscess drainage

RUSH rapid ultrasound in shock and hypotension, *FATE* focus assessed transthoracic echocardiography, *FUSA* focused ultrasound in surgical anesthesia, *STARS* subcostal to apical, respiratory to parasternal, *LVOT VTI* left ventricular outflow tract velocity time integral, *VExUS* venous excess ultrasound score

Key Ultrasound Findings

Clinical scenario	Cardiac POCUS	Lung POCUS	Other POCUS
Cardiac arrest	Evaluate for cardiac activity, LV/RV function and cavity size, PE, tamponade, thrombus, VF, PEA/asystole, hypovolemia, RWMA, compression efficacy	Evaluate for pneumothorax, effusions/hemothorax	Evaluate for AAA, aortic dissection, DVT, abdominal free fluid, ETT, pulse checks, procedural guidance
Undifferentiated shock	Cardiac arrest + Pulmonary artery occlusion pressure (mitral valve E/e′ velocities), LVOT VTI	Cardiac arrest + Pulmonary edema, effusions	Cardiac arrest + VExUS
Sepsis and septic shock	Undifferentiated shock + Endocarditis, cavity size, septal movement, Takotsubo cardiomyopathy, LVOTO	Undifferentiated shock + Pneumonia, ARDS	Undifferentiated shock + UTI, cholecystitis, liver abscess, appendicitis, diverticulitis, septic joint, abscess, necrotizing soft tissue infection

LV left ventricle, *RV* right ventricle, *PE* pulmonary embolism, *VF* ventricular fibrillation, *PEA* pulseless electrical activity, *RWMA* regional wall motion abnormality, *AAA* abdominal aortic aneurysm, *DVT* deep venous thrombosis, *ETT* endotracheal tube, *LVOT VTI* left ventricular outflow tract velocity time integral, *VExUS* venous excess ultrasound score, *LVOTO* left ventricular outflow tract obstruction, *ARDS* acute respiratory distress syndrome, *UTI* urinary tract infection

Pearls and Pitfalls

- In the cardiac arrest patient, POCUS can diagnose arrest etiology, guide treatment, identify ROSC, and estimate prognosis. However, this must be considered in the correct clinical context.
- When performing POCUS during cardiac arrest, minimize interruptions in chest compressions and consider early conversion to transesophageal echocardiography.
- Understand the limitations of VExUS and perform hepatic vein assessment with simultaneous ECG to avoid misidentifying severity.
- Use POCUS to evaluate the type of shock, diagnose etiologies, and tailor therapy according to hemodynamic profile, cluster, and phenotype.
- Consider using POCUS in serial assessments to evaluate progression of illness and changes in status (e.g., reduced fluid responsiveness, fluid overload).

References

1. Omoto R. Cardiac output monitoring in the intensive coronary care unit with the ultrasonic Doppler flowmeter. Kokyu To Junkan. 1974;22(7–8):565–8.
2. Barnes RW, Foster EJ, Janssen GA, Boutros AR. Safety of brachial arterial catheters as monitors in the intensive care unit–prospective evaluation with the Doppler ultrasonic velocity detector. Anesthesiology. 1976;44(3):260–4. https://doi.org/10.1097/00000542-197603000-00021.
3. Sauer W, Luft D, Risler T, Renn W, Eggstein M. Significance of ultrasonics in the placement of a central venous catheter. Dtsch Med Wochenschr 1946. 1988;113(37):1423–7. https://doi.org/10.1055/s-2008-1067829.
4. Lichtenstein D, Axler O. Intensive use of general ultrasound in the intensive care unit. Prospective study of 150 consecutive patients. Intensive Care Med. 1993;19(6):353–5. https://doi.org/10.1007/BF01694712.
5. Niendorff DF, Rassias AJ, Palac R, Beach ML, Costa S, Greenberg M. Rapid cardiac ultrasound of inpatients suffering PEA arrest performed by nonexpert sonographers. Resuscitation. 2005;67(1):81–7. https://doi.org/10.1016/j.resuscitation.2005.04.007.
6. Gottlieb M, Alerhand S. Managing cardiac arrest using ultrasound. Ann Emerg Med. 2023;81(5):532–42. https://doi.org/10.1016/j.annemergmed.2022.09.016.
7. Keikha M, Salehi-Marzijarani M, Soldoozi Nejat R, Sheikh Motahar Vahedi H, Mirrezaie SM. Diagnostic accuracy of rapid ultrasound in shock (RUSH) exam; a systematic review and meta-analysis. Bull Emerg Trauma. 2018;6(4):271–8. https://doi.org/10.29252/beat-060402.
8. Atkinson PR, Beckett N, French J, Banerjee A, Fraser J, Lewis D. Does point-of-care ultrasound use impact resuscitation length, rates of intervention, and clinical outcomes during cardiac arrest? A study from the sonography in hypotension and cardiac arrest in the emergency department (SHoC-ED) investigators. Cureus. 2019;11(4):e4456. https://doi.org/10.7759/cureus.4456.
9. Atkinson PR, Milne J, Diegelmann L, et al. Does point-of-care ultrasonography improve clinical outcomes in emergency department patients with undifferentiated hypotension? An international randomized controlled trial from the SHoC-ED investigators. Ann Emerg Med. 2018;72(4):478–89. https://doi.org/10.1016/j.annemergmed.2018.04.002.
10. Atkinson P, Taylor L, Milne J, et al. Does point of care ultrasound improve resuscitation markers in undifferentiated hypotension? An international randomized controlled trial from the sonography in hypotension and cardiac arrest in the emergency department (SHoC-ED) series. Cureus. 2020;12(8):e9899. https://doi.org/10.7759/cureus.9899.
11. Volpicelli G, Lamorte A, Tullio M, et al. Point-of-care multiorgan ultrasonography for the evaluation of undifferentiated hypotension in the emergency department. Intensive Care Med. 2013;39(7):1290–8. https://doi.org/10.1007/s00134-013-2919-7.
12. Bagheri-Hariri S, Yekesadat M, Farahmand S, et al. The impact of using RUSH protocol for diagnosing the type of unknown shock in the emergency department. Emerg Radiol. 2015;22(5):517–20. https://doi.org/10.1007/s10140-015-1311-z.
13. Shokoohi H, Boniface KS, Pourmand A, et al. Bedside ultrasound reduces diagnostic uncertainty and guides resuscitation in patients with undifferentiated hypotension. Crit Care Med. 2015;43(12):2562–9. https://doi.org/10.1097/CCM.0000000000001285.
14. Milne J, Atkinson P, Lewis D, et al. Sonography in hypotension and cardiac arrest (SHoC): rates of abnormal findings in undifferentiated hypotension and during cardiac arrest as a basis for consensus on a hierarchical point of care ultrasound protocol. Cureus. 2016;8(4):e564. https://doi.org/10.7759/cureus.564.
15. Javali RH, Loganathan A, Srinivasarangan M, et al. Reliability of emergency department diagnosis in identifying the etiology of nontraumatic undifferentiated hypotension. Indian J Crit Care Med Peer-Rev. 2020;24(5):313–20. https://doi.org/10.5005/jp-journals-10071-23429.
16. Yoshida T, Yoshida T, Noma H, Nomura T, Suzuki A, Mihara T. Diagnostic accuracy of point-of-care ultrasound for shock: a systematic review and meta-analysis. Crit Care. 2023;27(1):200. https://doi.org/10.1186/s13054-023-04495-6.
17. Grady KL, Dracup K, Kennedy G, et al. Team management of patients with heart failure: a statement for healthcare professionals from The Cardiovascular Nursing Council of the American Heart Association. Circulation. 2000;102(19):2443–56. https://doi.org/10.1161/01.cir.102.19.2443.
18. Kim KH, Jentzer JC, Wiley BM, et al. Diamond-Forrester classification using echocardiography haemodynamic assessment in cardiac intensive care unit patients. ESC Heart Fail. 2021;8(6):4933–43. https://doi.org/10.1002/ehf2.13527.
19. Kenny JÉS, Prager R, Rola P, Haycock K, Basmaji J, Hernández G. Unifying fluid responsiveness and tolerance with physiology: a dynamic interpretation of the Diamond-Forrester classification. Crit Care Explor. 2023;5(12):e1022. https://doi.org/10.1097/CCE.0000000000001022.
20. Bughrara N, Cha S, Safa R, Pustavoitau A. Perioperative Management of Patients with sepsis and septic shock, Part I: systematic approach. Anesthesiol Clin. 2020;38(1):107–22. https://doi.org/10.1016/j.anclin.2019.10.013.
21. Bughrara N, Diaz-Gomez JL, Pustavoitau A. Perioperative management of patients with sepsis and septic shock, part II: ultrasound support for resuscitation. Anesthesiol Clin. 2020;38(1):123–34. https://doi.org/10.1016/j.anclin.2019.11.001.
22. Bergum D, Haugen BO, Nordseth T, Mjølstad OC, Skogvoll E. Recognizing the causes of in-hospital cardiac arrest–a survival benefit. Resuscitation. 2015;97:91–6. https://doi.org/10.1016/j.resuscitation.2015.09.395.

23. Bergum D, Nordseth T, Mjølstad OC, Skogvoll E, Haugen BO. Causes of in-hospital cardiac arrest—incidences and rate of recognition. Resuscitation. 2015;87:63–8. https://doi.org/10.1016/j.resuscitation.2014.11.007.
24. Dewolf P, Wauters L, Clarebout G, Elen J. Timing and identification of the cause and treatment of a cardiac arrest: a potential survival benefit. Med Princ Pract Int J Kuwait Univ Health Sci Cent. 2022;31(4):384–91. https://doi.org/10.1159/000525553.
25. Breitkreutz R, Walcher F, Seeger FH. Focused echocardiographic evaluation in resuscitation management: concept of an advanced life support-conformed algorithm. Crit Care Med. 2007;35(5 Suppl):S150–61. https://doi.org/10.1097/01.CCM.0000260626.23848.FC.
26. Hernandez C, Shuler K, Hannan H, Sonyika C, Likourezos A, Marshall J. C.A.U.S.E.: Cardiac arrest ultra-sound exam–a better approach to managing patients in primary non-arrhythmogenic cardiac arrest. Resuscitation. 2008;76(2):198–206. https://doi.org/10.1016/j.resuscitation.2007.06.033.
27. Testa A, Cibinel GA, Portale G, et al. The proposal of an integrated ultrasonographic approach into the ALS algorithm for cardiac arrest: the PEA protocol. Eur Rev Med Pharmacol Sci. 2010;14(2):77–88.
28. Breitkreutz R, Price S, Steiger HV, et al. Focused echocardiographic evaluation in life support and peri-resuscitation of emergency patients: a prospective trial. Resuscitation. 2010;81(11):1527–33. https://doi.org/10.1016/j.resuscitation.2010.07.013.
29. Lichtenstein DA. How can the use of lung ultrasound in cardiac arrest make ultrasound a holistic discipline. The example of the SESAME-protocol. Med Ultrason. 2014;16(3):252–5. https://doi.org/10.11152/mu.2013.2066.163.dal1.
30. Lichtenstein D, Malbrain MLNG. Critical care ultrasound in cardiac arrest. Technological requirements for performing the SESAME-protocol–a holistic approach. Anaesthesiol Intensive Ther. 2015;47(5):471–81. https://doi.org/10.5603/AIT.a2015.0072.
31. Atkinson P, Bowra J, Milne J, et al. International Federation for Emergency Medicine Consensus Statement: sonography in hypotension and cardiac arrest (SHoC): an international consensus on the use of point of care ultrasound for undifferentiated hypotension and during cardiac arrest. CJEM. 2017;19(6):459–70. https://doi.org/10.1017/cem.2016.394.
32. Beckett N, Atkinson P, Fraser J, et al. Do combined ultrasound and electrocardiogram-rhythm findings predict survival in emergency department cardiac arrest patients? The second sonography in hypotension and cardiac arrest in the emergency department (SHoC-ED2) study. CJEM. 2019;21(6):739–43. https://doi.org/10.1017/cem.2019.397.
33. Lien WC, Liu YP, Chong KM, et al. A novel US-CAB protocol for ultrasonographic evaluation during cardiopulmonary resuscitation. Resuscitation. 2017;115:e1–2. https://doi.org/10.1016/j.resuscitation.2017.03.016.
34. Lien WC, Hsu SH, Chong KM, et al. US-CAB protocol for ultrasonographic evaluation during cardiopulmonary resuscitation: validation and potential impact. Resuscitation. 2018;127:125–31. https://doi.org/10.1016/j.resuscitation.2018.01.051.
35. Gardner KF, Clattenburg EJ, Wroe P, Singh A, Mantuani D, Nagdev A. The Cardiac Arrest Sonographic Assessment (CASA) exam – a standardized approach to the use of ultrasound in PEA. Am J Emerg Med. 2018;36(4):729–31. https://doi.org/10.1016/j.ajem.2017.08.052.
36. Chua MT, Chan GW, Kuan WS. Reversible causes in cardiovascular collapse at the emergency department using ultrasonography (REVIVE-US). Ann Acad Med Singap. 2017;46(8):310–6.
37. Ávila-Reyes D, Acevedo-Cardona AO, Gómez-González JF, Echeverry-Piedrahita DR, Aguirre-Flórez M, Giraldo-Diaconeasa A. Point-of-care ultrasound in cardiorespiratory arrest (POCUS-CA): narrative review article. Ultrasound J. 2021;13(1):46. https://doi.org/10.1186/s13089-021-00248-0.
38. Chu SE, Chang CJ, Chen HA, et al. Core ultrasound in REsuscitation (CURE): a novel protocol for ultrasound-assistant life support via application of both transesophageal and transthoracic ultrasound. Resuscitation. 2022;173:1–3. https://doi.org/10.1016/j.resuscitation.2022.01.031.
39. Wyckoff MH, Greif R, Morley PT, et al. 2022 international consensus on cardiopulmonary resuscitation and emergency cardiovascular care science with treatment recommendations: summary from the basic life support; advanced life support; pediatric life support; neonatal life support; education, implementation, and teams; and first aid task forces. Circulation. 2022;146(25):e483–557. https://doi.org/10.1161/CIR.0000000000001095.
40. Maite A Huis In 't Veld, Allison MG, Bostick DS, et al. Ultrasound use during cardiopulmonary resuscitation is associated with delays in chest compressions. Resuscitation. 2017;119:95–8. https://doi.org/10.1016/j.resuscitation.2017.07.021.
41. Clattenburg EJ, Wroe P, Brown S, et al. Point-of-care ultrasound use in patients with cardiac arrest is associated prolonged cardiopulmonary resuscitation pauses: a prospective cohort study. Resuscitation. 2018;122:65–8. https://doi.org/10.1016/j.resuscitation.2017.11.056.
42. Clattenburg EJ, Wroe PC, Gardner K, et al. Implementation of the Cardiac Arrest Sonographic Assessment (CASA) protocol for patients with cardiac arrest is associated with shorter CPR pulse checks. Resuscitation. 2018;131:69–73. https://doi.org/10.1016/j.resuscitation.2018.07.030.
43. Gaspari R, Harvey J, DiCroce C, et al. Echocardiographic pre-pause imaging and identifying the acoustic window during CPR reduces CPR pause time during ACLS – a prospective Cohort Study. Resusc Plus. 2021;6:100094. https://doi.org/10.1016/j.resplu.2021.100094.
44. Gaspari RJ, Gleeson T, Alerhand S, et al. A multicenter, prospective study comparing subxiphoid and parasternal views during brief echocardiography: effect on image quality, acquisition time, and visualized anatomy. J Emerg Med. 2022;62(5):648–56. https://doi.org/10.1016/j.jemermed.2021.10.032.
45. Gaspari R, Weekes A, Adhikari S, et al. Emergency department point-of-care ultrasound in out-of-hospital and in-ED cardiac arrest. Resuscitation. 2016;109:33–9. https://doi.org/10.1016/j.resuscitation.2016.09.018.
46. Kleber C, Giesecke MT, Lindner T, Haas NP, Buschmann CT. Requirement for a structured algorithm in cardiac arrest following major trauma: epidemiology, management errors, and preventability of traumatic deaths in Berlin. Resuscitation. 2014;85(3):405–10. https://doi.org/10.1016/j.resuscitation.2013.11.009.
47. Tayal VS, Kline JA. Emergency echocardiography to detect pericardial effusion in patients in PEA and near-PEA states. Resuscitation. 2003;59(3):315–8. https://doi.org/10.1016/s0300-9572(03)00245-4.
48. Reynolds JC, Nicholson T, O'Neil B, et al. Diagnostic test accuracy of point-of-care ultrasound during cardiopulmonary resuscitation to indicate the etiology of cardiac arrest: a systematic review. Resuscitation. 2022;172:54–63. https://doi.org/10.1016/j.resuscitation.2022.01.006.
49. Alerhand S, Adrian RJ, Long B, Avila J. Pericardial tamponade: a comprehensive emergency medicine and echocardiography review. Am J Emerg Med. 2022;58:159–74. https://doi.org/10.1016/j.ajem.2022.05.001.
50. Eisenberg MJ, Oken K, Guerrero S, Saniei MA, Schiller NB. Prognostic value of echocardiography in hospitalized patients with pericardial effusion. Am J Cardiol. 1992;70(9):934–9. https://doi.org/10.1016/0002-9149(92)90742-h.

51. Eke OF, Selame L, Gullikson J, Deng H, Dutta S, Shokoohi H. Timing of pericardiocentesis and clinical outcomes: is earlier pericardiocentesis better? Am J Emerg Med. 2022;54:202–7. https://doi.org/10.1016/j.ajem.2022.01.062.
52. Spodick DH. Acute cardiac tamponade. N Engl J Med. 2003;349(7):684–90. https://doi.org/10.1056/NEJMra022643.
53. Burlew CC, Moore EE, Moore FA, et al. Western Trauma Association critical decisions in trauma: resuscitative thoracotomy. J Trauma Acute Care Surg. 2012;73(6):1359–63. https://doi.org/10.1097/TA.0b013e318270d2df.
54. Seamon MJ, Haut ER, Van Arendonk K, et al. An evidence-based approach to patient selection for emergency department thoracotomy: a practice management guideline from the Eastern Association for the Surgery of Trauma. J Trauma Acute Care Surg. 2015;79(1):159–73. https://doi.org/10.1097/TA.0000000000000648.
55. Inaba K, Chouliaras K, Zakaluzny S, et al. FAST ultrasound examination as a predictor of outcomes after resuscitative thoracotomy: a prospective evaluation. Ann Surg. 2015;262(3):512–8; discussion 516–518. https://doi.org/10.1097/SLA.0000000000001421.
56. Schellenberg M, Inaba K. Critical decisions in the management of thoracic trauma. Emerg Med Clin North Am. 2018;36(1):135–47. https://doi.org/10.1016/j.emc.2017.08.008.
57. Bougouin W, Marijon E, Planquette B, et al. Pulmonary embolism related sudden cardiac arrest admitted alive at hospital: management and outcomes. Resuscitation. 2017;115:135–40. https://doi.org/10.1016/j.resuscitation.2017.04.019.
58. Hess EP, Campbell RL, White RD. Epidemiology, trends, and outcome of out-of-hospital cardiac arrest of non-cardiac origin. Resuscitation. 2007;72(2):200–6. https://doi.org/10.1016/j.resuscitation.2006.06.040.
59. Kuisma 1997_9243146_epidemiology and outcome pe.pdf.
60. Javaudin F, Lascarrou JB, Le Bastard Q, et al. Thrombolysis during resuscitation for out-of-hospital cardiac arrest caused by pulmonary embolism increases 30-day survival: findings from the French National Cardiac Arrest Registry. Chest. 2019;156(6):1167–75. https://doi.org/10.1016/j.chest.2019.07.015.
61. Lau V, Blaszak M, Lam J, German M, Myslik F. Point-of-care resuscitative echocardiography diagnosis of intracardiac thrombus during cardiac arrest (PREDICT study): a retrospective, observational cohort study. Resusc Plus. 2022;10:100218. https://doi.org/10.1016/j.resplu.2022.100218.
62. Alerhand S, Adrian RJ. What echocardiographic findings differentiate acute pulmonary embolism and chronic pulmonary hypertension? Am J Emerg Med. 2023;72:72–84. https://doi.org/10.1016/j.ajem.2023.07.011.
63. Lavonas EJ, Drennan IR, Gabrielli A, et al. Part 10: special circumstances of resuscitation: 2015 American Heart Association guidelines update for cardiopulmonary resuscitation and emergency cardiovascular care. Circulation. 2015;132(18 Suppl 2):S501–18. https://doi.org/10.1161/CIR.0000000000000264.
64. Konstantinides SV, Meyer G, Becattini C, et al. 2019 ESC Guidelines for the diagnosis and management of acute pulmonary embolism developed in collaboration with the European Respiratory Society (ERS). Eur Heart J. 2020;41(4):543–603. https://doi.org/10.1093/eurheartj/ehz405.
65. Berdowski J, Berg RA, Tijssen JGP, Koster RW. Global incidences of out-of-hospital cardiac arrest and survival rates: systematic review of 67 prospective studies. Resuscitation. 2010;81(11):1479–87. https://doi.org/10.1016/j.resuscitation.2010.08.006.
66. Gaspari R, Weekes A, Adhikari S, et al. Comparison of outcomes between pulseless electrical activity by electrocardiography and pulseless myocardial activity by echocardiography in out-of-hospital cardiac arrest; secondary analysis from a large, prospective study. Resuscitation. 2021;169:167–72. https://doi.org/10.1016/j.resuscitation.2021.09.010.
67. Teran F, Dean AJ, Centeno C, et al. Evaluation of out-of-hospital cardiac arrest using transesophageal echocardiography in the emergency department. Resuscitation. 2019;137:140–7. https://doi.org/10.1016/j.resuscitation.2019.02.013.
68. Buick JE, Drennan IR, Scales DC, et al. Improving temporal trends in survival and neurological outcomes after out-of-hospital cardiac arrest. Circ Cardiovasc Qual Outcomes. 2018;11(1):e003561. https://doi.org/10.1161/CIRCOUTCOMES.117.003561.
69. Kedan I, Ciozda W, Palatinus JA, Palatinus HN, Kimchi A. Prognostic value of point-of-care ultrasound during cardiac arrest: a systematic review. Cardiovasc Ultrasound. 2020;18(1):1. https://doi.org/10.1186/s12947-020-0185-8.
70. Tsao CW, Aday AW, Almarzooq ZI, et al. Heart disease and stroke Statistics-2023 update: a report from the American Heart Association. Circulation. 2023;147(8):e93–e621. https://doi.org/10.1161/CIR.0000000000001123.
71. Tomruk O, Erdur B, Cetin G, Ergin A, Avcil M, Kapci M. Assessment of cardiac ultrasonography in predicting outcome in adult cardiac arrest. J Int Med Res. 2012;40(2):804–9. https://doi.org/10.1177/147323001204000247.
72. Thandar S, Sahu AK, Sinha TP, Bhoi S. Role of initial cardiac activity assessed by point-of-care ultrasonography in predicting cardiac arrest outcomes: a prospective cohort study. Turk J Emerg Med. 2023;23(1):24–9. https://doi.org/10.4103/2452-2473.366482.
73. Zaki HA, Iftikhar H, Shaban EE, et al. The role of point-of-care ultrasound (POCUS) imaging in clinical outcomes during cardiac arrest: a systematic review. Ultrasound J. 2024;16(1):4. https://doi.org/10.1186/s13089-023-00346-1.
74. Gouveia E, Melo R, Machado C, Caldeira D, et al. Incidence of acute aortic dissections in patients with out of hospital cardiac arrest: a systematic review and meta-analysis of observational studies. Int J Cardiol Heart Vasc. 2022;38:100934. https://doi.org/10.1016/j.ijcha.2021.100934.
75. Gibbons RC, Smith D, Feig R, Mulflur M, Costantino TG. The sonographic protocol for the emergent evaluation of aortic dissections (SPEED protocol): a multicenter, prospective, observational study. Acad Emerg Med Off J Soc Acad Emerg Med. 2024;31(2):112–8. https://doi.org/10.1111/acem.14839.
76. Sutarjono B, Ahmed AJ, Ivanova A, et al. Diagnostic accuracy of transthoracic echocardiography for the identification of proximal aortic dissection: a systematic review and meta-analysis. Sci Rep. 2023;13(1):5886. https://doi.org/10.1038/s41598-023-32800-4.
77. Thomas W, Henry J, Chew JE, Premaratne M, Blecher G, Haji DL. Review article: accuracy of emergency physician performed point-of-care ultrasound of the thoracic aorta: a systematic review and narrative synthesis of the literature. Emerg Med Australas. 2023;35(5):720–30. https://doi.org/10.1111/1742-6723.14262.
78. Erbel R, Aboyans V, Boileau C, et al. 2014 ESC Guidelines on the diagnosis and treatment of aortic diseases: Document covering acute and chronic aortic diseases of the thoracic and abdominal aorta of the adult. The Task Force for the Diagnosis and Treatment of Aortic Diseases of the European Society of Cardiology (ESC). Eur Heart J. 2014;35(41):2873–926. https://doi.org/10.1093/eurheartj/ehu281.
79. Writing Committee Members, Isselbacher EM, Preventza O, et al. 2022 ACC/AHA Guideline for the Diagnosis and management of aortic disease: a report of the American Heart Association/American College of Cardiology Joint Committee on Clinical Practice Guidelines. J Am Coll Cardiol. 2022;80(24):e223–393. https://doi.org/10.1016/j.jacc.2022.08.004.
80. Gottlieb M. SPEED of sound: the role of ultrasound in aortic dissection. Acad Emerg Med Off J Soc Acad Emerg Med. 2024;31(2):201–3. https://doi.org/10.1111/acem.14885.
81. Harris DG, Garrido D, Oates CP, et al. Repair of ruptured abdominal aortic aneurysm after cardiac arrest. J Vasc Surg. 2016;64(5):1497–502. https://doi.org/10.1016/j.jvs.2016.05.085.

82. Broos PPHL, t'Mannetje YW, Loos MJA, et al. A ruptured abdominal aortic aneurysm that requires preoperative cardiopulmonary resuscitation is not necessarily lethal. J Vasc Surg. 2016;63(1):49–54. https://doi.org/10.1016/j.jvs.2015.08.061.
83. Darling RC, Messina CR, Brewster DC, Ottinger LW. Autopsy study of unoperated abdominal aortic aneurysms. The case for early resection. Circulation. 1977;56(3 Suppl):II161–II164.
84. Fernando SM, Tran A, Cheng W, et al. Accuracy of presenting symptoms, physical examination, and imaging for diagnosis of ruptured abdominal aortic aneurysm: systematic review and meta-analysis. Acad Emerg Med Off J Soc Acad Emerg Med. 2022;29(4):486–96. https://doi.org/10.1111/acem.14475.
85. Hendrickson RG, Dean AJ, Costantino TG. A novel use of ultra sound in pulseless electrical activity: the diagnosis of an acute abdominal aortic aneurysm rupture. J Emerg Med. 2001;21(2): 141–4. https://doi.org/10.1016/s0736-4679(01)00362-6.
86. Leigh-Smith S, Harris T. Tension pneumothorax–time for a re-think? Emerg Med J. 2005;22(1):8–16. https://doi.org/10.1136/emj.2003.010421.
87. Chan KK, Joo DA, McRae AD, et al. Chest ultrasonography versus supine chest radiography for diagnosis of pneumothorax in trauma patients in the emergency department. Cochrane Database Syst Rev. 2020;7(7):CD013031. https://doi.org/10.1002/14651858.CD013031.pub2.
88. Demi L, Wolfram F, Klersy C, et al. New international guidelines and consensus on the use of lung ultrasound. J Ultrasound Med. 2023;42(2):309–44. https://doi.org/10.1002/jum.16088.
89. American College of Surgeon Committee on Trauma. Advanced Trauma Life Support (ATLS) student course manual. 10th ed. American College of Surgeon Committee on Trauma; 2018.
90. Mojoli F, Bouhemad B, Mongodi S, Lichtenstein D. Lung ultrasound for critically ill patients. Am J Respir Crit Care Med. 2019;199(6):701–14. https://doi.org/10.1164/rccm.201802-0236CI.
91. Lichtenstein DA, Lascols N, Prin S, Mezière G. The "lung pulse": an early ultrasound sign of complete atelectasis. Intensive Care Med. 2003;29(12):2187–92. https://doi.org/10.1007/s00134-003-1930-9.
92. Gottlieb M, Holladay D, Peksa GD. Ultrasonography for the confirmation of endotracheal tube intubation: a systematic review and meta-analysis. Ann Emerg Med. 2018;72(6):627–36. https://doi.org/10.1016/j.annemergmed.2018.06.024.
93. Gottlieb M, Patel D, Sundaram T. Comparison of endotracheal tube location on ultrasound accuracy, time, and confidence. Am J Emerg Med. 2022;62:127–8. https://doi.org/10.1016/j.ajem.2022.08.048.
94. Gottlieb M, Patel D, Jung C, et al. Comparison of saline versus air for identifying endotracheal intubation with ultrasound. Am J Emerg Med. 2022;58:131–4. https://doi.org/10.1016/j.ajem.2022.05.053.
95. Gottlieb M, O'Brien JR, Ferrigno N, Sundaram T. Point-of-care ultrasound for airway management in the emergency and critical care setting. Clin Exp Emerg Med. 2024;11(1):22–32. https://doi.org/10.15441/ceem.23.094.
96. Gottlieb M, Berzins D, Hartrich M, et al. Diagnostic accuracy of ultrasound to confirm endotracheal tube depth. Am J Emerg Med. 2022;62:9–13. https://doi.org/10.1016/j.ajem.2022.09.033.
97. Gottlieb M, Cozzi N, Hartrich M, et al. Comparison of dynamic versus static ultrasound to confirm endotracheal tube depth. Am J Emerg Med. 2023;74:17–20. https://doi.org/10.1016/j.ajem.2023.09.014.
98. Pavlov CS, Casazza G, Semenistaia M, et al. Ultrasonography for diagnosis of alcoholic cirrhosis in people with alcoholic liver disease. Cochrane Database Syst Rev. 2016;3(3):CD011602. https://doi.org/10.1002/14651858.CD011602.pub2.
99. Yen YH, Kuo FY, Chen CH, et al. Ultrasound is highly specific in diagnosing compensated cirrhosis in chronic hepatitis C patients in real world clinical practice. Medicine (Baltimore). 2019;98(27):e16270. https://doi.org/10.1097/MD.0000000000016270.
100. Eberle B, Dick WF, Schneider T, Wisser G, Doetsch S, Tzanova I. Checking the carotid pulse check: diagnostic accuracy of first responders in patients with and without a pulse. Resuscitation. 1996;33(2):107–16. https://doi.org/10.1016/s0300-9572(96)01016-7.
101. Ochoa FJ, Ramalle-Gómara E, Carpintero JM, García A, Saralegui I. Competence of health professionals to check the carotid pulse. Resuscitation. 1998;37(3):173–5. https://doi.org/10.1016/s0300-9572(98)00055-0.
102. Deakin CD, Low JL. Accuracy of the advanced trauma life support guidelines for predicting systolic blood pressure using carotid, femoral, and radial pulses: observational study. BMJ. 2000;321(7262):673–4. https://doi.org/10.1136/bmj.321.7262.673.
103. Kang SY, Jo IJ, Lee G, et al. Point-of-care ultrasound compression of the carotid artery for pulse determination in cardiopulmonary resuscitation. Resuscitation. 2022;179:206–13. https://doi.org/10.1016/j.resuscitation.2022.06.025.
104. Cohen AL, Li T, Becker LB, et al. Femoral artery Doppler ultrasound is more accurate than manual palpation for pulse detection in cardiac arrest. Resuscitation. 2022;173:156–65. https://doi.org/10.1016/j.resuscitation.2022.01.030.
105. Cheung JCH, Yip YY. Pseudo-PEA: an easily overlooked player in cardiac arrest. Resuscitation. 2021;168:240–1. https://doi.org/10.1016/j.resuscitation.2021.08.051.
106. Rabjohns J, Quan T, Boniface K, Pourmand A. Pseudo-pulseless electrical activity in the emergency department, an evidence based approach. Am J Emerg Med. 2020;38(2):371–5. https://doi.org/10.1016/j.ajem.2019.158503.
107. Lalande E, Burwash-Brennan T, Burns K, et al. Is point-of-care ultrasound a reliable predictor of outcome during atraumatic, non-shockable cardiac arrest? A systematic review and meta-analysis from the SHoC investigators. Resuscitation. 2019;139:159–66. https://doi.org/10.1016/j.resuscitation.2019.03.027.
108. Lalande E, Burwash-Brennan T, Burns K, et al. Is point-of-care ultrasound a reliable predictor of outcome during traumatic cardiac arrest? A systematic review and meta-analysis from the SHoC investigators. Resuscitation. 2021;167:128–36. https://doi.org/10.1016/j.resuscitation.2021.08.027.
109. Hu K, Gupta N, Teran F, Saul T, Nelson BP, Andrus P. Variability in interpretation of cardiac standstill among physician sonographers. Ann Emerg Med. 2018;71(2):193–8. https://doi.org/10.1016/j.annemergmed.2017.07.476.
110. Rose JS, Bair AE, Mandavia D, Kinser DJ. The UHP ultrasound protocol: a novel ultrasound approach to the empiric evaluation of the undifferentiated hypotensive patient. Am J Emerg Med. 2001;19(4):299–302. https://doi.org/10.1053/ajem.2001.24481.
111. Perera P, Mailhot T, Riley D, Mandavia D. The RUSH exam: rapid ultrasound in SHock in the evaluation of the critically lll. Emerg Med Clin North Am. 2010;28(1):29–56, vii. https://doi.org/10.1016/j.emc.2009.09.010.
112. Seif D, Perera P, Mailhot T, Riley D, Mandavia D. Bedside ultrasound in resuscitation and the rapid ultrasound in shock protocol. Crit Care Res Pract. 2012;2012:503254. https://doi.org/10.1155/2012/503254.
113. Joseph MX, Disney PJS, Da Costa R, Hutchison SJ. Transthoracic echocardiography to identify or exclude cardiac cause of shock. Chest. 2004;126(5):1592–7. https://doi.org/10.1378/chest.126.5.1592.

114. Dunfield R, Ross P, Dutton D, et al. SHoC-IVC: does assessment of the inferior vena cava by point-of-care ultrasound independently predict fluid status in spontaneously breathing patients with undifferentiated hypotension? CJEM. 2023;25(11):902–8. https://doi.org/10.1007/s43678-023-00584-1.
115. Holm JH, Frederiksen CA, Juhl-Olsen P, Sloth E. Perioperative use of focus assessed transthoracic echocardiography (FATE). Anesth Analg. 2012;115(5):1029–32. https://doi.org/10.1213/ANE.0b013e31826dd867.
116. Díaz-Gómez JL, Via G, Ramakrishna H. Focused cardiac and lung ultrasonography: implications and applicability in the perioperative period. Rom J Anaesth Intensive Care. 2016;23(1):41–54. https://doi.org/10.21454/rjaic.7518.231.lus.
117. Nikravan S, Bughrara N, Klick J, Lanspa MJ, Rapoport L, Díaz-Gomez J. An echocardiographic approach for the management of shock: the subcostal to apical, respiratory to parasternal-cardiac to respiratory, aortic to stomach protocol. Semin Ultrasound CT MR. 2024;45(1):74–83. https://doi.org/10.1053/j.sult.2023.12.008.
118. Forrester JS, Diamond G, Chatterjee K, Swan HJ. Medical therapy of acute myocardial infarction by application of hemodynamic subsets (first of two parts). N Engl J Med. 1976;295(24):1356–62. https://doi.org/10.1056/NEJM197612092952406.
119. Weingart S. EMCrit 367 – panel: 4 quadrant hemodynamic ultrasound integration, IVC ultrasound and much more! EMCrit Blog2024. https://emcrit.org/emcrit/4-quadrant-hemodynamics/
120. Beaubien-Souligny W, Rola P, Haycock K, et al. Quantifying systemic congestion with point-of-care ultrasound: development of the venous excess ultrasound grading system. Ultrasound J. 2020;12(1):16. https://doi.org/10.1186/s13089-020-00163-w.
121. Banjade P, Subedi A, Ghamande S, Surani S, Sharma M. Systemic venous congestion reviewed. Cureus. 2023;15(8):e43716. https://doi.org/10.7759/cureus.43716.
122. Prager R, Arntfield R, Wong MYS, et al. Venous congestion in septic shock quantified with point-of-care ultrasound: a pilot prospective multicentre cohort study. Can J Anaesth J Can Anesth. 2024;71(5):640–9. https://doi.org/10.1007/s12630-024-02717-1.
123. Andrei S, Bahr PA, Nguyen M, Bouhemad B, Guinot PG. Prevalence of systemic venous congestion assessed by Venous Excess Ultrasound Grading System (VExUS) and association with acute kidney injury in a general ICU cohort: a prospective multicentric study. Crit Care. 2023;27(1):224. https://doi.org/10.1186/s13054-023-04524-4.
124. Torres-Arrese M, Mata-Martínez A, Luordo-Tedesco D, et al. Usefulness of systemic venous ultrasound protocols in the prognosis of heart failure patients: results from a prospective multicentric study. J Clin Med. 2023;12(4):1281. https://doi.org/10.3390/jcm12041281.
125. Bhardwaj V, Vikneswaran G, Rola P, et al. Combination of inferior vena cava diameter, hepatic venous flow, and portal vein pulsatility index: venous excess ultrasound score (VEXUS score) in predicting acute kidney injury in patients with Cardiorenal syndrome: a prospective cohort study. Indian J Crit Care Med Peer-Rev. 2020;24(9):783–9. https://doi.org/10.5005/jp-journals-10071-23570.
126. Longino A, Martin K, Leyba K, et al. Correlation between the VExUS score and right atrial pressure: a pilot prospective observational study. Crit Care. 2023;27(1):205. https://doi.org/10.1186/s13054-023-04471-0.
127. Beaubien-Souligny W, Galarza L, Buchannan B, et al. Prospective study of ultrasound markers of organ congestion in critically ill patients with acute kidney injury. Kidney Int Rep. 2024;9(3):694–702. https://doi.org/10.1016/j.ekir.2023.12.018.
128. Aslaner MA, Helvacı Ö, Haycock K, et al. Diagnostic accuracy of venous system ultrasound for subtypes of acute kidney injury. Emerg Med J. 2024;41(5):304–10. https://doi.org/10.1136/emermed-2023-213241.
129. Natraj R, Bhaskaran AK, Rola P, Haycock K, Siuba MT, Ranjit S. Venous congestion assessed by venous excess ultrasound (VExUS) and acute kidney injury in children with right ventricular dysfunction. Indian J Crit Care Med Peer-Rev. 2024;28(5):447–52. https://doi.org/10.5005/jp-journals-10071-24705.
130. Islas-Rodríguez JP, Miranda-Aquino T, Romero-González G, et al. Effect on kidney function recovery guiding decongestion with VExUS in patients with Cardiorenal syndrome 1: a randomized control trial. Cardiorenal Med. 2024;14(1):1–11. https://doi.org/10.1159/000535641.
131. Koratala A, Romero-González G, Soliman-Aboumarie H, Kazory A. Unlocking the potential of VExUS in assessing venous congestion: the art of doing it right. Cardiorenal Med. 2024:350. https://doi.org/10.1159/000539469.
132. Dalla Betta MB, Esener D, Swanson W, Kaddis A, Aguayo Romero F, Fields JM. The frequency of POCUS in the treatment of sepsis in the emergency department: a retrospective cohort study. POCUS J. 2023;8(1):71–80. https://doi.org/10.24908/pocus.v8i1.15683.
133. Vincent JL, De Backer D. Circulatory shock. N Engl J Med. 2013;369(18):1726–34. https://doi.org/10.1056/NEJMra1208943.
134. Cortellaro F, Ferrari L, Molteni F, et al. Accuracy of point of care ultrasound to identify the source of infection in septic patients: a prospective study. Intern Emerg Med. 2017;12(3):371–8. https://doi.org/10.1007/s11739-016-1470-2.
135. Haydar SA, Moore ET, Higgins GL, Irish CB, Owens WB, Strout TD. Effect of bedside ultrasonography on the certainty of physician clinical decisionmaking for septic patients in the emergency department. Ann Emerg Med. 2012;60(3):346–358.e4. https://doi.org/10.1016/j.annemergmed.2012.01.006.
136. L'Heureux M, Sternberg M, Brath L, Turlington J, Kashiouris MG. Sepsis-induced cardiomyopathy: a comprehensive review. Curr Cardiol Rep. 2020;22(5):35. https://doi.org/10.1007/s11886-020-01277-2.
137. Beesley SJ, Weber G, Sarge T, et al. Septic cardiomyopathy. Crit Care Med. 2018;46(4):625–34. https://doi.org/10.1097/CCM.0000000000002851.
138. Vieillard-Baron A, Prin S, Chergui K, Dubourg O, Jardin F. Hemodynamic instability in sepsis: bedside assessment by Doppler echocardiography. Am J Respir Crit Care Med. 2003;168(11):1270–6. https://doi.org/10.1164/rccm.200306-816CC.
139. Vieillard-Baron A, Prigent A, Repessé X, et al. Right ventricular failure in septic shock: characterization, incidence and impact on fluid responsiveness. Crit Care. 2020;24(1):630. https://doi.org/10.1186/s13054-020-03345-z.
140. Evans JS, Huang SJ, McLean AS, Nalos M. Left ventricular outflow tract obstruction-be prepared! Anaesth Intensive Care. 2017;45(1):12–20. https://doi.org/10.1177/0310057X1704500103.
141. Balik M, Novotny A, Suk D, et al. Vasopressin in patients with septic shock and dynamic left ventricular outflow tract obstruction. Cardiovasc Drugs Ther. 2020;34(5):685–8. https://doi.org/10.1007/s10557-020-06998-8.
142. Di Vece D, Silverio A, Bellino M, et al. Dynamic left intraventricular obstruction phenotype in Takotsubo syndrome. J Clin Med. 2021;10(15):3235. https://doi.org/10.3390/jcm10153235.
143. Pablo CR, David AO, Carlos V, et al. Beta blockers as salvage treatment in refractory septic shock complicated with dynamic left ventricular outflow tract obstruction: a rare case presentation. J Investig Med High Impact Case Rep. 2021;9:23247096211056491. https://doi.org/10.1177/23247096211056491.
144. Malbrain MLNG, Van Regenmortel N, Saugel B, et al. Principles of fluid management and stewardship in septic shock: it is time to consider the four D's and the four phases of fluid therapy.

Ann Intensive Care. 2018;8(1):66. https://doi.org/10.1186/s13613-018-0402-x.

145. Santa-Teresa P, Muñoz J, Montero I, et al. Incidence and prognosis of intra-abdominal hypertension in critically ill medical patients: a prospective epidemiological study. Ann Intensive Care. 2012;2(Suppl 1):S3. https://doi.org/10.1186/2110-5820-2-S1-S3.
146. Boyd JH, Forbes J, Nakada T-A, Walley KR, Russell JA. Fluid resuscitation in septic shock: a positive fluid balance and elevated central venous pressure are associated with increased mortality. Crit Care Med. 2011;39(2):259–65. https://doi.org/10.1097/CCM.0b013e3181feeb15.
147. Cherpanath TGV, Geerts BF, Lagrand WK, Schultz MJ, Groeneveld ABJ. Basic concepts of fluid responsiveness. Neth Heart J. 2013;21(12):530–6. https://doi.org/10.1007/s12471-013-0487-7.
148. Sweeney DA, Wiley BM. Integrated multiorgan bedside ultrasound for the diagnosis and management of sepsis and septic shock. Semin Respir Crit Care Med. 2021;42(5):641–9. https://doi.org/10.1055/s-0041-1733896.
149. Guerin L, Monnet X, Teboul JL. Monitoring volume and fluid responsiveness: from static to dynamic indicators. Best Pract Res Clin Anaesthesiol. 2013;27(2):177–85. https://doi.org/10.1016/j.bpa.2013.06.002.
150. Monnet X, Marik PE, Teboul JL. Prediction of fluid responsiveness: an update. Ann Intensive Care. 2016;6(1):111. https://doi.org/10.1186/s13613-016-0216-7.
151. Jabot J, Teboul JL, Richard C, Monnet X. Passive leg raising for predicting fluid responsiveness: importance of the postural change. Intensive Care Med. 2009;35(1):85. https://doi.org/10.1007/s00134-008-1293-3.
152. Boulain T, Achard JM, Teboul JL, Richard C, Perrotin D, Ginies G. Changes in BP induced by passive leg raising predict response to fluid loading in critically ill patients. Chest. 2002;121(4):1245–52. https://doi.org/10.1378/chest.121.4.1245.
153. Vignon P, Repessé X, Bégot E, et al. Comparison of echocardiographic indices used to predict fluid responsiveness in ventilated patients. Am J Respir Crit Care Med. 2017;195(8):1022–32. https://doi.org/10.1164/rccm.201604-0844OC.
154. Marik PE, Cavallazzi R. Does the central venous pressure predict fluid responsiveness? An updated meta-analysis and a plea for some common sense. Crit Care Med. 2013;41(7):1774–81. https://doi.org/10.1097/CCM.0b013e31828a25fd.
155. Muller L, Toumi M, Bousquet PJ, et al. An increase in aortic blood flow after an infusion of 100 ml colloid over 1 minute can predict fluid responsiveness: the mini-fluid challenge study. Anesthesiology. 2011;115(3):541–7. https://doi.org/10.1097/ALN.0b013e318229a500.
156. Wu Y, Zhou S, Zhou Z, Liu B. A 10-second fluid challenge guided by transthoracic echocardiography can predict fluid responsiveness. Crit Care. 2014;18(3):R108. https://doi.org/10.1186/cc13891.
157. Theerawit P, Touman N, Sutherasan Y, Kiatboonsri S. Transthoracic ultrasound assessment of B-lines for identifying the increment of extravascular lung water in shock patients requiring fluid resuscitation. Indian J Crit Care Med. 2014;18(4):195–9. https://doi.org/10.4103/0972-5229.130569.
158. Romano M, Viana E, Martins JD, Corga Da Silva R. Evaluation of congestion levels in septic patients admitted to critical care units with a combined venous excess-lung ultrasound score (VExLUS)—a research protocol. POCUS J. 2023;8(1):93–8. https://doi.org/10.24908/pocus.v8i1.16188.
159. Melo RH, Santos MHCD, da Ramos FJS. Beyond fluid responsiveness: the concept of fluid tolerance and its potential implication in hemodynamic management. Crit Care Sci. 2023;35(2):226–9. https://doi.org/10.5935/2965-2774.20230012-en.
160. Tullo G, Candelli M, Gasparrini I, Micci S, Franceschi F. Ultrasound in sepsis and septic shock-from diagnosis to treatment. J Clin Med. 2023;12(3):1185. https://doi.org/10.3390/jcm12031185.

Ultrasound Education

24

Paul Olszynski and Youyou Duanmu

Background

Point-of-care ultrasound (POCUS) education began largely ad hoc as ultrasound was brought to the bedside of emergency medicine in the 1980s. Since then, POCUS has become a core competency in emergency medicine residency training and an increasingly important clinical tool for many other medical specialties. Several medical schools have incorporated POCUS into their curricula because of its superiority to common physical examination maneuvers and the shift toward clinically grounded training. For those seeking to become leaders in the field of POCUS, dedicated ultrasound fellowships have been established to provide advanced training expanding beyond the clinical use of ultrasound to also include administrative, educational, and research aspects of POCUS. As POCUS continues to expand, it will also remain critically important to address continuing professional development among the post-residency physicians using it in practice.

POCUS is a uniquely multidimensional skill that requires knowledge of anatomy, hand–eye coordination, and image interpretation, all set upon a strong foundation in clinical assessment and decision-making. Teaching POCUS thus demands a deliberate approach to curriculum design and assessment to ensure learners are proficient in all domains of POCUS. This chapter reviews established learning principles and theories as well as recent innovations in medical education that can be applied to maximize the effectiveness of POCUS teaching efforts.

Curricular Design

Curriculum design typically starts with the end in mind, meaning educators should clearly identify the desired learning outcomes of the educational program (informed by the learners' needs). Then, they should build out the rest of the educational session or program from there. To do so efficiently, educators need a stepwise, reproducible, iterative, logical approach to developing a curriculum. One commonly used curriculum design model is Kern's six-step approach to curriculum design [1]. This model includes the following steps: (i) problem identification and general needs assessment, (ii) targeted needs assessment, (iii) goals and objectives, (iv) educational strategies, (v) implementation, and (vi) evaluation and feedback (Fig. 24.1).

P. Olszynski (✉)
Department of Emergency Medicine, University of Saskatchewan, Saskatoon, SK, Canada
e-mail: p.olszynski@usask.ca

Y. Duanmu
Department of Emergency Medicine, Stanford University, Palo Alto, CA, USA
e-mail: yduanmu@stanford.edu

M. Gottlieb, N. Panebianco (eds.), *Advanced Point-of-Care Ultrasound*, https://doi.org/10.1007/978-3-031-85308-1_24

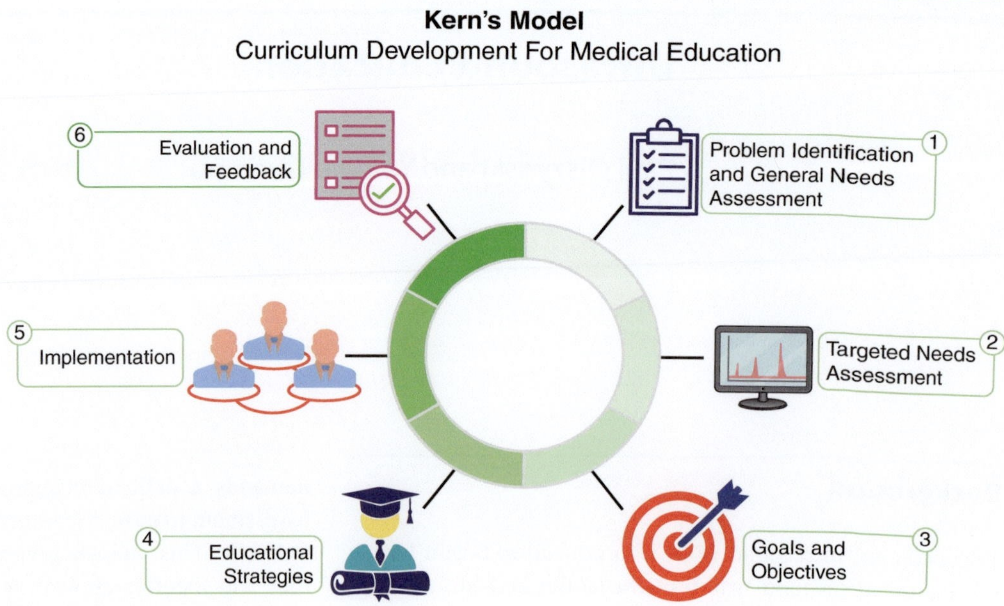

Fig. 24.1 Kern's model of curriculum design in medical education [1]

Problem Identification and Needs Assessment

It is important to begin with problem identification and both a general and targeted needs assessment. The general needs assessment process can start with a review of national standards and guidelines, such as the expectations for a graduating emergency medicine physician [2, 3]. Next, identify the targeted needs for the local context. This latter aspect should focus on the known stakeholders, including trainees (i.e., those who influence or are impacted by the curriculum), and may include informal discussions or more rigorous processes like surveys, focus groups, interviews, or assessment of annual training data (e.g., in-service examination scores, board examination pass rates) [4].

Goals and Objectives

When developing the educational session, identify what the goals (i.e., broader, overarching purpose) and objectives (i.e., discrete, measurable outcomes) of the program should be. This approach is also known as backward curriculum design since it starts with the desired outcomes, and then content, equipment, instructors, and space needs are planned accordingly [5]. A single-occurrence ultrasound training session will likely include more modest goals and learning objectives than a comprehensive longitudinal ultrasound program. While the former can focus on knowledge of indications, scan acquisition, and interpretation of common findings for a select ultrasound application, the latter will likely have more robust outcomes that go beyond knowledge and image acquisition skills. When developing goals and objectives, it is important to also reflect on what resources are available to ensure feasibility.

One model to help frame objectives is Bloom's taxonomy (Fig. 24.2) [6]. This model uses a pyramid ranging from simple recall to the creation of novel information by the trainee. While most curricula will not have objectives at all six levels, this can help inform a more robust set of objectives and avoid exclusively low-level (e.g., recall, describe) objectives. In addition to considering the level, educators should also ensure the objectives are clear and concrete enough to be adequately assessed. One approach to this is to use the SMART criteria: Specific, Measurable, Achievable, Relevant, and Time-Bound. For example, if one were seeking to create a learning objective for a cardiac ultrasound course, one could select "Understand cardiac ultrasound views." However, a better learning objective would be: "By the end of this course, learners will be able to generate parasternal long axis views of sufficient quality for interpretation."

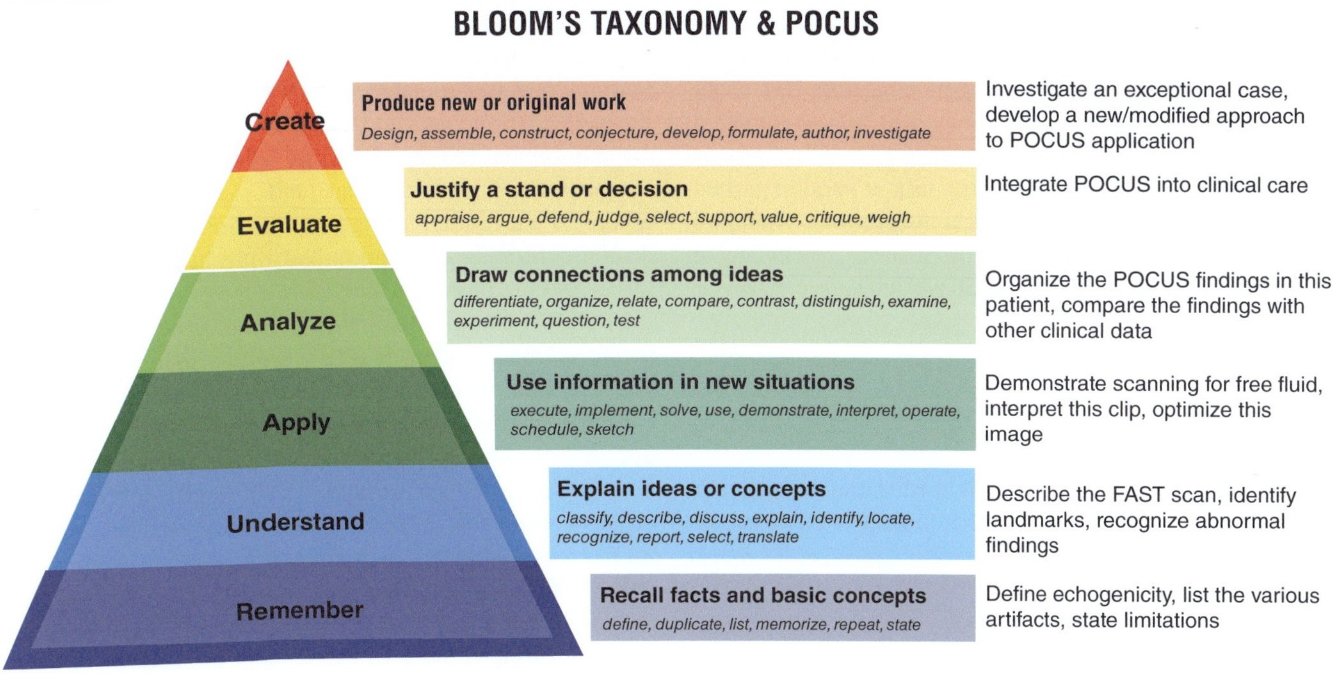

Fig. 24.2 Bloom's taxonomy of learning objectives and key terms as related to POCUS. (*Adapted from https://cft.vanderbilt.edu/guides-sub-pages/blooms-taxonomy/*)

Educational Strategies

After determining that the training request and goals are appropriate for the trainees, the next step is choosing how to best meet the goals. Teaching POCUS can be very resource intensive since proficiency includes cognitive domains (e.g., knowledge of indications, test characteristics, appropriate clinical integration) as well as psychomotor skill development (e.g., sonographic skills for image acquisition and optimization) (Table 24.1) [7]. In acute and critical care settings especially, proficiency in clinical integration also requires situational awareness, a rationale for employing a specific scan or technique at a given moment, and an ability to interpret the findings accurately and rapidly during resuscitation.

From a historical perspective, POCUS training started as in-person courses and workshops for physicians already in practice that included a mix of lectures and hands-on supervised scanning using simulated patients. These types of sessions are popular among physician learners but require significant resources (e.g., large number of instructors, ultrasound machines, standardized patients), making them difficult for many medical school and residency programs to afford. To address this cost barrier, didactic content has shifted to online platforms (e.g., podcasts, video tutorials, free open access medical education (FOAM) resources, and learning management systems), thus saving some of the time and money spent on these during workshops; however, the need for supervised scanning and longitudinal coaching persists. Technology-enhanced learning solutions, including image archival systems, enable remote, asynchronous supervision and feedback for trainees at sites with few qualified experts. POCUS simulation can also be used to safely introduce trainees to ultrasound-guided procedures and invasive diagnostic applications such as transvaginal and transesophageal ultrasound. These modalities can also help expose learners to a wide range of ultrasound-related pathology in a nonclinical setting, providing opportunities to explore and integrate findings into simulated clinical scenarios.

Table 24.1 The I-AIM model for clinical ultrasound [7]

Model component	Examples
Indications	Evidence-based, mechanism-specific, scope of practice
Acquisition	Patient positioning, probe type, probe and machine adjustments, image capture
Interpretation	Recognition of structures and relevant findings, identifying artifacts and pathology
Medical decision-making	Incorporating ultrasound into the clinical context and pretest probability, incorporating ultrasound test characteristics into the findings

Learning Theories

Before implementing a curriculum, it is helpful to understand some of the foundational learning theories that inform how learning happens. There are five main learning orientations from which many of the major contemporary learning theories are derived: behaviorist, cognitivist, social learning, constructivist, and humanist [8]. Few educators rely exclusively on a single orientation; many will use a number of these depending on the learner level (e.g., medical student versus POCUS fellow) and learning task at hand (e.g., bedside procedural skills versus clinical integration). Therefore, a working knowledge of these orientations, including an understanding of their strengths and weaknesses, can be very useful.

Behaviorist Orientation

Central to the behaviorist approach to education is the notion that educator feedback (or stimuli) directly impacts behavioral changes in the learner. By providing positive feedback, a correctly performed task is reinforced. By providing corrective feedback, a learner improves their performance in a safe educational environment. An example of this is deliberate practice, where repeated cycles of feedback are given to a learner who is motivated to improve and is provided with opportunities to improve over time.

Deliberate practice, rather than mere experience alone, has been shown to be a key contributor to expertise [9]. It is through a combination of dedicated practice over time and deliberate attention to specific aspects of the skill in question that one can achieve expertise. In other words, it is not "practice makes perfect," but rather "perfect practice makes perfect." More recent research has focused on using mastery learning within ultrasound, a theory built upon learner-centric progression using serial practice and structured feedback [10–12]. Emphasizing feedback for performance improvement, familiar to most medical educators, is based upon the behaviorist orientation. However, relying solely on the behaviorist orientation risks oversimplifying the learning process itself.

Cognitivist Orientation

Unlike the behaviorist orientation, the cognitivist orientation recognizes that learning is more complex than simple feedback loops and their resultant performance changes. The cognitivist orientation focuses on optimizing the learners' cognitive and information processing during the learning process itself. To optimize learning and to inform training strategies, cognitivist learning theories leverage hypotheses of how learners structure knowledge, how knowledge is transferred from their limited working memory into a long-term stable memory for storage, and how memory retrieval and automation subsequently occur.

Cognitive load theory is one commonly described learning theory rooted in the cognitivist tradition, whereby a learning task is associated with three types of cognitive load: intrinsic, extraneous, and germane [13]. Intrinsic load is directly related to the complexity of the task, relative to the learner's baseline knowledge and skills. Extraneous load relates to educational designs or environmental aspects that do not contribute to learning and may in fact distract from learning (e.g., receiving clinical care pages or messages during POCUS training, being posed questions that do not relate to the learning task at hand). Germane load relates to the actual cognitive load devoted to the task of learning itself. Effective learning occurs when the sum of these three loads does not exceed the learner's overall total cognitive capacity. For example, asking a learner to fan through a subcostal view of the heart may be associated with a very high intrinsic load for a novice completely unfamiliar with cardiac anatomy, but only moderately so for a learner who has reviewed the scan technique and relevant sonographic anatomy. This same task may pose little to no intrinsic load to an advanced learner familiar with this scan, who may be ready for additional learning in image optimization, interpretation, and clinical integration. The role of the educator is to determine how to structure the training session so that the intrinsic load is manageable for the target learner and that the extraneous load is kept to a minimum.

Social Learning Orientation

While both behaviorist and cognitivist learning orientations emphasize the individual aspect of the learning process, social learning theories view learning within a social context, where learning can occur through observations and interactions with others, even in the absence of any direct feedback. For example, a small group of POCUS fellows scanning together affords an excellent opportunity to learn from each other without a preceptor present. However, learning is only effective if the desired behavior or target performance is known to the group of learners. A group of novices who do not know where to begin will not be an effective learning exercise. They are also at risk of learning incorrect techniques from each other. Therefore, while potentially effective, educators need to keep these limitations in mind and provide clear learning objectives and resources to the group.

Constructivist Orientation

In the constructivist orientation, learning is an active process whereby knowledge is co-created by the learners themselves, where learners construct meaning for themselves. The role of the educator in this orientation would be to create a supported learning environment that can empower and encourage learners to build their own knowledge and skills. One example of this would be for learners to create a concept map. A concept map is a diagram or figure that can demonstrate relationships between different concepts. In this context, the learners could recreate the Rapid Ultrasound for Shock and Hypotension (RUSH) examination and then identify how the elements of this protocol overlap with other protocols (e.g., cardiac assessment, aorta assessment, focused assessment with sonography in trauma (FAST)).

Humanist Orientation

An educator with a humanist orientation emphasizes that learning is self-directed and a part of a learner's self-actualization process to fulfill their own potential and their own ideal self. The role of the educator in this orientation may therefore be as a facilitator for this growth or a role model. An example of this would be the self-determination theory, which is centered around learners' motivation. Self-determination theory involves three main components: autonomy, competence, and relatedness [14]. Autonomy is focused on freedom and intrinsic drive or motivation to learn. Notably, providing external rewards (extrinsic motivation) can actually detract from one's own motivation to learn (intrinsic motivation) [15]. Competence is built upon the idea of learners seeking mastery or expertise on a topic and can be enhanced with positive feedback [15]. Finally, relatedness refers to a sense of belonging and relation to others. If applying self-determination theory to an ultrasound rotation, educators might emphasize having small groups of learners (relatedness), providing positive feedback highlighting successes and growth (autonomy), and encouraging continued learning toward mastery (competence).

Assessment and Evaluation

The next step is to determine the approach to assessment and evaluation, which should always be considered prior to the curriculum being initiated. Assessment is learner-centric, whereas evaluation is more program-centric and informs how well the curriculum is performing in terms of meeting objectives. Moreover, assessment is further divided into assessment for learning (i.e., formative feedback) and assessment of learning (i.e., summative assessment of their learning). We will discuss each of the following separately below. However, it is important to note that these are often interrelated, such that assessment of learning across the group of learners can also serve as an outcome for evaluation of the program itself.

Feedback

Feedback is a critical element for learner improvement and integral to many education theories described above. Feedback should follow the same SMART criteria described earlier for learning objectives [16]. A number of feedback models commonly known and used in clinical medicine can also apply to POCUS teaching, including the Pendleton rules [17], the One-Minute Preceptor model [18], and R2C2 [19, 20] (Table 24.2).

Table 24.2 Common feedback models

Feedback model	Recommended steps	Example of POCUS-specific application
Pendleton rules	1. Ask the learner what went well 2. Tell the learner what went well 3. Ask if there was anything they would do differently 4. Share points for improvement	After a trauma resuscitation, the preceptor can ask the learner how the FAST performance and interpretation went, what went well, and what could be improved upon
One-minute preceptor model	1. Get a commitment from the learner 2. Probe for supporting evidence 3. Teach general rules 4. Reinforce what was done correctly 5. Correct mistakes	1. Get a commitment from the learner regarding their interpretation of findings from a cardiac scan 2. Ask the learner what made them determine that the systolic function was severely decreased 3. Teach general rules about decreased systolic function for that view 4. Reinforce what was done well 5. Correct any knowledge errors
R2C2 model	1. Build relationships 2. Explore reactions 3. Explore content 4. Coach for performance change	1. Preceptor builds rapport with the learner during a scan shift by clarifying their goals to work on image acquisition skills 2. Explore the learner's reaction to feedback given about their POCUS image acquisition skills 3. Help the learner understand the content of the feedback and what determinate/indeterminate criteria their scans are measured against 4. Coach the learner in identifying gaps and goal setting

FAST focused assessment with sonography in trauma

Assessment of Learning

Increasingly, POCUS educators are calling for programmatic assessment that involves several varied, low- and medium-stakes assessments [21, 22]. These include workplace-based assessments, quizzes, portfolios, objective structured clinical exams (OSCEs), and other assessment modalities and are considered the best-suited approach to determining proficiency in a given domain or skill (Fig. 24.3). Importantly, this should extend well beyond purely tracking the total number of scans performed, as this can be a poor surrogate for skill assessment [22].

While students should be held accountable for their learning through assessment, Kern specifically states educators are also accountable for the outcomes of their educational sessions. Specifically, educators can (and should) determine if the session resulted in the expected gains in knowledge, skills, or both.

> First, educational programs have aims or goals, whether or not they are clearly articulated. Second, medical educators have a professional and ethical obligation to meet the needs of their learners, patients, and society. Third, medical educators should be held accountable for the outcomes of their interventions. And fourth, a logical, systematic approach to curriculum development will help achieve these ends. [1]

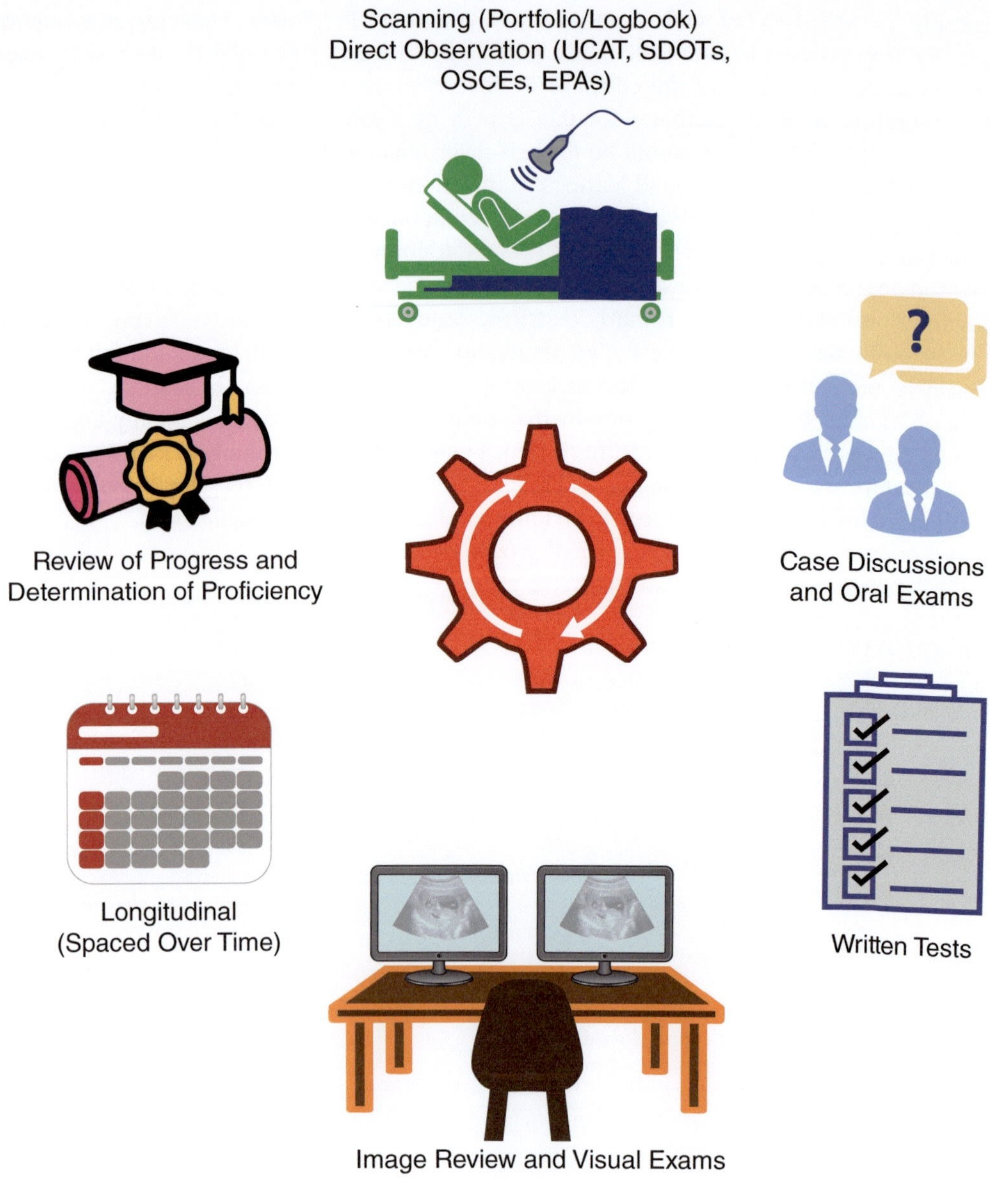

Fig. 24.3 Programmatic assessment for POCUS trainees. *UCAT* ultrasound competency assessment tool, *SDOT* standardized direct observation tool, *OSCE* objective structured clinical encounter, *EPA* entrustable professional activity

Educators can demonstrate these gains by measuring trainee performance using various assessment tools. Such assessments can include simple quizzes or structured encounters using validated checklists like the Ultrasound Competency Assessment Tool (UCAT) or Standardized Direct Observation Tests (SDOTs). More recently, there has also been an increasing focus on entrustable professional activities (EPAs), which are assessed through workplace-based assessments of tasks or actions that programs expect trainees to perform independently upon graduation of the program [23] (Table 24.3). POCUS as an EPA integrates well within a competency-based model of training, and efforts are ongoing to further develop and refine these for residency and fellowship programs. With programmatic assessment in mind, the more assessment points of various types, the more data educators have to make sound determinations of proficiency and readiness for independent practice [24, 25].

Program Evaluation

There are numerous models available for evaluating an educational session or program. One of the most widely used models for evaluating the effectiveness of an educational program is the Kirkpatrick model [26, 27]. This model applies four levels of training assessment: reaction, learning, behavior, and results (Table 24.4). Other common models for program evaluation include context, input, process, and product (CIPP); the logic model; the realist approach; and reach, effectiveness, adoption, implementation, and maintenance (RE-AIM) [28, 29]. Regardless of the specific program evaluation model selected, the key is to consider a broad array of inputs (e.g., preparatory time, costs, space, resources) and outputs (e.g., learner and system outputs, program resources created). By using a robust and inclusive model, educators can help to measure, refine, and ensure the quality of POCUS curricula, as well as to guide rigorous POCUS education research.

Table 24.3 O-score entrustability scale and point of care ultrasound

Level	Descriptor by assessor	Descriptor by assessor regarding POCUS
1	Requires complete hands-on guidance, did not do, or was not given the opportunity to do. *"I had to do"*	Not familiar with the POCUS application and is unable to perform it. *"I had to demonstrate all aspects of the scan"*
2	Able to perform tasks but requires constant direction. *"I had to talk them through"*	Familiar with some aspects of the scan including indications and key landmarks but needs consistent guidance/reminders. *"I had to talk them through transducer maneuvers and interpretation of the image"*
3	Demonstrates some independence but requires intermittent direction. *"I had to prompt them from time to time"*	Is able to perform most of the scan but requires occasional prompting to complete it. *"I had to remind them to adjust depth, gain and/or transducer position in order for the image to be adequate for interpretation"*
4	Independence but unaware of risks and still requires supervision for safe practice. *"I need to be in the room just I case"*	Performs the scan but fails to optimize the image and/or lacks confidence/efficiency. *"I had to reassure them that the scan was adequate and provided advice to improving scan efficiency"*
5	Shows complete independence, understands risks and performs safely, practice ready. *"I did not need to be there"*	Performs the scan proficiently with appropriate optimization and clinical integration. *"Performs the POCUS application efficiently"*

Table 24.4 Kirkpatrick model [26, 27]

Level	Summary	Example
1. Reaction	Learners' feelings toward the educational experience (e.g., teachers, materials, activities)	Survey assessing learners' overall experience with the ultrasound rotation and which components they found most versus least valuable
2. Learning	Changes in learners' knowledge, skills, and attitudes	Post-rotation multiple-choice test and SDOT
3. Behavior	Changes in learners' practice	Tracking of ultrasound examinations performed for clinical applications post-rotation
4. Results	Changes at the broader, system level	Tracking of improvement in throughput and patient-relevant outcomes resulting from the rotation or training

SDOT standardized direct observation tool

Training for Specific Learner Populations

POCUS in Undergraduate Medical Education

With a growing number of disciplines adopting an expanding number of POCUS applications, it is not surprising that many educators have turned their attention to medical schools. Data suggest that approximately 57% of medical schools have a POCUS curriculum, with the majority occurring in the first or second year [30]. Since proficiency in POCUS takes a significant amount of time and effort, it is a good idea to start early. However, scaling up POCUS training to include the hundreds of trainees enrolled in an undergraduate medical education (UME) program can require significant planning and effort.

There have been a few consensus statements aimed at identifying the knowledge and skills learners should be introduced to during their UME training [31, 32]. While these are very comprehensive, this may not be possible for all institutions. Therefore, POCUS educators should coordinate with UME leadership to understand how POCUS should fit within the existing UME curriculum objectives, training, and assessment. For example, trainees are expected to have a clinical approach to common medical presentations like shortness of breath and abdominal pain. POCUS can then be integrated into these existing training objectives. In building a UME POCUS program, consider starting with achievable objectives and early successes; then, build upon this to develop the program upward as access to POCUS equipment and resources increases.

The most common teaching modalities used in UME to date include lectures/tutorials (in-person or online) and hands-on scanning sessions [30]. However, as technology has advanced, portable devices and cloud-based image archiving have enabled a relatively small number of faculty to remotely supervise significantly more trainees [33]. Furthermore, learning management systems allow for asynchronous learning through video tutorials, assignments, and online quizzes. The next frontier in UME POCUS may involve using artificial intelligence (AI) to identify trends in learner skill deficiencies and areas for growth, as well as AI-guided scanning to reduce the need for instructor-based sessions, which remains a common barrier [34].

POCUS in Residency Education

The structure and content of POCUS education in residency are influenced by the practice needs and goals of trainees upon graduation. Emergency medicine was the first specialty in the United States and Canada to incorporate longitudinal POCUS training as a part of residency curricula. The Accreditation Council for Graduate Medical Education (ACGME) requires emergency medicine graduates to demonstrate proficiency in POCUS within multiple residency milestones, including diagnostic testing, resuscitation management, and procedural guidance [35]. These skills have been deemed necessary for providing a standard of care as a graduating emergency medicine attending. This has been evidenced by a rise in POCUS examinations performed over time within emergency medicine residency programs [36]. In recent years, specialties including internal medicine, family medicine, critical care, general surgery, obstetrics and gynecology, pediatrics, and others have proposed or implemented POCUS education in their residency training [37, 38].

For residencies incorporating POCUS training with the goal of independent practice, the mainstays of an ultrasound curriculum often include guided scanning shifts, didactic lectures, assigned online or textbook reading, hands-on workshops, quizzes, and quality assurance review through feedback of scans performed. Emergency medicine residencies generally require an ultrasound rotation lasting 2–4 weeks with the option for additional elective rotations later in residency training [39]. The required ultrasound rotation should provide a framework for core POCUS modalities, informed by societal guidelines. For example, the American College of Emergency Physicians recommends 15 core applications within the scope of practice for graduating emergency medicine physicians (Table 24.5) [2]. Ultrasound electives later in residency may include further training in advanced modalities such as resuscitative ultrasound, as well as options for pursuing further educational, research, or quality improvement projects [40].

Programs should track resident progress over time and provide regular updates and feedback on their progress. This should include both tracking of the number of POCUS scans performed (e.g., total number and distribution of POCUS examination type) as well as the quality of the images.

Table 24.5 List of core POCUS applications for emergency medicine

Aorta
Bowel
Cardiac/hemodynamic assessment
Deep vein thrombosis
Hepatobiliary
Musculoskeletal
Ocular
Pediatric (appendicitis, hypertrophic pyloric stenosis, intussusception, lung, musculoskeletal)
Pregnancy
Procedural guidance
Skin and soft tissue
Testicular
Thoracic/airway
Trauma
Ultrasound-guided nerve blocks
Urinary tract

Currently, this can be performed using middleware solutions, learning management systems, or during image review. However, as technology evolves, there may be a role for AI to identify growth trajectories and areas for remediation and focused skill interventions [34].

POCUS in Ultrasound Fellow Education

Clinical ultrasound fellowship training is geared toward both advanced clinical ultrasound skills as well as additional administrative, educational, and research skills [41]. The Emergency Ultrasound Fellowship Accreditation Council has instituted minimum requirements a program must meet in order to be designated as an accredited fellowship. At the time of writing, these minimum requirements for fellows include performing 1000 scans, having scans be reviewed for quality assurance by ultrasound-trained faculty, becoming proficient as an ultrasound educator, and taking part in ultrasound research and quality improvement endeavors [42]. The Royal College of Physicians and Surgeons of Canada has issued similar requirements for accreditation of Acute Care POCUS Fellowships. As ultrasound fellows often become leaders in POCUS within their future departments, their training should also include the knowledge necessary to train and credential POCUS trainees, enact quality assurance reviews, select and maintain ultrasound equipment, and incorporate POCUS billing into departmental finances.

Fellowship training beyond the minimum requirements is determined by the mission and areas of focus of specific institutions, as well as the goals of individual fellow trainees. Fellowship training often involves further instruction in medical education, including the skills for creating didactic lectures, running hands-on workshops, and developing ultrasound curricula. Fellows may also pursue further training in research methodology to gain the skills necessary to advance and expand the field of POCUS research.

In the United States, emergency medicine-trained clinical ultrasound fellowship graduates have the option to sit for the American Board of Emergency Medicine Focused Practice Designation in Advanced Emergency Medicine Ultrasonography [43, 44]. In Canada, ultrasound-trained physicians can obtain a practice-eligible designation of an Area of Focused Competence in Acute Care Point-of-Care Ultrasonography through the Royal College of Physicians and Surgeons of Canada [44]. POCUS certification options for physicians who are not boarded in emergency medicine remain limited. The National Board of Echocardiography provides a certification pathway in critical care echocardiography, and there are several certificate programs across the specialties, but a specialty-agnostic POCUS certification exam for all physicians currently does not exist in the United States. In Canada, the Canadian Point of Care Ultrasound Society (CPOCUS) does offer certification in POCUS for a range of disciplines based on the applications and skills acquired, regardless of specialty.

Faculty POCUS Training and Skill Maintenance

Faculty who trained prior to the implementation of structured POCUS education in residency may choose to follow a practice-based pathway to attain POCUS proficiency. A practice-based POCUS training program should include established course material covering POCUS indications, technique, and interpretation, as well as longitudinal hands-on practice and clinical experience including observed preceptorships and feedback.

Faculty may also be asked to complete periodic continuing education endeavors to maintain their certification and skills to practice POCUS in the clinical setting. These requirements are typically set by individual hospital credentialing boards but can involve quality review of a portion of scans performed as well as a specified number of continuing education hours at regular intervals.

As new indications for POCUS are often being introduced, clinical departments have an obligation to ensure faculty are given the opportunity to refresh their skills as well as gain familiarity with POCUS applications introduced after they complete residency training. Faculty development sessions are especially important in academic departments where faculty will be responsible for supervising residents in POCUS applications with which they may be less familiar.

Pearls and Pitfalls

- Curriculum design benefits from an iterative stepwise approach, including performing a needs assessment (general and targeted), setting appropriate learning goals and objectives, selecting appropriate educational strategies, implementing the curriculum, and then evaluating the learner, the curriculum, and the program.
- To teach across the continuum of medical education, an understanding of key learning theories can help educators select the most appropriate educational strategies.
- In the assessment of learner performance, educators should consider the level(s) of learning outcomes assessed and employ a programmatic approach to assessment.
- Feedback should be provided with the intention of fostering a safe and constructive learning environment.

References

1. Kern DE, Thomas PA, Hughes MT. Curriculum development for medical education: a six-step approach. Johns Hopkins University Press; 2009.
2. American College of Emergency Physicians. Ultrasound guidelines: emergency, point-of-care, and clinical ultrasound guidelines in medicine. Ann Emerg Med. 2023;82(3):e115–55. https://doi.org/10.1016/j.annemergmed.2023.06.005.
3. Atkinson P, Bowra J, Lambert M, Lamprecht H, Noble V, Jarman B. International Federation for Emergency Medicine point of care ultrasound curriculum. CJEM. 2015;17(2):161–70. https://doi.org/10.1017/cem.2015.8.
4. Gottlieb M, Wagner E, Wagner A, Chan T. Applying design thinking principles to curricular development in medical education. AEM Educ Train. 2017;1(1):21–6. https://doi.org/10.1002/aet2.10003. Published 2017 Jan 19
5. Wiggins G, McTighe J. Understanding by design. Expanded 2nd ed. Association for Supervision and Curriculum Development; 2005.
6. Anderson LW, Krathwohl DR. A taxonomy for learning, teaching and assessing: a revision of bloom's taxonomy of educational objectives. Complete ed. New York: Longman; 2001.
7. Bahner DP, Hughes D, Royall NA. I-AIM: a novel model for teaching and performing focused sonography. J Ultrasound Med. 2012;31(2):295–300. https://doi.org/10.7863/jum.2012.31.2.295.
8. Torre DM, Daley BJ, Sebastian JL, Elnicki DM. Overview of current learning theories for medical educators. Am J Med. 2006;119(10):903–7. https://doi.org/10.1016/J.AMJMED.2006.06.037.
9. Ericsson KA. Deliberate practice and acquisition of expert performance: a general overview. Acad Emerg Med. 2008;15(11):988–94. https://doi.org/10.1111/J.1553-2712.2008.00227.X.
10. Rider AC, Miller DT, Ashenburg N, Duanmu Y, Lobo V, Schertzer K, Sebok-Syer SS. Using a simulated model and mastery learning approach to teach the ultrasound-guided serratus anterior plane block to emergency medicine residents: a pilot study. AEM Educ Train. 2020;5(3):e10525. https://doi.org/10.1002/aet2.10525. PMID: 34041432; PMCID: PMC8138100.
11. Smith S, Lobo V, Anderson KL, Gisondi MA, Sebok-Syer SS, Duanmu Y. A randomized controlled trial of simulation-based mastery learning to teach the extended focused assessment with sonography in trauma. AEM Educ Train. 2021;5(3):e10606. https://doi.org/10.1002/aet2.10606. PMID: 34141999; PMCID: PMC8190510.
12. Bailitz J, O'Brien J, McCauley M, Murray D, Jung C, Peksa G, Gottlieb M. Development of an expert consensus checklist for emergency ultrasound. AEM Educ Train. 2022;6(4):e10783. https://doi.org/10.1002/aet2.10783. PMID: 35936814; PMCID: PMC9348840.
13. van Merrienboer JJ, Sweller J. Cognitive load theory in health professional education: design principles and strategies. Med Educ. 2010;44(1):85–93.
14. Ryan RM, Deci EL. Self-determination theory and the facilitation of intrinsic motivation, social development, and well-being. Am Psychol. 2000;55(1):68–78. https://doi.org/10.1037/0003-066x.55.1.68.
15. Deci EL. Effects of externally mediated rewards on intrinsic motivation. J Pers Soc Psychol. 1971;18(1):105–15. https://doi.org/10.1037/h0030644.
16. Buckley C, Natesan S, Breslin A, Gottlieb M. Finessing feedback: recommendations for effective feedback in the emergency department. Ann Emerg Med. 2020;75(3):445–51. https://doi.org/10.1016/j.annemergmed.2019.05.016.
17. Pendleton D. The consultation: an approach to learning and teaching. Oxford: Oxford University Press; 1984.
18. Neher JO, Gordon KC, Meyer B, Stevens N. A five-step "microskills" model of clinical teaching. J Am Board Fam Pract. 1992;5(4):419–24.
19. Sargeant J, Lockyer J, Mann K, Holmboe E, Silver I, Armson H, Driessen E, MacLeod T, Yen W, Ross K, Power M. Facilitated reflective performance feedback: developing an evidence- and theory-based model that builds relationship, explores reactions and content, and coaches for performance change (R2C2). Acad Med. 2015;90(12):1698–706. https://doi.org/10.1097/ACM.0000000000000809. PMID: 26200584
20. Natesan S, Jordan J, Sheng A, et al. Feedback in medical education: an evidence-based guide to best practices from the Council of Residency Directors in emergency medicine. West J Emerg Med. 2023;24(3):479–94. https://doi.org/10.5811/westjem.56544. Published 2023 May 5
21. DeBiasio C, Pageau P, Shefrin A, Woo MY, Cheung WJ. Point-of-Care-ultrasound in undergraduate medical education: a scoping review of assessment methods. Ultrasound J. 2023;15(1):30.
22. Gottlieb M, Duanmu Y. Beyond the numbers: assessing competency in point-of-care ultrasound. Ann Emerg Med. 2023;81(4):427–8. https://doi.org/10.1016/j.annemergmed.2023.01.020. Epub 2023 Feb 17
23. Amiel JM, Andriole DA, Biskobing DM, et al. Revisiting the core entrustable professional activities for entering residency. Acad Med. 2021;96(7S):S14–21. https://doi.org/10.1097/ACM.0000000000004088.
24. Damewood SC, Leo M, Bailitz J, et al. Tools for measuring clinical ultrasound competency: recommendations from the ultrasound competency work group. AEM Educ Train. 2019;4(Suppl 1):S106–12. https://doi.org/10.1002/aet2.10368. Published 2019 Jul 30.
25. Gottlieb M, Jordan J, Siegelman JN, Cooney R, Stehman C, Chan TM. Direct observation tools in emergency medicine: a systematic review of the literature. AEM Educ Train. 2020;5(3):e10519. https://doi.org/10.1002/aet2.10519. Published 2020 Sep 4.
26. Kirkpatrick DL. Evaluating Training Programs. San Francisco: Tata McGraw-Hill Education/Berrett-Koehler Publishers; 1975.
27. Kirkpatrick D, Kirkpatrick J. Evaluating training programs: the four levels. San Francisco: Berrett-Koehler Publishers; 2006.
28. Frye AW, Hemmer PA. Program evaluation models and related theories AMEE guide no. 67. Med Teach. 2012;34(5):e288–99. https://doi.org/10.3109/0142159X.2012.668637.
29. Hosseini S, Yilmaz Y, Shah K, et al. Program evaluation: an educator's portal into academic scholarship. AEM Educ Train. 2022;6(Suppl 1):S43–51. https://doi.org/10.1002/aet2.10745. Published 2022 Jun 23
30. Russell FM, Zakeri B, Herbert A, Ferre RM, Leiser A, Wallach PM. The state of point-of-care ultrasound training in undergraduate medical education: findings from a National Survey. Acad Med. 2022;97(5):723–7. https://doi.org/10.1097/ACM.0000000000004512. Epub 2022 Apr 27
31. Ma IWY, Steinmetz P, Weerdenburg K, Woo MY, Olszynski P, Heslop CL, Miller S, Sheppard G, Daniels V, Desy J, Valois M, Devine L, Curtis H, Romano MJ, Martel P, Jelic T, Topping C, Thompson D, Power B, Profetto J, Tonseth P. The Canadian medical student ultrasound curriculum: a statement from the Canadian ultrasound consensus for undergraduate medical education group. J Ultrasound Med. 2020;39(7):1279–87. https://doi.org/10.1002/jum.15218. Epub 2020 Jan 13. PMID: 31943311; PMCID: PMC7317450.
32. Hoppmann RA, Mladenovic J, Melniker L, et al. International consensus conference recommendations on ultrasound education for undergraduate medical students. Ultrasound J. 2022;14:31. https://doi.org/10.1186/s13089-022-00279-1.

33. Panebianco NL, Liu RB, Alerhand S, et al. Joint recommendations and resources for clinical ultrasound education amidst the COVID-19 era. AEM Educ Train. 2020;4(4):438–42. https://doi.org/10.1002/aet2.10506. Published 2020 Sep 4.
34. Kayarian F, Patel D, O'Brien JR, Schraft EK, Gottlieb M. Artificial intelligence and point-of-care ultrasound: benefits, limitations, and implications for the future. Am J Emerg Med. 2024; https://doi.org/10.1016/j.ajem.2024.03.023. Published online March 25
35. Accreditation Council for Graduate Medical Education (ACGME) Emergency Medicine Supplemental Guide. Accessed 12 Dec 2023. Available at: https://www.acgme.org/globalassets/pdfs/milestones/emergencymedicinesupplementalguide.pdf.
36. Gottlieb M, Cooney R, King A, Mannix A, Krzyzaniak S, Jordan J, Shappell E, Fix M. Trends in point-of-care ultrasound use among emergency medicine residency programs over a 10-year period. AEM Educ Train. 2023;7(2):e10853. https://doi.org/10.1002/aet2.10853. PMID: 37008649; PMCID: PMC10061573.
37. LoPresti CM, Schnobrich D, Novak W, Fondahn E, Bardowell R, O'Connor AB, Uthlaut B, Ortiz J, Soni NJ. Current point of care ultrasound use and training among internal medicine residency programs from the 2020 APDIM program director's survey. Am J Med. 2022;135(3):397–404.
38. Hall JWW, Holman H, Barreto T, Bornemann P, Vaughan A, Bennett KJ, Chamberlain J, Micks T, Maurer DM, Bergus GR. Point-of-care ultrasound in family medicine residencies 5-year update: a CERA study. Fam Med. 2020;52(7):505–11. https://doi.org/10.22454/FAMMED.2020.223648.
39. Gottlieb M, Arno K, Kuhns M, Chan TM. Distribution of clinical rotations among emergency medicine residency programs in the United States. AEM Educ Train. 2018;2(4):288–92. https://doi.org/10.1002/aet2.10117. Published 2018 Aug 10.
40. Alerhand S, Situ-Lacasse E, Ramdin C, Gottlieb M. National Survey of point-of-care ultrasound scholarly tracks in emergency medicine residency programs. West J Emerg Med. 2021;22(5):1095–101. https://doi.org/10.5811/westjem.2021.5.52118. Published 2021 Aug 21.
41. Adhikari S, Leo M, Liu R, et al. The 2023 Core content of advanced emergency medicine ultrasonography. J Am Coll Emerg Phys Open. 2023;4(4):e13015. https://doi.org/10.1002/emp2.13015. Published 2023 Aug 9.
42. Emergency Ultrasound Fellowship Accreditation Council AEMUS Program Requirements. Accessed 12 Dec 2023. Available at: https://eufacouncil.org/wp-content/uploads/2023/08/AEMUS-Program-Requirements_2023.pdf
43. American Board of Emergency Medicine. Advanced EM Ultrasonography. Available at: https://www.abem.org/public/become-certified/focused-practice-designation/advanced-em-ultrasonography. Last accessed 25 Apr 2024.
44. Gottlieb M, Duran-Gehring P, Coneybeare D, Lema P. Creation of a novel course for the advanced emergency medicine ultrasound focused practice designation examination. AEM Educ Train. 2022;6(5):e10810. https://doi.org/10.1002/aet2.10810.
45. Royal College of Physicians and Surgeons of Canada. Standards of Accreditation for Areas of Focused Competence Programs in Acute Care Point-of-Care Ultrasonography. Available at: https://www.royalcollege.ca/content/dam/documents/ibd/acute-care-point-of-care-ultrasonography-(pocus)/acute-care-pocus-sa-e.pdf. Last accessed 25 Apr 2024.

Ultrasound Research

25

Hamid Shokoohi, Srikar Adhikari, and Anthony J. Weekes

Introduction

Point-of-care ultrasound (POCUS) has rapidly evolved from a novel technology to an essential component of medical imaging and clinical care across various specialties. The vast proliferation of research projects, dedicated journals, and a wide range of publications and scientific presentations underscore this remarkable success. POCUS technological advancements, a growing emphasis on evidence-based medicine, and the development of standardized training programs and certification processes have all played important roles in driving this success. In this evolution, clinician scientists and researchers have been instrumental in advancing this field by continuously testing and validating its applications and assessing their impact on clinical practice and patient care. The substantial increase in academic positions and the development of training modules, including a rise in fellowship programs within emergency medicine and beyond, have further launched scientific progress in this field [1, 2].

Given the increase in advanced emergency medicine ultrasound fellowships, with research requirements for training program accreditation, along with increasing expansion of POCUS within other specialties, we anticipate a greater urgency for generating research ideas and an increase in research proposals being presented to institutional review boards and submitted for publication. As with all disciplines, generating high-quality research is more important than having a high quantity of research reports. Dissemination of high-quality and clinically relevant research findings to a wide audience can have a positive impact on patient-centered outcomes and clinical practice across multiple disciplines.

As fellows and faculty begin to work on their research initiatives, understanding the unique challenges inherent to POCUS research, and the dynamic between ultrasound technology and its expanding applications, is vital for scientific advancements and improving patient care. Depending on one's prior experience and training in research skills, attending a research skills workshop may be beneficial to gain a solid foundation in study design, research methods, data analysis, and to network with other researchers. This educational step can significantly enhance one's ability to conduct rigorous research and contribute valuable insights to the field of POCUS. Seeking research collaborations is essential for expanding one's publication portfolio. Initially, these don't have to be large, multicenter studies; even small scholarly projects can substantially enrich one's research portfolio. Engaging in collaborations opens opportunities for learning, sharing ideas, and broadening one's research impact across various domains. Early in one's career, it is critical to regularly assess and reevaluate their research portfolio, progress, and achievements at least every 3 months to gauge their impact on career goals and make necessary adjustments [3]. This ongoing self-evaluation is extremely beneficial for advancing a research career, helping to identify strengths and areas for growth. Adjusting strategies based on these reflections can significantly enhance one's research trajectory.

This chapter serves as a guide to help fellows, faculty, and other researchers in navigating a successful path in POCUS research. It offers insights, practical tips, and focused research strategies tailored to this field. Notably, it does not cover finer details of epidemiology, biostatistics, research ethics, and regulation, as these topics are extensively covered in other dedicated publications and textbooks. From main principles to cutting-edge advancements, this chapter

H. Shokoohi (✉)
Department of Emergency Medicine, Massachusetts General Hospital, Harvard Medical School, Boston, MA, USA
e-mail: hshokoohi@mgh.harvard.edu

S. Adhikari
Department of Emergency Medicine, University of Arizona, Tucson, AZ, USA
e-mail: sadhikari@aemrc.arizona.edu

A. J. Weekes
Department of Emergency Medicine, Atrium Health's Carolinas Medical Center, Wake Forest School of Medicine, Charlotte, NC, USA
e-mail: anthony.weekes@atriumhealth.org

M. Gottlieb, N. Panebianco (eds.), *Advanced Point-of-Care Ultrasound*, https://doi.org/10.1007/978-3-031-85308-1_25

explores the key steps in the journey of conducting and reporting research projects effectively. To emphasize these elements, we provide specific examples relevant to POCUS research to accompany recommendations and offer suggestions based on lessons learned from our collective experiences, incorporating both successes and mistakes encountered along the way. Whether new to POCUS research or looking to refine your research expertise, this chapter is designed to provide researchers with essential principles to optimize the quality of their research effort, improve their chances of successful publication, and foster impactful contributions in the field of POCUS research.

The Landscape of Pocus Research

POCUS and Patient-Centered Outcome Research

While POCUS is often seen primarily as a diagnostic imaging tool, rather than as an intervention or a predictor of alternative outcomes, researchers in the field must also understand its potential positive impact on overall patient outcomes. However, existing reports and clinical guidelines primarily focus on traditional patient-centered outcomes, such as mortality, return of spontaneous circulation, and neurological status. While projects centered on these outcomes are effective and impactful, they may not always capture the specific impacts of POCUS. This scarcity of patient-centered outcome-related POCUS research exists because most reports evaluate it solely as a diagnostic tool, rather than as an intervention. Moreover, among the few outcome studies published, POCUS has often demonstrated no significant impact [4–8]. However, this lack of impact is likely due to the inappropriate choice of outcomes studied. For instance, asking whether performing POCUS 30 min into the care of a patient with septic shock affects mortality may not be the right question, as numerous other factors and decisions also influence this outcome.

To address this, researchers should consider a wider range of outcome measures. These include procedural safety, reduction in morbidity, time to treatment, downstream use of imaging, throughput improvement, and patient satisfaction. These metrics can serve as additional patient-oriented outcomes providing valuable insights for clinicians. Ultrasound-guidance for procedures, especially for vascular access, is one of the best examples of a POCUS application having a positive impact on patient-centered outcomes. This practice is prominently featured in evidence-based healthcare recommendations and policies [9, 10].

Despite its benefit in various scenarios, such as cardiopulmonary resuscitation or polytrauma, POCUS has yet to be fully integrated into mainstream clinical protocols like Advanced Cardiovascular Life Support and Advanced Trauma Life Support [11–13]. This lack of incorporation can be attributed to several factors. However, providing further evidence of its efficacy and cost-effectiveness, compared to traditional diagnostic methods, would help this integration.

Finally, there is a clear need for high-quality, multi-institutional, and large-scale prospective research in the field of POCUS to address these challenges and advance the field. When developing ultrasound research projects, researchers should prioritize identifying patient-centered outcomes. This can lead to a greater likelihood of obtaining funding and the ability to conduct more impactful research.

Comparative Diagnostic Accuracy in POCUS Research

In comparison to other imaging modalities, like plain film radiography and computed tomography (CT), POCUS offers the advantage of real-time, rapid diagnosis at the bedside, potentially streamlining downstream testing, and reducing the need for invasive procedures and additional imaging. Consequently, it can substantially impact outcomes such as time to diagnosis, interventions, disposition decisions, radiation exposure, and healthcare costs. While observational studies primarily highlight the diagnostic accuracy of POCUS, their impact on patient-centered outcomes remains uncertain. Thus, focusing exclusively on diagnostic accuracy— compared to other imaging modalities or feasibility studies—may not necessarily yield impactful research, given the existing evidence. For example, while numerous studies have focused on the diagnostic accuracy of POCUS in detecting intra-abdominal free fluid in trauma, small bowel obstruction, pericardial effusion, and pediatric pneumonia, they may lack bigger impact and broader scale implementation unless outcomes extend beyond accuracy. More recently, research has increasingly focused on POCUS in critical illnesses where other imaging may not be feasible or immediately available (e.g., trauma, cardiac arrest, septic shock, undifferentiated hypotension). In these cases, diagnostic accuracy is more meaningful, as there are no alternate options [5, 6, 8, 11, 12, 14, 15]. While diagnostic accuracy remains important when assessing new modalities, it is critical to move beyond feasibility and accuracy assessment once these have been adequately demonstrated across multiple types of operators. As such, it is important to prioritize research that explores the broader implications of POCUS findings on patient management, treatment decisions, procedural outcomes, and healthcare delivery.

POCUS Research in Healthcare Delivery

Presenting data on the cost-effectiveness assessment of specific POCUS applications and their impact on clinical workflow is highly valuable for informing its clinical adoption and integration. Research studies focusing on procedural safety and throughput provide valuable insights into optimizing patient care delivery and resource utilization. Moreover, prioritizing research projects focused on integration and measuring outcomes that effectively impact disposition, shorten length-of-stay, reduce imaging and ancillary test use, cut costs, and enhance resource utilization, underscores the potentially transformative impact of POCUS on healthcare delivery. It is also crucial to expand the focus of POCUS research projects to facilitate service delivery, especially in situations where access to 24-h radiology services is limited or challenging. For instance, demonstrating that POCUS use in outpatient settings can reduce patient referrals and expedite care could help identify additional relevant patient- and system-level metrics, particularly in the current value-based payment era. Research projects focused on integrating POCUS into healthcare systems in lower-resourced communities and austere environments can also facilitate high-impact integration and broaden access to quality care.

By strategically focusing research efforts on understanding the integration of POCUS into clinical workflows, and its impacts on patient outcomes, healthcare systems can achieve substantial improvements in efficiency and resource allocation. Projects aimed at evaluating the incorporation of POCUS into standard protocols (e.g., hypotension, trauma), while measuring healthcare-oriented outcomes (e.g., reduced length of stay through timely diagnosis, expedited disposition decisions enabled by accurate POCUS findings, and a reduction in unnecessary and more expensive imaging), offer great promise. Furthermore, research initiatives that explore the cost-effectiveness, patient safety, resource utilization, and population health benefits of POCUS-guided interventions offer invaluable information for healthcare administrators. Examples include nerve blocks which influence pain reduction and decreased opioid use; reduced central venous access through ultrasound-guided peripheral lines placement; and improved patient safety with ultrasound-guided central vascular catheter placement [16–22].

Moreover, research should further evaluate the role of implementation science to enhance knowledge translation and incorporation of evidence-based recommendations into practice. Implementation science research focuses on identifying barriers and building upon facilitators to enhance use on a broader scale, which is particularly well-suited for POCUS.

POCUS Educational Research

Numerous studies have investigated POCUS education and training programs aimed at enhancing proficiency in image acquisition, interpretation, and integration into clinical decision-making processes. These initiatives typically encompass diverse training and education platforms, including structured learning modules, hands-on instruction sessions, preceptorships, gamification approaches, simulation-based learning, and virtual reality methods tailored for physicians-in-training, medical students, nurses, and non-medical providers. As POCUS faculty explore innovative teaching methods for learners of various levels, early consideration of study design and publication of these educational efforts is essential. This should include the systematic collection of data and assessment of outcomes, ensuring that new educational strategies are not just applied but are also thoroughly evaluated for their impact and shared across the academic community.

In evaluating educational interventions, it is crucial to consider some of the unique components of education research. First, one must consider the educational framework, which serves as the theoretical underpinning to inform the proposed educational intervention [23, 24]. Second, educational interventions often operate in uncontrolled environments, which can lead to numerous confounding factors (e.g., concomitant training or on-shift experiences, variations in clinical learning opportunities) that can influence the eventual outcomes. As such, many educational programs may benefit from more expansive program evaluation frameworks, which are less commonly used in other research settings [25, 26]. Third, education researchers need to consider a wider range of outcomes, such as learner preferences, knowledge, skills, attitudes, behaviors, and healthcare results [27, 28]. They should also consider a broader range of research methodologies, including qualitative, quantitative, and mixed-method approaches. Surveys and assessment tools should be well-developed, and sufficient validity evidence gathered before being used in the study [29, 30]. For those who will be developing or using tools for assessment, it is critical to ensure raters receive sufficient training, and their consistency in rating be evaluated by measuring inter- and intra-rater reliability. Finally, it is important to also consider longer-term outcomes (e.g., retention, application to practice), rather than focusing exclusively on initial knowledge or skill acquisition. As many of these components can be complex for novice education researchers, it is advisable to engage an education research expert early in the process to avoid common errors and improve the study's rigor [31].

POCUS Technology Research

As POCUS technology evolves, with advancements like handheld ultrasound devices, tele-ultrasound, and artificial intelligence (AI) integration, researchers must adapt their methodologies. For example, the use of handheld ultrasound devices allows for more convenient and accessible imaging in various clinical settings, ranging from EDs to remote areas with limited resources. Examples of technology-based POCUS research include evaluating the diagnostic accuracy and clinical outcomes of handheld devices, or assessing the role and impact of tele-ultrasound.

Studies focusing on the integration of AI in POCUS can explore AI algorithms' performance in image interpretation, automation of measurements, predictive models, and even real-time decision support [32–34]. AI POCUS projects often have the potential to be multi-institutional and multi-disciplinary by including scientists, clinicians, and entrepreneurs that can increase opportunities for statistical and programming support, equipment loans, or funding for multicenter studies. Some studies may benefit from a large database to centralize data from various institutions and allow researchers to conduct large-scale studies with diverse patient populations and standardized imaging protocols.

Practical considerations include staying updated on technological trends, understanding the capabilities and limitations of new devices, and exploring AI's role in enhancing diagnostic accuracy. Advances in technology and connectivity can be helpful in teaching POCUS to students and expanding its use to more health care environments (e.g., prehospital care, resource limited settings). Collaborating with industry partners can provide access to the latest technologies and insights into future developments. Success in technology-based POCUS research hinges on blending clinical insight with technical expertise, ensuring the research remains relevant and impactful in the rapidly changing landscape of POCUS.

In technology-based POCUS research, it is important to prioritize patient-centered outcomes over technological advancements in isolation. While innovation is important, the primary objective should always be to enhance patient care and clinical practice. While industry partners may sponsor projects, governmental grants and other sponsors may hesitate to support research solely focused on technological enhancements without addressing some components of clinical outcomes. For example, a potential project solely focused on ultrasound technology improvements to enhance image quality by scanning deeper structures, enhancing contrast resolution, or reducing artifacts may benefit clinicians in their interpretations but the project's primary focus would be on advancing ultrasound technology, rather than directly impacting patient care outcomes.

Choosing a Research Topic

The backbone of any research project lies in its research question, illuminating the path through the research process. Developing a clear and precise research question can significantly impact the quality and efficacy of a research project. Therefore, we propose several key considerations when developing and refining the research question. While many factors can influence the success and feasibility of a research topic in POCUS, individual circumstances and institutional infrastructure often dictate the feasibility of the project. Therefore, carefully evaluating institutional resources and consulting local experts before finalizing the research question is also important.

The PICO Framework

The PICO (patient, intervention, comparison, outcome) format is a widely known strategy for framing a focused research question. The PICO format breaks down the four main components of a study question, making it easier to identify the relevant information. This is particularly important in POCUS research to ensure the relevant intervention and outcomes are clearly defined and properly aligned. For example, when seeking to evaluate the effectiveness of POCUS versus palpation for identifying a pulse during cardiac arrest, the following format could be used:

P: *Among patients in cardiac arrest,*
I: *does POCUS*
C: *compared with manual pulse palpation*
O: *reduce time to resumption of chest compressions?*

Modifications of PICO have also been described which include additional elements, such as time (PICOT) or study design (PICOS). While not required for the traditional PICO question format, these remain additional critical elements to consider when designing the study.

There are several reasons why it is important for current and future POCUS research to address focused research questions that carefully include or represent the PICO framework for specific clinical conditions. First, decision making on clinical guidelines, recommendations, and healthcare policy is based on expert consensus of available evidence in the research literature. Expert panels or task forces use the PICO approach to assemble evidence-based recommendations about the integration of POCUS application into clinical care. Second, this can inform the trial design by narrowing the study population (which will inform the inclusion and exclusion criteria) and identifying what the specific comparator is to ensure it is an appropriate control or comparison group. Third, this can help ensure the outcomes are sufficiently discrete and measurable.

The FINER Criteria

In evaluating a potential research project, considering the FINER (feasibility, interest, novelty, ethics, and relevance) criteria is very helpful. The criteria for FINER assessment and tips for using this scoring system are outlined in Table 25.1.

Feasibility emerges as one of the most pivotal factors for fellows, given the time constraints in their fellowship year. It is essential to acknowledge that, while high-quality, long-term studies with transformative outcomes are desirable, they may not always be feasible within fellowship time-frames. Prioritizing research projects that a fellow can complete within 1–2 years is very different from what faculty can accomplish over many years and with dedicated research funding (Table 25.2).

Brainstorming and identifying current research trends in POCUS can be accomplished through various avenues. Searching medical databases (e.g., PubMed, Scopus) using keywords related to POCUS research in specific areas of interest can yield valuable information on the current state of the literature and generate ideas for potential research projects. Another method is to explore POCUS abstracts presented at national meetings and recent journal publications. By reviewing these abstracts and papers, researchers can gain insights into the latest research topics, methodologies, and advances in the field of POCUS. Focusing on limitations and controversies highlighted in the existing literature and under-researched areas, where there is a lack of sufficient studies and new developments can help to refine the research question. However, one must always consider why an area has been understudied and whether this presents an opportu-

Table 25.1 The FINER criteria for the purpose of selecting POCUS research topic

Item	Criteria to be evaluated	Tips for researchers
Feasibility	• Study population • Funding • Resource availability • Time constraints • Technical knowledge • Scope of research • Institutional support	• Begin with pilot studies to assess feasibility, and to trial at your institution • Opt for studies needing less time, resources, and money unless grant funding available • Choose a sample population with easy access and a high volume • Collaborate with others to reduce workload and increase completion chances • Recruit medical students to assist with data collection; can train them to do POCUS • Identify the theme of research at your program
Interest	• Interest to POCUS researchers • Interest to multiple specialties • Potential impact on the medical community • Alignment with funding bodies' priorities • Potential for future research to build upon this • Potential for publication	• Ensure project alignment with your passions and curiosity • Prioritize projects that match educational objectives or program strengths • Select teammates with personal interests and motivations for participating in and completing the project • Identify topics that are priority items for the field of POCUS or beyond • Select topics that are straightforward and require minimal explanation • Opt for topics that team members readily understand and support
Novelty	• Uniqueness of the research question • Contribution to the cutting-edge applications • Exploring new methodologies • Merging scopes of science and clinical research • Translational research	• Novelty can include extensions or advancements of prior research and does not have to reflect a completely new construct • Prioritize validating previous studies in different settings • Consider different methodologies to view data through a novel lens • Prioritize gaps in knowledge or areas requiring further exploration by conducting pilot and proof-of-concept projects
Ethics	• Respect for participants • Harm minimization • Informed consent • Data privacy • Equity of care	• Assure the project will meet IRB requirements • Minimize risks with a comprehensive plan • Balance educational needs with subject safety • Ensure ethical integrity throughout the research process
Relevance	• Alignment with the clinical scope of POCUS • Potential impact on clinical outcomes • Potential for changing practices • Potential for optimizing resource utilization • Alignment for POCUS priorities in researcher's specialty • Potential to fill knowledge gaps	• Choose a focused and attainable project scope • Prioritize topics with clear relevance and consensus among the team • Assess if results will meaningfully contribute to the medical literature • Evaluate generalizability of findings • Determine if results are patient-oriented evidence • Identify which group(s) being helped (e.g., patients, hospitals, ultrasound companies, the healthcare system)

IRB institutional review board, *POCUS* point-of-care ultrasound

Table 25.2 Comparing potential research projects to demonstrate application of the FINER criteria

Project title	F	I	N	E	R
A randomized, multicenter trial comparing POCUS with HIDA scan in patients with high probability of cholecystitis	+	++	+++	++	++
Cardiac and carotid ultrasound in patients with reduced neurologic function after cardiac arrest	+	++++	+++++	+++++	++++
Impacts of body habitus on successful completion of ultrasound protocols	++	++	++	++	++
Randomized controlled trial on the success rate of PIV insertion with or without ultrasound	++	+++	+	+++	++++
A national survey on QA processes in clinical ultrasound fellowship programs	+++	+++	+++	+++	+++

POCUS point-of-care ultrasound, *HIDA* hepatobiliary iminodiacetic acid scan, *PIV* peripheral intravenous line, *QA* quality assurance

nity for more novel research or a topic that has consistently failed to meet the FINER criteria.

It is crucial to discuss the proposed research question with mentors, advisors, or peers whose area of interest is not necessarily ultrasound. They can provide valuable feedback on the clarity, focus, and broader significance of the question and suggest further refinements. They can also speak to the broader significance and ensure that interest extends beyond just the investigators to have a broader impact, thereby enhancing the likelihood of successful publication.

It is important to recognize that conducting POCUS research poses unique methodological challenges, due to variability in protocols for ultrasound scans. Other challenges include variations in skill sets among the clinician sonographers, differences in ultrasound machines, and diverse patient populations. An important characteristic of ultrasound studies is the variation in test characteristics at different stages of disease progression. Typically, the ability of POCUS to detect more advanced diseases or those with more extreme cutoffs yields better diagnostic or prognostic accuracy compared with POCUS for detection of lesser disease severity or milder abnormalities [35]. Therefore, setting up the enrollment criteria to consider these limitations and challenges is critical. Moreover, factors such as limited research support, lack of funding, institutional restrictions, the unpredictable nature of the acute care environment, and cooperation of ancillary staff further compound these challenges. Adaptability in research strategies tailored to the diverse settings and various nuances of POCUS research is essential. Therefore, considering the research landscape and identifying gaps or areas of significance are crucial steps in selecting a research project.

Before Starting a Research Project

Research Planning

Research requires patience, thoughtful planning, attention to detail, resilience, and transparency. It may take days or weeks to contemplate an idea before shaping a research question into a viable project. The next step is delving into the specifics of the project and assessing its feasibility. It is common for a robust plan to require countless hours of work. Embrace writing as a tool to enhance one's critical thinking process. In addition to organizing and clarifying the project, this writing often serves as the backbone of the manuscript. As the background, methods, and discussion take form for the initial study concept, the literature search will serve as the foundation for the eventual paper and future references.

Team-Building

Building a research team is paramount for expanding one's research productivity. A unified team, sharing common goals in research and publishing, accelerates the publication process. A well-functioning, cohesive team can significantly enhance the productivity and reach of one's research outputs, making teamwork a priority for research productivity. Building a successful POCUS research team requires a strategic approach, emphasizing task design, collaboration, and diversity of skills. In addition to recruiting individuals with specific expertise, it is beneficial to create tasks and include individuals who can help complete specific tasks (e.g., proposal/protocol writing, subject enrollment, database design, statistical analysis, manuscript writing). It is important to recruit individuals who have the skill sets to complete their roles and have a reputation for being responsive and timely in meeting deadlines. Also, consider recruiting a representative from groups of individuals who may be impacted by your study. For example, if conducting an educational POCUS study on emergency medicine residents, recruiting an emergency medicine resident as a co-investigator may add tremendous value to the project in regards to having their perspective and facilitating communications.

In the early stages of the project, it can be helpful to use smaller teams to avoid lengthy delays with scheduling and reaching consensus. Typically, the team will expand as the project progresses. Statistical support should also be considered when building the team. Consultation with institutional biostatisticians or other sources should be done if team members or the research mentor are unable to provide this service. As the team leader, it is important that one has a system to keep everything organized and communicate with the team at timely intervals to ensure that the project is moving forward and on track. Team leaders should also help ensure all team members are supported and have a voice in the study.

Throughout the research process, it is important to maintain an updated task list and timeline as part of the team charter. This document delineates the roles and responsibilities of the research team members, ensuring that each individual is aware of their specific duties within the project. Incorporating a schedule and timeline is also valuable, especially if the project is sponsored. Starting with the end goal (e.g., presenting at a particular national conference) and working backward to assign timelines for different tasks helps keep the team and the project on track for success. Without a clear deadline, research projects often lose priority.

Authorship

It is necessary to clearly communicate the roles and expectations for authorship within the research team. Discuss expectations, deliverables, author listing, and timeline upfront at the planning stage of research. The primary investigator or senior researcher should take the lead in initiating these conversations. Determining authorship roles should include first, second, and last author positions, with the remaining authors typically listed by role or alphabetically [36]. A senior faculty member who is also tasked with overseeing the project and ensuring the accuracy of the work is typically the last author. Consider sponsoring others and emphasizing their value, especially those who are underrepresented, early in their career, or near promotion.

As the research process unfolds and right before submission, it is important to revisit authorship based on individual contributions. Acknowledge all contributors, even if they are not listed as authors. Encourage an ethical authorship culture, rejecting gift or ghost authorship practices. Ensure alignment with authorship criteria outlined by the International Committee of Medical Journal Editors (ICMJE) [37]. ICMJE's four key criteria for authorship are: (1) substantial contributions to the conception or design of the work; or the acquisition, analysis, or interpretation of data for the work; (2) drafting the work or reviewing it critically for important intellectual content; (3) final approval of the version to be published; and (4) agreement to be accountable for all aspects of the work in ensuring that questions related to the accuracy or integrity of any part of the work are appropriately investigated and resolved. Those investigators or contributors not meeting all four of the above-mentioned criteria should be acknowledged but would not qualify as authors. Address any discrepancies in authorship with professionalism, and provide a rationale with supporting evidence when possible. Beware of authors overestimating their contributions and demonstrate impartiality in assessing individual contributions to scientific work [38].

Research Mentorship

Research mentors play a critical role in guiding novice researchers through research steps. This mentorship is not just for those interested in research and academics as a career focus but is essential for anyone seeking to complete a research project. In most instances, a junior researcher may have more than one mentor for different aspects of their research. Regardless of the topic, format, and type of study, setting up a mentor-mentee relationship is key to the success of any project [39].

Starting a mentorship relationship typically involves an unwritten contract in which roles, commitments, goals, and expectations are clearly defined. This foundational agreement ensures that both the mentor and mentee are aligned in their objectives and responsibilities. Mentors commit to providing guidance, expertise, and support, while mentees commit to actively engaging in the learning process and applying the knowledge gained. Clearly defining these roles helps prevent misunderstandings and sets a clear path for the project's progression.

Commitments include regular meeting schedules, timely feedback, and mutual accountability. Mentors may dedicate specific weekly hours to the mentee, while mentees agree to meet deadlines and prepare adequately for discussions.

Mentorship goals should be specific, measurable, attainable, relevant, and time-bound (SMART). Both parties should agree on the project's scope and objectives, with the mentee making a substantial contribution. Clear communication and mutual understanding of roles, expectations, and deliverables are key to a successful collaboration. Emphasizing this contract-based approach ensures that the mentorship is productive, structured, and beneficial for both the mentor and mentee. It also provides a framework to ensure that both parties remain on track and committed to their agreed-upon objectives.

Ideally, mentees should identify a mentor who takes a personal and professional interest in their overall academic development. The value of interactions and learning from these mentors cannot be overstated, as they play a significant role in shaping one's research career, offering diverse perspectives and expertise that contribute to comprehensive research skills and knowledge. Trainees may collaborate with faculty mentors by assisting in ongoing projects or proposing their own research ideas. When joining existing projects, it is essential to utilize the experience to grow additional research skills in that arena and, ideally, develop a subsequent study to build upon those research findings. This can also serve as an opportunity to develop a research track record and preliminary data for future grants, as discussed further below.

It is important to choose a mentor whose research expertise aligns with what the mentee is trying to accomplish and establish a professional relationship based on respect and clear communication. Review faculty research accomplishments, clearly gauge their interest in your project, and assess their availability to dedicate time to it. It is advisable to approach more than one mentor based on complementary interests and expertise.

Mentors should also understand the objectives of their mentees and what they hope to gain from the mentorship. It is crucial for mentors to listen, observe, provide constructive feedback, and share their experiences and perspectives while respecting the mentee's experience. Mentors should avoid being judgmental and maintain confidentiality, supporting mentees in all aspects of their project. Mentors are not necessarily from one's own institution or limited to their own specialty. The modern digital environment (e.g., social media, virtual conference platforms) has significantly expanded this and offered access to external mentors in unprecedented ways [40, 41]. In many instances, peer mentorship plays an important role in specific areas, such as peers with significant statistical, informatics, and study design expertise [42].

Research Process Steps

Developing a Project Timeline

Each research project is unique. Efforts and activities are continuous, not mutually exclusive, and may overlap. How you start, what you do during the process, and how you finish are all important to the outcome of the research project and the experience of the team of investigators. Table 25.3 provides an example of a potential POCUS research timetable. Time frames (shaded) shown in the table can be condensed or expanded based on the scope of the project, feasibility, and specific deadlines (e.g., periods of performance for grant funding, conference abstract due dates). Budget your time wisely, as each step in the research process often takes longer than anticipated. Take good notes, keep track of all communications, and have an organized method to hold yourself and team members accountable for tasks and deadlines. Plan for routinely scheduled meetings with the study team and mentors for updates on progress, action items (e.g., data cleaning, institutional review board submission, manuscript writing), and to troubleshoot problems or challenges.

Writing a Study Protocol

After considering the nascent research question, perform a thorough literature review to identify similar research on the population of interest, using a similar methodology, or measuring relevant outcomes. Incorporate elements that were effective and build upon barriers identified in prior work to develop the protocol. When drafting the research protocol, ensure it aligns with relevant reporting guidelines (Table 25.4) [43]. Consult with the research mentor, other experts, relevant or influential parties who will be affected by the project, team members, and the statistician to optimize the ability to successfully answer your research question.

This foundational document should outline the study's objectives, methodology, expected outcomes, data collection techniques, and analytic plan (Table 25.5). It should include a clear hypothesis and the rationale for the study, supported by the literature review. It must detail the POCUS application to be studied, the patient population, and the criteria for inclusion and exclusion. It should also describe the POCUS image acquisition protocol, POCUS equipment and probe settings, and POCUS user group(s). Ensure the POCUS training for the study staff is explicitly defined and consistent throughout the protocol to avoid variability in image acquisition and interpretation. Similarly, if multiple institutions are involved, make sure the data collection, transfer, and storage methods are explicitly stated and consistent across sites. Multi-institutional studies often require some form of data-sharing agreement as well.

The overall sample size should be reported, along with a justification for the proposed number of participants. Typically, a sample size justification will include the power (80% or 90% for most studies), level of significance (alpha = 0.05), and the anticipated incidence, expected difference, or acceptable standard deviation for the primary outcome. The latter aspects can be informed by prior literature or local data. Providing a 10–20% buffer over the calculated sample size allows for participants who drop out, incomplete cases, and redistribution of inconclusive results to avoid being underpowered for the primary outcome.

The study protocol serves as a roadmap for the research, ensuring that the study is systematically organized and adheres to ethical and scientific standards. A well-crafted protocol is crucial for guiding the research team, obtaining institutional review board (IRB) approvals, and securing funding.

Before finalizing the research protocol, it is helpful to conduct a very brief pilot study on at least one sample subject, whose data will not be included in any analysis, to ensure that the protocol does what it is intended to do and the data collection form contains all of the elements needed to conduct the study.

Table 25.3 Potential POCUS research timetable

POCUS Research Timeline												
ACTIVITIES	July	Aug	Sept	Oct	Nov	Dec	Jan	Feb	Mar	Apr	May	June
	Year 1											
Review literature to understand the area of interest, generate hypotheses, explore study design ideas.	■	■	■									
Define a concise research question. Identify content experts, mentor(s), and stakeholders.			■	■	■	■						
Define a research hypothesis and objectives.					■	■	■	■	■			
Define exposure/testing or intervention.					■	■	■	■	■			
Define and select variables and outcomes. Provide rationale and citations.								■	■	■		
Identify options for study design.								■	■	■		
Define independent variables predictors of interest, source documents, and enrollment strategy (for prospective studies)								■	■	■		
Identify key stakeholders and resources required (e.g., skill set, time). Confirm team members/co-investigators and their roles.								■	■	■		
Conduct brief pilot study or research workflow rehearsal to assess feasibility and refine the approach.								■	■	■		
Develop the research and analytic plan with a biostatistician.									■	■		
Discuss with a local research review committee of peers prior to IRB submission.										■	■	■
Consult with research staff abstractors. Develop informed consent and surveys.										■	■	■
Define a plan to collect data.											■	■
Submit to the IRB.											■	■
Select a short list of target journals.											■	■
Start writing the manuscript.											■	■
Begin data collection/enrollment phase.												■

(continued)

Table 25.3 (continued)

	Year 2											
Continue data collection/enrollment phase.	■	■	■	■	■	■	■	■	■	■	■	■
	Year 3											
Complete data collection/enrollment phase.	■	■	■	■	■	■						
Clean/compile data and set up guard rails in coding variables (e.g., max/min values, outliers, look for nonsensical responses, interim data cleaning, reports for missingness and verification/validation with source document).					■	■	■					
Analyze data and create figures and tables.						■	■	■	■			
Update manuscript with results and interpretation.								■	■			
Review literature to update discussion.									■	■		
Format sections and tables to follow author instructions of the specific journal.									■	■		
Submit abstract and/or manuscript for peer review.										■	■	
Respond to itemized peer reviewers' comments and revise												■

IRB institutional review board, *POCUS* point-of-care ultrasound

Institutional Review Board

The next step is to submit an IRB application. Prior to submission, the team needs to prepare the application, which involves gathering all necessary documents, protocols, consent forms, and any additional information required by the IRB. Often there are variations in criteria and guidelines among institutions. Therefore, it is important to check past local IRB submissions and talk to the ultrasound division and research directors before submitting to ensure alignment and enhance the likelihood of IRB approval.

The IRB process involves a thorough review of the research protocol to ensure ethical standards are met, particularly regarding patient safety and informed consent. The application should provide a detailed risk assessment and describe measures to protect patient data and privacy. Specifically, for POCUS projects, the IRB application should address the non-invasiveness of the technique, the plan for incidental findings, and the overall minimal risk associated with the studies.

The IRB proposal must be written in clear and simple language, as there are often several individuals without medical experience who will either process your application to prepare it for review or sit on the IRB committee that will review it. Keep in mind that the purpose of the IRB is to assure that appropriate steps are being taken to protect the rights and

Table 25.4 Reporting guidelines by type of study and methods

Study type	Reporting guidelines
Case reports	CAse REport (CARE [46]
Study protocols	Standard Protocol Items: Recommendations for Interventional Trials (SPIRIT) [47]/(SPIRIT-AI) [48]
Animal preclinical studies	Animal Research: Reporting of In Vivo Experiment (ARRIVE) [49]
Diagnostic studies	Standards for Reporting of Diagnostic Accuracy Studies (STARD) [50]
Observational studies	The Strengthening the Reporting of Observational Studies in Epidemiology (STROBE) [51]
Prognostic studies	Transparent Reporting of a Multivariable Prediction Model for Individual Prognosis or Diagnosis (TRIPOD) [52]
Quality improvement studies	Standards for Quality Improvement Reporting Excellence (SQUIRE) [53]
Artificial intelligence	Checklist for Artificial Intelligence in Medical Imaging (CLAIM) [54]
Randomized control trials	Consolidated Standards of Reporting Trials (CONSORT) [55]
Systematic reviews	Preferred Reporting Items for Systematic Reviews and Meta-Analyses (PRISMA/PRISMA-Scr) [56, 57]. Meta-analysis of Observational Studies in Epidemiology (MOOSE) [58]
Scoping reviews	Preferred Reporting Items for Systematic Reviews and Meta-Analyses - Extension for Scoping Reviews (PRISMA-ScR) [56, 57]
Qualitative research	Standards for Reporting Qualitative Research (SRQR) [59]
Economic evaluations	Consolidated Health Economic Evaluation Reporting Standards (CHEERS) [60]
Clinical practice guidelines	The International Appraisal of Guidelines Research and Evaluation (AGREE) [61]

Table 25.5 Study protocol summary

Protocol
Principal investigator
Faculty mentor
Co-investigator(s)
Brief study description
Primary objective(s)
Secondary objective(s)
Hypothesis
Study design
Study population
Inclusion criteria
Exclusion criteria
Independent variables *with definitions and rationale*
Dependent variables *with definitions and rationale*
Statistical analysis
Image storage/data privacy and security
Study scheduling of subject participation

Table 25.6 IRB approval types and estimated timeline

Approval type	Description	Estimated timeline
Exempt	Minimal risk studies that fit specific criteria defined by individual IRBs may be eligible for exemption from continuous IRB oversight.	2–4 weeks
Expedited	Research involving no more than minimal risk (which typically involves most observational studies). Meeting the specific regulatory criteria set by the institutional IRB may qualify your study for an expedited review process, which is quicker than the full IRB review.	1–2 months
Full board	Interventional studies and those that involve more than minimal risk to participants (including many studies of investigational devices), that typically do not qualify for exempt or expedited review, require review by the full IRB committee.	2–3 months

IRB institutional review board

welfare of humans participating as subjects in the research. IRB approval or exemption is required for most studies; therefore, it is very important that you carefully review this application before submission. The IRB staff can also be contacted if needed for assistance. Notably, some institutions will also include non-human subjects determinations, which would not warrant IRB review. These typically reflect publicly available data or information that does not involve human or animal subjects (e.g., distribution of POCUS topics published in a medical journal).

Typically, the IRB process will take several weeks to months, depending upon the complexity of the study, documents required, completeness of the initial submission, and the individual institution. Table 25.6 describes three common forms of IRB review. We recommend using this "down time", as an opportunity to start writing while the study is fresh in your mind. This initial draft can then be updated once the data collection and analysis are completed at a later stage.

Data Collection

Data collection in POCUS research should be systematic from image acquisition to storage, and transfer of images and videos (e.g., DICOM, MP3, AVI). It is essential to adhere to the protocol to ensure the consistency and reliability of the data. The research team must be trained in POCUS techniques to capture high-quality images that can be analyzed effectively. Details should be provided regarding who obtained the images, their training, and the process for assessing proficiency or competency in the examination before enrolling (if applicable). If a study includes secondary review of images by ultrasound faculty, the rubric or protocol used to evaluate the images needs to be explicitly described, along with the training and number of reviewers.

Study staff involved in data gathering must be trained in the study methods to ensure consistency in data collection. Notably, data collection in POCUS research is distinct from many other methodologies due to the reliance on obtaining actual images, which demands a thorough standardization of ultrasound protocols and the need for operator proficiency. Additionally, capturing and storing ultrasound images for analysis poses technical challenges that require careful planning. The data collection process should be monitored regularly to identify any issues early on (e.g., redundant variables that may lead to discrepancies, the need for built-in instructions to data extractors for determining responses for key variables). It is also important to maintain accurate records and logs of the POCUS scans, including patient demographics, clinical settings, and any deviations from the protocol. This step is critical for the validity of the research findings.

All data should be carefully entered into a data collection form that should be specifically created or tailored for the study. Ideally, the data should be entered directly into an online database (as opposed to writing it on a paper document and transcribing it into an online database at a later time), that can be easily transferred when statistical analyses need to be performed. Involving the statistician in the data collection process can also help ensure the data are reported using the correct scales and able to be easily translated into the statistical software for analysis.

Data Analysis

Collaboration between clinical investigators and statisticians is essential to plan, execute, and disseminate successful research studies. Although investigators do not need to be experts in statistical analyses, understanding some fundamental concepts is essential to knowing how to communicate effectively with statisticians and ensures appropriate selection or execution of analyses tailored to the study's needs. Table 25.7 provides a summary of common statistical methods. Figure 25.1 provides a flowchart for selecting statistical tests. Figure 25.2 and Table 25.8 provide a review of common test characteristics. Importantly, statisticians also rely on the investigators' clinical expertise to provide context and to identify relevant predictors, confounders, and outcomes of

Table 25.7 Common statistical methods used in POCUS studies

Statistical method	Description and examples
Descriptive statistics	Describe demographic or characteristics data using: Frequencies and proportions for categorical variables Mean (standard deviation) or median (interquartile range) for continuous variables Carefully consider whether to report means or medians: Use mean and standard deviation if the data distribution is symmetric (i.e., normally distributed) Use median and interquartile range if significant outliers are present and the distribution is not normal (i.e., skewed deviation) Example: report the age distribution of patients undergoing POCUS for gallbladder disease using mean and standard deviation if ages are normally distributed, or median and interquartile range if they are skewed Ensure that the chosen descriptive statistics accurately represent the central tendency and spread of the data
Bivariate analysis	Determine differences between binary outcome groups using: Number or frequency for categorical variables Median (interquartile range) or mean (standard deviation) for continuous variables For bivariate analyses: Use chi-square tests for categorical variables Use t-tests, or a non-parametric equivalent for continuous variables Example: compare the frequency of positive findings in ultrasound versus CT scans for diagnosing appendicitis using Chi-square tests and t-tests for patient age distributions Ensure sample size is adequate to achieve reliable results
Correlation analysis	Subtype of bivariate analysis: Both variables are continuous Evaluate the strength and direction of the relationship between two continuous variables Example: Correlation between pulmonary artery pressure and troponin level in patients with pulmonary embolism Use Pearson's correlation coefficient for normally distributed data, and spearman's rank correlation for non-normally distributed data
Analysis of variance (ANOVA)	Subtype of bivariate analysis: Compare means across multiple groups to identify statistically significant differences between cohorts Example: use ANOVA to compare mean B-line values across three patient cohorts with mild, moderate, and severe heart failure based on their ejection fractions Ensure assumptions of ANOVA (e.g., homogeneity of variances, normality) are met before applying the test

Table 25.7 (continued)

Statistical method	Description and examples
Multivariable analysis / regression analysis	Assess the relationship between independent variables (predictors) and a dependent variable (outcome): Example: relationship between POCUS cardiac findings and short-term mortality in patients with pericardial tamponade Use regression analyses for: Examining associations Predicting outcomes For prediction models during multivariable analyses: Include performance metrics for discrimination, and calibration Ideally, test models in an external database Consider potential confounders and interaction effects among variables
Survival analysis	Analyze time-to-event data: Example: compare POCUS and CT regarding the time to diagnosis of diverticulitis or time to disposition Use Kaplan-meier curves and Cox proportional hazards methods for these analyses Ensure to check the proportional hazards assumption when using Cox proportional hazards models
Receiver operating characteristic (ROC) analysis	Common test for evaluating the accuracy of POCUS compared to other diagnostic images: Example: evaluate the accuracy of POCUS in diagnosing pneumothorax compared to chest X-ray Use ROC curve ROC curve: Plots sensitivity against 1-specificity Calculate the area under the ROC curve (AUC) Interpretation: The closer the ROC curve is to the upper left corner of the graph, the higher the test accuracy Ideal ROC curve has an AUC = 1.0 (sensitivity = 1, false positive rate = 0, specificity = 1) Consider the clinical context and the balance between sensitivity, and specificity when interpreting the AUC
Kappa coefficients	Assess interrater reliability and agreement among different interpretations (e.g., presence or absence of B-lines, pericardial effusion, right ventricular dilatation) Use the intraclass correlation coefficient when more than two responses are available Note: The Kappa statistic can be biased despite high overall agreement (kappa paradox) Consider alternatives like Gwet's AC1 in such situations Example: Evaluate the agreement between multiple clinician sonographers on the presence of pleural effusion in POCUS images using the intraclass correlation coefficient or Gwet's AC1 Ensure the chosen statistic appropriately reflects the level of agreement and reliability among raters

POCUS point-of-care ultrasound, *CT* computed tomography

interest. This is particularly relevant given the unique nature of POCUS data and research (Table 25.9). For instance, clinical investigators must communicate to statisticians about potential image interpretation variability, so that the statistician can account for this when choosing appropriate methodology.

It is important to clarify the statistician's role upfront in a study, including whether they will assist with planning the analyses, performing the analyses, or both aspects. Agreeing on a detailed analytic plan beforehand is vital for executing the study and budgeting the statisticians' time. Acknowledging statisticians' contributions in research publications and presentations is essential, ensuring their due credit and potential authorship. This discussion should take place at the early stages to secure proper recognition. As a general guide, if the study could not have been presented or published without the statistician's input, then authorship is warranted (provided they meet the ICMJE criteria), regardless of whether the statistician was paid for their services or not.

By articulating research goals early, statisticians can help investigators to develop a tailored and detailed statistical analysis plan, verify that the data necessary to answer the research question are being collected and coded in a usable format, and ensure proper data analysis and reliable presentation of findings. Early and frequent involvement of statisticians in project development is crucial, as they can provide invaluable input and review of study proposals.

It is also important to note that the statistical analysis of image-based data has greatly evolved, thanks to advancements in computational statistics, machine learning, and the availability of sophisticated software tools, and online modules. Looking forward, we can expect the development of even more efficient and user-friendly software and algorithms. These future tools are likely to offer improved accuracy, speed, and usability of statistical software making advanced image analysis techniques available to both experts and non-experts.

Submitting the Manuscript

When determining where to submit your manuscript, it is important to consider several factors. Start by searching for journals specializing in POCUS-related research, such as

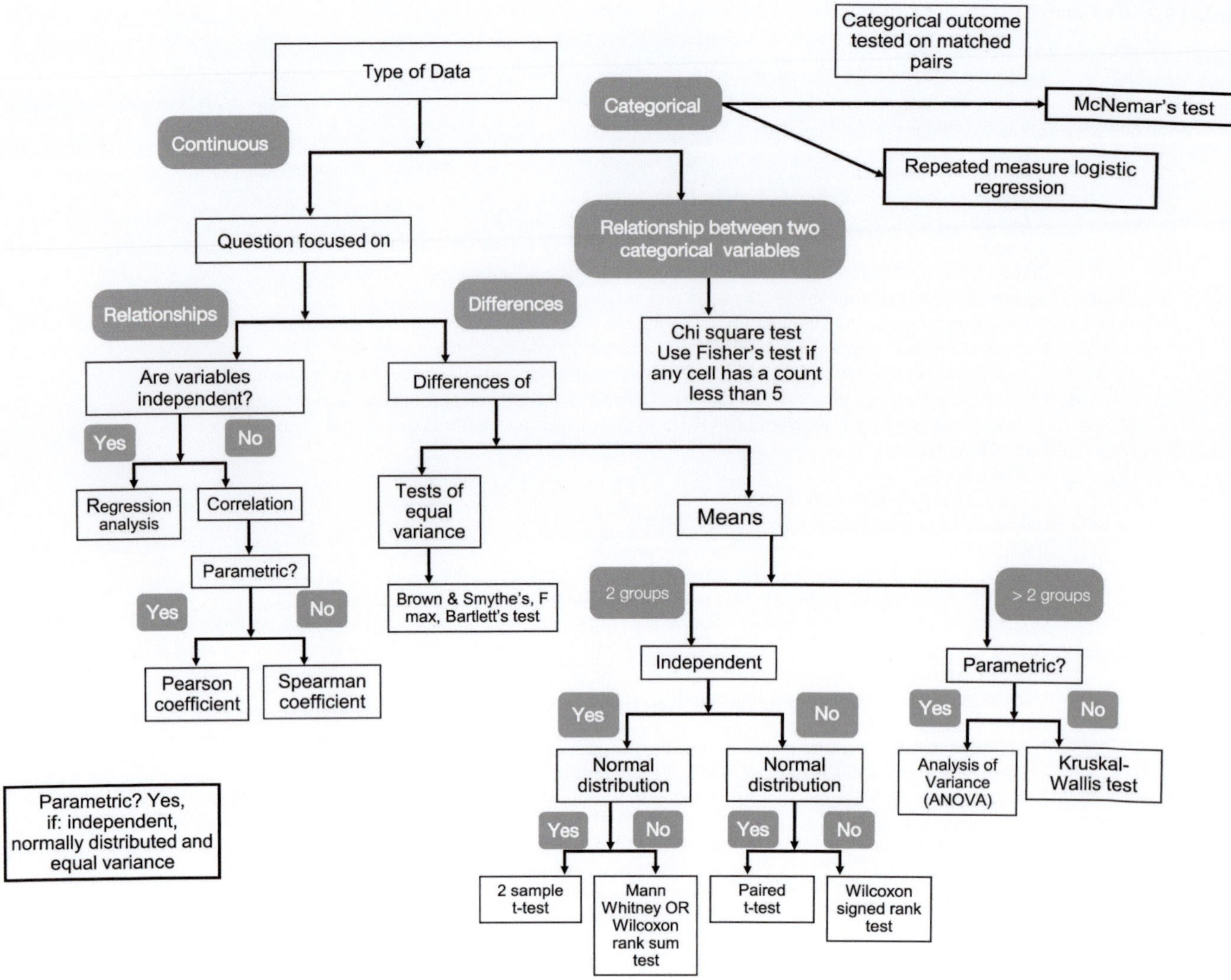

Fig. 25.1 Statistical analysis pathways for common image-based original research [44, 45]

Fig. 25.2 Assessment of true positives, true negatives, false positives, and false negatives

	Presence of Outcome/Disease	Absence of Outcome/Disease
Positive Test	True Positive (TP)	False Positive (FP)
Negative Test	False Negative (FN)	True Negative (TN)

Table 25.8 Formulas for common test characteristics

Test characteristic	Calculation
Sensitivity	TP/(TP + FN)
Specificity	TN/(TN + FP)
Positive predictive value	TP/(TP + FP)
Negative predictive value	TN/(TN + FN)
Positive likelihood ratio	Sensitivity/(100 – specificity)
Negative likelihood ratio	(100 – sensitivity)/(specificity)

TP true positive, *FP* false positive, *FN* false negative, *TN* true negative

those focusing on clinical ultrasound, emergency medicine, critical care, or the specific medical specialty relevant to the study. Reviewing PubMed Journal Selector can help by listing relevant articles and their associated journals based on your keywords. Additionally, examining the journals cited in your references, or related to your clinical care setting may help identify potential targets for submission. Supplementing your search with journal selector sites that suggest journals based on your abstract and keywords can also be helpful (Table 25.10).

Table 25.9 Specific challenges in POCUS research methodology

Challenge	Description	Impact	Solutions
Lack of controlled trials	POCUS research often relies on observational studies due to ethical or practical challenges in conducting randomized controlled trials	Observational studies, while valuable, may lack the rigor and control of experimental designs, potentially limiting causal inference	Leveraging quasi-experimental designs (e.g., interrupted time series, comparative effectiveness studies) Using methods like propensity score matching or instrumental variable analysis
Operator dependency	The clinician's experience significantly impacts the quality and reliability of POCUS imaging	Variability among clinicians performing the examination can introduce bias, while reliance on primarily expert users can limit study generalizability	Using histograms to visualize each operator's performance (TP/TN/FP/FN) Providing standardized research training for POCUS users to ensure uniform competence
Convenience sampling	Enrolling consecutive patients in POCUS studies is challenging due to the limited number of physicians with the requisite POCUS skills	This often results in reliance on convenience samples, decreasing study robustness, generalizability, and overall sample size.	Broader POCUS training among clinicians is needed to support more rigorous research methodologies
Inconclusive results	POCUS findings may sometimes yield inconclusive results, complicating data analysis	Factors, such as image quality, patient factors, and operator skill level, can contribute to interpretation uncertainty, affecting sensitivity, specificity, and predictive values	Careful study design, sample size calculations, and statistical power considerations should be in place Include inconclusive results in data analysis and conducting sensitivity analyses
Interrater reliability in image interpretations	Ensuring consistency and agreement among different interpreters in POCUS image analysis is essential.	Variability in interpretation can affect the validity of study results	Including an interrater reliability assessment in the methods Using consensus reviews, standardized scoring systems, or image interpretation criteria

POCUS point-of-care ultrasound, *TP* true positive, *TN* true negative, *FP* false positive, *FN* false negative

Table 25.10 List of common journal selector sites

Journal selector site	Description	Website
Elsevier Journal Finder	Identify Elsevier journals that may be suitable based on your abstract/keywords	https://journalfinder.elsevier.com/
Journal/Author Name Estimator (JANE)	Uses text mining to suggest journals based on your manuscript	https://jane.biosemantics.org/
JournalGuide	Database of journals with detailed information, and search functionality	https://www.journalguide.com/
Springer Journal Suggester	Recommends Springer journals based on your article's title, and abstract	https://journalsuggester.springer.com/
IEEE Publication Recommender	Find IEEE journals that may be suitable for their research	https://publication-recommender.ieee.org/
PubMed Journal Selector	Finds journals indexed in PubMed based on keywords or your manuscript	https://www.ncbi.nlm.nih.gov/pmc/journals/
Taylor & Francis Journal Suggester	Recommends Taylor & Francis journals based on your article's abstract	https://authorservices.taylorandfrancis.com/publishing-your-research/choosing-a-journal/journal-suggester/
Wiley Journal Finder	Matches your paper's abstract to Wiley journals using artificial intelligence	https://journalfinder.wiley.com/
Scopus Journal Analyzer	Analyzes your abstract, and suggest journals indexed in Scopus	https://www.scopus.com/sources

Prioritize journals that adhere to reporting guidelines and maintain high editorial and peer review standards. Consider factors such as scope, relevance, timeframes for decisions, impact factor, and criteria for evaluation when selecting potential journals. Begin with a "reach" journal (i.e., a more prestigious journal for which the article has a lower likelihood of acceptance), while keeping back-up options with a higher likelihood of success. Even if the "reach" journal does not accept the manuscript, they often provide comments that make the manuscript better for the next submission.

Develop a strategy for resubmission and revisions, including assigning tasks and responsibilities to authors [62].

Select the top five journals you plan to submit to and prepare for resubmission upon receiving a rejection. Rejection is part of the process, and you should be always ready for that. Therefore, have a backup plan and consider the feedback received on your article evaluation before submitting the next journal.

Be realistic about the suitability of your study for each journal, aiming for a high-quality submission that closely aligns with the journal's standards. When selecting journals, consider publication fees (also known as article processing charges) and the business model of each journal, ensuring alignment with your budget and publication goals.

Be wary of solicitations from predatory journals requesting POCUS articles. When approached by these journals, it is essential to be cautious and do a thorough assessment before engaging with them. Predatory journals often lack rigorous peer review processes, editorial oversight, and academic credibility, which can damage your credibility, and impact your research. When journals promise rapid publication, charge extremely high fees, or offer to waive fees without providing transparent information about their review process, this should raise a red flag [63].

The rise of internet-only and non-traditional publication platforms offer significant advantages such as rapid dissemination and wider reach of research findings. These platforms encourage interactive discourse and immediate feedback. However, some may lack the rigorous peer review seen in traditional PubMed-indexed journals, potentially impacting the perceived credibility and thoroughness of the research. When in doubt, seek guidance from mentors and local researchers before submitting to a particular journal or alternate publication platform.

Grants and Funding

Obtaining grant funding for POCUS research is crucial to promote high-quality research, including multicenter trials, and to make a broader impact on patient care through changes in clinical practice. Grant funding not only provides the financial resources necessary for conducting extensive research but also enables the development of innovative technologies and methodologies. Funding facilitates the exploration and widespread implementation of new protocols and procedures, ensuring that clinical practice evolves with the latest scientific evidence. Moreover, high-quality POCUS research funded through grants can address critical gaps in knowledge, leading to a deeper understanding of complex medical conditions, and the development of novel diagnostic approaches. Multicenter trials, which are often resource-intensive, benefit significantly from grant funding, allowing for collaborative research that can validate findings across diverse populations and settings. Funding can also support more robust initiatives aimed at improving diversity, equity, and inclusion in recruitment, and eliminating bias in research involving diverse patient populations, including historically underrepresented groups. This not only enhances the quality and relevance of patient care but also fosters an inclusive environment where biases are actively identified and addressed. Ultimately, grant funding is essential for propelling the POCUS field forward, fostering innovation, and translating research findings into tangible benefits for patients, and the broader healthcare system.

When seeking grant and funding opportunities, POCUS investigators should focus on identifying high-priority projects that will attract resources from federal agencies, industry partners, or foundations. This may include greater emphasis on patient-centered outcomes, cost-effectiveness, or the development of novel technologies. Projects with a primary focus on POCUS accuracy, educational proficiency, comparative research, and well-established applications are less likely to receive funding. The key elements in a grant submission are included in Table 25.11. However, it is critical to review the individual request for proposal (RFP) or request for application (RFA) to ensure all required grant elements are included. Table 25.12 provides examples of sources for POCUS research funding.

Having a well-defined specific aims page is crucial, as it serves as a synopsis of the research proposal and highlights the rationale, objectives, and potential impact of the study. A

Table 25.11 The outline of the different sections of a grant proposal

Section	Summary
Project summary	A concise summary of the entire project, including its aims, methodology, and potential impact
Specific aims	Concise and clear listing of the aims of the research project including hypotheses
Research plan	Detailed description of the research, including background, significance, innovation, outcomes, approach, sample size, data analysis, potential problems, solutions, and bibliography
Facilities and other resources	Description of the facilities and resources available that will support the project
Equipment	Description of the equipment essential for the project
Biosketch	A brief professional biography, contributions to science, and list of publications of the principal investigator(s) and key personnel
Budget	A line-by-line account of the funding required for the project, categorized by expense type
Budget justification	Explanation of the budget, detailing the necessity of each expense for the project's success
Supplemental forms	Additional forms that may be required (data sharing plans, inclusion of children, women, and minorities, study timeline, protection of human subjects), depending on the grant and funding agency
Letters of support	Letters from collaborators, institutional leaders, or others who support the project

Table 25.12 Sources of grants and financial sponsorship for POCUS research

Federal
National Institutes of Health (NIH) https://grants.nih.gov/
National Institute of Biomedical Imaging and Bioengineering (NIBIB) https://www.nibib.nih.gov/research-funding/opportunities
Agency for Healthcare Research and Quality (AHRQ) https://www.ahrq.gov/funding/fund-opps/index.html
Biomedical Advanced Research and Development Authority (BARDA) https://medicalcountermeasures.gov/barda/
Defense Advanced Research Projects Agency (DARPA) https://www.darpa.mil/
Department of Defense (DOD) https://www.grants.gov/
Foundations
American Heart Association (AHA) https://professional.heart.org/en/research-programs/aha-funding-opportunities
Robert Wood Johnson (RWJ) https://www.rwjf.org/en/grants/active-funding-opportunities.html
Society for Academic Emergency Medicine (SAEM) https://www.saem.org/about-saem/academies-interest-groups-affiliates2/saem-foundation/apply-for-a-grant/what-we-fund
American Institute of Ultrasound in Medicine (AIUM) https://www.aium.org/
Emergency Medicine Foundation (EMF) https://www.emfoundation.org/grants/apply-for-a-grant

well-crafted specific aims page is essential for effectively communicating with the program officials of funding agencies, as it clearly outlines the objectives, significance, innovation, and approach of the proposed research to grant reviewers, aiming to secure a competitive overall score and increase the chances of funding success. Table 25.13 features an example specific aims page for POCUS research.

The specific aims section, typically on a single page, consists of three parts [64]. The introductory paragraph outlines the research topic, and rationale, and identifies critical knowledge gaps, particularly focusing on the new information or guidance provided by the POCUS application. The sentence, "There is a critical unmet need to …" should be at the end of the first paragraph in bold. Secondly, the proposed solution is introduced, including the approach, main hypotheses derived from previous reports, potential project impact, and alignment with funding agency goals. Finally, two to four aims are presented, each detailing its title, strategy, and anticipated outcome or impact. These aims are designed to be independent, ensuring that each can yield results on its own.

Collaboration with a multidisciplinary team, including senior mentors or collaborators, enhances the feasibility and impact of the proposed research, especially in securing support for projects involving multiple institutions or disciplines. Establishing sustainable, long-term relationships and openly discussing expectations and deliverables with collaborators fosters a complementary workflow and accelerates the development and completion of high-quality research projects.

Table 25.13 Example of specific aims page from a research proposal featuring POCUS in pulmonary embolism [65]

Specific Aim 1	To determine the incidence of primary outcome (composite of death, circulatory or respiratory deterioration, or administration of reperfusion therapy), within 5 days in patients with acute pulmonary embolism. We will risk-stratify each patient using the sPESI ESC approaches. For each risk category, as determined by each prognostic model, we will compare the proportions of patients with the primary outcomes within 5 days of PE diagnosis and the sensitivity, specificity, and positive and negative predictive values. The proportion of misclassifications will be determined
Specific Aim 2	To evaluate the sensitivity, specificity, and positive and negative predictive values of each right ventricular assessment modality. The presence of abnormality will be considered a candidate predictor of increased risk for clinical deterioration within 5 days Approach: We will use predetermined definitions of the presence of RV dilatation for each of the different modalities: CT, cardiac POCUS, natriuretic peptide, and troponin. We will compare the sensitivity, specificity, and positive and negative predictive values for each different RV dysfunction assessment modality for primary, and secondary outcomes at 5 days
Specific Aim 3	To derive a prediction model for PE patients for the primary outcome of clinical deterioration within 5 days Approach: We will then use logistic regression to determine variables associated with primary outcomes, and determine RVD inclusive prediction models. We will then internally and externally validate the prognostic model

CT computed tomography, *ESC* european society of cardiology risk stratification of pulmonary embolism, *PE* pulmonary embolism, *RV* right ventricle, *sPESI* simplified pulmonary embolism severity index, *RVD* right ventricular dilation

Non-funded research related to the same research question serves as an essential foundation for securing funding, offering researchers a platform to hone their methods and gather preliminary data, which is crucial to demonstrate the project's feasibility and impact.

Securing federal funding for research is a marathon, not a sprint. It often involves years of effort and facing multiple rejections before achieving success. Persistence, continuous improvement, and a dedicated approach are essential. Having a strong, supportive team is crucial, enhancing your chances of successfully obtaining federal funding by pooling resources, expertise, and resilience.

Pearls and Pitfalls

- Seek out mentors and colleagues to review the study to ensure it meets the FINER criteria. These external reviewers should ideally not be members of the study team so as to provide a stepped-back viewpoint.
- Begin writing the manuscript during the IRB submission process, rather than waiting until the study is complete.
- Engage a statistician early in the research process, including the data collection, analytic plan, and interpretation of statistical analyses.
- Discuss authorship at the start of the project and reassess as the study progresses.
- Ensure you use a standardized protocol and training for all POCUS users.
- Use the pilot data as preliminary findings to strengthen your grant application.

References

1. American College of Emergency Physicians. Ultrasound guidelines: emergency, point-of-care, and clinical ultrasound guidelines in medicine. Ann Emerg Med. 2023;82:e115–55.
2. Barron KR, Wagner MS, Hunt PS, et al. A primary care ultrasound fellowship: training for clinical practice and future educators. J Ultrasound Med. 2019;38:1061–8.
3. Gottlieb M, Promes SB, Coates WC. A guide to creating a high-quality curriculum vitae. AEM Educ Train. 2021;5:e10717.
4. Atkinson P, Hunter S, Banerjee A, et al. Does point-of-care ultrasonography change emergency department care delivered to hypotensive patients when categorized by shock type? A post-hoc analysis of an international randomized controlled trial from the SHoC-ED investigators. Cureus. 2019; https://doi.org/10.7759/cureus.6058.
5. Kim DJ, Bell C, Jelic T, et al. Point of care ultrasound literature primer: key papers on focused assessment with Sonography in trauma (FAST) and extended FAST. Cureus. 2022;14:e30001.
6. Gaspari R, Weekes A, Adhikari S, et al. Emergency department point-of-care ultrasound in out-of-hospital and in-ED cardiac arrest. Resuscitation. 2016;109:33–9.
7. Gaspari R, Weekes A, Adhikari S, et al. Comparison of outcomes between pulseless electrical activity by electrocardiography and pulseless myocardial activity by echocardiography in out-of-hospital cardiac arrest; secondary analysis from a large, prospective study. Resuscitation. 2021; https://doi.org/10.1016/j.resuscitation.2021.09.010.
8. Frankel HL, Kirkpatrick AW, Elbarbary M, et al. Guidelines for the appropriate use of bedside general and cardiac ultrasonography in the evaluation of critically ill patients—part I: general ultrasonography. Crit Care Med. 2015;43:2479.
9. UCSF-Stanford E, McDonald KM. Making health care safer a critical analysis of patient safety practices. Am J Health Syst Pharm. 1995;52:2543–9.
10. Franco-Sadud R, Schnobrich D, Mathews BK, et al. Recommendations on the use of ultrasound guidance for central and peripheral vascular access in adults: a position statement of the Society of Hospital Medicine. J Hosp Med. 2019;14:E1–E22.
11. Levitov A, Frankel HL, Blaivas M, et al. Guidelines for the appropriate use of bedside general and cardiac ultrasonography in the evaluation of critically ill patients-part II: cardiac ultrasonography. Crit Care Med. 2016;44:1206–27.
12. Kim DJ, Atkinson P, Sheppard G, et al. POCUS literature primer: key papers on POCUS in cardiac arrest and shock. CJEM. 2024;26:15–22.
13. Gottlieb M, Alerhand S. Managing cardiac arrest using ultrasound. Ann Emerg Med. 2022; https://doi.org/10.1016/j.annemergmed.2022.09.016.
14. Shokoohi H, Boniface KS, Pourmand A, Liu YT, Davison DL, Hawkins KD, Buhumaid RE, Salimian M, Yadav K. Bedside ultrasound reduces diagnostic uncertainty and guides resuscitation in patients with undifferentiated hypotension. Crit Care Med. 2015;43:2562–9.
15. Gaspari R, Weekes A, Adhikari S, et al. A retrospective study of pulseless electrical activity, bedside ultrasound identifies interventions during resuscitation associated with improved survival to hospital admission. A REASON study. Resuscitation. 2017;120:103–7.
16. Lentz B, Fong T, Rhyne R, Risko N. A systematic review of the cost-effectiveness of ultrasound in emergency care settings. Ultrasound J. 2021;13:16.
17. Brass P, Hellmich M, Kolodziej L, Schick G, Smith AF. Ultrasound guidance versus anatomical landmarks for internal jugular vein catheterization. Cochrane Database Syst Rev. 2015;1:CD006962.
18. Shokoohi H, Boniface K, McCarthy M, et al. Ultrasound-guided peripheral intravenous access program is associated with a marked reduction in central venous catheter use in noncritically ill emergency department patients. Ann Emerg Med. 2013;61:198–203.
19. Blaivas M, Adhikari S, Lander L. A prospective comparison of procedural sedation and ultrasound-guided interscalene nerve block for shoulder reduction in the emergency department. Acad Emerg Med. 2011;18:922–7.
20. Morrison RS, Dickman E, Hwang U, et al. Regional nerve blocks improve pain and functional outcomes in hip fracture: a randomized controlled trial. J Am Geriatr Soc. 2016;64:2433–9.
21. Ablordeppey EA, Drewry AM, Beyer AB, Theodoro DL, Fowler SA, Fuller BM, Carpenter CR. Diagnostic accuracy of central venous catheter confirmation by bedside ultrasound versus chest radiography in critically ill patients: a systematic review and meta-analysis. Crit Care Med. 2017;45:715.
22. Guay J, Kopp S. Peripheral nerve blocks for hip fractures in adults. Cochrane Database Syst Rev. 2020;11:CD001159.
23. Gottlieb M, Krzyzaniak SM, Natesan S, Quinn A, Robinson D, Fant A, Sherbino J, Chan TM. Education theory made practical: creating open educational resources via an apprenticeship model. AEM Educ Train. 2022;6:e10802.
24. Bordage G. Conceptual frameworks to illuminate and magnify. Med Educ. 2009;43:312–9.
25. Frye AW, Hemmer PA. Program evaluation models and related theories: AMEE guide no. 67. Med Teach. 2012;34:e288–99.
26. Hosseini S, Yilmaz Y, Shah K, Gottlieb M, Stehman CR, Hall AK, Chan TM. Program evaluation: an educator's portal into academic scholarship. AEM Educ Train. 2022;6:S43–51.
27. Kirkpatrick DL. Evaluating training programs. 3rd ed. McGraw-Hill Education (India) Pvt Limited; 2006.
28. Kirkpatrick D, Kirkpatrick J. Evaluating training programs: the four levels. Berrett-Koehler Publishers; 2006.
29. Hill J, Ogle K, Gottlieb M, Santen SA, Artino AR Jr. Educator's blueprint: a how-to guide for collecting validity evidence in survey-based research. AEM Educ Train. 2022;6:e10835.
30. Hill J, Ogle K, Santen SA, Gottlieb M, Artino AR Jr. Educator's blueprint: a how-to guide for survey design. AEM Educ Train. 2022;6:e10796.
31. Gottlieb M, Dehon E, Jordan J, Bentley S, Ranney ML, Lee S, Khandelwal S, Santen SA. Getting published in medical education:

overcoming barriers to scholarly production. West J Emerg Med. 2018;19:1–6.
32. Marozzi MS, Cicco S, Mancini F, et al. A novel automatic algorithm to support lung ultrasound non-expert physicians in interstitial pneumonia evaluation: a single-center study. Diagnostics (Basel). 2024; https://doi.org/10.3390/diagnostics14020155.
33. Gottlieb M, Patel D, Viars M, Tsintolas J, Peksa GD, Bailitz J. Comparison of artificial intelligence versus real-time physician assessment of pulmonary edema with lung ultrasound. Am J Emerg Med. 2023;70:109–12.
34. Shokoohi H, LeSaux MA, Roohani YH, Liteplo A, Huang C, Blaivas M. Enhanced point-of-care ultrasound applications by integrating automated feature-learning systems using deep learning. J Ultrasound Med. 2019;38:1887–97.
35. Shokoohi H, Duggan NM, Adhikari S, Selame LA, Amini R, Blaivas M. Point-of-care ultrasound stewardship. J Am Coll Emerg Physicians Open. 2020;1:1326–31.
36. Gottlieb M, Lotfipour S, Murphy L, Kraus CK, Langabeer JR 2nd, Langdorf MI. Scholarship in emergency medicine: a primer for junior academics part I: writing and publishing. West J Emerg Med. 2018;19:996–1002.
37. ICMJE. https://icmje.org/news-and-editorials/updated_recommendations_may2023.html. Accessed 2 Apr 2024.
38. Herz N, Dan O, Censor N, Bar-Haim Y. Opinion: authors overestimate their contribution to scientific work, demonstrating a strong bias. Proc Natl Acad Sci USA. 2020;117:6282–5.
39. Jordan J, Berger M, Curato M, Ilgen JS, Hopson LR, Clarke SO, Chipman AK, Janicki A, Gottlieb M. "Not just a checkbox": a qualitative study of the resident scholarly experience. AEM Educ Train. 2022;6:e10824.
40. Gottlieb M, Fant A, King A, Messman A, Robinson D, Carmelli G, Sherbino J. One click away: digital mentorship in the modern era. Cureus. 2017;9:e1838.
41. Yarris LM, Chan TM, Gottlieb M, Juve AM. Finding your people in the digital age: virtual communities of practice to promote education scholarship. J Grad Med Educ. 2019;11:1–5.
42. Paetow G, Zaver F, Gottlieb M, Chan TM, Lin M, Gisondi MA. Online mastermind groups: a Non-3 for professional development. Cureus. 2018;10:e3013.
43. EQUATOR network. https://www.equator-network.org/. Accessed 2 Apr 2024.
44. Appendix I. Flow chart to determine appropriate statistical test to analyze data. McGraw Hill Medical.
45. Mishra P, Pandey CM, Singh U, Keshri A, Sabaretnam M. Selection of appropriate statistical methods for data analysis. Ann Card Anaesth. 2019;22:297–301.
46. Gagnier JJ, Kienle G, Altman DG, Moher D, Sox H, Riley D, CARE Group. The CARE guidelines: consensus-based clinical case reporting guideline development. BMJ Case Rep. 2013; https://doi.org/10.1136/bcr-2013-201554.
47. Chan A-W, Tetzlaff JM, Altman DG, et al. SPIRIT 2013 statement: defining standard protocol items for clinical trials. Rev Panam Salud Publica. 2015;38:506–14.
48. Rivera SC, Liu X, Chan A-W, Denniston AK, Calvert MJ, SPIRIT-AI and CONSORT-AI Working Group. Guidelines for clinical trial protocols for interventions involving artificial intelligence: the SPIRIT-AI extension. BMJ. 2020;370:m3210.
49. Percie du Sert N, Hurst V, Ahluwalia A, et al. The ARRIVE guidelines 2.0: updated guidelines for reporting animal research. BMC Vet Res. 2020;16:242.
50. Bossuyt PM, Reitsma JB, Bruns DE, et al. STARD 2015: an updated list of essential items for reporting diagnostic accuracy studies. BMJ. 2015;351:h5527.
51. von Elm E, Altman DG, Egger M, Pocock SJ, Gøtzsche PC, Vandenbroucke JP, Initiative STROBE. Strengthening the reporting of observational studies in epidemiology (STROBE) statement: guidelines for reporting observational studies. BMJ. 2007;335:806–8.
52. Collins GS, Reitsma JB, Altman DG, Moons KGM. Transparent reporting of a multivariable prediction model for individual prognosis or diagnosis (TRIPOD): the TRIPOD statement. Br J Surg. 2015;102:148–58.
53. Ogrinc G, Davies L, Goodman D, Batalden P, Davidoff F, Stevens D. SQUIRE 2.0 (standards for QUality improvement reporting excellence): revised publication guidelines from a detailed consensus process. BMJ Qual Saf. 2016;25:986–92.
54. Mongan J, Moy L, Kahn CE Jr. Checklist for artificial intelligence in medical imaging (CLAIM): a guide for authors and reviewers. Radiol Artif Intell. 2020;2:e200029.
55. Schulz KF, Altman DG, Moher D, CONSORT Group. CONSORT 2010 statement: updated guidelines for reporting parallel group randomised trials. BMJ. 2010;340:c332.
56. Page MJ, McKenzie JE, Bossuyt PM, et al. The PRISMA 2020 statement: an updated guideline for reporting systematic reviews. BMJ. 2021;372:n71.
57. Tricco AC, Lillie E, Zarin W, et al. PRISMA extension for scoping reviews (PRISMA-ScR): checklist and explanation. Ann Intern Med. 2018;169:467–73.
58. Stroup DF, Berlin JA, Morton SC, Olkin I, Williamson GD, Rennie D, Moher D, Becker BJ, Sipe TA, Thacker SB. Meta-analysis of observational studies in epidemiology: a proposal for reporting. Meta-analysis of observational studies in epidemiology (MOOSE) group. JAMA. 2000;283:2008–12.
59. O'Brien BC, Harris IB, Beckman TJ, Reed DA, Cook DA. Standards for reporting qualitative research: a synthesis of recommendations. Acad Med. 2014;89:1245–51.
60. Husereau D, Drummond M, Augustovski F, et al. Consolidated health economic evaluation reporting standards 2022 (CHEERS 2022) statement: updated reporting guidance for health economic evaluations. BMJ. 2022;376:e067975.
61. Brouwers MC, Kerkvliet K, Spithoff K, AGREE Next Steps Consortium. The AGREE reporting checklist: a tool to improve reporting of clinical practice guidelines. BMJ. 2016;352:i1152.
62. Garg N, Gottlieb M. Resident research tips: surviving and thriving within the peer review process. Ann Emerg Med. 2018;71:247–51.
63. Hansoti B, Langdorf MI, Murphy LS. Discriminating between legitimate and predatory open Access Journals: report from the International Federation for Emergency Medicine Research Committee. West J Emerg Med. 2016;17:497–507.
64. Monte AA, Libby AM. Introduction to the specific aims Page of a Grant proposal. Acad Emerg Med. 2018;25:1042–7.
65. Weekes AJ, Raper JD, Lupez K, et al. Development and validation of a prognostic tool: pulmonary embolism short-term clinical outcomes risk estimation (PE-SCORE). PLoS One. 2021;16:e0260036.

Diversity, Equity, and Inclusion in Point-of-Care Ultrasound

26

Almaz Dessie and Jodi Jones

Background

In recent years, global social justice movements and a growing awareness of health inequities have made the principles of diversity, equity, inclusion, belonging, and anti-racism major priorities in all industries, including academic medicine [1, 2]. It is increasingly recognized that promoting health equity, as well as workforce diversity and inclusion, is essential to achieve clinical excellence in medicine [3–6]. Accordingly, we believe that successful leadership in point-of-care ultrasound (POCUS) requires understanding and championing these principles in research, education, professional development, and clinical practice.

The acronym DEI (diversity, equity, and inclusion) is often condensed into a single concept but encompasses three distinct principles. To frame the content of this chapter, we must first define these key terms [7, 8].

Diversity is a property of groups of people rather than individuals. When we promote diversity in our workspace or our community, we are purposefully including and engaging people of different backgrounds and experiences. Diversity can exist across every spectrum of identity: race, ethnicity, sex, gender, sexual orientation, socioeconomic status, religion, nationality and immigration status, age, physical ability, and many other indices. Studies show that diverse groups produce better work in terms of innovation, fiscal performance, and scholarship [9–12]. In medicine, diverse groups are also associated with better communication and healthcare utilization, as well as overall improved outcomes with reduced health disparities [13–22].

A. Dessie (✉)
Department of Emergency Medicine, Warren Alpert Medicine School of Brown University, Providence, RI, USA
e-mail: almaz@brown.edu

J. Jones
Department of Emergency Medicine, University of Texas Southwestern Medical Center, Dallas, TX, USA
e-mail: jodi.jones@utsouthwestern.edu

Equity refers to fair treatment for all people, so that individuals or groups are given appropriate resources and opportunities to allow them to be successful, or in the case of health equity, to thrive. Equity differs from equality, which provides the same resources to all without consideration or acknowledgment that people have unique advantages and disadvantages based on background, experiences, and identity (Fig. 26.1). Health equity requires valuing all lives equally and addressing injustices that affect health [23]. An equitable work environment or health equity-conscious clinical practice includes policies, actions, and culture that ensure that one's identity does not dictate outcomes [24].

Inclusion is the culture created by an institution, whether a hospital, ultrasound division, national society, or editorial board, in which members are actively supported and valued. When policies, practices, attitudes, and cultures are successfully inclusive, all individuals and groups will feel a sense of belonging, allowing them to be themselves, perform their best, and, in the case of healthcare, provide the best possible care.

Data from 2019 reported that 64% of physicians in the United States were men, despite the majority of medical school graduates being women in recent years. The majority of physicians are also White (56%), and United States medical schools have struggled to increase matriculation of students from historically excluded racial and ethnic groups [25]. The field of POCUS has mirrored this culture in medicine and has lacked racial, ethnic, and gender diversity in terms of leadership, scholarship, and recognition [26, 27]. However, POCUS is a relatively new subspecialty of medicine, growing in popularity and influence in an era of increasing diversity of the physician workforce and increasing prioritization of DEI. This provides an opportunity to shape the subspecialty to make larger, systemic changes toward equity.

POCUS is uniquely positioned as a tool for health equity due to its accessibility and affordability across nearly all healthcare environments, from quaternary care hospitals to rural community hospitals, low- and middle-income

M. Gottlieb, N. Panebianco (eds.), *Advanced Point-of-Care Ultrasound*, https://doi.org/10.1007/978-3-031-85308-1_26

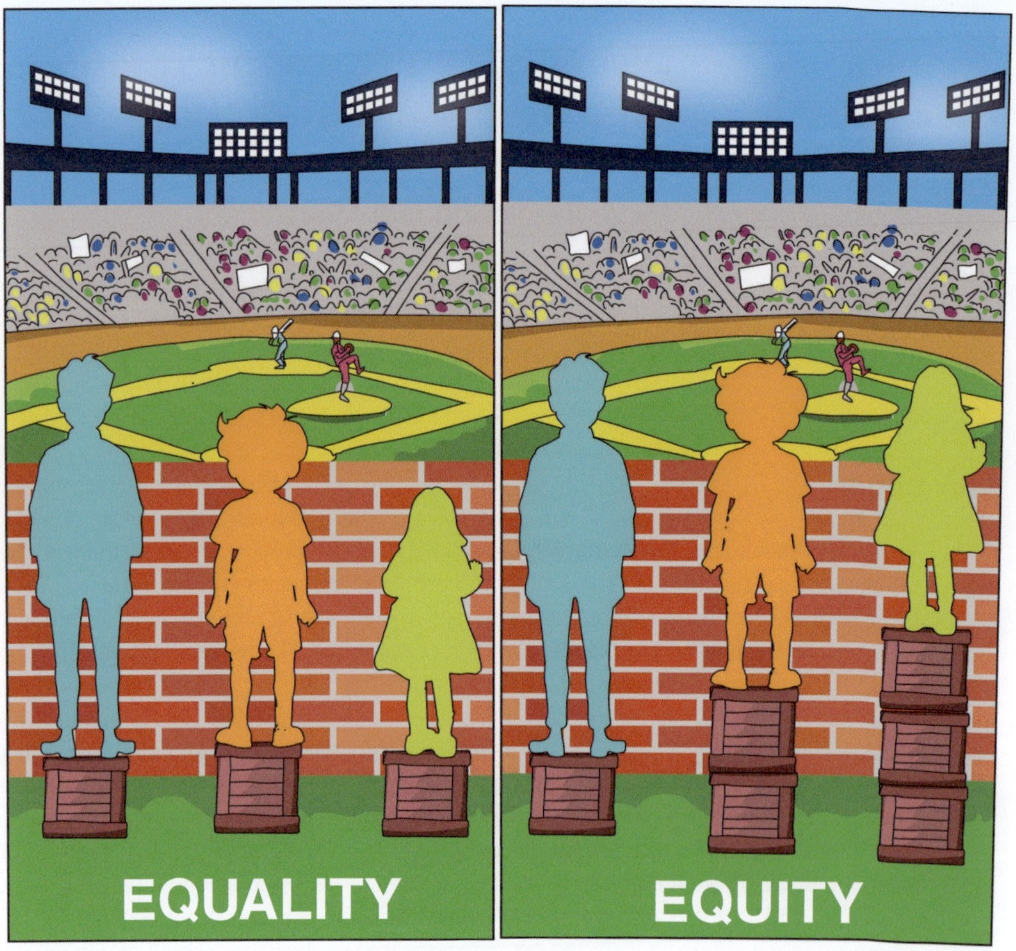

Fig. 26.1 Equality versus equity.

countries, emergency medical services, tele-ultrasound, and beyond. As such, centering DEI as core tenets when expanding POCUS access globally is paramount. We, as POCUS leaders in education, research, innovation and technology, health policy, and clinical care, are uniquely positioned to be champions of DEI in all that we do.

Strategies to Promote DEI in the POCUS Workforce

Increasing diversity in the ultrasound workforce starts with the purposeful recruitment of applicants of varied backgrounds across all levels of medical training. Numerous successful programmatic efforts to improve diversity have been described in the literature from pre-medical pathway programs to medical schools and residencies [28–31]. Similar strategies to diversify programs at the fellow and faculty level are applicable to POCUS [32, 33]. For example, when reviewing applicants using an equity lens, biased assessments—such as awards and board scores—should be deprioritized [34–37]. This can be accompanied by assessing other holistic metrics, such as the structural or individual barriers an applicant has overcome, or specific attributes that may benefit the patient population (e.g., fluency in a relevant language or growing up in the surrounding community) [34–41].

Other strategies include the strategic recruitment of historically excluded groups, standardizing interview processes to reduce biases, ensuring diverse representation in selection committees, and providing underrepresented applicants an opportunity to meet and candidly converse with peers within the program [28–33]. If the ultrasound program is lacking in diversity of a particular type, this should be acknowledged, and programmatic efforts to correct this should be made public to all applicants. Due to the overall low numbers of underrepresented groups in medicine, additional resources for recruiting those from underrepresented backgrounds may be required. For example, many programs have sponsored visiting clerkships for underrepresented medical students applying for residency, which are effective in increasing the matriculation of Black and Hispanic/Latino/Latinx residents; similar initiatives could be created for fellowship programs [42].

Specific considerations for the POCUS community have already been described in the literature with regard to equity and inclusion for gender, race, and ethnicity [26, 27].

Essential first steps for any POCUS division or national organization include rigorous data collection and reporting regarding gender, racial, and ethnic demographics across all institutions, accompanied by programmatic processes: recruitment/hiring, promotion, salary, award distribution, and leadership positions. Such data reporting allows for transparent assessment of current trends, targeted efforts to increase diversity, and measurement of progress and efficacy [32, 43].

Individual leaders in POCUS should be engaged in continuous self-work to mitigate their own biases and internalized racism [44, 45]. Additionally, POCUS leaders have a duty to promote DEI in their collaborations, speaking opportunities, conference planning, and leadership position recruitment. Those from privileged backgrounds or with professional social capital can practice allyship by avoiding participation in any professional groups, including teaching ultrasound courses, that lack gender parity, racial/ethnic diversity, or other types of diversity. For example, POCUS leaders, when invited to participate in a panel, course, or collaboration, should inquire about the other participants [46]. If diversity is lacking, they should advise the organizers and suggest other individuals who may help bring more diversity. This will bring a more engaging range of perspectives to the table. Further, POCUS leaders can encourage efforts to overcome barriers to participation for underrepresented groups, such as scholarships to attend meetings, reduced registration fees, childcare resources, and lactation-supportive conference spaces [47].

Efforts to diversify the ultrasound workforce are meaningless without simultaneous, comprehensive strategies to promote retention of historically minoritized groups by creating a culture of inclusion that fosters belonging. Conversations and concerns about equity and inclusion should be encouraged and never stifled or met with punitive actions. Numerous published strategies can help POCUS experts develop additional expertise in responding to overt and subtle racism, microaggressions, sexism, transphobia, and homophobia in clinical medicine and within their ultrasound division. These may take the form of workshops, simulations, reading/book clubs to facilitate conversations, and continuing medical education [48–52].

Given that many ultrasound divisions are small and training programs may only have one or two fellows, leaders need to consider how to best support their fellows and division members to report any unacceptable behavior such as bullying, discrimination, harassment, or retaliation for pointing out inequity. Every ultrasound division needs a clear structure of reporting and oversight for such behavior that is transparent and accessible to its members. We suggest building a structure of third-party oversight, such as a designated ombudsperson outside of the immediate department or division, to ensure neutral mediation, accountability, and restorative justice whenever possible [53, 544].

Underrepresented trainees and faculty in POCUS need ample mentorship and sponsorship to be successful. Specific mentorship programs and targeted opportunities recognizing individual needs and challenges are advisable, such as professional development programs for underrepresented faculty [55]. Leaders can also encourage individuals from historically excluded groups to apply for leadership positions as well as sponsor them for awards and professional opportunities. Peer mentorship is an effective approach when a program lacks diversity in higher ranks [56–58]. Due to the smaller size of many POCUS divisions, peer mentorship can be structured across other small academic divisions based on academic roles, identities, or life experiences. For example, programs could create a peer mentorship group that includes early career faculty who are parents of young children across the simulation, medical education, injury prevention, and clinical ultrasound divisions. The structure of peer mentorship programs should take into account the needs of the individual mentees and group members' expertise. This may include check-ins at regular intervals, facilitated discussions focused on relevant personal or professional topics, opportunities to practice presentations or share works in progress and receive feedback, and help setting goals with accountability [58, 59]. Additionally, given the robust network of POCUS leaders worldwide and our increasingly virtual collaborations, POCUS organizations can connect underrepresented individuals across academic institutions and medical specialties to provide effective mentorship when local identity-concordant mentorship is not possible.

Strategies to Promote DEI in POCUS Education

DEI principles should be incorporated into POCUS training programs to ensure learners feel welcomed, valued, and respected. In addition to recruiting a diverse faculty to deliver the education, a POCUS training program should include a curriculum that considers the diversity of the patient populations served by learners. An effective POCUS curriculum that is representative, equitable, inclusive, and accessible while addressing the needs of the learners fosters a sense of belonging for everyone, including standardized and clinical patients [60–62].

Curricular design (or redesign) involves strategic planning to determine the content and evaluative methods for the learner to achieve course objectives [61]. This requires a stepwise process of evaluating the current curriculum, identifying any gaps or opportunities that may be present, redesigning content to address these gaps, and eliciting feedback from learners on the success of the curricular changes [63]. Opportunities to improve a current curriculum could include adjusting course materials to be sourced from a diversity of authors, addressing any content delivery disparities, and employing evaluative processes that are equitable. Examples of content delivery disparities are lack of access to required technology to view the content for all students, small print on handouts for learners with low vision, or excessive reliance on a single mode of instruction (e.g. oral vs. visual). In considering equitable evaluative processes, utilizing multiple forms of learner assessment (e.g. multiple-choice tests, standardized direct observational assessment tools, objective structured clinical assessments, and multiple sources for evaluations including patients and peers) may provide more holistic forms of measuring POCUS competency [64]. After the implementation of these changes in the curriculum, it is necessary to evaluate the outcomes of the redesign to ensure effectiveness. This is not a one-time process but one that should be repeated periodically, incorporating learner feedback with continued refinement [61, 63]. Equity-centered pedagogy inherently values the input and feedback of all learners in curricular design [61].

Diverse learning environments offer distinct challenges and opportunities that must be addressed to fully maximize learning potential [65]. When learners are exposed to new ideas and situations, it compels them to move beyond their routine learning patterns and engage in mindful thinking [65]. These benefits are gleaned when there is active engagement, allowing for an exchange between different people and ideas. In an increasingly interconnected world, exposure to diversity is more possible than ever and will prepares learners to interact with people from different backgrounds, cultures, and traditions. This global perspective is essential for breaking down stereotypes and creating a more inclusive and compassionate society. Because of this, we emphasize that education on diversity and equity, as it relates to POCUS, should be included in the curriculum with the same emphasis as traditional skills such as image acquisition and ultrasound billing.

While ultrasound images may be thought of as "colorblind" shades of gray, white, and black, lectures and textbooks include images of probe placement on real people, and inclusion of different skin tones and body types is important to promote equity in teaching materials. Similarly, incorporating a wide range of patient models in hands-on ultrasound education, including various body types, genders, ethnicities, and medical conditions, is pivotal to preparing POCUS learners for real-world, diverse patient encounters [4]. For instance, patients with obesity may have different acoustic windows or image quality due to attenuation [66–68]. However, this patient population can also be subject to stigma, bias, and disparities in utilization of ultrasound based on the perceived difficulty of exams. This can lead to excessive usage of computed tomography and unnecessary radiation exposure. By gaining experience with POCUS in this population, users can address some of the perceived technical challenges by decreasing the transducer frequency and applying increased pressure directly over the organ of interest to reduce the depth of adipose tissue and generate better quality images [69]. This can then lead to increased appropriate and equitable use of POCUS in this population.

Strategies to Promote DEI in Clinical POCUS Practice

The effectiveness of ultrasound practice is not solely dependent on technical proficiency but also on the ability to provide patient-centered care that considers the cultural backgrounds and needs of patients. Incorporating DEI principles in clinical POCUS practice includes recognition of cultural nuances during sensitive procedures and mindful interactions with patients who have experienced trauma. Cultural humility entails recognizing the intricacies of identities and acknowledging that, even when similarities exist, there are nuances that differentiate individuals' lived experiences [70]. It emphasizes the understanding that a clinician can never attain complete competence regarding the ever-changing and dynamic nature of a patient's experience [71].

Cultural humility and communication skills are essential for working with diverse patient populations. Cultural humility in POCUS practice involves understanding and respecting the cultural beliefs, values, and practices of patients when performing POCUS. It requires clinicians to adapt their approach to patient care to ensure POCUS examinations are conducted in a culturally sensitive manner. This can be accomplished in many different forms, including but not limited to clear communication, respect for modesty and privacy, and seeking consent for physical contact. Effective communication is essential for building trust and rapport with patients, particularly when explaining the examination process and the results. Clinicians should communicate clearly and respectfully, considering language barriers, literacy levels, and cultural norms. Using interpreters or language services—instead of friends and family members—is the standard of care for effective communication with patients with limited English proficiency.

Physical contact during ultrasound exams can be perceived differently across identities and cultures. Seeking verbal consent before touching patients and explaining the purpose of each step in the examination process can help promote comfort and trust between provider and patient. Whenever possible, ask the patient to reposition their body to improve images rather than moving their body yourself (e.g. ask the patient to lift their arm up overhead to perform the right upper quadrant FAST view rather than moving their arm yourself). Additionally, one area of particular importance is the care of transgender patients who have historically been dehumanized and stigmatized in healthcare settings. It is critical to ensure adequate training in the care of transgender and gender diverse patients to create patient-provider interactions that are appropriate and affirming. For example, the use of testosterone can cause anatomical changes to any vaginal tissues, if present [72]. The use of a transabdominal ultrasound might be necessary for evaluation, as transvaginal ultrasound may exacerbate gender dysphoria, increase traumatic injury to atrophic vaginal tissue, or not be feasible after gender-affirming surgery [73].

As with all aspects of the physical examination, clinicians should be sensitive to the patient's preferences regarding exposure of the body during ultrasound examinations and take steps to ensure patient comfort. Sensitive examinations require healthcare professionals to approach patients with respect, empathy, and cultural sensitivity. This may include providing privacy screens, alternative clothing options or additional drapes for modesty, and allowing ample time for the exam to be conducted at a comfortable pace for the patient.

Ultrasound examinations should utilize a trauma-informed care approach, which emphasizes physical, psychological, and emotional safety for both patients and clinicians [74]. Trauma-informed care involves being sensitive to the potential psychological impact of trauma the patient may have already experienced while minimizing further harm that may arise from conducting examinations.

To create a safe and supportive environment, the physician should allow the patient to have control over the ultrasound examination when possible. This may include accomodating the patient's preferences regarding the gender of the physician, allowing family members to be present, and truncating examinations, if necessary. In addition to direct communication, this is accomplished by paying attention to nonverbal cues, including body language, facial expressions, and gestures, as these may convey information about the patient's comfort level and emotional state. While certain routine POCUS examinations such as cardiac or deep venous thrombosis may not be considered a sensitive examination for the sonographer, a patient may feel uncomfortable with the exposure of the groin or chest. Highly sensitive exams, such as transvaginal ultrasound, should be performed slowly, explain all maneuvers, and allow the patient to control the procedure as much as possible, including the ability to insert the probe themselves, if desired, and inform the physician if they need the examination to be stopped. The use of chaperones when learning and practicing ultrasounds allows the learner to practice through a trauma-informed lens. Importance should be placed on providing a full explanation, allowing the clinical patient or standardized patient to ask questions prior to performing the ultrasound, and only exposing the area of immediate interest while performing the examination [75].

If consent is not given to perform POCUS as part of a patient's clinical care, it is essential to remain composed and professional. Avoid reacting emotionally or defensively, and instead demonstrate empathy and understanding, which can help diffuse tension and foster constructive dialogue. Take the time to actively listen and understand the reasons behind the rejection, if given. Acknowledge the patient's right to make their own choices and express gratitude for their honesty and transparency, without pressuring or attempting to change their mind. Documentation should reflect this patient-centered mindset, noting that a patient "declined" a POCUS exam rather than "refused".

In closing, POCUS leaders must understand diversity, equity, and inclusion as central principles informing every aspect of their work. No individual or POCUS program is able to incorporate every action item listed in this chapter and certainly not all at once. However, incremental changes are possible by individuals, divisions, and organizations. By applying a DEI lens to recruitment and retention, POCUS education, and hands-on scanning and interactions with patients, POCUS experts can promote equity and foster sustainable positive change for our discipline.

Pearls and Pitfalls

- Diversity exists across a broad spectrum of identities. Diverse teams lead to better outcomes.
- Increasing diversity requires programmatic and sustained efforts with reporting, transparency, and accountability.
- Use holistic review processes to consider the broader view of the applicant's lived experiences and the unique attributes and skills they bring to the program.
- Utilize standardized interviewing processes and diverse selection committees.
- Engage in continuous self-work to identify and mitigate internal biases.
- Be an ally and sponsor for those underrepresented in medicine, and encourage appropriate diversity and parity in author groups and speaker panels.
- Ensure the curriculum is designed or restructured to be inclusive and accessible.
- Utilize cultural humility and trauma-informed care when performing ultrasound education and examinations.

References

1. Association of American Medical Colleges. Addressing and eliminating racism in the AAMC and beyond. Accessed 16 Oct 2024 https://www.aamc.org/addressing-and-eliminating-racism-aamc-and-beyond
2. Rosenkranz KM, Arora TK, Termuhlen PM, et al. Diversity, equity and inclusion in medicine: why it matters and how do we achieve it? J Surg Educ. 2021;78(4):1058–65. https://doi.org/10.1016/j.jsurg.2020.11.013.
3. Parker RB, Stack SJ, Schneider SM. ACEP diversity summit 2016 attendees. Why diversity and inclusion are critical to the American College of Emergency Physicians' future success. Ann Emerg Med. 2017;69(6):714–7. https://doi.org/10.1016/j.annemergmed.2016.11.030. PMID: 28139303
4. O'Leary K. Advancing diversity, equity and inclusion in medicine. Nat Med. 2021;27(12):2056. https://doi.org/10.1038/s41591-021-01612-2.
5. Cohen JJ, Gabriel BA, Terrell C. The case for diversity in the healthcare workforce. Health Aff (Millwood). 2002;21(5):90–102. https://doi.org/10.1377/hlthaff.21.5.90.
6. Vereen RJ, Wolf MF. Physician workforce diversity is still necessary and achievable if it is intentionally prioritized. J Racial Ethn Health Disparities. 2024; https://doi.org/10.1007/s40615-024-01953-x. Epub ahead of print. PMID: 38466513.
7. Mckinsey & Company. What is diversity, equity, and inclusion? Accessed 16 Oct 2024. https://www.mckinsey.com/featured-insights/mckinsey-explainers/what-is-diversity-equity-and-inclusion
8. American Psychology Society. Equity, diversity, and inclusion framework. Accessed 16 Oct 2024. https://www.apa.org/about/apa/equity-diversity-inclusion/framework
9. Hunt V, Layton D, Prince S. Why diversity matters. Accessed 16 Oct 2024. https://www.mckinsey.com/capabilities/people-and-organizational-performance/our-insights/why-diversity-matters
10. Rock D, Grant H. Why diverse teams are smarter. Harvard Business Review. Accessed 1 Dec 2023. https://hbr.org/2016/11/why-diverse-teams-are-smarter
11. Hunt V, Yee L, Prince S, Dixon-Fyle S. Delivering through diversity. Accessed 16 Oct 2024. https://www.mckinsey.com/capabilities/people-and-organizational-performance/our-insights/delivering-through-diversity
12. Nielsen MW, Alegria S, Börjeson L, et al. Gender diversity leads to better science. Proc Natl Acad Sci. 2017;114(8):1740–2. https://doi.org/10.1073/pnas.1700616114.
13. Alsan M, Garrick O, Graziani G. Does diversity matter for health? Experimental evidence from Oakland. Am Econ Rev. 2019;109(12):4071–111.
14. Blanchard J, Nayar S, Lurie N. Patient–provider and patient–staff racial concordance and perceptions of mistreatment in the health care setting. J Gen Intern Med. 2007;22:1184–9.
15. Cooper LA, Roter DL, Johnson RL, et al. Patient-centered communication, ratings of care, and concordance of patient and physician race. Ann Intern Med. 2003;139(11):907–15. https://doi.org/10.7326/0003-4819-139-11-200312020-00009. PMID: 14644893.
16. Gomez LE, Bernet P. Diversity improves performance and outcomes. J Natl Med Assoc. 2019;111(4):383–92. https://doi.org/10.1016/j.jnma.2019.01.006. Epub 2019 Feb 11. PMID: 30765101.
17. Greenwood BN, Hardeman RR, Huang L, Sojourner A. Physician-patient racial concordance and disparities in birthing mortality for newborns. Proc Natl Acad Sci. 2020;117(35):21194–200. https://doi.org/10.1073/pnas.1913405117. PMID: 32817561
18. Nguyen AM, Siman N, Barry M, et al. Patient-physician race/ethnicity concordance improves adherence to cardiovascular disease guidelines. Health Serv Res. 2020;55(Suppl 1):51. https://doi.org/10.1111/1475-6773.13398.
19. Persky S, Kaphingst KA, Allen VC Jr, Senay I. Effects of patient-provider race concordance and smoking status on lung cancer risk perception accuracy among African-Americans. Ann Behav Med. 2013;45(3):308–17. https://doi.org/10.1007/s12160-013-9475-9. PMID: 23389688
20. Saha S, Komaromy M, Koepsell TD, Bindman AB. Patient-physician racial concordance and the perceived quality and use of health care. Arch Intern Med. 1999;159(9):997–1004. https://doi.org/10.1001/archinte.159.9.997.
21. Snyder JE, Upton RD, Hassett TC, et al. Black representation in the primary care physician workforce and its association with population life expectancy and mortality rates in the US. JAMA Netw Open. 2023;6(4):e236687. https://doi.org/10.1001/jamanetworkopen.2023.6687. PMID: 37058307.
22. Takeshita J, Wang S, Loren AW, et al. Association of Racial/ethnic and gender concordance between patients and physicians with patient experience ratings. JAMA Netw Open. 2020;3(11):e2024583. https://doi.org/10.1001/jamanetworkopen.2020.24583. PMID: 33165609.
23. Jones CP. Systems of power, axes of inequity: parallels, intersections, braiding the strands. Med Care. 2014;52:S71–5. https://doi.org/10.1097/MLR.0000000000000216.
24. National Center for Family Philanthropy. Catalytic change: Lessons learned from the racial justice grantmaking assessment. Accessed 16 Oct 2024. https://www.ncfp.org/knowledge/catalytic-change-lessons-learned-from-the-racial-justice-grantmaking-assessment/
25. Association of American Medical Colleges. Diversity in medicine facts and figures 2019. Accessed 16 Oct 2024. https://www.aamc.org/data-reports/workforce/report/diversity-medicine-facts-and-figures-2019
26. Dessie AS, Lewiss RE, Stolz LA, et al. The state of gender inclusion in the point-of-care ultrasound community. Am J Emerg Med. 2022;56:283–5. https://doi.org/10.1016/j.ajem.2021.07.021.
27. Rosario J, Lewiss RE, Stolz LA, et al. Creating a more racial-ethnic inclusive clinical ultrasound community. Am J Emerg Med. 2022;54:208–11. https://doi.org/10.1016/j.ajem.2022.02.015.
28. Lall MD, Backster A, White MH, et al. Recruitment of a diverse emergency medicine residency program: creating and maintaining a culture of diversity, equity, and inclusion. AEM Educ Train. 2021;5(Suppl 1):S112–5. https://doi.org/10.1002/aet2.10674. PMID: 34616983
29. Garrick JF, Perez B, Anaebere TC, et al. The diversity snowball effect: the quest to increase diversity in emergency medicine: a case study of highland's emergency medicine residency program. Ann Emerg Med. 2019;73(6):639–47. https://doi.org/10.1016/j.annemergmed.2019.01.039. PMID: 30902450.
30. Capers Q, McDougle L, Clinchot DM. Strategies for achieving diversity through medical school admissions. J Health Care Poor Underserved. 2018;29(1):9–18. https://doi.org/10.1353/hpu.2018.0002.
31. Parsons M, Caldwell MT, Alvarez A, et al. Physician pipeline and pathway programs: an evidence-based guide to best practices for diversity, equity, and inclusion from the Council of Residency Directors in Emergency Medicine. West J Emerg Med. 2022;23(4):514–24. https://doi.org/10.5811/westjem.2022.2.54875. PMID: 35980420
32. Boatright D, Branzetti J, Duong D, et al. Racial and ethnic diversity in academic emergency medicine: how far have we come? Next steps for the future. AEM Educ Train. 2018;2(Suppl 1):S31–9. https://doi.org/10.1002/aet2.10204.

33. Davenport D, Alvarez A, Natesan S, et al. Faculty recruitment, retention, and representation in leadership: an evidence-based guide to best practices for diversity, equity, and inclusion from the council of residency directors in emergency medicine. West J Emerg Med. 2022;23(1):62–71. https://doi.org/10.5811/westjem.2021.8.53754.
34. Nguyen M, Mason HRC, O'Connor PG, et al. Association of socioeconomic status with alpha omega alpha honor society membership among medical students. JAMA Netw Open. 2021;4(6):e2110730. https://doi.org/10.1001/jamanetworkopen.2021.10730. PMID: 34076702
35. Boatright D, Ross D, O'Connor P, et al. Racial disparities in medical student membership in the alpha omega alpha honor society. JAMA Intern Med. 2017;177(5):659–65. https://doi.org/10.1001/jamainternmed.2016.9623.
36. Edmond MB, Deschenes JL, Eckler M, Wenzel RP. Racial bias in using USMLE step 1 scores to Grant internal medicine residency interviews. Acad Med. 2001;76(12):1253–6. https://doi.org/10.1097/00001888-200112000-00021.
37. Sajadi-Ernazarova K, Ramoska E, Saks M. USMLE scores do not predict the clinical performance of emergency medicine residents. MedJEM. 2020;1(2):4–7. https://doi.org/10.52544/2642-718.
38. Association of American Medical Colleges, Advancing Holistic Principles Advisory Committee. Holistic review. Accessed 5 Jan 2024. https://www.aamc.org/services/member-capacity-building/holistic-review
39. Gallegos M, Landry A, Alvarez A, et al. Holistic review, mitigating bias, and other strategies in residency recruitment for diversity, equity, and inclusion: an evidence-based guide to best practices from the Council of Residency Directors in emergency medicine. West J Emerg Med. 2022;23(3):345–52. https://doi.org/10.5811/westjem.2022.3.54419.
40. Diamond L, Izquierdo K, Canfield D, et al. A systematic review of the impact of patient-physician non-English language concordance on quality of care and outcomes. J Gen Intern Med. 2019;34(8):1591–606. https://doi.org/10.1007/s11606-019-04847-5. Epub 2019 May 30. PMID: 31147980
41. Gottlieb M, Davenport D, Landry A, et al. Holistic review in applicant selection: a scoping review. Acad Med. 2024; https://doi.org/10.1097/ACM.0000000000005891. Epub ahead of print. PMID: 39348144
42. Duong DK, Samuels EA, Boatright D, Wilson T. Association between emergency medicine clerkship diversity scholarships and residency diversity. AEM Educ Train. 2020;5(3):e10547. https://doi.org/10.1002/aet2.10547. PMID: 34099994.
43. Yousif H, Ayogu N, Bell T. The path forward – an anti racist approach to academic medicine. N Engl J Med. 2020;383(15):e91. https://doi.org/10.1056/NEJMpv2024535.
44. Chapman EN, Kaatz A, Carnes M. Physicians and implicit bias: how doctors may unwittingly perpetuate health care disparities. J Gen Intern Med. 2013;28(11):1504–10. https://doi.org/10.1007/s11606-013-2441-1.
45. Hall WJ, Chapman MV, Lee KM, et al. Implicit racial/ethnic bias among health care professionals and its influence on health care outcomes: a systematic review. Am J Public Health. 2015;105(12):e60–76. https://doi.org/10.2105/AJPH.2015.302903.
46. Collins FS, National Institute of Health. Time to end the Manel tradition. Accessed 15 June 2021. https://www.nih.gov/about-nih/who-we-are/nih-director/statements/time-end-manel-tradition
47. Cleveland Manchanda EC, Vogel LD, et al. Best practices for lactation support at conferences and standardized testing centers. Obstet Gynecol. 2020;135(2):475–8. https://doi.org/10.1097/AOG.0000000000003661.
48. Mundo W, Vaughn J, Odetunde A, et al. A national pilot study on simulation-based upstander training for emergency medicine clinicians. AEM Educ Train. 2024;8(3):e10990. https://doi.org/10.1002/aet2.10990. PMID: 38800608
49. Neves da Silva HV, Heery LM, et al. What happened and why: responding to racism, discrimination, and microaggressions in the clinical learning environment. MedEdPORTAL. 2022;18:11280. https://doi.org/10.15766/mep_2374-8265.11280. PMID: 36381136.
50. Washington EF, Hall Birch A, Morgan Robert L. When and how to respond to microaggressions. Harvard Business Review. Accessed 16 Oct 2024. https://hbr.org/2020/07/when-and-how-to-respond-to-microaggressions
51. Cruz M, Fong-Olivares Y, Davi WC. Brave dialogues: an essential leadership practice to Foster diversity, equity, and inclusion in organizations. In: Marques J, Dhiman S, editors. Leading with diversity, equity and inclusion. Future of business and finance. Cham: Springer; 2022. https://doi.org/10.1007/978-3-030-95652-3_8.
52. Sulistio MS, Chen CL, Eleazu I, et al. Personal actions to create a culture of inclusion: navigating difficult conversations with medical colleagues. Ann Intern Med. 2023;176(11):1520–5. https://doi.org/10.7326/M23-1374.
53. Sukhera J, Goez H, Brown A, Haddara W, Razack S. Codesigning policy-based solutions to discrimination and harassment in academic medicine: an inclusive approach. Acad Med. 2023;98(12):1356–9. https://doi.org/10.1097/ACM.0000000000005466. PMID: 37801596
54. Acosta D, Karp DR. Restorative justice as the Rx for mistreatment in academic medicine: applications to consider for learners, faculty, and staff. Acad Med. 2018;93(3):354–6. https://doi.org/10.1097/ACM.0000000000002037.
55. Beech BM, Calles-Escandon, et al. Mentoring programs for underrepresented minority Faculty in Academic Medical Centers: a systematic review of the literature. Acad Med. 2013;88(4):541–9. https://doi.org/10.1097/ACM.0b013e31828589e3.
56. Prendergast HM, Heinert SW, Erickson TB, et al. Evaluation of an enhanced peer mentoring program on scholarly productivity and promotion in academic emergency medicine: a five-year review. J Natl Med Assoc. 2019;111(6):600–5. https://doi.org/10.1016/j.jnma.2019.07.001.
57. Mayer AP, Blair JE, Ko MG, et al. Long-term follow-up of a facilitated peer mentoring program. Med Teach. 2014;36(3):260–6. https://doi.org/10.3109/0142159X.2013.858111.
58. Yeung EM, Zia A. Facilitated peer mentoring to close the gender gap in academic emergency medicine. CJEM. 2022;24(4):359–61. https://doi.org/10.1007/s43678-022-00331-y.
59. Fleming GM, Simmons JH, Xu M, et al. A facilitated peer mentoring program for junior faculty to promote professional development and peer networking. Acad Med. 2015;90(6):819–26. https://doi.org/10.1097/ACM.0000000000000705. PMID: 25830537
60. Corsino L, Fuller AT. Educating for diversity, equity, and inclusion: a review of commonly used educational approaches. J Clin Transl Sci. 2021;5(1):e169. https://doi.org/10.1017/cts.2021.834. PMID: 34733545
61. Gamrat C, Tiwari S, Bekiroglu, SO. Inclusive addie: initial considerations for DEI pedagogy. Diversity, Equity and Inclusion (DEI) Teaching and learning. Accessed 16 Oct 2024. https://er.educause.edu/articles/2022/3/inclusive-addie-initial-considerations-for-dei-pedagogy
62. Verbree AR, Isik U, Janssen J, Dilaver G. Inclusion and diversity within medical education: a focus group study of students' experiences. BMC Med Educ. 2023;23(1):61. https://doi.org/10.1186/s12909-023-04036-3. PMID: 36698110
63. Henry TL, Rollin FG, Olakuni OE. How to create a diversity, equity and inclusion curriculum: more than checking a box. Ann Family Med. 2024;22(2):154–60. https://doi.org/10.1370/afm.3078.
64. Damewood SC, Leo M, Bailitz J, et al. Tools for measuring clinical ultrasound competency: recommendations from the ultrasound competency work group. AEM Educ Train. 2019;4(Suppl 1):S106–12.

65. Smedley BD, Stith Butler A, Bristow LR. Institute of Medicine (US) Committee on Institutional and Policy-Level Strategies for Increasing the Diversity of the U.S. Healthcare Workforce. In: The Nation's Compelling Interest: Ensuring Diversity in the Health-Care Workforce. Washington (DC): National Academies Press (US); 2004. Paper Contribution D, Diversity Considerations in Health Professions Education. Accessed 16 Oct 2024. https://www.ncbi.nlm.nih.gov/books/NBK216014/.
66. Mavrogeni SI, Bacopoulou F, Markousis-Mavrogenis G, et al. Cardiovascular imaging in obesity. Nutrients. 2021;13(3):744. https://doi.org/10.3390/nu13030744. PMID: 33652678
67. Shashaty MG, Stapleton RD. Physiological and management implications of obesity in critical illness. Ann Am Thorac Soc. 2014;11(8):1286–97. https://doi.org/10.1513/AnnalsATS.201404-159FR. PMID: 25172506
68. Singh M, Sethi A, Mishra AK, et al. Echocardiographic imaging challenges in obesity: guideline recommendations and limitations of adjusting to body size. J Am Heart Assoc. 2020;9(2):e014609. https://doi.org/10.1161/JAHA.119.014609. PMID: 31914879
69. Uppot RN. Technical challenges of imaging & image-guided interventions in obese patients. Br J Radiol. 2018;91(1089):20170931. https://doi.org/10.1259/bjr.20170931. PMID: 29869898.
70. Stubbe DE. Practicing cultural competence and cultural humility in the care of diverse patients. Focus. 2020;18:49–51. https://doi.org/10.1176/api.focus.20190041.
71. Lekas HM, Pahl K, Fuller LC. Rethinking cultural competence: shifting to cultural humility. Health Serv Insights. 2020;20(13):1178632920970580. https://doi.org/10.1177/1178632920970580. PMID: 33424230.
72. Zwickl S, Burchill L, Wong AFQ, et al. Pelvic pain in transgender people using testosterone therapy. LGBT Health. 2023;10(3):179–90. https://doi.org/10.1089/lgbt.2022.0187.
73. Obedin-Maliver J. Pelvic Pain and persistent menses in transgender men. https://transcare.ucsf.edu/guidelines/pain-transmen. Accessed 25 June 2024.
74. Kuehn BM. Trauma-informed care may ease patient fear, clinician burnout. JAMA. 2020;323(7):595–7.
75. Australian Sonographers Association Guideline: Intimate examinations, consent and chaperones. Accessed 15 Oct 2024. https://www.sonographers.org/publicassets/cc28b72c-2985-ea11-90fb-0050568796d8/Intimate_Examination_Guidelines.pdf.

Administration of Ultrasound Programs

27

Robert Strony and Amie Hall Woods

Introduction

The quality assurance and quality improvement process for point-of-care ultrasound (POCUS) is pivotal in ensuring the delivery of high-quality, safe, and effective diagnostic imaging at the bedside. Central to the success of a POCUS program is the implementation of comprehensive and continuous training for healthcare providers, coupled with strong leadership to guide and sustain the initiative. Effective training programs should encompass not only technical proficiency but also adherence to protocols and standards. Leadership, on the other hand, must advocate for, and allocate resources to maintain high standards, foster a culture of continuous quality improvement, and ensure compliance with regulatory requirements. Furthermore, meticulous record-keeping and robust data strategies are essential for documenting clinical encounters, supporting quality improvement initiatives, and facilitating reimbursement. Accurate and detailed documentation helps demonstrate the value of POCUS, streamline billing processes, and providing a foundation for ongoing performance evaluation.

Securing funding from hospital leadership for POCUS programs requires a strategic approach, emphasizing the clinical, and financial benefits of the technology. This includes presenting data on improved patient outcomes, reduced diagnostic times, and potential cost savings. Standards for safety and infection control are integral to POCUS practice, necessitating adherence to guidelines for equipment cleaning and disinfection to prevent healthcare-associated infections. Peer-reviewed quality oversight is another cornerstone of a successful POCUS program, involving regular case reviews, feedback sessions, and adherence to best practice guidelines. By fostering an environment of continuous learning and quality enhancement, clinicians can ensure the reliable and effective use of POCUS, ultimately improving patient care and outcomes.

POCUS Leadership

Clearly defined leadership and collaboration are crucial for the successful integration and utilization of a departmental POCUS program, and system-wide POCUS programs across healthcare institutions. Organizational team building plays a pivotal role in fostering interdisciplinary collaboration, and ensuring alignment of goals and priorities. In a system-wide program, creating a multidisciplinary POCUS leadership team with representatives from various clinical specialties, administrative leadership, and ultrasound experts has demonstrable importance [1]. Single-department programs should likewise utilize the knowledge base available, which may include other local POCUS leaders. This team serves as the driving force behind the development, implementation, and oversight of POCUS initiatives.

At the helm of this leadership team is the medical director of ultrasound, whose responsibilities encompass a broad range of duties critical to the effective functioning of the program. The director serves as the primary liaison between clinical departments, administrative leadership, and external stakeholders, advocating for resources, support, and institutional buy-in. This role requires strong leadership skills, clinical expertise in ultrasound, and a keen understanding of healthcare system dynamics. The director is responsible for overseeing all aspects of the POCUS program development, including protocol development, quality assurance, training, and credentialing [2].

Awareness of the complex roles and relationships of key players within the healthcare institution is essential for effective POCUS leadership. This involves building relationships

R. Strony (✉)
Department of Emergency Medicine, University of Pittsburgh Medical Center, North Central Region, Pittsburgh, PA, USA
e-mail: stronyrj@upmc.edu

A. H. Woods
Department of Emergency Medicine, UVA School of Medicine, Inova Campus - Inova Fairfax Hospital, Annandale, VA, USA
e-mail: amie.woods@inova.org

M. Gottlieb, N. Panebianco (eds.), *Advanced Point-of-Care Ultrasound*, https://doi.org/10.1007/978-3-031-85308-1_27

with departmental chairs, hospital administrators, quality improvement committees, and regulatory bodies to garner support and facilitate collaboration. Engaging stakeholders early and communicating the value proposition of POCUS in improving patient care, enhancing diagnostic accuracy, and reducing healthcare costs are essential [1]. Savvy POCUS leaders can navigate institutional politics and secure resources necessary for program success by establishing rapport, and providing data demonstrating tangible benefits.

Advising the departmental or hospital-wide leadership on best practices for standardizing POCUS credentialing and privileging is a key role of a POCUS leader [1]. While emergency medicine has traditionally led the way in POCUS training and utilization, the expansion of POCUS into other specialties necessitates collaboration in credentialing and privileging processes. Standardized credentialing criteria based on competency assessment, training, and ongoing proficiency evaluation are important [3]. This ensures that clinicians across specialties meet uniform standards of proficiency and competency in POCUS [1, 3]. The American College of Emergency Physicians (ACEP) 2023 Ultrasound Guidelines describe a stepwise process in both residency training and post-residency clinical practice that allows for clinical ultrasound training, credentialing, and incorporation of new applications [3].

Fostering a culture of continuous quality improvement and innovation is central to effective POCUS leadership. This entails implementing mechanisms for ongoing performance evaluation, feedback, and outcome measurement to ensure the delivery of high-quality care. Establishing quality metrics aligned with departmental or institutional goals and clinical outcomes, such as length of stay, diagnostic accuracy, and patient satisfaction is paramount [4]. By tracking these metrics and leveraging data-driven insights, POCUS leaders can identify areas for improvement, refine protocols, and drive practice evolution.

POCUS leadership is critical for maximizing impact on patient care delivery. Through organizational team-building, effective leadership, standardized credentialing processes, and strategic navigation of key stakeholders, healthcare institutions can successfully integrate POCUS into clinical practice. By fostering a culture of collaboration, continuous quality improvement and innovation, POCUS leadership can drive positive outcomes, enhance patient care, and optimize healthcare delivery.

Documentation and Reimbursement

Documentation and reimbursement play integral roles in the successful implementation and sustainability of POCUS programs, ensuring financial viability and regulatory compliance. Central to this process are Current Procedural Terminology (CPT) codes, which facilitate billing for POCUS services rendered. The American Medical Association (AMA) regularly updates and revises CPT codes to reflect advancements in medical practice and technology. A key milestone in POCUS reimbursement was the establishment of specific CPT codes for ultrasound-guided procedures, enabling clinicians to bill for these examinations accurately [5].

Ultrasound billing is divided into two distinct areas: professional and technical fees. The professional component refers to the interpretation of the ultrasound images and the generation of a report by a qualified healthcare provider. The technical component involves the use of ultrasound equipment, the acquisition of images, and any necessary technical support. When billing for these components, separate CPT codes represents each part. A "limited" study refers to an ultrasound examination that targets a specific area or addresses a specific clinical question. "Limited" studies typically involve fewer images and are less comprehensive than a "complete" study, which covers an entire anatomical region or evaluates multiple aspects within the scope of examination. Table 27.1 lists commonly used POCUS CPT codes by anatomical location/modality with descriptions.

CPT modifiers indicate specific circumstances affecting the service provided, such as when a procedure has both professional and technical components. A common modifier used in POCUS billing is modifier "26", which specifies billing for only the professional component of a service when the technical component is billed separately. In addition to CPT codes, reimbursement for POCUS services may be influenced by Diagnosis Related Groups (DRGs), a classification system used by the Centers for Medicare & Medicaid Services (CMS) and other payers to determine payment for inpatient hospital stays. DRGs categorize patients into groups based on their diagnoses, procedures performed, age, and other factors, with each group assigned a predetermined payment rate. While DRGs primarily affect inpatient reimbursement, they indirectly impact outpatient services by influencing hospital finances and resource allocation. POCUS charges in the inpatient realm will almost invariably be bundled into the global hospital DRG. While increasing relative value units (RVUs), the overall revenue impact will be nominal for POCUS performed as an inpatient. Thus, there is greater opportunity for direct POCUS revenue in the outpatient or ambulatory setting, where POCUS is billed as a separate charge.

Distinguishing between hard and soft revenue streams is essential for assessing the financial impact of POCUS programs. Hard revenue streams refer to direct income generated from POCUS services, such as reimbursements from payers, patient copayments, and out-of-pocket expenses. Soft revenue streams encompass indirect benefits, such as cost savings, improved patient outcomes, and enhanced operational efficiency. While hard revenue streams are easier to quantify and track, soft revenue streams may have a more

Table 27.1 Commonly Used CPT (Current Procedural Terminology) Codes Used for POCUS (Point-Of-Care-Ultrasound) Based on Anatomic location/modality and CPT Code Descriptors. American Medical Association (AMA). CPT Professional 2024 1st Edition

CPT code	Anatomical location/modality	Code description
76512	Ocular	B-scan (with or without superimposed non-quantitative A-scan)
76604	Chest/lung	Ultrasound chest (includes mediastinum), real time with image documentation
76604 76705 93308	EFAST	Requires at least one view of the heart, bilateral lung views, and RUQ, LUQ, and suprapubic views
76705	Abdomen	Ultrasound, abdominal limited (e.g., single organ, quadrant, follow up)
76706	Abdominal aortic aneurysm	Ultrasound abdominal aorta, real-time with image documentation, screening study for AAA
76775	Retroperitoneum	Ultrasound, retroperitoneal (e.g., renal, aorta, nodes), real-time with image documentation limited
76815	OB transabdominal	Ultrasound pregnant uterus, real-time with image documentation, limited (e.g., fetal heartbeat, placental location, fetal position and/or qualitative amniotic fluid volume), 1 or more fetuses
76817	OB transvaginal	Ultrasound, pregnant uterus, real-time with image documentation, transvaginal. If a transvaginal examination is done in addition to transabdominal obstetric ultrasound exam, use 76817 *in addition to the* appropriate transabdominal code.
76830	Non-OB transvaginal	Ultrasound, transvaginal. If a transvaginal examination is done in addition to transabdominal non-ob ultrasound exam, use 76830 *in addition to* appropriate transabdominal exam code
76857	Pelvic transabdominal female Pelvic transabdominal male Urinary bladder quantitative, (bladder volume) and qualitative	Ultrasound pelvic (non-obstetric), limited or follow-up. Can be used for limited evaluation of male pelvis, including evaluation and measurement of urinary bladder, prostate, seminal vesicles, and any pelvic pathology (e.g., bladder tumor, enlarged prostate, free pelvic fluid, pelvic abscess). Code 76857, *instead of* 76770, should be used if the urinary bladder alone (not including kidneys) is imaged. It should also be used if measuring bladder volume with direct bladder imaging
76870	Male genitalia	Ultrasound, scrotum, and contents.
76882	Musculoskeletal (extremity and joint) limited	Ultrasound, limited, joint or focal evaluation of other non-vascular extremity structure(s) (e.g., joint space, particular tendon, muscle, nerve, other soft tissue structures or masses), real-time with image documentation
76886	Pediatric hip	Ultrasound, limited, static (not requiring physician, or other qualified health care professional manipulation)
76937	Vascular access	Ultrasound guidance for vascular access, requiring ultrasound evaluation of potential access sites, documentation of selected vessel patency, concurrent real time ultrasound visualization of vascular needle entry, with permanent recording and reporting (list separately in addition to code for primary procedure)
93308	Transthoracic echocardiography (TTE)	Echocardiography, transthoracic, real-time with image documentation (2D), including M-mode recording when performed; follow-up, or limited study
93312	Transesophageal echocardiography (TEE)	Echocardiography, transesophageal, real-time with image documentation (2D) (with or without M-mode recording, including probe placement, image acquisition, interpretation, and report)
93971	Extremity venous duplex	Duplex scan of extremity veins, including responses to compression and other maneuvers; unilateral, or limited study
93979	Duplex aorta, IVC, Iliac, or bypass grafts.	Duplex scan of aorta, inferior vena cava, iliac vasculature, or bypass grafts; unilateral or limited study (screening study for AAA, use code 76706, as above)
20604	Ultrasound-guided arthrocentesis/injection small	Arthrocentesis, aspiration, and/or injection of small joint or bursa (e.g., fingers, toes); with ultrasound guidance, with permanent recording, and reporting.
20606	Ultrasound-guided arthrocentesis/injection medium	Arthrocentesis, aspiration, and/or injection, intermediate joint or bursa (e.g., temporomandibular, acromioclavicular, wrist, elbow or ankle, olecranon bursa); with ultrasound guidance, with permanent recording, and reporting
20608	Ultrasound-guided arthrocentesis/injection large	Arthrocentesis, aspiration, and/or injection, major joint or bursa (e.g.,shoulder, hip, knee, subacromial bursa) with ultrasound guidance, with permanent recording, and reporting
32555	Ultrasound-guided thoracentesis	Thoracentesis, needle or catheter, aspiration of the pleural space with imaging guidance.
32557	Ultrasound-guided pigtail catheter insertion	Pleural drainage, percutaneous, with insertion of an indwelling catheter, with imaging guidance.
49083	Ultrasound-guided paracentesis	Abdominal paracentesis (diagnostic or therapeutic) with imaging guidance
76942	Ultrasound-guided aspiration (non-joint) or nerve block	Ultrasound guidance for needle placement (e.g., biopsy, aspiration, injection, localization device), imaging supervision, and interpretation. Please reference the current CPT code book for nerve blocks, as some blocks include imaging guidance inherent in the CPT code, and others use the 76942 in addition to the separate nerve block CPT code

significant long-term impact on the financial viability and sustainability of POCUS programs [6].

Comprehensive documentation of POCUS examinations is essential for accurate billing, quality assurance, and medicolegal purposes. POCUS reports should include pertinent clinical information, examination findings, interpretations, and recommendations. The Society of Radiographers (SoR) and the British Medical Ultrasound Society (BMUS) provide guidelines for standardized reporting of ultrasound examinations, emphasizing the importance of clear, concise, and comprehensive documentation [7]. Additionally, saving images obtained during POCUS examinations is essential for quality assurance, peer review, billing, and educational purposes. Healthcare institutions must establish protocols for image storage, archiving, and retrieval, ensuring compliance with regulatory requirements and data security standards. CMS has specific requirements for documentation of POCUS studies, including the following key elements:

1. *Clinical Indication*: Clearly state the reason for performing the ultrasound. This should align with the patient's symptoms, clinical presentation, or differential diagnosis.
2. *Description of the Procedure*: Document the type of ultrasound performed, including the anatomical area or system evaluated. It is also crucial to specify whether the study is limited or complete.
3. *Findings*: Provide a detailed interpretation of the ultrasound images. This should include any significant findings, such as abnormalities or pertinent negatives, as well as a conclusion or diagnostic impression.
4. *Clinical Correlation*: Describe how the ultrasound findings correlate with the patient's clinical presentation. This helps establish the relevance of the study to the patient's care.
5. *Images and Retention*: Ensure that ultrasound images are saved and stored in accordance with CMS guidelines and hospital policy. This includes retaining images for a specific period, and ensuring they are accessible for review and auditing.
6. *Date, Time, and Provider Information*: Record the date and time of the ultrasound examination, and clearly identify the healthcare provider who performed and interpreted the study.
7. *Medical Necessity*: Demonstrate that the ultrasound was medically necessary for patient care, as CMS may scrutinize studies that appear to lack a clear indication or justification.

The proliferation of handheld ultrasound devices has expanded access to POCUS across clinical settings, presenting unique documentation, and reimbursement challenges. While handheld devices offer portability, affordability, and ease of use, they may lack advanced features and functionality compared to traditional ultrasound machines. Additionally, billing for POCUS services performed using handheld devices requires adherence to the same documentation and reimbursement guidelines as conventional ultrasound examinations. Therefore, clinicians must ensure that handheld POCUS examinations meet the same standards of quality, accuracy, and documentation as those performed using traditional cart-based equipment.

The Stark Law, also known as the "physician self-referral law", is a United States federal regulation aimed at preventing conflicts of interest in healthcare. The primary focus of the law is to prohibit physicians from referring patients for designated health services to entities with which they have a financial relationship. This relationship can be through ownership, investment, or compensation arrangements. The Stark Law's connection with POCUS lies in its regulation of referrals and financial interests involving imaging services. If a physician has a financial stake in an entity that provides ultrasound services, they must ensure that their referral practices do not violate the Stark Law. For example, if a hospital owns its ultrasound equipment and employs physicians to use it, this arrangement is generally permissible because the physicians are not profiting from the referrals themselves. However, if a physician owns an external imaging center and refers patients there for ultrasound services, this could create a conflict of interest under the Stark Law. While POCUS is often practiced within hospitals and doesn't typically raise Stark Law concerns, it is important for healthcare providers and administrators to be aware of the law's provisions, particularly in contexts where financial relationships could influence referrals for imaging services. As POCUS utilization increases in the outpatient clinics, attention to rules and regulations unique to that setting will be necessary.

Documentation and reimbursement are critical considerations in the development and operation of POCUS programs. Understanding CPT codes, DRGs, hard and soft revenue streams, and the requirements for POCUS reports and image storage is essential for maximizing financial performance and regulatory compliance. By implementing robust documentation processes, leveraging appropriate reimbursement mechanisms, and adapting to technological advancements, such as handheld ultrasound devices, departments and healthcare institutions can optimize the financial sustainability and clinical impact of their POCUS programs.

Budget Planning

Budget planning for a POCUS program is a multifaceted endeavor that requires careful consideration of various factors, including equipment procurement, training, maintenance, and ongoing support. Payment structures and budgetary allocations may vary depending on the organizational structure, size, and scope of the healthcare institution. Understanding the financial landscape and identifying sources of revenue, and other financial support, are essential for the sustainability of a POCUS program.

One approach to budget planning involves categorizing expenses into distinct buckets, each representing different aspects of the POCUS program. There are three main expense categories: capital expenses, operational expenses, and revenue expenses [8]. Capital expenses encompass the initial investment in ultrasound equipment, including the purchase of machines, probes, and bundled accessories. These typically have a set monetary threshold (e.g., the total cost must exceed $5000). Operational expenses include ongoing costs, such as training, maintenance, supplies, and software licenses. Revenue expenses are any costs for work, or services required to obtain reimbursement for POCUS services rendered.

Sources of revenue and support for a POCUS program may include direct reimbursements from payors, patient copayments, grants, philanthropic donations, and institutional subsidies. POCUS charges (including professional and technical fees) will overestimate actual collected revenue. Collected revenue will rely heavily on payor mix and line of business (e.g., Medicaid vs. Medicare vs. commercial plans vs. uninsured). Collected revenue can be a fraction of actual billed charges depending on the payor. For example, Medicare reimburses for POCUS services performed in various clinical settings, including hospitals, physician offices, and ambulatory surgery centers, under specific CPT codes. Additionally, some private insurers may offer separate reimbursement rates for technical and professional components of POCUS examinations.

Understanding the nuances of technical and professional fee structures is essential for accurate billing and reimbursement, as the technical fee is often significantly greater than the professional fee. This nuance is particularly important with the rise of low-cost handheld devices, as the facility fee cannot be charged if the device is personally owned by the billing physician, per Stark Law, as described above. Finally, developing a relationship with a preferred vendor or vendors may improve negotiation options for warranties, equipment trade-ins, and loaners. Similarly, having a preferred vendor reduces the number of machine makes and models that the information systems technology, and biomedical engineering teams need familiarity with.

Expenses associated with a system-wide POCUS program extend beyond direct costs related to equipment and operations. Indirect expenses, such as staff time, administrative support, and infrastructure upgrades, must also be factored into budget planning. The importance of allocating resources for ongoing training and education to ensure competency among healthcare providers performing POCUS examinations should not be underestimated. Investments in quality assurance initiatives, data analytics, middleware software, and program evaluation are essential for optimizing clinical outcomes and demonstrating the value of POCUS to stakeholders. Programs looking to increase validity and exposure of their group may consider pursuing one of several pathways to accreditation, such as via ACEP Clinical Ultrasound Accreditation Program (CUAP) or the American Institute of Ultrasound in Medicine (AIUM). Budget planning for a POCUS program requires a comprehensive understanding of expenses, revenue sources, and reimbursement mechanisms to ensure financial sustainability. However, most studies demonstrate that POCUS allows for cost-effective care in the acute care setting [9].

Safety and Infection Control

Ensuring adequate safety and infection control measures for POCUS machines and probes is essential to mitigate the risk of healthcare-associated infections (HAIs) and protect both patients and healthcare providers. POCUS machines and probes can serve as potential vectors for the transmission of pathogens if proper infection control measures are not followed. Comprehensive guidelines and protocols have been established to minimize the risk of contamination and ensure the safe use of POCUS equipment across various clinical settings [10].

Transesophageal echocardiography (TEE), and endocavitary probes pose unique infection control challenges due to their direct contact with mucous membranes and bodily fluids, thus requiring high-level disinfection. Stringent cleaning and disinfection protocols are essential to prevent cross-contamination and transmission of infectious agents. The American Society of Echocardiography (ASE) provides recommendations for the cleaning and disinfection of TEE probes, emphasizing the use of high-level disinfectants, and adherence to manufacturer instructions [11]. Similarly, endocavitary probes, such as transvaginal and transrectal probes, require thorough cleaning and disinfection between each use to prevent the spread of infection.

Several key principles guide the safe handling and disinfection of POCUS machines and probes. The Centers for Disease Control and Prevention (CDC) recommends adhering to standard precautions, including hand hygiene, personal protective equipment, and environmental cleaning, to minimize the risk of contamination. Additionally, the use of appropriate disinfectants with proven efficacy against common HAI pathogens is essential. The CDC provides guidance on disinfection practices for non-critical medical equipment, including ultrasound probes, to prevent the transmission of multidrug-resistant organisms, and other infectious agents [12].

Proper storage and maintenance of POCUS equipment are crucial to prevent microbial growth and ensure the effectiveness of disinfection protocols. Ultrasound probes should be stored in a clean, dry environment to minimize the risk of contamination between uses. Regular inspection and maintenance of POCUS machines and probes are essential to identify any defects or issues that may compromise their safety or performance. The Joint Commission emphasizes the importance of equipment maintenance and biomedical engineering support in healthcare facilities, to ensure the safe and effective use of medical devices.

In addition to cleaning and disinfection protocols, the use of disposable probe covers, or barriers can provide an additional layer of protection against contamination. Disposable covers are commonly used with endocavitary and TEE probes to prevent direct contact with mucous membranes, and bodily fluids. However, it is essential to ensure that probe covers are compatible with the specific type of probe being used, and do not compromise image quality or diagnostic accuracy.

Education and training are critical components of infection control initiatives for POCUS equipment. Healthcare providers should receive comprehensive training on proper cleaning and disinfection techniques, as well as the importance of adhering to infection control protocols. The World Health Organization (WHO) emphasizes the role of education and awareness in preventing HAIs, and promoting safe healthcare practices [13].

Safety and infection control of POCUS machines and probes are essential to prevent HAIs, and ensure the delivery of high-quality patient care. Comprehensive cleaning and disinfection protocols, including the use of appropriate disinfectants, and disposable probe covers, are necessary to minimize the risk of contamination. Additionally, proper storage, maintenance, and education are critical components of infection control initiatives for POCUS equipment. By adhering to established guidelines and protocols, healthcare facilities can mitigate the risk of infection transmission and promote the safe use of POCUS technology in clinical practice.

Quality Oversight

Quality assurance in a POCUS program works to ensure the accuracy, reliability, and diagnostic utility of ultrasound examinations and provider skill across diverse clinical settings, while quality improvement seeks to elevate the skill and education of practicing providers. Robust quality assurance policies and procedures should be implemented to maintain the highest standards of image quality and interpretation. Comprehensive image review protocols are key aspect of quality assurance, while feedback mechanisms and ongoing skills maintenance are vital for quality improvement.

Principles of image review encompass a systematic evaluation of appropriate indication, image acquisition, interpretation, and documentation to identify areas for improvement and ensure adherence to established standards. The ACEP ultrasound guidelines recommend regular peer review of POCUS images by qualified practitioners to assess technical adequacy, diagnostic accuracy, and clinical relevance. This process involves comparing images against predefined criteria, such as image clarity, anatomical landmarks, and pathology visualization, to identify discrepancies or areas for improvement. One useful tool is the POCUS Image Quality (POCUS IQ) scale [14]. The POCUS IQ scale was developed by POCUS-trained physicians and assesses sonographers' image acquisition skills by evaluating image quality for any POCUS application.

An effective quality improvement program provides constructive feedback to healthcare providers based on the results of image review. Middleware programs can vastly enhance the ability to perform quality assurance on images, give feedback, track number of performed exams, and provide in-depth analytics. The ACEP ultrasound guidelines highlight the importance of delivering feedback in a timely, objective, and non-punitive manner to facilitate learning, and continuous improvement [3]. Feedback should be tailored to the individual needs and skill levels of practitioners, focusing on specific areas of strength and areas requiring improvement [15]. Additionally, incorporating peer-to-peer feedback and case-based discussions can enhance collaborative learning and knowledge sharing among providers.

Maintenance of skills is a critical aspect of quality assurance in POCUS programs, ensuring ongoing proficiency and competency among healthcare providers. Structured training programs, continuing education opportunities, and regular proficiency assessments need to support skill development and retention. This includes participation in hands-on workshops, simulation training, online courses, and attendance at conferences or seminars focused on POCUS education and best practices.

A quality assurance program that incorporates elements of image review, feedback, and skill maintenance enhances the quality and consistency of POCUS examinations. Continuous feedback to healthcare providers, based on image review findings, with an emphasis on identifying opportunities for improvement and promoting best practices are essential. Ongoing education and training initiatives should be implemented to support skill development and ensure proficiency among clinicians performing POCUS examinations.

Quality assurance and quality improvement are integral components of a POCUS program. Optimizing diagnostic accuracy, and maintaining provider proficiency and competency will lead to improved patient outcomes and minimization of risk. By adhering to established guidelines, implementing robust image review protocols, providing constructive feedback, and supporting ongoing skills maintenance initiatives, healthcare institutions can ensure the delivery of high-quality POCUS services across diverse clinical settings. Collaboration among multidisciplinary teams, utilization of feedback mechanisms, and commitment to continuous learning are essential for achieving excellence in POCUS imaging and enhancing patient care.

Pearls and Pitfalls

- Ensure clear delineation of roles and responsibilities among POCUS leaders at different levels (e.g., departmental, institutional).
- Foster interdisciplinary collaboration to leverage expertise and resources across specialties.
- Establish standardized protocols and guidelines to promote consistency and efficiency in POCUS implementation.
- Develop robust training programs to equip healthcare providers with requisite skills and knowledge.
- Regularly assess and reassess the needs of the program, and interface with institutional leadership for support of those needs.
- Emphasize documentation of POCUS findings, including images and interpretations consistent with published guidelines.
- Educate providers on appropriate billing and coding practices to optimize reimbursement, including the role of personally-owned vs. hospital-acquired devices. Implement systems for auditing documentation practices to ensure compliance and mitigate billing errors.
- Stay abreast of evolving regulatory requirements, such as Stark Law, and reimbursement policies related to POCUS at the division, department, and national level.
- Conduct a comprehensive needs assessment to determine equipment and resource requirements at the division, department, and enterprise level.
- Prioritize investment in high-quality, versatile ultrasound machines that meet diverse clinical needs, and standardize machines to reduce costs.
- Consider long-term maintenance and upgrade costs when budgeting for equipment procurement. Explore potential cost-saving measures, such as bulk purchasing agreements or equipment leasing arrangements.
- Allocate resources for ongoing training, quality assurance initiatives, and program expansion.
- Implement rigorous cleaning and disinfection protocols in accordance with infection control guidelines. Encourage adherence to hand hygiene practices, before and after performing POCUS examinations.
- Regularly inspect equipment for signs of wear or damage, and promptly address any issues.
- Utilize quality assurance software tools to track and analyze POCUS data for trends and patterns. Develop mechanisms for addressing discrepancies or concerns raised during image review processes.

References

1. Strony R, Marin JR, Bailitz J, et al. Systemwide clinical ultrasound program development: an expert consensus model. West J Emerg Med. 2018;19(4):649–53.
2. Hoppmann R, Blaivas M, Elbarbary M, et al. Goals and objectives for fellowship training in point-of-care ultrasound. J Grad Med Educ. 2019;11(1):1–18. https://doi.org/10.4300/JGME-D-18-00816.1.
3. American College of Emergency Physicians. Ultrasound guidelines: emergency, point-of-care, and clinical ultrasound guidelines in medicine. Ann Emerg Med. 2023;82(3):e115–55.
4. Moore CL, Molina AA, Lin H. Ultrasonography in community emergency departments in the United States: access to timely and high-quality care. Acad Emerg Med. 2000;7(9):963–8.
5. American College of Emergency Physicians. Ultrasound-Guided Procedure Codes. Available at: https://www.acep.org/siteassets/uploads/uploaded-files/acep/membership/sections-of-membership/ultra/acep-us-cpt-update-2024_edit.pdf. Last accessed 8/31/2024.
6. Van Schaik GWW, Van Schaik KD, Murphy MC. Point-of-Care Ultrasonography (POCUS) in a community emergency department: an analysis of decision making and cost savings associated with POCUS. J Ultrasound Med. 2019;38(8):2133–40.
7. SoR and BMUS. Guidelines for professional ultrasound practice. 8th ed. Society of Radiographers and British Medical Ultrasound Society; 2023. ISBN: 978-1-909802-89-6.
8. Whitson MR, Mayo PH. Ultrasonography in the emergency department. Crit Care. 2016;20(1):227.
9. Lentz B, Fong T, Rhyne R, Risko N. A systematic review of the cost-effectiveness of ultrasound in emergency care settings. Ultrasound J. 2021;13(1):16.
10. American Institute of Ultrasound in Medicine. AIUM Official Statement: guidelines for cleaning and preparing external- and internal-use ultrasound transducers and equipment between patients as well as safe handling and use of ultrasound coupling gel. J Ultrasound Med. 2023;42(7):E13–22.
11. American Society for Echocardiography. Transesophageal Transducer Cleaning and Care Guide. Available at: https://www.asecho.org/wp-content/uploads/2020/03/8257134-ABS-001-08-08_TEE_Care_Guide_ENG.pdf. Last accessed 8/31/2024.

12. Centers for Disease Control and Prevention. Guidelines for Environmental Infection Control in Health-Care Facilities Recommendations of CDC and the Healthcare Infection Control Practices Advisory Committee (HICPAC). Available at: https://www.cdc.gov/infection-control/media/pdfs/guideline-environmental-h.pdf. Last accessed 8/31/2024.
13. World Health Organization. World Health Organization Global Report on Infection Prevention and Control. 23 May 2022. Available at: https://www.who.int/publications/i/item/9789240051164. Last accessed 8/31/2024.
14. Dessie AS, Calhoun AW, Kanjanauptom P, et al. Development and validation of a point-of-care-ultrasound image quality assessment tool: the POCUS IQ scale. J Ultrasound Med. 2023;42(1):135–45.
15. Buckley C, Natesan S, Breslin A, Gottlieb M. Finessing feedback: recommendations for effective feedback in the emergency department. Ann Emerg Med. 2020;75(3):445–51.

System Management and Information Technology

28

Robinson M. Ferre and Jason T. Nomura

Introduction

Ultrasound is a well-established imaging tool used in modern healthcare environments. Traditional imaging departments, such as the department of radiology, have a robust imaging infrastructure that includes ultrasound devices, imaging software systems, information technology (IT) experts, and support systems designed to minimize errors and maximize efficiency. These systems were designed for consultative imaging studies, in a workflow where diagnostic image acquisition and interpretation occur separately.

Point-of-care ultrasound (POCUS) is different from the traditional consultative imaging paradigm. POCUS is not only unique in how it incorporates into patient care but also how it requires unique system management and imaging workflows. Having knowledge of traditional imaging systems and their requirements is essential to thoughtfully building a sustainable POCUS program. POCUS experts must understand both the traditional imaging systems, as well as the unique requirements of a clinician-centric POCUS workflow, to be able to collaborate with local IT experts to build, maintain, and improve their own POCUS programs.

Unique Aspects of POCUS Systems

Any ultrasound system can be utilized in a POCUS environment; however, there are specific factors that can make an ultrasound system better optimized for use in a POCUS program. These features can help facilitate rapid deployment to the bedside, switching between diagnostic and procedural imaging, multiple patient management, data retention, disinfection, and reduction in machine damage.

Ultrasound systems targeted for use in the POCUS environment have a variety of features that make them more ideal for a busy acute care setting. Larger ultrasound systems, traditionally designed for radiology and cardiology departments, include advanced features that require additional space for hardware. This translates into a bulky system footprint that can be harder to move between and within patient care rooms on a rapid basis. Some of the more esoteric features that require more space for physical components may be limited in POCUS systems, in favor of implementing features and workflows that are more conducive to POCUS implementation. When selecting ultrasound systems, prioritized features should be weighed against availability for purchase, implementation, cost, and equipment limitations. Features to consider in ultrasound system selection are further described in Table 28.1.

Ultrasound systems can be divided into categories based on their form factors, which can impact other elements, ergonomics, and user interactions. The main categories of ultrasound systems are cart-based systems (similar to traditional machines), hand-carry or laptop configurations, tablet-style, and handheld systems (Fig. 28.1) [1]. Laptop and tablet format systems may include a mounting cart that they can be docked into, and removed from for more portability. Tablet systems may also be mounted in specified rooms or locations. Handheld or pocket ultrasound systems will commonly require an additional display device (e.g., smartphone, tablet) for use.

R. M. Ferre (✉)
Department of Emergency Medicine, Indiana University School of Medicine, Indianapolis, IN, USA
e-mail: rferre@iu.edu

J. T. Nomura
Department of Emergency Medicine, Christiana Care Health System, Newark, DE, USA
e-mail: jnomura@christianacare.org

M. Gottlieb, N. Panebianco (eds.), *Advanced Point-of-Care Ultrasound*, https://doi.org/10.1007/978-3-031-85308-1_28

Table 28.1 Key features for POCUS systems to target acute care environments

System feature	Justification
Critically important *Features that are key for successful routine use in acute critical environments*	
Battery power	Mobility to move between patient encounters and locations
DICOM encoding software	Conform to medical imaging formatting standards for archiving
Durable multidirectional wheels	Portable systems should be nimble to mobilize between locations quickly
Large screen with wide viewing angle	Ease of visualization of exam images by the care team
Machine durability	Durability of the hardware, screens, and probes to accommodate frequent and high-volume use
Probe features	Probe(s) capable of broad frequency scanning (1-15mHz), and footprint appropriate for all requisite scan types
Rapid boot-up/wake time	Quick access to use for acute unexpected events
Server-based date and time	To account for daylight savings time changes to avoid errors
Small footprint	Crowded environment with multiple providers and equipment in patient rooms
Uniform disinfectant compatibility of components	Uniform disinfectant for probes and systems, outside of high-level disinfection, to ensure patient safety
Warranty	Warranty with coverage for the ultrasound machine, battery, and probes. While the length of the warranty for each will often differ, the length should be reasonable for each component
Wireless data transmission	Data transmission and reception occur immediately during the encounter, instead of periodically when attached to a hard wire connection
Moderately important *Features that improve user interface and operation in acute care settings*	
Automated calculations	Assistance for users to avoid errors
Backlit keyboard	Improved visualization in varied light environments
Multi-probe connector	Ease and reduced time for probe switching for multiple POCUS exam indications
Simplified keyboard	Removal of extraneous or less used functions and keys for ease of use
Sealed keyboard	Reduction in potential contamination or damage to internal components
Optional *Features that can be helpful but would have to be balanced against resources, other features, and program goals*	
Image acquisition guidance	For new user education and image optimization
Needle guidance software/hardware	To improve procedure safety and success
Physical storage space on the ultrasound system	Ease of access to necessary supplies
Reference image library	For new user education
Retractable power cord	Reduction in potential cord damage
Touch screen	Reduction in potential mechanical failure of keys or contamination
Wireless charging	Reduction in power cord damage and potential improved charging

DICOM digital imaging and communications in medicine, *POCUS* point-of-care ultrasound

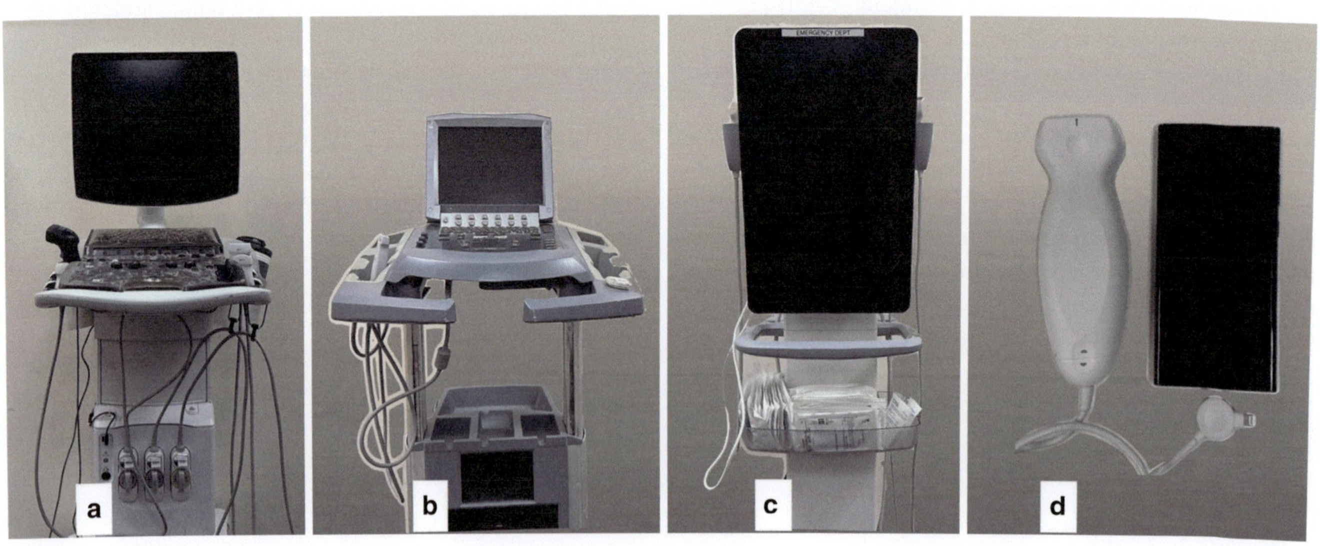

Fig. 28.1 Ultrasound system categories. (**a**) cart-based, (**b**) laptop or hand-carry configuration with mounting cart, (**c**) tablet-style with mounting cart, (**d**) handheld with a smartphone

Handheld Systems

There has been an increasing array of handheld ultrasound systems in recent years. This is partially fueled by hardware miniaturization and an expanding variety of clinical environments where POCUS can be used. Handheld systems can have different feature priorities than traditional systems (e.g., portability versus screen size), and selection should be based on the intended clinical use and deployment model.

One way that current handheld systems can differ from traditional probes is the transducer technology used. All probes rely on a process to convert electrical energy into acoustic energy and its reversal to generate an image. The majority of modern probes utilize synthetic piezoelectric crystals, the most common being lead zirconate titanate (PZT), with different additives and formats to create proprietary probe arrays [2]. Newer technology can incorporate microelectromechanical systems (MEMS) to create micromachined ultrasound transducers (MUT) [3]. These MUTs can be integrated with a complementary metal-oxide semiconductor (CMOS) to improve transducer-to-electronics connection to produce chip-based ultrasound transducers [4]. This has led to probes that can vary their imaging format and frequency to function as a single multi-purpose transducer. The key element of a MUT is the mobile membrane layer that vibrates and creates the ultrasound pressure wave. There are two main types of MUTs in current use: capacitive (CMUT) and piezoelectric (PMUT) [3]. CMUTs contain capacitors that cause the vibration of the membrane layer to produce the pressure wave [5]. PMUTs contain piezoelectric crystals in a layer or plate format, responding to electrical stimulation to vibrate the membrane, producing the pressure wave; the ultrasound wave is not created directly by the piezoelectric elements [3]. When the ultrasound wave returns to the probe, it deforms the membrane which creates a signal in the capacitor or piezoelectric layer that is interpreted into an image on the system.

When evaluating handheld systems, care should be taken to evaluate the imaging capability and probe format availability. Image quality may not match the traditional systems, even from the same manufacturer, and not all transducer formats may be available. Operational details of handheld systems can vary by manufacturer and should be considered in relation to the goals of the ultrasound program and infrastructure (Table 28.2).

Table 28.2 Handheld system options that can vary between systems and manufacturers

Feature	Options
Battery charging	Wired by device
	Wired to outlet power
	Wireless charging of transducer
	Wireless charging of removable battery
	Proprietary cradle for removable battery
	Multiple methods available for the device
Data storage	On-device
	Personal cloud storage
	Commercial/proprietary cloud storage
	DICOM server transfer
	Multiple simultaneous storage targets
	Multiple single storage targets
Display device/ connected device	Tablet
	Smart phone
	Mini-laptop
	Proprietary device
Patient information source	Manual entry
	Barcode scanning with the device camera
	Modality worklist function, local
	Modality worklist function, cloud
	Combination of methods
Transducer to device connection	Removable wire (lightning, USB-C, micro-USB, proprietary)
	Bluetooth
	WiFi
	Nonremovable proprietary wires
	Multiple options available with or without adapters
Transducer power	Rechargeable battery
	Disposable battery
	Powered by device
	Multiple methods available

DICOM digital imaging and communications in medicine

Mobile Device Management

An important component of the handheld system is the accompanying mobile device. This usually takes the form of a personal format smartphone or tablet device; these can be either the clinician's personal device or an institution-issued device. Institutions may have restrictions on personal devices being utilized in this capacity, so it is wise to confirm which approach may be best at a given institution. Unless a proprietary device is paired with the ultrasound probe, rendering it a single-use medical device, a mobile device must be chosen and managed in conjunction with the handheld probe. Commonly, the mobile device will be required to run the software interface to operate the probe and view the images. Because the software both functions for medical care and the control of a medical hardware device, it is considered a medical device or a mobile medical application [6].

Whether an institution-owned device or a personal device is used, mobile device management (MDM) solutions should be used for operational and security purposes. Hospital-owned devices may be easier for a POCUS program, as the control and oversight are deferred to IT. MDM solutions are generally software-based and allow the IT department a certain level of control over the device (Table 28.3). Not all elements of an MDM may be employed by the system, as

Table 28.3 Mobile device management elements and examples

Mobile device management elements	Examples
Application installation	Custom version of application install, or enabling restrictions on connection and function of application
Application update	Central timing of application updates to match other infrastructure elements
Automatic device locking	Time out; required passcode or password
Data transfer restrictions	Disabled screen capture; cut and paste ability
Device location	GPS
On-device storage restrictions	Disabled data saving on the storage device
Remote locking or disabling	Ability for security to remotely disable the device
Remote wiping	Ability for security to remotely wipe devices of information
Secure connections	VPN
User restrictions	User directory, password formats

GPS global positioning system, *VPN* virtual private network

customization and configuration will vary by institution. An institution may choose to have a specific operating system for their mobile devices; however, if using a personal device, the MDM plan should account for both Android and iOS devices, given the current device market share.

Security concerns for handheld devices usually center around protected health information (PHI), including access to PHI through the device and avoidance of inadvertent PHI release. Impermissible use and lack of safeguards to prevent release are the most common violations related to the Health Insurance Portability and Accountability Act (HIPAA) [7]. Another concern is a non-intended individual accessing the device and viewing PHI. The level of security, device access, and restrictions will be based on institutional policies and MDM implementation. User testing should occur to ensure that security restrictions do not impede POCUS workflow, leading to errors in workflow and data capture. This includes working with collaborators in IT to ensure that appropriate security standards are met for the network and cloud-based storage.

Life Cycle and Warranty

Ultrasound systems are subjected to regular wear and tear in a dynamic acute care environment. Technological equipment, such as ultrasound systems, have a projected life cycle or lifespan with routine use. The life cycle of a traditional cart-based ultrasound system is estimated to be 7 years with an annual volume of over 4000 scans per year, or 9 years if less than 2000 scans per year [8]. However, these data are based on radiology devices, so this is likely shorter when considering the harsher environment for POCUS. Use of the device beyond its life cycle may lead to increased breakdowns, impaired imaging, increased costs for repairs, and prolonged downtime. It is important to identify what entity manages equipment lifecycle records at each institution (often this falls under clinical engineering), and meet at regularly scheduled intervals to review when devices will need replacement. Capital requests can take months to process and are not guaranteed to be funded, so an organized central inventory of ultrasound assets can inform purchasing plans before equipment failure requires an emergent replacement.

Warranty contracts can help to cover issues that arise with routine use and can vary from 1 to 5 years, depending upon ultrasound system manufacturers. Some warranties offer extensions and riders to expand coverage. Typically, additional warranty coverage is available for ultrasound system repair and replacement through the manufacturer. User damage (e.g., probe damage from being dropped) is not generally covered; however, some companies may offer a reduced price for replacements due to user damage during the warranty period. Product line retirement by the manufacturer is also a concern, as it can make obtaining replacement parts to maintain a system difficult or impossible.

Many POCUS devices rely on battery power for function. Batteries generally have shorter life cycles and warranty periods than the rest of the ultrasound system. User actions that can reduce battery life include how close to 0% power the battery is discharged, referred to as depth of discharge [9]. Repeated full discharges of the battery will reduce the performance and life cycle of the battery. Automated power-down options are available on many systems to help reduce full battery discharges when not in use. To help reduce repeated full or near-full discharges, some manufacturers have implemented docking charge stations or wireless charging stations to make charging easier in a busy environment.

Device Maintenance

Routine system maintenance is important to optimize ultrasound system imaging. The POCUS program end-users can attend to some aspects of maintenance, such as cleaning, damage inspection, and performance evaluation. These activities can be a formal scheduled process (e.g., machine rounding checklists), occur during routine use, or a combination of both [10]. When performing image review, the

Table 28.4 Terms related to device maintenance as defined by the United States Food and Drug Administration [11]

Term	Definition
Recondition, refurbish, rebuild	Restore a medical device to original specifications from the OEM
Remanufacture	Work done to a finished product that significantly changes the product's safety, performance, or intended use
Remarket	Transfer of the device to another owner; can be by sale, donations, or lease
Repair	Servicing non-working or damaged elements to original specifications, outside of upkeep
Service	Repair, preventative, or routine maintenance of a device for original intended use according to original safety and performance specifications defined by the OEM

OEM original equipment manufacturer

ultrasound images should be assessed for quality degradation or missing image components which could suggest potential transducer malfunction or damage.

There are several terms that are related to device maintenance as defined by the United States Food and Drug Administration (Table 28.4) [11]. Typically, the institution will engage in the service and repair of ultrasound equipment, depending on available resources and expertise. Some servicing tasks may be outsourced to the original equipment manufacturer (OEM) staff or third-party companies. Replacement parts—either OEM, refurbished OEM, or equivalent third-party parts—can be purchased for use. Care should be taken to note what is required to maintain the system warranty if using third-party or refurbished parts.

The ultrasound system has a modality display used during image acquisition. This is different from a diagnostic display which is used solely to view and interpret medical images (e.g., a computer workstation) [12]. Currently, most system displays utilize liquid crystal display (LCD), or light-emitting diodes (LED). Standardized test pattern images with varying degrees of grayscale in the image are used to evaluate the display performance to ensure appropriate image display and the ability to differentiate grayscale levels for clinical interpretation. Probes should be evaluated regularly through the use of a standardized phantom for quality assurance regarding image quality, uniformity, and resolution [13]. These servicing tasks are generally managed by the institution through clinical engineering or medical physicists.

With the development of handheld ultrasound systems, there is less certainty around device servicing, especially for individually-owned devices. Mobile device screen technology usually incorporates newer technology sooner than standard medical devices, such as organic light-emitting diode (OLED) technology. Personal smartphones can incorporate screen protectors or cases that could affect the display quality. Personal smartphone devices may also acquire screen damage more frequently and be used with damage for a longer time before repair or replacement, than medical devices. While there is little standardization of guidance in this area, the POCUS program should take these factors into consideration when selecting and maintaining handheld devices.

Workflow Solutions

In addition to the hardware, a functional workflow solution is a core component of any POCUS program. It is important for POCUS program leaders to have a core knowledge of relevant workflow terminology and a basic understanding of how hospital imaging systems work. Table 28.5 contains common workflow-related key terms and definitions that POCUS leaders should be familiar with. Having knowledge of these items will form the basis of a productive conversation with members of the IT team.

Core Systems in POCUS Workflows

POCUS Manager / Middleware

When POCUS first began being utilized in emergency medicine, it centered around the clinical management of the patient and procedural guidance. There was limited infrastructure around image archiving or image reports outside of information included in the patient encounter note. As the use of POCUS has expanded and matured as an imaging modality, there has been greater focus on exam, image, and report management. Because of the differences in the clinical paradigm for POCUS from traditional consultative imaging and educational programs, various alternative management strategies were developed. This led to the development and use of middleware systems, so named because they sat in the middle between the ultrasound system, the picture archiving and communication systems (PACS), and electronic health record (EHR) programs. However, with efforts to standardize workflow elements and evolution of the field, there has been a greater focus on the abilities of these programs to expand their scope and functionality. Because of the need for expanded capabilities and integration into workflow processes, a more appropriate designation for these software programs would be a POCUS manager.

POCUS managers serve a function analogous to a PACS, with unique features that POCUS programs need. Most importantly, they have the capability to receive and transmit messages using Digital Imaging and Communications in Medicine (DICOM), and Health Level-7 (HL7) standards.

Table 28.5 Common terms and definitions in information technology workflows

Common terms and definitions	
AD	Active Directory. Database of all users that allows the identification and authentication of the user when accessing the system. This also allows the authorization of the user's level of access.
ADT	Admission, discharge, and transfer. When a patient is registered within the EHR, their information is made available to other programs through an ADT notification system. This system contains patient demographics, as well as unique healthcare encounter information. This database is made available to other software programs (e.g., PACS) to ensure that the correct patient demographics and unique healthcare encounter match between the EHR and the interfacing software program.
DICOM	Digital Imaging and Communications in Medicine. DICOM is the standard protocol for handling and sharing image data and files within healthcare. It defines the image file format and network protocol to store and retrieve patient's imaging data within a PACS or VNA.
EBIW	Encounter-based imaging workflow. EBIW is a type of imaging workflow that associates a patient's demographics and unique healthcare encounter information with images obtained in clinical care before an order is generated. The necessary patient information is usually acquired directly from the registration information and not from an order generated within the EHR.
EHR	Electronic health record. An EHR is a digital record of a patient's medical history.
HL7	Health Level-7. HL7 is a standard format for exchanging information between health information systems.
LDAP	Lightweight directory access protocol. A mechanism that allows a user to be identified within a directory database. For example, the hospital creates a single directory of all employees. LDAP allows many different software programs used within the hospital to use that same directory database to validate the user and their credentials.
MWL	Modality worklist (also known as a DICOM modality worklist). A MWL is a database of pending orders for imaging modalities that contain the appropriate patient demographic information and study information. This ensures that the correct patient demographics are associated with the images that will be obtained on the imaging modality.
PACS	Picture archiving and communications system. A medical image storage system that can store, transmit, and retrieve images and reports from multiple imaging modalities in a healthcare setting. Unlike a VNA, the workflow, display configurations, and storage are done differently by different vendors.
OBIW	Order-based imaging workflow (also known as scheduled workflow). OBIW is a type of workflow that begins when an order is first placed for an imaging exam to be completed. This is the standard workflow for radiology- or cardiology-based imaging studies where an order is placed and then scheduled to occur.
POCUS manager	A POCUS manager (also known as middleware) is software that acts as a bridge between a database and applications. Frequently, this includes functionality for creation, management, and transmission of images and worksheets for archiving along with imaging quality assurance capability.
Use case	A use case is a concept used in software design and implementation. A use case describes a desired task that requires software, and how it will be used within a given context. The use case usually details how a user will interact with the software and the necessary transactions that must occur between different systems to accomplish the desired task.
VNA	Vendor neutral archive. A medical image storage system that can store images and documents in a standard format with a standard interface, that allows them to be accessed in a vendor-neutral manner. Unlike a PACS system, the VNA stores all medical images in the same format with a vendor-neutral interface. It is often used to manage all images within healthcare, and not just those taken for traditional radiologic imaging modalities.
Workflow	A sequence of processes or steps needed to take a piece of work from initiation to completion.

This allows them to interact with both the ultrasound machine, the EHR, and any long-term archive system, such as a vendor neutral archive (VNA) or PACS. POCUS manager products also have built-in features that are unique and highly desirable to POCUS workflows, such as the ability to perform quality assurance and track various outputs, such as exams performed or tasks needing completion. POCUS manager products allow users without POCUS privileges to perform and complete POCUS reports, and send them to privileged POCUS users for review and finalization. This type of workflow is unique to POCUS imaging workflows and is not found in traditional consultative imaging workflows. POCUS manager solutions allow for this workflow by creating different types of users (i.e., users with POCUS privileges and users without POCUS privileges), each with different permissions (e.g., can finalize POCUS reports that are sent to the EHR, can complete POCUS reports and route to a user with POCUS privileges). Depending on the type of POCUS manager program and its unique configuration, user-level permissions can also be tied to individual worksheets, exam types, or exam groups. This is highly desirable for enterprise-level uses where the POCUS manager is shared across multiple specialties, each with their own unique POCUS exams that they are privileged to perform.

POCUS managers, while highly valuable for POCUS programs, can be prohibitively expensive for smaller organizations. In some cases, institutions may be able to leverage their PACS and EHR to come up with a workable solution in collaboration with other imaging departments [14]. For those desiring an encounter-based imaging workflow, which is valuable in the acute care setting with unscheduled patient encounters where a clinician can decide in real-time what exam(s) to perform, the POCUS manager is essential, as it allows for an automated order to be placed and completed after the POCUS exam has been completed (See section below on encounter- vs. order-based workflows).

Lightweight Directory Access Protocol (LDAP)

A unique aspect of POCUS workflows is the need to identify the operator performing the exam and communicate that information back to the POCUS manager. Identifying the operator on the ultrasound machine gives the manager system the ability to create an assignment task list for that user and track any steps needed within the workflow of the study (e.g., worksheet completion, finalizing the worksheet, sending for quality assurance). If no such task list exists, identifying the operator on the machine at a minimum allows the operator to easily sort through studies in the POCUS manager, to find their exams, and complete a report. A common mechanism used to identify and verify a user's credentials is using LDAP, an open-source protocol for accessing a list of users in a directory server. Hospital systems maintain a directory of authorized users including their login credentials. If mapped correctly, a user may put their username into a specific field on the patient information screen and have their credentials verified in the PACS or VNA, when the study is sent by the ultrasound machine. Leveraging the institutional active directory (AD) can reduce the administrative burden of having to create and maintain accounts for users, and removing their credentials from a system when the individual is no longer active. More sophisticated systems have leveraged LDAP to allow for the completion of POCUS reports directly on the ultrasound machine itself.

Admission, Discharge, and Transfer (ADT)

When patients present to a healthcare facility, they are registered in the health information system (HIS). Demographic data are collected or updated within the HIS system at that time. In addition, a unique visit or healthcare encounter is created at the time of registration. A part of the HIS is the ADT notification system. The ADT system provides patient demographics, as well as the unique healthcare encounter information, to other software programs in the local healthcare IT ecosystem. The ADT system shares this information to ensure that the correct patient's demographics and unique healthcare encounter information match between all systems that may be involved in the patient's care for that particular visit. For an encounter-based imaging workflow, it is the ADT notification system that provides the necessary information to create, populate, and update a modality worklist (MWL) when a patient encounter starts, ends, or their information is updated.

Vendor Neutral Archive (VNA)

While PACS systems are proprietary systems that store and retrieve information in a way that is unique to a particular vendor, a VNA completes these same tasks in an open-source, vendor-neutral way. PACS systems have specific requirements that are optimized for radiology- or cardiology-based imaging workflows. However, imaging data have become increasingly ubiquitous in modern healthcare. Traditionally, these images have been siloed in unique applications and generally do not use a DICOM standard. However, as EHRs have become more common in healthcare, IT systems have also become more mature and have sought to bring all images captured within the healthcare environment into an enterprise-level solution. This enterprise-level approach seeks to take images captured in silos and bring them into a common application that can archive, retrieve, and categorize images in a standard way. VNAs were developed to meet this need. POCUS workflows are easily integrated into a VNA, allowing for easier long-term retrieval and storage of images, rather than relying on the POCUS manager to provide the long-term storage needed by modern healthcare systems.

Picture Archiving and Communication System

PACS systems are integral to imaging workflows. PACS systems use the DICOM standard for communication with different imaging modalities and storage systems. However they also have integration engines that allow them to communicate with the EHR which uses an HL7 communication standard. In addition to storing images, PACS systems also receive order requests from the EHR, schedule those requests to be completed, and then manage documentation workflows for reports to be completed. These management tasks are completed using the radiology information system (RIS) which is a proprietary feature for different PACS systems. MWL serves as a core component of the PACS system where order information including patient demographics and visit data is shared with the correct imaging modality (e.g., ultrasound machine). POCUS managers function similarly to PACS systems with unique features needed by POCUS users and programs.

IT Standards

While each hospital or healthcare system is unique, international standards exist that define how IT systems should operate and interact with each other [15]. These standards ensure that device manufacturers and software developers will create products that can operate within any healthcare environment. Despite being highly technical, these standards also contain a use case that describes the context in which the standard exists.

Integrating the Healthcare Enterprise (IHE) is an international organization that creates standards that describe how different healthcare software systems should interact with each other [16]. IHE has published a standard for both encounter-based and order-based imaging workflows. These standards describe how a modality (e.g., an ultrasound machine), the EHR, and the image archiver (e.g., VNA or

PACS), should interact with each other to associate ultrasound images to a particular patient and then store those images in an accessible manner with an associated report in the EHR [16, 17]. POCUS workflows are heavily dependent on how different systems interact. IHE publishes these standards as technical frameworks and integration profiles, which are reviewed and updated as new technology arises and requirements change. Technical frameworks are dense technical documents designed for developers and engineers. Integration profiles are driven by use cases that outline specific clinical examples and provide a high-level summary of the systems involved and how they should be integrated with each other.

DICOM is a standard that was created to manage medical images, including their format, storage, and communication between devices in a non-proprietary way [18]. These standards set rules around how the ultrasound machines interact with storage servers and scheduling services. It established the MWL, which enabled a scheduling system to communicate patient and order information to the modality. DICOM uses tags and stores these as metadata. The fields seen on the patient information screen are examples of these DICOM tags. Because there are no DICOM tags displayed on ultrasound machines to differentiate between a user with POCUS privileges (e.g., attending physician) and a user without POCUS privileges (e.g., trainee), these attributes cannot be conveyed to other software solutions that have been built for POCUS workflows. As a result, these software solutions built for POCUS will often use the data from another DICOM field on the patient information screen (e.g., reading doctor), and input that data into a desired field (e.g., attending physician) within the software system.

Knowing that DICOM and IHE standards exist is important when working with different stakeholders in creating and improving a program's POCUS workflow. Knowing and referencing an international standard can remove objections from local IT leadership and help to coordinate efforts with the ultrasound machine vendor and POCUS manager developer or VNA provider to create the best POCUS workflow for a particular work environment. Having a working knowledge of how these systems operate will also allow POCUS leaders to find creative solutions to existing barriers.

Order-Based and Encounter-Based Imaging Workflows

The integration of these IT systems and the user interactions are the basis of an imaging workflow from study initiation to completion. Several different POCUS workflows have been described [14, 16, 17, 19]. However, any imaging workflow can be classified as either an order-based or an encounter-based workflow. Regardless of the type of workflow used, the purpose of the workflow is to get the ultrasound report into the EHR and the images into a long-term storage system (e.g., PACS or VNA). The workflow should allow a clinician to perform a POCUS exam on a registered patient, associate the saved images with an interpretive report, file the report within the patient's EHR, and archive the images in a long-term storage system in a retrievable manner. To understand how software systems must interact to accomplish this workflow, it is best to consider this workflow from the clinician's viewpoint, where the workflow progresses from the start of a POCUS exam and ends when the interpretive report is finalized by applying a digital signature (Fig. 28.2). It is also important to remember that imaging devices (e.g., ultrasound machines) and healthcare imaging systems (e.g., PACS, VNA) use DICOM as the communication standard, whereas

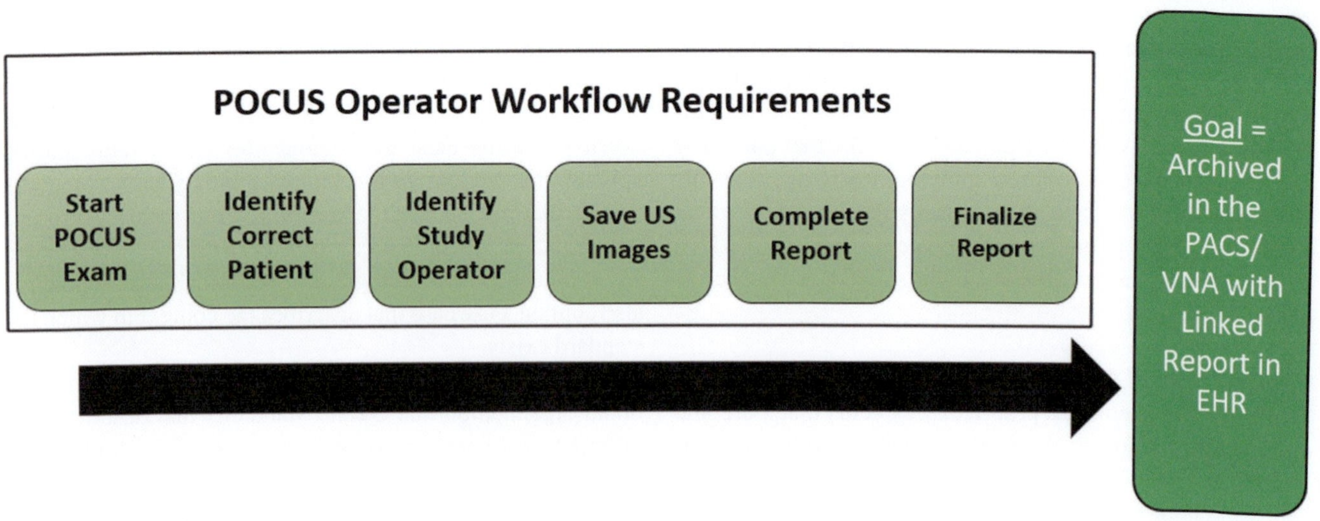

Fig. 28.2 Core elements of a POCUS workflow. *EHR* electronic health record, *POCUS* point-of-care ultrasound

EHRs and patient registration systems (e.g., ADT) use HL7 as their communication standard. For this reason, the ultrasound machine cannot directly communicate with the EHR and requires an interface (e.g., POCUS manager) to share information between systems.

Order-based imaging workflows (OBIW), also known as schedule-based workflows, begin when an order is placed to perform a specific ultrasound exam on a particular patient. This type of workflow involves the clinician placing an order for an imaging study to be performed on a patient who has already been registered in the HIS. If we consider the use case of a POCUS exam to be done in the emergency department, the order placed in the EHR causes a cascade of things to occur. The EHR sends a message to the archiver (e.g., PACS or VNA) that an exam is to be performed through an HL7 message. The PACS or VNA is then able to create a unique identifier for that exam, known as the accession number. This information is then relayed to a DICOM MWL in a specific area (e.g., emergency department) and for a specific modality (e.g., ultrasound). The person responsible for performing the exam, can find the correct patient and begin the correct study that has been ordered by searching the MWL on the ultrasound machine. Once the study has been completed, the study is sent back to the PACS or VNA, and a communication is sent back to the EHR that the order has been completed. Because an accession number was previously created by the PACS or VNA and associated with the correct patient through the MWL, the study can easily be archived in the PACS or VNA and linked back to the order that was originally placed in the EHR. Figure 28.3 contains an overview of the steps and systems involved in an OBIW. Because a POCUS manager can function as an archiving replacement for PACS, the POCUS manager system may be used in place of a traditional radiology PACS in

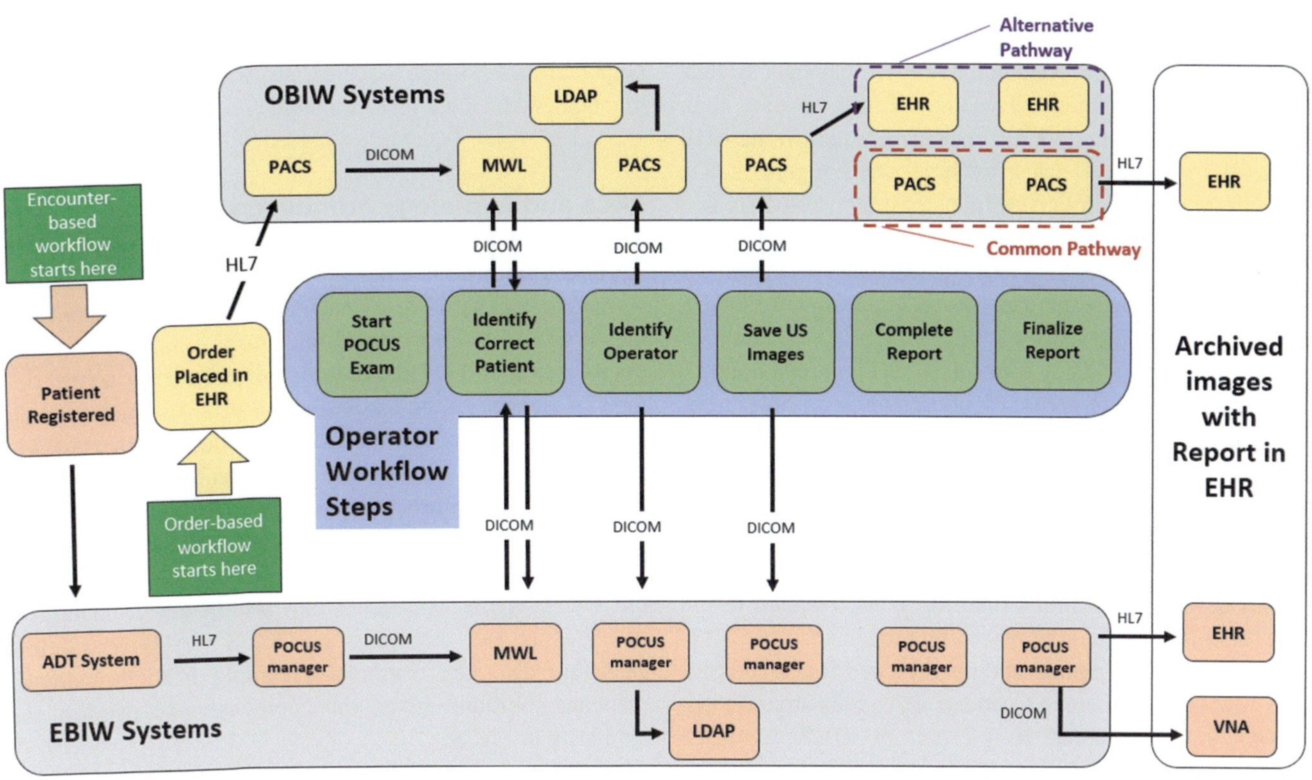

Fig. 28.3 Overview of order-based and encounter-based POCUS workflows and systemsOrder-based and encounter-based imaging workflows, use similar IT systems but interact with these systems in unique ways. EBIW uses its own MWL that is populated, not by order, but when a patient is registered at a unique location (e.g., emergency department at West Hospital). This is the starting place of an EBIW. In contrast, OBIW begins when an order is placed and populates the same MWL that radiology-based studies use. A POCUS manager functions similarly to a PACS system for image management and interacts with the ultrasound machine in similar ways using DICOM communication standards. In EBIW, the images are saved to the POCUS manager system where a report is generated, and an order, report, and linked images are sent to the EHR. Images are sent to the VNA for long-term storage. An OBIW that uses a POCUS manager system as its PACS will also use the POCUS manager to complete and finalize the report. However, an OBIW may also be set up to use the same PACS system used for radiology-based studies. In this case, the report is completed in the EHR and linked to the order and images in the PACS system. *OBIW* order-based imaging workflow, *EBIW* encounter-based imaging workflow, *EHR* electronic health record, *PACS* picture archiving and communication system, *VNA* vendor neutral archive, *LDAP* lightweight directory access protocol, *ADT* admission discharge and transfer, *DICOM* digital imaging and communications in medicine, *HL7* health level 7

an OBIW. An advantage of the OBIW is that it can leverage existing systems easily found in most healthcare systems.

In contrast, an encounter-based imaging workflow (EBIW) requires a unique infrastructure and a POCUS manager application. The EBIW more closely matches how work is accomplished in the clinical environment, where a pre-existing order is not required for a clinician to perform a POCUS exam. The EBIW begins when the POCUS exam starts. However, in order for the study to meet the requirements of a VNA and EHR, patient information from the ADT must be associated with the ultrasound images. While this task can be completed in the POCUS manager after the study has been completed, the ideal workflow utilizes a MWL that is populated based on registration information conveyed via the ADT notification system to the POCUS manager. Once the MWL is populated, the operator can select the correct patient on the ultrasound machine before beginning the exam. Similar to an OBIW, the user should be identified using a mapped DICOM field with an integrated LDAP interface within the POCUS manager product. Once the images are saved and the study is completed, images are found in the POCUS manager system, and a report is completed and finalized. Exams that are finalized are sent from the POCUS manager system to the EHR via an HL7 message. Because the order was not generated in the EHR first, an unsolicited order message (ORM) is first sent to the EHR. The EHR acknowledges this message, and the final report—with a link to the study images—is sent via an HL7 observation result message (ORU) from the POCUS manager to the EHR.

An advantage of EBIW over OBIW is that it can improve efficiency and ease of access by not requiring an order to be placed prior to use. A disadvantage of an EBIW is that the workflow is not visible in the EHR until a study appears within the EHR. POCUS workflows face the unique challenge of getting clinicians to complete all the steps of the workflow. While there are fewer requirements in EBIW, the entire workflow process is not visible until a final report has resulted within EHR. In contrast, the order placed by the clinician in OBIW "announces" that a clinical study will be performed and provides visibility to others (e.g., coders and administrators) that a POCUS exam should be present. In EBIW, no such "announcement" is made, making accountability to finish the remaining steps of the workflow more challenging using existing mechanisms (e.g., coders, IT administrators). This means that the important clinical information from the exam, and any ability for revenue capture, are unavailable until the entire workflow has been completed.

Interdisciplinary Collaborations

To create and maintain a successful POCUS workflow and program, requires collaboration among different relevant parties within an institution. Outside the clinical stakeholders, key collaborators for a successful POCUS program include IT and clinical engineering. These partners will help to establish the behind-the-scenes infrastructure to support the ultrasound systems with a smooth clinical interface and end-user experience.

Information Technology

For a program to flourish, IT infrastructure and services are vital for POCUS operations. Ultrasound imaging workflows rely on several IT systems to be able to communicate with the ultrasound device. This involves information flowing both to and from the ultrasound system. This integration for workflow will rely on several applications and processes for final archiving and clinical information communication, with minimal effort from the clinical end-user. Interactions can be with program analysts, managers, project managers, or combinations of them, depending on the necessary task or project. For ongoing maintenance, a specific IT manager will help facilitate routine updates, software patches, improvements, new device integration, and resolution of problems.

PACS and Radiology Administration

Administrators of a healthcare system's PACS are essential team members for IT and imaging departments. Not only are they responsible for the daily operations, image linking, and maintenance of the PACS but also data integrity across systems. A portion of the institution's PACS administrators are responsible for the reconciliation of studies with workflow errors, such as missing or erroneous identifiers (e.g., patient name, patient identifier number, date of service, accession number). They identify workflow failures to improve infrastructure and prevent further errors. Because of their expertise with imaging workflows, they will be key collaborators in choosing and managing a POCUS workflow solution. They are also key resources regarding POCUS manager software solutions, given the components of overlap and similarity to PACS.

Radiology administration can be an invaluable collaborator given the many elements of radiology infrastructure that can be leveraged for POCUS, including coding, billing, orders, worklists, and study reconciliation. Working with radiology administration can prevent redundant work and provide access to resources for the advancement of POCUS workflow infrastructure.

Security

IT security protocols, regulations, and standards are very complex and far-reaching, making the security team a vital role in controlling access to POCUS hardware, connectivity, and software. Security concerns center around PHI and access to the institution's networked devices and software. Access security is generally accomplished by a login process with user databases and passwords. The integration of POCUS elements with the institution's security infrastructure is key to reducing the burden on users and administrators. For example, utilizing the institution's active directory to have uniform user login and passwords across systems, including the POCUS devices and POCUS manager, improves the user experience. This also allows the use of a single sign-on user authentication method to reduce the user's having to repeatedly enter their passwords. They are also key in developing a remote access pathway to POCUS software when outside the institution's network. The security team is also a key player in the MDM plan for handheld devices discussed earlier, and ensuring adequate safeguards.

Clinical Engineering

The biomedical equipment technicians and the clinical or biomedical engineers are responsible for the servicing and repair of medical devices. In addition to performing maintenance of the ultrasound systems, they can offer insight into the life cycle, work with the manufacturer on servicing equipment, and help inform equipment selection and purchasing for replacements. Clinical engineering is also responsible for elements of machine maintenance that are outside the experience of the general clinician administrator for a POCUS program.

Regardless of the type of ultrasound system and workflow used within a program, the decision should incorporate clinical end-users in the decision making process. The ultrasound systems selected should be able to perform within the intended environment and for the intended purposes, and integrate into the chosen POCUS workflow. Ultimately, this means that the POCUS program leadership, who have a broad viewpoint including clinical, administrative, and operational elements, should be responsible for the final decision on machine acquisition [20].

Pearls and Pitfalls

- Ultrasound systems should be matched to the planned clinical use. The difference between traditional systems and handheld systems can impact their integration.
- Early testing and collaboration with IT for handheld mobile device management is important to ensure that handheld devices are able to be integrated into the IT infrastructure and POCUS workflow.
- Life cycle estimates for ultrasound machines are typically 7–9 years, depending on case volume. However, these are based on radiology literature. POCUS systems used within a harsh environment likely will have a shorter life cycle.
- Maintenance and adherence to regulatory requirements for ultrasound hardware, include elements outside the usual POCUS clinical leader. Collaborate with clinical engineering for regulatory quality assurance requirements.
- Order-based imaging workflows are already in use in most radiology departments. Developing an encounter-based imaging workflow will require IT collaboration and will integrate better within the clinical workflow.
- Every specialty has a unique lexicon. Understanding IT terminology and vocabulary will aid in collaboration, meeting productivity, and achieving your goals.
- Communication standards between healthcare systems and devices are not universal; ultrasound systems utilize DICOM, while the EHR utilizes HL7. This means that without an interface between them, such as the POCUS manager, PACS, or a VNA, the data cannot be translated to allow transfer from the ultrasound to the EHR.
- User identification is important in a POCUS workflow; integrate the institution's active directory and LDAP system into the workflow. Utilize existing resources and systems instead of replicating work.

Disclosures/Conflicts of Interest

Robinson M. Ferre: Advisory Board, FujiFilm SonoSite, Inc., Course Director, 3rd Rock Ultrasound, LLC. Consulting, Philips, Vave Health, Inc.

Jason T. Nomura: Consulting: Philips, Caption AI. Research Funding: Bristol Myers Squibb, Bayer.

References

1. Tayal VS, Blaivas M, Foster TR, editors. Ultrasound program management. Springer; 2018.
2. Shung KK. Diagnostic ultrasound imaging and blood flow measurements. 2nd ed. CRC Press; 2015.
3. Roy K, Lee JE, Lee C. Thin-film PMUTs: a review of over 40 years of research. Microsyst Nanoeng. 2023;9:95.
4. Rothberg JM, Ralston TS, Rothberg AG, Martin J, Zahorian JS, Alie SA, Sanchez NJ, Chen K, Chen C, Thiele K, Grosjean D, Yang J, Bao L, Schneider R, Schaetz S, Meyer C, Neben A, Ryan

B, Petrus JR, Lutsky J, McMahill D, Corteville G, Hageman MR, Miller L, Fife KG. Ultrasound-on-chip platform for medical imaging, analysis, and collective intelligence. Proc Natl Acad Sci USA. 2021;118(27):e2019339118.
5. Wang J, Zheng Z, Chan J, Yeow JTW. Capacitive micromachined ultrasound transducers for intravascular ultrasound imaging. Microsyst Nanoeng. 2020;6:73.
6. US Food and Drug Administration. Policy for device software functions and mobile medical applications. US Food and Drug Administration; 2022.
7. US Department of Health and Human Services. Enforcement Highlights – Current. Accessed April 2024, https://www.hhs.gov/hipaa/for-professionals/compliance-enforcement/data/enforcement-highlights/index.html.
8. European Society of Radiology (ESR). Renewal of radiological equipment. Insights Imaging. 2014;5(5):543–6.
9. Preger Y, Barkholtz HM, Fresquez A, Campbell DL, Juba BW, et al. Degradation of commercial lithium-ion cells as a function of chemistry and cycling conditions. J Electrochem Soc. 2020;167:120532.
10. Prats MI, Nelson BP, Gold DL, Branditz LD, Boulger CT, Bahner DP. CLEAR: a novel approach to ultrasound equipment homeostasis. J Ultrasound Med. 2019;38(3):767–73.
11. US Food and Drug Administration. FDA report on the quality, safety and effectiveness of service of medical devices. US Food and Drug Administration; 2018.
12. American Association of Physicists in Medicine. Display Quality Assurance Report of AAPM Task Group 270. AAPM; 2019.
13. American College of Radiologists and American Association of Physicists in Medicine. ACR-AAPM technical standard for diagnostic medical physics performance monitoring of real time ultrasound equipment. ACR; 2021.
14. Rong K, Chimileski B, Kaloudis P, Herbst MK. Impact of an epic-integrated point-of-care ultrasound workflow on ultrasound performance, compliance, and potential revenue. Am J Emerg Med. 2021;49:233–9.
15. Roth CJ, Lannum LM, Persons KR. A foundation for enterprise imaging: HIMSS-SIIM collaborative white paper. J Digit Imaging. 2016;29(5):530–8.
16. Integrating the Healthcare Enterprise. Available at https://www.ihe.net. Accessed February 2024.
17. IHE Radiology Technical Framework, supplements for trial implementation, encounter based imaging workflow. Available at: https://www.ihe.net/resources/technical_frameworks/#radiology. Accessed February 2024.
18. Bidgood WD Jr, Horii SC, Prior FW, Van Syckle DE. Understanding and using DICOM, the data interchange standard for biomedical imaging. J Am Med Inform Assoc. 1997;4(3):199–212.
19. Thompson B, Schoenfeld E, Westafer L, Visintainer P, Budhram G. Implementation of an automated, user-centered point-of-care ultrasound workflow improves documentation and billing. Acad Emerg Med. 2023;30(3):180–6.
20. AIUM Official Statement: ultrasound system and transducer specifications used in purchasing decisions. J Ultrasound Med. 2023;42(7):E8–9.

29 Emerging Applications in Point-of-Care Ultrasound

Laura Oh, Andrew W. Kirkpatrick, and Rachel B. Liu

Background

As technology advances in the twenty-first century, innovation has led to exciting new possibilities for point-of-care ultrasound (POCUS) users. These leaps forward have offered a glimpse of new applications, improved diagnostic capabilities, and novel tools for the end-user. The association with advances in technology, changing how POCUS is used by clinicians is a familiar one. In the past, POCUS has benefited from technological leaps forward, including the miniaturization of POCUS machines to handheld devices, post-processing techniques that have improved image quality, wireless hardware that allows cordless experiences, and cloud-based storage that has connected POCUS users across the globe. As technology progresses, new ideas will impact how clinicians are utilizing POCUS to care for patients. Three emerging applications are highlighted below to demonstrate how today's advances are shaping new uses of POCUS. While this list is not comprehensive, it shows how new technologies are broadening POCUS horizons from our current conception.

L. Oh (✉)
Department of Emergency Medicine, Emory University, Atlanta, GA, USA
e-mail: laura.oh@emory.edu

A. W. Kirkpatrick
Departments of Critical Care Medicine and Surgery, University of Calgary, Calgary, AB, Canada
e-mail: andrew.kirkpatrick@ahs.ca

R. B. Liu
Department of Emergency Medicine, Yale School of Medicine, New Haven, CT, USA
e-mail: rachel.liu@yale.edu

Artificial Intelligence in POCUS

Artificial Intelligence (AI) in medicine is expanding at a rapid pace, with most United States Food and Drug Administration (FDA)-authorized, AI-enabled medical devices residing in the field of radiology [1]. AI is an umbrella term that encompasses both machine learning and deep learning; it refers to computer systems performing tasks that typically require human cognition [2]. The term machine learning (ML) describes the creation of algorithms that learn from and make predictions based on patterns of data [2]. A further subsect of ML is deep learning (DL), which passes data through layers of neural networks (similar to neuronal organization in the human brain) that lead to object recognition and classification in a more robust fashion than traditional ML [3]. Most current advances in POCUS AI use DL techniques [4].

Algorithm-based ML is performed in three main ways: supervised, unsupervised, and reinforcement learning. Supervised learning is the most common method for ultrasound ML development [2, 3], and uses labeled datasets established by expert-defined "ground truths". These ground truths are established in a process where experts attest to the efficacy of an algorithm compared to what is known in reality [4]. For example, in a dataset examining the pleural line, an expert panel may determine the number of frames in which B lines are either present or absent. The experts' results are established as the gold standard "truths." The same dataset is presented to the algorithm with the goal of close agreement to the ground truth, and iterative adjust-

M. Gottlieb, N. Panebianco (eds.), *Advanced Point-of-Care Ultrasound*, https://doi.org/10.1007/978-3-031-85308-1_29

ments are made to increase its accuracy, reliability, and validity. This type of ML can be labor intensive because there are few expert-reviewed, patient-level, labeled datasets. Additionally, the quality of the ML output is defined by the human expert input. However, it presents opportunities for POCUS experts to form research partnerships with AI companies in developing prospective datasets for training, validation, and testing to further advance the field.

AI software targeting POCUS users has demonstrated good diagnostic accuracy for several clinical conditions. A prolific area of AI development has been lung ultrasound, with algorithms showing high sensitivity and specificity for B-line detection, quantification, and severity scoring [5, 6]. Differences found in performance parameters between physicians and AI algorithms for pulmonary edema highlight the need for continuous refinement and research development [7]. Similarly, cardiac AI for the classification of ejection fraction has been shown to match cardiologist and POCUS expert visual estimation [8]. More recent data also demonstrate accuracy for diastolic assessment using POCUS [9].

There has been a rapidly growing interest in bladder volume AI since urinary retention is a common presentation, and current devices can misidentify ascites, cysts, fibroids, and other pelvic structures as the bladder. One early study reported high sensitivity and specificity of AI software compared to sonographer-performed measurement [10], which potentially offers cost savings when offered on less expensive handheld devices versus traditional bladder scanners. Some devices also have an "auto-sweep" feature, which steers a sound beam in multiple planes from a single view, minimizing the need to obtain multiple views for volume calculation.

At this time, many of the AI tools for POCUS are in the research and development stages, although several commercial products have been released for clinical use in select abdominal, cardiac, lung, musculoskeletal, and vascular applications [11]. The advancement of AI in ultrasound has been slower than other modalities within diagnostic imaging because of its operator-dependent nature, variability in image quality due to patient and machine factors, lack of standardized protocols in image acquisition, frequent presence of artifacts, use of dynamic video cine clips instead of high-resolution static frames, subjectivity in interpretation, and unavailability of large labeled datasets [4, 12]. However, some of these barriers are also driving the need for POCUS AI growth.

Currently, the main benefits of POCUS AI stem from its use in *detection* (organ or structure identification—e.g., ascites, pulmonary edema; Fig. 29.1), *classification* (categorization of disease stage—e.g., ejection fraction determination; Fig. 29.2), and *segmentation* (discriminating the borders of distinct structures—e.g., diaphragm, rib shadows, pleural

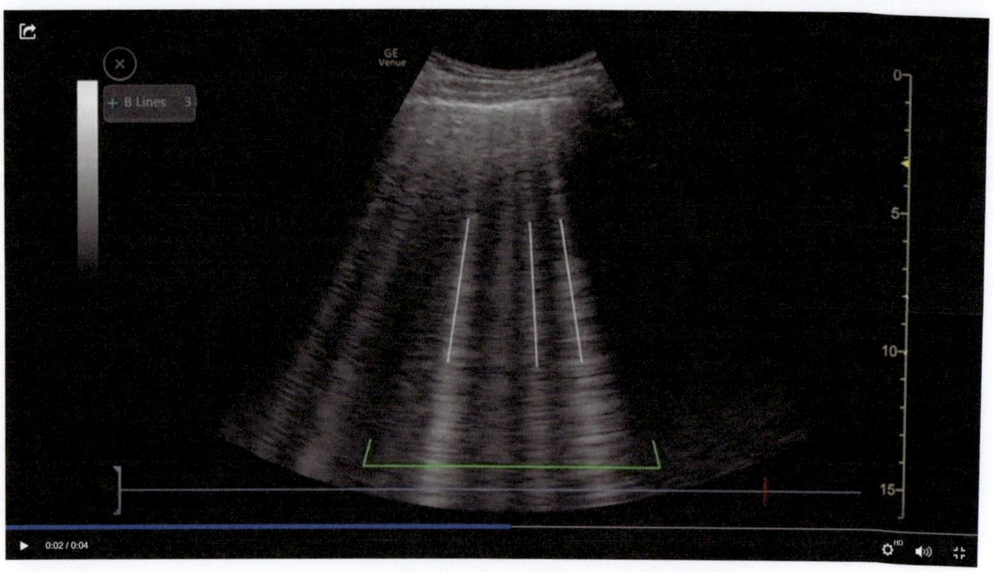

Fig. 29.1 Example of artificial intelligence for detection. The software has placed white lines where it has detected B lines

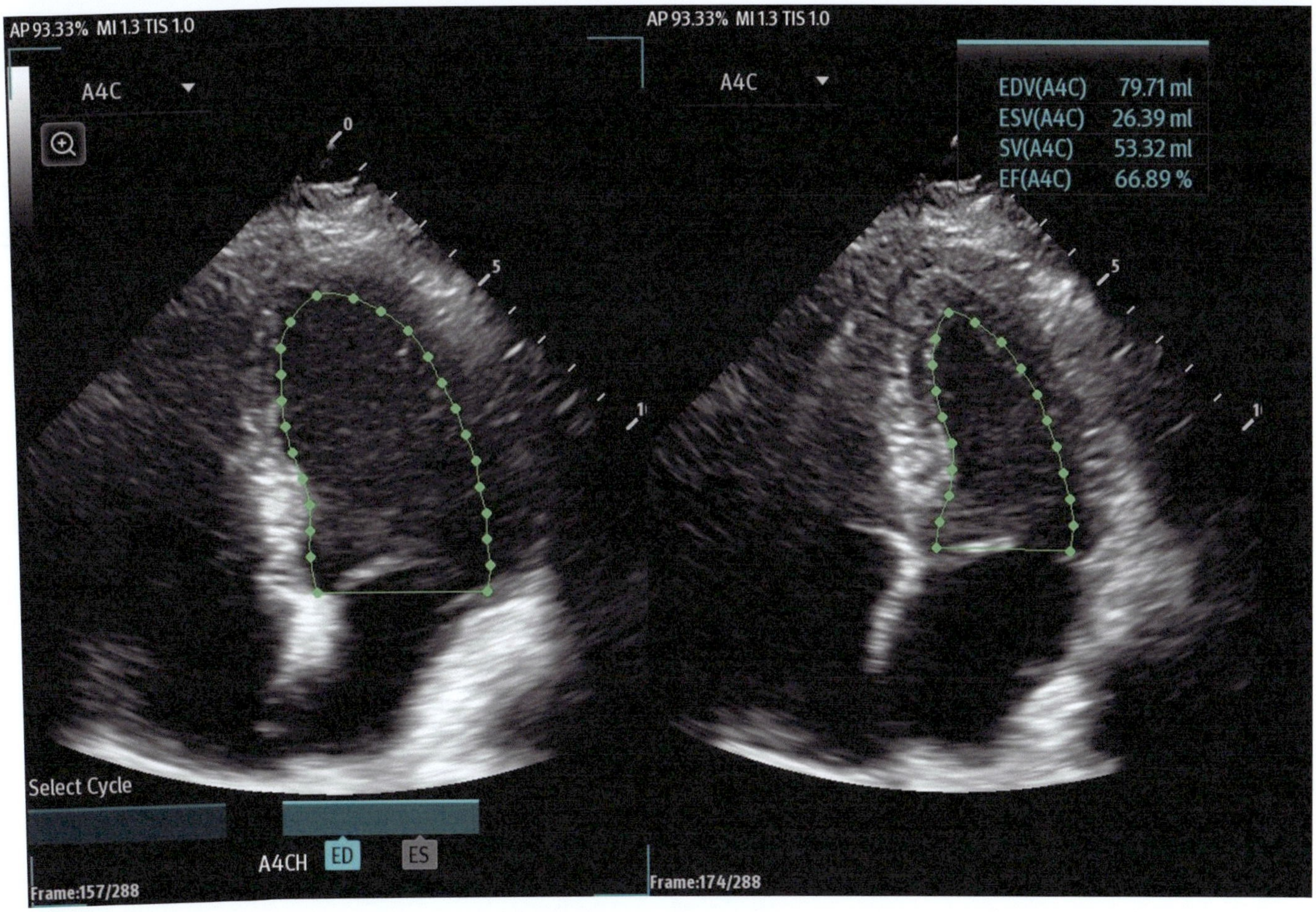

Fig. 29.2 Example of artificial intelligence for classification, allowing auto-calculation of ejection fraction. (*Image courtesy of Michael Gottlieb, MD*)

line; Fig. 29.3) [13]. Newer AI tools can also perform functions, such as highlighting or auto-labeling of anatomic and pathologic structures (Fig. 29.4).

Other novel features include assistance in image acquisition, such as auto-capture, image quality meters, and machine guidance of probe maneuvers that can lead to optimal image capture (Fig. 29.5). In this way, POCUS AI can enhance efforts to educate novice users without time-intensive direct human supervision, while providing real-time feedback and consistency in image acquisition and interpretation [14]. It may also aid in decreasing variation within and across operators, and increasing standardization in image quality.

AI may also provide benefits in workflow and program administration. This includes the immediate delivery of quality improvement feedback to individuals, which is traditionally a time-consuming manual process provided by expert ultrasound faculty [5]. Auto-capture features may facilitate the archiving of images. For example, some commercial products auto-detect examination types based on the selected probe or preset, combined with auto-identification of scanned structures. Auto-documentation can streamline chart completion and billing processes and may be used to track metrics required for credentialing, privileging, and continuous quality improvement.

AI shows increasing promise in POCUS for assistance with image acquisition, interpretation, diagnosis, education, and administration. With increasing computer processing power and improvements in approaches to DL, growth in this area will cause AI to become integrated into everyday POCUS use.

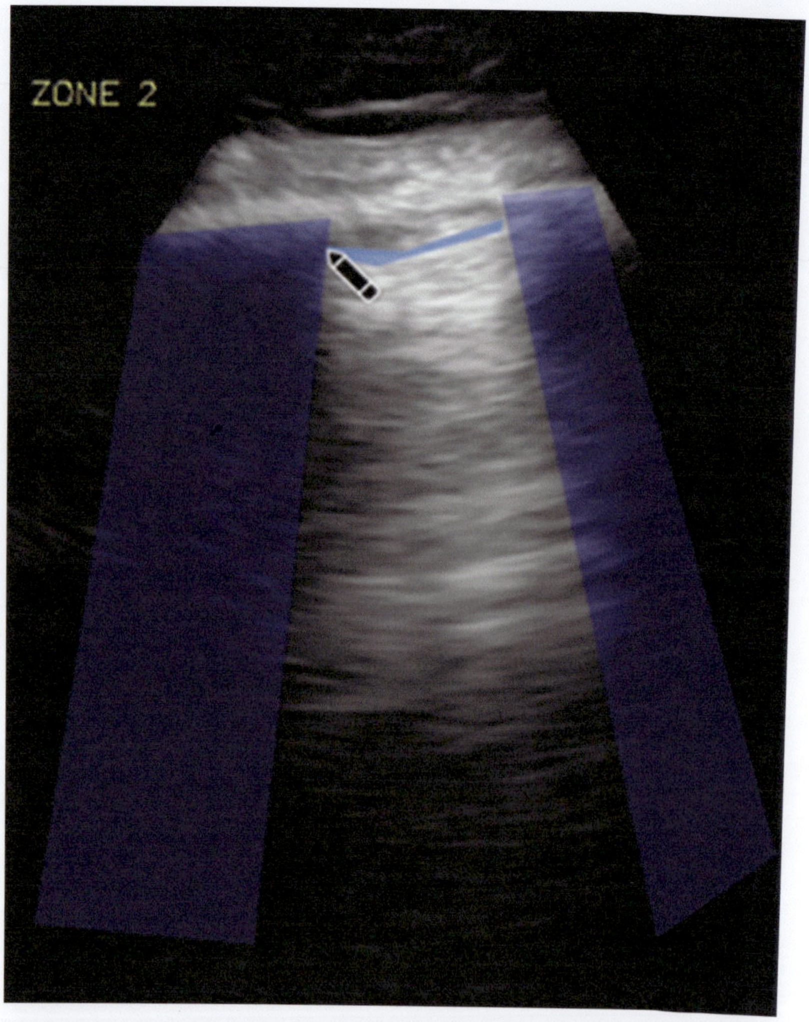

Fig. 29.3 Example of artificial intelligence (AI) for segmentation performed by a POCUS expert to train an AI algorithm. The dark blue segments were labeled by the expert as rib shadow, and the light blue segment was labeled as the pleural line. This may help the AI software perform labeling functions and identify landmark structures

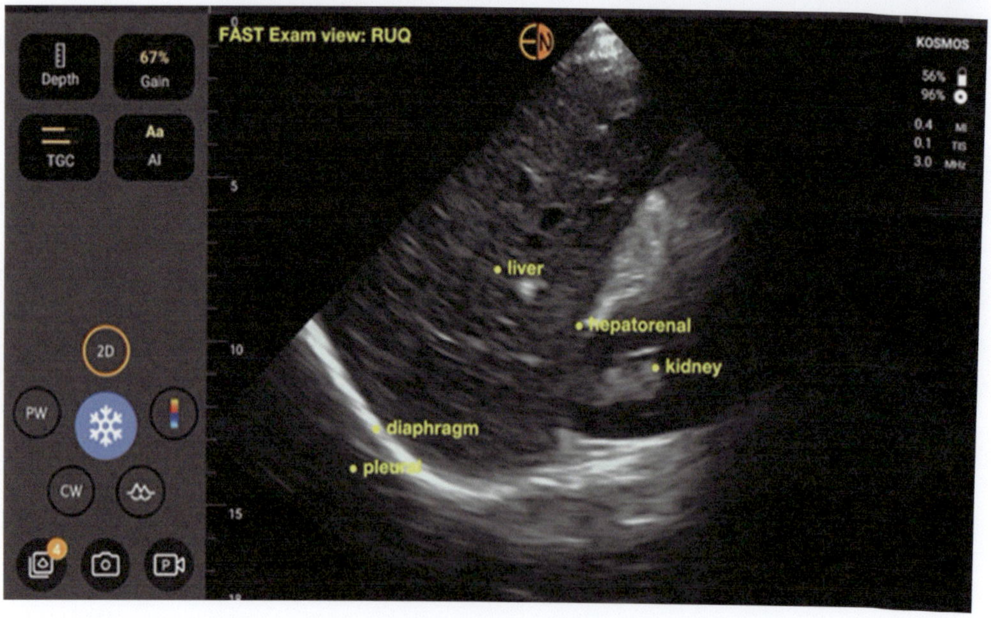

Fig. 29.4 An example of auto-labeling as the operator obtains a right upper quadrant view

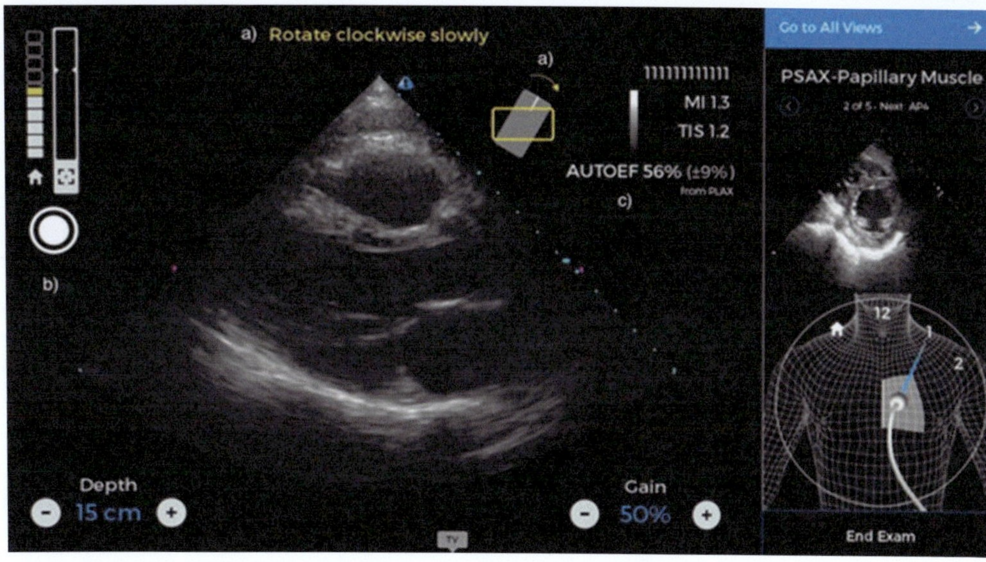

Fig. 29.5 Example of image guidance using auto-assistance. The software has detected that the operator has performed a parasternal long-axis view, and is guiding the operator to obtain a parasternal short-axis view. There is a meter assessing image quality, which will trigger auto-saving of the image when the quality is deemed high. The software has given an auto-calculated measurement of ejection fraction

Contrast-Enhanced Ultrasound

Contrast-enhanced ultrasound (CEUS) is the use of ultrasound contrast agents (UCAs) to augment traditional medical ultrasonography. In the 1960s, it was observed that the presence of small air bubbles in injected solutions could increase ultrasound signal intensity [15]. The technique of agitated saline continues to have use in the evaluation of right-to-left intracardiac shunts and central line confirmation [16]; however, UCAs have evolved over time. The microbubbles of second-generation UCAs are more stable, utilizing a phospholipid shell to encapsulate an inert gas, perfluorocarbon, or sulfur hexafluoride. These agents can last in circulation for at least 5 minutes, and since they are similar to (or smaller in size than) a red blood cell, they are blood-pool agents confined to the intravascular space [15]. When a microbubble comes into contact with an ultrasound beam at low acoustic power (mechanical index of 0.2–0.4), it produces a non-linear harmonic response that can be separated from tissue signal using contrast harmonic ultrasound; this allows for evaluation of tissue perfusion at the capillary level [17].

Although the use of CEUS for trauma is an off-label indication in the United States, it has been researched in Europe for decades [17]. While the focused assessment with sonography in trauma (FAST) examination focuses on indirect evidence of injury by assessing for free fluid in potential spaces, the contrast-enhanced FAST examination can look for direct evidence of injury, such as lacerations or extravasation (Fig. 29.6). Since UCAs are metabolized from the body within 15 minutes and are not nephrotoxic, the use of contrast has several advantages, including that it is easily repeatable and blood testing (e.g., creatinine level) do not need to be obtained prior to use. Although CEUS has potential as a trauma evaluation tool, it does not fully replace computed tomography, which is better at evaluating structures such as the adrenal glands, renal collecting system, bowel, and diaphragm. Opportunities for use of CEUS may be particularly relevant for special populations, such as pediatric patients, where a radiation-sparing diagnostic modality may be preferred [18].

Another emerging application of CEUS is its use pre- and post-percutaneous intervention for acute occlusive myocardial infarction [19, 20]. When a microbubble is insonated with high power (i.e., using a high mechanical index setting), the microbubble expands and collapses. This acoustic response results in fluid jets that can erode a nearby thrombus. Sonothrombolysis, the intentional destruction of microbubbles using high acoustic power to fragment a thrombus, is a promising area of CEUS research. Preliminary data from small trials indicate that sonothrombolysis may improve long-term outcomes for patients who have suffered an acute myocardial infarction by reducing myocardial infarction size and preserving left ventricular systolic function [21]. Other applications for CEUS include, but are not limited to evaluation of aortic aneurysm rupture and endoleak, actively bleeding soft-tissue hematomas, testicular and adnexal torsion, infectious processes, and ectopic pregnancy [22–26].

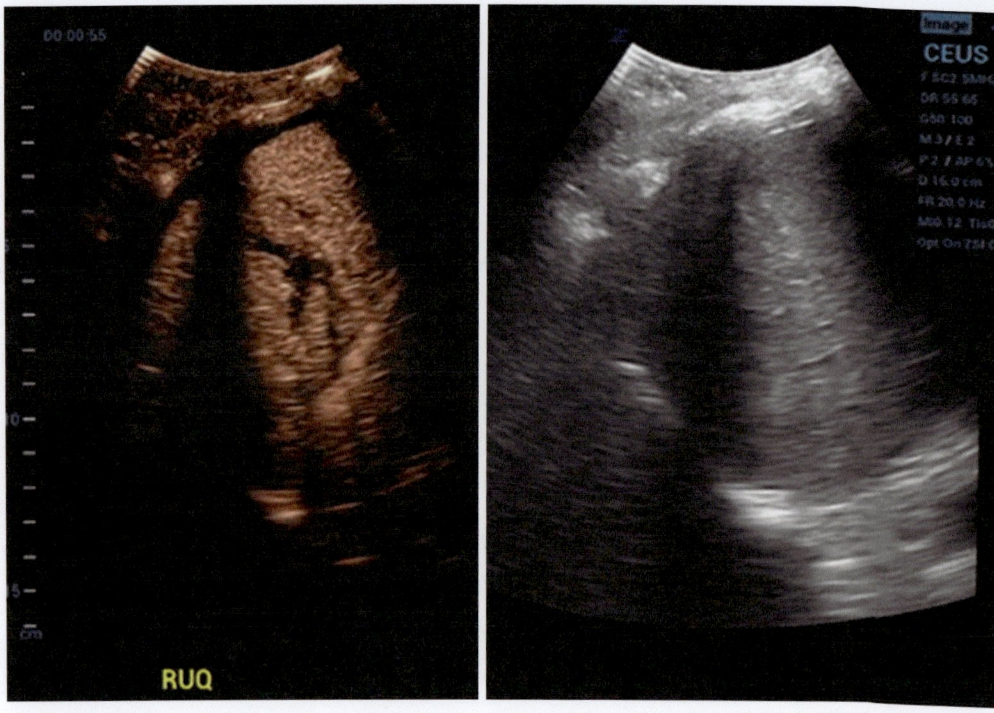

Fig. 29.6 Liver laceration demonstrated with contrast-enhanced ultrasound (left), compared with a grayscale image (right). (*Image courtesy of Tobias Kummer, MD*)

Remote Telementored Ultrasound

Remote telementored ultrasound (RTMUS) is a form of telemedicine in which a remote expert guides a distant end-user to obtain meaningful images that can be interpreted by the expert asynchronously or in real-time. It is a rapidly evolving field where almost anybody willing to take direction may be remotely guided to image a patient while following a remote expert's guidance using common communicative technologies [27]. There are many related acronyms, such as remotely-supported ultrasound, tele-ultrasound, telesonography, or telementoring, all of which combine use of ultrasound with telemedicine [28–30]. This paradigm of a remote guide has a multitude of potential uses across and above the planet, thereby improving access to healthcare for remote and underserved areas. In space medicine, RTMUS has become a backbone of healthcare onboard the International Space Station, as there are no other imaging modalities available in space [30, 31]. Despite the immense potential of RTMUS on Earth, its effectiveness has yet to be fully proven in robust clinical trials [28, 30].

Remote Tele-mentored Self-Performed Ultrasound

Remote tele-mentored self-performed ultrasound (RTMSPUS) is a specific subset of RTMUS that involves the virtual interpretation of ultrasound images obtained by variably experienced sonographers on their own bodies (Fig. 29.7). Self-imaging techniques may also lead to the empowerment of patients as they take a more direct role in the diagnosis and management of their own health conditions. RTMSPUS was first described for supporting health care on the International Space Station [32, 33]. Ground-based experts were able to guide astronauts in space to position probes on themselves in order to generate images that could be remotely interpreted. Astronauts demonstrated the feasibility of RTMSPUS in the performance of the FAST examination, echocardiography, and the evaluation of central vasculature, among other examinations [32, 34–37]. RTMSPUS is one example of how telemedicine can be leveraged as a way to improve physical examination during a remote encounter and extend the physician-patient relationship into arenas outside the traditional hospital setting [34–36].

At the present time, self-performed ultrasound may be either guided by a remote expert or completely autonomous, based on just-in-time education, asynchronous feedback, or AI. A recent case report showed that ultrasound naïve, non-physicians users were capable of obtaining expert-quality lung ultrasound clips with minimal training (15-minute training tutorial). This study had a younger population and a high study refusal rate, which may limit the generalizability of this technique [38]. Another case report described the self-imaging of pregnant women for maternal wellness and noted that the image quality was adequate for assessing amniotic fluid in most participants. However, the identification of fetal heartbeat and fetal facial profile was more challenging [39]. The authors thus concluded that the next step in advancing

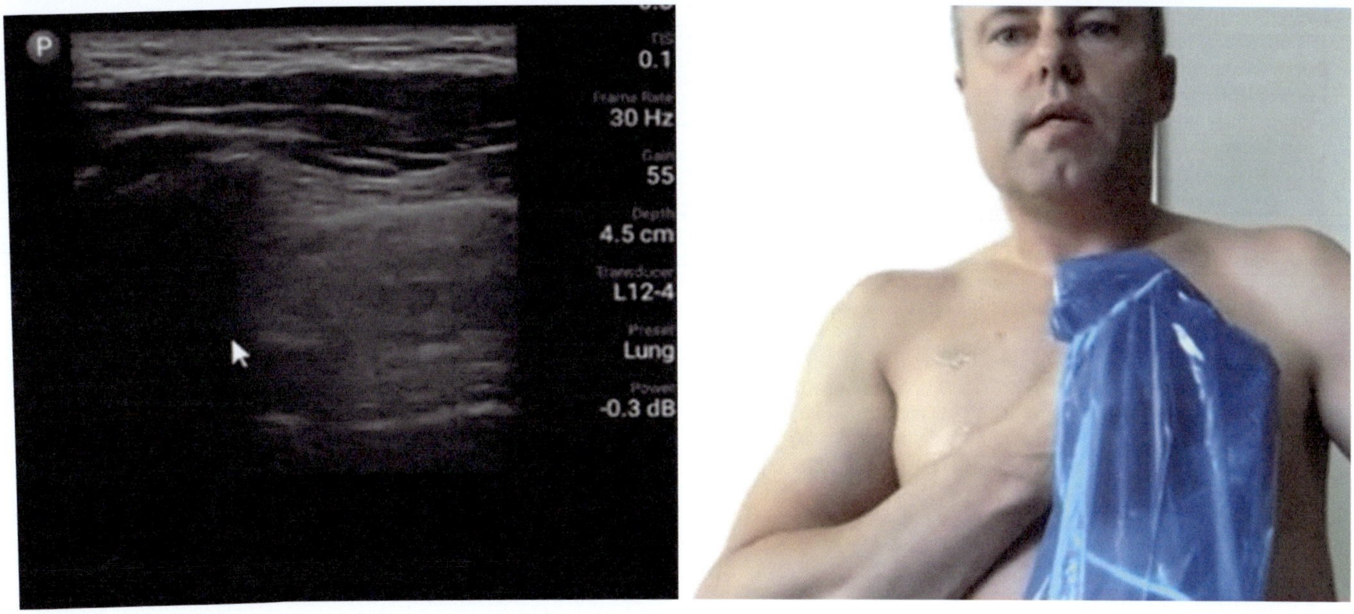

Fig. 29.7 Ultrasound-naïve patient performing remote tele-mentored, self-performed ultrasound under the guidance of a remote lung ultrasound expert, giving step-by-step guidance over a social media application

Table 29.1 Examples of self-performed ultrasound

Indication	Existing or theoretical status
Remotely tele-mentored self-performed ultrasound	
Space medicine	Assessing central venous pressure, cardiac function, and muscle mass [35–37]
COVID-19 lung examinations	Diagnosis and monitoring of the disease during the COVID-19 pandemic [42]
Maternal wellness examination	Fetal assessment during pregnancy [39]
Appendicitis	Self-diagnosis of appendicitis at home [41]
Self-performed autonomous ultrasound	
Heart failure	Patients have self-imaged after 15-minute tutorials with acceptable accuracy [38]
Lung examinations	Patients have self-imaged after self-education with online presentations with acceptable accuracy [43]
Fetal wellness	Patients have performed self-imaging after direct instruction on how to use ultrasound, with the pertinent examination details explained over 5–10 min using example images [40]

self-performed ultrasound for fetal wellness should involve an evaluation of remotely mentored examinations in the same cohort. Additional case series have demonstrated the ability of non-clinicians to self-image under remote guidance to assess for fetal wellbeing and appendicitis [40, 41]. Self-performed ultrasound may be greatly enhanced and could potentially be autonomously performed by patients with advances in artificial and augmented intelligence. These modest examples of current applications of self-performed ultrasound are summarized in Table 29.1, although we expect this table to become outdated as the field continues to rapidly expand. As ultrasound technology becomes cheaper and more powerful, future medicine cabinets may contain a smartphone-powered ultrasound next to the thermometer and home blood pressure cuff.

Disclosures/Conflicts of Interest
Andrew W. Kirkpatrick: Consulting for Zoll Medical and Innovative Trauma Care; Grant funding by 3M/Acelity.
Rachel B. Liu: Consulting for Caption Health, Inc. (GE).

References

1. Health C for D and R. Artificial Intelligence and Machine Learning (AI/ML)-Enabled Medical Devices. FDA. Published online December 6, 2023. Accessed 10 Apr 2024. https://www.fda.gov/medical-devices/software-medical-device-samd/artificial-intelligence-and-machine-learning-aiml-enabled-medical-devices
2. Brattain LJ, Telfer BA, Dhyani M, Grajo JR, Samir AE. Machine learning for medical ultrasound: status, methods, and future opportunities. Abdom Radiol (NY). 2018;43(4):786–99. https://doi.org/10.1007/s00261-018-1517-0.

3. Mueller B, Kinoshita T, Peebles A, Graber MA, Lee S. Artificial intelligence and machine learning in emergency medicine: a narrative review. Acute Med Surg. 2022;9(1):e740. https://doi.org/10.1002/ams2.740.
4. Issues. Ground Truths Are Human Constructions. Issues in Science and Technology. January 16, 2024. Accessed 3 Aug 2024. https://issues.org/ai-ground-truths-human-constructions-jaton/
5. Sonko ML, Arnold TC, Kuznetsov IA. Machine learning in point of care ultrasound. POCUS J. 7(Kidney):78–87. https://doi.org/10.24908/pocus.v7iKidney.15345.
6. Baloescu C, Toporek G, Kim S, et al. Automated lung ultrasound B-line assessment using a deep learning algorithm. IEEE Trans Ultrason Ferroelectr Freq Control. 2020;67(11):2312–20. https://doi.org/10.1109/TUFFC.2020.3002249.
7. Gottlieb M, Patel D, Viars M, Tsintolas J, Peksa GD, Bailitz J. Comparison of artificial intelligence versus real-time physician assessment of pulmonary edema with lung ultrasound. Am J Emerg Med. 2023;70:109–12. https://doi.org/10.1016/j.ajem.2023.05.029.
8. Asch FM, Mor-Avi V, Rubenson D, et al. Deep learning-based automated echocardiographic quantification of left ventricular ejection fraction: a point-of-care solution. Circ Cardiovasc Imaging. 2021;14(6):e012293. https://doi.org/10.1161/CIRCIMAGING.120.012293.
9. Gottlieb M, Schraft E, O'Brien J, Patel D. Diagnostic accuracy of artificial intelligence for identifying systolic and diastolic cardiac dysfunction in the emergency department. Am J Emerg Med. 2024;86:115–9. https://doi.org/10.1016/j.ajem.2024.10.019.
10. Alpert EA, Gold DD, Kobliner-Friedman D, Wagner M, Dadon Z. Revolutionizing bladder health: artificial-intelligence-powered automatic measurement of bladder volume using two-dimensional ultrasound. Diagnostics. 2024;14(16):1829. https://doi.org/10.3390/diagnostics14161829.
11. Blaivas M, Arntfield R, White M. DIY AI, deep learning network development for automated image classification in a point-of-care ultrasound quality assurance program. J Am Coll Emerg Physicians Open. 2020;1(2):124–31. https://doi.org/10.1002/emp2.12018.
12. Moore CL, Wang J, Battisti AJ, et al. Interobserver agreement and correlation of an automated algorithm for B-line identification and quantification with expert sonologist review in a handheld ultrasound device. J Ultrasound Med. 2022;41(10):2487–95. https://doi.org/10.1002/jum.15935.
13. Park SH. Artificial intelligence for ultrasonography: unique opportunities and challenges. Ultrasonography. 2021;40(1):3–6. https://doi.org/10.14366/usg.20078.
14. Kayarian F, Patel D, O'Brien JR, Schraft EK, Gottlieb M. Artificial intelligence and point-of-care ultrasound: benefits, limitations, and implications for the future. Am J Emerg Med. 2024;80:119–22. https://doi.org/10.1016/j.ajem.2024.03.023.
15. Kummer T, Oh L, Phelan MB, Huang RD, Nomura JT, Adhikari S. Emergency and critical care applications for contrast-enhanced ultrasound. Am J Emerg Med. 2018;36(7):1287–94. https://doi.org/10.1016/j.ajem.2018.04.044.
16. Smit JM, Raadsen R, Blans MJ, Petjak M, Van de Ven PM, Tuinman PR. Bedside ultrasound to detect central venous catheter misplacement and associated iatrogenic complications: a systematic review and meta-analysis. Crit Care. 2018;22(1):65. https://doi.org/10.1186/s13054-018-1989-x.
17. Miele V, Piccolo CL, Galluzzo M, Ianniello S, Sessa B, Trinci M. Contrast-enhanced ultrasound (CEUS) in blunt abdominal trauma. Br J Radiol. 2016;89(1061):20150823. https://doi.org/10.1259/bjr.20150823.
18. Paltiel HJ, Barth RA, Bruno C, et al. Contrast-enhanced ultrasound of blunt abdominal trauma in children. Pediatr Radiol. 2021;51(12):2253–69. https://doi.org/10.1007/s00247-020-04869-w.
19. Porter TR, Mathias W. Cardiovascular Sonothrombolysis. Curr Cardiol Rep. 2019;21(8):86. https://doi.org/10.1007/s11886-019-1167-z.
20. El Kadi S, Porter TR, Verouden NJW, van Rossum AC, Kamp O. Contrast ultrasound in cardiovascular ischemic disease: shifting to theragnostic clinical trials. JACC Cardiovasc Imaging. 2022;15(2):345–60. https://doi.org/10.1016/j.jcmg.2021.07.028.
21. Mathias W, Tsutsui JM, Tavares BG, et al. Sonothrombolysis in ST-segment elevation myocardial infarction treated with primary percutaneous coronary intervention. J Am Coll Cardiol. 2019;73(22):2832–42. https://doi.org/10.1016/j.jacc.2019.03.006.
22. Nakanishi K, Watanabe R, Shimizu S, Nakai M. Efficacy of contrast-enhanced ultrasonography in detecting graft rupture sites after abdominal aortic aneurysm repair. Interact Cardiovasc Thorac Surg. 2014;18(2):250–2. https://doi.org/10.1093/icvts/ivt485.
23. Catalano O, Lobianco R, Cusati B, Siani A. Contrast-enhanced sonography for diagnosis of ruptured abdominal aortic aneurysm. Am J Roentgenol. 2005;184(2):423–7. https://doi.org/10.2214/ajr.184.2.01840423.
24. Kummer T, Mohn KJ, Bardwell AJ, Boyum JH. Evaluation of soft-tissue hematomas with real-time, contrast-enhanced ultrasound: a pilot study with preliminary findings. Ultrasound Q. 2023;39(3):179. https://doi.org/10.1097/RUQ.0000000000000621.
25. Yusuf GT, Rafailidis V, Moore S, et al. The role of contrast-enhanced ultrasound (CEUS) in the evaluation of scrotal trauma: a review. Insights Imaging. 2020;11:68. https://doi.org/10.1186/s13244-020-00874-7.
26. Valentino M, Bertolotto M, Derchi L, et al. Role of contrast enhanced ultrasound in acute scrotal diseases. Eur Radiol. 2011;21(9):1831–40. https://doi.org/10.1007/s00330-010-2039-5.
27. McBeth P, Crawford I, Tiruta C, et al. Help is in your pocket: the potential accuracy of smartphone- and laptop-based remotely guided resuscitative telesonography. Telemed E-Health. 2013;19(12):924–30. https://doi.org/10.1089/tmj.2013.0034.
28. Duarte ML, dos Santos LR, Iared W, Peccin MS. Telementored ultrasonography: a narrative review. São Paulo Med J. 2022;140(2):310. https://doi.org/10.1590/1516-3180.2020.0607.R2.15092021.
29. Pian L, Gillman LM, McBeth PB, et al. Potential use of remote telesonography as a transformational technology in underresourced and/or remote settings. Emerg Med Int. 2013;2013:986160. https://doi.org/10.1155/2013/986160.
30. Alhussein M. Use of real-time remote tele-mentored ultrasound echocardiography for cardiovascular disease diagnosis in adults: a systematic review. Ultrasound Med Biol. 2024;50(6):779–87. https://doi.org/10.1016/j.ultrasmedbio.2024.01.073.
31. Dulchavsky SA, Sargsyan AE, Garcia KM, Melton SL, Ebert D, Hamilton DR. Intuitive ultrasonography for autonomous medical care in limited-resource environments. Acta Astronaut. 2011;68(9):1595–607. https://doi.org/10.1016/j.actaastro.2009.08.024.
32. Sargsyan AE, Hamilton DR, Jones JA, et al. FAST at MACH 20: clinical ultrasound aboard the international space station. J Trauma Acute Care Surg. 2005;58(1):35. https://doi.org/10.1097/01.TA.0000145083.47032.78.
33. Martin DS, South DA, Garcia KM, Arbeille P. Ultrasound in space. Ultrasound Med Biol. 2003;29(1):1–12. https://doi.org/10.1016/S0301-5629(02)00692-0.
34. Jones JA, Sargsyan AE, Barr YR, et al. Diagnostic ultrasound at MACH 20: retroperitoneal and pelvic imaging in space. Ultrasound Med Biol. 2009;35(7):1059–67. https://doi.org/10.1016/j.ultrasmedbio.2009.01.002.
35. Hamilton DR, Sargsyan AE, Martin DS, et al. On-orbit prospective echocardiography on international space station crew. Echocardiography. 2011;28(5):491–501. https://doi.org/10.1111/j.1540-8175.2011.01385.x.

36. Zamboni P, Sisini F, Menegatti E, et al. Ultrasound monitoring of jugular venous pulse during space missions: proof of concept. Ultrasound Med Biol. 2018;44(3):726–33. https://doi.org/10.1016/j.ultrasmedbio.2017.11.001.
37. Scott JM, Downs M, Martin DS, et al. Teleguided self-ultrasound scanning for longitudinal monitoring of muscle mass during spaceflight. iScience. 2021;24(4):102344. https://doi.org/10.1016/j.isci.2021.102344.
38. Chiem AT, Lim GW, Tabibnia AP, Takemoto AS, Weingrow DM, Shibata JE. Feasibility of patient-performed lung ultrasound self-exams (Patient-PLUS) as a potential approach to telemedicine in heart failure. ESC Heart Fail. 2021;8(5):3997–4006. https://doi.org/10.1002/ehf2.13493.
39. Pontones CA, Titzmann A, Huebner H, et al. Feasibility and acceptance of self-guided mobile ultrasound among pregnant women in routine prenatal care. J Clin Med. 2023;12(13):4224. https://doi.org/10.3390/jcm12134224.
40. Hadar E, Wolff L, Tenenbaum-Gavish K, et al. Mobile self-operated home ultrasound system for remote fetal assessment during pregnancy. Telemed E-Health. 2022;28(1):93–101. https://doi.org/10.1089/tmj.2020.0541.
41. Kim C, Kang BS, Choi HJ, Lim TH, Oh J, Chee Y. Clinical application of real-time tele-ultrasonography in diagnosing pediatric acute appendicitis in the ED. Am J Emerg Med. 2015;33(10):1354–9. https://doi.org/10.1016/j.ajem.2015.07.048.
42. Omboni S, Padwal RS, Alessa T, et al. The worldwide impact of telemedicine during COVID-19: current evidence and recommendations for the future. Connect Health. 2022;1:7–35. https://doi.org/10.20517/ch.2021.03.
43. Duggan NM, Jowkar N, Ma IWY, et al. Novice-performed point-of-care ultrasound for home-based imaging. Sci Rep. 2022;12:20461. https://doi.org/10.1038/s41598-022-24513-x.

Ultrasound Applications in Global Health

30

Andrea Dreyfuss, Jessica Schmidt, and Melissa Villa

Background

In 2021, *The Lancet* reported that 47% of the world had little to no access to diagnostics, including ultrasound [1]. Ultrasonography allows for rapid diagnosis, triage, and management of patients in resource-limited environments. With the evolution of ultra-portable ultrasound technology and lower costs per unit, devices can be easily carried around the globe to boost diagnostic capacity. A landmark report from the World Health Organization (WHO) in 1985 concluded that there are real advantages to be gained from the use of ultrasound in low- and middle-income countries (LMICs), and noted the potential for improved patient care [2].

The health care and diagnostic needs of each community are unique, and the specific needs of one resource-limited environment may differ from another. Thus, it is important to assess the needs of the community prior to program implementation. While there are disease entities that one may not encounter frequently in higher-income countries, many of the ultrasound needs are similar. In addition to infectious illnesses, LMICs experience a high burden of non-communicable diseases and a disproportionate burden of trauma morbidity, and mortality [3, 4]. Cardiac ultrasound, as a screening tool in patients with chest pain, and the extended focused assessment with sonography in trauma (eFAST) for patients with traumatic injuries, can be useful regardless of where one practices. Other applications, such as musculoskeletal ultrasound for fracture assessment, are particularly useful in regions where plain film radiography is not readily accessible. There are also unique indications for POCUS in the global health setting, such as evaluation of region-specific diseases like rheumatic heart disease, late-presentation congenital heart diseases, extrapulmonary tuberculosis, and dengue, among others [5, 6].

A. Dreyfuss (✉)
Department of Emergency Medicine, Hennepin County Medical Center, Minneapolis, MN, USA
e-mail: andrea.dreyfuss@hcmed.org

J. Schmidt
Department of Emergency Medicine, University of Wisconsin, Madison, WI, USA
e-mail: jschmidt@medicine.wisc.edu

M. Villa
Department of Emergency Medicine, University of Pennsylvania, Philadelphia, PA, USA
e-mail: melissa.villa@pennmedicine.upenn.edu

Technical Considerations

POCUS in LMICs incurs several unique challenges. While some challenges will be site-specific, there are certain technical challenges common to nearly all sites. This section will cover some of the technical aspects unique to global health settings, as well as a review of the importance of appropriate preparation.

Initial Preparation

Prior to traveling to a new location, a local needs assessment should be performed [7]. In this assessment, consideration should be given to the clinical environment, patient population, and physical space, acknowledging that ultrasound applications may be broader than typical uses in high-resource settings due to a lack of other diagnostic modalities [8]. While some of this needs assessment can be performed at a distance in collaboration with local partners, it is best practice to also include a site visit.

The needs assessment should include an understanding of the local burden of diseases unique to the geographic area (e.g., tuberculosis, dengue, intestinal parasites, rheumatic heart disease), an assessment of the prevalence of advanced disease states, complications of underdiagnosed congenital abnormalities, and the effects of under- or untreated chronic medical conditions. Trauma is a leading cause of death in many limited-resource settings, and special attention should be paid to common traumatic injuries, and how POCUS can

M. Gottlieb, N. Panebianco (eds.), *Advanced Point-of-Care Ultrasound*, https://doi.org/10.1007/978-3-031-85308-1_30

be used in their diagnosis and management [9]. Beyond the traditional eFAST protocol, one could consider adding musculoskeletal, ophthalmic, and neurologic POCUS applications to the initial sonographic trauma survey, in collaboration with surgical and other specialty stakeholders. Similarly, obstetric complications in the setting of limited prenatal care are also common emergency presentations, and ultrasound can be invaluable in the assessment of obstructed or breech labor, hemorrhage, and sepsis from retained products of conception [10, 11].

In addition to the clinical environment, the needs assessment should include an evaluation of local staffing. Due to reduced numbers of healthcare providers in limited-resource settings, task-shifting may be commonplace [12]. Understanding who cares for patients, how patients are triaged, and what specialty services are available is important. If a radiology department exists, consider exploring partnerships with radiologists or technicians who may be interested in expanding ultrasound applications. Investment in ultrasound training for conditions that can be managed locally or regionally should be emphasized.

An assessment of the physical space is important as well. This includes understanding what facilities are available, including other diagnostic modalities, with the caveat that some of the equipment may be out of service or nonfunctional [13]. Even with functioning equipment, additional challenges may include intermittent power outages, lack of electricity, limited or no access to the internet, extremes of weather, or limited staffing [14]. Extra batteries, wireless machines, and machines that do not require frequent software updates are important considerations. Finally, cost and availability of renewable resources, such as gel, need to be considered (Table 30.1, Fig. 30.1) [15].

Table 30.1 Ultrasound gel alternatives for resource-limited settings

Medium	Recipe
Cassava [16]	8 parts ground cassava root 1 part salt 32 parts water Boil and cool
Cornstarch [17]	1 part cornstarch 10 parts water Boil and cool
Glucomannan [18]	1 tsp glucomannan powder 8 oz water Heat and cool
Guar Gum [19]	1 cup water 1.5 tsp guar gum 1 tbsp isopropyl alcohol Shake to mix
Oil [20]	Olive oil

Machine Selection

Lack of access to an ultrasound machine is one of the most common barriers cited by healthcare providers in LMIC settings [21, 22]. The selection of an appropriate ultrasound machine should be heavily informed by the needs assessment. Considerations include not only the cost of the machine but also the size, image quality, durability, and serviceability. Handheld ultrasound machines are becoming more commonplace in resource-limited environments, with the advantage of portability and longer battery life. However, disadvantages of handheld devices include the potential for machines to become misplaced or stolen, and limitations in image quality and machine features (e.g., color Doppler, calculation packages) [23]. Refurbished machines can help reduce costs; however, all donations should adhere to WHO guidelines [24]. Ultrasound-specific considerations for donation include the machine's anticipated shelf-life, provision of spare parts not locally available, provision of a physical copy of the user manual (as internet may not be universally available), appropriate

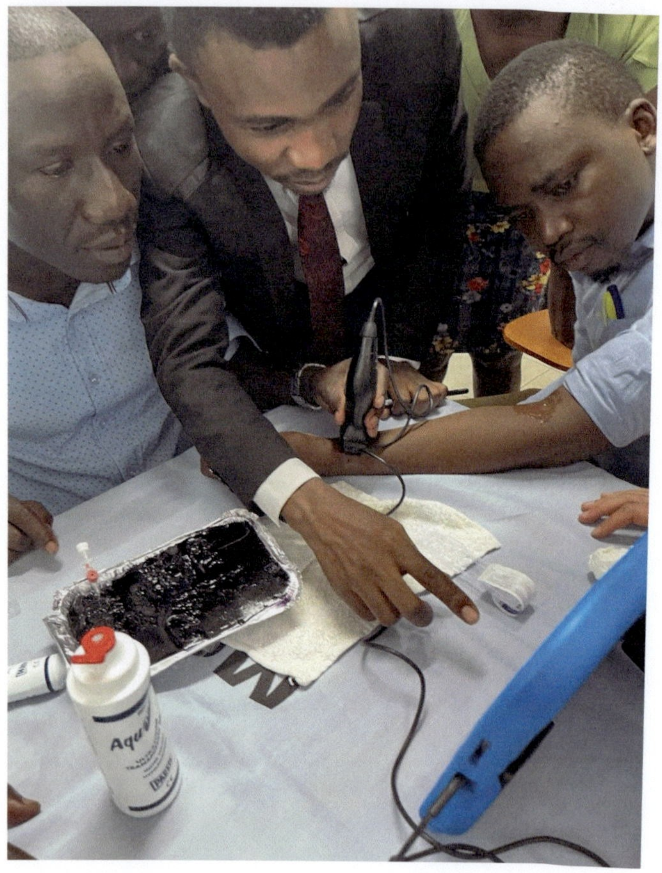

Fig. 30.1 Training in Mbale, Uganda using a locally-made peripheral intravenous access gelatin model

region-specific power voltage and adaptors, availability of service centers, and the cost of transport [25]. Given these complexities and nuances, machine selection decision-making should always be completed in conjunction with local partners.

Image Storage and Quality Assurance

Image storage is an important component of ultrasound education and quality assurance. Traditionally, ultrasound images were printed as still images with thermal printers, which were then attached to patients' medical charts. While printers may still be in use in some international settings, disadvantages of printers include the inability to capture video, the cost of printer paper and ink, and the risk of printer malfunction. Local machine storage can be considered but should include encrypted and password-protected drives. More contemporary image storage systems include electronic picture archiving and communications systems (PACS), which can be digitally stored on local systems or cloud-based storage systems. The advantages of a cloud-based storage system include the ability to remotely review images and having a larger storage capacity. However, with any image storage system, care should be taken to ensure patient privacy and to respect local laws regarding protected health information.

Strategies for Successful Global POCUS Education

While there exists a pressing need to enhance ultrasound capabilities and, consequently, healthcare outcomes in LMICs, lack of ultrasound training remains an important obstacle [22, 26, 27]. Concerted efforts should be directed toward developing a cadre of skilled POCUS practitioners, who can themselves then serve as expert trainers in a "train-the-trainer" model. Speaking with local or international experts who have created POCUS training programs in similar geographic areas can be insightful, and these experts are often receptive to discussing their own successes and challenges.

Developing Local Partnerships

After completing the local needs assessment that delves into the burden of disease, clinical environment, and potential learners, the next step involves establishing collaborative partnerships with international organizations, non-governmental organizations (NGOs), local hospitals, medical schools, and local healthcare providers—each of which will play an important and complementary role. For local healthcare providers, collaboration may provide insight into local adaptations due to resource constraints or unique cultural practices, in addition to building local networks for resource sharing and referral. Working with local healthcare providers also increases engagement and develops leadership skills (see "Training the Trainers" section below). International organizations and NGOs can provide financial and administrative support, in addition to an ongoing community presence. Examples of POCUS-NGO collaborative partnerships, include Medicins San Frontiers, Point-of-care Ultrasound in Resource Limited Environments (PURE), Ondas de Latinoamerica, and Global Emergency Care [28–32]. Engaging with local entities facilitates knowledge exchange, capacity building, and helps to ensure the sustainability of educational programs. These collaborations play a crucial role in shaping POCUS curricula to align with the healthcare priorities of the local community.

Adapting to Practice Locations

Ideally, training and education will integrate into existing systems and will include buy-in from local administration. Using local translators may be essential for effective communication (Fig. 30.2). Learners should be free of other clinical responsibilities and compensated for time and travel, if possible [33]. Other ultrasound-specific considerations for teaching include finding a space with minimal environmental light for better image quality, identifying adequate private space for patient scanning, and respecting cultural norms for ultrasound patient models [34]. Additional awareness should be paid to the possibility that the local population may have had limited previous exposure to electronic devices, such as standard keyboards, measurement tools, and concepts of ultrasound physics. In this scenario, additional training may be needed on machine operation.

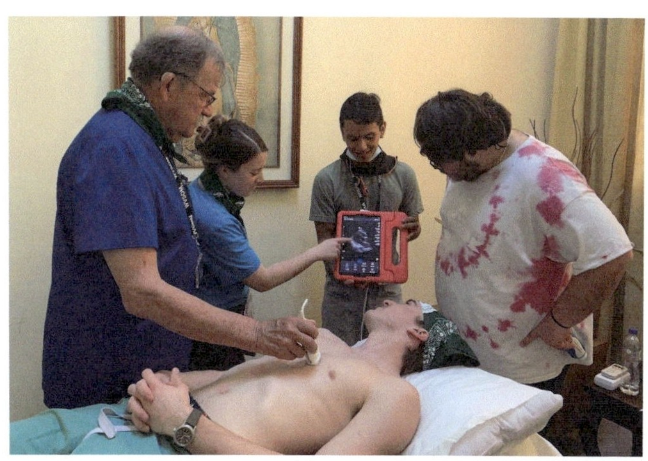

Fig. 30.2 A local Peruvian translator holding the iPad and engaging with medical student ultrasound education

Training the Trainers

Recognizing local champions who can engage in long-term train-the-trainer educational programs is crucial. While short ultrasound courses or workshops can provide immediate training and spark interest, continued education is essential for long-term skill retention [31, 35]. A well-structured train-the-trainer program ensures that healthcare professionals in regions with limited access to specialized training gain comprehensive knowledge and practical skills in ultrasound. Empowering a cohort of trained educators establishes a sustainable framework for disseminating ultrasound expertise (Fig. 30.3). This model can improve diagnostic capabilities and strengthen healthcare infrastructure, particularly in underserved communities. These programs have demonstrated success even when training non-physician learners [12, 36].

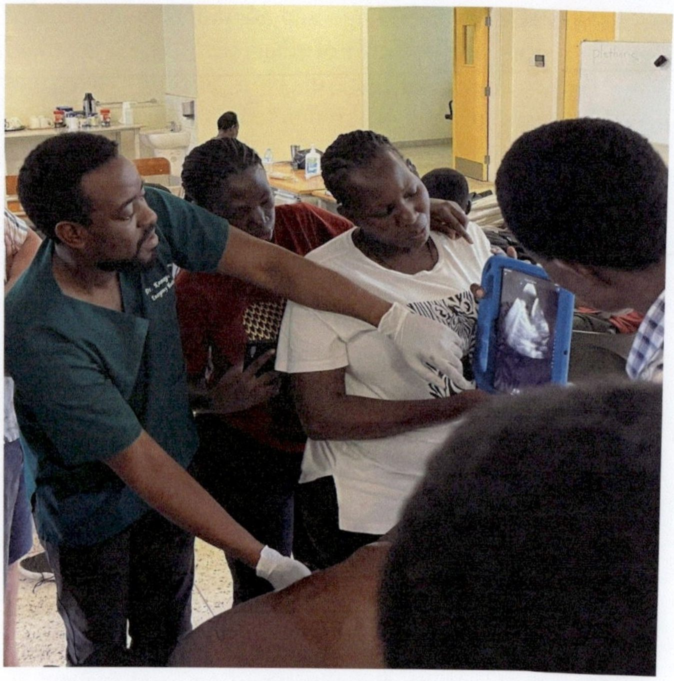

Fig. 30.3 Peer-teaching in Kampala, Uganda

Tele-Ultrasound

Tele-ultrasound is the electronic transfer of images from one location to another and is increasingly used either for acute medical decision-making or quality assurance [37]. Beyond cloud-based sharing, other solutions to remote image transfer, include transmission over private messaging, sharing images on web-based platforms via USB drives, and real-time image sharing over video platforms (Fig. 30.4). The use of lower-cost or readily available technology, such as smartphones and web cameras can expand the capacity of real-time remote mentorship and clinical support. However, a major potential barrier to tele-ultrasound in limited-resource settings is the lack of access to high-speed, stable, and affordable internet [37].

One example of a longitudinal multimodal educational program was conducted in Peru, which demonstrated the effective use of tele-ultrasound for physician learners, alongside other didactic strategies [38]. Ultrasound experts from the United States and Latin America, participated in a group chat with learners, facilitating communication and providing tele-ultrasound support. Additionally, monthly scheduled tele-ultrasound scanning sessions were held to offer targeted feedback and assistance on scans where learners need the most support. This model's cost-effectiveness has enabled its successful replication in multiple other Latin American countries without the need for extensive travel. Further studies present compelling evidence for the feasibility and effectiveness of tele-ultrasound for training in diverse healthcare settings [39–42].

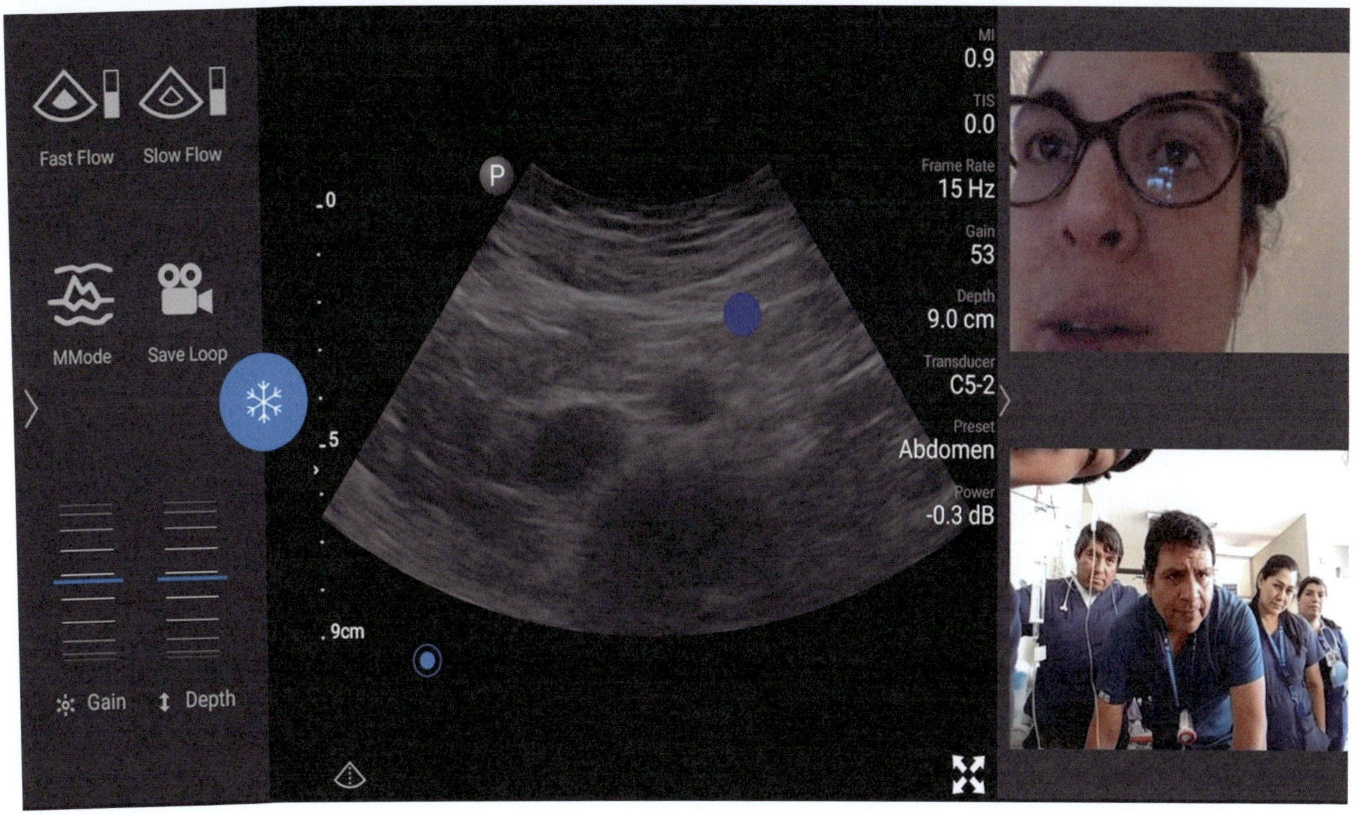

Fig. 30.4 Tele-ultrasound using real-time image sharing

Artificial Intelligence

The integration of artificial intelligence (AI) into ultrasound education in resource-limited settings holds immense promise, as suggested by emerging literature [43]. Novice sonographers can benefit from AI in image acquisition and interpretation. Comparing the diagnostic use of lung ultrasound to chest radiographs for suspected pneumonia in resource-limited settings indicates that ultrasound, potentially enhanced by AI, can serve as a reliable and cost-effective tool [44]. This is especially important in areas with limited traditional imaging resources. Other teaching applications using AI to help novice learners identify sonographic structures or probe positions are also promising [45].

Research

Research in global ultrasound is an important and growing field. Building health research capacity has been identified by the WHO, among others, as a key driver to healthcare development [46, 47]. Building health research capacity involves developing infrastructure including, formalized training, innovative funding, and building partnerships with institutions in high-income settings. Research outcomes can then be used to support POCUS programming by demonstrating its impact to policymakers and funders.

Several areas of global POCUS research are worth highlighting. First and foremost, research is needed to understand the feasibility and acceptability of ultrasound in LMICs [48, 49]. As noted above, working in LMICs has its own sets of unique challenges. Research in this area should focus on barriers, facilitators, and structural needs [21]. This includes understanding patient and provider attitudes toward POCUS, scalability, and the impact on the healthcare system.

A second key area of global POCUS research is focused on clinical care, including diagnosis and management of common diseases affecting LMICs. This is especially relevant as there is often a lack of ancillary diagnostic testing, and diagnosis is often delayed, making pathologies and management strategies different in LMICs compared with higher-resourced settings [50, 51]. Examples include investigations into challenging diagnostic dilemmas, such as tuberculosis in immunocompromised patients [52], or the distinction between viral and bacterial pneumonia in children [53]. Research should also include developing and evaluating POCUS protocols for the management of diseases more prevalent in LMICs (e.g., fluid management for patients with shock in dengue or severe malaria) [54–58].

Finally, it is important to evaluate the effects of POCUS on patient outcomes. Previous research has demonstrated that POCUS improves diagnostic accuracy, reduces time to diagnosis, identifies the need for procedures or interventions, and changes practice in patient referrals in LMIC emergency care settings [59–62]. In other fields of medicine, however, it is less clear that ultrasound is universally beneficial. In obstetrics, some research has suggested that the use of ultrasound may have a neutral or potentially negative outcome [63]. Further research is needed to evaluate patient-centered outcomes including morbidity and mortality, and to explore unintended consequences, such as financial implications to patients and health systems [64, 65].

Ethical and Technical Considerations

There are several components of conducting global research that make it more challenging both ethically and technically. These include avoiding "parachute" research, where researchers from high-income countries visit a host country for only short periods of time without respecting local priorities or recognizing local expertise [66]. Research should instead reflect an academic partnership, including asking for an invitation to perform research in an international setting, partnering throughout the research process with a local team to develop priorities and design, building local capacity through training, and ensuring equitable authorship [67, 68].

This partner-based approach will also be useful in other challenges inherent to performing global research, including addressing international institutional review board (IRB) requirements, country-specific prohibitions, and language considerations. Where an IRB does not exist, another institution or ethics board may be needed for research approval and clearance. The investigator may need IRB approval both in the study country and at their home institution. This process can take months and should be initiated very early in project development. Additional considerations include language interpreters, local language consent, culturally-appropriate research design, community engagement, and data sharing [69].

Scaling Up

Scaling up refers to the process of expanding and enhancing successful local initiatives to a larger scale, from single institutions to broader regional or national programs. This approach includes, educational, administrative, and clinical endeavors. For example, in Africa, several studies have explored the role of POCUS education tailored to specific regions [8, 70]. In 2014, the African Ultrasound Committee within the African Federation of Emergency Medicine (AFEM) was established, fostering collaboration, support, and growth among emergency medicine POCUS educators across the continent [8]. Similarly, during the first Federation of Latin American Emergency Medicine (FLAME) Conference in April 2024, a subcommittee of POCUS in the region was established. This subcommittee also shared the goal of fostering collaboration across Latin America and has been tasked with developing a unified POCUS curriculum for emergency medicine residents across the continent. This initiative addresses the challenge that educational resources often come from more affluent areas with access to advanced imaging technologies and differing disease burdens. These partnerships and insights are critical, as core POCUS competencies may vary from region to region.

Effective scaling requires thorough preparation and strategic partnership to integrate these initiatives into local systems. The American College of Emergency Physicians (ACEP) has developed a model for scaling up POCUS education through regional workshops and training programs, demonstrating how successful educational models can be adapted and expanded [71]. Integrating local physicians as trainers and using technology to bridge educational gaps can facilitate wider adoption and training [38]. Expansion strategies should concentrate on replicating successful POCUS education models in diverse settings, ensuring adaptability to local contexts, and being mindful of resource constraints. Leveraging technology, including online platforms and tele-ultrasound, is vital to reaching a wider audience, especially in areas with limited access to traditional educational resources. For example, telemedicine and e-health have emphasized the role of tele-ultrasound in extending POCUS training to remote areas using online platforms for training and consultations [72].

Specific Diseases for Ultrasound Application in Resource-Limited Settings

Tuberculosis

Tuberculosis (TB) is the leading cause of death due to a single infectious bacterial agent globally [73]. The diagnosis is challenging due to a lack of access to diagnostic testing and overlap with other clinical diseases [74]. Chest radiography is the first-line imaging modality in the diagnosis of pulmonary TB with common findings including upper-lobe nodules or consolidations, cavitary lesions, lymphadenopathy, and pleural effusions [75, 76]. As with radiographic findings, sonographic findings of pulmonary TB can be non-specific and include subpleural nodules, a miliary pattern, consolidations, cavitations, and pleural effusions (Fig. 30.5) [77]. The most specific finding includes cavitations (89–100% specific, 30–39% sensitive), whereas subpleural nodules and consolidations are more sensitive (72–80%) but less specific [78–80].

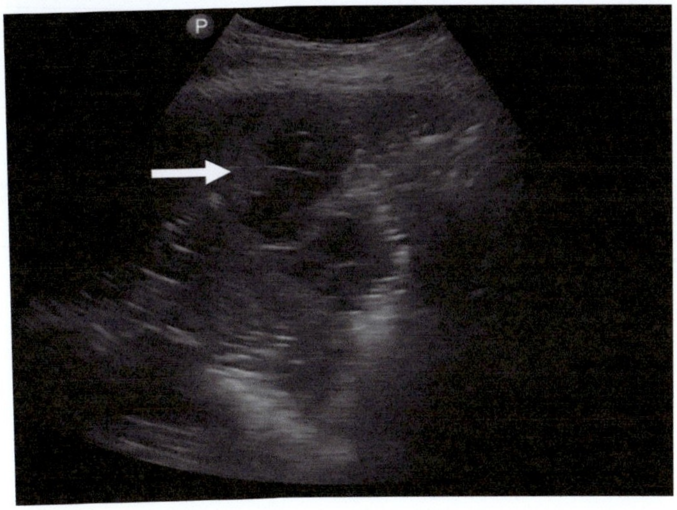

Fig. 30.5 Cavitary lesions with internal septations are visualized with a curvilinear probe. (*Image courtesy of Jackeline Estofarnero Huancollo, MD*)

While extrapulmonary TB is less common, it often affects vulnerable populations, such as children and immunocompromised patients [81]. The Focused Assessment with Sonography for HIV-associated TB (FASH) is a multicomponent examination protocol to identify common findings, such as pericardial and pleural effusions, ascites, focal liver and splenic lesions, and enlarged periaortic lymph nodes (Fig. 30.6) [52]. First described in South Africa, the FASH exam was developed to identify extrapulmonary TB in patients living with HIV. The FASH examination is performed using the curvilinear or phased array probe and the patient is scanned in six different locations. In resource-limited communities, where access to chest radiography and computed tomography is limited, the FASH protocol has been shown to aid in a more rapid diagnosis of extrapulmonary TB [82]. In South Africa, the Emergency Medicine Association adopted FASH as a module in their POCUS training curriculum, and it is one of the most frequently used modules [70].

Dengue

Dengue infection is a mosquito-borne viral disease that is a leading cause of illness in at-risk areas [83]. While many patients have a self-limited febrile illness, in some patients, severe complications can occur including plasma leakage into serosal cavities resulting in life-threatening hypovolemic shock [84]. This vascular leakage is a key component in the pathophysiology of severe dengue and can be detected with ultrasound. POCUS is highly sensitive for diagnosing the small pleural effusions, ascites, hepatomegaly (liver diameter > 15 cm), splenomegaly (spleen diameter > 12 cm), and gallbladder wall thickening (wall thickness diameter > 3 mm) seen in severe dengue infections [55]. Abnormal POCUS findings can identify fluid leakage before laboratory derangements and, when present, are associated with an increased risk of thrombocytopenia, and the development of severe infection [85, 86]. Despite characteristic sonographic findings in severe dengue, some authors have cautioned that these features alone cannot rule out dengue fever [87]. However, while ultrasound may not exclude dengue, serial exams can augment clinical care and identify patients at risk of developing severe disease [54].

Rheumatic Heart Disease

Rheumatic heart disease (RHD) is one of the most prevalent acquired cardiovascular diseases worldwide [88]. RHD disproportionately affects those living in more resource-limited settings [89]. Although most cases are acquired in childhood, it is a lifelong disease, leading to a high prevalence of heart failure in both pediatric and adult populations, often with severe gaps in screening and detection [90]. POCUS features of RHD include thickened mitral valves with restricted movement (hockey stick appearance), mitral regurgitation, and atrial enlargement (Fig. 30.7) [91]. The aortic valve can also be involved, resulting in regurgitation or stenosis. Decompensated heart failure can be seen with B-lines and pleural effusions. Several authors have proposed targeted and general screening approaches that have resulted in significant changes in patient management [6, 92].

Other Diseases

Table 30.2 describes several other common disease entities seen in global settings, as well as typical presentations and sonographic features. This table is not intended to represent a comprehensive list but rather to provide a few additional select examples.

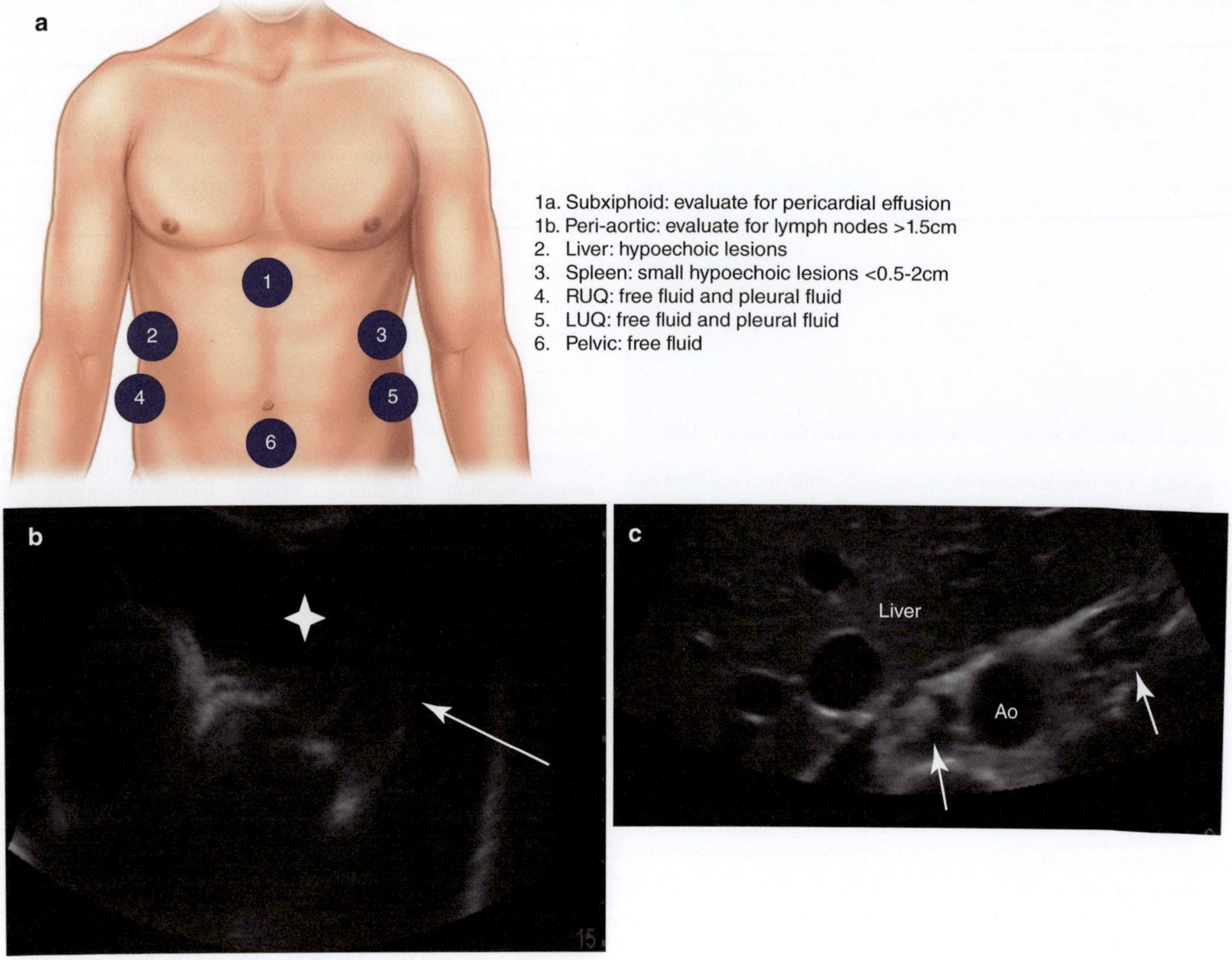

Fig. 30.6 (**a**) FASH exam probe positions and representative images. (**b**) Pericardial effusion (star) with fibrinous bands (arrow). (**c**) Peri-aortic lymph nodes (arrows) next to aorta (Ao)

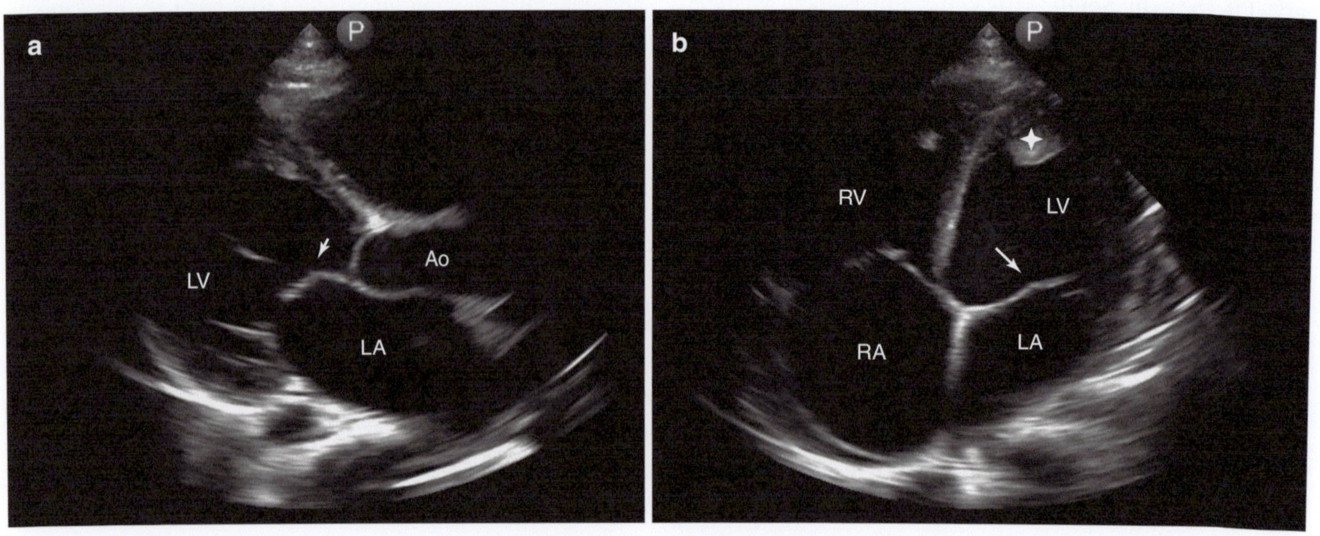

Fig. 30.7 Rheumatic heart disease. (**a**) parasternal long-axis view of rheumatic heart disease with a characteristic hockey stick (arrow) mitral valve leaflet, along with additional pathology, including left atrial (LA) enlargement. (**b**) apical 4-chamber view with hockey stick (arrow) mitral valve leaflet and left ventricular thrombus (star)

Table 30.2 Common global diseases and associated sonographic findings

Disease	Organism	Clinical presentation	Global distribution	Sonographic features
Amebic liver abscess [93, 94]	Protozoa entamoeba histolytica	Fever, right upper quadrant abdominal pain, jaundice	Central and South Africa, India, Mexico	Single round, or oval hypoechoic lesions
Hydatid disease [95, 96]	Echinococcus tapeworm	Abdominal pain, nausea, and vomiting (liver cysts) Chronic cough (pulmonary) Many are asymptomatic	Worldwide (especially Middle East, Mediterranean, Central Asia, China, East Africa, South America, Australia, and New Zealand)	Single, or multiple cysts with daughter vesicles, "wheel spoke" "Water lily" sign: floating membranes in anechoic cyst 'Eggshell' calcified cysts
Leishmaniasis [97–99]	Protozoan parasites transmitted through sandfly bites	Visceral/Kala-azar (fever, weight-loss, hepatosplenomegaly, anemia) Cutaneous (ulcers) Mucocutaneous (destruction of nose/mouth/throat)	Visceral: Brazil, East Africa, India Cutaneous: Central and South America, Mediterranean, Middle East, Asia Mucocutaneous: Peru, Bolivia, Brazil, Ethiopia	Visceral: hepatosplenomegaly, ascites, splenic lesions [81] Cutaneous: thick, hypoechoic, irregular dermis, may have enhanced vascularity
Lymphatic filariasis [100–102]	Filarial nematode parasites transmitted by mosquitoes	Painful lymphedema, and elephantiasis of limbs Hydrocele of scrotum	Africa, Asia, Middle East, Caribbean, South America, Pacific Islands	Nests: serpiginous calcifications in lymphatic tissue "Filarial dance" sign: moving echogenic structures in dilated lymphatic channels, typically scrotal but also seen in axilla or breast
Schistosomiasis/ Bilharzia [103–106]	Trematode flatworms (snails intermediate hosts)	Rash (cercarial dermatitis) Katayama disease: fever, cough, myalgia, headache, hematuria, and abdominal pain (early) Chronic: liver failure, bladder pain, obstructive uropathy, and bladder cancer	Africa, Brazil	Bladder wall thickening, pseudo-polys, and calcifications Periportal fibrosis "bull's eye," left liver lobe hypertrophy, gallbladder wall thickening, splenomegaly, and splenic nodules

Pearls and Pitfalls

- A pre-departure needs assessment is critical and should include an understanding of local disease burden, the clinical environment (physical and personnel), and available diagnostic modalities.
- Trauma and non-communicable diseases represent a high burden of disease in LMIC, which should be recognized prior to travel.
- Machine selection should include considerations of cost, image-quality, durability, and serviceability.
- Donated equipment should follow WHO guidelines including provision of spare parts and user manuals.
- Lack of electricity and non-functioning equipment are common challenges.
- Successful education is founded on strong local partnerships and integration into local health networks.
- A train-the-trainer model creates sustainability.
- Tele-ultrasound may be used for quality assurance as well as real-time medical decision-making; however, connectivity may be a limitation.

References

1. Yadav H, Shah D, Sayed S, Horton S, Schroeder LF. Availability of essential diagnostics in ten low-income and middle-income countries: results from national health facility surveys. Lancet Glob Health. 2021;9(11):e1553–60. https://doi.org/10.1016/S2214-109X(21)00442-3.
2. WHO. Future use of new imaging technologies in developing countries, vol. 723. Report of a WHO Scientific Group World Health Organ Tech Rep Ser.; 1985. p. 1–67.
3. Shanthakumar D, Payne A, Leitch T, Alfa-Wali M. Trauma care in low- and middle-income countries. Surg J (N Y). 2021;7(4):e281–5. https://doi.org/10.1055/s-0041-1732351.
4. IHM. Global Burden of Disease Study 2019 (GBD 2019) Results. 2020. https://vizhub.healthdata.org/gbd-results/.
5. Lu JC, Sable C, Ensing GJ, et al. Simplified rheumatic heart disease screening criteria for handheld echocardiography. J Am Soc Echocardiogr. 2015;28(4):463–9. https://doi.org/10.1016/j.echo.2015.01.001.
6. Muhame RM, Dragulescu A, Nadimpalli A, et al. Cardiac point of care ultrasound in resource limited settings to manage children with congenital and acquired heart disease. Cardiol Young. 2021;31(10):1651–7. https://doi.org/10.1017/S1047951121000834.
7. Henwood PC, Mackenzie DC, Rempell JS, et al. A practical guide to self-sustaining point-of-care ultrasound education programs in resource-limited settings. Ann Emerg Med. 2014;64(3):277–285.e2. https://doi.org/10.1016/j.annemergmed.2014.04.013.
8. Salmon M, Landes M, Hunchak C, et al. Getting it right the first time: defining regionally relevant training curricula and provider

core competencies for point-of-care ultrasound education on the African Continent. Ann Emerg Med. 2017;69(2):218–26. https://doi.org/10.1016/j.annemergmed.2016.07.030.
9. Network GBoDC. Global Burden of Disease Study 2019 (GBD 2019) Results. 2020. https://vizhub.healthdata.org/gbd-results/.
10. Girum T, Wasie A. Correlates of maternal mortality in developing countries: an ecological study in 82 countries. Matern Health Neonatol Perinatol. 2017;3:19. https://doi.org/10.1186/s40748-017-0059-8.
11. Stefanovic V. Role of obstetric ultrasound in reducing maternal and neonatal mortality in developing countries: from facts to acts. DSJUOG. 2020;14(1):43. https://doi.org/10.5005/jp-journals-10009-1617.
12. Abrokwa SK, Ruby LC, Heuvelings CC, Bélard S. Task shifting for point of care ultrasound in primary healthcare in low- and middle-income countries-a systematic review. EClinicalMedicine. 2022;45:101333. https://doi.org/10.1016/j.eclinm.2022.101333.
13. Perry L, Malkin R. Effectiveness of medical equipment donations to improve health systems: how much medical equipment is broken in the developing world? Med Biol Eng Comput. 2011;49(7):719–22. https://doi.org/10.1007/s11517-011-0786-3.
14. WHO. Energizing health: accelerating electricity access in health-care facilities: executive summary. 2023. https://who.int/publications/i/item/9789240066984.
15. Vinograd AM, Fasina A, Dean AJ, et al. Evaluation of noncommercial ultrasound gels for use in resource-limited settings. J Ultrasound Med. 2019;38(2):371–7. https://doi.org/10.1002/jum.14697.
16. Salmon M, Salmon C, Bissinger A, et al. Alternative ultrasound gel for a sustainable ultrasound program: application of human centered design. PLoS One. 2015;10(8):e0134332. https://doi.org/10.1371/journal.pone.0134332.
17. Binkowski A, Riguzzi C, Price D, Fahimi J. Evaluation of a cornstarch-based ultrasound gel alternative for low-resource settings. J Emerg Med. 2014;47(1):e5–9. https://doi.org/10.1016/j.jemermed.2013.08.073.
18. Milton SC, Cronin AJ, Monti JD. Evaluation of glucomannan powder as an ultrasound transmission gel alternative for resource-constrained environments: a prospective, comparative study. Wilderness Environ Med. 2018;29(4):446–52. https://doi.org/10.1016/j.wem.2018.06.007.
19. Cherukuri AR, Lane L, Guy D, Perusse K, Keating DP, DeStigter KK. Shake no bake: a homemade ultrasound gel recipe for low-resource settings. J Ultrasound Med. 2019;38(4):1069–73. https://doi.org/10.1002/jum.14788.
20. Luewan S, Srisupundit K, Tongsong T. A comparison of sonographic image quality between the examinations using gel and olive oil, as sound media. J Med Assoc Thail. 2007;90(4):624–7.
21. Ginsburg AS, Liddy Z, Khazaneh PT, May S, Pervaiz F. A survey of barriers and facilitators to ultrasound use in low- and middle-income countries. Sci Rep. 2023;13(1):3322. https://doi.org/10.1038/s41598-023-30454-w.
22. Shah S, Bellows BA, Adedipe AA, Totten JE, Backlund BH, Sajed D. Perceived barriers in the use of ultrasound in developing countries. Crit Ultrasound J. 2015;7(1):28. https://doi.org/10.1186/s13089-015-0028-2.
23. Le MT, Voigt L, Nathanson R, et al. Comparison of four handheld point-of-care ultrasound devices by expert users. Ultrasound J. 2022;14(1):27. https://doi.org/10.1186/s13089-022-00274-6.
24. WHO. Medical device donations: considerations for solicitation and provision: WHO Medical device technical series. 2011.
25. McDonald S, Fabbri A, Parker L, Williams J, Bero L. Medical donations are not always free: an assessment of compliance of medicine and medical device donations with World Health Organization guidelines (2009-2017). Int Health. 2019;11(5):379–402. https://doi.org/10.1093/inthealth/ihz004.
26. Becker DM, Tafoya CA, Becker SL, Kruger GH, Tafoya MJ, Becker TK. The use of portable ultrasound devices in low- and middle-income countries: a systematic review of the literature. Trop Med Int Health. 2016;21(3):294–311. https://doi.org/10.1111/tmi.12657.
27. Boniface KS, Raymond A, Fleming K, et al. The Global Health Service Partnership's point-of-care ultrasound initiatives in Malawi, Tanzania and Uganda. Am J Emerg Med. 2019;37(4):777–9. https://doi.org/10.1016/j.ajem.2018.08.065.
28. Terry B, Polan DL, Nambaziira R, Mugisha J, Bisanzo M, Gaspari R. Rapid, remote education for point-of-care ultrasound among non-physician emergency care providers in a resource limited setting. Afr J Emerg Med. 2019;9(3):140–4. https://doi.org/10.1016/j.afjem.2019.05.004.
29. Nadimpalli A, Tsung JW, Sanchez R, et al. Feasibility of training clinical officers in point-of-care ultrasound for pediatric respiratory diseases in Aweil, South Sudan. Am J Trop Med Hyg. 2019;101(3):689–95. https://doi.org/10.4269/ajtmh.18-0745.
30. Shokoohi H, Raymond A, Fleming K, et al. Assessment of Point-of-Care Ultrasound Training for Clinical Educators in Malawi, Tanzania and Uganda. Ultrasound Med Biol. 2019;45(6):1351–7. https://doi.org/10.1016/j.ultrasmedbio.2019.01.019.
31. Henwood PC, Mackenzie DC, Rempell JS, et al. Intensive point-of-care ultrasound training with long-term follow-up in a cohort of Rwandan physicians. Trop Med Int Health. 2016;21(12):1531–8. https://doi.org/10.1111/tmi.12780.
32. Ondas. Ondas de Latinoamerica: advancing point-of-care ultrasound education in Latin America. Accessed 20 Apr 2024, https://www.ondasdelatinoamerica.org/.
33. Vogt A, Wang S. Twelve tips for medical teaching in low-resource settings. Med Teach. 2017;39(10):1029–32. https://doi.org/10.1080/0142159X.2017.1327041.
34. Davis NR, Alade KH. Twelve tips for point-of-care ultrasound teaching in low-resource settings. Med Teach. 2021;43(10):1134–8. https://doi.org/10.1080/0142159X.2020.1845307.
35. Wanjiku GW, Bell G, Wachira B. Assessing a novel point-of-care ultrasound training program for rural healthcare providers in Kenya. BMC Health Serv Res. 2018;18(1):607. https://doi.org/10.1186/s12913-018-3196-5.
36. Stolz LA, Muruganandan KM, Bisanzo MC, et al. Point-of-care ultrasound education for non-physician clinicians in a resource-limited emergency department. Trop Med Int Health. 2015;20(8):1067–72. https://doi.org/10.1111/tmi.12511.
37. Britton N, Miller MA, Safadi S, Siegel A, Levine AR, McCurdy MT. Tele-ultrasound in resource-limited settings: a systematic review. Front Public Health. 2019;7:244. https://doi.org/10.3389/fpubh.2019.00244.
38. Dreyfuss A, Martin DA, Farro A, et al. A novel multimodal approach to point-of-care ultrasound education in low-resource settings. West J Emerg Med. 2020;21(4):1017–21. https://doi.org/10.5811/westjem.2020.4.45928.
39. Robertson TE, Levine AR, Verceles AC, et al. Remote tele-mentored ultrasound for non-physician learners using FaceTime: a feasibility study in a low-income country. J Crit Care. 2017;40:145–8. https://doi.org/10.1016/j.jcrc.2017.03.028.
40. Levine AR, Buchner JA, Verceles AC, et al. Ultrasound images transmitted via FaceTime are non-inferior to images on the ultrasound machine. J Crit Care. 2016;33:51–5. https://doi.org/10.1016/j.jcrc.2016.02.019.
41. Levine AR, McCurdy MT, Zubrow MT, Papali A, Mallemat HA, Verceles AC. Tele-intensivists can instruct non-physicians to acquire high-quality ultrasound images. J Crit Care. 2015;30(5):871–5. https://doi.org/10.1016/j.jcrc.2015.05.030.
42. Martin DA, Guillen M, Farro A, Condori M, Dreyfuss A, Nagdev A. Role of tele-ultrasound for teaching ultrasound-guided nerve

blocks in the emergency department: a case series from Peru. Clin Pract Cases Emerg Med. 2022;6(3):204–7. https://doi.org/10.5811/cpcem.2022.2.55417.
43. Kayarian F, Patel D, O'Brien JR, Schraft EK, Gottlieb M. Artificial intelligence and point-of-care ultrasound: benefits, limitations, and implications for the future. Am J Emerg Med. 2024;80:119–22. https://doi.org/10.1016/j.ajem.2024.03.023.
44. Nti B, Lehmann AS, Haddad A, Kennedy SK, Russell FM. Artificial intelligence-augmented pediatric lung POCUS: a pilot study of novice learners. J Ultrasound Med. 2022;41(12):2965–72. https://doi.org/10.1002/jum.15992.
45. Mor-Avi V, Khandheria B, Klempfner R, et al. Real-time artificial intelligence-based guidance of echocardiographic imaging by novices: image quality and suitability for diagnostic interpretation and quantitative analysis. Circ Cardiovasc Imaging. 2023;16(11):e015569. https://doi.org/10.1161/CIRCIMAGING.123.015569.
46. Minja H, Nsanzabana C, Maure C, et al. Impact of health research capacity strengthening in low- and middle-income countries: the case of WHO/TDR programmes. PLoS Negl Trop Dis. 2011;5(10):e1351. https://doi.org/10.1371/journal.pntd.0001351.
47. Lansang MA, Dennis R. Building capacity in health research in the developing world. Bull World Health Organ. 2004;82(10):764–70.
48. Riaz A, Cambaco O, Ellington LE, et al. Feasibility, usability and acceptability of paediatric lung ultrasound among healthcare providers and caregivers for the diagnosis of childhood pneumonia in resource-constrained settings: a qualitative study. BMJ Open. 2021;11(3):e042547. https://doi.org/10.1136/bmjopen-2020-042547.
49. Okiror W, Namayanja C, Okalebo C, et al. Acceptability and feasibility of using point of care ultrasound scan among health care professionals in Eastern Uganda: a cross-sectional study. Research Square. 2024.
50. The Lancet Global Health. Essential diagnostics: mind the gap. Lancet Glob Health. 2021;9(11):e1474. https://doi.org/10.1016/S2214-109X(21)00467-8.
51. Driban M, Dissak-Delon FN, Carvalho M, et al. Failure to receive prescribed imaging is associated with increased early mortality after injury in Cameroon. PLOS Glob Public Health. 2023;3(8):e0001951. https://doi.org/10.1371/journal.pgph.0001951.
52. Heller T, Wallrauch C, Goblirsch S, Brunetti E. Focused assessment with sonography for HIV-associated tuberculosis (FASH): a short protocol and a pictorial review. Crit Ultrasound J. 2012;4(1):21. https://doi.org/10.1186/2036-7902-4-21.
53. Buonsenso D, De Rose C. Implementation of lung ultrasound in low- to middle-income countries: a new challenge global health? Eur J Pediatr. 2022;181(1):1–8. https://doi.org/10.1007/s00431-021-04179-9.
54. Michels M, Sumardi U, de Mast Q, et al. The predictive diagnostic value of serial daily bedside ultrasonography for severe dengue in Indonesian adults. PLoS Negl Trop Dis. 2013;7(6):e2277. https://doi.org/10.1371/journal.pntd.0002277.
55. Dewan N, Zuluaga D, Osorio L, Krienke ME, Bakker C, Kirsch J. Ultrasound in Dengue: a scoping review. Am J Trop Med Hyg. 2021;104(3):826–35. https://doi.org/10.4269/ajtmh.20-0103.
56. Pugliese CM, Adegbite BR, Edoa JR, et al. Point-of-care ultrasound to assess volume status and pulmonary oedema in malaria patients. Infection. 2022;50(1):65–82. https://doi.org/10.1007/s15010-021-01637-2.
57. Kotlyar S, Olupot-Olupot P, Nteziyaremye J, et al. Assessment of myocardial function and injury by echocardiography and cardiac biomarkers in African children with severe plasmodium falciparum Malaria. Pediatr Crit Care Med. 2018;19(3):179–85. https://doi.org/10.1097/PCC.0000000000001411.
58. Wegener A, Holm AE, Gomes LC, et al. Prevalence and dynamic changes in lung ultrasound findings among adults with uncomplicated malaria and controls in the Amazon Basin, Brazil. Am J Trop Med Hyg. 2022;106(6):1637–45. https://doi.org/10.4269/ajtmh.21-1107.
59. Becker TK, Tafoya CA, Osei-Ampofo M, et al. Cardiopulmonary ultrasound for critically ill adults improves diagnostic accuracy in a resource-limited setting: the AFRICA trial. Trop Med Int Health. 2017;22(12):1599–608. https://doi.org/10.1111/tmi.12992.
60. Wanjiku GW, Bell G, Kapadia S, Wachira BW. Impact of point-of-care ultrasound use on patient referral decisions in rural Kenya: a mixed methods study. BMC Health Serv Res. 2024;24(1):212. https://doi.org/10.1186/s12913-024-10673-1.
61. Kolbe N, Killu K, Coba V, et al. Point of care ultrasound (POCUS) telemedicine project in rural Nicaragua and its impact on patient management. J Ultrasound. 2015;18(2):179–85. https://doi.org/10.1007/s40477-014-0126-1.
62. Shah SP, Epino H, Bukhman G, et al. Impact of the introduction of ultrasound services in a limited resource setting: rural Rwanda 2008. BMC Int Health Hum Rights. 2009;9:4. https://doi.org/10.1186/1472-698X-9-4.
63. Kurjak A, Medjedovic E, Stanojević M. Use and misuse of ultrasound in obstetrics with reference to developing countries. J Perinat Med. 2023;51(2):240–52. https://doi.org/10.1515/jpm-2022-0438.
64. Kim ET, Singh K, Moran A, Armbruster D, Kozuki N. Obstetric ultrasound use in low and middle income countries: a narrative review. Reprod Health. 2018;15(1):129. https://doi.org/10.1186/s12978-018-0571-y.
65. Edzie EKM, Dzefi-Tettey K, Gorleku PN, et al. Audit of the appropriateness of the indication for obstetric sonography in a tertiary facility in Ghana. Pan Afr Med J. 2021;40:35. https://doi.org/10.11604/pamj.2021.40.35.26349.
66. Odeny B, Bosurgi R. Time to end parachute science. PLoS Med. 2022;19(9):e1004099. https://doi.org/10.1371/journal.pmed.1004099.
67. Garbern SC, Hyuha G, González Marqués C, et al. Authorship representation in global emergency medicine: a bibliometric analysis from 2016 to 2020. BMJ Glob Health. 2022;7(6):e009538. https://doi.org/10.1136/bmjgh-2022-009538.
68. Kumar R, Khosla R, McCoy D. Decolonising global health research: shifting power for transformative change. PLOS Glob Public Health. 2024;4(4):e0003141. https://doi.org/10.1371/journal.pgph.0003141.
69. Pratt B. Sharing power in global health research: an ethical toolkit for designing priority-setting processes that meaningfully include communities. Int J Equity Health. 2021;20(1):127. https://doi.org/10.1186/s12939-021-01453-y.
70. van Hoving DJ, Lamprecht HH, Stander M, et al. Adequacy of the emergency point-of-care ultrasound core curriculum for the local burden of disease in South Africa. Emerg Med J. 2013;30(4):312–5. https://doi.org/10.1136/emermed-2012-201358.
71. Ultrasound guidelines: emergency, point-of-care and clinical ultrasound guidelines in medicine. Ann Emerg Med. 2017;69(5):e27–54. https://doi.org/10.1016/j.annemergmed.2016.08.457.
72. Recker F, Hohne E, Damjanovic D, Schafer V. Ultrasound in telemedicine: a brief overview. Appl Sci. 2022;12(3):958.
73. WHO. Global tuberculosis report 2020 2020. Global Tuberculosis Programme. https://who.int/publications/i/item/9789240013131
74. Singh S, Dey B, Sachdeva KS, et al. Challenges in tuberculosis diagnosis and management: recommendations of the expert panel. J Lab Physicians. 2015;7(1):1–3. https://doi.org/10.4103/0974-2727.154778.

75. WHO. Systematic screening for active tuberculosis principles and recommendations. 2013.
76. Bhalla AS, Goyal A, Guleria R, Gupta AK. Chest tuberculosis: radiological review and imaging recommendations. Indian J Radiol Imaging. 2015;25(3):213–25. https://doi.org/10.4103/0971-3026.161431.
77. Montuori M, Casella F, Casazza G, et al. Lung ultrasonography in pulmonary tuberculosis: a pilot study on diagnostic accuracy in a high-risk population. Eur J Intern Med. 2019;66:29–34. https://doi.org/10.1016/j.ejim.2019.06.002.
78. Fentress M, Henwood PC, Maharaj P, et al. Thoracic ultrasound for TB diagnosis in adults and children. Public Health Action. 2022;12(1):3–6. https://doi.org/10.5588/pha.21.0072.
79. Cozzi D, Bartolucci M, Giannelli F, et al. Parenchymal cavitations in pulmonary tuberculosis: comparison between lung ultrasound, chest X-ray and computed tomography. Diagnostics (Basel). 2024;14(5):522. https://doi.org/10.3390/diagnostics14050522.
80. Bigio J, Kohli M, Klinton JS, et al. Diagnostic accuracy of point-of-care ultrasound for pulmonary tuberculosis: a systematic review. PLoS One. 2021;16(5):e0251236. https://doi.org/10.1371/journal.pone.0251236.
81. Sharma SK, Mohan A, Kohli M. Extrapulmonary tuberculosis. Expert Rev Respir Med. 2021;15(7):931–48. https://doi.org/10.1080/17476348.2021.1927718.
82. Patel MN, Beningfield S, Burch V. Abdominal and pericardial ultrasound in suspected extrapulmonary or disseminated tuberculosis. S Afr Med J. 2011;101(1):39–42. https://doi.org/10.7196/samj.4201.
83. CDC. About Dengue: What You Need to Know. 2023. https://www.cdc.gov/dengue/about/index.html#:~:text=Almost%20half%20of%20the%20world's,infected%20by%20a%20dengue%20virus.
84. Guzman MG, Halstead SB, Artsob H, et al. Dengue: a continuing global threat. Nat Rev Microbiol. 2010;8(12 Suppl):S7–16. https://doi.org/10.1038/nrmicro2460.
85. Santhosh VR, Patil PG, Srinath MG, Kumar A, Jain A, Archana M. Sonography in the diagnosis and assessment of dengue fever. J Clin Imaging Sci. 2014;4:14. https://doi.org/10.4103/2156-7514.129260.
86. Donaldson CD, de Mel S, Clarice CSH, et al. Admission ultrasonography as a predictive tool for thrombocytopenia and disease severity in dengue infection. Trans R Soc Trop Med Hyg. 2021;115(12):1396–402. https://doi.org/10.1093/trstmh/trab064.
87. Parmar J, Mohan C, Kumar GP, Vora M. Ultrasound is not useful as a screening tool for dengue fever. Pol J Radiol. 2017;82:693–700. https://doi.org/10.12659/PJR.902861.
88. Nascimento BR, Nunes MCP, Lima EM, et al. Outcomes of echocardiography-detected rheumatic heart disease: validating a simplified score in cohorts from different countries. J Am Heart Assoc. 2021;10(18):e021622. https://doi.org/10.1161/JAHA.121.021622.
89. Beaton A, Okello E, Lwabi P, Mondo C, McCarter R, Sable C. Echocardiography screening for rheumatic heart disease in Ugandan schoolchildren. Circulation. 2012;125(25):3127–32. https://doi.org/10.1161/CIRCULATIONAHA.112.092312.
90. Kotit S, Said K, ElFaramawy A, Mahmoud H, Phillips DIW, Yacoub MH. Prevalence and prognostic value of echocardiographic screening for rheumatic heart disease. Open Heart. 2017;4(2):e000702. https://doi.org/10.1136/openhrt-2017-000702.
91. Seitler S, Zuhair M, Shamsi A, et al. Cardiac imaging in rheumatic heart disease and future developments. Eur Heart J Open. 2023;3(2):oeac060. https://doi.org/10.1093/ehjopen/oeac060.
92. Mirabel M, Celermajer DS, Ferreira B, et al. Screening for rheumatic heart disease: evaluation of a simplified echocardiography-based approach. Eur Heart J Cardiovasc Imaging. 2012;13(12):1024–9. https://doi.org/10.1093/ehjci/jes077.
93. Anesi JA, Gluckman S. Amebic liver abscess. Clin Liver Dis (Hoboken). 2015;6(2):41–3. https://doi.org/10.1002/cld.488.
94. Ralls PW, Barnes PF, Radin DR, Colletti P, Halls J. Sonographic features of amebic and pyogenic liver abscesses: a blinded comparison. AJR Am J Roentgenol. 1987;149(3):499–501. https://doi.org/10.2214/ajr.149.3.499.
95. Alshoabi SA, Alkalady AH, Almas KM, et al. Hydatid disease: a radiological pictorial review of a great neoplasms mimicker. Diagnostics (Basel). 2023;13(6):1127. https://doi.org/10.3390/diagnostics13061127.
96. WHO. Echinococcosis. 2021. Fact Sheet. https://www.who.int/news-room/fact-sheets/detail/echinococcosis#:~:text=Abdominal%20pain%2C%20nausea%20and%20vomiting,exerted%20on%20the%20surrounding%20tissues.
97. Saavedra AC, Valencia BM, Tueros P, Wortsman X, Llanos-Cuentas A, Lavarello RJ. Ultrasonographic characteristics of cutaneous leishmaniasis. J Eur Acad Dermatol Venereol. 2020;34(4):e193–5. https://doi.org/10.1111/jdv.16111.
98. Sechi A, Neri I, Patrizi A, et al. Ultrasound patterns of localized cutaneous leishmaniasis and clinical correlations. J Ultrasound. 2022;25(2):343–8. https://doi.org/10.1007/s40477-020-00537-9.
99. WHO. Leishmaniasis. 2023. https://www.who.int/news-room/fact-sheets/detail/leishmaniasis#:~:text=Leishmaniasis%20is%20caused%20by%20protozoan,and%20lack%20of%20financial%20resources.
100. Prevention CfDCa. Lymphatic Filariasis. https://www.cdc.gov/parasites/lymphaticfilariasis/index.html.
101. Dreyer G, Santos A, Noroes J, Amaral F, Addiss D. Ultrasonographic detection of living adult Wuchereria bancrofti using a 3.5-MHz transducer. Am J Trop Med Hyg. 1998;59(3):399–403. https://doi.org/10.4269/ajtmh.1998.59.399.
102. Dietrich CF, Chaubal N, Hoerauf A, et al. Review of dancing parasites in lymphatic filariasis. Ultrasound Int Open. 2019;5(2):E65–74. https://doi.org/10.1055/a-0918-3678.
103. Cozzi D, Bertelli E, Savi E, et al. Ultrasound findings in urogenital schistosomiasis: a pictorial essay. J Ultrasound. 2020;23(2):195–205. https://doi.org/10.1007/s40477-019-00405-1.
104. Cimini A, Ricci M, Gigliotti PE, et al. Medical imaging in the diagnosis of schistosomiasis: a review. Pathogens. 2021;10(8):1058. https://doi.org/10.3390/pathogens10081058.
105. Pereira LM, Domingues AL, Spinelli V, McFarlane IG. Ultrasonography of the liver and spleen in Brazilian patients with hepatosplenic schistosomiasis and cirrhosis. Trans R Soc Trop Med Hyg. 1998;92(6):639–42. https://doi.org/10.1016/s0035-9203(98)90794-5.
106. WHO. Schistosomiasis. 2023. Fact Sheet. https://www.who.int/news-room/fact-sheets/detail/schistosomiasis.

Index

M. Gottlieb, N. Panebianco (eds.), *Advanced Point-of-Care Ultrasound*, https://doi.org/10.1007/978-3-031-85308-1

T

U

V

W

Y

Z

MIX
Papier aus verantwortungsvollen Quellen
Paper from responsible sources
FSC® C105338

If you have any concerns about our products,
you can contact us on
ProductSafety@springernature.com

In case Publisher is established outside the EU,
the EU authorized representative is:
Springer Nature Customer Service Center GmbH
Europaplatz 3, 69115 Heidelberg, Germany

Printed by Libri Plureos GmbH
in Hamburg, Germany